The Scientific Basis of Urology

Third Edition

Edited by

Anthony R. Mundy, MS, FRCP, FRCS
Professor of Urology, Institute of Urology,
University College Hospital, London, UK

John M. Fitzpatrick, MCh, FRCSI, FRC(Urol), FRCSGlas, FRCS
Professor of Surgery, Surgical Professorial Unit,
University College Dublin, Ireland

David E. Neal, FMed Sci, MS, FRCS
Professor of Surgery, Department of Surgery,
School of Surgical and Reproductive Science,
University of Cambridge, UK

Nicholas J. R. George, MD, FRCS
Consultant Urologist, Withington Hospital,
and Senior Lecturer, Department of Urology,
University Hospitals of South Manchester, UK

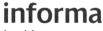

informa
healthcare

New York   London

First published in 1999 by Isis Medical Media, Ltd, Oxford, UK
This edition published in 2010 by Informa Healthcare, Telephone House, 69-77 Paul Street, London EC2A 4LQ, UK.

Simultaneously published in the USA by Informa Healthcare, 52 Vanderbilt Avenue, 7th floor, New York, NY 10017, USA.

A CIP record for this book is available from the British Library.

ISBN-13: 978-1-84184-679-8

Orders may be sent to: Informa Healthcare, Sheepen Place, Colchester, Essex CO3 3LP, UK
Telephone: +44 (0)20 7017 5540
Email: CSDhealthcarebooks@informa.com
Website: http://informahealthcarebooks.com/

For corporate sales please contact: CorporateBooksIHC@informa.com
For foreign rights please contact: RightsIHC@informa.com
For reprint permissions please contact: PermissionsIHC@informa.com

Typeset by MPS Limited, A Macmillan Company
Printed and bound in the United Kingdom

Preface

It is 10 years since the first edition, and 5 years since the second edition of this book. We are pleased that there is demand for a third edition. Once again, we have included some new chapters, but more importantly, the whole book has been revised to reflect a changing understanding of the scientific basis of urology over the last few years. When the editors—senior gentlemen all!—completed their training in urology and became consultants, there was a tacit assumption that our knowledge base would last us through for the rest of our careers. Now, instead of reckoning on a 25-year life expectancy for our knowledge base, it is probably nearer 2.5 years. One considerable benefit from editing this book is that the four of us have managed to keep up to date, and we hope that other readers will benefit in the same way. We all believe that a sound scientific basis is essential for a good clinical practice and therefore hope that this book will be of interest to all urologists.

Tony Mundy

Contents

Contributors

Hashim U. Ahmed   Department of Urology, Division of Surgical and Interventional Sciences, University College London, London, U.K.

Daniela E. Andrich   Institute of Urology, University College Hospital, London, U.K.

Ken M. Anson   Department of Urology, St. George's Hospital, London, U.K.

Manit Arya   Department of Urology, Division of Surgical and Interventional Sciences, University College London, London, U.K.

Haley L. Bennett   Beatson Institute for Cancer Research, Glasgow, U.K.

Pierre-Marc G. Bouloux   Department of Endocrinology, Royal Free and University College Hospital Medical School, Royal Free Hospital, London, U.K.

John R. Bradley   Cambridge University Hospitals NHS Foundation Trust, Cambridge, U.K.

John Bridgewater   University College London Cancer Institute, University College London Medical School, London, U.K.

Judith Cave   Southampton General Hospital, Southampton, U.K.

Michael Craggs   London Spinal Cord Injuries Centre, Royal National Orthopaedic Hospital, Stanmore, U.K.

Anne C. Cunningham   Faculty of Applied Sciences, University of Sunderland, Sunderland, U.K.

Neil G. Docherty   The Conway Institute, University College Dublin, Ireland

Mark Emberton   Department of Urology, Division of Surgical and Interventional Sciences, University College London, London, U.K.

Mark Feneley   Institute of Urology, University College Hospital, London, U.K.

John M. Fitzpatrick   Mater Misericordiae Hospital and University College Dublin, Ireland

Christopher H. Fry   Postgraduate Medical School, University of Surrey, Guildford, U.K.

Giulio Garaffa   Department of Urology, University College London Hospitals, London, U.K.

Nicholas J. R. George   Department of Urology, Withington Hospital, University Hospitals of South Manchester, Manchester, U.K.

Vincent J. Gnanapragasam   Uro-oncology Group, Department of Oncology, Hutchinson MRC Research Centre, University of Cambridge, Cambridge, U.K.

T. R. Leyshon Griffiths   Urology Group, Department of Cancer Studies and Molecular Medicine, University of Leicester, Leicester, U.K.

Thiru Gunendran   Department of Urology, University Hospital of South Manchester, Manchester, U.K.

Freddie C. Hamdy   Nuffield Department of Surgery, University of Oxford, Oxford, U.K.

Thang S. Han   Department of Endocrinology, Royal Free and University College Hospital Medical School, Royal Free Hospital, London, U.K.

George B. Haycock   Academic Department of Paediatrics, Guy's Hospital, London, U.K.

John A. Kirby   Institute of Cellular Medicine, Newcastle University, Newcastle upon Tyne, U.K.

Sarah Knight   London Spinal Cord Injuries Centre, Royal National Orthopaedic Hospital, Stanmore, U.K.

Hing Leung   Beatson Institute for Cancer Research, Glasgow, U.K.

Rachel Lewis   Department of Oncology, University College Hospitals, London, U.K.

Iain M. J. Mackenzie   Department of Anaesthesia and Critical Care, University Hospital Birmingham NHS Foundation Trust, Edgbaston, Birmingham, U.K.

Patrick H. Maxwell   Division of Medicine, University College Hospital, London, U.K.

Nick Mayer   University Hospitals of Leicester, Leicester, U.K.

Danish Mazhar   Department of Medical Oncology, Addenbrooke's Hospital, Cambridge, U.K.

Mary McCormack   Department of Oncology, University College Hospitals, London, U.K.

Suks Minhas   Department of Urology, University College London Hospitals, London, U.K.

Caroline Moore   Department of Urology, Division of Surgical and Interventional Sciences, University College London, London, U.K.

Anthony R. Mundy   Institute of Urology, University College Hospital, London, U.K.

David E. Neal   Department of Oncology, University of Cambridge, Addenbrooke's Hospital, Cambridge, U.K.

Graeme O'Boyle   Institute of Cellular Medicine, Newcastle University, Newcastle upon Tyne, U.K.

Tim O'Brien   Department of Urology, Guy's and St Thomas' Hospital, London, U.K.

Kieran J. O'Flynn   Department of Urology, Salford Royal Foundation Trust, Salford, Manchester, U.K.

Sanjay Ojha   Cambridge University Hospitals NHS Foundation Trust, Cambridge, U.K.

Uday Patel   St George's Hospital and Medical School, London, U.K.

Heather Payne   Department of Oncology, University College Hospitals, London, U.K.

David J. Ralph   Department of Urology, University College London Hospitals, London, U.K.

William G. Robertson   Physiology Department, Royal Free and University College Medical School, London, U.K.

Craig N. Robson   Northern Institute for Cancer Research, The Medical School, University of Newcastle, Newcastle, U.K.

Rashmi Singh   Department of Urology, Kingston and St. George's Hospital, London, U.K.

Rona Smith   Cambridge University Hospitals NHS Foundation Trust, Cambridge, U.K.

Naeem Soomro   Department of Urology, Freeman Hospital, Newcastle upon Tyne, U.K.

Angela Swampillai   Department of Oncology, University College Hospitals, London, U.K.

Andy Symes   Department of Urology, St George's Hospital, London, U.K.

David Talbot   Department of Hepatobiliary and Transplant Surgery, Freeman Hospital, Newcastle upon Tyne, U.K.

Christina Thirlwell   University College London Cancer Institute, University College London Medical School, London, U.K.

David F. M. Thomas   Department of Paediatric Urology, St James's University Hospital, Leeds, U.K.

Maxine G. B. Tran   Department of Urology, Addenbrooke's Hospital, Cambridge, U.K.

Miles Walkden   University College Hospital, London, U.K.

Michael Williams   Department of Clinical Oncology, Addenbrooke's Hospital, Cambridge, U.K.

Nicholas A. Wisely   Department of Anaesthesia, University Hospital of South Manchester, Manchester, U.K.

Neville Woolf   Medical School Administration, University College London, London, U.K.

Introduction to Cell Biology

Haley L. Bennett and Hing Leung
Beatson Institute for Cancer Research, Glasgow, U.K.

INTRODUCTION

Cell biology is a discipline that is no longer solely the domain of the bench-bound scientist. Mainstream awareness of the concepts that this discipline entails is increasing, and while many a patient may not know what DNA stands for, they will be well aware of the impact of genetics. As the field of cell biology has expanded and diversified, so have its translational applications within the clinic. Cell biologists are identifying novel key drug targets and gaining a more thorough understanding of the cellular action of currently available therapies. In turn, medical professionals can design therapeutic regimes specifically targeted to the needs of the individual patient, thus narrowing the gap between the bench and the bedside.

How then is cell biology important to urologists? Like in any branch of medicine, a keen knowledge of the biology of the cell allows for an appreciation of the molecular basis of pathologies and the resulting cellular dysfunction, and how this dysfunction can manifest at the level of the tissue and/or organ. Within the field of urology, many recent developments have stemmed from better understanding of the molecular and cellular processes in disease, including urological oncology and andrology.

The aim of this chapter is to present a thorough overview of the main aspects of cell biology as they relate to cellular behavior. The reader should gain an appreciation of structural and molecular components of the cell and how these components interact to govern cellular growth, proliferation, differentiation, and other key biological behaviors. Finally, using cancer as an example, this chapter will evaluate the mechanisms whereby normal cellular behaviors can be manipulated or subverted, resulting in a pathological state.

THE MOLECULES OF LIFE

The cell is the fundamental unit of all organisms. In essence, it is a fluid-filled sac enclosed by a lipid membrane, yet this sac possesses the ingredients and machinery to drive its own replication, react to its external environment, and control its energy expenditure. To gain a full understanding of cell biology and the mechanisms that underlie cellular behavior, we must first be familiar with the molecules that make up the cell. The cell is 90% water, and the remaining 10% comprises 50% protein, 15% DNA and RNA, 15% carbohydrate, and 10% lipid. The structure and function of these classes of biomolecules will be discussed in the following section.

Proteins

Proteins are macromolecules comprising a chain of amino acids (Fig. 1A). There are 20 different amino acids that can be stringed together in any order by peptide bonds to make up an almost infinite number of proteins. Usually, proteins are of 100 to 1000 amino acids in length. The *primary* structure of a protein refers to its amino acid sequence. Once assembled, small sections of a protein will fold into a *secondary* structure stabilized by hydrogen bonding between neighboring or proximal amino acids. These secondary structures include α-helices, β-sheets, and turns, and a protein may contain many regions with different secondary structures that stabilize each other. The overall three-dimensional or *tertiary* structure of a protein in its entirety is determined by the intramolecular bonds between local and distant amino acids. These bonds are weaker than those maintaining secondary structure, and thus the tertiary structure can be manipulated or altered in certain conditions. This propensity for flexibility has allowed proteins to assume enumerable functional roles in the cell, as will be discussed later. Finally, a single protein, or monomer, can assemble with other monomers to form multimeric structures, and in many cases, multimeric assembly is required for protein function. This *quaternary* structure is defined by the number and relative order of protein monomers within a multimeric complex.

The relative abundance of proteins in a cell compared with that of other biomolecules suggests the necessity of this class in all aspects of cellular function. In fact, most cellular tasks are executed by proteins. Some functional classes of proteins include structural components (cytoskeletal, matrix), enzymatic components (catalytic), control of gene expression (transcription factors), and intercellular communication (growth factors, hormones). Proteins are classified into families on the basis of structural homology. As a protein's structure governs its function, generally these classifications translate into functional divisions.

Deoxyribonucleic Acid

Deoxyribonucleic acid (DNA) is a polymer of single nucleotides linked by phosphodiester bonds. Nucleotides consist of a five-carbon sugar with a phosphate group attached to carbon 5 and a purine or pyrimidine base attached to carbon 2 (Fig. 1B). There are four nucleotide bases—thymine, cytosine, adenine, and guanine—and the nucleotide itself is often referred to as the base subunit that it contains. RNA, or ribonucleic acid, also comprises these bases except for thymine, which is replaced by uracil. Nucleotides are arranged as two complimentary antiparallel strands in a double helix and the order in which they are linked is referred to as its primary structure. In the cell nucleus, DNA helices are tightly coiled into protein-associated chromosomes, whereas RNA exists predominantly as single-stranded polymers and are found both in the nucleus and cytoplasm.

Sections of DNA contain genes, which are regions of the molecule that code for a protein. The process whereby genes are manufactured into proteins is known as gene expression, and is described in detail in chapter 2. Briefly, gene expression is initiated

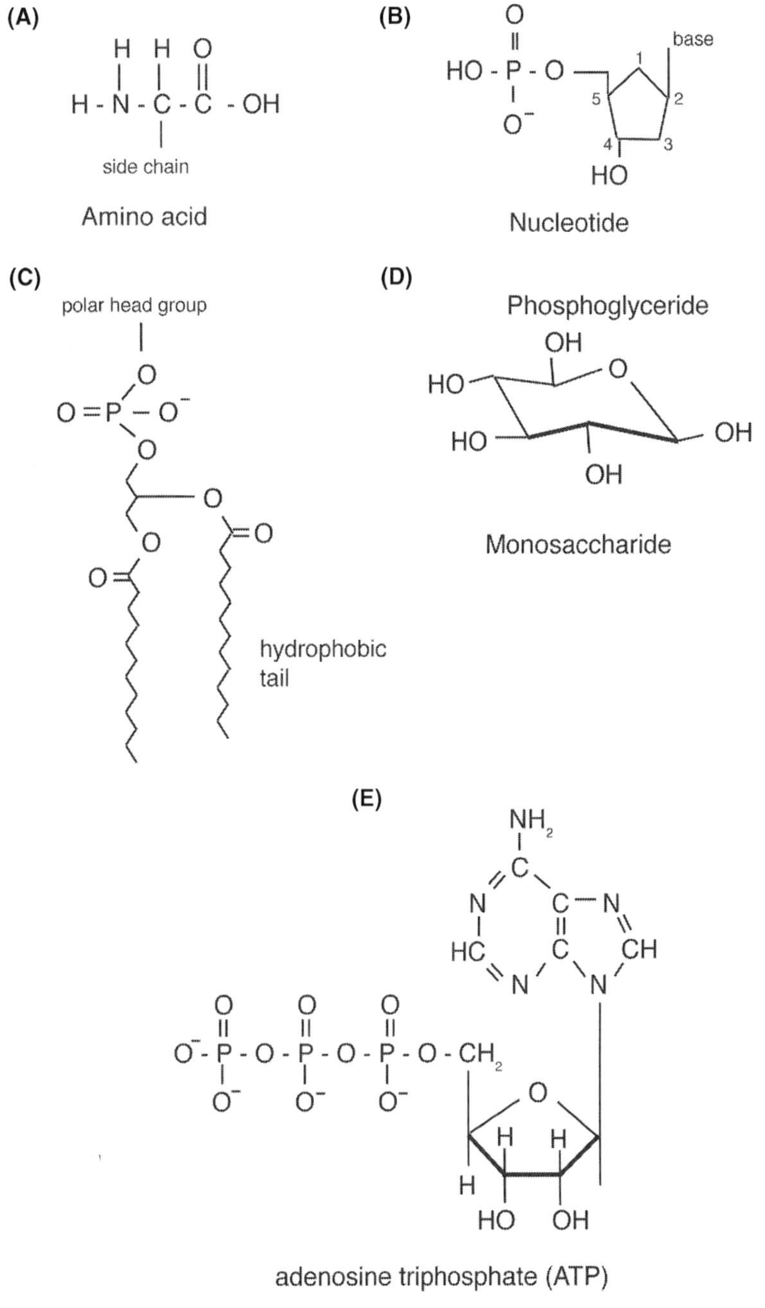

Figure 1 Chemical structures of some key classes of biomolecules: (**A**) amino acid, (**B**) phosphoglyceride, (**C**) nucleotide, (**D**) monosaccharide, and (**E**) ATP.

when protein-coding regions of DNA are copied into messenger RNA by RNA polymerases, an event known as transcription. Messenger RNA then guides the manufacture of protein by specifying the sequence of amino acids to be joined to make up the protein. This process, known as translation, takes place on ribosomes on rough endoplasmic reticulum.

Lipids

Fatty acids are a vital energy resource and can be modified to generate numerous types of lipids with a variety of functions. Fatty acids comprise a hydrocarbon chain attached to a carboxyl group. The length of the hydrocarbon chain can vary, and the longer the chain, the lower the solubility in water. Saturated fatty acids contain no double bonds between carbon atoms in the hydrocarbon chain, whereas those that do are referred to as unsaturated. Fatty acids used for energy are stored in the cell in the form of triacylglycerols.

Phospholipids, another fatty acid derivative, are the building blocks of the plasma membrane, a water-impermeable phospholipid bilayer that surrounds the cell and protects its contents from the external environment. The membrane itself is composed of two layers of phospholipid molecules that are arranged with their hydrophobic fatty acyl tails buried within the bilayer, forming a hydrophobic core, while the hydrophilic polar ends are in contact with the cell interior (cytosol) or exterior (exoplasmic). Phosphoglycerides are the most abundant phospholipid found in membranes, followed by sphingolipids and cholesterol (Fig. 1C). Proteins are also found embedded within or attached to the membrane and play vital roles in cell-cell and cell-matrix communication as well as facilitating the transport of molecules in and out of the cell. All membrane components can move laterally along the plane of the membrane, allowing both stability and fluidity.

Carbohydrates

Sugars, or monosaccharides, are the smallest unit of carbohydrates (Fig. 1D). Monosaccharides comprise up to seven carbon atoms bound to an equal ratio of water molecules, the most common being hexoses and pentoses. Monosaccharides polymerize into disaccharides, such as sucrose and lactose, or can form short or long chains known as oligosaccharides or polysaccharides, respectively. These chains are held together by glycosidic bonds. Oligosaccharide chains can also be covalently linked to proteins and lipids. Glucose, a hexose sugar, is the main fuel source used in animal cells and can be stored in the form of glycogen, a multibranched polymer.

Adenosine Triphosphate

The small molecule adenosine triphosphate (ATP) is utilized by all cells in the body as a means to transfer energy harvested from the breakdown of glucose, a process known as respiration (Fig. 1E). The conversion of ATP, which contains three phosphate groups attached to adenosine, to ADP involves the transfer of a phosphate group to a substrate protein. This releases energy required to catalyze energetically unfavorable reactions within the cell. This process mediates a multitude of cellular events such as the synthesis of new macromolecules, the transport of molecules against their concentration or electrochemical gradient, cellular movement, or signal transduction.

HOW CELLS RESPOND TO THEIR ENVIRONMENT

Every eukaryotic cell shares a number of key features—a plasma membrane enclosing its contents, a cytoskeleton that maintains shape and structure, a nucleus that contains the genetic material, and organelles that each have a unique function that contributes to normal cellular activity. The key architectural components of the cell are discussed in greater detail in chapter 2.

The main aim for any cell is to generate the biomolecules required to maintain a homeostatic environment and to perform its required function at the level of the tissue or organ. The requirement of the cell may be to differentiate, to proliferate, or to undergo programmed cell death, to name some examples. Such cellular behaviors are directed or modified by external cues, detected by molecules that "sense" alterations to the cells' environment. How these cues are detected and how they drive changes to the cell by utilizing or synthesizing the biomolecules, discussed in the previous section, is the focus of the remainder of this chapter.

Detection of Changes in the Extracellular Environment

Because of the relative impermeability of the plasma membrane, specific transmembrane proteins are embedded within it that can detect conditions outside the cell. These integral proteins can respond to chemical signals by the binding of ligand to their extracellular domain. These receptors have exquisite sensitivity for specific ligands, which can be soluble (e.g., growth factors, cytokines, neurotransmitters) or insoluble (e.g., collagen, fibronectin, and other components of the extracellular matrix). Binding of their cognate ligand alters the conformation of the receptor and drives the formation of a multiprotein signaling complex. This complex, via specific protein-protein interactions and enzymatic activation, initiates a cascade of signaling events. Thus, the "message" that originated at the cell surface by ligand-receptor binding is passed from protein to protein by a series of enzymatic reactions and eventuates in a particular cellular event, such as gene transcription or ion flux. This process is known as signal transduction.

Other transmembrane proteins function to regulate the flow of molecules between the cell's exterior and the cytosol. Although gases and lipophilic molecules, such as steroids, can passively diffuse through

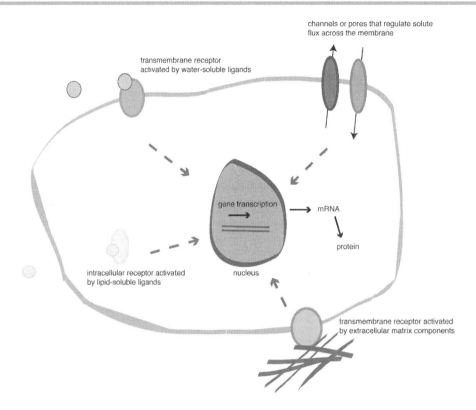

Figure 2   Detection of changes in the extracellular environment. Receptors bind ligands that are present in the extracellular space, diffuse the plasma membrane, or enter the cell by transmembrane pores. These signals initiate a cellular response such as gene transcription, which in turn can lead to protein production.

the membrane, most ions, proteins, and small molecules, such as glucose and amino acids, require assistance to gain entry or exit. Transmembrane protein complexes form hydrophilic pores or channels that facilitate flow of molecules either down their electrochemical or concentration gradient, or alternatively against the gradient, at the expense of ATP. In this manner, cells maintain fine control over their membrane potential by the regulated transport of ions and over their energy status by monitoring the flow of nutrients. Receptors for lipophilic ligands that can diffuse the membrane, such as steroids, reside in the cytoplasm rather than being presented on the cell surface. Steroid receptors are activated upon binding of their ligand in a manner homologous to transmembrane receptors. Upon activation, these receptors enter the nucleus and assume their role as transcription factors (Fig. 2).

Mechanisms of Signal Transduction

Protein-Protein Interactions

The cascade of signaling events initiated by an extracellular cue is facilitated by a number of types of relay molecules that are recruited to form the multimeric signaling complex (Fig. 3). These molecules are divided

into three main classes—adapter, docking, and catalytic proteins. Adapters act to bridge proteins of various classes to the activated receptor but do not possess enzymatic activity (e.g., Shc and the p85 subunit of PI3-kinase). Similarly, docking proteins do not contain catalytic domains and rather provide a scaffold on which proteins of various classes can assemble and maintain proximity (e.g., insulin receptor substrates 1–4). Finally, catalytic proteins contain an enzymatic activity, such as kinase, lipase, or phosphatase. However, within the sea of molecules available, how does a protein recognize its specific binding partner? Proteins contain various functional modules, unique sequences of amino acids that fold into a specific conformation that links two proteins together. By directing particular protein-protein interactions, these modules determine subsequent signal specificity. A brief outline of some of the well-characterized functional modules is given in the following paragraph.

Proteins containing Src-homology (SH)2 domains or phosphotyrosine-binding (PTB) domains bind to specific phosphorylated tyrosine residues on other proteins. Examples include the adapters Shc and the catalytic protein tyrosine kinase Src. SH3 domains recognize sequences on target proteins that are rich in the amino acid proline. Src, for example, also contains SH3 domains. In addition to protein-protein interactions,

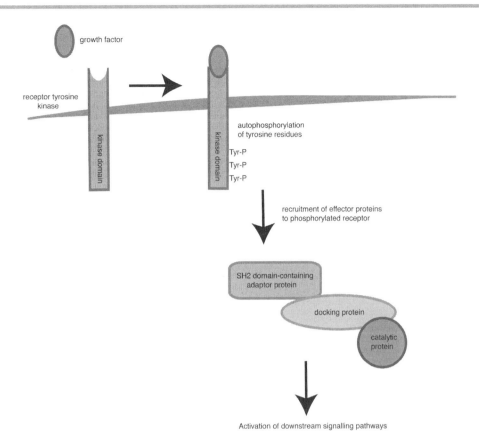

Figure 3 Mechanisms of signal transduction by receptor tyrosine kinases. Growth factor binding to the extracellular domain of the receptor induces autophosphorylation of tyrosine residues within the kinase domain. These residues provide binding sites for SH2 domain–containing proteins, allowing for recruitment of effector proteins to the activated receptor. Interactions between effector proteins are maintained by specific functional domains and may be transient or constitutive. Proteins with catalytic activity then propagate the membrane-initiated signal to other downstream cellular effectors.

other protein modules allow for recognition of certain lipids, DNA sequences, or other molecules. Examples include the pleckstrin homology domain, which recognizes specific membrane phospholipids and thus plays a key role in determining intracellular localization (e.g., Akt) and DNA-binding domains (DBD), which allow for transcription factors to recognize particular regions on DNA and thus regulate transcription.

Posttranslational Modifications

For a cell to propagate a signal initiated by an extracellular cue to the subcellular target, for example, to the nucleus to drive the transcription of certain genes, a series of chemical reactions must occur. These reactions commonly result in the posttranslational modification of proteins within the signal cascade—that is, a chemical alteration or addition made to a protein that changes its function or activity without altering its primary amino acid sequence. These modifications allow a protein (the activator) to "talk" to the next protein in the sequence (the effector) and pass on the message downstream. There are several types of posttranslational modifications, some of which are discussed below.

Phosphorylation. Phosphorylation of proteins refers to the transfer of a phosphate group, commonly from ATP, by a class of enzymatic proteins called kinases to a substrate. This supplies the substrate with high potential energy. Phosphorylation can both activate and inhibit a protein substrate, depending on its energy status. If the protein exists predominantly in a conformation that does not favor activation, then phosphorylation can drive the protein into a high-energy state. On the other hand, energy may be required to "switch off" a protein, and in this case phosphorylation is needed to induce an energy-unfavorable inhibitory conformation.

Specific amino acid residues within a protein act as acceptors of phosphate groups. Phosphorylation occurs at tyrosine, serine, or threonine residues, and the kinases that catalyze this transfer are highly specific. Kinases can have a transmembrane localization [e.g., receptor tyrosine kinases, which include the epidermal growth factor receptor (EGFR) family] or can be found intracellularly [Src family kinases, mitogen-activated protein (MAP) kinases, Akt]. The target proteins of kinases include both catalytic proteins such as other kinases, or noncatalytic proteins such as adapters or scaffolding proteins that form the skeleton of multi-protein signaling complexes. Another class of enzymes known as phosphatases can remove the phosphate group from a particular residue of a protein, thereby altering its activity. The antagonistic action of kinases and phosphatases thus tightly regulates both the duration and magnitude of signal transduction by phosphorylation (Fig. 4A).

Ubiquitylation. Another key posttranslational modification is ubiquitylation, a process whereby a small molecular weight protein called ubiquitin is covalently attached to lysine residues on a target protein (Fig. 4B). This is achieved by the sequential action of ubiquitin-activating (E1), ubiquitin-conjugating (E2), and ubiquitin-ligating (E3) enzymes. The mechanism of ubiquitylation is analogous to phosphorylation in that it can be activated by cell surface ligands, is reversible, and can determine protein-protein interactions. However, unlike phosphorylation, multiple types of ubiquitylation can occur, rendering it a more complex system. Ubiquitin can be ligated as a single molecule (monoubiquitylation) or as a polymeric chain (polyubiquitylation). The biological effects of different forms of ubiquitylation are diverse, but the best characterized is endocytosis. In this process, transmembrane proteins tagged with ubiquitin are internalized by the cell into a vesicle known as endosome. The type of ubiquitylation then determines whether the protein is recycled back to the membrane, or whether it proceeds to the lysosome where it is degraded into its constituent amino acids. Ubiquitylation can also play a role in the nucleus, for example, by decreasing the stability of transcription factors, and in DNA repair pathways.

SUMOylation, acetylation, and other posttranslational modifications. SUMO (small ubiquitin-related modifier) is a small molecular weight protein that is structurally related to ubiquitin, and indeed many similarities exist between the two in terms of ligation and lysine attachment. The role of SUMOylation appears to be substrate specific; however, it has been implicated as a negative regulator of transcription, potentially by promoting the interaction of transcription factors with corepressors. Cross talk with another

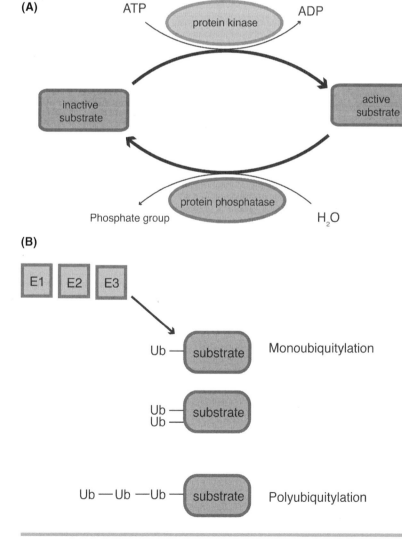

(A)

ATP — protein kinase — ADP

inactive substrate — active substrate

Phosphate group — protein phosphatase — H_2O

(B)

E1 E2 E3

Ub — substrate   Monoubiquitylation

Ub — / Ub — substrate

Ub — Ub — Ub — substrate   Polyubiquitylation

Figure 4 Proteins are subject to posttranslational modifications. (**A**) Phosphorylation is the process whereby a phosphate group is transferred from ATP to a substrate. This process is catalyzed by protein kinases and reversed by protein phosphatases. (**B**) Ubiquitylation describes the ligation of one or several ubiquitin molecules to a substrate by a series of reactions catalyzed by E1, E2, and E3 enzymes. The outcomes of ubiquitylation (mono- or polyubiquitylation) are diverse and include endocytosis or proteosomal degradation of the substrate protein.

mechanism of posttranslation modification, acetylation, may compete with SUMO for binding, and many have antagonistic effects. Acetylation occurs when an acetyl group (CH_3CO) is covalently attached to lysine and this process is catalyzed by a group of enzymes known as acetyl transferases. Acetylation protects proteins from rapid digestion by intracellular proteases, although other functions for this modification are being revealed.

In addition, other protein modifications exist that not only add to the diversity of protein function but also play key roles in controlling their degradation or intracellular localization. These include methylation, glycosylation, biotinylation, and ribosylation. Posttranslational modifications can be overlapping, antagonistic, or cooperative, and both the functional outcomes and mechanisms underlying their individual and combined regulation are an emerging field within cell biology.

Key Signaling Cascades

Although there is an enormous variety of extracellular stimuli that elicit a cellular response, they commonly share the same signaling pathways within the cell. Examples of frequently utilized signaling cascades include the MAP kinase, PI3-kinase/Akt, IKK/NFκ-B, and JAK/STAT pathways. The cascades activated by certain ligands are cell-type specific, although there may be common preferences. For example, one MAP kinase cascade, the Ras/Erk (extracellular-regulated kinase) pathway, is activated by epidermal growth factor (EGF) in many cell types. In the most basic model, a number of known proteins are recruited and activated in a particular sequence, which, for simplification, occurs in this order: EGFR → Grb2 → Sos → Ras → Raf → Mek → Erk1/2 → transcription factors → gene expression. Of course, in reality the system is much more complex; the signal is not propagated in such a linear fashion and rarely is only one cascade activated by one stimulus. Rather, signal cascades cross talk can be synergistic or antagonistic and, at any given time, can be activated by a variety of stimuli.

Given that many signaling pathways utilize the same proteins, activated in the same sequence, how does the cell generate specific outcomes to different extracellular cues? This specificity is often achieved by the regulation of the *duration* and *magnitude* of the signal. For example, the aforementioned kinases Erk1/2 are activated by a variety of extracellular signals, such as growth factors, lipid hormones, and insoluble matrix components. However, the length of time that Erk1/2 remain activated after stimulation is a vital determinant in the cellular response, as is the strength, or magnitude, of activation. In addition, the shuttling of proteins such as Erk1/2 to different locations around the cell determines its access to substrates; thus, intracellular trafficking is another mechanism that is utilized to govern signal specificity. In these ways, although many signaling pathways may intersect at particular effector proteins like Erk1/2, the cellular response can be as diverse as proliferation, differentiation, or migration.

Signal Termination

Once a cell has received a cue from its environment and has utilized the cellular machinery to elicit a behavioral response, it must then deactivate the signaling cascade. Termination of the signal is crucial for cellular homeostasis and disruption to this process is a key hallmark of oncogenesis. Numerous mechanisms exist that lead to signal termination. Initially, the deactivation of key enzymes that facilitate phosphorylation or other posttranslational modifications that positively mediate signaling are countered by the action of negative mediators, such as phosphatases. In addition, the levels of proteins themselves are regulated, and there are many examples of activated proteins that become targeted for degradation by ubiquitylation, such as EGFR. Ubiquitin moieties attached to a targeted protein are recognized by adapters that deliver them to proteosomes, resulting in their degradation by hydrolysis. This latter mechanism is also used to turn over long-lived proteins that are no longer required for normal cellular function, by lysosomal degradation.

CELLULAR BEHAVIORS

The previous section highlighted the ways in which individual cells can respond to the extracellular environment and the mechanisms that facilitate signal propagation through a cell. This section will describe the aspects of cellular behavior that can be affected by various signals and how this can impact on tissue homeostasis (Fig. 5).

Proliferation

Many mitogenic signals, such as hormones and growth factors, can stimulate cell replication. Some cell types, such as epithelia, are constantly being renewed and thus are highly responsive to mitogenic cues. These cues can be blood-borne (endocrine), be produced by neighboring or nearby cells (paracrine), or be secreted by an individual cell for self-stimulation (autocrine). For a cell to divide, it must make the machinery required to replicate its DNA, breakdown the nuclear envelope, segregate the new chromosomes, reform the nuclear membrane, and divide the cytoplasm. This is an enormous task and numerous checkpoints exist along the way to ensure the cell can commit to the next stage of division.

The sequence of events that underlies cell division is called the cell cycle. Cells that are actively moving through the cell cycle are known as proliferating cells. Cells that are nondividing are referred to as quiescent and are maintained in G0 phase. The start of the cycle occurs at G1 phase, a rest period that prepares the cells for a period of DNA synthesis, known as the S phase. This is followed by G2, which leads to mitosis (M phase) whereby cells undergo active division. The cell cycle and the proteins that control its progression, namely the cyclins and the cyclin-dependent kinases, are discussed in detail in chapter 2.

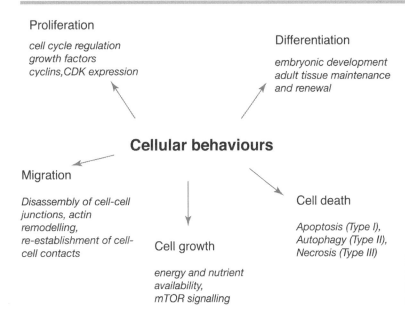

Proliferation

cell cycle regulation
growth factors
cyclins,CDK expression

Differentiation

embryonic development
adult tissue maintenance
and renewal

Cellular behaviours

Migration

Disassembly of cell-cell
junctions, actin
remodelling,
re-establishment of cell-
cell contacts

Cell growth

energy and nutrient
availability,
mTOR signalling

Cell death

Apoptosis (Type I),
Autophagy (Type II),
Necrosis (Type III)

Figure 5 Summary of cellular behaviors elicited by changes in the extracellular environment. All contribute to the maintenance of tissue homeostasis and are subject to deregulation in pathologies such as cancer.

It is vital that proliferation be tightly regulated to maintain tissue homeostasis. Indeed, tumor cells subvert the normal cell cycle regulatory checkpoints to obtain a capacity for uncontrolled proliferation. This ability can be achieved by a number of mechanisms. A frequent event in many cancers in the deregulation of growth factor signaling, either by amplification or mutation of surface receptors (e.g., EGFR) or positive effector proteins (e.g., Ras), or loss of negative regulators (e.g., PTEN) that lie within the signaling transduction cascade. This leads to the upregulation of proproliferative genes, pushing cells through the cell cycle. If this increase in proliferation outweighs cell death, then hyperplasia or tumor growth will result.

Cell Growth

Cell growth refers to an increase in physical size of an individual cell, as opposed to the larger tissue mass that results from proliferation. This process, known as hypertrophy, reflects an increase in metabolism of an individual cell in the condition of high nutrient availability and the absence of environmental cellular stressors. In this event a cell is free to drive de novo RNA and protein synthesis, and these macromolecules constitute the increased cellular bulk. As this is an anabolic event, it is crucial that the cell has at its disposal not only sufficient energy but also the building blocks required for synthesis.

A cell ascertains its nutrient and energy availability (glucose, amino acids, oxygen, and ATP) by various intracellular sensors, which initiate signal cascades that culminate at a key protein known as mammalian target of rapamycin (mTOR). A multitude of signaling pathways feed in to the mTOR pathway, and thus this master regulator integrates many inputs informing the cellular environment. For example, the

binding of insulin to the transmembrane insulin receptor signals via the Akt pathway to mTOR, reflecting an abundance of glucose for energy production. Conversely, low ATP levels are detected by AMP kinase, an enzyme that is activated by AMP and negatively regulates mTOR activity. Free amino acids activate mTOR signaling via the class III PI3-kinase, hVsp43; however, the precise mechanisms underlying this activation are still to be elucidated. The level of mTOR activity is determined by the relative strength of these various inputs. Downstream targets of mTOR include S6 kinase, which activates ribosomal protein S6, and 4E-BP1, an inhibitor of cap-dependent translation. These proteins in turn directly regulate the synthesis and translation of mRNA to create new protein.

Environmental stressors negatively impact on mTOR signaling and act to halt protein synthesis and conserve energy. Such stressors include starvation, hypoxia, DNA damage, oxidative or osmotic stress, and heat shock. In certain conditions such as starvation, cells can increase available nutrients by the degradation of existing proteins, membrane components, or entire organelles. Free amino acids, carbohydrates, and lipids can be generated for reuse by proteolytic or lysosomal degradation. Once the levels of available biomolecules are sufficient, then mTOR signaling can be switched back on and protein synthesis reinitiated. In this way, cells can maintain a degree of autonomy from the extracellular environment when under stress to allow for greater chance of survival. This capacity for adaptation when under metabolic or environmental stress is a key feature of cancer cells, and the mTOR pathway is frequently hyperactivated in cancer. Given its role as a key integrator of numerous cascades, mutation or overexpression of upstream regulators renders this protein vulnerable to deregulation.

Cell Death

Cell death is an event vital for normal embryonic and neonatal development as well as for proper maintenance of adult tissues. In development, certain cells are genetically programmed to die to permit the formation of glandular and ductal lumen and this same program is utilized in adult tissue for morphogenetic remodeling in response to injury or cellular stressors. Programmed cell death, otherwise known as apoptosis or type I cell death, is defined by a cascade of molecular events that results in a characteristic morphological appearance—cellular shrinkage, the breakdown of organelles, the condensation of DNA into chromatin, and the leakage of cytosol into the extracellular space (blebbing). Two mechanisms referred to as the extrinsic and intrinsic pathways lead to apoptotic cell death. The extrinsic pathway is initiated by the activation of transmembrane receptors of the tumor necrosis factor receptor (TNFR) superfamily by soluble ligands such as Fas or TRAIL, whereas the intrinsic pathway is activated by cellular stressors such as ionizing radiation or chemotherapeutic drugs. These pathways utilize intracellular proteins from the Bcl-2 family to permeabilize the mitochondrial membrane, releasing cytochrome C into the cytosol and activating a family of proteolytic enzymes, known as caspases, to degrade intracellular substrates. Alternatively, these pathways can promote cell death by a caspase-independent mechanism by the permeabilization of lysosomes and the subsequent generalized degradation of cytosolic proteins and organelles by the lysosomal proteases cathepsins. Dead cells are then cleared from tissue by macrophages.

Type II, or autophagic, cell death is a process whereby a cell "eats itself." Damaged or long-lived proteins, cytoplasm, or entire organelles are engulfed by vacuoles called autophagosomes, which fuse with lysosomes wherein their contents are degraded. A cell can eventually die via the digestion of its entire contents and be cleared from tissue by macrophages, and thus autophagy is used as a mechanism to maintain tissue homeostasis and remodeling alongside apoptosis. Intriguingly, autophagy is also used as a survival mechanism to generate nutrients from preexisting proteins and organelles in periods of starvation or stress. However, the point at which nutrient generation ends and death by self-digestion begins is a complex story that is only starting to be elucidated. Many key molecules utilized during autophagy overlap with apoptotic pathways, such as p53 and Bcl-2. It was suggested that the two processes are mutually exclusive and inhibitory; however, evidence suggests that they can occur simultaneously, adding further complexity to the mechanisms that underlie cell death.

Finally, type III, or necrotic, cell death describes the process when cells are killed by damage that is beyond repair and usually affects large numbers of cell within a tissue. It is characterized by cellular swelling, irreversible plasma membrane and organelle damage, and random DNA cleavage. Cellular contents are extruded into the extracellular space, and this, unlike during apoptosis, provokes an inflammatory response. Like apoptosis and autophagy, necrosis is controlled by molecular signaling cascades that overlap, and indeed, in certain cases, this form of cell death can be recruited upon failure of apoptotic or autophagic induction. Given the extensive cross talk between the death cascades, it has been difficult to describe specific necrotic effectors; however, the kinase RIP1 as well as reactive oxygen species (ROS) and calcium have been implicated in this process.

As previously mentioned, the evasion of cell death by cancer cells is a key factor for tumorigenesis. Many oncogenes have been implicated in such evasion by their disruption of apoptotic signaling and/or promotion of survival, for example, overexpression of antiapoptotic proteins Bcl-2 or Bcl-XL, the increased Akt signaling due to PTEN deletion, or the loss of the autophagy regulatory gene Beclin-1. Prosurvival signaling is essential for cancer cells to endure the lack of proper vascularization within early tumors and the onslaught of chemotherapeutic drugs, or to form secondary tumors within new microenvironments.

Differentiation

The process of differentiation entails the expression of particular genes within a precursor cell that drives its functional specialization. This process underlies embryonic development and is also vital for the homeostatic functioning and maintenance of adult tissues via the differentiation of stem cells. Stem cells themselves can divide to form other stem cells, or can be committed to a pathway of differentiation—from a restricted potential stem cell, to a progenitor cell and finally to a terminally differentiated cell. This process is usually determined by the presence of extracellular factors that drive expression of certain genes. Once differentiated, most cells are committed to serve that function and are unable to dedifferentiate.

Numerous signaling pathways are implicated in driving differentiation, or alternatively in maintaining the stem cell population. Soluble extracellular factors such as transforming growth factor (TGF) α and β, stem cell factor (SCF)/kit or certain cytokines have all been shown to activate differentiation in particular settings. Similarly, specific transcription factors have been implicated in differentiation including β-catenin via the Wnt pathway, Hedgehog, and Notch.

As with other cell behaviors discussed in this chapter, the process of differentiation can be used by cancer cells to promote tumorigenesis. Genes that are switched off in a terminally differentiated cell can be reexpressed because of oncogenic activity and this can alter the differentiation status of that cell. A key histological marker of aggressive disease is the degree of dedifferentiation within tumor tissue. Altered differentiation also underlies the ability of tumor cells to form metastases. During development, mesenchymal cells migrate to their respective positions within tissues where many then undergo terminal epithelial differentiation. Tumor cells can reverse this process by reexpressing mesenchymal genes and allowing epithelial cells to obtain a migratory phenotype. It is a hotly debated issue within the cancer field, however, as to whether de- or transdifferentiated cells actually represent the altered state of preexisting cells that were terminally differentiated, or whether these populations are derived from a stem cell or progenitor that had acquired oncogenic characteristics. Evidence suggests cancer stem cells may exist in certain tumor types and, if definitively proven, has far-reaching implications on the development of future cancer therapies.

Migration

The capacity for cells to actively move around the body or locally within tissues is necessary for development, wound healing, and the regular tissue maintenance. Migration through tissue is facilitated by a number of mechanisms involving the de-adhesion of a cell to its neighbors (in the case of cells originating within a given tissue), the remodeling of the actin cytoskeleton to push the cell forward, coupled with the release of extracellular proteases that degrade the surrounding extracellular matrix. Migration can be stimulated by a number of cytokines and guidance factors, which can either act as chemoattractive/repulsive agents or alternatively to promote the disassembly of cell-cell or cell-matrix interactions.

Cells that are structurally bound within a tissue must first disassemble their cell-cell contacts to become motile. Between neighboring cells, a number of junctions exist that facilitate adhesion, communication, and structural support. *Adherens junctions* are supported by the calcium-regulated binding of the extracellular domain of cadherin molecules of adjacent cells. The expression pattern of cadherins is highly specific for different cell types, for example, epithelial cells express E-cadherin and vascular endothelial cells express VE-cadherin. Cadherin molecules are bound by their cytoplasmic domain to β-catenin and via interactions with α-catenin and other actin-binding molecules; the complex is bridged to the actin cytoskeleton. *Tight junctions* are portions of plasma membrane between adjacent cells that appear to be fused together at points, providing an impermeable barrier to small hydrophilic molecules and ions. Tight junctions also prevent the diffusion of membrane-bound proteins between the apical and basolateral surface; thus they maintain functional polarity. *Gap junctions* are small pores between adjacent cells that allow for diffusion of small molecules and ions. Finally, *desmosomes* comprise specific cadherins known as desmoglein and desmocollin that are bound to intermediate filaments via the cytosolic plakoglobin and desmoplakins, providing mechanical strength. Likewise, intermediate filament bundles secure adhesion to the extracellular matrix through structures called *hemidesmosomes*.

Once detached from its neighbors, a cell migrates by the formation of transient sites of interaction with the extracellular matrix, called focal adhesions. The focal adhesion complex comprises a multitude of different proteins such as Fak, Src, and paxillin, and acts to bridge extracellular matrix–bound integrins to the actin cytoskeleton. Focal adhesions are linked to stress fibers composed of actin and myosin, which in turn provide the mechanical contractility to promote cell migration. The coordinated activity of proteins of the Rho family of GTPases act at the leading edge of the migrating cell to reorganize actin filaments, generating protrusive finger-like (filopodia) and sheet-like (lamellipodia) structures, while also stimulating contraction at the rear of the cell by regulating the assembly of acto-myosin filaments. In this manner, the signals generated at focal adhesions promote the directional migration of the cell. Migrating cells can also secrete proteases such as matrix metalloproteases (MMPs) to degrade the local matrix and provide space into which the cell can move.

Understanding the processes that regulate cell migration is vital as it is the acquisition of this behavior that underlies invasive, and therefore lethal, forms of cancer. Various oncogenes have been shown to increase motility by the alteration of actin dynamics. In addition, the disassembly of cell-cell junctions by the deregulation or loss of E-cadherin and the switch to its mesenchymal counterpart is frequently observed in epithelial cancers. Similarly, changes in integrin expression can promote migration and survival of metastatic cells in unfamiliar microenvironments. Cancer therapeutics that specifically undermine invasive potential are thus a key mechanism to combat metastatic disease.

SUMMARY

This chapter has presented the basic concepts of cell biology—the ways in which cells use biomolecules to maintain structure, sense their environment, and react accordingly. The molecular mechanisms underlying the main cellular behaviors—proliferation, growth, death, differentiation, and migration—will be discussed in greater detail in the next chapter.

SUGGESTED READING

1. Lodish H, Baltimore D, Berk A, et al. Molecular Cell Biology. 5th ed. New York: Scientific American Books, 2004.
2. Hanahan D, Weinberg RA. The hallmarks of cancer. Cell 2000; 100(1):57–70.
3. Seet BT, Dikic I, Zhou MM, et al. Reading protein modifications with interaction domains. Nat Rev Mol Cell Biol 2006; 7(7):473–483.

The Cell and Cell Division

David E. Neal

Department of Oncology, University of Cambridge, Addenbrooke's Hospital, Cambridge, U.K.

STRUCTURE OF THE CELL

Cell Membrane

The cell membrane confines the contents of the cell. It consists of a continuous bilayer of phospholipid with the polar hydrophilic ends forming the outer and inner layers and the hydrophobic tails forming the central core of the bilayer. The hydrophilic heads on the two sides of the cell membrane are of different composition, those on the outside often being modified by glycosylation: a process that involves the addition of various sugar residues. Embedded in this lipid bilayer are proteins whose function can be classified as follows:

- *Signal transduction.* These proteins mediate the action of external ligands such as growth factors and neurotransmitters). These receptor proteins cross the cell membrane and may have intrinsic enzyme functions (such as the tyrosine kinase activity of the receptor for epidermal growth factor) or may be linked to other proteins such as G proteins (e.g., the muscarinic acetylcholine receptor) (Fig. 1).
- *Cell-cell or cell-matrix contact.* Specialized junctions between cells and between cells and the intercellular matrix occur, involving transmembrane proteins such as integrins and cadherins that interact on the outside with molecules such as fibronectin, and on the inside with molecules such as catenin, talin, and vinculin that act as intermediate links to the cell skeleton, which is made of actin fibers. These proteins form specialized cellular contacts, such as desmosomes and tight junctions.
- *Carrier proteins.* These are involved in the transport of small molecules and ions across the cell membrane (as in glucose, the Na^1/K^1 pump or the multidrug resistance pump). These proteins may be energy dependent or passive—if they are active, they usually utilize adenosine triphosphate (ATP) as a source of energy. These carrier proteins often transport other molecules at the same time in the opposite direction (Fig. 2).
- *Channel proteins.* These are involved in the transport of ions across the cell membrane. These function in a passive way and effectively are hydrophilic pores; they function more efficiently than carrier proteins and can carry ions more than 1000-fold faster. They are selective for certain ions and may be closed or open. The stimuli for opening these channels may be electrical current, ligand binding (as with acetylcholine binding to nicotinic receptors), or mechanical deformation.
- *Intracellular organelles.* These are also bounded by membranes and include rough and smooth endoplasmic reticulum (ER), Golgi apparatus, and nuclear membranes. These intracellular membranes compartmentalize the cell into functionally distinct units (Fig. 3) and are extensive, having a surface area 10- to 25-fold greater than the cell membrane itself. Intracellular proteins are synthesized on free cytosolic ribosomes and remain in the cytoplasm, but proteins for export begin their life by being synthesized on ribosomes that have special signaling molecules that dock with receptors on the ER, Golgi apparatus, lysosomes, etc., which mediate transport to their final destination.
- *There are specialized areas of the cell membrane.* These include the structure of the synapse or neuromuscular junction, which are dealt with elsewhere in the book. In addition, cells have small vesicles that can be involved in the storage of neurotransmitters. Calveolae are small vesicles formed by budding off the cell membrane. Clathrin-coated pits are other specialized areas of the cell membrane that are responsible for internalization of activated ligand-bound receptors, thereby reducing the intensity of the associated signaling cascade. In such areas of the cell, adapter proteins are found, which may act as signal transduction molecules.

Endoplasmic Reticulum

The ER is convoluted and may occupy up to 10% of the cell volume; it plays a central role in protein and lipid biosynthesis and is the site for synthesis of proteins and lipids that are destined to be incorporated in other cell organelles such as mitochondria (Fig. 4).

Ribosomes are found free in the cytosol or attached to the ER (rough ER) when making a protein destined for export. In the latter circumstance, a signaling molecule targets the ribosome with its mRNA to the ER, into which it secretes its protein (Fig. 5).

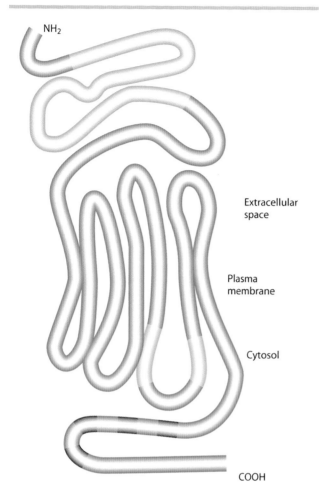

NH₂

Extracellular
space

Plasma
membrane

Cytosol

COOH

Figure 1 A schematic drawing of a G-protein-linked receptor. Receptors that bind protein ligands have a large, extracellular, ligand-binding domain formed by the part of the polypeptide chain shown in light green. Receptors for small ligands such as adrenaline (epinephrine) have small extracellular domains, and the ligand-binding site is usually deep within the plane of the membrane, formed by amino acids from several of the trans-membrane segments. The parts of the intracellular domains that are mainly responsible for binding to trimeric G proteins are shown in orange, while those that become phosphorylated during receptor desensitization (discussed later) are shown in red.

Smooth ER is abundant in some cells. It is involved in the storage of calcium ions and therefore has a role in the contraction of smooth muscle cells, which is brought about by calcium release from these structures as well as transmembrane influx. Together with the Golgi apparatus, it is involved in the synthesis of lipoproteins. In liver and some other cells, it contains the cytochrome p450 enzymes, which detoxify lipid-soluble drugs by converting them into water-soluble forms.

Golgi Apparatus

This system of flattened sacs, which lie in continuity with the ER, is involved in sorting, packaging, and modifying macromolecules for secretion or for delivery to other intracellular organelles (Fig. 6). It consists of a stack of four to six flattened cisternae with an entry (cis) and exit (trans) surface. Glycosylation of proteins such as mucin takes place in the Golgi apparatus. Other proteins are sorted for differential transport to certain organelles; for instance, acid hydrolase is transported from here to the lysosomes, and if the cell synthesizes hormones or neurotransmitters, these are excreted by small, smooth vesicles budding off from the Golgi apparatus before transport to the cell membrane, where exocytosis takes place.

Mitochondria

These are the powerhouse of the cell and are responsible for the production of most of the high-energy phosphate intermediates, such as ATP. They are present in virtually all cells and mediate oxidative respiration, in which pyruvate is converted to carbon dioxide and water with the production of about 30 molecules of ATP. Mitochondria consist of an outer membrane and a convoluted inner membrane containing the inner space or matrix, which is packed with hundreds of enzymes. Acetyl coenzyme A is the central intermediate produced by fatty acid oxidation and glycolysis (Fig. 7), and the citric acid cycle takes place in the mitochondria (Fig. 8). In the mitochondria,

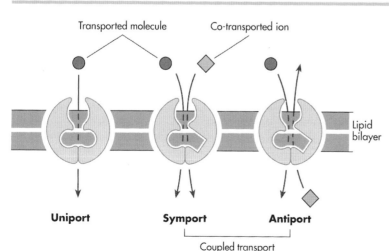

Transported molecule   Co-transported ion

Lipid
bilayer

Uniport   **Symport**   **Antiport**

Coupled transport

Figure 2 Three types of carrier-mediated transport. The schematic diagram shows carrier proteins functioning as uniports, symports and antiports.

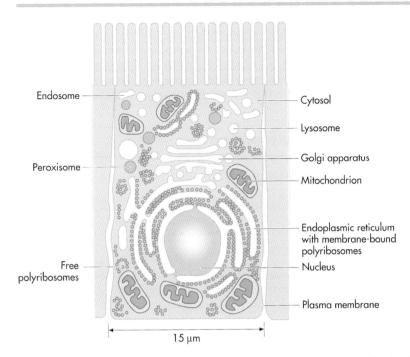

Figure 3 The major intracellular compartments of an animal cell. The cytosol, endoplasmic reticulum, Golgi apparatus, nucleus, mitochondrion, endosome, lysosome, and peroxisome are distinct compartments isolated from the rest of the cell by at least one selectively permeable membrane.

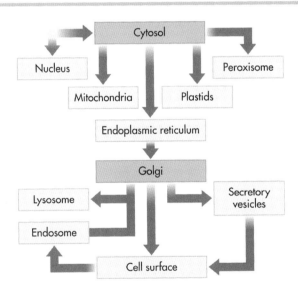

Figure 4 The intracellular compartments of the eukaryotic cell involved in the biosynthetic-secretory and endocytic pathways. Each compartment encloses a space that is topologically equivalent to the outside of the cell, and they all communicate with one another by means of transport vesicles. In the biosynthetic-secretory pathway, protein molecules are transported from the ER to the plasma membrane or (via late endosomes) to lysosomes. In the endocytic pathway, molecules are ingested in vesicles derived from the plasma membrane and delivered to early endosomes and then (via late endosomes) to lysosomes. Many endocytosed molecules are retrieved from early endosomes and returned to the cell surface for reuse; similarly, some molecules are retrieved from the late endosome and returned to the Golgi apparatus, and some are retrieved from the Golgi apparatus and returned to the ER. All of these retrieval pathways are shown with arrows. *Abbreviation*: ER, endoplasmic reticulum.

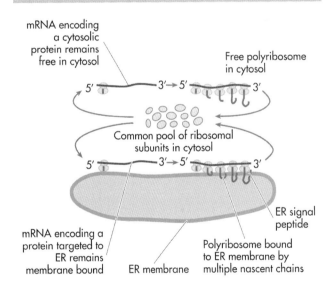

Figure 5 Free and membrane-bound ribosomes. A common pool of ribosomes is used to synthesize both the proteins that stay in the cytosol and those that are transported into the ER. It is the ER signal peptide on a newly formed polypeptide chain that directs the engaged ribosome to the ER membrane. The mRNA molecule may remain permanently bound to the ER as part of a polyribosome, while the ribosomes that move along it are recycled; at the end of each round of protein synthesis, the ribosomal subunits are released and rejoin the common pool in the cytosol. *Abbreviation*: ER, endoplasmic reticulum.

high-energy electrons from NADH and FADH2 are passed to oxygen during oxidative phosphorylation by the respiratory chain, which is situated on the inner membrane of the mitochondria (Fig. 9). There are

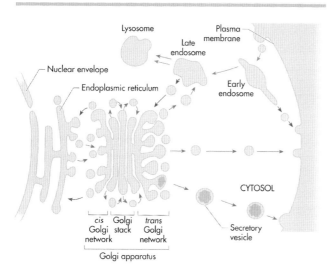

Figure 6 The major intracellular compartments of an animal cell. The cytosol, endoplasmic reticulum, Golgi apparatus, nucleus, mitochondrion, endosome, lysosome and peroxisome are distinct compartments isolated from the rest of the cell by at least one selectively permeable membrane.

three large enzyme groups embedded in the inner membrane (Fig. 10).

1. The NADH dehydrogenase complex, which contains a flavin and ubiquinone
2. The cytochrome b-c_1 complex, which contains three hemes and iron-sulfur protein
3. The cytochrome oxidase complex, which contains two cytochromes and copper

It is thought that ATP is formed by a process of chemiosmotic coupling. The passage of electrons down each of the three parts of the respiratory chain results in H^1 being pumped into the intermembrane space of the mitochondria to set up an electrochemical proton gradient. The subsequent backflow of H^1 into the matrix provides the energy to drive the enzyme ATP synthase. Mitochondria are also actively involved in the induction of caspases during the process of apoptosis (Fig. 11).

Mitochondrial DNA

Mitochondria and chloroplasts contain the DNA that encodes the crucial structural and functional proteins, which permit the mitochondria to divide during cell division. Mitochondrial DNA utilizes biochemically distinct pathways from those of nuclear DNA. For instance, protein synthesis taking place in the cytoplasm but directed by nuclear DNA is blocked by cyclohexidine, whereas protein synthesis directed by mitochondrial DNA is blocked by chloramphenicol, erythromycin, and tetracycline. Mitochondria are not synthesized de novo, but arise from division of the organelle, which occurs during mitosis and is driven by mitochondrial DNA. Mitochondrial DNA is a circular structure like that of bacteria; in mammalian cells, it contains around 16.5 kbp. It synthesizes 2 ribosomal RNAs, 22 transfer RNAs (tRNAs), and 13 peptides. Unlike nuclear DNA, most of the nucleotides are direct coding sequences with little or no space left for regulatory codons (Table 1). Analysis of the genetic code shows that the codon sequence is relaxed, allowing many tRNA molecules to recognize

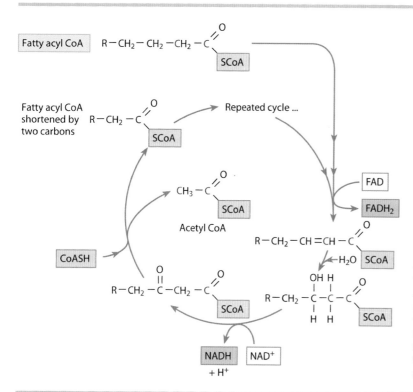

Figure 7 The fatty acid oxidation cycle. The cycle is catalyzed by a series of four enzymes in the mitochondrial matrix. Each turn of the cycle shortens the fatty acid chain by two carbons (*red*), as indicated, and generates one molecule of acetyl CoA and one molecule each of NADH and FADH2. The NADH is freely soluble in the matrix. The FADH2, in contrast, remains tightly bound to the enzyme fatty acyl-CoA dehydrogenase; its two electrons will be rapidly transferred to the respiratory chain in the mitochondrial inner membrane, regenerating FAD.

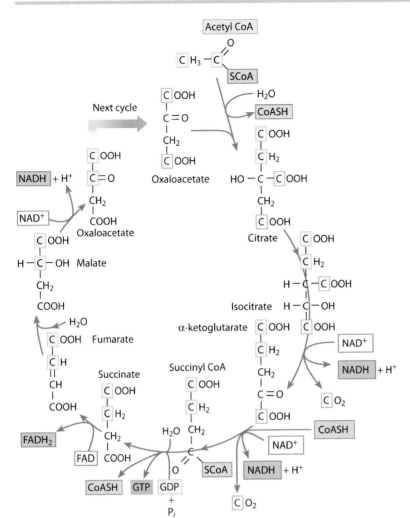

Figure 8 The citric acid cycle. The intermediates are shown as their free acids, although the carboxyl groups are actually ionized. Each of the indicated steps is catalyzed by a different enzyme located in the mitochondrial matrix. The two carbons from acetyl CoA that enter this turn of the cycle (*shadowed in red*) will be converted to CO_2 in subsequent turns of the cycle: it is the two carbons shadowed in blue that are converted to CO_2 in this cycle. Three molecules of NADH are formed. The GTP molecule produced can be converted to ATP by the exchange reaction GTP + ADP → GDP + ATP. The molecule of FADH2 formed remains protein-bound as part of the succinate dehydrogenase complex in the mitochondrial inner membrane; this complex feeds the electrons acquired by FADH2 directly to ubiquinone (see below). *Abbreviations*: ATP, adenosine triphosphate; GTP, guanosine triphosphate.

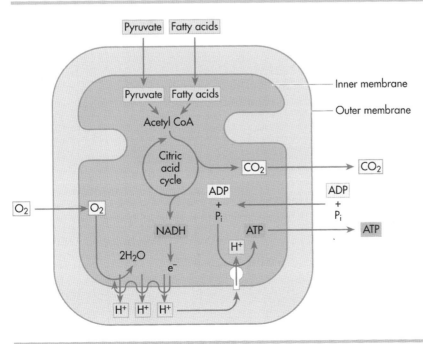

Figure 9 A summary of mitochondrial energy metabolism. Pyruvate and fatty acids enter the mitochondrion, are broken down to acetyl CoA, and are then metabolized by the citric acid cycle, which produces NADH (and FADH2, which is not shown). In the process of oxidative phosphorylation, high-energy electrons from NADH (and FADH2) are then passed to oxygen by means of the respiratory chain in the inner membrane, producing adenosine triphosphate by a chemiosmotic mechanism. NADH generated by glycolysis in the cytosol also passes electrons to the respiratory chain (not shown). Since NADH cannot pass across the mitochondrial inner membrane, the electron transfer from cytosolic NADH must be accomplished indirectly by means of one of several 'shuttle' systems that transport another reduced compound into the mitochondrion; after being oxidized, this compound is returned to the cytosol, where it is reduced by NADH again.

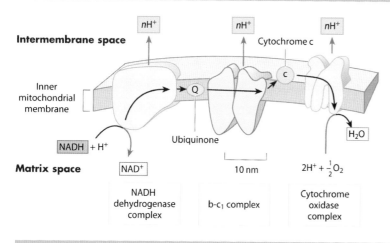

Figure 10 The path of electrons through the three respiratory enzyme complexes. The size and shape of each complex is shown, as determined from images of two-dimensional crystals (crystalline sheets) viewed in the electron microscope at various tilt angles. During the transfer of two electrons from NADH to oxygen (*red lines*), ubiquinone and cytochrome c serve as carriers between the complexes.

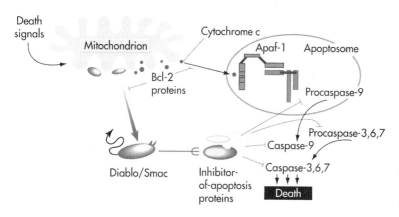

Figure 11 Factors in apoptosis. This diagram shows that DNA-damaging agents result in induction of apoptosis through release of cytochrome c from mitochondria.

Table 1 Differences Between Nuclear and Mitochondrial Coding

Codon	Standard	Mitochondrial
UGA	STOP	Trp (tryptophan)
AUA	Ile (isoleucine)	Met (methionine)
AGA/AGG	Arg (arginine)	STOP

any one of four nucleotides in the third or "wobble" position. In addition, in man, 3 of the 64 codons have different meanings from the standard codons.

Because mitochondrial inheritance is cytoplasmic, one would expect mitochondria to be inherited from the maternal side because the sperm has little cytoplasm. It is thought that both mitochondria and chloroplasts evolved from endosymbiotic bacteria more than a billion years ago. However, over time, some mitochondrial genes have been transferred to nuclear DNA; for instance, lipoproteins in the mitochondrial membranes are synthesized from nuclear genes and modified in the cell's Golgi apparatus.

THE NUCLEUS

This is the most striking organelle in the cell. It is separated from the rest of the cell by the nuclear membrane, which consists of a lipid bilayer fenestrated by multiple nuclear pores. Inside the nucleus is the nucleolus, which is the factory that produces ribosomes. All chromosomal DNA is held in the nucleus, but it is associated with an equal mass of histone proteins. The dense nucleolus is the site for the assembly of ribosomes.

Nuclear pores (Fig. 12) are highly specialized structures, which mediate the transfer of macromolecules across the nuclear membrane. Many proteins (e.g., the androgen receptor) contain a nuclear localization signal (NLS), which comprise short sequences of highly basic amino acids such as lysine. This NLS binds to importin-α and is actively transported into the nucleus. This whole process is driven by a concentration gradient of RAN-GTP.

Arrangement of DNA

Each DNA molecule in the nucleus is packaged as a chromosome, which, in essence, is an enormously long molecule arranged as two strands of a double helix. There are 23 pairs of chromosomes (22 autosomes and 1 sex chromosome: X or Y), which contain about 6×10^9 nucleotide pairs. Each DNA molecule not only has to be able to code for many different proteins (Fig. 13), but also has to be able to replicate itself reliably during mitosis and to be able to repair itself when damaged

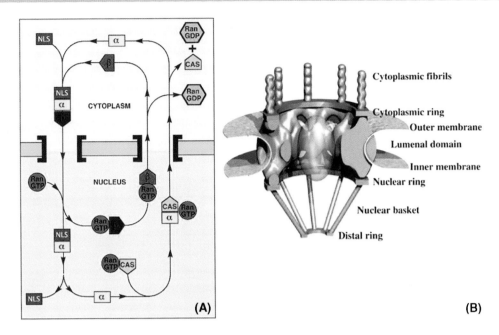

(A)

(B)

Figure 12 (**A**) Translocation of nuclear hormone receptors from the cytoplasm into the nucleus using the importin alpha (*yellow box*) and importin beta (*orange box*) components. This process is under the control of RanGTP, which causes the dissociation of importin beta from the process. (**B**) Structure of the nuclear pore through which this process takes place.

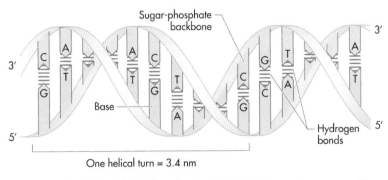

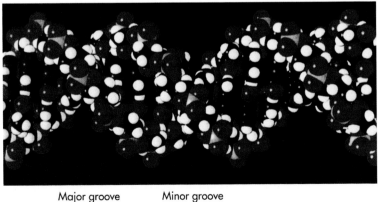

Figure 13 DNA double helix. In a DNA molecule, two antiparallel strands that are complementary in their nucleotide sequence are paired in a right-handed double helix with about 10 nucleotide pairs per helical turn. A schematic representation (*top*) and a space-filling model (*bottom*) are illustrated here.

by chemicals or radiation. At the ends of each chromosome are the telomeres and at the center is the centromere, which serves to anchor the chromosome via the kinetochore to the mitotic spindle during cell division.

Not all DNA in the chromosomes is used to produce mRNA; indeed, most of it is arranged into regulatory elements (noncoding sequences) found in "introns." The function of much of the DNA sequence structure is

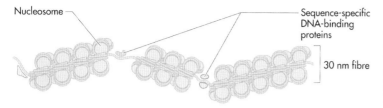

Figure 14 Nucleosome-free regions in 30-nm fibers. A schematic section of chromatin illustrating the interruption of its regular nucleosomal structure by short regions where the chromosomal DNA is unusually vulnerable to digestion by DNase I. At each of these nuclease-hypersensitive sites, a nucleosome appears to have been excluded from the DNA by one or more sequence-specific DNA-binding proteins.

not understood. It used to be known as "junk DNA," but some of these sequences encode small segments of RNA, known as short hairpin (because of its shape) RNA, which can act to regulate the half-life of other messenger RNA, and hence protein synthesis. Totally unknown until a few years ago, this system is now known to be an important means of regulating cell function in most organisms.

Histone Proteins

These proteins allow formal packaging of DNA in the nucleus; without them, DNA in mammalian cells would not be arranged in a regular way, and cell division and gene transcription would not be possible. They are small proteins with a large amount of dibasic amino acids, such as arginine and lysine, which bind to DNA because of their positive charges. There are of five types: the H1 histones and the nucleosomal histones (H2A, H2B, H3, and H4), which are highly evolutionarily conserved. The nucleosomal histones are responsible for the coiling of DNA into nucleosomes (Fig. 14), which are essential to the accommodation of DNA in the nucleus. It is thought that nucleosome histones are preferentially bound to areas of DNA that are adenine/thymine (AT) rich; these proteins can be prevented from binding by the attachment of inhibitory proteins. Nucleosomes are themselves packed together even more tightly by H1 histone proteins.

Figure 15 shows how DNA within chromosomes is ordered. DNA that is actively being transcribed into mRNA is unfolded, but is at its most condensed during mitosis, when individual chromosomes can be recognized by their specific banded structure. Histone acetylation and deacetylation (mediated by histone acetylases, deacetylases, and their inhibitors) are crucial to the process of transcription, as acetylation allows unwinding of the chromatin and access to general and specific transcription factors (Fig. 16).

DNA Replication

Replication of DNA requires that it is unwound at so-called replication forks, each strand acting as a template for synthesis. DNA polymerase α is used on the lagging strand and DNA polymerase δ on the leading strand (Fig. 17). Both sections are synthesized in the 5′ to the 3′ direction (on the new strand), and the lagging strand is initially synthesized as short segments called

Okazaki segments. In man, each molecule of DNA (the full length of the chromosome) is so long that several replication forks are required; these are often clustered together in areas of DNA that are transcriptionally active. For instance, in women whose second X chromosome is condensed as heterochromatin (Barr body), the active X chromosome replicates throughout each S phase, which lasts for about eight hours, whereas the heterochromatin replicates only late in the S phase. During mitosis, a huge amount of histone protein has to be synthesized (histone protein forms an equal mass to DNA), and in man there are 20 replicated sets of histone protein genes arranged as tandem repeats on several chromosomes, each set of which contains all five histone proteins.

DNA Replication Errors

Errors can arise during DNA replication owing to insertion of the wrong base or the insertion of a run of microsatellite repeats (replication errors). These are normally repaired by nucleotide excision enzymes or replication error repair enzymes, respectively. Errors in DNA repair are a common feature of most human cancer.

Telomeres and Telomerase

Because of its structure and the way that it synthesizes nucleotides, DNA polymerase cannot replicate the very ends of chromosomes, which are modified into special regions called telomeres. In many species, these consist of tandem repeats rich in G (in man, GGGTTA). This region is replicated by a special enzyme called telomerase, which recognizes the GGGTTA sequence. Because there is no complementary DNA strand to replicate, telomerase uses an RNA template, which is structurally part of the telomerase, as a temporary extension for replication of the other strand. After several rounds of extension, one strand is longer and therefore can be used in turn as a template for replication of the second strand by DNA polymerase. It is thought that the telomeres shorten after each round of cell division and that this may limit the lifespan of a cell (senescence). Some malignant tumors are known to have high levels of telomerase, a feature that may mean that the cell can divide without the lengths of the telomeres being a limiting factor.

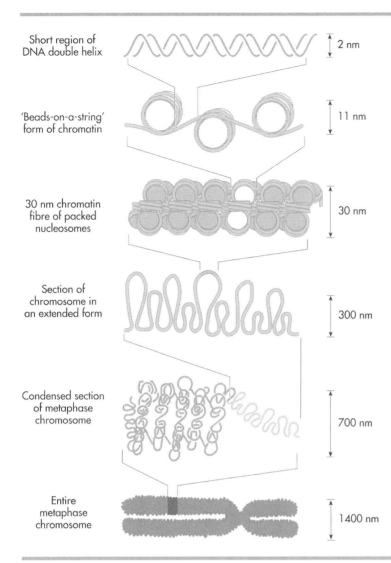

Short region of
DNA double helix — 2 nm

'Beads-on-a-string'
form of chromatin — 11 nm

30 nm chromatin
fibre of packed
nucleosomes — 30 nm

Section of
chromosome in
an extended form — 300 nm

Condensed section
of metaphase
chromosome — 700 nm

Entire
metaphase
chromosome — 1400 nm

Figure 15 Model of chromatin packing. This schematic drawing shows some of the many orders of chromatin packing postulated to give rise to the highly condensed mitotic chromosome.

This rather simplistic view has been replaced by one in which "capping" of the telomeres is important. It is true that during aging of the cell, the telomeres become shorter, but while the telomeres are capped, cell division can carry on. If the capping process fails, senescence and apoptosis can occur, but, more importantly, fusion of chromosomes can occur. This process is thought to be important in carcinogenesis (Fig. 18).

CELL DIVISION AND SENESCENCE

Senescence

Normal human cells cannot go on dividing forever in tissue culture; eventually, they senesce and will not divide further in response to mitogens. This process is accompanied by loss of telomerase, failure to phos-phorylate the retinoblastoma protein in response to mitogens, and high levels of p21 (WAF1) and p16, which are cyclin-dependent kinase inhibitors that profoundly inhibit cell division.

Cell Division

Cell division (Fig. 19) involves duplication of DNA, mitosis (nuclear division), and cytokinesis (division of the cytoplasm). Following replication of DNA, the centrosome divides to form the mitotic spindle, and the chromosomes condense and align in the center of the cell, where they are pulled apart by the mitotic spindle.

Mitosis: the "M" Phase

Prophase. The chromatin condenses into chromosomes that have duplicated and hence are formed

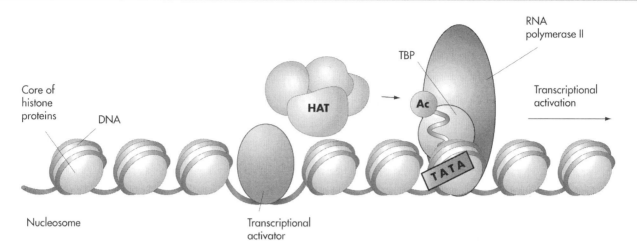

Figure 16 Conventional view of how histone acetylases interact with DNA. This cartoon shows how the acetylation of histone residues 'opens up' the DNA by release of histone proteins. A more dynamic process is the current view.

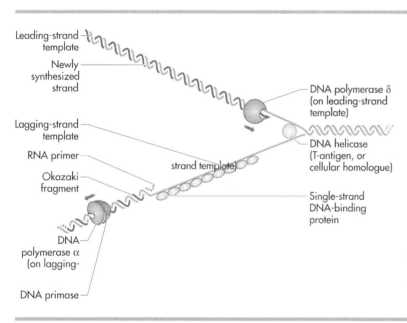

Figure 17 A mammalian replication fork. The mammalian replication fork is important in several respects. First, it makes use of two DNA polymerases, one for the leading strand and one for the lagging strand. It seems likely that the leading-strand polymerase is designed to keep a tight hold on the DNA, whereas that on the lagging strand must be able to release the template and then rebind each time that a new Okazaki fragment is synthesized. Second, the mammalian DNA primase is a subunit of the lagging-strand DNA polymerase, while that of bacteria is associated with the DNA helicase.

of sister chromatids held together by the centromere. The centrosome divides to form the mitotic spindle. The nucleolus disperses.

Prometaphase. The nuclear membrane disrupts. The kinetochores begin to form. These are specialized proteins attached to the centromere to which the microtubule proteins of the spindle pole bind. Patients with scleroderma form autoantibodies to kinetochore protein.

Metaphase. The chromosomes are aligned at the metaphase plate at the center of the cell.

Anaphase. The paired kinetochores suddenly separate, allowing the chromosomes to separate and to be pulled toward each spindle pole in a matter of minutes. Contraction of the microtubules pulls the chromosomes toward the spindle pole.

Telophase. The nuclear membrane begins to reform and the microtubules disappear. The nucleolus reappears.

Cytokinesis. The cytoplasm separates at a specialized contractile ring situated at the center of the cell, actively cutting the cytoplasm into two parts.

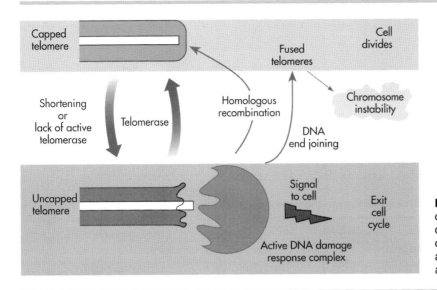

Figure 18 Telomeres. Telomeres are normally capped. Even shortened telomeres can be associated with normal cell cycling—provided they are capped. If the capping is lost, cells either undergo apoptosis or may be prone to chromosome fusion and malignancy.

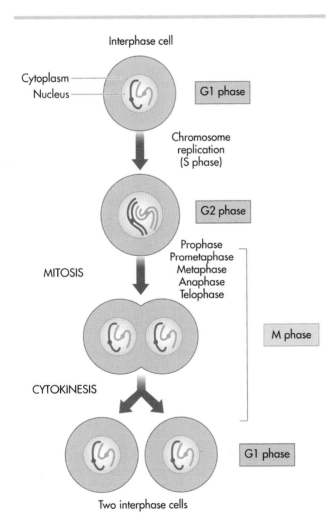

Figure 19 The four successive phases of a standard eukaryotic cell cycle. During interphase, the cell grows continuously; during M phase, it divides. DNA replication is confined to the part of Interphase known as S phase. G1 phase is the gap between M phase and S phase; G2 is the gap between S phase and M phase.

THE CELL CYCLE

In the adult human, cells are continuously being lost by the process of planned, programmed cell death (apoptosis). Some cells do not divide at all, although they can be destroyed (neurons and skeletal muscle fibers; however, recent work on stem cells suggest that these continue to exist in brain and muscle into adult life): some divide slowly, and others have to divide rapidly (such as cells in the bone marrow and lining of the gut). During cell division, DNA is replicated and reproduction of intracellular organelles takes place. Replication of DNA takes place during a specific part of mitosis known as the S phase. G2 is the period of rest before the prophase part of the M phase starts. The G1 phase occupies the period between the completion of the previous mitosis and the S phase; some mature cells, however, enter a specialized period of rest, G0, which can last for months or years.

The proportion of dividing cells can be measured by a number of different tests. Administration of radiolabelled thymidine or bromodeoxyuridine can allow labeling of cells in the S phase to be demonstrated by the use of photographic plates or monoclonal antibodies, respectively. Other antibodies can be used to measure the Ki67 antigen (Ki67 or MIB1) or proliferating cell nuclear antigen, which are expressed during particular parts of the cell cycle; these are useful in measuring cell proliferation within tumors. The amount of DNA within a population of cells can be estimated by the use of fluorescent stains such as ethidium bromide measured in a fluorescence-activated cell sorter.

The Control of Cell Division

This process is tightly controlled at certain critical points of the cell cycle, which are known as cell cycle checkpoints, at which certain brakes can be applied to stop the process if conditions are unfavorable (Fig. 20). Checkpoints are found at the G1/S

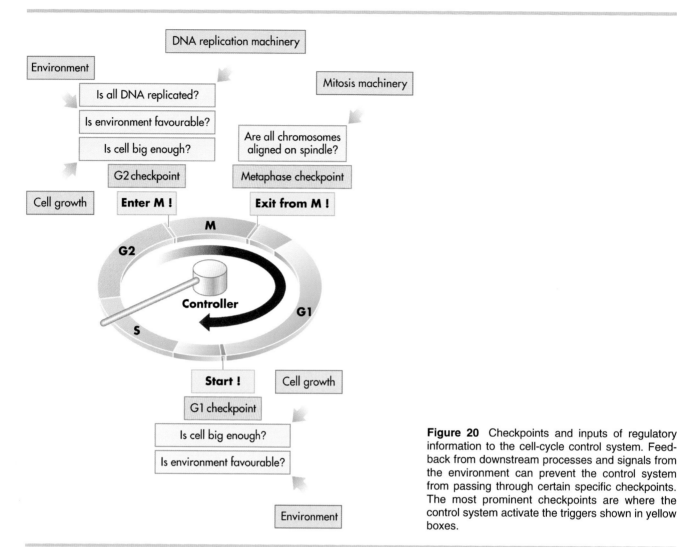

Figure 20 Checkpoints and inputs of regulatory information to the cell-cycle control system. Feedback from downstream processes and signals from the environment can prevent the control system from passing through certain specific checkpoints. The most prominent checkpoints are where the control system activate the triggers shown in yellow boxes.

transition (the start checkpoint); another is found at G2/M. Most studies have concentrated on the G2/M transition (the mitosis checkpoint). This cell cycle control mechanism is based on two series of proteins: the cyclin-dependent protein kinases (CDKs), which phosphorylate a series of downstream proteins on serine and threonine residues, and the cyclins, which along with other regulatory proteins bind to CDKs to alter their activity. Different cyclins are synthesized during different parts of the cell cycle (mitotic cyclins and G1 cyclins) (Fig. 21). In mammalian cells, there are at least six types of cyclin (A, B, C, D, E, and F). Entry into mitosis is stimulated by activation of a CDK by mitotic cyclin; in amphibians, this is known as maturation promotion factor (MPF) and consists of a cyclin and a cyclin-dependent kinase called cdc2—another is known as cdc4. Repetitive synthesis and degradation of cyclins is associated with the cell cycle. Activation of MPF drives mitosis, and degradation of cyclin then allows the cell to enter the S phase. As we shall see later, there is a set of proteins that can inhibit CDK known as cyclin-dependent kinase inhibitors (or inhibitors of cyclin-dependent kinases—INKs). The

activity of the CDK can therefore be abruptly switched on and off during different parts of the cell cycle.

In part, this process is controlled by the synthesis and degradation of the cyclins, but it is also affected by phosphorylation of the CDK on two sites (Fig. 22), which is controlled by two phosphatases known as Wee1 and MO15. Removal of one of the phosphate residues by means of another phosphatase—Cdc25— is then needed for activation of MPF. It is thought that the MPF autocatalytically activates itself, resulting in a steady rise in MPF levels during the cell cycle until the critical point when an explosive increase in activity takes place and drives the cell irretrievably into the M phase. Cdc2 is associated with the G1/S, and the G2/M transitions and cdc4 and cdc6 are associated with start, but are bound to different cyclins (cyclin B at mitosis and cyclin E and A at start at G1/S). The Kip/cip family of cyclin-dependent kinases, which include p21, p27 and p57, are capable of binding to and inhibiting most cyclin/CDK complexes. The expression of these CDK inhibitors is often dependent on upstream events that are activated by physiological signals, such as DNA damage, serum deprivation, or contact inhibition.

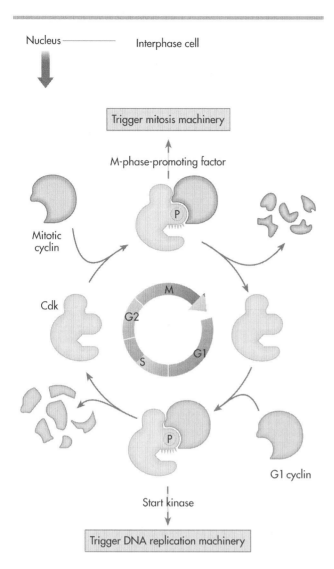

Figure 21 The core of the cell cycle control system. CDK is thought to associate successively with different cyclins to trigger downstream processes of the cycle. CDK activity is terminated by cyclin degradation. *Abbreviation*: CDK, cyclin-dependent protein kinase.

In contrast, the INK4 family of CDK inhibitors, including p15, p16, p18, and p19, bind to and inactivate D-type cyclins.

Growth Factors and the Control of the Cell Cycle

In mammalian cells, many peptide growth factors are potent inducers of cell division. These include platelet-derived growth factor; epidermal growth factor (EGF); insulin and insulin-like growth factors I and II; acidic and basic fibroblast growth factors (a-FGF and b-FGF); transforming growth factor α (TGF-α), which binds to the EGF receptor; and transforming growth factor β (TGF-β), which is structurally unrelated to TGF-α and is generally inhibitory. Many of these growth factors also act as proto-oncogenes.

These growth factors act over very short distances and may act on the cell that produces them (autocrine action) or on neighboring cell types (paracrine action). Many are found in serum, and this is one reason why serum is required to maintain cells in culture. High-affinity receptors for these growth factors are found on the cell membrane, and, in culture, cells compete for growth factors. As well as requiring growth factors for cell division, many cells require signals produced by intercellular contact and adherence (anchorage) mediated by means of adhesion molecules before they divide (anchorage-dependent growth).

Many growth factor receptors contain an endogenous tyrosine kinase, which is activated by ligand binding (Fig. 23). These receptors interact with proto-oncogenes, such as G proteins (such as ras), because tyrosine phosphorylation of the receptors facilitates binding of intermediate adapter proteins with so-called SH2 domains, which then link with other proteins (SOS, GRB2) that activate the ras pathway. Phosphorylation of downstream protein by growth factor receptors activates several early-response genes, which are stimulated within a few minutes of adding growth factor. In contrast, delayed-response gene activation requires protein synthesis. Many early-response genes activated by growth factor receptors control gene transcription; they include myc, jun, and fos, which are known to be crucial for gene transcription. In particular, myc is thought to be closely linked to activation of cell division.

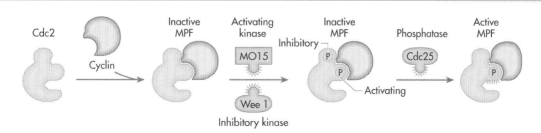

Figure 22 Genesis of MPF activity. Cdc2 becomes associated with cyclin as the level of cyclin gradually increases; this enables Cdc2 to be phosphorylated by an activating kinase on an 'activating' site, as well as by Wee1 kinase on Cdc2's catalytic site. The latter phosphorylation inhibits Cdc2 activity until this phosphate group is removed by the Cdc25 phosphatase. Active maturation promotion factor (MPF) is thought to stimulate its own activation by activating Cdc25 and inhibiting Wee1, either directly or indirectly.

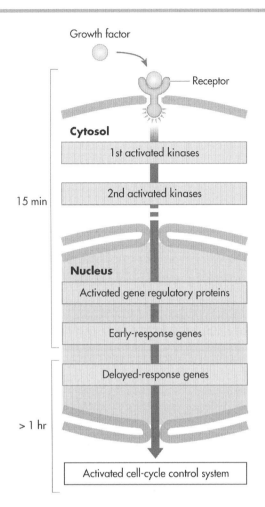

Growth factor

Receptor

Cytosol

| 1st activated kinases |

| 2nd activated kinases |

15 min

Nucleus

| Activated gene regulatory proteins |

| Early-response genes |

| Delayed-response genes |

> 1 hr

| Activated cell-cycle control system |

Figure 23 Typical signaling pathway for stimulation of cell proliferation by a growth factor. This greatly simplified diagram shows some of the major steps. It omits many of the intermediate steps in the relay system.

APOPTOSIS OR PROGRAMMED CELL DEATH

In many tissues, such as those of the hematopoietic system and the lining of the gut wall, proliferation and cell division are balanced by a process of planned cell death, the control of which is every bit as important as that involved in cell division. Programmed cell death also occurs in tumors, but the control of it is disrupted.

Apoptosis is a carefully orchestrated event in which the cell is programmed to die. The nucleus becomes shrunken and pyknotic, and the cytoplasm shrinks. The nucleus is sometimes extruded and may be engulfed by neighboring cells. No inflammatory reaction is excited by the process. This process is characterized by disintegration of the nuclear envelope and marked condensation of DNA into chromatin. On electrophoresis, the DNA assumes a characteristic banding pattern, implying that it has been cut by endonuclease enzymes. Nearby macrophages recognize the apoptotic cell and begin

to engulf and digest it. How this recognition process is mediated is unclear. The macrophages do not secrete inflammatory cytokines and chemokines; therefore, inflammation does not occur: apoptosis is quite different from necrosis.

Several genes are involved in this process. For instance, in thymic cells damaged by radiation, p53 is upregulated, an effect that increases the level of p21 (an inhibitor of cyclin-dependent kinase). This, in turn, slows down cell division, placing the cell in G1 arrest and allowing DNA repair to take place. It is thought that p21 is not directly concerned with the onset of apoptosis. In some cell types, such DNA damage initiates apoptosis, which is also associated with the upregulation of p53. There are a number of proteins known to promote apoptosis, including the bax family. Bax binds to and is inhibited by Bcl2. Homodimers of bax, which is upregulated by p53, bring on apoptosis. The Bcl2 protein binds and inactivates bax homodimers, thereby preventing apoptosis. Some types of apoptosis are not activated through p53. It is thought that the end point of apoptosis is the activation of a set of ICE-like cysteine proteases. Production of activated caspases is crucial to this process and may occur as a consequence of DNA damage. Detection of DNA damage and determination of the outcome, whether repair, apoptosis or carcinogenesis, is the responsibility of several genes, including BRCA1, BRCA2, ATM (ataxia telangiectasia), and p53. It is a highly complex process, which as noted above is frequently disrupted in cancer.

Aberrant expression of p53 and upregulation of Bcl2 will decrease the rate of apoptosis (although apoptosis is often higher in tumors with mutated p53 and upregulated Bcl2, because other mechanisms are activated). The point is that, in many tumors, DNA damage and the presence of mutated tumor suppressors and oncogenes will stimulate cell division, which will be in excess of the rate of apoptosis, so continued deregulated proliferation will probably lead to more DNA mutations occurring with each cell cycle.

STRUCTURE OF DNA AND RNA

Nucleic acids form the essential basis of DNA and RNA. These are made of the following three compounds:

1. *Bases*: Nitrogenous ring compounds called purines (adenine and guanine) or pyrimidines [cytosine, thymine (DNA), or uracil (RNA)].
2. *Pentose sugars*: Two types—ribose (β-D-ribose: RNA) and deoxyribose (β-D-2 deoxyribose: DNA).
3. *Phosphate*: The phosphate bond is attached to the 5′ C hydroxyl group, and in a nucleic acid, it bonds to the 3′ C position of the adjacent sugar residue.

The nucleoside is defined as a base plus a sugar (adenosine, guanosine, cytidine, thymidine, or uridine). The nucleotide is defined as a base plus a sugar plus a phosphate (Fig. 24). In addition to being the building blocks of DNA and RNA, nucleotides are used.

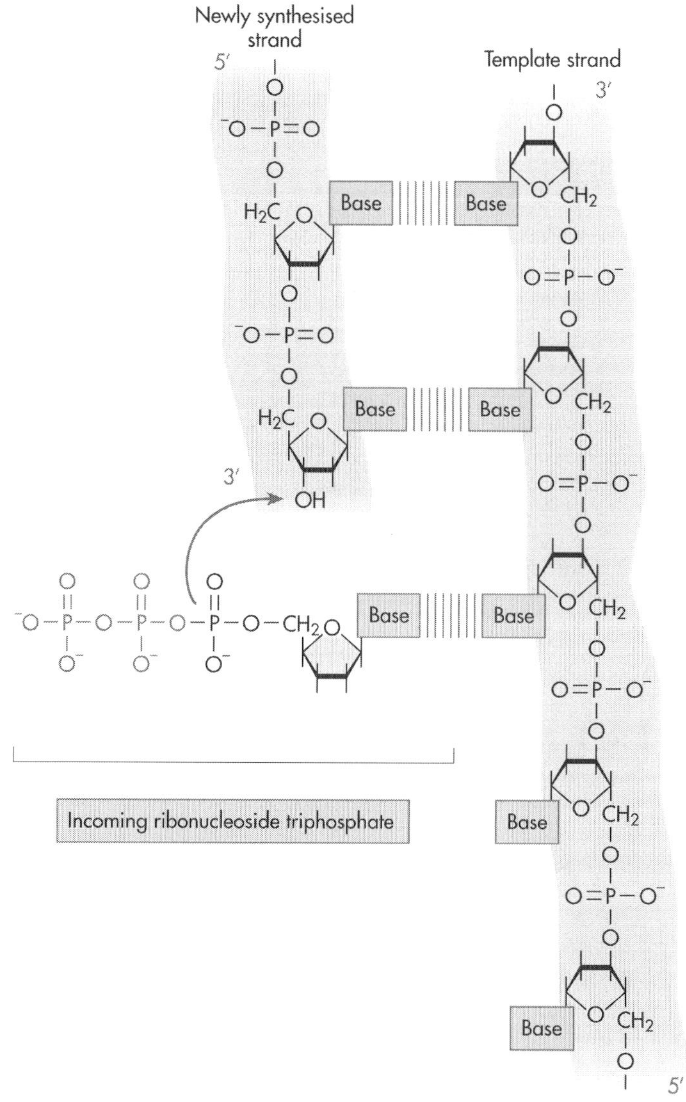

Figure 24 DNA synthesis. The addition of a deoxyribonucleotide to the 3′ end of a polynucleotide chain is the fundamental reaction by which DNA is synthesized. As shown, base-pairing between this incoming deoxyribonucleotide and an existing strand of DNA (template strand) guides the formation of a new strand of DNA with a complementary nucleotide sequence.

- As high-energy intermediates (such as ATP or guanosine triphosphate—GTP)
- In combination with other structures to form enzymes (coenzyme A)
- As signaling molecules (such as cyclic adenosine monophosphate—AMP)

RNA forms a single chain, whereas DNA forms a double helix held together by hydrogen bonding between bases on opposing strands; the individual nucleotides are held together by phosphate linkages between sugar residues (Fig. 24), the individual bases being suspended from the other end of the sugar residue. The sequence of bases forms the basis for all genetic information and is organized as a series of triplets, which code for individual amino acids. The hydrogen bonding between bases on opposing strands is not random, and on opposite sides of DNA, the following bases are always matched as complementary pairs (or Watson-Crick base pairs):

- G with C
- A with T (or A with U in RNA)

The triplet code for DNA and the corresponding amino acids are shown in Tables 2 and 3. A section of DNA can be read in a number of different "reading frames," depending on which particular nucleotide is the start of the reading frame.

The double helix formed by DNA occupies 3.4 nm for one complete turn, which contains 10 nucleotide pairs per turn and has a major and a minor groove. A single strand of DNA acting as a template will induce the formation of a second complementary strand if the appropriate nucleoside triphosphates and DNA polymerase are present in solution. Errors introduced by such complementary replication will induce a "point

Table 2   The Genetic Code

1st position (5' end)	U	C	A	G	3rd position (3' end)
U	Phe	Sea	Tyr	Cys	U
	Phe	Sea	Tyr	Cys	C
	Leu	Sea	STOP	STOP	A
	Leu	Sea	STOP	Trp	G
C	Leu	Pro	His	Arg	U
	Leu	Pro	His	Arg	C
	Leu	Pro	Gln	Arg	A
	Leu	Pro	Gln	Arg	G
A	Ile	Thr	Asn	Sea	U
	Ile	Thr	Asn	Sea	C
	Ile	Thr	Lys	Arg	A
	Met	Thr	Lys	Arg	G
G	Val	Ala	Asp	Gly	U
	Val	Ala	Asp	Gly	C
	Val	Ala	Glu	Gly	A
	Val	Ala	Glu	Gly	

Table 3   Amino Acids and Their Symbols

Letter	Symbols	Amino acid	Codons
A	Ala	Alanine	GCA, GCC, GCG, GCU
C	Cys	Cysteine	UGC, UGU
D	Asp	Aspartic acid	GAC, GAU
E	Glu	Glutamic acid	GAA, GAU
F	Phe	Phenylalanine	UUC, UUU
G	Gly	Glycine	GGA, GGC, GGG, GGU
H	His	Histidine	CAC, CAU
I	Ile	Isoleucine	AUA, AUC, AUU
K	Lys	Lysine	AAA, AAG
L	Leu	Leucine	UUA, UUG, CUA, CUC, CUG, CUU
M	Met	Methionine	AUG
N	Asn	Asparginine	AAC, AAU
P	Pro	Proline	CCA, CCC, CCG, CCU
Q	Gln	Glutamine	CAA, CAG
R	Arg	Arginine	AGA, AGG, CGA, CGC, CGG, CGU
S	Sea	Serine	AGC, AGU, UCA, UCC, UCG, UCU
T	Thr	Threonine	ACA, ACC, ACG, ACU
V	Val	Valine	GUA, GUC, GUG, GUU
W	Trp	Tryptophan	UGG
Y	Tyr	Tryosine	UAC, UAU

Table 4   The Size of Some Human Genes

Protein	Gene size (in kb)	MRNA size (in kb)	Number of introns
β-globulin	1.5	0.6	2
Insulin	1.7	0.4	2
Protein kinase C	11	1.4	7
Albumin	25	2.1	14
Catalase	34	1.6	12
LDL receptor	45	5.5	17
Factor VIII	186	9	25
Thyroglobulin	300	8.7	36
Dystrophin	>2000	17	>50

not quite correct because, in some organisms, several species of RNA may be produced from one gene, and spliced variants of mRNA in higher organisms are commonly tissue specific (such as splice variants for FGF receptors and p15, which is an alternative spliced variant of p16). The size of genes varies a great deal depending partly on the size of the protein to be produced (Table 4). Even within a gene sequence, although all of it is transcribed as primary RNA, not all sections are exported as mature RNA (Fig. 25). The gene is arranged into exons, which are exported from the nucleus as mature mRNA, and introns, which are excised from the primary transcript mRNA (Fig. 25) by means of RNA splicing and degraded in the nucleus.

Each gene produces messenger RNA (mRNA), and most genes (except those encoding ribosomes and tRNA) eventually produce proteins, some of which control the synthesis and modification of other compounds, such as nucleic acids, lipids, and carbohydrates. Less than 1% of DNA is transcribed into mature mRNA. Proteins have myriad functions, ranging from structural proteins, such as actins, right through to those that precisely control the rate of gene transcription.

mRNA Synthesis

After the opening up of the chromatin structure that occurs as a result of acetylation of histones, the next step is the synthesis of primary or heterogeneous mRNA (hnRNA), which is initiated by RNA polymerase type II, a large multiunit enzyme (Fig. 26). This enzyme binds to the promoter unit of the gene that is to be transcribed in conjunction with several other proteins called transcription factors.

The promoter region contains the site at which transcription factors bind and that is rich in TATA sequences (the so-called TATA box); it is situated about 25 nucleotides upstream of the start site of the gene. An AUG codon (methionine) always represents the start of each gene. RNA polymerase opens up the double-stranded helix, and RNA is synthesized by the polymerase, moving from the 3' to the 5' direction of DNA (i.e., the RNA is extended from the 5' to the 3' direction) (Fig. 26). This elongation continues until the polymerase reaches a STOP signal (UAA; UAG).

mutation'' where a single inappropriate base is inserted.

BASIC GENETIC MECHANISMS

Genes

Certain sections of DNA are arranged into genes, which are defined as lengths of DNA that produce specific mRNA and protein, although this definition is

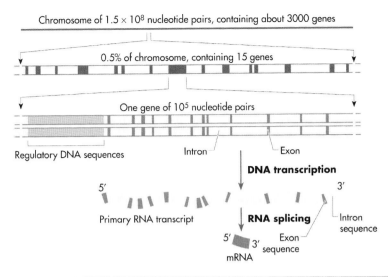

Figure 25 The organization of genes on a typical vertebrate chromosome. Proteins that bind to the DNA in regulatory regions determine whether a gene is transcribed; although often located on the 5′ side of a gene, as shown here, regulatory regions can also be located in introns, in exons, or on the 3′ side of a gene. Intron sequences are removed from primary RNA transcripts to produce messenger RNA (mRNA) molecules. The figure given here for the number of genes per chromosome is a minimal estimate.

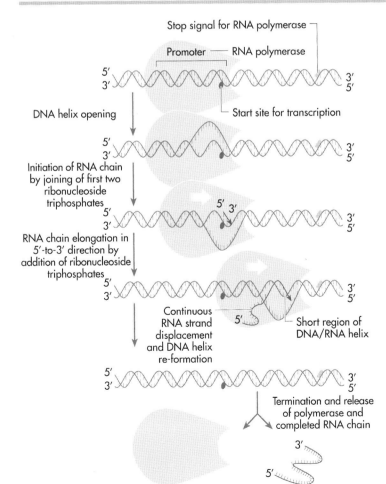

Figure 26 The synthesis of an RNA molecule by RNA polymerase. The enzyme binds to the promoter sequence on the DNA and begins its synthesis at a start site within the promoter. It completes its synthesis at a STOP (termination) signal, whereupon both the polymerase and its completed RNA chain are released. During RNA chain elongation, polymerization rates average about 30 nucleotides per second at 37°C. Therefore, an RNA chain of 5000 nucleotides takes about three minutes to complete.

Thirty nucleotides are added per second, so a chain of 5000 nucleotides will take about three minutes to make. Each strand of the double helix could, in theory, be used to copy into RNA, but, in any one section of DNA, only one strand is used, although, in any one chromosome, different strands are used in different parts.

There are three types of RNA polymerase (types I, II, and III). Type I RNA polymerase makes large ribosomal RNA and type III makes tRNA and the small 5S ribosomal RNA. Type II RNA polymerase is responsible for synthesis of the other types of RNA. Both ends of mRNA are modified. The 5′ end is "capped" by a methylated G nucleotide, whereas to the 3′ end a polyadenylated (poly-A) tail is added. The 5′ cap plays an important part in protein synthesis and protects the mRNA from degradation. The poly-A tail aids the export of mRNA, it may stabilize mRNA in the cytoplasm, and it serves a recognition signal for the ribosome. The primary RNA transcript from the gene is known as hnRNA, most of which is rapidly destroyed by removal and splicing of the remaining mRNA. The presence of the poly-A tail allows purification of the mRNA from other types of RNA, a fact that is useful in purifying mRNA for studies.

Introns and Exons: mRNA Processing

Early evidence for the presence of introns was the finding that mature RNA is relatively short and when, in experiments, it was annealed to DNA containing the gene of interest, it was found that the DNA formed several large loops, only short sections of DNA being adherent to mRNA. Primary mRNA transcribed

from the loops of DNA not bound to the mature mRNA does not form part of mature mRNA and is excised as introns. hnRNA, which is the primary transcript of the gene, is much longer than the mature mRNA; although it has the 5′ cap and poly-A tail, it also contains several introns. The hnRNA in the nucleus is coated with proteins and small nuclear ribonucleoproteins (snRNPs), which are somewhat similar to ribosomes, but much smaller (250 kDa compared with 4500 kDa); they are crucial to the excision of introns. Patients with systemic lupus erythematosas form autoantibodies against one or more snRNPs. As pointed out above (Table 4), introns form much of the largest part of hnRNA and of the genome itself. Introns can accumulate several mutations without necessarily affecting protein function (i.e., they comprise the so-called junk DNA). However, point mutations near the exon/intron junction can have disastrous effects on protein function if they result in introns not being removed (as in thalassemia) and in the formation of longer sections of mRNA and therefore of new types of protein. Spliceosomes are formed by aggregation of several snRNPs, ATP, and other proteins onto the exon/intron junction—they remove the intron as a "lariat" or noose-like structure (Fig. 27). Most genes contain several introns. After excision of introns, the exons are spliced together to form mature mRNA, which is then exported from the nucleus via the nuclear pores.

In the formation of some proteins, differential RNA splicing is the norm, producing different forms of RNA and hence different proteins. This is achieved by differential binding of distinct repressors or activators to the primary RNA transcript, which can alter the splice site and therefore alter the exact structure of

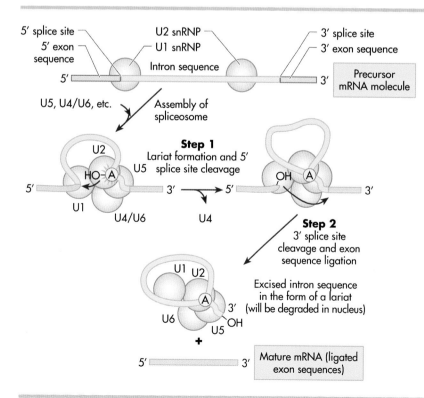

Figure 27 The RNA splicing mechanism. RNA splicing is catalyzed by a spliceosome formed from the assembly of U1, U2, U5 and U4/U6 snRNPs (green circles) plus other components (not shown). After assembly of the spliceosome, the reaction occurs in two steps: in step 1, the branch-point A nucleotide in the intron sequence, which is located close to the 3′ splice site, attacks the 5′ splice site and cleaves it; the cut 5′ end of the intron sequence thereby becomes covalently linked to this A nucleotide, forming the branched nucleotide. In step 2, the 3′-OH end of the first exon sequence, which was created in the first step, adds to the beginning of the second exon sequence, cleaving the RNA molecule at 3′ splice site; the two exon sequences are thereby joined to each other and the intron sequence is released as a lariat. The spliceosome complex sediments at 60S, indicating that it is nearly as large as a ribosome. These splicing reactions occur in the nucleus and generate mRNa molecules from primary RNA transcripts (mRNA precursor molecules).

the final mature mRNA. This occurs with the fibroblast growth factor receptors, which have several different spliced variants and different affinities for various members of the FGF family.

Control of Transcription

Following histone acetylation, various proteins bind to the promoter regions of genes to act as promoters and repressors. These can be classified into the following types:

- *Helix-turn-helix proteins.* These solely comprise amino acids and have a structure that facilitates binding into the major groove of DNA—their binding may block transcription or, conversely, may force bending of the DNA molecule facilitating transcription. The homeo-domain proteins are a type of helix-turn-helix protein involved in sequential embryonic development. Each of these homeo-domain proteins contains an identical section of 60 amino acids.
- *Zinc finger proteins.* Some transcription factors are rich in histidine and cysteine residues, which can bind zinc, thereby bending the protein into a finger-like shape. Steroid hormone receptors also contain several zinc fingers and are thought to function as transcription factors.
- *Proteins with a leucine zipper motif.* Certain α protein chains can form Y-shaped dimmers, which can attach to DNA; the two chains are held together by interactions between hydrophobic regions that are rich in leucine.
- *Helix-loop-helix proteins.* These form structures similar to leucine zippers.

These protein regulators of gene transcription can turn genes on or off depending on how they link with other transcription factors and RNA polymerase. It is also clear that many gene-regulatory proteins act at a distance upstream or downstream of the gene itself (Fig. 28); in some instances this can be a considerable distance from the promoter. These gene-regulatory proteins can have their function changed by increased de novo synthesis when needed, by ligand binding, by phosphorylation, or by combination with a second agent.

In addition to these specific transcription factors, general transcription factors are also required. Several proto-oncogenes are transcription factors. Fos and jun combine when phosphorylated to form the AP-1 protein, which functions as a transcription factor. Several growth factors interact through ras to activate MAP kinase (mitogen-activated kinase). MAP kinase phosphorylates a protein called Elk-1, which itself activates the transcription of fos.

Modification of DNA Can Alter Transcription

DNA that is tightly packaged around nucleosomes or the type that is packaged into heterochromatin is not easily transcribed. Unwinding of chromatin is controlled by acetylation of histone residues (deacetylation producing chromatin condensation). Condensation of the second X chromosome in women may affect the maternal or paternal copy at random, but small zones of neighboring cells in tissues will have the same X chromosome inactivated as a mosaic pattern. Another method of inactivating genes is heavy methylation of cytosine bases, which can result in inactivation of either the maternal or the paternal copies of particular genes. For instance, only the paternal insulin-like growth factor II gene is active; the maternal copy is inactivated or "imprinted" throughout the whole body. Recent data have suggested that some tumor suppressor genes can be inactivated—not through mutations or deletions, as in the case of retinoblastoma or p53—but through heavy methylation [such as the MTS (multitumor suppressor) gene, which encodes the p16 protein].

Posttranscriptional Modifications in mRNA Stability

Another method of controlling how much protein is produced by mRNA is to alter the stability of mRNA, which is normally a nascent molecule with a half-life of around 30 minutes to 10 hours. Some mRNAs have lengths of AU-rich noncoding sequences at the 3' end, which stimulate the removal of the poly-A tail, making the mRNA more stable. Some

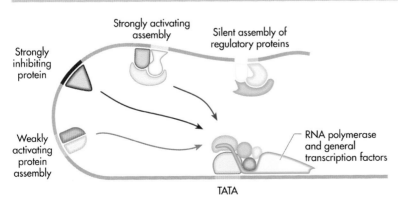

Figure 28 Integration at a promoter. Multiple sets of gene regulatory proteins can work together to influence a promoter, as they do in the eve stripe 2 module. It is not yet understood in detail how the integration of multiple inputs is achieved.

steroid hormones also increase the stability of certain mRNA molecules. Modification of the mRNA molecule can be mediated by proteins or, in some instances, can be mediated by RNA sequences that have intrinsic enzymic activity (i.e., they are RNA-ases). Posttranslational modifications in peptide chains can also lead to increased protein stability and increased duration of action.

Short Hairpin RNA

Some years ago it was found in plants and some primitive organisms that short sequences of RNA forming a hairpin shape could regulate the half-life of mRNA. Such short regulatory sequences are in fact used in cell biology experiments to "knock down" the function of certain genes. It was then found that the production of such short hairpin RNA (shRNA) sequences is an important part of the regulation of mammalian gene function. The expression of such shRNA sequences is now being actively studied in human health and disease.

Ribosomal RNA

During cell division, a large number of new ribosomes are required, and because the amplification process involved in protein synthesis (mRNA being translated into many protein molecules) is not available, most cells contain tandemly arranged multiple copies of ribosomal genes (around 200 per cell) on five pairs of different chromosomes. A tandem repeat is formed when duplicated DNA segments are joined head to tail. The initial ribosomal RNA (rRNA) (Fig. 29) transcript is 13,000 nucleotides long and is cut into three to form the 28S rRNA (5000 nucleotides), the 18S rRNA (2000 nucleotides), and the 5.8S rRNA (160 nucleotides) components of the ribosome. The 5S component of the large ribosomal subunit is transcribed separately by RNA polymerase III, and there are 2000 copies of the 5S rRNA genes arranged as a single cluster.

Packaging of ribosomal RNA occurs in the nucleolus, in which we find several large loops of DNA containing the tandem repeats for rRNA, which are known as nucleolar organizer regions. Here rRNA is transcribed by RNA polymerase I.

PROTEIN SYNTHESIS

When the mature mRNA reaches the cytoplasm after passing through the nuclear pores, it becomes attached to ribosomes, which catalyze the production of a peptide chain. Each amino acid is brought to the ribosome by its own specific small molecule of RNA, the tRNA (Fig. 30), which has an "anticodon" at its base corresponding to the codon for that particular amino acid. Specific enzymes couple specific amino acids to their particular tRNA molecule after the amino acid is activated by the attachment of AMP, after which it is known as adenylated amino acid. The

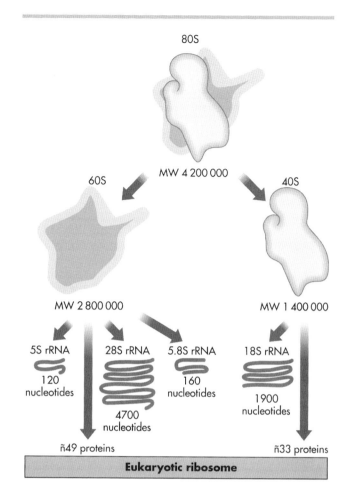

Figure 29 Eukaryotic ribosomes. Ribosomal components are commonly designated by their 'S values', which indicate their rate of sedimentation in an ultracentrifuge. Despite the differences in the number and size of their rRNA and protein components, both types of ribosomes have nearly the same structure, and they function in very similar ways. Although the 18S and 28S rRNAs of the eukaryotic ribosome contain many extra nucleotides not present in their bacterial counterparts, these nucleotides are present as multiple insertions that are thought to protrude as loops and leave the basic structure of each rRNA largely unchanged.

tRNA connected to its amino acid is referred to as an aminoacyl tRNA because of the bond between the amino acid and the tRNA. These mechanisms ensure that the right amino acid is brought by the correct tRNA to its specified position within the peptide chain. The genetic code is degenerate because most amino acids are coded for by more than one triplet, so that there is more than one tRNA for each amino acid, and a single tRNA can bind with more than one codon. Many amino acids require that the codon is accurate only in its first two positions (Table 2) and will tolerate "wobble" in the third position. Each incoming amino acid is attached to the carboxy end of the growing peptide chain.

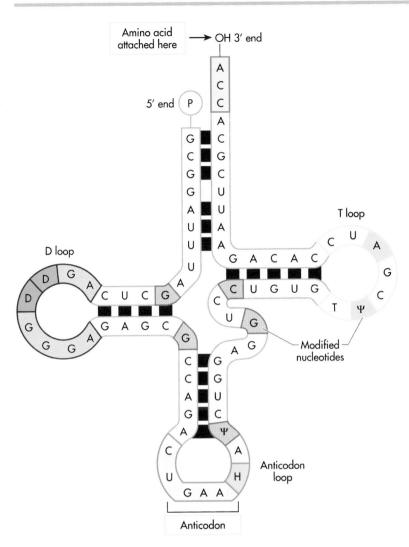

Figure 30 The 'cloverleaf' structure of tRNA. This is a view of a molecule after it has been partially unfolded. There are many different tRNa molecules, including at least one for each kind of amino acid. Although they differ in nucleotide sequence, they all have the three stem loops shown plus an amino acid-accepting arm. The particular tRNA molecule shown binds phenylalanine and is therefore denoted tRNA-Phe. In all tRNa molecules, the amino acid is attached to the A residue of a CCA sequence at the 3' end of the molecule. Complementary base-pairings are shown by red bars. *Abbreviation*: tRNa, transfer RNA.

Each ribosome consists of two major parts: the 60S and 40S subunits. The large 60S subunit comprises three separate parts: a 28S rRNA, a 5.5S rRNA, and a 5S rRNA (Fig. 31). These two subunits dock separately (the small subunit attaches first) on the mRNA at the AUG start codon (Fig. 31) and dock separately when the STOP codon (UAG) is reached (Fig. 32). Identification of the initiation site is important because, in principle, the mRNA can be read in any one of the reading frames, depending on the exact start site. Initiation factors assemble with the methionine tRNA at the start site before translation occurs.

Usually, there are several ribosomes attached to each mRNA molecule, so that at any one time there are several peptide chains in various stages of completion of synthesis. About 50% of the weight of the ribosome is RNA; the remainder comprises several types of proteins. Initially, it was thought that these proteins carried out the catalytic reactions of the RNA, but it is now clear that the RNA itself has these properties, and the function of the proteins is to modify these enzymatic functions. The ribosome has three binding sites for RNA; one for mRNA, one for incoming tRNA (A site), and one for outgoing tRNA and peptide chain (P site). On binding of an incoming tRNA, the aminoacyl-RNA bond is lysed, and the peptide bond is formed between the new amino acid and the peptide chain. The peptidyl-RNA in the A site is then moved to the P site by means of an energy-dependent reaction (GTP driven), freeing the A site for a new amino acid.

Obviously, recognition of the correct amino acid attached to the correct tRNA molecule is important. Firstly, the attachment of the amino acid to the tRNA is specific, and if an incorrect amino acid is bound to the aminoacyl synthetase enzyme, it is removed by hydrolysis. Secondly, the tRNA is attached to the mSteRNA as a complex with elongation factors,

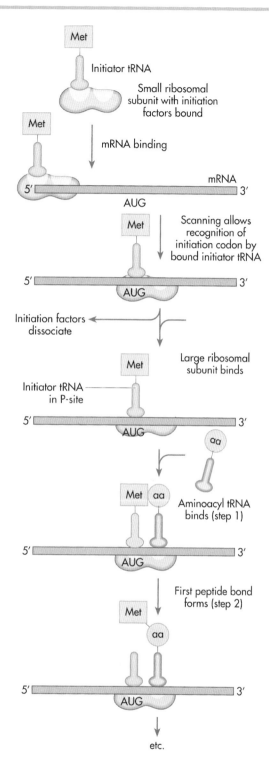

Figure 31 The initiation phase of protein synthesis in eukaryotes.

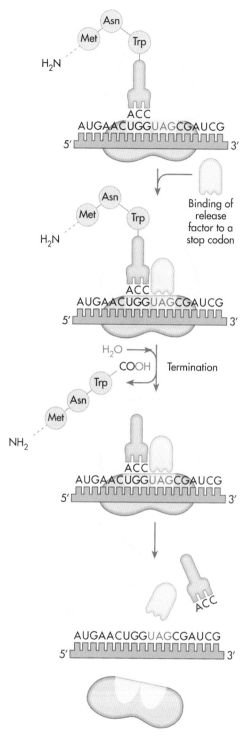

Figure 32 The final phase of protein synthesis. The binding of release factor to a STOP codon terminates translation. The completed polypeptide is released, and the ribosome dissociates into its two separate subunits.

which prevent the amino acid from immediately undergoing attachment to the peptide chain; and there is a short delay, which allows an incorrect tRNA to exit from the codon. It should be noted that the control of the levels of protein formation is achieved by the following three factors:

1. Controlling over gene transcription
2. Controlling the speed of mRNA degradation
3. Controlling posttranslational peptide and altering protein stability

For instance, upregulation of p53 in epidermal cells following exposure to sunlight is achieved by increasing the stability of protein that has already been made.

Inflammation

Neville Woolf

Medical School Administration, University College London, London, U.K.

INTRODUCTION

Inflammation is a reaction to injury in living tissue resulting in the accumulation of phagocytic cells and components of circulating plasma in the injured area. The inflammatory response is mediated via two biological pathways: the first involves changes in the caliber and permeability of the vessels constituting the microcirculation; the second is a complex series of operations leadingtoactivationof leukocytes. Basically, the inflammatory reaction is a protective one elicited by tissue injury or by the entry into a host of nonself elements such as pathogenic microorganisms. Inflammationacts to digest the components of dead tissue and to destroy and isolate the nonself elements just alluded to. It should not be forgotten, however, that the same functions which protect can also have devastating consequences, as, for example, when the inflammatory process becomes inappropriately activated in a systemic context, as in septic shock.

Changes in the Microcirculation

Injury is followed by an increase in caliber of arterioles, capillaries and venules at the site of its application. Arterioles dilate as a result of a chemically mediated relaxation of smooth muscle; capillaries and venules do so passively as a result of the increased flow mediated by arteriolar dilatation. This increase in local blood flow leads to two of the classic signs of acute inflammation: redness and heat.

Inflammation is characterized also by an increase in permeability of the microvessels, thus allowing more water and electrolyte, derived from plasma, to escape into the interstitial tissue, as well as the escape of high-molecular-weight proteins, such as fibrinogen, not normally found in extravascular interstitial fluid. This process, termed "exudation," causes another of the classic signs of inflammation, swelling, which may be localized, or may be the accumulation of edema fluid within serosa-lined spaces, such as the pericardial sac or peritoneal cavity.

Leukocyte Activation

This is a complex set of sequential processes, which include

- adhesion of leukocytes to microvascular endothelium in affected areas,
- migration of leukocytes through gaps between endothelial cells and across the basement membranes to reach the extravascular compartment,
- attachment of phagocytes to infecting microorganisms, to dead or injured cells or to foreign material at the site of injury,
- engulfment (phagocytosis) by the leukocytes of microorganisms or cell/tissue debris,
- microbial killing or digestion of cellular debris by phagocytes, and
- effects on surrounding cells/tissues of chemical mediators, either secreted or otherwise released from leukocytes.

CAUSES OF INFLAMMATION

The causes of inflammation are as follows:

- Mechanical trauma such as cutting or crushing
- Injury caused by living organisms
- Chemical injury (exogenous or endogenous)
- Excess ultraviolet or X-radiation
- Injury due to extremes of heat (burns) or cold (frostbite)
- Ischemia sufficiently severe to cause death or underperfused tissues
- Injury caused by excessive or inappropriate operation of the immune system

THE FORMATION OF THE INFLAMMATORY EXUDATE

Inflammatory edema and the formation of exudates are the expression of a net increase in the volume of water and electrolyte moving from the vascular to the extravascular compartment in the injured area,

Table 1 Patterns of Increased Vascular Permeability in Acute Inflammation

	Immediate transient	Delayed persistent	Immediate persistent
Injury	Mild	Moderate	Severe
Onset	Almost immediately	Up to 24 hr	Within a few minutes
Peak time	5 min	4–24 hr	15–60 min in experimental circumstances
Site of leakage	Postcapillary venules	Capillaries (relatively early peaking); venules plus capillaries in later peaking	
Duration	±15 min	Hours or days	Microvessels of all types
Mechanism	Histamine-induced interendothelial gap formation	Gap formation plus mild endothelial cell injury	Severe damage to endothelial cells and pericytes
Example	Mild type 1 hypersensitivity	Sunburn	Serious burns, major mechanical trauma

this being associated with the escape also of large-molecular-weight proteins (such as fibrinogen) that are normally held within the vascular compartment.

This process can be looked at in two ways. First, we need to consider the forces that determine the normal relationship between intra- and extravascular fluid and, second, the anatomical routes via which transfer of fluid and protein occurs.

Water, Solute, and Protein Leakage

Transport of water and solute across the microvascular endothelium shows many of the characteristics of ultrafiltration. Here, physical forces control the movement of fluid and electrolytes. The two forces normally acting (in opposition to each other) in this context are as follows:

- Intravascular hydrostatic pressure, which tends to push fluid out into the extravascular compartment
- Plasma oncotic pressure exerted by proteins, most notably albumin

An increase in the first force and a decrease in the second greatly increase fluid loss from the vascular compartment, a situation that is by no means confined to the context of inflammation. Normally, the result of interaction between these opposing forces is a small net outflow of fluid from the microcirculation. This excess fluid then drains from the extravascular compartment via the lymphatics. The importance of this last step is dramatically illustrated in patients with lymphoedema.

Chemical analysis of inflammatory exudates shows a protein concentration and pattern that is simply not attainable by the mechanisms mentioned above and for which other explanations must be canvassed. Such an explanation is readily found in the many data indicating that injury is followed by an increase in the permeability of microvessels. The patterns of exudate formation that we see in mammalian inflammation are the functional expressions of the severity and duration of injury and of the effects that such injury has on microvascular endothelium.

In mild injury, such as that caused by histamine, serotonin, or bradykinin, Majno and Palade proposed that plasma leakage was due to the formation of gaps between the endothelial cells of postcapillary venules. Recent studies have confirmed this and show that these gaps are coterminous with the sites of plasma leakage.

Patterns of increased vascular permeability are usually characterized in terms of two variables: the time between the injury and the first recordable changes in microvascular permeability, and the duration of the increase in such permeability. These patterns are described briefly in Table 1.

Neutrophil and Leukocyte Actions and Activation in Acute Inflammation

One of the most important components in defense against "nonself" elements is phagocytosis, first described by the Nobel laureate Élie Metchnikoff. If there is a lack of phagocytic cells or if those cells cannot seek out, engulf and destroy infectious organisms, the life of the affected individual will be endangered by increased susceptibility to infection.

The pivotal cell in the early phases of any inflammatory reaction is the neutrophil, which is present in relatively high concentrations in the blood, rapidly replaceable from bone marrow precursors and able to move more quickly than other leukocytes.

The two sets of lysosomal granules, that have led to their being called by some *granulocytes* contain enzymes such as muramidase (lysozyme), proteases, cationic proteins which act as reinforcing signals, peroxidase, lactoferrin (an iron-binding protein that inhibits bacterial multiplication) and alkaline phosphatase.

The operations necessary for effective neutrophil function have been listed on page 34. Few are more intriguing than the first of these: the adhesion between neutrophils and the microvascular endothelium, without which emigration of phagocytes from the blood into areas of tissue injury cannot occur. Failure to achieve a bond between neutrophils and endothelium occurs in some rare inherited syndromes and is associated with repeated episodes of bacterial infection.

Adhesion between leukocytes and endothelium is a two-stage process. In the first of these, the neutrophils move to the periphery of the column of flowing blood, adhere momentarily to the endothelial surface and then roll along that surface. In the second phase, the cells bind to the endothelial surface and flatten out before migrating through interendothelial cell gaps.

These two phases are mediated by two distinct sets of ligands and receptors. In the rolling phase, the microvascular endothelial cells in an injured area express molecules known as selectins because of their structural resemblance to lectins, a set of proteins, widely distributed in nature, that can distinguish with exquisite sensitivity between different complex sugars. Two types of selectin are known. One, E-selectin, is synthesized and expressed only after injury. This occurs about 30 minutes after the injury and usually reaches its peak in two to four hours. E-selectin binds to a complex sugar on the surface of white cells known as *sialy Lewis X*. Its expression is triggered by several signals, including the important cytokines interleukin-1 (IL-1) and tumor necrosis factor (TNF)-α.

The second, P-selectin, is synthesized constitutively and is stored in organelles, the Weibel-Palade bodies, within the endothelial cytoplasm. Following stimulation by appropriate triggers, the P-selectin is translocated to the endothelial surface, where it binds to another leukocyte surface sugar, lacto-*N*-fucopentaose III.

In the second phase of leukocyte adhesion, the endothelial components in the ligand-receptor interaction belong to a set of proteins known as the immunoglobulin gene superfamily. These include heavy and light chains of immunoglobulin, the a and β chains of the T-lymphocyte receptor, major histocompatibility peptides of both classes, β$_2$-microglobulin, CD4 and CD8 molecules on T lymphocytes and adhesion molecules on endothelium. The last-named comprise intercellular adhesion molecule (ICAM) 1 and 2, vascular cell adhesion molecule (VCAM)-1, and platelet-endothelial cellular adhesion molecule (PECAM)-1. ICAM 1 and 2 play a significant role in the binding of leukocytes to the endothelial surface. PECAM-1 contributes to the egress of leukocytes from the microvessels, and treatment with antibodies raised against PECAM inhibits leukocyte emigration, despite adhesion being perfectly normal. ICAM 1 and 2 are expressed constitutively on endothelium, but at very low levels. Release of the cytokines IL-1 and TNF-α upregulates IC expression, which reaches its peak about 24 hours after injury.

The leukocyte components belong to a family of two-chained transmembrane proteins known as integrins, which are expressed in many cell types. Some integrins are cell specific; this is the case with leukocytes, which express LFA-1, Mac1 and p150,95. These have a common β chain (CD18), and it is absence of this chain that underlies leukocyte adhesion syndromes.

Adhesion of leukocytes is followed by emigration from the small vessels, a process taking two to nine minutes. Leukocyte pseudopodia are inserted into interendothelial cell gaps, and the cells then move across the vessel wall into the surrounding tissues. As already mentioned, PECAM-1 plays an important part in this process, as does C-X-C chemokine known as IL-8.

Movement of leukocytes out of the microvasculature and through the extravascular compartment uses the same mechanisms that are involved in both phagocytosis and intracellular granule movement. They involve the plasma membrane of activated leukocytes and the peripheral zone of the leukocyte cytoplasm.

As with any cell capable of movement, leukocytes move as a result of interaction between the contrac-tile proteins actin and myosin. Stimulation of leukocytes by chemical signals results in an increasing proportion of the intracellular actin becoming arranged in a filamentous form, a process which is controlled by the expression of various proteins that can be stimulated or inhibited by calcium fluxes within the cells.

Phagocytes are stimulated not merely to move in the course of inflammatory reactions but also to move in a directed and purposive manner toward areas of tissue injury or of invasion by microorganisms. This is termed "chemotaxis," which, as its name implies, is controlled by a series of chemical messengers. For such a system to work, there must be adequate

- generation of signals that attract leukocytes to the site of injury,
- reception of these signals by protein or glycoprotein molecules on the surfaces of leukocytes, and
- transduction of the received signals so that the target leukocytes translate the former into action.

These signals, the chemical mediators of inflammation, are discussed in a later section of this chapter.

Reception and transduction of chemotactic signals is likely to start with the binding of the signal to a transmembrane receptor protein on the surface of the phagocyte. This is known to be true in the case of both the 5a component of the complement system and the formylated peptides released from bacteria in the course of bacterial protein synthesis. Occupation of a ligand-binding site on a surface receptor produces conformational changes that activate a G protein lying just beneath the plasma membrane and connected to the latter by a farnesyl bond. This in turn activates phospholipase, which cleaves phosphoinositol diphosphate (PIP$_2$). Cleavage of this molecule releases diacyglycerol and inositol triphosphate. The former activates protein kinase C, and the resulting protein cascade causes degranulation and secretion of granule contents; the latter produces calcium fluxes within the cell, which mediate chemotactic movement, and also releases arachidonic acid from cell membranes, with synthesis of prostaglandins and leukotrienes.

Cyclic nucleotides also play an important role in initiating leukocyte movement. cAMP and cGMP act in an opposing manner and may constitute a control system for regulating chemotactic movement and degranulation. cGMP enhances chemotactic movement, the release of histamine and leukotrienes from mast cells, the release of lymphokines from activated

T lymphocytes and the release of granule contents from neutrophils. In this context, the main effect of the cyclic nucleotides is probably exerted on the microtubules. cGMP promotes assembly of microtubules from tubulin, and cAMP has the opposite effect. Thus, drugs (such as levamisole) that raise the intracellular content of cGMP enhance the movement of phagocytes toward the source of chemoattractant substances and reverse the depression in chemotaxis that may follow a number of viral infections.

PHAGOCYTOSIS

Phagocytosis is the biological raison d'être of neutrophils. Before it can occur, the neutrophils traveling up their chemotactic gradient must recognize the particles, living or dead, which are to be engulfed and attach to them by means of ligand-receptor interactions. It has long been known that bacteria coated with immunoglobulin or dead tissue particles that have been exposed to fresh serum are more readily phagocytosed than those that have not. This coating of particles with protein is called *opsonization.*

Opsonins are either of the following:

- Immunoglobulins of the IgG class. For successful attachment of phagocytes to take place, the Fc fragment of the immunoglobulin must be intact.
- The C3b component of complement. This is of great biological value in defense against infection since complement activation by the alternate pathway does not require interaction between bacterial antigens and specific antibody.

The apparent restriction of opsonization to these two protein classes indicates that the phagocyte plasma membrane is the site of receptors both for the Fc fragment of immunoglobulin and the C3b component of complement.

For engulfment of bacteria, nonliving "foreign" particles, or cell and tissue debris, finger-like pseudopodia project from the plasma membrane of the phagocyte and fuse on the "far" side of the object to be engulfed, thus enclosing it within a vesicle formed of plasma membrane (the phagosome). The phagosome then buds off from the inner surface of the plasma membrane and migrates into the cytoplasm of the neutrophil or macrophage. The boundaries of the phagosome are formed of inverted plasma membrane, the inner lining of the phagosome being composed of the outer layer of the phagocyte plasma membrane.

Phagocytosis is an energy-dependent process that is inhibited by anything that interferes with ATP production. It is likely that the same mechanisms that "power" phagocyte movement are involved in phagocytosis and substances that inhibit chemotactic movement also inhibit phagocytosis.

Lysosomal Fusion and Degranulation

Phagosome formation is followed by movement of the lysosomes and fusion of the phagosome/lysosome membranes, this being associated with disappearance of the intralysosomal granules. The process is extremely rapid, and, again, as is the case with phagocytosis, is inhibited by any chemical substance that interferes with phagocyte movement.

BACTERIAL KILLING

The principal method of bacterial killing is oxygen-dependent. Phagocytosis is associated with a burst of oxidative activity known as the respiratory burst. This results in a stepwise reduction of molecular oxygen, ending in the formation of hydrogen peroxide, as follows:

- The respiratory burst is associated with a 2- to 20-fold increase in oxygen consumption, compared with a resting phagocyte, and there is a significant increase in glucose metabolism via the hexose monophosphate shunt.
- The reduction of molecular oxygen is catalyzed by a nonheme protein oxidase believed to be localized in the phagocyte plasma membrane. The presence of this oxidase is crucial for this type of bacterial killing; its absence leads to the congenital disorder known as chronic granulomatous disease of childhood.
- The hydrogen donor for oxygen reduction is either reduced nicotinamide adenine dinucleotide (NADH) or reduced nicotinamide adenine dinucleotide phosphate (NADPH). The presence of one of these is an essential link in the chain because hydrogen peroxide formation requires regeneration of NAD to NADP. The logical correlate of this is a requirement for adequate amounts of intracellular glucose-6-phosphate dehydrogenase if bacterial killing is to proceed normally.
- The reduction of molecular oxygen involves the gain of only one electron, resulting in the formation of an oxygen free radical, the superoxide anion (O_2^-). About 90% of the molecular oxygen consumed in the respiratory burst is converted into superoxide anion.
- The reaction of two superoxide anions in the presence of water results in the formation of hydrogen peroxide and molecular oxygen. This is termed a dismutation reaction and is catalyzed by the enzyme superoxide dismutase. Other highly reactive oxygen species formed in association with phagocyte activation include the highly reactive hydroxyl radical (OH), singlet oxygen and hypochlorous acid.

It is now believed that the most potent oxygen-dependent bactericidal activity in phagocytes is associated with hydrogen peroxide. This molecule, by itself, has significant bactericidal activity, but this is very markedly potentiated by a reaction occurring between hydrogen peroxide and intracytoplasmic halide ions that is catalyzed by the lysosomal enzyme, myeloperoxidase. The bactericidal effect is probably mediated by halogenation or oxidation of cell-surface components.

Other Mechanisms of Bacterial Killing

While oxygen-dependent killing is pivotal in defense against infection, it is not the only bactericidal mechanism. Some are related to the character of lysosomes and include the following:

- Low pH within the lysosome (3.5–4.0). This in itself may be bactericidal or bacteriostatic. In addition, the acid milieu promotes the production of hydrogen perioxide.
- Lysosomes containing lysozyme (muramidase), a low–molecular weight cationic protein that attacks the mucopeptide cell walls of some bacteria.
- Lactoferrin, an iron-binding protein found within lysosomes that inhibits the growth of several microorganisms.
- Lysosomal cationic proteins and hydrolases.

DEFECTS IN NEUTROPHIL FUNCTION

These defects may be quantitative or qualitative.

Even if all the operations described above are carried out normally, successful neutrophil defense against microorganisms requires an adequate number of these cells. Thus, neutropaenia from any cause confers a major increment of risk of infection. This situation can occur in any form of marrow failure such as may be caused by the following:

- Drugs, chemotherapeutic agents and toxins
- Bone marrow infiltration by large numbers of tumor cells
- Bone marrow fibrosis

Qualitative defects, of which there are many, can be considered most conveniently in relation to the specific functions which are defective. This is set out in Table 2.

Table 2 Defects in Neutrophil Function

Function affected	Disorder	Characteristics
Migration and chemotaxis	"Lazy leukocyte" syndrome	Defective response to chemotactic signals; nature of defect not yet elucidated.
	Job's syndrome	Typically affects fair-skinned, red-haired females; patients suffer from recurrent "cold" staphylococcal abscesses.
	Poorly controlled diabetes mellitus	Poor leukocyte movement reversed by insulin and glucose.
	Chédiak-Higashi syndrome	Rare autosomal recessive syndrome occurring in humans, cattle, mink, and certain strains of mouse; characterized by partial albinism, giant lysosomal granules in neutrophils and enhanced susceptibility to infection; believed to be related to failure of assembly of microtubules from tubulin; can be reversed (ex vivo) by agents that increase intracellular cGMP.
	Leukocyte adhesion deficiency syndrome	Because of absence of the CD18 β subunit of the integrins expressed on neutrophil surface; affects neutrophils only since other leukocytes express and adhesion molecule binding to Vascular cell adhesion molecule on endoethelium.
	Drug-related inhibition of leukocyte movement	Can occur after steroids or phenylbutazone
	Deficiencies in release of chemotactic signals	Affects mainly the complement system.
Disorders of phagocytosis	Opsonin deficiencies	Deficiencies in complement or IgG; some patients with sickle-cell disease show opsonin deficiency believed to be due to failure to activate the alternate pathway of complement activation.
	Failure of engulfment	Can occur in hyperosmolar states; may also be caused by drugs such as morphine analogues.
	Failures in lysosomal fusion	May be caused by drugs (steroids, colchicine, certain antimalarial agents).
Disorders of bacterial killing	Chronic granulomatous diseases of childhood	A rare disorder of childhood, sometimes X-linked and sometimes occurring as an autosomal recessive disorder; characterized by recurrent bacterial infections involving skin, bones, lungs and lymph nodes; lymph nodes draining infected areas are often enlarged and show sinusoids packed with mononuclear phagocytes and focal granuloma-like aggregates of mononuclear cells.
		The functional defect is failure of the respiratory burst (see page 37) and thus failure of oxygen-dependent killing.
		This reflects a defect in the cytochrome b-245 oxidase system that has two subunits. The X-linked syndrome is due to a mutation in the gene encoding the larger subunit, and in most cases, no gene product at all is produced.
		About one-third of patients with CGD have the autosomal recessive form, and here the defect arises as the result of a mutation in the gene encoding the smaller subunit or in the cytosolic components of the nicotinamide adenine dinucleotide phosphate oxidase system.

CHEMICAL MEDIATORS OF ACUTE INFLAMMATION

The process involved in acute inflammation, especially those controlling the activation of neutrophils, are under the control of a very large number of chemical signals. These mediators can be broadly classified under the rubrics exogenous and endogenous.

Only one group of exogenous mediators is recognized—the formylated peptides. These are low–molecular weight compounds produced by microorganisms in the course of protein synthesis, and all have methionine as the N-terminal residue. The most powerfully acting of these peptides is formylated methionine-leucyl-phenylalanine (*FMet-Leu-Phe*), for which neutrophils possess a surface receptor. FMet-Leu-Phe can also cause the expression of some adhesion molecules by microvascular endothelium.

Endogenous Mediators

The endogenous mediators of inflammation are grouped as shown in Table 3.

While it is impossible in a chapter of this length to comment in any detail on these multiple signaling systems, a few points are worth making.

Complement

The complement system consists of about 20 different proteins, functionally interlinked to play a significant part in immune responses and inflammation. Activation of complement may be achieved in two ways. In the first, the "classical" pathway, the union of antibody and antigen leads to the binding of a protein known as C1q. This step initiates the whole complement activation cascade. An "alternate" pathway exists in which no antibody/antigen union is required, and which can be triggered in many ways, including the presence of many strains of bacteria. The existence of the alternate pathway is clearly of great biological importance in the defense against infection.

Whichever pathway is involved, activation of complement yields chemical species that

* coat microorganisms, thus functioning as opsonins;
* lead to lysis of cell membranes via the formation of a membrane-attack complex; and
* influence both the vascular and cellular components of the inflammatory reaction.

Protein Mediators: Cytokines and Chemokines

Activation of cells involved in inflammation and in the immune response is associated with the release of many low–molecular weight proteins—the cytokines and chemokines. Only a few of the most important will be mentioned here.

Tumor Necrosis Factor α

This molecule derives its name from the fact that the serum of animals given bacterial endotoxin causes necrosis when injected into tumors. The active principle of such serum is the cytokine TNF-α. It is synthesized and secreted by activated macrophages, mast cells and T lymphocytes. At low concentrations, TNF-α upregulates the inflammatory response. It induces expression of adhesion molecules, thus promoting adhesion and migration of leukocytes from the microvessels to the extravascular compartment. It enhances the killing of intracellular organisms such as *Mycobacterium tuberculosis* and *Leishmania* and acts as a positive feedback loop for the production of a variety of cytokines.

At high concentrations (such as we may see in endotoxin shock), TNF-α acts systemically. In this context, it acts as a pyrogen, activates the clotting system, stimulates production of acute-phase proteins by the liver, inhibits myocardial contractility by stimulating nitric oxide production and causes inappropriate vasodilatation by the same mechanism.

Interleukin-1

The principle sources of IL-1 are monocytes and macrophages, but other cell types, such as endothelial cells and certain epithelial cells, may also produce this cytokine. IL-1 is a potent regulator of both local inflammatory events and many systemic ones. Its synthesis is stimulated by various microbial products, most notably bacterial endotoxin, and also by various cytokines. Locally, it upregulates adhesion molecule expression by endothelial cells, thus promoting adhesion of both leukocytes and platelets. Systemically, IL-1 produces fever and promotes the release of prostaglandins, glucocorticoids and acute-phase proteins. While it shares some of the functions of TNF-α, it lacks certain others, such as the ability to produce hemorrhagic necrosis in tumors.

This commonality of some functions between two molecules as different from each other as IL-1

Table 3 Endogenous Mediators of Inflammation.

Source	Mediators
Activated plasma protein cascades	The complement system The kinin system The intrinsic blood-clotting pathway The fibrinolytic system
Amines and proteins stored within cells and released on demand	Histamine 5-hydroxytryptamine Lysosomal enzymes and other proteins
Newly synthesized in cells and released from them on demand	**Lipids** Prostaglandins Leukotrienes Platelet-activating factor **Proteins** Cytokines such as interleukin-1 and tumor necrosis factor α and α and β chemokines

and TNF-α is not without interest. Many genes that are "switched on" in inflammatory diseases have their expression induced by IL-1 and TNF-α and, in some cases, TNF-neutralizing antibodies have had a beneficial effect in certain inflammatory disorders, such as rheumatoid arthritis. The link between these two cytokines appears to be that, after binding to their individual cell-surface receptors, both TNF and IL-1 activate a cytoplasmic form of the transcription factor NF-κB. DNA-binding motifs for NF-κB are found in the promoters and enhancers of more than 50 genes that are known to be activated in inflammation.

Chemokines

Chemokines are low–molecular weight proteins (8–11 kDa) that are important in initiating and sustaining inflammatory reactions. Some preferentially attract neutrophils; others attract monocytes. They are divided into two families: α and β.

The a family is encoded by genes located on chromosome 4. They are characterized by an amino acid sequence in which two terminal cysteines are separated by some other amino acid, thus giving the sequence Cys-X-Cys. Included in this group are IL-8, β-thromboglobulin, *gro-α*, *gro-β*, and *gro-γ*, and platelet factor 4.

The main source for the a chemokines is the monocyte, though some are produced also by T lymphocytes and endothelial cells. IL-8 mediates the rapid accumulation of neutrophils in inflamed tissues by inducing the expression of neutrophil-binding adhesion molecules on the surface of endothelial cells in the microvessels in injured areas. The chemokine *gro* acts also as a neutrophil chemoattractant as well as promoting the release of lysosomal enzymes. β thromboglobulin and platelet factor 4 are released from activated platelets and stimulate fibroblasts.

β chemokines are encoded by genes located on chromosome 17. They are potent attractants for memory T cells and monocytes.

Monocytes and Macrophages in Acute Inflammation

The cellular component of acute inflammation includes another type of phagocyte, the mononuclear phagocyte, which exists in two forms. An intermediate form known as the monocyte circulates in the blood; after migration into the tissues, it differentiates into the macrophage.

Monocytes have a half-life of about 222 hours, three times as long as that of the neutrophil. They are derived from bone marrow, and bone marrow destruction leads to a failure of injury to elicit a mononuclear cell response. Maturation from monocyte to macrophage within the tissues is accompanied by considerable structural and functional increase in the phagocytic, lysosomal and secretory apparatus, so that

- the cell becomes larger,
- the plasma membrane becomes more convoluted,

- lysosomes increase in number, and
- both the Golgi apparatus (secretion) and the endoplasmic reticulum (protein synthesis) become more prominent.

Like the neutrophil, the macrophage possesses surface receptors for the Fc component of immunoglobulin as well as for complement components. Again, like the neutrophil, the macrophage depends on anaerobic glycolysis for its energy needs during phagocytosis and has a respiratory burst after engulfment. Macrophages have certain advantages over neutrophils in that they

- have a longer life span,
- can synthesize and membranes and intracellular enzymes expended during phagocytosis (as the neutrophil cannot),
- can ingest particles far larger than those that can be engulfed by neutrophils, and
- can undergo mitotic division.

Many pathogenic microorganisms are engulfed within macrophages. Some of these parasitize the macrophages and multiply within phagosomes. Such organisms include *Listeria*, *Brucella*, *Salmonella*, *Mycobacteria*, *Chlamydia*, *Rickettsia*, *Leishmania*, *Toxoplasma*, *Trypanosoma*, and *Legionella*. This symbiotic relationship is destroyed as a result of what is effectively a dialogue between macrophages and T lymphocytes. Macrophage activation via this route leads to destruction of the "guest" organisms.

Chemical Signals That Influence Macrophage Function

Factors chemotactic for macrophages include those already mentioned in relation to neutrophils. In addition, however, there is an important group of chemical signals that trigger a wide range of macrophage functions other than chemotaxis. These are the lymphokines, secreted by T lymphocytes activated as a consequence of encountering specific antigens. T lymphocytes synthesize and secrete many products. Noteworthy in the context of macrophage activation is interferon-c; this is the most powerful enhancer of the ability of macrophages to kill intracellular parasites.

It should not be forgotten that macrophages also play a dominant role in the natural history of both healing and chronic inflammation. Their importance in relation to both of these processes rests on the fact that these cells have the power to

- phagocytose living and nonliving foreign material (including tissue debris, old or abnormal red blood cells, immune complexes and modified lipoprotein),
- kill many microorganisms,
- synthesize and release tissue-damaging products,
- synthesize and release mediators of acute inflammation and fever,
- present antigens to both T and B lymphocytes and in this way initiate immune responses,

- become activated by signals released from activated lymphocytes,
- release mediators that are chemoattractant for cells involved in repair and new blood vessel formation,

- synthesize and release growth factors that are important in healing, and
- regulate their own activities to a certain extent through the operation of autocrine loops.

4

Immunology

Anne C. Cunningham
Faculty of Applied Sciences, University of Sunderland, Sunderland, U.K.

Graeme O'Boyle and John A. Kirby
Institute of Cellular Medicine, Newcastle University, Newcastle upon Tyne, U.K.

INTRODUCTION

The immune system plays a key role in maintaining health and preventing disease. It has the capacity to destroy a very wide range of pathogens to prevent infection. In addition, it plays a key role in the recognition and destruction of transformed body cells and the prevention of cancer. To do that, it has to sense "danger" and respond by unleashing an effective and flexible arsenal to fight disease-causing organisms and cancerous cells. The immune system is not a discrete organ but a whole body system. To be effective, it must have the ability to respond to anything "dangerous" anywhere in the body. In reality, the immune system faces "outward" toward our barriers with the environment (musosal surfaces, skin) and is a highly dynamic, well-organized system.

This chapter will discuss the structure, function, and regulation of the immune system. It will explain the role of inflammation in the activation of immune effector mechanisms capable of destroying intracellular and extracellular pathogens. A well-functioning immune system represents a balance between making effective responses against dangerous agents while ignoring harmless things such as normal body components, food, and commensal organisms. This is a very exciting area of research in immunology, and it is clear that regulatory mechanisms exist to moderate the destructive capacity of immune responses. This harmful potential of immune responses are well demonstrated by the damage associated with immunopathologies seen in diseases such as glomerulonephritis, rheumatoid arthritis, and the extreme vigor of acute allograft rejection. The morbidity associated with genetic or induced immunodeficiency is also indicative of the importance of effective immune responses. The chapter concludes with a specific discussion of immunological examples drawn from the fields of clinical transplantation and cancer immunobiology.

STRUCTURE AND ORGANIZATION

There are two systems of immunity: the innate (or natural) responses that are phylogenetically older and present in all multicellular organisms and the acquired (or adaptive) responses, which are only present in vertebrates (with a jaw, including fish, reptiles, birds, and mammals) and evolved approximately 400 million years ago. The key difference between these responses is how they recognize danger. Innate receptors are not "specific" but recognize unique microbial structures found on pathogens. They are commonly referred to as "pattern recognition receptors" and they recognize "pathogen associated molecular patterns" (PAMPs), generally carbohydrates and lipids (1). These receptors can be most simply described as being biased to the enemy. Pathogens generally have a short cell cycle (minutes or hours) and can evolve rapidly to avoid recognition and destruction. However, we also possess adaptive receptors, which are produced by combining a diverse range of antigen receptor genes randomly (2). Each individual, therefore, also has many different rearranged antigen receptors and they can be most simply described as nonbiased. They are only expressed by T and B lymphocytes and generally recognize proteins.

Innate responses sense danger and coordinate the most effective adaptive immune responses for a particular pathogen. They lead to the activation of immune response genes and the activation of a specialized group of white blood cells, the antigen-presenting cells (APC). Once recognition and activation has taken place, then appropriate effector mechanisms remove the offending pathogen from the body. This does not happen everywhere in the body but is coordinated into different compartments. All white blood (immune) cells are produced in the bone marrow. This is the "primary" lymphoid organ. In addition, T lymphocytes mature in the thymus (where they undergo receptor rearrangement and a very important selection process). Innate recognition takes place in tissues (inductive sites), and inflammatory responses are generated. The purpose of inflammation is to focus on responses where they are needed. It results in an increase in immune cell/mediator recruitment to the site of infection. Ultimately, it is followed by the repair process. Figure 1 illustrates the principle behind

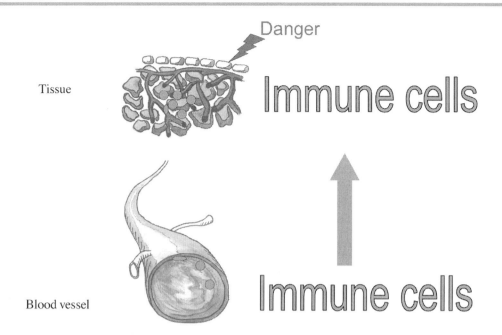

Figure 1 Relationship of innate and adaptive immune system.

inflammation; when danger is sensed, signals are released that lead to the recruitment of immune cells and mediators from the blood into tissue.

Adaptive immune responses take place in lymph nodes ("secondary" lymphoid organs). These unique structures are essentially "antigen" capture devices. Following inflammation, specialized APC in tissue (dendritic cells) drain to the regional lymph nodes where they activate T lymphocytes. Armies of effector lymphocytes are generated, which then home back to the inductive site to destroy pathogens/cancerous cells. Blood contains many immune cells traveling around the body; however, the really interesting action is taking place in the tissue and lymph nodes.

INNATE IMMUNITY

Nonspecific barriers to infection are the first obstacles a pathogen must overcome to achieve successful invasion of its host. These barriers are not acquired, do not change, and allow the specific immune system time to mount a response. The innate system of immune defense is, therefore, fast-acting but relatively nonspecific and nonadaptive. However, it is increasingly clear that the type of innate response influences the quality and quantity of the subsequent specific immune response. At the simplest level, the innate immune system consists of physical and biochemical barriers such as the skin, mucus, acid in the stomach, and lysozyme in many secretions, which all help to prevent the entry of microorganisms into the body. In addition, a battery of complex mechanisms designed to eliminate microbes that have penetrated normal body tissues also exists. More recently, the receptors

by which danger is sensed by the innate immune system have been described.

- C-type lectin receptors (CLRs)
- Toll-like receptors (TLRs)
- Nod-like receptors (NLRs)
- Retinoid acid–inducible gene-1 (Rig-1)-like receptors (RLRs)

Danger signals can be derived from pathogens, or from damaged tissue (endogenous signals), which enable the function of recognition and activation to take place. Each family of "sensors" has a distinct structure, which facilitates recognition and ultimately activation of immune responses. Recent evidence indicates that mutations in innate sensors can contribute to disease (3).

C-type Lectin Receptors

The structure of CLRs enables them to recognize repeating sugars found on yeasts, bacteria, and fungal cell walls. They consist of a collagen stalk, a neck region, and multiple carbohydrate recognition domains. They have multivalent binding domains, which increase the affinity and avidity of these molecules. This also explains why innate responses are broadly reactive rather than specific. These receptors exist as soluble molecules such as the mannan-binding lectin (MBL) and surfactant proteins A and D, or as receptors such as the mannose receptors expressed by macrophages. MBL is a very interesting molecule in that it can not only sense danger by its carbohydrate recognition domains but also activate the complement system (see later) (4).

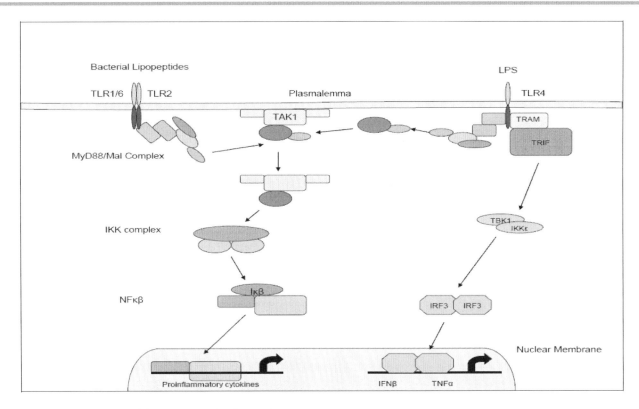

Figure 2 Features of the toll-like receptor signaling pathway.

Toll-like Receptors

TLRs represent a highly conserved gene family, which are very important in transducing signals via the transcription factor NFκβ and activating immune response genes. Each TLR is a type 1 membrane protein, and ligand recognition takes place via an extracellular leucine-rich domain complex. Signaling occurs via the intracellular tail, which activates nuclear transcription factors (NFκβ) and leads to the transcription of immune response genes (Fig. 2). There are 10 TLRs in humans, and they recognize a range of distinct cell wall and nucleic acid structures found in microbes and a range of endogenous molecules (Table 1).

In general, TLR1, 2, and 6 "sense" gram-positive bacteria and fungi, TLR4 senses gram-negative bacteria, TLR5 senses flagellum, and TLR3, TLR7, and TLR8 sense viruses (5).

Nod-like Receptors

The NLR family consists of 22 cytoplasmic proteins, which are primarily expressed by leukocytes but can also be present in many other cell types, including epithelial cells. These receptors generally recognize specific bacterial molecules, although viral nucleic acids can also stimulate some of these receptors. Following activation, the NLRs and TLRs can cooperate

Table 1 Ligand Specificity of Human TLRs

TLR	Ligand
1	(heterodimer with TLR2) triacylated bacterial lipopeptides, mycobacterial lipomannans
2	Lipoproteins, peptidoglycan, zymosan, liposaribomannan, staphylococcal enterotoxin B, HMGB-1, biglycan
3	Double-stranded RNA, poly(I:C)
4	LPS, heat shock proteins, taxol (mouse), RSV fusion protein, pneumolysin, fibronectin, lipotechoic acid, oligosaccharides from heparan sulfate and hyaluronic acid, β-defensin 2 (mouse), HMGB-1, saturated fatty acids (lauric acid) biglycan (with TLR2)
5	Flagellin
6	(heterodimer with TLR2) mycoplasmal lipopeptide, MALP-2, diacetylated lipoproteins, zymosan
7	Imidazoquinolines (anti viral compounds) single-stranded RNA (mouse)
8	Small synthetic antiviral compounds, single-stranded RNA (human)
9	Unmethylated CpG DNA
10	Pseudogene in mouse
11	Not present in humans, uropathogenic bacteria in mouse

Abbreviation: TLR, toll-like receptor.

through some common signaling systems leading to proinflammatory cell activation. However, activation of some NLRs also results in production of a macromolecular "inflammasome," which activates the proapoptotic enzyme caspase 1, which also generates active proinflammatory cytokines, including IL-1β and IL-18 (6).

Rig-1-like Receptors

Rig-1-like intracellular receptors primarily sense infection by some viruses, including influenza, by recognition of a characteristic 5'-triphosphate moiety associated with single-strand RNA sequences. Activation of these receptors leads to the production of the antiviral cytokine, interferon-β (IFN-β) (7).

To summarize, these innate sensors recognize danger in nature and often exploit differences between mammalian cells and pathogens (e.g., repeating sugars or distinct nucleic acid structures) and coordinate inflammatory responses by activation of distinct immune response genes (8).

Complement Activation

The complement system consists of up to 20 serum proteins that are involved in three interrelated enzyme cascades termed the "classical," the "alternative," and the "lectin" pathways. The end result of these cascades is the generation of a "membrane attack complex," which forms a potentially lethal membrane pore and a series of proinflammatory mediators, which recruit and activate other effector cells including neutrophils, macrophages, and mast cells. The alternative pathway may be activated directly, but nonspecifically, by a range of bacterial or yeast cell wall components, such as lipopolysaccharide (Fig. 3). The lectin pathway is initiated by MBL, which recognizes repeating mannose residues in bacterial cell walls. Once bound, this associates with a family of MBL-associated serine proteases, which activate serum C4 in a way similar to the classical pathway (see later), resulting in bacterial cell lysis and the generation of inflammatory mediators (C3a, C4a, and C5a).

Natural Killer Cells

Natural killer (NK) cells are frequently termed large granular lymphocytes on the basis of their morphology. The key feature of NK cells is their ability to kill virally infected or transformed body cells. For example, patients with defective NK cells frequently suffer severe infection by viruses such as cytomegalovirus. In many ways, they are related to cytotoxic T cells. However, their recognition of targets and control of killing are clearly different. NK cells possess receptors that can recognize class I major histocompatibility (MHC) antigens (see section on Cancer Immunotherapy), which deliver a strong inhibitory signal to the NK cell, preventing the lysis of healthy cells (9). Many tumors have defective genes or defective genetic regulation, which causes a lowering of the expression of MHC antigens. This reduces the classical immunogenicity of these cells but appears to enhance their susceptibility to NK cell-mediated cytolysis. Furthermore, infected or transformed cells express abnormal proteins, which can then be recognized by NK-activating receptors, and stimulate the delivery of a lethal hit.

Phagocytic Leukocytes

Phagocytes engulf and digest microorganisms and particles that are harmful to the body. Cells in this category can be divided into polymorphonuclear and mononuclear, but are all derived from common stem cells within the bone marrow. Neutrophils, the most common white blood cell, are generally the first cellular components to respond to tissue injury. They migrate from the blood across the endothelium and into the tissues within seconds of the recognition of a chemotactic stimulus. These stimuli may be chemicals specifically produced by bacteria, factors produced by damaged body cells, or peptides produced during the activation of complement.

Other phagocytic cells include tissue macrophages, such as mesangial cells in the kidney, Kupffer cells in the liver, alveolar macrophages in the lung, histiocytes in connective tissue, and microglial cells in the nervous system. Macrophages are highly phagocytic and contain numerous lysosomes and endocytic vesicles. They possess an enhanced antimicrobicidal capacity following activation. Phagocytes are also capable of secreting soluble agents able nonspecifically to damage cells and pathogens within the microenvironment. The most active of these factors are oxygen radicals, which are produced during the "respiratory burst" that follows cell activation.

Dendritic Cells

A specific class of mononuclear phagocytic cells forms a link between the innate and adaptive immune systems (10). These dendritic cells are named for the network of dendrite-like processes, which penetrate tissues to capture and phagocytose extracellular material. In normal situations, this phagocytosis is an immunologically silent process, which may contribute to the maintenance of immunological tolerance. However, following activation as a consequence of the innate system "sensing danger" by recognition of PAMPs, these cells acquire expression of a series of costimulatory molecules, which are required for induction of an adaptive immune response and also respond to chemokines by migration to regional lymph nodes. Crucially, dendritic cells break down proteins acquired by phagocytosis into short peptides, which can be presented in the context of MHC antigens to the antigen receptor on T lymphocytes.

Chemokines

The ability of cells to migrate is a highly regulated and specific biology. Leukocytes act to defend against infection and maintain balance. It is insufficient for leukocytes to merely react subsequent to gross tissue damage during infection; mechanisms exist to institute active surveillance of organs and tissues. The chemokine family of chemotactic cytokines is small

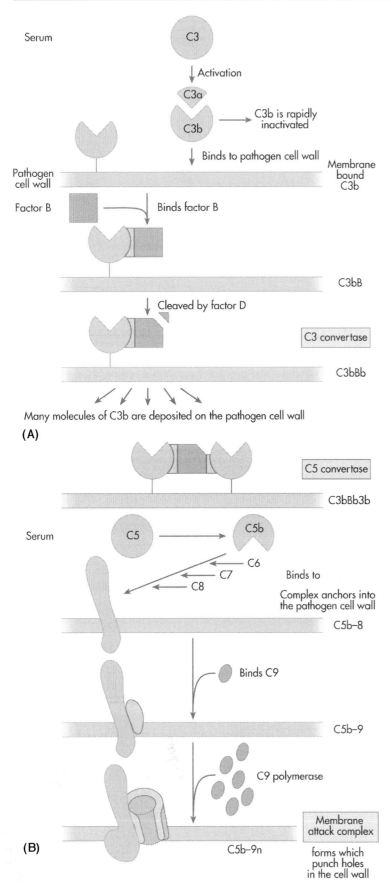

Figure 3 Complement activation.

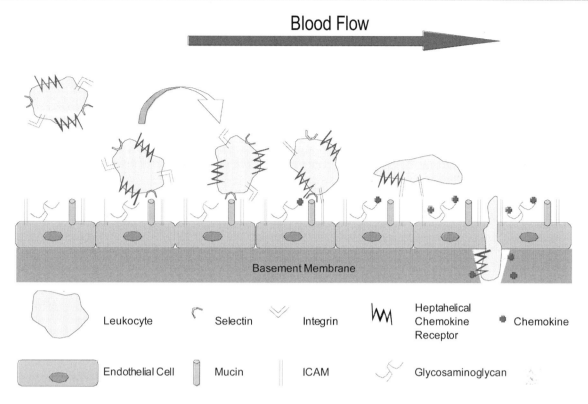

Figure 4 Stages of chemokine-stimulated leukocyte transendothelial migration.

(8–10 kDa); cytokines have a crucial role in leukocyte trafficking (11).

Leukocytes travel through the blood at high speed, and to penetrate a tissue, the multistep process of transendothelial migration must occur (Fig. 4). Shear forces in the blood causes leukocytes to roll along the surface of the vasculature because of weak adhesion between selectins on the leukocyte and endothelial surface. Chemokine receptors found on the cell membrane of the leukocyte may then encounter their chemokine ligand, causing activation of the adhesion process. Integrins on the leukocyte are activated within milliseconds, firmly tethering the leukocyte to the vessel wall. The leukocyte then migrates across the vessel surface toward a docking structure on the endothelial cell. Once leaving the high-pressure blood stream, chemokines then direct the leukocyte to migrate within the tissue along a chemokine gradient.

Over 45 different chemokines have been described, and they bind to over 22 different receptors. Chemokines can be subdivided on the basis of their functional role. CXCL12 is an example of a homeostatic chemokine; it is widely expressed and is important in immune surveillance by naïve lymphocytes. During disease or infection, inflammatory chemokines, such as CCL2, are produced and these direct activated leukocytes from the blood into the tissue. Inflammatory chemokines are typically stored within the endothelial cells lining blood vessels and are rapidly released upon endothelial stress or activation by cytokines. The chemokine system is thought to

consist of a complex network with a large degree of cross talk and redundancy. This is because individual chemokines can bind a number of chemokine receptors expressed on a range of leukocytes. In turn, each receptor may bind a range of chemokine. For example, the chemokine CCL7 is able to activate four different chemokine receptors, and up to 11 different chemokines bind the chemokine receptor CCR1, which is expressed by lymphocytes and mononuclear phagocytes. Because of this redundancy, targeting chemokines in human disease has proven difficult, although animal models have suggested a number of possible approaches, such as blocking groups of receptors at once to limit inflammation. Chemokine nomenclature is based around their structure and the position of highly conserved cysteine residues. C-chemokines have a single cysteine, CC-class chemokine have two conserved cysteines, CXC chemokines have two conserved cysteines with an intervening amino acid, and CX3C chemokine have three amino acids between their conserved cysteines.

Aside from their role in leukocyte migration, chemokines are also able to direct some immune effector mechanisms. Some chemokines, particularly those that act to attract polymorphonuclear cells, are able to cause respiratory burst and degranulation, while also influencing the movement of these cells. Chemokines play a role in the activation of lymphocytes by APC, and can influence the polarization of the immune response toward antibody- or cell-based responses. Chemokines are also involved in the metastasis of cancer cells. Cancers are characterized by a distinct metastatic pattern involving the regional lymph nodes, and tissues such as bone marrow, lung, and liver. For example, it has been demonstrated that the chemokine receptor CCR7 is highly expressed in many human cancer cells, malignant tumors, and metastases. Its ligand CCL21 is expressed in organs representing the first destinations of cancer metastasis.

ADAPTIVE IMMUNITY

The adaptive immune system has evolved to provide a versatile defense mechanism against infectious pathogens. The innate immune system is able to hold pathogens at bay for a time, but infectious microorganisms rapidly evolve to bypass these defenses. Each process of adaptive immunity is dependent on the function of lymphocytes and is characterized by an escalating response with a high degree of specificity. Furthermore, adaptive responses are characterized by immunological memory, which enables a more vigorous reaction after secondary exposure to a specific agent.

Resting lymphocytes are small mononuclear cells with little cytoplasm. However, following exposure to an antigen, a small proportion of antigen-specific cells expand rapidly and begin to divide. This process of clonal expansion is an essential feature of adaptive immunity. Lymphocytes may be divided functionally into T and B cells.

T cells and Cellular Immunity

The T-cell precursor is generated within the bone marrow but migrates to the thymus before maturing and developing the ability to recognize foreign antigen. Each newly formed T cell expresses numerous copies of an identical T-cell antigen receptor (TCR). However, the receptor on each different T cell varies in sequence and antigen specificity. This seemingly random variability enables at least a few cells within the total T-cell population to respond to antigens on any given pathogen. Following antigen encounter, these few specific cells divide to generate a sufficient number of responsive cells to mount a useful immune response. Estimates show that a single antigen-specific T cell can proliferate to generate a clone of over 1000 identical cells. This mechanism is termed clonal selection.

In recent years, the process by which maturing T cells generate their enormous receptor diversity has been determined. The TCR is a heterodimer and, for more than 90% of the cells, consists of an α and a β chain. Each chain is composed of a variable region, a constant region, a transmembrane region, and a cytoplasmic tail. The initial genomic sequence of DNA encoding each chain contains a large number of possible variable sequences followed by multiple diversity and joining sequences. Each mature chain is produced after a genetic rearrangement process that involves extensive deletion of genomic DNA and the resplicing of single, variable, joining, and diversity regions. It has been estimated that this process can yield a total of 10^{17} different αβ T-cell receptors.

A proportion of T cells, particularly those found close to the epithelial cells of the mucosa (including the genitourinary tract), express an alternative form of the TCR. This consists of a γ and δ chain heterodimer. The function of these γδ T cells is not clear. They appear to be less variable than αβ T cells, and are thought to represent an older, more primitive lineage.

Receptors expressed by each T cell are generated by a random process, and it is therefore likely that some newly formed cells will recognize antigens produced by healthy, or "self," body cells. The capacity to discriminate between self and nonself, and to prevent a response to self, is vital for normal immune function. This important requirement is fulfilled by the thymus, which is essential for the generation of T-cell self-tolerance. Equally essential to normal immune function is the thymus' other function—to provide a microenvironment suitable for T-cell maturation.

Thymic Tolerance

T-cell function is regulated by the affinity of the antigen receptor for a given ligand. The T cell will be activated by interaction with an antigen only if the affinity is sufficiently high. Essentially, the thymus selects newly formed cells that show no more than a low affinity for all self-antigens but deletes any cell-bearing receptors that recognize self-antigens with a dangerously high affinity (12). It has been estimated that only 3% of newly formed T cells survive this selection process and escape the thymus to join the recirculating pool.

T-Cell Recirculation

T cells that have not encountered their specific antigen, and are therefore naive, migrate from the circulation across specialized high endothelial venules to secondary lymphoid sites, such as the spleen, lymph nodes, and Peyer's patches in the genitourinary tract. These sites provide the ideal environment for contact with foreign antigens, and enable antigen-specific clonal expansion and the generation of effector/memory subsets. If a naive lymphocyte is not activated after 10 to 20 hours, it recirculates from the lymph node, through the lymphatic system and back into the blood at the thoracic duct. However, during an immune response, the blood flow through a lymph node rises dramatically and increases the number of lymphocytes within the node. Nonspecific resting cells leave the node followed, after three to four days, by a large number of activated antigen-specific T cells. These cells recirculate to the site of primary inflammation and to local lymphoid tissues. Finally, after a week or so, small, long-lived memory cells begin to leave the lymph node to join the recirculating pool. It has been estimated for adults that almost 50% of recirculating T cells are memory cells. These memory cells migrate differently from naive T cells and recirculate through the peripheral tissue where they first encountered their specific antigen (such as the skin, genitourinary, gastrointestinal, or respiratory system).

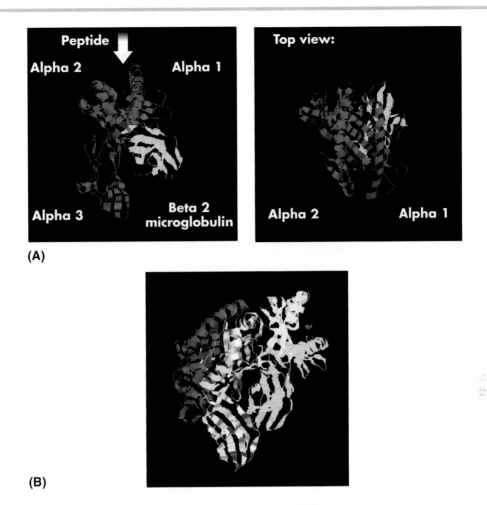

Figure 5 Crystal structures of (**A**) class I and (**B**) class II major histocompatibility antigens.

Major Histocompatibility Antigens

Human cells can express two classes of MHC antigen. The class I antigens are expressed constitutively on most cells, whereas the class II antigens are generally induced by stimulation with proinflammatory cytokines such as IFNγ or tumor necrosis factor-α (TNFα). Class II MHC antigens are generally only expressed constitutively by specialized cells of the immune system that are adapted for antigen presentation (such as dendritic cells). MHC molecules are essentially peptide receptors. They are specialized glycoproteins that bind a diverse array of peptides and present them to T cells.

Resolution of the structure of the MHC antigens (Fig. 5) has been one of the most significant advances in immunology during the past few years (13). Class I and class II MHC antigens have a similar three-dimensional structure but a different subunit structure. Class I MHC consists of a transmembrane α-chain that has three domains and a noncovalently attached β2-microglobulin. Class II MHC is a heterodimer of two transmembranous glycoproteins. A remarkable feature of these molecules is the prominent groove on their membrane-distal surface, which is always occupied by short peptide sequences. Class I MHC molecules typically contain nine amino acid peptides, whereas class II molecules can accommodate much larger peptides of up to 25 amino acid residues.

The genes encoding MHC antigens are extremely polymorphic within the human population. This polymorphism is generally restricted to the region of the groove and allows different forms of the MHC molecule to bind different families of short peptides. Table 2 shows the number of polymorphisms for the human class I (HLA-A, HLA-B, and HLA-C) and class II (HLA-DR, HLA-DP, and HLA-DQ) MHC alleles.

T-Cell Antigens

The TCR can recognize only short peptide "epitopes" bound in the groove of MHC antigens. Evidence suggests that the T-cell receptor interacts simultaneously with the MHC molecule and the peptide. In general, peptides from intracellular proteins are loaded into class I antigens, and peptides from phagocytosed extracellular proteins are loaded into class II antigens. However, a "cross-priming" pathway in specialized APC such as dendritic cells can allow

Table 2 Polymorphism of Human MHC Antigens

MHC	Class I			Class II		
Name	HLA-A	HLA-B	HLA-C	HLA-DR	HLA-DP	HLA-DQ
Number of allelic variants	697	1109	381	693	129	158

Data from the Anthony Nolan Trust, 2008.
Abbreviation: MHC, major histocompatibility.

extracellular proteins to yield peptides, which are loaded into class I MHC antigens.

T-cell self-tolerance is vital, given the inability of MHC molecules to discriminate between loading peptides from normal self-proteins and peptides from, for example, a pathogenic organism. The lymphocyte is activated only when the T-cell receptor binds to an MHC-peptide complex with an affinity greater than a triggering level. Thus, thymic deletion of all T cells that recognize MHC-self-peptide complexes with an affinity above this level will produce cells that can reach the required affinity only by interaction with complexes formed with nonself peptides.

Helper or CD4 T Cells

Approximately 60% of human peripheral T cells express the CD4 antigen on their cell surface. This antigen binds to a domain on the class II MHC antigen during interaction between the T-cell receptor and the class II MHC-peptide complex. Formation of this complex plays an important role in T-cell activation and has an additional implication for the immune response. As class II MHC antigens primarily form complexes with peptides derived from extracellular proteins, CD4 T cells are activated, albeit indirectly, by extracellular antigens (Fig. 6).

It is now clear that CD4 T cells are responsible for the regulation of most phases of the adaptive immune response. These cells are generally not directly cytotoxic, but produce a range of soluble mediators, or cytokines, able to affect other cells in the local environment. For this reason, they are often termed helper cells. Recent studies of individual clones of activated helper cells have shown that they can be divided functionally into several subpopulations. These are termed T_h1, T_h2, T_h17, and immunoregulatory T cells (Treg) cell types and are distinguished

from each other by the range of cytokines they produce or by their biological functions (14).

The T_h2 subpopulation is generated in the presence of IL-4 and produces a range of cytokines that are involved in antibody responses mediated by B cells and in mast-cell proliferation, eosinophilia and granuloma formation. These cytokines include IL-3, IL-4, IL-5, and IL-10. Significantly, IL-4 stimulates B cells to produce the IgE class of antibody, and these antibodies are involved in the release of histamine by degranulating mast cells.

The T_h1, T_h17, and Treg subpopulations may share a common precursor and are increasingly thought to be closely related, with a possibility for cytokine-induced transformation between these phenotypes (Fig. 7).

The T_h1 lymphocyte subpopulation appears to direct delayed-type hypersensitivity reactions by the production of cytokines such as IFNγ and TNFβ. These factors enhance the local recruitment and activation of phagocytes and stimulate the division of antigen-specific lymphocytes, including the CD8 cytotoxic cells described in the next section.

The T_h17 phenotype was only named in 2005, but is already recognized as playing a major role during the early stages of a number of inflammatory disease processes. These cells produce IL-17, which induces many body cells to secrete a range of chemokines, which recruit and activate innate immune cells, leading to further inflammatory damage.

Treg can reduce T cell–mediated immune processes. While TGFβ and IL-10 are known to modulate T-cell activity and T_h1 cell differentiation, the precise mechanism through which Treg function is not clear. An important subset of Treg can be identified by the transcription factor foxp3, which appears to be a master switch for regulatory function. Study of immunoregulation is one of the most exciting areas of

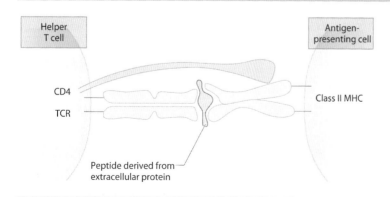

Figure 6 The presentation of antigen to CD4$^+$ T cells.

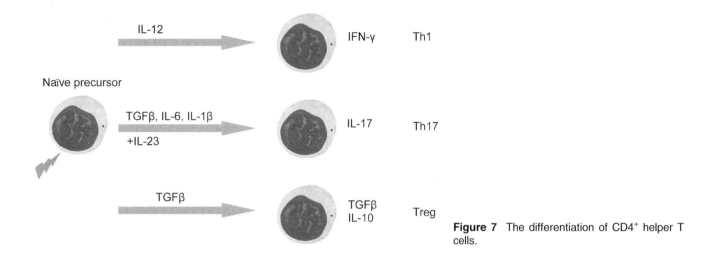

Figure 7 The differentiation of CD4$^+$ helper T cells.

immunological research and holds great promise for the understanding and treatment of immunopathologies, and even cancer.

Cytotoxic or CD8 T Cells

Approximately 40% of peripheral T cells express the CD8 antigen. This molecule binds to a domain on the class I MHC antigen during interaction between the T-cell receptor and the class I MHC–peptide complex. The formation of this complex plays an important role in the activation of CD8 T cells. As class I MHC antigens primarily form complexes with peptides derived from intracellular proteins, it follows that CD8 T cells are activated by intracellular antigens (Fig. 8). However, the cross-priming pathway in dendritic cells can allow presentation of, for example, viral peptides from the extracellular milieu to CD8 T cells, which can then recognize other cells infected with the same virus.

The CD8 lymphocyte subpopulation fulfills two roles. Its primary role is its involvement in the process of antigen-specific target cell lysis followed by cytokine secretion. Following activation, the CD8 T cell differentiates from a resting, or precursor, state to form a cytotoxic effector cell. This cell efficiently kills target cells that express the specific class I MHC–peptide complex. The direct lytic process involves lymphocyte degranulation and the secretion of agents including perforin, which forms pores in the target cell membrane, and granzymes, which induce the fragmentation of DNA within the target cell by a process termed apoptosis.

The ability of CD8 cytotoxic cells to lyse target cells containing nonself proteins is consistent with their involvement in the prevention of the spread of viruses by killing virally infected cells. Virally infected cells are recognized by the cytotoxic lymphocyte because nonself viral peptides are expressed in the peptide-binding groove of their class I MHC antigens. A similar mechanism may allow cytotoxic cells to kill class I MHC antigen–expressing tumor cells that produce novel tumor-associated antigens (see section on Cancer Immunotherapy).

B Cells and Humoral Immunity

In humans, B cells constitute approximately 10% of the circulating lymphocytes and are produced within the bone marrow. Resting B cells are morphologically similar to T cells despite being functionally distinct from them. B cells use a membrane-bound form of

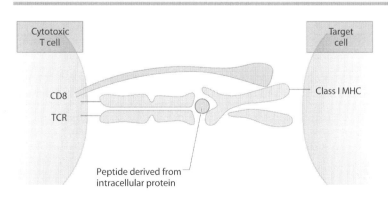

Figure 8 The presentation of antigen to CD8$^+$ T cells.

immunoglobulin to recognize antigen. The receptor can also be secreted as an immunoglobulin molecule or antibody following B-cell activation. Like T cells, B cells also have a clonal specificity for antigen, with each activated cell producing soluble immunoglobulins with a single specificity. B cells also express class II MHC antigens constitutively, and can therefore present foreign peptide to CD4 T cells, which can then help further in B cell maturation and potentiate immunoglobulin production.

Immunoglobulins

The immunoglobulins (Igs), or antibodies, are a group of five glycoproteins that are divided into five classes, termed IgM, IgG, IgA, IgD, and IgE. These classes differ from each other in structure and molecular weight, but their functions are broadly similar. One portion of the molecule, the variable region, binds to a specific site on an antigen, whereas the constant region may interact with, and regulate the function of, additional components of the immune system, such as complement, phagocytes, or cytotoxic cells. Unlike the T-cell receptor, immunoglobulins are not restricted to peptide binding and are able to bind efficiently to carbohydrates, nucleic acids, proteins, and a range of chemical and biochemical compounds.

Approximately 10% of the total immunoglobulin pool consists of IgM, which is a large, pentameric structure normally restricted to the blood. After primary infection, IgM is the first immunoglobulin produced by antigen-specific B cells. It has a low affinity for antigen, but the multivalency confers a relatively high avidity of overall binding. IgM is able to activate complement efficiently. Activated helper T cells, particularly of the T_h2 phenotype, produce cytokines that are able to stimulate B cells to class-switch from production of IgM to IgG. This smaller immunoglobulin makes up about 75% of the immunoglobulin pool, can diffuse more rapidly than IgM and, in addition to the activation of complement, can bind to a range of cellular components of the innate immune system.

IgA makes up about 15% of the total immunoglobulin pool and is generally restricted to mucosal sites. It is present in colostrum, saliva, and tears. Nearly all the IgD is associated with antigen recognition on the surface of B cells, whereas IgE is found on the surface of mast cells.

Immunoglobulin Diversity

The diversity of immunoglobulin specificities is generated by genetic splicing in a manner analogous to that of the rearrangement of the genes encoding the TCR. In the case of human immunoglobulins, it has been estimated that this process can produce up to 10^{11} different immunoglobulin molecules. However, unlike T cells, B cells supplement this process by rearranging immunoglobulin genes after antigen recognition by "somatic hypermutation." The mutated B cells, which, coincidentally, have a higher affinity for the antigen than the original clone, survive. The overall immunoglobulin response tends to become more specific as the immunoglobulins produced by the mutant cells possess an increased affinity for their antigen. This process is termed affinity maturation.

Classical Pathway of Complement Activation

The classical pathway of complement is activated by the interaction between subunit q of the complement C1 complex and the constant region of IgM or IgG molecules bound to their specific antigen. The activated C1 complex initiates the classical pathway of complement activation, in which classical C3 and C5 convertase are produced (Fig. 9). Beyond this point, both the alternative and classical pathways are identical and cause cell damage in a similar way.

Opsonization

Many human leukocytes express one or more of three classes of Fc receptor for domains on the constant region of IgG molecules. These cells include mononuclear phagocytes, neutrophils, eosinophils, and NK cells. These Fc receptors enable the leukocytes to recognize antibody-coated antigens by a process known as opsonization. This greatly enhances the efficiency of phagocytosis and increases the specificity of cellular elements of the innate immune response.

Antibody-Dependent, Cell-Mediated Cytotoxicity

Many NK cells express a relatively low-affinity Fc receptor for IgG. This receptor enables these cells to bind to IgG-coated targets and triggers a process that results in target cell lysis. As the receptor has a low IgG affinity, it binds aggregated IgG more readily than monomeric immunoglobulin in the plasma. This appears to prevent the inappropriate activation of NK cells in the blood.

ADHESION MOLECULES

A series of specialized adhesion and signaling molecules is involved in the migration of leukocytes across vascular endothelium and into body tissues and also in the regulation of T-cell activation.

Ligands and Receptors

Three main families of molecules are involved in binding and supporting the migration of leukocytes. These are the selectins and members of the integrin and immunoglobulin superfamilies. The involvement of selectins is mainly restricted to an initial low-affinity interaction typified by leukocytes "rolling" across the vascular endothelium. Members of the other two families are of importance during leukocyte stimulation, tight adhesion to endothelium, and extravasation into tissues (15).

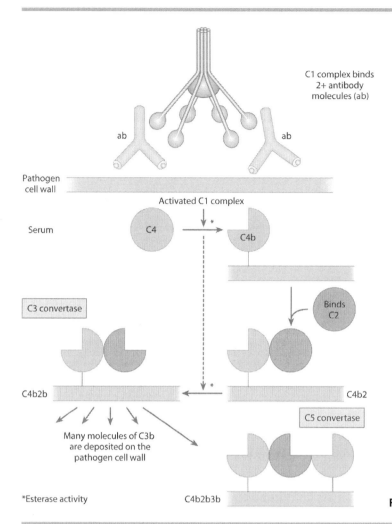

C1 complex binds
2+ antibody
molecules (ab)

ab   ab

Pathogen
cell wall

Activated C1 complex

Serum   C4 ———→ * C4b

C3 convertase   Binds
C2

C4b2b   ←———— * C4b2

C5 convertase

Many molecules of C3b
are deposited on the
pathogen cell wall

*Esterase activity   C4b2b3b

Figure 9 The classical pathway of complement activation.

Selectins

The three members of the selectin family are designated L-selectin, E-selectin, and P-selectin after the lymphocyte, endothelial cell, and platelet on which they were respectively identified. These molecules contain three structural regions and a cytoplasmic tail. The N-terminal domain is closely related to calcium-dependent lectins, whereas the central domain shares characteristics with an epidermal growth factor sequence. The third domain contains a number of repeating sequences homologous to a sequence found in proteins that regulate the activity of complement. Each selectin is thought to possess the ability to bind to a number of carbohydrate ligands.

Integrins

Integrins are a superfamily of transmembrane glycoproteins consisting of noncovalently linked α and, generally smaller, β subunits. They are widely expressed by cells of the body and are usually grouped by virtue of their common b chains into eight subfamilies. At least 14 discrete α subunits have been identified, and it is clear that a given α chain may associate with more than one β chain

(Table 3). The extracellular portion of the α chain contains three or four sites that bind divalent cations essential for integrin function. Both chains generally have short cytoplasmic regions able to interact with the cytoskeleton, and these may be phosphorylated. Phosphorylation is often associated with cell activation and can enhance the affinity of adhesion to the ligand (inside-out signaling).

Integrins play a key role in both cell-cell and cell-matrix adhesion. They bind to components of the extracellular matrix, such as collagen, fibronectin, laminin, and vitronectin. Some integrins have affinity for specific peptide domains, such as the well-characterized arginine-glycine–aspartic acid sequence, which is present in a number of extracellular matrix components. Three subfamilies of integrins are of particular importance for leukocyte adhesion. These include a member of the $\beta1$ family of "very late antigens" (VLA)-4 ($\alpha_4\beta1$), $\beta2$ integrins termed the leukocyte cell adhesion molecules (LCAM; $\alpha_L\beta2$, $\alpha_M\beta2$, and $\alpha_X\beta2$), and $\beta7$ integrins ($\alpha_4\beta7$ and $\alpha_e\beta7$).

The $\beta1$ integrin VLA-4 is expressed by many mononuclear leukocytes and binds to the immunoglobulin superfamily member vascular cell adhesion molecule (VCAM)-1 in addition to fibronectin. The $\beta2$

Table 3 The Integrin Family

Integrin	β subunit	Other names	α subunit	Other common name	Ligands
VLA-1	β1	CD29	α1	CD49a	Laminin (collagen)
VLA-2	β1	VLAb	α2	CD49b	Collagen (laminin)
VLA-3	β1	gpIIa	α3	CD29c	Fibronectin, laminin, collagen
VLA-4	β1		α4	CD49d	VCAM-1, fibronectin
VLA-5	β1		α5	CD49e	Fibronectin
VLA-6	β1		α6	CD49f	Laminin
β1α7			α7		Laminin
β1α8			α8		
β1αV			αV	CD51	Fibronectin
LFA-1	β2	CD18	αL	CD11a	ICAM-1, ICAM-2, ICAM-3 ICAM-1, C3bi,
Mac-1			αM	CD11b	fibrinogen C3bi
p150, 95			αX	CD11c	
CD41a	β3	CD61	αIIb	CD41	Fibrinogen, fibronectin, vitronectin, Von
b3aV		or	αV	CD51	Willebrand factor
		gpIIIa			As above 1-thrombospondin
b4a6	β4		α6	CD49f	Laminin
b5aV	β5	bX, bS	αV	CD51	Vitronectin, fibronectin
b6aV	β6		αV	CD51	Fibronectin; activation of latent TGFβ
LPAM-1	β7	Bp	α4	CD49d	VCAM-1, MadCam1, fibronectin
CD103			αe		E-cadherin
b8aV	β8		αV	CD51	Activation of latent TGFβ by dendritic cells

Abbreviations: VLA, very late antigen; LFA, lymphocyte function–associated antigen; VCAM, vascular cell adhesion molecule; ICAM, intercellular adhesion molecule.

subfamily is restricted to cells of the leukocyte lineage and includes lymphocyte function–associated antigen-1 (LFA-1) and Mac-1, which both serve to anchor leukocytes to cells that express intercellular adhesion molecule (ICAM)-1. The β7 family is expressed by mucosal lymphocytes. The $\alpha_4\beta_7$ integrin has recently been demonstrated to be the gut-homing receptor, enabling gut-trophic lymphocytes to enter the Peyer's patches. The αEβ7 (CD103) integrin is expressed by nearly all lamina propria lymphocytes in the gut, and by many intraepithelial lymphocytes in mucosal surfaces, including the gut, airways, and the urogenital system.

Immunoglobulin Superfamily Members

ICAM-1 is a large transmembrane glycoprotein bearing five domains containing the folded β sheet characteristic of immunoglobulins. The molecule is expressed constitutively by endothelial cells but is significantly upregulated by stimulation with IL-1, TNFα, and IFNγ. The cytokines TNFα and IFNγ also induce and upregulate the expression of ICAM-1 on a range of parenchymal cells, including fibroblasts and epithelial cells in the skin, lung, and liver. This process enhances the adhesion of β2 integrin–expressing leukocytes.

Structural studies have shown that VCAM-1 contains seven immunoglobulin domains. The first and fourth of these regions are homologous and function during lymphocyte adhesion. VCAM-1 is constitutively expressed on endothelial cells at a low level, but expression is upregulated within 12 hours and then maintained at high levels by stimulation with the cytokines IL-1 and TNFα. Immunocytochemical studies

have also demonstrated the presence of VCAM-1 on a variety of nonvascular cells, including renal epithelial cells, neural cells, and the synovial cells of inflamed joints.

Costimulation

Ligation of a T-cell receptor with its specific MHC-peptide ligand is insufficient to activate the T cell. This observation has generated the two-signal hypothesis for lymphocyte activation. Signal one is defined as interaction with specific MHC and peptide, and signal two is a nonspecific costimulatory signal.

Studies have indicated that the TCR has only a very modest affinity for its specific MHC-peptide ligand. This has been estimated as between 1×10^{-5} M and 5×10^{-5} M, which is considerably lower than the value for a typical IgG molecule, which is of the order of 1×10^{-9} M. This affinity is too low to allow stable conjugates to form between T-cell receptors and the 210 to 340 specific MHC-peptide ligands required for lymphocyte activation. The multiplicity of antigen-independent adhesion molecule interactions plays a vital role in stabilizing the T-cell and antigen-presenting cell complex sufficiently to allow T-cell receptor signal transduction to take place. This adhesion is rapidly increased following T-cell receptor ligation by an increase in the affinity of LFA-1 (inside-out signaling).

Appropriate ligation of the lymphocyte adhesion molecules LFA-1 and VLA-4 is known to generate costimulatory signals able to augment lymphocyte activation. Furthermore, monoclonal antibodies specific for LFA-1 have been shown to stimulate the proliferation of resting lymphocytes. The best characterized costimulatory molecule is the T-cell-surface molecule

CD28, which interacts with members of the B7 ligand family (CD80, CD86) on antigen-presenting cells, leading to the generation of a signal important for the activation and proliferation of antigen-specific T cells (16). Expression of the B7 family of ligands is restricted to a small group of specialized mononuclear cells, including dendritic cells and B cells. Other costimulatory molecules contribute to the response, including CD40 ligand (CD40L), which binds to CD40 on antigen-presenting cells. This leads to upregulation of B7 and therefore further T-cell stimulation. Antigen presentation in the absence of satisfactory costimulatory signal transduction may even produce stable lymphocyte hyporeactivity. Indeed, the therapeutic elimination of CD28 signaling by the blockade of B7 molecules with the soluble receptor-like construct CTLA4-Ig has resulted in partial cardiac allograft tolerance in a murine model.

EXAMPLES OF CLINICAL IMMUNOLOGY

Acute Allograft Rejection

The extreme vigor of allograft rejection can be explained by the process termed alloreactivity. Although mature T cells have been selected in the thymus for specific tolerance of all potential self-MHC antigen-self-peptide complexes, the cells have not been selected for tolerance of the subtly different MHC molecule–peptide complexes expressed on the surface of donor cells. It has been estimated that up to 2% of all recipient T cells may respond to the allogeneic MHC molecules expressed by graft tissues. Furthermore, as this situation reflects an artificial cross-reaction, a significant proportion of the responsive lymphocytes are present as memory cells, which facilitate the rapid initiation of the rejection response.

It is not clinically feasible to match the organ donor and recipient for identical MHC antigens, given the enormous polymorphism of MHC alleles (Table 2). Consequently, it has been necessary to develop drugs to suppress the immune response. One of the most successful immunosuppressive drugs is cyclosporin A, a calcineurin inhibitor, which revolutionized organ transplantation in the 1980s. This cyclic peptide blocks the production of IL-2 during T-cell activation. The function of this cytokine is best illustrated by its original name, which was "T-cell growth factor." Without IL-2, the graft-specific lymphocytes are unable to divide and cannot initiate the rejection response.

Cancer Immunotherapy

The prospects for successful cancer immunotherapy depend on the ability of T cells to recognize tumor antigens. During the 1950s, some chemically induced tumors were shown to express specific, "nonself" antigens that allowed sensitized animals to reject transplanted tumor cells. More recent studies have shown that T cells are able to recognize tumor-derived peptides complexed in the groove of MHC molecules.

A range of tumor-specific antigens have been detected, including the MAGE family (MAGE-1), which is found in 37% of human melanomas, a smaller proportion of other tumors, and no normal tissues except the immunologically privileged testis. Peptides from MAGE-1 associate with the class I molecules HLA-A1 and HLA-Cw16 and can be recognized by cytotoxic lymphocytes. The related molecule MAGE-3 is associated with a greater proportion of cancers and yields immunogenic peptides that complex with HLA-A1 and HLA-A2. Studies have demonstrated that up to 35% of transitional bladder cancers express MAGE antigens, with the proportion increasing to 61% of invasive tumors. Further tumor-associated proteins have been identified, including BAGE, and GAGE-1 and GAGE-2, which also yield peptides that can be recognized by cytotoxic T cells and are expressed by 10% to 20% of bladder cancers. In addition to the identification of proteins expressed by a range of cancer cells, tumors also express unique peptide epitopes derived from mutated genes. Recent work has identified such mutations in murine cancers, which yield peptides recognizable by both CD8 CTL and CD4 "helper" T cells.

It is, however, becoming increasingly clear that many cancer cells evolve a capacity to "evade" a local immune response (17). Not only do some cells express reduced levels of MHC molecules, the primary T-cell receptor ligand, but some also acquire a capacity to actively kill specific "effector" T cells by the "Fas counterattack." In this system, the cancer cell develops expression of Fas-ligand, which can engage the Fas receptor on local T cells, thereby initiating a proapoptotic cycle, which results in T-cell death. Another potential example of an immune evasion strategy is loss of the expression of E-cadherin by many epithelial cancer cells. It is now known that this molecule is an effective adhesion receptor for intraepithelial T cells, which are thought to be responsible for normal immune surveillance of mucosal surfaces. It is possible that the acquisition of these successful phenotypic attributes (from the cancer's point of view!) is a reflection of microevolution within the developing cancer, leading to selection of phenotypic variants that can evade an otherwise cancer-clearing immune response.

BCG Treatment of Bladder Cancer

The treatment of superficial bladder cancer by intravesical administration of BCG is almost a unique example of successful cancer "immunotherapy." The mechanism by which BCG can cause bladder cancer regression is not clear (18). However, it is known that BCG is an effective agent for the activation of dendritic cells in vitro, presumably by a mechanism involving ligation of multiple PAMPs, including the TLRs. Furthermore, model systems have shown that both activated T cells and NK cells are potentially involved in the clearance of bladder cancer cells. A challenge remaining in this area is the precise definition of optimal ways to induce immunological clearance of bladder cancer cells without resorting to the administration of viable, and often harmful, BCG bacteria. Indeed, current research is focusing on methods to induce an intravesical immune response by administration of defined subfractions of BCG by ligation of an optimal repertoire of PAMPs.

REFERENCES

1. Janeway CA Jr. Presidential address to the American association of immunologists. The road less traveled by: the role of innate immunity in the adaptive immune response. J Immunol 1998; 161:539–544.

2. Cooper MD, Alder MN. The evolution of adaptive immune systems. Cell 2006; 124:815–822.

3. McDermott MF, Tschopp J. From inflammasomes to fevers, crystals and hypertension: how basic research explains inflammatory diseases. Trends Mol Med 2007; 13:381–388.

4. Holmskov UL. Collectins and collectin receptors in innate immunity. APMIS Suppl 2000; 100:1–59.

5. Mitchell JA, Paul-Clark MJ, Clarke GW, et al. Critical role of toll-like receptors and nucleotide oligomerisation domain in the regulation of health and disease. J Endocrinol 2007; 193:323–330.

6. Delbridge LM, O'Riordan MX. Innate recognition of intracellular bacteria. Curr Opin Immunol 2007; 19:10–16.

7. Saito T, Gale M Jr. Principles of intracellular viral recognition. Curr Opin Immunol 2007; 19:17–23.

8. Creagh EM, O'Neill LA. TLRs, NLRs and RLRs: a trinity of pathogen sensors that co-operate in innate immunity. Trends Immunol 2006; 27:352–357.

9. Bottino C, Castriconi R, Moretta L, et al. Cellular ligands of activating NK receptors. Trends Immunol. 2005; 26:221–226.

10. Watts C, Zaru R, Prescott AR, et al. Proximal effects of toll-like receptor activation in dendritic cells. Curr Opin Immunol 2007; 19:73–78.

11. Jin T, Xu X, Hererld D. Chemotaxis, chemokine receptors and human disease. Cytokine 2008; 44:1–8.

12. Naeher D, Daniels MA, Hausmann B, et al. A constant affinity threshold for T cell tolerance. J Exp Med 2007; 204:2553–2559.

13. Bjorkman PJ. Finding the groove. Nat Immunol 2006; 7:787–789.

14. Chen Z, O'Shea JJ. Th17 cells—a new fate for differentiating helper T cells. Immunol Res 2008; 41:87–102.

15. Rose DM, Alon R, Ginsberg MH. Integrin modulation and signaling in leukocyte adhesion and migration. Immunol Rev 2007; 218:126–134.

16. Bour-Jordan H, Bluestone JA. Regulating the regulators: costimulatory signals control the homeostasis and function of regulatory T cells. Immunol Rev 2009; 229:41–66.

17. Pettit SJ, Seymour K, O'Flaherty E, et al. Immune selection in neoplasia: towards a microevolutionary model of cancer development. Br J Cancer 2000; 82:1900–1906.

18. Brandau S, Suttmann H. Thirty years of BCG immunotherapy for non-muscle invasive bladder cancer: a success story with room for improvement. Biomed Pharmacother 2007; 61:299–305.

5

The Nature of Renal Function

George B. Haycock
Academic Department of Paediatrics, Guy's Hospital, London, U.K.

HOMEOSTASIS

Homeostasis is the regulation of the volume and composition of the intracellular fluid (ECF), the "internal environment" that bathes the cells. The kidney is the preeminent organ of homeostasis, although the lungs, gut, and skin also contribute to it. One component of homeostasis is excretion of products of metabolism: failure of excretion leads to accumulation of these products with progressive pollution of the ECF. A second component is conservation of ECF solutes (mainly nutrients) that are too valuable to be allowed to escape into the urine. The third component is constant adjustment of the urinary excretion rate of water and inorganic solutes to maintain their concentrations in the ECF within the normal range, in the face of unpredictably changing input from the diet and from other body water compartments. This last might be called homeostasis proper. To achieve it, the kidney must

1. detect small changes in ECF volume, or in the concentration of any of its many constituents, before such changes become serious; and
2. respond by altering the volume or composition of the urine so as to correct the tendency to abnormality.

This is achieved by negative feedback: a rise in the ECF concentration of, say, potassium leads to an increase in its excretion rate with a consequent return of the ECF concentration to normal, while a fall in its concentration leads to a decrease in excretion rate, defending the ECF against hypokalemia. The kidney's capacity to alter the volume of urine and the concentration of its constituent solutes in urine is very large. An adult can vary daily urine volume between a minimum of about 500 mL and a maximum of more than 20 L, while the urinary concentration and excretion rate of the major ECF cation, sodium, can vary by at least three orders of magnitude.

The Concept of External Balance

Homeostasis requires (in the nongrowing organism) that net input of any substance into the ECF be exactly equal to net output from it. In health, body composition remains constant because output, mainly via the kidney, can be varied continuously in response to changes in input. The net external balance (NEB) for any substance is the algebraic difference between input and output over any specified period of time; that is,

$$NEB = input - output \qquad (1)$$

Balance may be positive (input > output), negative (output > input), or zero (input = output). Normally, NEB for all nonmetabolized substances is zero, except in growing individuals, in whom it is continuously positive. Since the main determinant of input is food intake, an obvious survival advantage enjoyed by an animal with a large reserve of renal function is the ability to eat a varied diet. As renal function is lost, dietary freedom becomes constrained. In advanced renal failure, survival is possible only on a rigorously controlled diet, reversing the normal physiological state of affairs: homeostasis is achieved by adjusting intake to match a relatively constant urinary output.

Growth and Renal Function

The size of the kidneys, and therefore their functional capacity, increases with growth of the body as a whole. Between the age of two years and maturity, glomerular filtration rate (GFR) and renal plasma flow in healthy humans are approximately proportional to body surface area (BSA) at about 120 mL/min/1.73 m^2 (range 90–150) and 600 mL/min/1.73 m^2 (range 450–750), respectively. The association between renal function and BSA is empirical, and probably does not reflect any underlying physiological principle. Some have argued that it should be standardized to ECF volume or body weight: the latter undoubtedly gives a better fit than BSA in newborn infants (Fig. 1) (1). GFR in healthy, term, newborn infants is about 30 mL/min/1.73 m^2, rising to 50 mL/min/1.73 m^2 at 1 month, 80 mL/min/1.73 m^2 at 6 months, and 100 mL/min/1.73 m^2 at one year, and attaining the adult value by 18 months to two years.

Whatever standardizing factor is applied, renal function is low at birth and during the first few months of extrauterine life, even corrected for body size. Despite this, normal infants thrive and show no clinical or biochemical evidence of failure of excretion

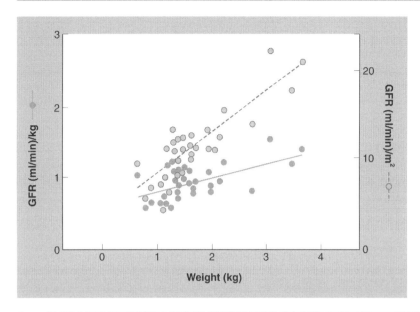

Figure 1 GFR corrected for body surface area (*interrupted line*) and weight (*continuous line*) in newborn infants. Within the range studied, GFR factored by surface area increases threefold while GFR factored by weight less than doubles. *Abbreviation*: GFR, glomerular filtration rate. *Source*: From Ref. 1.

or homeostasis. This can be explained by the fact that the infant is growing very rapidly at this stage, increasing body weight by up to 5% per week. This results in a strongly positive NEB for most nutrients, particularly since they are supplied by the baby's normal diet (human milk) in quantities that provide only just enough energy, protein, and minerals to support normal growth and activity. The residue remaining for excretion is, therefore, very small: growth provides the infant with a "third kidney" (2). A major advantage to the infant of constraining glomerular filtration at a low level is conservation of energy by the mother-infant dyad. Approximately 99% of filtered sodium is absorbed, with its attendant anions, by the renal tubule. This is an active process (see below) and accounts for almost all of the energy expenditure of the kidney. The additional energy cost of reabsorbing the sodium filtered at an "adult" level of glomerular filtration would be significant, given the marginal sufficiency provided by human milk, amounting to about 3% of basal metabolic rate (3,4). The negative aspect of the low GFR of the newborn is its lack of reserve. If growth is interrupted for any reason (such as intercurrent infection), or if an unphysiological diet containing too much protein (such as unmodified cow's milk) is given, the solute load presented for excretion can overwhelm the kidney, leading to a form of acute renal insufficiency with resulting metabolic imbalance. This principle is illustrated by the syndrome of late metabolic acidosis of prematurity (5).

The Concept of Renal Clearance

It follows from the above that, in a steady state, the composition of the urine is determined by dietary and metabolic input to the ECF, and not by renal function: individuals with a GFR of 100 and 10 mL/min,

respectively, will produce identical urine if they are eating identical diets. Since the function of the kidneys is to regulate the ECF, one way of quantifying renal function is to measure the rate of processing of ECF (plasma). For any substance (x) present in both plasma and urine, it is simple to calculate the volume of plasma containing the quantity of x excreted in the urine in a specified period of time. This volume is the renal clearance of x, the volume of plasma (not urine) cleared of x per unit of time. Renal clearance is given by the formula

$$C_x = \frac{U_x \times V}{P_x} \quad (2)$$

where C, U, and P represent clearance, urine, and plasma concentrations, respectively, and V is the urine flow rate. C is expressed in the same units as those chosen to express V (e.g., mL/min, L/day).

In the special case of a substance that is freely filtered by the glomerulus, such that its concentrations in plasma water and glomerular filtrate are the same, and which is not secreted or reabsorbed by the tubule or metabolized by the kidney, the filtration rate of x (F_x) must equal its excretion rate (E_x). The renal clearance of such a substance is equal to the GFR. No endogenous substance has been described that fulfills these criteria exactly in humans. Inulin, a starch-like polymer of fructose, does meet them, and is therefore an ideal marker for measurement of GFR. The chelating agents EDTA and DTPA, which can be labeled with radioisotopes for easy assay in plasma and urine, and the radio contrast chemical, sodium iothalamate, are excellent alternatives. Creatinine is an ideal marker for GFR in dog; unfortunately, in humans, it is secreted by the tubule to a small extent when renal function is normal but to a considerably greater extent when renal function is reduced. Despite this limitation, a carefully performed creatinine clearance test is an adequate measure of GFR for most clinical purposes (6).

Any substance whose clearance is greater than GFR must be secreted by the tubule. Conversely, any freely filtered substance with a clearance less than GFR must be reabsorbed by the tubule. Dividing C_x by GFR gives the fractional excretion of x (FE_x). If creatinine clearance (C_{cr}) is taken as GFR,

$$FE_x(\%) = \left(\frac{U_x \times P_{cr}}{U_{cr} \times P_x}\right) \times 100 \qquad (3)$$

Note that it is not necessary to measure V to calculate FE_x: simultaneously obtained blood and urine samples are sufficient.

A substance that is completely cleared by the kidney, that is, its concentration in renal venous plasma is zero, has a clearance equal to renal plasma flow (RPF). The organic anions paraaminohippurate (PAH) and orthoaminohippurate (hippuran) are almost ideal markers for measurement of RPF in most circumstances. An exception is in the newborn, in whom renal extraction of PAH is incomplete (7). Dividing GFR by RPF gives the filtration fraction (FF), the proportion of renal arterial plasma removed from the circulation as glomerular filtrate.

$$FF = \frac{GFR}{RPF} = \frac{C_{inulin}}{C_{PAH}} = \frac{U/P_{inulin}}{U/P_{PAH}} = \frac{U_{inulin} \times P_{PAH}}{U_{PAH} \times P_{inulin}} \qquad (4)$$

Typical normal values after infancy for GFR, RPF, and FF are 120 ± 30 mL/min/1.73 m^2, 600 ± 150 mL/min/1.73 m^2, and 0.2, respectively.

FUNCTIONAL SEGMENTATION OF THE NEPHRON

Each nephron consists of a glomerulus and a tubule (Fig. 2). The tubule is divided into two major segments: the proximal and distal tubules. The proximal tubule is further divided into the early (S_1) and late (S_2) proximal convoluted tubule, the proximal straight tubule (pars recta, S_3), and the loop of Henle. About 90% of the human nephron population (superficial cortical nephrons) have short loops of Henle that descend only into the outer medulla before bending and returning toward the surface of the cortex. The remaining 10% have long loops of Henle that descend deep into the inner medulla and bend at or near the papillary tip. These are the tubules that arise from those glomeruli situated in the deepest layer of the cortex, the juxtamedullary nephrons: they form an important part of the mechanism for urinary concentration and dilution. The parts of the loop that extend into the inner medulla are thin-walled and are called the thin descending and thin ascending limbs. The cortical part of the ascending limb is relatively thick-walled and is referred to as the thick ascending limb (TAL). The TAL of each nephron passes through the vascular pole of its own glomerulus where it is intimately related to the afferent and efferent arterioles in a structure called the juxtaglomerular apparatus (JGA). The JGA marks the functional division between the proximal and distal tubules.

The distal tubule is also divided into distal convoluted tubule, connecting tubule, cortical collecting duct (CCD), and medullary collecting duct. The different segments of the nephron are identifiable not only by their anatomical relationships but also by the ultrastructural and histochemical characteristics of their epithelia. Details may be found in relevant anatomical and pathological studies (8–10).

The Function of the Glomerulus

The glomerulus is a network of specialized capillaries that act as a size- and electrical charge–selective ultrafilter, retaining large molecules such as proteins within the lumen while allowing the passage of small molecules (water, electrolytes, and other crystalloid

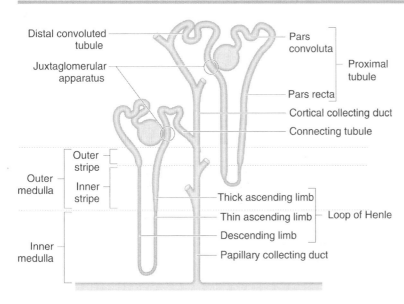

Figure 2 Schematic diagram of two nephrons, one of which is a juxtamedullary nephron (long loop of Henle) and one a superficial cortical nephron (short loop of Henle). The figure is not drawn to scale—the loop of Henle of the juxtamedullary nephron is actually much longer in proportion to the rest of the nephron than represented here.

solutes) into Bowman's space. The concentration of these solutes in glomerular filtrate is almost identical with that in plasma, with a small correction for the Gibbs-Donnan effect (because of the fact that negatively charged proteins are at much higher concentration within the capillary lumen than in glomerular filtrate). Ultrafiltration is a passive process, and the concentrations of small solutes in glomerular filtrate depend entirely on their concentrations in plasma and whether they are bound to plasma albumin. Glomerular filtrate is, therefore, the precursor of urine, the final composition of which is extensively modified by tubular reabsorption and secretion. Some important waste products of protein metabolism are entirely (e.g., urea) or mainly (e.g., creatinine) excreted by glomerular filtration. Although the excretion rate of these compounds is maintained at reduced levels of GFR, this is at the cost of sustained elevation of their plasma concentrations.

The Function of the Proximal Tubule

Pars Convoluta and Pars Recta

Two-thirds of the volume of the glomerular filtrate is reabsorbed in the proximal tubule. The nature of the reabsorptive process can be summarized as follows:

1. It is isotonic.
2. Some solutes (bicarbonate, glucose and amino acids) are preferentially reabsorbed in the initial segments of the proximal tubule, leading to their almost complete removal from the tubular fluid and a rise in the concentration of chloride (Cl^-).
3. It is energy and oxygen dependent.
4. Some solutes (such as inulin, creatinine, and urea) are reabsorbed little or not at all, and are therefore concentrated about threefold with respect to plasma by the end of the proximal tubule.

Organic anions such as PAH and penicillin are actively secreted in this segment. The fluid delivered into the loop of Henle is therefore the following:

1. Isotonic with plasma.
2. Chloride-rich and bicarbonate-poor.
3. At a pH lower than that of plasma (more acid).
4. More concentrated than plasma with respect to substances excreted solely or principally by glomerular filtration. The ratio of the tubular fluid inulin concentration to the plasma inulin concentration ($TF:P_{inulin}$) at any point along the tubule is a measure of the volume of filtrate that has been absorbed at that point. For example, if $TF:P_{inulin}$ is 10, 90% of filtered water has been reabsorbed at that point. Similarly, the urine-to-plasma inulin ratio ($U:P_{inulin}$) is a measure of the amount of filtered water that is reabsorbed between glomerular filtrate and the final urine (as is, approximately, $U:P_{creatinine}$).

Loop of Henle

Net reabsorption continues in the loop so that about 85% of filtered sodium and 70% of filtered water have been reabsorbed at entry into the distal tubule. The major function of the loop is concentration and dilution of urine: reabsorption in this segment is, therefore, no longer isotonic.

Concentration and dilution of urine are both powered by the same energy-dependent process: absorption of salt without water in the TAL. The fluid entering the distal tubule is hypotonic with respect to plasma, irrespective of whether the final urine is concentrated or dilute at the time. Salt reabsorption in the TAL also generates hypertonicity in the interstitium surrounding the TAL. This hypertonicity is amplified by countercurrent exchange and multiplication in the loops of Henle and vasa recta, leading to the establishment of an osmotic gradient in the medulla with the highest osmolality at the papillary tip. In the presence of antidiuretic hormone (ADH), the collecting duct becomes permeable to water, which is osmotically extracted from the lumen by the hypertonic medulla, leading to the formation of concentrated urine.

The Function of the Distal Tubule

The distal tubule adjusts the composition of the final urine by selectively reabsorbing or secreting individual solutes according to the need of the moment. For example, reabsorption of Na from the tubular fluid is virtually complete in Na depletion, while in Na repletion exactly sufficient Na escapes reabsorption to balance dietary input. Many substances (such as sodium, chloride, calcium, and phosphate) are normally filtered in amounts greatly exceeding dietary input, and the excretion rate is regulated by varying the amount reabsorbed. Other important substances, notably hydrogen ion and potassium, generally enter the distal tubule in very small amounts, and the rate of excretion depends mainly on varying the rate of active secretion into the tubular fluid. The rate of water excretion is determined by ADH, which increases the water permeability of the collecting duct and thus regulates the rate of osmotic reabsorption of water into the hypertonic medullary and papillary interstitium.

GLOMERULAR FILTRATION

GFR is determined by the interaction of the physical forces driving filtration and the permeability of the filtration barrier (the glomerular capillary wall) to water and small solutes. The composition of the filtrate in health is that of a protein-free ultrafiltrate of plasma, because of the almost complete impermeability of the glomerular capillaries to protein.

The Glomerular Capillary Wall

Structure

The glomerular capillary wall consists of three layers: a lining endothelium composed of thin, fenestrated polygonal squames, a basement membrane, and an outer epithelium consisting of cells (podocytes) each of which possesses a central body from which radiate fern-like foot processes (pedicels) that interdigitate with those of adjacent cells. In section, the transected foot processes appear as islands of cytoplasm intimately attached to the basement membrane and connected to one another by a fine membrane. The view afforded by scanning electron microscopy shows these islands to be sections through alternating processes from adjacent cells (11). The basement membrane is a hydrated proteoglycan gel with a thickness of about 3200 Å in the adult and rather less in the infant. Ultrastructural examination reveals a central relatively electron dense lamina densa, sandwiched between a lamina rara interna and a lamina rara externa. The thin squames of the endothelium contain numerous fenestrae of 700 Å diameter. This differentiates them from the endothelium of capillaries in other tissues. All three layers take up cationic stains, indicating that they are negatively charged.

Location of the Filtration Barrier

All three layers of the glomerular capillary wall probably contribute to the retention of macromolecules in the capillary lumen. Ultrastructural studies using macromolecular tracers of different sizes and electrical charge suggest that very large molecules are completely excluded from the basement membrane, while smaller ones penetrate it to varying degrees (12). Small quantities of molecules of approximately the size of albumin appear to traverse the basement membrane but are retained at the filtration slits between the epithelial foot processes (13). The electrical charge, as well as the size, of molecules is an important determinant of their ability to cross the capillary wall into Bowman's space (14). Proteinuric states are associated with loss of negative charge from one or more layers of the capillary wall. The passage of large amounts of protein from the plasma into the glomerular filtrate is prevented partly by the physical structure of the proteoglycan mesh of the basement membrane and partly by its electronegativity. The small amount of albumin that crosses the basement membrane is further contained by the polyanionic coat surrounding the epithelial cells and extending to the filtration slits between them. The relative importance of charge and size selectivity is still controversial. The filtration slits between foot processes are bridged by a fine membrane, the slit diaphragm, which consists mainly of a specialized membrane protein, nephrin (15). Nephrin molecules from adjacent foot processes interdigitate to form a zipper-like structure, which is thought to be the limiting part of the filtration complex for albumin. Mutations in the gene for nephrin cause a severe form of recessively inherited congenital nephrotic syndrome (CNS), known as CNS of the Finnish type (16). Other specialized proteins expressed in the foot processes are also essential to the proper formation of the filtration barrier, and mutations in the genes that code for them cause other, even rarer, forms of CNS. The role of these proteins, if any, in the pathogenesis of acquired forms of nephrotic syndrome is unknown.

Dynamics of Glomerular Filtration

Starling Forces

Glomerular filtration is driven by the balance between the hydrostatic pressure gradient between capillary and Bowman's space, generated by myocardial contraction, and the oncotic pressure (colloid osmotic pressure) gradient generated by the protein concentration gradient between the same two compartments. Hydrostatic pressure favors, and oncotic pressure opposes, filtration. These forces are referred to as Starling forces. Starling forces govern the movement of fluid between the intravascular and extravascular compartments of the extracellular fluid throughout the body as a whole, glomerular filtration being a special example of their application. The net ultrafiltration pressure (P_{UF}) is, therefore, the algebraic sum of the hydrostatic (P) and oncotic (π) pressure gradients between capillary (C) and Bowman's space (BS).

$$P_{UF} = (P_C - P_{BS}) - \sigma(\pi_C - \pi_{BS}) \qquad (5)$$

Since π_{BS} is insignificant and σ (the reflection coefficient for albumin) has a value of unity,

$$P_{UF} = P_C - P_{BS} - \pi_C \qquad (6)$$

P must be higher at the arterial than at the venous end of the glomerular capillary plexus, or blood would not flow. The pressure drop is small, however, since the glomerular capillaries are low-resistance vessels between two high-resistance components (the afferent and efferent arterioles). As plasma passes through the glomerulus, filtration occurs and the plasma proteins are progressively concentrated toward the venous end by removal of water. The force opposing filtration (π_C) therefore increases. The combination of falling P_C and rising π_C causes P_{UF} to diminish toward the venous end of the capillary. These pressures have been directly measured in several species. At least in the Munich-Wistar rat and the squirrel monkey, P_{UF} at the venous end of the circuit is zero (17) This means that filtration actually stops before the efferent arteriole is reached, a condition referred to as filtration equilibrium. A normalized plot of filtration pressure gradients can therefore be drawn (Fig. 3). The mean ultrafiltration pressure is shown as the integrated area between the curves for P and π. For technical reasons, it is not possible in filtration equilibrium to measure at what point along the notional distance between afferent and efferent arteriole equilibrium is achieved. If all other variables are held constant, and plasma flow is increased or decreased, this point will move to the right or the left, respectively: there is an infinite family of curves yielding pressure equilibrium at the efferent arteriole. Under these conditions, filtration fraction is constant, and

$$GFR \sim GPF \qquad (7)$$

That is, GFR is plasma flow dependent (18). It is not known whether filtration equilibrium is the normal condition in humans.

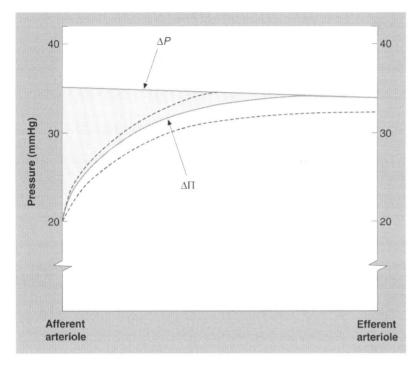

Figure 3 Hydrostatic (*P*) and oncotic (Π) pressure profiles along an idealized glomerular capillary. Δ*P* and ΔΠ refer, respectively, to the hydrostatic and oncotic pressure gradients between the capillary lumen and Bowman's space. As plasma traverses the capillary bed from afferent to efferent arteriole, removal of fluid by filtration causes the plasma protein concentration to rise, with a consequent increase in ΔΠ. In filtration equilibrium (*unbroken lines*), ΔΠ rises to equal Δ*P*, and filtration stops before the efferent arteriole is reached. An infinite number of lines (e.g., *upper interrupted line*) can be drawn that yield filtration equilibrium: these cannot be experimentally distinguished. As flow increases, the point of intersection of Δ*P* and ΔΠ moves to the right, eventually producing filtration disequilibrium (*lower interrupted line*). In filtration disequilibrium, measurements of afferent and efferent arteriolar pressures allow a unique curve for ΔΠ to be plotted, from which K_f can be calculated (see text). The shaded area represents P_{UF}. *Source*: From Ref. 20.

The Ultrafiltration Coefficient

At any given P_{UF}, filtration rate is inversely proportional to the resistance offered by the filtering membrane. The reciprocal of this resistance is the ultrafiltration coefficient (K_f). K_f is the product of the surface area of the membrane (*S*) and its hydraulic permeability or conductivity (*k*), the latter being expressed as rate of flow (*Q*) per unit *S* per unit P_{UF}.

$$k = Q \times S^{-1} \times P_{UF}^{-1} \quad (8)$$

Although *S* can be estimated morphometrically, it is difficult or impossible to measure effective *S*, the area participating in filtration at any given time. In the absence of a reliable value for *S*, *k* cannot be calculated. The composite term K_f is, therefore, preferred for most purposes. Thus,

$$GFR = P_{UF} \times k \times S = P_{UF} \times K_f \quad (9)$$

In filtration equilibrium, K_f is not limiting to GFR and cannot be calculated from experimental measurements. When filtration disequilibrium is induced by massive volume expansion, K_f becomes rate limiting, and a unique value can be calculated for it from measurements of hydrostatic and oncotic pressures in the afferent and efferent arterioles and in Bowman's space, and single nephron GFR. Identical values for single nephron K_f of 0.08 nL/sec/mmHg have been found experimentally in both rat and dog, despite the fact that filtration equilibrium probably does not obtain in the latter species (19,20). Depending on the value taken for *S*, this yields an estimate for *k* in the range 25 to 50 nL/sec/mmHg/cm². This is 10 to 100 times higher than that found in capillaries from other tissues, enabling filtrate to be formed at a very high rate despite quite low values for P_{UF} (<10 mmHg). It is evident from equation (9) that GFR may change as a result of changes in factors affecting one or more of the components of P_{UF} (changes of glomerular plasma flow, and changes of plasma albumin concentration or urinary tract obstruction), changes in *S* (reduction of nephron numbers), or changes in *k* (diffuse glomerular disease). More than one of these may be involved in progressive renal disease.

Regulation of Glomerular Filtration

Factors affecting P_{UF}. As discussed above, GFR is plasma flow dependent if

1. filtration equilibrium exists,
2. Δ*P* − Δπ at the afferent arteriole does not change, and
3. K_f is constant.

Under physiological conditions, these requirements are probably met, at least approximately. Plasma flow is determined by arterial pressure and renal vascular resistance, which resides mostly in the afferent and efferent glomerular arterioles. Angiotensin II (AII) and norepinephrine (noradrenaline, NE) constrict both afferent and efferent arterioles; these hormones are released in ECF volume contraction and other conditions in which arterial filling, and therefore renal perfusion pressure is reduced. Efferent arteriolar constriction raises P_C, and therefore P_{UF}, more than it reduces glomerular blood flow, leading to maintenance of GFR by an increase in FF. Conversely, vasodilators such as prostaglandins E_2 and I_2

(prostacyclin) and bradykinin, despite a lowering of arterial blood pressure, cause renal plasma flow to rise because of dilatation of both afferent and efferent arterioles. Here again, GFR remains relatively constant with an associated fall in FF. It is likely that both vasodilator and vasoconstrictor hormones also affect K_f (see below). Obstruction of the flow of urine causes reduction or abolition of glomerular filtration because of a rise in P_{BS}.

Factors affecting K_f. The mesangial cells that support the glomerular capillaries are contractile (21). Their contraction causes constriction of the capillaries, with a resulting fall in S and therefore K_f. AII, NE, and prostaglandins all alter K_f to the degree necessary to offset their effects on P_{UF}; in other words, the glomerular hemodynamic response to vasoactive substances is nicely balanced by changes in K_f, maintaining GFR approximately constant. Both AII and ADH cause cultured mesangial cells to contract, and this may be a physiologically important effect in vivo.

Autoregulation. In common with other vital organs such as the brain, the kidneys can regulate their own blood flow, even in an artificial perfusion system where systemic humoral and nervous controlling factors cannot operate. This is because of differential constriction of the afferent and efferent arterioles. Analysis of the determinants of GFR in this model system suggests that the damping effect on GFR is mediated in part by autoregulation of plasma flow and partly by compensatory changes in P_C, producing parallel changes in P_{UF}. As mentioned in the previous section, a role for mesangial cell contraction in autoregulation is likely, probably by altering K_f; locally produced AII may be involved in this process. Autoregulation fails at extremes of blood pressure. In severe hypertension, the exposure of the kidney to excessive pressure overwhelms the resistance of the afferent arterioles, causing the phenomenon of pressure natriuresis. When blood pressure falls below the autoregulatory range, RPF and GFR decline and prerenal failure develops.

PROXIMAL TUBULAR FUNCTION

About two-thirds of filtered salt and water is reabsorbed in the proximal tubule. Other solutes including glucose, amino acids, bicarbonate, and low–molecular weight proteins are almost completely reclaimed in this tubule segment, as is about 90% of filtered inorganic phosphate. Epithelial transport of many of these is linked to sodium transport and dependent on it for its energy supply. Exceptions include some classes of amino acid, which are transported without sodium by a complicated series of co- and countertransporters.

Salt and Water Reabsorption in the Proximal Tubule

Sodium Reabsorption

The proximal tubular epithelial cells are arranged in a single layer lining the cylindrical basement membrane. They exhibit polarity: the membranes on

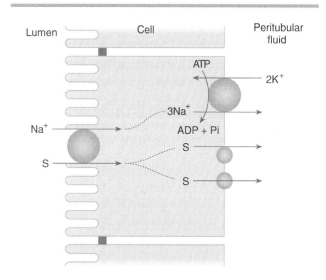

Figure 4 Schematic view of a proximal tubular cell. The apical (*brush border*) membrane (*left*) is depicted as a wavy line. The basolateral membrane (*right* and lining the intercellular space) is separated from the apical membrane by the tight junction (*dark squares*). S represents any substance that enters the cell across the apical membrane by secondary active transport via a sodium-S cotransporter. The enzyme Na+, K+-ATPase (*upper right*) maintains a steep gradient for sodium across the apical membrane by constantly extruding sodium across the basolateral membrane.

opposite sides of the cells have different characteristics. The part of the cell membrane that faces the tubular lumen is called the *apical membrane*; the part that faces the basement membrane and the intercellular space is the *basolateral membrane*. Adjacent cells are attached to one another at the tight junction, which separates the apical from the basolateral membranes (Fig. 4).

The enzyme sodium, potassium adenosine triphosphatase (Na+, K+-ATPase, also known as the sodium pump) is located in the basolateral membrane. Powered by energy released by the hydrolysis of ATP, it transports sodium out of the cell interior and potassium into it, with a stoichiometry of 3 Na+: 2 K+. This process is called *primary active transport*. A consequence of the action of Na+, K+-ATPase is a very low intracellular sodium concentration, establishing a steep concentration gradient between the tubular fluid and the cell interior that favors sodium entry across the apical membrane. This membrane is impermeable to sodium, but contains proteins of several different types that act as specialized sodium channels. Each of these not only allows sodium entry but also transports another solute into or out of the cell. This is called *secondary active transport*, since the energy driving it is provided indirectly by Na+, K+-ATPase at a site remote from the transport process itself. Inhibition of Na+, K+-ATPase by ouabain blocks sodium reabsorption in all nephron segments (22).

One of these proteins is NHE3, a member of a family of transporters called Na+, H+-exchangers (23).

Ion exchangers or antiporters are so called because they transport two species of ions, in this case sodium and hydrogen ions (protons), in opposite directions. Sodium entry, therefore, leads to alkalinization of the cell interior and acidification of the tubular fluid. By an indirect process described later in this chapter, this effectively causes reabsorption of bicarbonate in an amount chemically equivalent to the amount of sodium entering via NHE3. This takes place early in the proximal tubule, and because bicarbonate, in common with other solutes described below, is reabsorbed in preference to chloride (24), the concentration of chloride in the tubular fluid increases to a level substantially higher than that in the peritubular fluid. Chloride, therefore, moves down its concentration gradient from tubular fluid to peritubular space, partly by simple diffusion across the tight junction (which is not really chemically tight) and partly via chloride channels in the apical and basolateral membranes. Diffusion across the tight junction, bypassing the cell interior, is referred to as reabsorption via the paracellular shunt pathway. Because chloride is an anion, its movement from the luminal to the peritubular aspects of the tubule generates an electrical voltage, lumen positive, across the epithelium that acts as a further driving force for sodium reabsorption (25). At least some of this also occurs through the paracellular shunt pathway.

Other apical membrane proteins transport sodium and another solute (the cotransportate) in the same direction, and are called *cotransporters*. For example, the sodium-glucose cotransporter is activated when one sodium ion and one glucose molecule attach to specific receptors on the protein on the luminal side of the membrane. The molecule then either rotates in the membrane or alters its configuration in such a way that the sodium and glucose are transferred to the cytoplasmic side of the apical membrane, where they are released. Other cotransporters include a sodium phosphate transporter and a whole set of specific transporters for different amino acids. The general mode of operation of secondary active transport in the apical membrane of the proximal tubule is schematized in Figure 4. Both the antiporter and the cotransporters are potentially bidirectional. It is only the maintenance of the steep concentration gradient favoring sodium entry, resulting from sodium removal by Na^+, K^+-ATPase, that causes them to transport protons out of the cell and the various cotransportates to the cell interior. The antiporter and several of the apical membrane cotransporter proteins have now been sequenced and the corresponding genes mapped and cloned.

Water Reabsorption in the Proximal Tubule

Water is reabsorbed by osmosis, diffusing down the osmotic gradient established by solute reabsorption. The epithelium is freely permeable to water so that osmotic equilibration is virtually instantaneous, and the osmolality of the tubular fluid at all points in the proximal tubule is not measurably different from that of plasma. An unknown, but probably substantial,

proportion of water reabsorption takes place through the paracellular shunt pathway and provides yet another mechanism promoting sodium reabsorption. Active transport of sodium across the basolateral membrane into the lateral intercellular spaces leads to a small, transient osmotic water gradient favoring water reabsorption across the tight junction. The resulting water flux causes salt to be transported passively by a process known as convection or solvent drag, given that the tight junction is permeable to sodium and chloride. The relative importance of transcellular and paracellular reabsorption of sodium and water is uncertain.

Effect of Physical Forces on Proximal Tubular Reabsorption

Water and solute reabsorbed from the tubular lumen is returned to the blood in the peritubular capillary plexus, which is perfused by blood draining from glomerular efferent arterioles. The peritubular capillaries are therefore in series with and downstream from the glomerulus. The rate of reabsorption of tubular fluid is governed by the Starling forces across the peritubular capillary wall (26). The importance of the peritubular oncotic pressure in this process has been demonstrated both by micropuncture in the intact animal and by studies in the isolated, perfused rabbit proximal tubule (27,28). The effect of changes in peritubular hydrostatic pressure is less clear. Since the protein concentration of postglomerular plasma is proportional to the filtration fraction [eq. (4)], it follows that changes in glomerular function may induce secondary changes in proximal tubular reabsorption rate; this may be important in maintenance of glomerulotubular balance (GTB) (see below).

Proximal Tubular Reabsorption of Other Solutes

Glucose

Glucose is reabsorbed by cotransport with sodium, chiefly in the early proximal tubule. Glucose is not merely acting as an energy source for sodium transport, since the nonmetabolized glucose analogue α-methyl-D-glucoside can be substituted for it, but its transport is dependent on sodium reabsorption. At least two sodium-glucose cotransporters have been identified in mammalian proximal tubule; they have been named SGLT-1 and SGLT-2, respectively. SGLT-1 binds one sodium ion and one glucose molecule, while SGLT-2 has a stoichiometry of $2Na^+$:1 glucose. SGLT-2 is probably the more important of the two (29). It is saturable, and when the filtered load of glucose exceeds its maximal transporting capacity (T_m), the excess is excreted in the urine. The relationship between glucose filtration, reabsorption and excretion is shown in Figure 5. Glycosuria occurs in hyperglycemia (as in diabetes mellitus) because the filtered load of glucose exceeds the T_m of the transport system. Glycosuria because of abnormalities of the tubular glucose transport system (renal glycosuria) occurs when the renal threshold for glucose is less than the normal

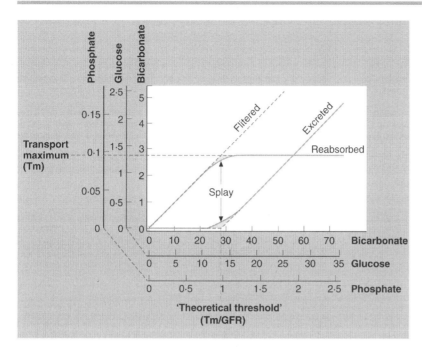

Figure 5 Curves of filtration, excretion, and reabsorption of three solutes reabsorbed actively from glomerular filtrate, plotted against the plasma concentration of the solute. Values plotted on the abscissa (x-axis) are plasma concentrations (mmol/L); those on the ordinate (y-axis) are the quantities filtered, excreted, and reabsorbed (mmol/100 mL glomerular filtration rate).

blood glucose concentration and is because of mutations in the gene for SGLT-2 (30).

Phosphate

The majority of filtered phosphate is reabsorbed with sodium in the early proximal tubule. Studies of phosphate excretion at different plasma phosphate concentrations show that the ion is handled in a manner similar to glucose, that is, by a saturable transport system with a T_m and a threshold; hence, a similar set of titration curves can be drawn (Fig. 5). In contrast to glucose, some degree of phosphaturia is normally present, since dietary phosphate in excess of requirement must be excreted: in the adult (nongrowing) subject, dietary intake and urinary excretion are equal (NEB = 0). Thus, the normal plasma phosphate concentration is just above the threshold value, and is indeed defined by it, whereas, in health, the plasma glucose concentration is always below the renal threshold. The mechanism of proximal tubular phosphate reabsorption is discussed in more detail later in this chapter.

Amino Acids

Amino acids are reabsorbed in the same general manner as glucose and phosphate. At least five transport proteins exist, some of which transport sodium and one of the major subclasses of amino acids with high specificity, while others operate as exchangers, transporting one group of amino acids out of the cell in exchange for entry of another (31). The normal plasma concentrations of all the amino acids are below threshold in health, so that normal urine contains virtually no amino acids of any kind. Several inherited defects of proximal tubular amino acid

transport systems have been described. By far, the commonest is cystinuria. This is caused by mutations in an apical membrane system that operates as an amino acid exchanger. It transports cystine and the dibasic amino acids arginine, lysine, and ornithine into the cell in exchange for exit of neutral amino acids. This is another form of secondary active transport. The driving force for exchange is the steep cell-to-lumen gradient for neutral amino acids generated by sodium-coupled entry of the latter, also across the apical membrane. The exchanger is a heterodimer of two components, labeled rBAT and $b^{o,+}AT$, respectively (32). The mutations that cause cystinuria affect rBAT, and numerous loss of function mutations have so far been identified in different families (33). The only clinical significance of cystinuria is the tendency to form cystine stones in the urinary tract: affected individuals are otherwise healthy.

Proteins

Several low–molecular weight proteins are present in normal plasma in measurable concentrations. Examples are α-1 microglobulin, β-2 microglobulin, and retinol-binding protein (RBP). Because they are smaller than the size barrier of the glomerular ultrafilter, significant amounts are present in glomerular filtrate and enter the proximal tubule, where they are reabsorbed by pinocytosis into the tubular epithelial cells where they are digested to their component amino acids and returned to the body protein pool. They are therefore virtually absent from normal urine. Proximal tubular dysfunction, however, leads to a urinary leak of these proteins and a characteristic pattern of low–molecular weight proteinuria known as *tubular proteinuria*. Measurement of urinary excretion of β-2 microglobulin and RBP, usually expressed as fractional excretion rates, is a useful means of distinguishing between proteinuria of glomerular and nonglomerular (tubulo-interstitial) origin (34).

Only very small amounts of albumin and other large plasma proteins normally pass the glomerular filter. These are essentially completely reabsorbed by a mechanism similar to that for low–molecular weight proteins. At low filtered loads, the system behaves as a high-affinity, low-capacity transporter with virtually complete clearance of albumin from the tubular fluid, while at high filtered loads this mechanism becomes saturated and a high-capacity, low-affinity mode operates, so that reabsorption continues to rise with increasing load, but about one-third of the filtered albumin escapes reabsorption and appears in the urine (35). In such conditions of glomerular proteinuria, the urinary albumin excretion rate is always considerably less than the amount filtered and catabolized. This probably explains why proteinuria of apparently trivial amounts (<10 g/day) may cause hypoalbuminaemia in some cases of the nephrotic syndrome.

Proximal Tubular Secretion of Organic Anions

Many organic substances, anionic at physiological pH, are actively secreted by the proximal tubule. These include endogenous substances such as hippurate and exogenous substances such as penicillin, probenecid, and derivatives of hippuric acid such as orthoamino-hippurate (hippuran) and paraaminohippurate (PAH). The renal clearance of these compounds exceeds GFR, and in the case of hippuran and PAH extraction is almost complete. The secretory site is the proximal convoluted tubule, especially the middle and late segments. The small amount of PAH that escapes secretion is accounted for by blood perfusing the deepest (juxtamedullary) nephrons, in which the postglomerular blood flows directly into the medullary vasa recta system without passing through the cortical peritubular capillary plexus, bypassing the secretory site for PAH. In the adult, only about 10% of nephrons are of this type, so the underestimation of renal plasma flow by PAH clearance is small. In the newborn infant, in contrast, the superficial cortical nephrons (the last to be formed) function little or not at all, and the juxtamedullary nephrons provide the lion's share of renal function. Clearance of PAH and similar substances is, therefore, an unreliable measure of renal plasma flow in babies and newborn animals. PAH secretion is saturable and T_m-limited; below the renal threshold, excretion increases in parallel with rising plasma concentration, while above this value, there is no further rise in excretion. A similar, but separate, transport system exists for the secretion of organic cations.

GLOMERULOTUBULAR BALANCE

Delivery of fluid to the distal tubule is, by definition, the difference between GFR and proximal tubular reabsorption rate. Since the rate of distal fluid delivery is an important determinant of distal tubular function, and therefore of homeostasis, it is important that glomerular and proximal tubular function are coupled together. This coupling is known as GTB: changes in GFR are partially offset by parallel and proportional changes in proximal tubular reabsorption (36). GTB has been shown experimentally to exist: When GFR is manipulated by altering renal perfusion pressure, changes in proximal tubular reabsorption take place as the theory predicts. At least three mechanisms are involved.

Peritubular Physical Forces

The protein concentration in postglomerular plasma is determined by arterial plasma protein concentration and filtration fraction. If GFR increases without a parallel increase in plasma flow, filtration fraction rises and peritubular capillary oncotic pressure is increased. This alters the balance of Starling forces in the peritubular environment in a direction that favors reabsorption. Conversely, a fall in GFR and filtration fraction leads to a reduction in the pressure gradient for reabsorption (37). The oncotic pressure of the peritubular capillary plasma has been shown to be a powerful, and possibly rate-limiting, factor in proximal tubular reabsorption (27).

Filtration of Preferentially Reabsorbed Substances

Sodium is reabsorbed in the early proximal tubule with bicarbonate, phosphate, amino acids, lactate and citrate in preference to chloride; glucose is also absorbed by cotransport. The more these substances are presented to the tubule, the more sodium (and therefore water) will be reabsorbed. At any plasma concentration, a change in GFR will produce a parallel and proportionate change in the rate of filtration of these substances, inducing a change in proximal tubular reabsorption rate in the same direction. This effect will be amplified by the secondary effect on downstream, passive sodium reabsorption described in a previous section. Thus, any random fluctuation in GFR will cause secondary changes in both active proximal tubular sodium reabsorption and in the peritubular environment, reinforcing one another in the preservation of GTB.

Tubuloglomerular Feedback

The ascending limb of the loop of Henle passes through the vascular pole of its own glomerulus, where it is intimately associated with the afferent and efferent arterioles in the JGA. There is strong evidence that delivery of some solute, probably chloride, is sensed at the JGA, where it provides the afferent stimulus for regulation of GFR by negative feedback (38). In experiments where the loop of Henle was perfused in both orthograde and retrograde directions with solutions of various NaCl concentrations and at various rates, a clear inhibitory effect was seen on RPF and GFR as concentration (or flow rate) was increased (39). The effect is probably mediated at least in part by local production and conversion of angiotensin, producing glomerular vasoconstriction (especially of the efferent arteriole) and increasing vascular resistance. TGF may provide an emergency defense against drastic salt and water depletion in tubular injury. If proximal tubular NaCl reabsorption were severely impaired by anoxia or the action of a nephrotoxic drug, the resulting flood of sodium-rich urine would lead rapidly to fatal dehydration and electrolyte depletion unless GFR were to fall by some means. The oliguria of acute renal failure may be seen, in this light, as a life-preserving response rather than an undesirable feature of the syndrome. Recognition that the TAL of the loop of Henle is the most vulnerable part of the nephron to ischemic injury (40) is entirely consistent with this view, since the TAL is included in the anatomical feedback loop consisting of glomerulus–proximal tubule–loop of Henle–JGA.

SODIUM EXCRETION AND EXTRACELLULAR FLUID VOLUME

Sodium and Extracellular Fluid Volume

The major osmotically active solute in the ECF is sodium chloride: 90% of the sodium in the body, and almost all the chloride, is located in the extracellular compartment. Since the tonicity of body fluids is held within very narrow limits by regulation of water intake and excretion, it follows that a gain or loss of total body NaCl leads to expansion or contraction of ECF volume. Conversely, ECF volume is the major determinant of sodium excretion rate. In subjects on a salt-restricted diet, a tiny increase in ECF volume is followed by an immediate natriuresis (41). ECF volume expansion beyond a certain threshold volume is a stimulus to sodium excretion, the magnitude of the natriuresis being proportionate to the amount by which this volume is exceeded. Conversely, sodium-free urine is produced when ECF volume is below this threshold, while sodium appears in the urine as soon as this volume is even slightly exceeded. The relationship between ECF volume and sodium excretion is shown in Figure 6. It is evident that the stimulus producing the increase in sodium excretion cannot be plasma sodium concentration, which does not change, but ECF volume. How changes in this volume are sensed and whether it is the total ECF volume or a particular component or function of it that is important have been the subject of much investigation.

Control of Sodium Excretion

The control system regulating sodium excretion and, therefore, ECF volume is in three parts: an afferent (sensory) component, which detects a signal indicating the need to excrete or conserve sodium; an effector organ (the kidney); and a means of transmitting the

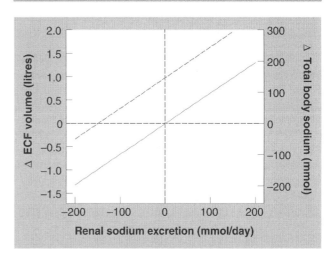

Figure 6 The relationship between ECF volume, total body sodium and urinary sodium excretion rate, assuming that a gain or loss of 1 L of ECF corresponds to a gain or loss of 150 mmol sodium, and that the ECF sodium concentration does not change. Negative values for sodium excretion indicate the magnitude of the sodium deficit that must be made up before sodium appears in the urine, which is actually sodium free at points to the left of the vertical zero line. The solid oblique line describes the relationship as observed in recumbent subjects; the interrupted line shows the relationship in the upright (quiet standing) position. The line is displaced upward, indicating sodium retention, but the slope of the relationship is unchanged. *Abbreviation*: ECF, extracellular fluid. *Source*: From Ref. 41.

response to the afferent stimulus to the kidney, the efferent (messenger) component.

The Afferent Stimulus

Both acute (saline loading) and chronic (high dietary sodium intake) volume expansion are natriuretic stimuli. Maneuvres that expand intrathoracic blood volume, such as head-out water immersion, are natriuretic even though total ECF volume becomes contracted as natriuresis continues (42). The magnitude of the response is correlated with left atrial volume, and left atrial stretch receptors probably mediate the effect. Stimulation of carotid sinus baroreceptors by underfilling of the arterial tree, as by hypotension or vasodilatation, is antinatriuretic; observations in subjects with arteriovenous fistulae indicate that underfilling of the high-pressure (arterial) compartment overrides the effect of overfilling of the low-pressure (venous) compartment, so that the net response is antinatriuretic (43). Volume or sodium receptors have been postulated in the liver or portal venous system, following the observation that saline infused into the portal vein or ingested orally is more natriuretic than the same amount infused into a peripheral vein. The presence of baroreceptors in the interstitial space is suggested by the differential natriuretic effects of saline infusions of different oncotic pressures; the fluid that expands intravascular volume the least and the interstitial compartment the most (isotonic saline) is much more natriuretic than an equivalent volume of plasma or hyperoncotic albumin (44). Receptors in the pulmonary interstitium may subserve this function.

Changes in the perfusion pressure perceived by the kidney itself, in consequence of changes in arterial blood pressure, lead to changes in urinary sodium excretion both by intrarenal mechanisms and by affecting the rate of renin secretion. It is likely that most or all of these receptors play a part in determining the natriuretic status of the kidney, perhaps via a (hypothetical) integrating mechanism located in the hypothalamus or elsewhere. In general, reduction in effective arterial volume, that is, underfilling of the arterial tree in relation to its holding capacity, seems to engender a sodium-retaining response sufficient to override conflicting or interfering stimuli from elsewhere. Examples include congestive cardiac failure, the nephrotic syndrome, and some cases of cirrhosis of the liver.

Renal Effector Responses

Theoretically, the renal sodium excretion rate could be altered either by changing GFR without an accompanying change in tubular reabsorption, or by the reverse. In fact, changes in tubular reabsorption are undoubtedly responsible for physiological regulation of this function. Patients with chronic renal failure are able to remain in external sodium balance on a fixed sodium intake despite progressively falling GFR; an adjustment of tubular reabsorption must have taken place. It has been shown in many experimental models that the natriuretic response to volume expansion is not abolished if GFR is prevented from increasing, or even artificially decreased. Furthermore, experimental manipulations, which produce large increases in GFR are not necessarily natriuretic. For example, in dogs, protein feeding, dexamethasone administration, dopamine infusion, and saline infusion all increase GFR by up to 30%: of these, only saline loading is consistently natriuretic (45).

If sodium excretion is modulated by changes in tubular reabsorption, which part of the tubule is mainly responsible? Experimental studies favor the distal nephron as the important effector. Natriuresis can be dissociated not only from GFR (see above) but also from absolute and fractional proximal tubular sodium reabsorption (46). Humoral factors known to influence sodium reabsorption rate [such as aldosterone and atrial natriuretic peptide (ANP)] act mainly on distal nephron segments. In rats, saline loading causes marked changes in sodium reabsorption in the collecting duct, resulting in apparent sodium secretion in response to extreme volume expansion. Newborn infants, in whom fractional proximal tubular sodium reabsorption is lower than that in adults, maintain sodium balance perfectly well, presumably by distal tubular compensation. Furthermore, it appears logical that the most distal part of the nephron is responsible for the final adjustment of the sodium excretion rate since, by definition, further downstream adjustments are not possible.

It should be emphasized that the response to saline volume expansion is normally a reduction in sodium reabsorption in both proximal and distal nephron segments, and that the dissociation between these mentioned above was produced by unphysiological experimental manipulations. The fact that the distal parts of the nephron can maintain a degree of sodium homeostasis in the absence of parallel responses in the proximal tubule probably reflects the extreme importance of control of ECF volume; if proximal tubular reabsorption is impaired or abnormal, external balance for sodium can still be maintained. However, the cost of maintaining sodium balance in these circumstances may be secondary disturbances of potassium and hydrogen ion excretion, as in Bartter's syndrome.

Intrarenal Control of Sodium Excretion

Sodium excretion is correlated with renal artery pressure. ECF volume is an important determinant of renal artery pressure, with resulting effects on intrarenal haemodynamics. The main resistance vessels in the renal microcirculation are the afferent and efferent glomerular arterioles. The latter are interposed between the glomerular and peritubular capillary plexuses. The hydrostatic pressure in the peritubular capillaries, therefore, varies in proportion to renal artery pressure and in inverse proportion to renal arteriolar resistance. Volume expansion directly increases perfusion pressure and, partly by inhibition of the rennin-angiotensin-aldosterone system (RAAS), reduces arteriolar resistance: volume contraction has the reverse effects. Thus, volume expansion leads to an increase, and volume contraction to a decrease, in peritubular capillary pressure. The effect of angiotensin II on the renal circulation is complex. It causes both preglomerular (afferent arteriole) and postglomerular (efferent arteriole) vasoconstriction, but the postglomerular effect predominates, largely because of the production of vasodilator prostaglandins in the afferent arteriole that offset the vasoconstrictor action of angiotensin II. Conditions in which the RAAS is stimulated, such as volume contraction, therefore increase glomerular capillary pressure, leading to an increase in filtration fraction and postglomerular plasma oncotic pressure. Suppression of the RAAS (volume expansion) has the opposite effect. In sum, volume expansion causes an increase in hydrostatic pressure and a decrease in oncotic pressure in the peritubular capillaries. This reduces the Starling pressure gradient for fluid reabsorption from the peritubular interstitium and hence from the proximal tubule, favoring natriuresis. Volume contraction initiates the opposite sequence of events and is therefore antinatriuretic. These processes are schematized in Figure 7 (47).

Although the above discussion has focused on the proximal tubule, the rate of fluid absorption in the distal nephron is also influenced by Starling forces, since the cortical part of the distal tubule is supplied by the same peritubular capillary network that supplies the proximal tubule, and the medullary part by

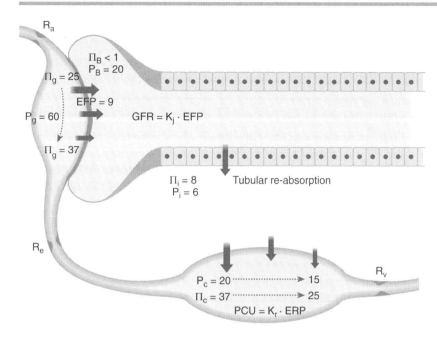

$\Pi_B < 1$
$P_B = 20$

$\Pi_g = 25$

$EFP = 9$

$P_g = 60$

$GFR = K_j \cdot EFP$

$\Pi_g = 37$

$\Pi_i = 8$
$P_i = 6$

Tubular re-absorption

$P_c = 20 \cdots\!\rightarrow 15$

$\Pi_c = 37 \cdots\!\rightarrow 25$

$PCU = K_r \cdot ERP$

R_a

R_e

R_v

Figure 7 Schematic diagram of the forces responsible for filtration of fluid from the glomerular capillaries and reabsorption of fluids into the peritubular capillaries. The forces are expressed in mmHg and are considered representative of those found in normal humans. *Source*: From Ref. 47.

capillaries that receive part of their blood supply from the efferent arterioles of juxtamedullary (deep cortical) nephrons. It has sometimes been argued that physical forces alone are sufficient to explain the regulation of renal sodium excretion, but this hypothesis is rendered untenable by other observations, notably by the fact that saline expansion is natriuretic even if renal perfusion pressure is artificially prevented from rising or even reduced. It follows that extrarenal factors are also involved.

The Efferent Limb in the Regulation of Sodium Excretion

The fact that sodium excretion is influenced by changes in the apparent volume of ECF subcompartments remote from the kidney indicates not only that volume sensors exist at those sites, but also that there must be some means of altering renal sodium excretion in response to the signals they receive. This message ("increase or decrease sodium excretion") may be transmitted from sensor to effector by a number of efferent pathways.

The Renal Nerves

The renal nerve supply contains efferent postganglionic fibers located in the splanchnic nerves: stimulation of these is antinatriuretic while denervation is natriuretic. α-Adrenergic endings have been identified in close approximation to proximal and distal tubules as well as blood vessels; a direct effect on epithelial transport seems likely. Denervation of one kidney causes natriuresis in the ipsilateral and antinatriuresis in the contralateral kidney, suggesting a role also for the afferent fibers in the control of sodium excretion, perhaps by integrating the responses of the two kidneys via a renorenal reflex (48).

Aldosterone

The mineralocorticoid aldosterone is an important regulator of tubular sodium handling. Released in response to activation of the renin-angiotensin system, which in turn is stimulated by volume contraction, it acts on the distal convoluted tubule and collecting duct to stimulate sodium reabsorption, where it also promotes secretion of K^+ and H^+ (see below). Although other factors undoubtedly interact with aldosterone and can even override it in the *mineralocorticoid escape phenomenon*, its importance in sodium homeostasis is illustrated by the finding that adrenalectomized animals, on a fixed replacement dose of mineralocorticoid, achieve sodium balance only at the cost of greatly exaggerated changes in ECF volume, body weight, blood pressure, and potassium concentration (49).

Catecholamines

Catecholamines affect sodium excretion, noradrenaline (norepinephrine) being antinatriuretic and dopamine natriuretic; both α-adrenergic and dopaminergic receptors have been identified in the kidney. It has been suggested that dopamine is an important mediator of sodium excretion, particularly in chronic renal failure; however, it is likely that the major effects of these amines are mediated via their action as locally released neurotransmitters, rather than as circulating hormones proper. The fact that L-dopa, a precursor of dopamine, is natriuretic when infused into the renal artery further supports the view that local synthesis accounts for the origin of most or all of the dopamine present in the kidney. This does not exclude an important role for the amine as a second messenger, that is, a locally acting vasoactive and natriuretic factor, the activity of which may be increased by other, circulating, substances.

Prostaglandins

The vasodilator prostaglandins PGE$_2$ and PGI$_2$ (prostacyclin) are synthesized within the kidney and are natriuretic. Inhibitors of prostaglandin synthase such as indomethacin and ibuprofen cause RPF and GFR to fall and the fractional proximal tubular sodium reabsorption to increase. These effects are partly offset by volume expansion and greatly exaggerated by volume contraction; the combination of volume contraction and a nonsteroidal antiinflammatory agent may lead to acute renal failure. Angiotensin II stimulates renal release of prostaglandins: The main physiological role of renal prostaglandins may be to maintain glomerular plasma flow and filtration rate in volume-contracted states, when AII levels are high.

The Kallikrein-Kinin System

The kinins, bradykinin and kallidin, are another class of vasodilator and natriuretic substances produced locally within the kidney. They are formed by the action of the proteinase kallikrein, produced in the distal tubule, on a circulating precursor. The renin-angiotensin-aldosterone system, prostaglandins, and kinins all interact in complex ways. AII and aldosterone both stimulate kallikrein production, while kinins promote prostaglandin synthesis. Angiotensin-converting enzyme (ACE) not only converts AI to AII but also inactivates bradykinin; it is also known as kininase II. ACE therefore causes vasoconstriction and antinatriuresis by both AII production and bradykinin degradation; ACE inhibition has the opposite effects, accounting for the fact that ACE inhibitors lower blood pressure even when the RAAS is not activated. Catecholamines, the RAAS, prostaglandins, and kinins can be regarded as components of a complex intrarenal paracrine system that normally act synchronously to regulate and stabilize renal blood flow and GFR in response to changes in extrarenal influences such as ECF volume and circulating hormones.

Natriuretic Peptides

Volume expansion causes natriuresis in dogs even when GFR is artificially constrained and supramaximal doses of mineralocorticoid and vasopressin are given (50). The design of the experiments in which this was demonstrated excluded all feasible explanations for the natriuresis except the action of a natriuretic hormone. In the 1980s, a new class of peptide hormones was identified (51). The first of these was ANP, so called because it is synthesized in the cardiac atria and released in response to atrial stretch. Related peptides are produced elsewhere in the body, including the brain, probably the anterior hypothalamus. Human ANP is composed of 28 amino acids, including a 17–amino acid ring formed by a disulfide bridge. It is formed by cleavage of a 126–amino acid prohormone. At least three other fragments of the same prohormone have hormonal activity and are known, respectively, as long-acting natriuretic peptide (amino

acids 1–30), vessel dilator hormone (31–67) and kaliuretic hormone (79–98). ANP is a systemic and renal vasodilator, and also reduces pulmonary vascular resistance. It acts directly on arteriolar smooth muscle by a pathway not involving prostaglandins or nitric oxide. Its actions on the renal vasculature include dilatation of the arcuate arteries and afferent arterioles, and antagonism of mesangial cell contraction induced by both AII and vasopressin. These effects combine to cause an increase in GFR and a reduction in fractional proximal tubular sodium reabsorption, probably because of altered physical (Starling) forces. It also has direct effects on the distal renal tubule, decreasing sodium reabsorption by inhibiting both its entry into the tubular cells through sodium channels in the apical membrane and its exit from the cell across the basolateral membrane by reducing Na^1, K^1-ATPase activity. At the cellular level, the actions of ANP are mediated by cyclic guanosine monophosphate (c-GMP) and c-GMP-dependent protein kinase (52). Other actions of ANP include suppression of renin release, inhibition of aldosterone synthesis, and antagonism of AII-mediated vasoconstriction. Natriuretic peptides are the subject of much ongoing research, and are beginning to be used experimentally as therapeutic agents. Further details are available from recent reviews (53–55).

There is a compelling logic in atrial distension being an important natriuretic stimulus, since in most circumstances atrial stretch is a sensitive indicator of circulating volume. The right atrium is the main source of ANP, suggesting that the observed pulmonary effects of the hormone may be physiologically important. In pathological states such as congestive heart failure, atrial distension may become dissociated from ECF and circulatory volume. It is theorized that ANP release is beneficial in heart failure both by reducing afterload and by mitigating the salt and water retention characteristic of that condition. ANP is involved, and may be preeminent, in the natriuresis of the syndrome of inappropriate secretion of antidiuretic hormone (SIADH). The major actions of ANP are schematized in Figure 8.

SODIUM REABSORPTION BEYOND THE PROXIMAL TUBULE

About one-third of filtered sodium is reabsorbed distal to the proximal tubule. As in the proximal tubule, active extrusion of sodium by Na^+, K^+-ATPase across the basolateral membrane accounts for the exit step of sodium from the cell interior, and also generates a steep concentration gradient across the apical membrane. Entry from tubular fluid to cell interior takes place by secondary active transport down this gradient via a family of Na^+-K^+-Cl^- cotransporters, coded for by genes collectively named SLC12, at least three of which are expressed in different segments of the distal nephron, and an amiloride-sensitive sodium channel. In contrast to events in the proximal tubule, where reabsorption is isotonic, salt and water reabsorption are dissociated in more distal segments.

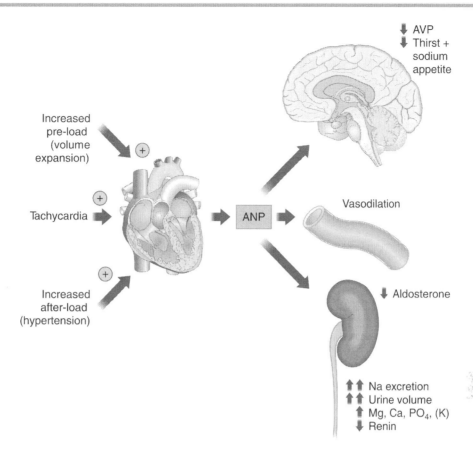

Figure 8 Schematic outline of the major actions of atrial natriuretic peptide.

The Loop of Henle

About 25% of filtered sodium is reabsorbed in the loop of Henle, all of it in the TAL. Entry into the cell here is effected by the transporter NKCC2 (the corresponding gene is SLC12A2; see above), which as its name suggests transports 1 Na^+, 1 K^+, and 2Cl^-. Since the number of positively and negatively charged ions transported is equal, transport is electroneutral. Ammonium (NH_4^+), if present in the tubular fluid, can substitute for K^+. NKCC2 is inhibited by bumetanide and furosemide (frusemide), a fact that accounts for the diuretic action of these drugs. The gene is located on chromosome 15q, and mutations of it cause one form of Bartter's syndrome of hypokalemia, alkalosis, hypercalciuria and hyper-reninaemia with normal blood pressure, (56) as had been predicted from the close similarity between Bartter's syndrome and the effect of chronic administration of loop diuretics. The very large amount of sodium reabsorbed by this transport system, and its relatively distal location, accounts for the great pharmacological power of the loop diuretics. The activity of NKCC2 causes large amounts of potassium and chloride, as well as sodium, to enter the cell from the tubular fluid. The absorbed potassium is recycled back into the tubule lumen via another apical membrane transporter, ROMK, and the chloride leaves the cell across the basolateral membrane via a chloride channel, ClC-Kb. Mutations in both ROMK and ClC-Kb can also cause forms of Bartter's syndrome (57,58) since NKCC2 can operate efficiently only if the absorbed potassium and chloride are prevented from accumulating within the cell. The relationship between the various transporters in the TAL cell is shown in Figure 9.

The Distal Convoluted Tubule

About 5% to 8% of filtered sodium is reabsorbed in the DCT. Apical sodium entry in this segment takes place via an electroneutral, thiazide-sensitive Na^+-Cl^- cotransporter (TSC). The gene is SLC12A3, located at 16q12–13. Mutations of this gene cause Gitelman's syndrome, a variant of Bartter's syndrome distinguished from the classical forms by milder clinical course, hypocalciuria and hypomagnesemia (59). As would be expected, inhibition of the TSC by thiazide diuretics mimics the features of Gitelman's syndrome precisely. Because much less sodium is reabsorbed by the TSC than by NKCC2, thiazides are much weaker diuretics than loop diuretics. However, if a loop diuretic [such as furosemide (frusemide)] and a thiazide (such as metolazone) are used together, the two effects reinforce one another and massive diuresis results.

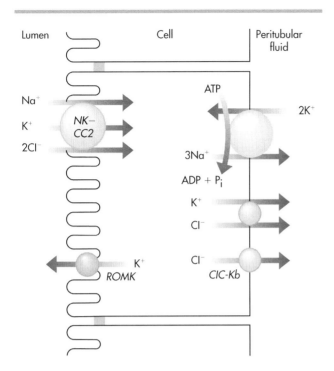

Lumen   Cell   Peritubular fluid

Figure 9 Membrane transporters in the thick ascending limb (TAL) of the loop of Henle. Orientation as in Figure 4. Sodium, potassium, and chloride enter the cell via NKCC-2 (*upper left*). Sodium is then returned to the peritubular fluid by the action of Na$^+$, K$^+$-ATPase (*upper right*); chloride is returned to the peritubular fluid by ClC-Kb (*lower right*) and potassium is recycled to the tubular lumen via the potassium channel ROMK (*lower left*). Mutations in any of these three transport proteins (NKCC-2, ROMK, or ClC-Kb) cause Bartter's syndrome (see text).

The Collecting Duct

Only 3% to 5% of filtered sodium enters the CCD in most circumstances. However, the filtered load of sodium is so large that this amounts to 750 to 1250 mmol/day, several times the normal daily intake. Regulation of sodium reabsorption in this terminal nephron segment is therefore crucial to homeostasis, since no further adjustment of urine composition can occur at a more distal site. Sodium enters the cell in this segment via a highly sodium-selective, low-conductance, amiloride-sensitive sodium channel located in the apical membrane of the principal cells, commonly abbreviated to ENaC (epithelial sodium channel). Opening of ENaC is under the control of aldosterone, and therefore volume contraction promotes, and volume expansion inhibits, sodium reabsorption through it. Entry of sodium across the apical membrane, without an accompanying anion, creates a lumen-negative voltage across the epithelium, which promotes the movement of H$^+$ and K$^+$ in the opposite direction. Blockade of this channel with amiloride therefore leads to H$^+$ and K$^+$ retention, as does aldosterone deficiency. The channel consists of three subunits, designated α-, β-, and γ-ENaC, respectively,

coded for by three separate genes. The gene for α-ENaC is on chromosome 12, while those for β- and γ-ENaC are close together on 16p. Two distinct hereditary diseases are caused by mutations in ENaC genes. Liddle's syndrome, a form of dominantly inherited hypertension with hypokalemia and suppression of renin and aldosterone, was first shown to be because of mutations in the β-ENaC gene that cause the channel to be constitutively open even in the absence of mineralocorticoid (60). The consequence is overabsorption of sodium, volume expansion, and increased potassium excretion. It was subsequently shown that the syndrome could also be caused by mutations in the gene for γ-ENaC. The rare disorder pseudohypoaldosteronism type 1 (PHA1) is physiologically the mirror image of Liddle's syndrome with salt wasting, hyperkalemia, and acidosis despite high levels of renin and aldosterone. It is because of loss of function mutations in the genes for ENaC (61). The inheritance of PHA1 is recessive in some pedigrees and dominant in others. Some families with PHA1 have mutations in the α-ENaC gene; others in that for β-ENaC. The three subunits of ENaC have considerable sequence homology and structural similarity, suggesting descent from a common ancestor gene.

RENAL CONTROL OF POTASSIUM AND HYDROGEN ION SECRETION

Potassium Excretion

On a normal diet and at normal levels of renal function, the rate of potassium filtration exceeds that of potassium excretion 5- to 10-fold. At first sight, this might suggest that excretion is controlled by varying the rate of tubular reabsorption of filtered potassium, as is the case for sodium. In fact, almost all the filtered potassium is reabsorbed in the proximal tubule; potassium excretion depends on distal tubular secretion of the ion.

Proximal Tubular Potassium Reabsorption

Potassium is reabsorbed isotonically throughout the length of the proximal convoluted tubule, a process apparently continued in the proximal straight tubule. As described above, it is absorbed by NKCC2 in the TAL but recycled to the lumen via ROMK; the loop of Henle probably makes little or no net contribution to potassium reabsorption or secretion. The fluid issuing from the loop into the early distal convoluted tubule contains relatively little potassium (5–15% of the filtered load); this fraction remains constant while urinary potassium excretion varies from minimum to maximum, a 200-fold range. It is therefore logically necessary that changes in potassium excretion are effected at a more distal site.

Potassium Transport in the Distal Tubule and Collecting Duct

Potassium is secreted in the distal tubule in potassium repletion and reabsorbed in potassium depletion; the latter case is unusual. The major site of potassium

Table 1 The Effects of Various Conditions on the Factors Determining Renal Potassium Excretion

Condition	Δ Distal sodium delivery	Δ Aldosterone	Δ Intracellular (K^+)	$\Delta U_K V$	ΔP_K
Volume expansion	↑	↓	–	–	–
Volume contraction	↓	↑	–	–	–
K^+ loading	–	–	↑	↑	↑
K^+ depletion	–	–	↓	↓	↓
Acute metabolic acidosis	–	–	↓	↓	↑
Chronic metabolic acidosis	↑	–	–	↑	↓
Metabolic alkalosis	–	–	↑	↑	↓
Mineralocorticoid deficiency	↓	↓	?↓	↓	↑
Mineralocorticoid excess	↑	↑	?↑	↑	↓
Proximal tubulopathies	↑	↑	?↑	↑	↓
Loop diuretics, thiazides	↑	↑	–	↑	↓
K^+-sparing diuretics	↓	↑	?↓	↓	↑

Notes: ↓ Direction of change in UkV produced to restore Pk to normal. ? shows the direction of change indicated by the relevant arrows is probable but not certain. Data from references cited in the text.
Abbreviations: UkV, urinary potassium excretion rate; Pk, plasma potassium concentration.

secretion is the late distal convoluted tubule and CCD, corresponding to the location of ENaC (see the section on sodium reabsorption in the collecting duct). There are two major cell types in the CCD: principal cells and intercalated cells. Potassium secretion is a function of the former—reabsorption, of the latter. The driving force for potassium secretion is the lumen-negative voltage resulting from sodium reabsorption. Although perhaps 90% of this potential difference is effaced by secondary, passive chloride reabsorption, the remaining 10% or so is associated with counter-movement of potassium and H^+. Electrophysiological studies indicate that epithelial potassium transport is a complex process involving several component steps.

Intracellular potassium concentration is an important modulator of potassium secretion into the tubular lumen. Like all cells, distal tubular cells transport sodium out and potassium in across both basolateral and apical membranes. The apical (luminal) membrane of principal cells, however, allows potassium to leave the cell down its electrochemical gradient by two mechanisms: one is the potassium channel ROMK and the other a potassium chloride symporter (cotransporter). A rise in the peritubular (ECF) potassium concentration stimulates Na^+, K^+-ATPase in the basolateral membrane, thus increasing potassium entry. The net force driving potassium secretion is therefore made up of two components: a *concentration gradient*, resulting mainly from intracellular potassium concentration, and an *electrical potential gradient*, resulting from sodium reabsorption, as described above. The electrical driving force is proportional to the rate of sodium reabsorption. This is determined by two main factors. The first is the rate of sodium entry into the CCD: anything that increases distal sodium delivery, such as inhibition of its reabsorption in more proximal segments, stimulates sodium entry into principal cells and hence potassium secretion. The second is aldosterone, which increases both sodium entry across the apical membrane via ENaC and sodium-potassium exchange across the basolateral membrane by upregulating Na^+, K^+-ATPase (62,63).

The interaction between distal sodium delivery and aldosterone is crucially important in the normal control of potassium excretion in response to changes in ECF volume. Volume expansion increases distal sodium delivery by inhibition of reabsorption at more proximal sites, and suppresses activity of the RAAS and therefore aldosterone secretion. The resulting effects on distal sodium reabsorption, and thus on potassium secretion, are mutually opposed and cancel one another. Volume contraction produces opposite effects (reduced distal Na delivery, increased aldosterone secretion). Therefore, physiological changes in sodium excretion rate because of changes in ECF volume do not cause inappropriate secondary effects on potassium excretion. Conditions in which the normal relationship between distal sodium delivery and aldosterone release are disrupted, however, cause predictable disturbances of potassium balance: some examples are given in Table 1.

Acute and chronic changes in acid-base status exert important effects on potassium balance. Acute metabolic alkalosis enhances, and metabolic acidosis inhibits, tubular potassium secretion, leading to hypokalemia and hyperkalemia, respectively. This is probably secondary to changes in intracellular potassium concentration: alkalosis promotes potassium entry into cells, thus increasing the cell-to-tubular lumen potassium gradient, while acidosis has the opposite effect. The rate of secretion of H^+ may have a further effect on potassium secretion: in acidosis, increased H^+ flux attenuates the potential difference between cell and tubular fluid, reducing the driving force for potassium extrusion. Chronic metabolic acidosis, in contrast to acute, is accompanied by increased potassium secretion and eventual potassium depletion. This is probably because of increased distal delivery of sodium secondary to hyperchloraemia: bicarbonate deficiency inhibits proximal sodium reabsorption by mechanisms discussed in an earlier section. The fact that chronic respiratory acidosis, in which bicarbonate levels are elevated, is not accompanied by potassium wasting lends support to this view. Diuretics that inhibit sodium reabsorption at sites proximal to the CCT cause urinary potassium wasting because of the simultaneous induction of increased distal sodium delivery and hyperaldosteronism secondary to volume contraction. These include loop diuretics such as mercurials, furosemide (frusemide), and ethacrynic acid, as well as thiazides, carbonic anhydrase inhibitors and osmotic diuretics. Diuretics such as spironolactone, triamterene, and amiloride, which work by inhibiting sodium reabsorption at the potassium-secreting site, cause potassium retention and hyperkalemia.

Hydrogen Ion Excretion

Volatile and Nonvolatile Acids

The pH of the ECF is regulated within a very narrow range (7.40 ± 0.04) despite a number of perturbing influences. By far, the largest of these is the continuous generation of carbonic acid as the end product of carbohydrate metabolism. Because carbonic acid can be dehydrated to CO_2 and water by the enzyme carbonic anhydrase (CA) in the lungs, and the resulting CO_2 excreted in expired air, it is known as volatile acid (VA). Regulation of CO_2 excretion, therefore, depends on pulmonary function, and its retention or excessive loss result in respiratory acidosis and alkalosis, respectively. In addition, a much smaller amount of nonvolatile acid (NVA), acid that cannot be dehydrated to anhydrides in the lung, is generated from other metabolic pathways. The principal components of NVA are as follows:

1. Sulfuric acid, from combustion of sulfur-containing amino acids
2. Phosphoric acid, mainly from dietary organic phosphate
3. Organic acids (OA), such as lactic and aceto-acetic acids, from incomplete combustion of carbohydrate and fat, respectively

Organic acids usually form only a small component of NVA but may become important in disease states (diabetic ketoacidosis, lactic acidosis and hereditary organic acidemias). The amount of sulfuric acid produced depends on the intake of animal protein: strict vegetarians (vegans), who eat no animal products at all, generate predominantly alkaline products of metabolism and therefore excrete alkaline urine. Since, by definition, NVA cannot be excreted via the lungs it must be excreted by the kidney if the pH of the ECF is not to become progressively, and eventually fatally, lowered. The disproportion between the production rates of VA and NVA is enormous. An adult human on a mixed Western diet produces about 14,000 mmol of carbonic acid daily but only about 50 to 100 mmol of NVA. This fact is dramatically illustrated by the difference in the rate of development of acidosis following total obstruction of the trachea, as opposed to total obstruction of the urinary tract.

Intracellular Fluid Buffers

A quantity of acid added to plasma or whole blood lowers the pH far less than it would if added to a similar volume of water. This is because of the presence of powerful buffer systems in both plasma and red cells.

The most important of the ECF buffers is the carbonic acid–bicarbonate buffer system.

$$pH = 6.1 + \log \frac{[HCO_3^{\,-}]}{[H_2CO_3]} \qquad (10)$$

Addition of H^+ depletes (HCO_3^-) by titrating it to H_2CO_3 with a consequent fall in pH. The role of the kidney is to regenerate HCO_3^- (buffer base) by excreting H^+, thus back-titrating or recharging the buffer system. Addition of 1 mol of HCO_3 (as $NaHCO_3$) is equivalent to the excretion of 1 mmol of H^+; loss of 1 mmol of HCO_3^- (as in diarrhea or bicarbonaturia) causes metabolic acidosis quantitatively equivalent to the addition of 1 mol of H^+ (e.g., as hydrochloric acid) to the ECF.

Reabsorption of Filtered Bicarbonate

The bicarbonate concentration in glomerular filtrate is the same as that in plasma. At normal GFR (180 L/day) and normal plasma bicarbonate (26 mmol/L) this represents a potential daily loss of more than 4500 mmol of bicarbonate, equivalent to adding 4500 mmol of acid to the ECF. All, or very nearly all, of this filtered bicarbonate must be reabsorbed to prevent severe acidosis. This takes place almost entirely in the proximal tubule(64), according to the scheme shown in Figure 10. Note (a) that bicarbonate reabsorption is dependent on H^+ secretion, (b) that it is accompanied by reabsorption of an equivalent amount of sodium, and (c) that the HCO_3^- ion restored to the ECF is synthesized in the proximal tubular cell, and is not the same one that is titrated by secreted H^+ in the tubular lumen. The process is dependent on intracellular CA to provide a source of H^+ and HCO_3^- ions by hydration of CO_2, and intraluminal CA (derived from the brush border of the apical cell membrane) to remove the H_2CO_3 formed there by dehydration to CO_2; the high diffusibility of CO_2 leads to its rapid movement down its concentration into the cell, completing the cycle and preventing the intraluminal reaction from coming to equilibrium and stopping.

Titration curves similar to those for glucose and phosphate (Fig. 5) can be plotted for bicarbonate and a T_m and threshold value identified. An abnormally low threshold defines proximal renal tubular acidosis (RTA), in which urinary acidification capacity is normal but only when the plasma bicarbonate has fallen below the (low) threshold value, that is, at the cost of sustained metabolic acidosis (Fig. 11). Proximal RTA is most commonly seen as part of a generalized disorder of proximal tubular function (the Fanconi syndrome), but has been described as an isolated tubular defect in at least two forms (65,66).

Distal Tubular Hydrogen Ion Secretion

Proximal reabsorption of filtered HCO_3^- does not contribute to the excretion of ingested or endogenously formed NVA and is therefore irrelevant to external H^+ balance: it merely prevents acidosis because of renal HCO_3^- wasting. To achieve acid balance, H^+ must be secreted into the urine in a quantity exactly

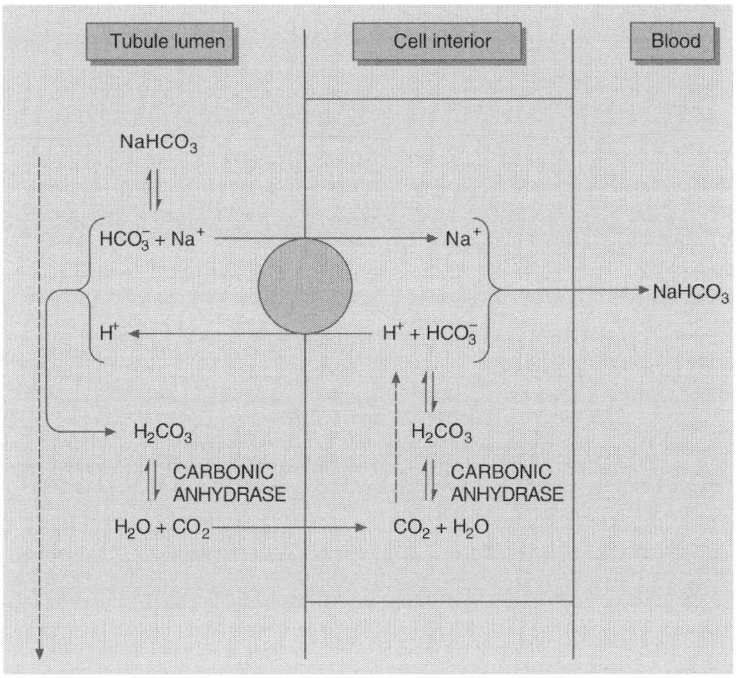

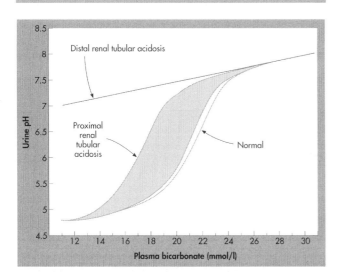

Figure 10 Proximal tubular reabsorption of filtered bicarbonate. The process is dependent on carbonic anhydrase present in the apical membrane of the proximal but not the distal tubule.

Figure 11 Urine pH plotted against plasma bicarbonate concentration in normal subjects and patients with proximal and distal RTA. In distal RTA, much commoner of the two kinds, urine pH does not fall below that of plasma, even in severe metabolic acidosis. In proximal RTA, normal urine acidification is achieved but only at abnormally low plasma bicarbonate concentrations. The curve of the relationship in proximal RTA shows the same sigmoid form as in normal subjects but is shifted to the left to varying degrees depending on the severity of the condition, passing through the shaded area. *Abbreviation*: RTA, renal tubular acidosis. *Source*: From Ref. 65.

equivalent to dietary and metabolic input of NVA, typically 50 to 100 mmol/day for an adult (depending on diet). This requires that the pH of the urine be lowered below that of ECF; that is, the tubule must pump hydrogen ions "uphill" from high pH [low (H^+)] to low pH [high (H^+)]. This takes place in the distal nephron, particularly the collecting duct. The reaction whereby H^+ is generated for secretion is the same as that operating in the proximal tubule: intracellular synthesis and ionization of H_2CO_3 from CO_2 and water. The process of secretion is, however, different utilizing an active, energy-dependent H^+ transporter (proton pump). The tubular H^+ pump can sustain a maximum pH gradient of about 10^3 (ECF pH 7.4, urine pH 4.4). At pH 4.4, 1 L of water contains only about 0.4 mmol H^+: at a daily urine flow rate of 2 to 3 L, this is clearly inadequate to achieve H^+ balance. The ability to do so depends on the presence of urinary buffers.

Urinary Buffers

The principal buffer in normal urine is inorganic phosphate. The buffering reaction is as follows:

$$H^+ + Na_2HPO_4 \leftrightarrow Na^+ + NaH_2PO_4 \qquad (11)$$

The pK of this reaction is 6.8, leading to the following version of the Henderson-Hasselbalch equation:

$$pH = 6.8 + \log \frac{[NaHPO_4{}^-]}{[Na_2HPO_4]} \qquad (12)$$

The pK of 6.8 is well suited to the normal ECF pH of 7.4, since maximal buffering will take place within one pH unit of 7.4, that is, well within the capacity of the H^+ pump.

The other important means of accommodating a large amount of secreted H^+ within the available range of urinary pH is by the formation of ammonium ($NH_4{}^+$). This is formed in the urine from secreted H^+

and ammonia (NH_3), the latter being synthesized from glutamine by the tubular cells. Thus,

$$NH_3 + H^+ + NaCl = NH_4Cl + Na^+ \qquad (13)$$

The Na^+ ion is reabsorbed in exchange for the secreted H^+ and restored to the ECF as $NaHCO_3$. The reactions between secreted H^+ and urinary phosphate and ammonia are illustrated in Figure 12. Unlike urinary phosphate excretion, ammonia synthesis can be upregulated in response to increased need to secrete H^+; this is a very important adaptive response to chronic acidosis. The classical (distal) type of RTA is because of inability to lower urinary pH significantly below that of plasma; an acquired form of distal RTA may be seen in obstructive uropathy (67).

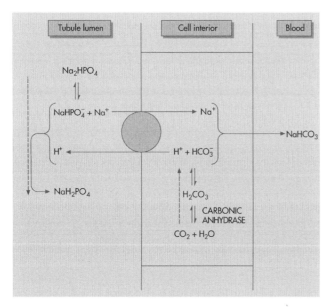

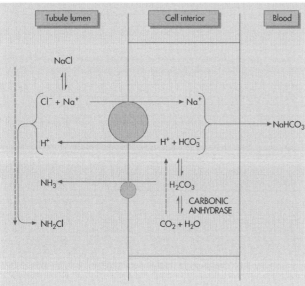

Figure 12 Distal tubular hydrogen ion secretion (urinary acidification). (**A**) Titration of urinary phosphate buffer. (**B**) Buffering by secreted ammonia. See text for details.

Relationship Between Hydrogen Ion Secretion and Sodium Ion Reabsorption

As discussed above, H^+ secretion requires the reabsorption of an equivalent amount of sodium. Conversely, failure of H^+ secretion is associated with impairment of Na^+ reabsorption: Patients with proximal and distal RTA have proximal and distal Na^+ wasting, respectively. Control of H^+ secretion is fundamentally dependent on changes in Na^+ reabsorption at different nephron sites (68).

DIVALENT CATIONS, PHOSPHATE, AND VITAMIN D

Renal Handling of Calcium

Calcium is filtered in amounts greatly exceeding its rate of dietary intake and therefore of excretion; it is reabsorbed in all the actively transporting segments of the tubule by a variety of mechanisms. Reabsorption occurring in the distal tubule is responsive to changes in calcium intake and to other factors known to influence calcium excretion; that in more proximal segments is not.

Glomerular Filtration

Calcium is present in plasma in three forms: protein bound, complexed to anions (principally phosphate), and ionized (Ca^{2+}). The last two together form ultra-filterable calcium (Ca_{UF}). The concentration of calcium in glomerular filtrate is the same as that of plasma Ca_{UF}, approximately 1.58 mmol/L (6.3 mg/dL).

Proximal Tubule

Calcium is reabsorbed approximately isotonically in the proximal tubule: A slight rise in tubular fluid concentration occurs in the initial (S1) segment, with little or no change in the remainder of the proximal tubule. Reabsorption is partly passive and dependent on sodium transport, but an active transport system also exists in the basolateral membrane probably involving sodium-calcium countertransport; that is, calcium is extruded from the cell as sodium enters. The interdependence of proximal sodium and calcium reabsorption is very close: factors such as changes in ECF volume that affect sodium absorption produce proportionate and parallel changes in calcium absorption. As with sodium, about 60% of filtered calcium is reabsorbed in the proximal tubule (69).

Loop of Henle

Calcium reabsorption continues in parallel with that of sodium in the TAL; factors affecting the delivery of sodium out of the loop produce proportionate changes in calcium delivery. The reabsorption of both is markedly inhibited by furosemide (frusemide) (70). As previously explained, the NKCC2 transporter is electroneutral, but back-leak of potassium into the tubular fluid takes place through potassium channels (ROMK) in the apical membrane. This recycling of potassium creates a lumen-positive voltage across the epithelium, which drives other positively charged ions, including calcium, into the peritubular space via the paracellular shunt pathway, accounting for calcium reabsorption in this part of the tubule.

Distal Tubule

Calcium ions are actively reabsorbed in the distal convoluted tubule and collecting duct. Transport in this segment varies independently of sodium reabsorption: It is probable that homeostatic changes in calcium excretion are effected here. Factors increasing calcium reabsorption include parathyroid hormone, hypocalcemia (probably by PTH-independent mechanisms as well as by promoting PTH release), metabolic alkalosis, and hyperphosphatemia. Hypoparathyroidism, hypercalcemia, chronic metabolic acidosis, and phosphate depletion are inhibitory (i.e., they increase calcium excretion). Vitamin D has been reported to have both enhancing and inhibiting effects on calcium excretion: a physiologically important role for vitamin D in renal calcium excretion has not been demonstrated in man. The apparent discrepancies among these reports may be because of species differences. Calcium enters distal tubular cells across the apical membrane through nifedipine-sensitive calcium channels. The driving force appears to be the electrical polarization of the membrane, which is strongly influenced by intracellular chloride concentration. Measures that decrease intracellular chloride (such as thiazide diuretics) cause hyperpolarization of the membrane and enhance calcium uptake, thus decreasing its excretion. This explains why thiazides decrease calcium excretion while increasing sodium excretion (71).

Renal Handling of Magnesium

Magnesium is processed by the kidney in a manner similar, but not identical, to calcium. The major difference is that the proximal tubule is proportionally less important and Henle's loop more important in the case of magnesium. Moreover, unlike calcium, overall renal magnesium handling is of the T_m-threshold type (Fig. 5).

Glomerular Filtration

Like calcium, magnesium is present in plasma in protein-bound, complexed, and ionized (Mg^{2+}) forms. Mg_{UF} is about 80% of total plasma magnesium, a rather higher fraction than for calcium.

Proximal Tubule

Magnesium is absorbed less avidly in the proximal tubule than sodium and calcium, so that its concentration rises along the length of the segment to a value about 1.6 times that in glomerular filtrate. This probably reflects a lower epithelial permeability to magnesium than to calcium, the forces driving reabsorption of the two being similar. Proximal magnesium reabsorption changes in parallel with that of sodium in

response to changes in factors influencing the latter, but to a lesser extent.

Loop of Henle

Eighty percent of the magnesium delivered into the loop is reabsorbed there; this segment, therefore, accounts for quantitatively the most important fraction of magnesium reabsorption. To what extent active and passive (voltage-dependent) transport is responsible is not known. Furosemide (frusemide) strongly inhibits magnesium reabsorption, suggesting that the same mechanism that accounts for calcium reabsorption in the loop is involved.

Distal Tubule

Only a small proportion (<5%) of filtered magnesium is reabsorbed in the distal tubule and collecting duct. The mechanism responsible has not been identified. Although it is tempting to dismiss distal tubular reabsorption as unimportant because the amount involved is small, this is misleading because 5% of the filtered load represents a large quantity of magnesium in relation to dietary intake, and the final regulation of magnesium excretion is presumably effected at the most distal site capable of magnesium reabsorption, probably the distal convoluted tubule.

Renal Handling of Phosphate

Inorganic phosphate (P) is filtered and reabsorbed by a T_m-limited transport system (Fig. 5). Although FEP can be calculated by equation (3), marked variability in T_{mP} secondary to changes in GFR makes FEP an imprecise way of describing tubular P reabsorption. The quotient T_{mP}/GFR defines the theoretical P threshold, that is, the intercept on the x-axis of Figure 5 obtained by extending to the left the horizontal segment of the $\dot{P}$ excretion curve and ignoring the splay. It is this quantity that is altered by changes in circulating PTH and other modulators of tubular P transport. T_{mP}/GFR can be calculated from the equation (72)

$$\frac{T_{mP}}{GFR} = P_P - \left(\frac{U_P \times P_{creatinine}}{U_{creatinine}} \right) \qquad (14)$$

Segmental Tubular Phosphate Reabsorption

The bulk of filtered P is reabsorbed in the proximal tubule, where it is responsive to influences such as changes in ECF volume, which alter sodium reabsorption. Entry into the cell is via sodium phosphate cotransporters (NPT) in the apical membrane. Two families of such transporters have now been characterized in renal cortex from several species, including man. Designated as type I and type II transporters, respectively, both are present in proximal tubular apical membranes. Type II transporters are thought to be the main physiologically important regulators of P reabsorption. NPT IIa is a protein of 635 amino acids, probably has eight transmembrane-spanning domains and has sites for protein phosphorylation that probably regulate transporter activity via protein kinase C. It transports with a stoichiometry of 3Na:1P. The gene is located on chromosome 5 (that for the type I transporter is on chromosome 6).

PTH and Phosphate Reabsorption

PTH inhibits P reabsorption in both proximal and distal segments. Changes in proximal P reabsorption are paralleled by changes in sodium reabsorption, as would be expected from the nature of the transport process, whereas in the distal tubule, PTH has no effect on sodium transport. PTH binds to proximal tubular cell receptors that activate the adenylate cyclase and protein kinase C pathways. Acute changes in transporter activity are mediated by activation of protein kinase C, which reduces activity of the sodium phosphate cotransporter (NPT IIa). Chronic changes probably involve alterations in gene transcription and translation. PTH release is controlled directly and indirectly by phosphate intake. Increasing P intake leads to transient hyperphosphatemia, which in turn causes hypocalcemia. Hypocalcemia stimulates PTH release both directly and by altering vitamin D metabolism (see below). The increased level of PTH inhibits P reabsorption, leading to phosphaturia that compensates for the increase in dietary P.

Phosphatonin, Phex, Dmp1, Klotho, and Phosphate Reabsorption

The activity of NPT IIa is inhibited by not only PTH, but also a recently described protein of the fibroblast growth factor family, FGF23(73), produced in osteocytes. FGF23 is also secreted by some tumors that cause *tumor-induced osteomalacia*, a paraneoplastic syndrome leading to renal phosphate wasting, hypophosphatemia, and rickets/osteomalacia (74). FGF23 is inactivated by a yet unidentified peptidase that cleaves it into two inactive fragments. Mutations in FGF23 that render it resistant to enzymatic cleavage but do not inhibit its activity cause a rare, autosomal dominant, form of hypophosphatemic rickets (75). Two other proteins are also expressed in osteocytes, and are believed to be involved in the regulation of expression of the gene for FGF23. The gene for the first of these to be described is called PHEX (a phosphate-regulating gene with homologies to genes for endopeptidases on the X chromosome), and is mutated in patients with the relatively common X-linked hypophosphatemic rickets (76). The second is called DMP-1 (dentin matrix protein-1) and the gene for it is mutated in the very rare autosomal recessive hypophosphatemic rickets (77). The phenotypes of all these forms of hereditary hypophosphatemia are similar, and are caused by inhibition of NPT IIa either by the uncontrolled release of FGF23 or by failure of its enzymatic degradation, leading to inhibition of P reabsorption by NPT IIa, phosphaturia, and hypophosphatemic rickets. Yet another gene, rather quaintly called *klotho* in honor of the Greek goddess who spins the thread of life, is mutated in transgenic mice with a premature aging syndrome. Further studies have shown that klotho is expressed in the renal tubule and is an essential coreceptor for FGF23. Klotho-deficient mice

and FGF-deficient mice develop identical phenotypes, indicating that klotho expression in the renal tubules is necessary for the renal effect of FGF23. These interrelationships are reviewed at greater length by Kurosu and Kuro-o (78).

Renal Metabolism of Vitamin D

The active end product of vitamin D metabolism is the hormone 1,25-dihydroxycholecalciferol (1,25-DHCC, 1,25-dihydroxyvitamin D_3). It is produced from vitamin D by 25-hydroxylation, which takes place in the liver, and subsequent 1α-hydroxylation, which takes place in the mitochondria of the proximal tubular cells. In conditions of 1,25-DHCC repletion, 1α-hydroxylation is suppressed and the inactive metabolite 24,25-DHCC is produced instead (79). The kidney is thus an endocrine organ producing a hormone under negative feedback control: According to need, conversion of 25-HCC oscillates between 1α- and 24-hydroxylation. Apart from the circulating concentration of 1,25-DHCC, other factors promoting 1α-hydroxylation include, in descending order of power, hypocalcemia, hypophosphatemia, and PTH. As well as regulating the production of 1,25-DHCC, the kidney is one of its target organs, along with intestine and bone. Localization of the hormone to the nuclei of distal tubular cells occurs (80) and presumably mediates its renal action, which is to enhance tubular calcium reabsorption, reinforcing the elevation of ECF Ca and P concentrations mediated by its other major actions: stimulation of intestinal Ca and P transport and mobilization of bone mineral. Failure of renal 1α-hydroxylation of vitamin D is one of the three main processes that result in bone disease because of chronic renal failure, the other two being secondary hyperparathyroidism and chronic metabolic acidosis.

CONCENTRATION AND DILUTION OF URINE

Osmolality and Tonicity of Body Fluids

In health, the osmolality of body fluids is controlled within narrow limits (291 $\pm$ 4 mosmol/kg H_2O) by regulation of water intake and excretion. Osmolality is a physical property of solutions that depends on the total molar concentration of all solutes present, in other words the number of solute particles dissolved in 1 kg of solvent (water), and is measured in the laboratory by various techniques such as freezing point depression. Tonicity refers to effective osmolality, that is, that part of the total osmolality of the fluid in question (e.g., ECF) that is contributed by solutes to which the cell membrane is impermeable. Normally sodium and its attendant anions make up nearly all of the tonicity of the ECF, urea and glucose being relatively permeant, although in insulin deficiency (type 1 diabetes mellitus) glucose is impermeant and does contribute to tonicity. Some exogenous solutes can contribute to tonicity (alcohol, mannitol) in special circumstances, but these are not present in the body fluids in normal conditions. In the absence of exogenous, osmotically active substances, osmolality of plasma can be approximated by the formula

$$Osmolality = (2 \times P_{Na}) + P_{Urea} + P_{Glucose} \qquad (15)$$

where the plasma concentrations of sodium, urea, and glucose are all expressed in mmol/L. If the osmolality as measured in the laboratory is significantly greater than the result of equation (15), this is evidence for the presence of an abnormal osmolyte (most commonly alcohol in the comatose or confused adult patient).

Changes in ECF tonicity are sensed by osmoreceptors located in the anterior hypothalamus. ECF hypertonicity produces thirst, leading to increased water intake (providing the subject has access to water), and release of ADH, leading to a reduction in water excretion: hypotonicity has the opposite effects. Mammals in the wild state drink in response to thirst: they therefore oscillate between isotonicity, the point at which thirst disappears, and marginal hypertonicity, which stimulates further water intake. They rarely, if ever, need to excrete dilute urine but may need to excrete highly concentrated urine if water is not available in response to the thirst stimulus. Civilized man, in contrast, frequently drinks in excess of biological need for social and cultural reasons and because of the availability of flavored (and otherwise adulterated) drinks. The ability to excrete urine more dilute than ECF is therefore essential to the avoidance of dilutional hypotonicity.

The Diluting Segment

As previously discussed, proximal tubular fluid reabsorption is isotonic. The dissociation between water and solute reabsorption necessary for the production of urine with osmolality different from that of ECF takes place in more distal parts of the nephron. Micropuncture studies showed that the fluid in the early distal convoluted tubule is hypotonic to plasma (about 100 mosmol/kg H_2O) irrespective of whether the final urine was concentrated or dilute at the time (81). Solute is therefore actively reabsorbed without water in this segment. This is now known to be via the Na^+-K^+-$2Cl^-$ transporter NKCC2 (see above). The TAL and early distal convoluted tubule therefore comprise the obligate diluting segment. Further dilution occurs in the early distal convoluted tubule via the thiazide-sensitive Na^+Cl^- cotransporter TSC. When maximally dilute urine is being produced, the late distal tubule and collecting duct also becomes water impermeable in the absence of ADH, and continuing solute (NaCl) reabsorption in the late distal convoluted tubule and the collecting duct leads to the elaboration of urine of osmolality about 40 mosmol/kg H_2O. The production of concentrated urine depends on the establishment of interstitial hypertonicity in the medulla, a process that ingeniously utilizes the same transporting process that is responsible for dilution, that is, active electrolyte reabsorption in the TAL.

Countercurrent Multiplication and Exchange

The processes of countercurrent multiplication and exchange convert the hyperosmolality of the interstitium surrounding the TAL, and resulting from NaCl reabsorption, into an axial concentration gradient maximal at the papillary tip. The elements of the countercurrent system are the loops of Henle (multipliers) and the vasa recta (exchangers), the collecting duct being the site of final osmotic water reabsorption. The mechanism was described in principle many years ago, but a more detailed understanding of the process required methods of investigation not available until much later. A general description of the medullary countercurrent system is beyond the scope of this chapter: the reader is referred to an authoritative symposium published in 1983 (82), and to a lucid account of the properties of such systems in biology (83). A recurring difficulty has been to account for concentration of solute in the inner medullary and papillary interstitium (where the tonicity is highest) in the apparent absence of active solute reabsorption in the thin (inner medullary) segment of the ascending limb (Fig. 2). This probably depends on passive recycling of urea through facilitated diffusion in the medulla. Various models have been constructed to account for the observed hypertonicity in the inner medulla without the need to postulate active solute reabsorption in the thin ascending limb, but none has been unequivocally validated to date.

The Antidiuretic Hormone

The human ADH is the cyclic nonapeptide arginine vasopressin (AVP):

$$Cys - Tyr - Phe - Glu - Asp - Cys - Pro - Arg - Gly - NH_2$$

A ring structure is formed by a disulfide bridge between the two cysteine residues. AVP is synthesized in cells whose bodies lie in the supraoptic and paraventricular nuclei of the anterior hypothalamus, and is released from their axonal endings in the posterior pituitary. It is released in response to both osmoreceptor stimulation and carotid sinus and aortic arch baroreceptor stimulation (84). The former is responsible for maintaining tonicity of body fluids in the normal range, while the latter causes renal water retention in the face of underfilling of the high-pressure compartment of the circulation because of, for example, volume depletion, vasodilatation or left ventricular failure. Baroreceptor-mediated AVP release is not suppressible by hypotonicity, and so hyponatremia is commonly seen in conditions associated with it. A much larger proportional volume change is needed than osmolar change to initiate an AVP response (Fig. 13). An increase of only 1% to 2% in plasma osmolality suffices to elicit a maximally antidiuretic plasma level (5 pg/mL), while a reduction in blood volume or pressure of about 7% to 8% is needed before a significant AVP response is seen (85). However, very high AVP levels are produced when hypovolemia or hypotension become more severe than this.

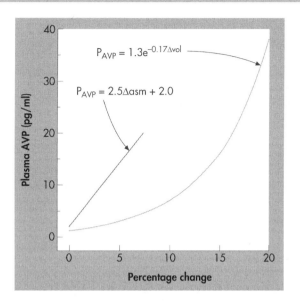

Figure 13 The antidiuretic response to isovolemic decrease in plasma osmolality (*straight line*) and isotonic depletion of plasma volume (*curved line*). The negative value of the exponent of the equation relating P_{AVP} to volume arises from the fact that the volume change (Δvol) is in a negative direction. *Source*: From Ref. 85.

Antidiuretic Hormone Receptors

AVP binds to specific receptors (V_2 receptors) on the collecting duct cells, causing activation of adenylate cyclase and conversion of ATP to cyclic AMP. This initiates a chain of intracellular events that culminate in the insertion of water channels in the apical membrane of the cell, rendering it permeable to water. The gene for the V_2 receptor is on the long arm of the X chromosome: loss of function mutations in it is responsible for the disease X-linked diabetes insipidus (86). As recently as 2005 a new syndrome was described, termed nephrogenic syndrome of inappropriate antidiuresis (87), shown to be because of gain of function mutations in the same gene. The clinical features are similar to those seen more commonly in the syndrome of inappropriate secretion of ADH: the production of inappropriately concentrated urine in the presence of hyponatremia and normovolemia, but with low, rather than high, ADH levels. The condition has since been described in neonates (88).

Aquaporins

The water channels referred to in the previous paragraph belong to a family of proteins known as *aquaporins*, of which different members are expressed in different cell types. The human collecting duct aquaporin is aquaporin 2, and the gene that codes for it is located on chromosome 12 in the region 12q13. Mutations in the gene for aquaporin 2 cause a form of diabetes insipidus clinically indistinguishable from that caused by mutations in the V_2 receptor gene except that, as would be expected, it is inherited as

an autosomal recessive condition and affects both sexes equally (89).

Free Water Clearance and Reabsorption

The urinary solute excretion rate is determined by dietary and metabolic factors, but is usually in the region of 500 to 1500 mosmol/day for an adult on an average diet. Taking a notional value of 580 mosmol/day, and assuming a plasma osmolality of 290 mosmol/kg H_2O, it is evident that 2 L of isotonic urine would suffice to excrete this amount of solute. Any additional water excretion will render the urine hypotonic to plasma: such additional water excretion is called free water clearance, C_{H_2O}. Osmolar clearance (C_{OSM}) can be calculated by the following equation:

$$C_{OSM} = \frac{U_{OSM} \times V}{P_{OSM}} \quad (16)$$

where V is urine flow rate, OSM is osmolality, and U and P refer to urine and plasma, respectively. When urine is isotonic with plasma, $U_{OSM} = P_{OSM}$ (by definition), and therefore $C_{OSM} = V$. When urine is hypotonic to plasma, $C_{OSM} < V$, and

$$C_{H_2O} = V - C_{OSM} \quad (17)$$

When urine is hypertonic, $C_{OSM} > V$, and therefore the calculated value for C_{H_2O} is negative. Reversing the sign, negative free water clearance becomes free water reabsorption, usually designated Tc_{H_2O}.

$$Tc_{H_2O} = C_{OSM} - V \quad (18)$$

C_{H_2O} and Tc_{H_2O} define the limiting values for renal water excretion, and therefore for tolerated water ingestion. At a solute excretion rate of 580 mosmol/day, C_{OSM} is 2 L a day. Rearranging equation (15),

$$V = \frac{C_{OSM} \times P_{OSM}}{U_{OSM}} \quad (19)$$

and taking values of 40 and 1200 mosmol/kg H_2O as minimal and maximal U_{OSM}, respectively, yields limiting values for V of about 15 and 0.5 L daily. Corresponding maximum values for C_{H_2O} and Tc_{H_2O} are 12.5 and 1.52 L/day. Thus, at any given solute excretion rate, the defense against overhydration and dilution (C_{H_2O}) is much more effective than that against dehydration and concentration (Tc_{H_2O}), a conclusion borne out by clinical experience. This huge capacity to protect the body fluids from dilution may be an evolutionary inheritance from our fishy and amphibian ancestors, to whom (in fresh water) osmotic dilution is a constant threat.

REFERENCES

1. Coulthard MG, Hey EN. Weight as the best standard for glomerular filtration in the newborn. Arch Dis Child 1984; 59:373–375.
2. McCance RA. The maintenance of stability in the newly born. 1. Chemical exchange. Arch Dis Child 1959; 34: 361–370.

3. Dugdale AE. Evolution and infant feeding. Lancet 1986; 1:1441–1442.

4. Manz F, Kalhoff H, Remer T. Renal acid excretion in early infancy. Pediatr Nephrol 1997; 11:231–243.

5. Kildeberg P. Disturbances of hydrogen ion balance occurring in premature infants. II. Late metabolic acidosis. Acta Paediatr 1964; 53:517–526.

6. Arant BS Jr, Edelmann CM Jr, Spitzer A. The congruence of creatinine and inulin clearances in children: use of the technicon autoanalyzer. J Pediatr 1972; 81:559–561.

7. Calcagno PL, Rubin MI. Renal extraction of para-amino-hippurate in infants and children. J Clin Invest 1963; 42:1632–1639.

8. Tisher CC, Bulger RE, Trump BF. Human renal ultrastructure. I. Proximal tubule of healthy individuals. Lab Invest 1966; 15:1357–1394.

9. Bulger RE, Tisher CC, Myers CH, et al. Human renal ultrastructure. II. The thin limb of Henle's loop and the interstitium in healthy individuals. Lab Invest 1967; 16:124–141.

10. Tisher CC, Bulger RE, Trump BF. Human renal ultrastructure. 3. The distal tubule in healthy individuals. Lab Invest 1968; 18:655–668.

11. Arakawa M. A scanning electron microscopic study of the human glomerulus. Am J Pathol 1970; 64:457–466.

12. Kanwar YS, Farquar MG. Anionic sites in the glomerular basement membrane. In vivo and in vitro localization in the laminae rarae by cationic probes. J Cell Biol 1979; 81:137–153.

13. Venkatachalam MA, Karnovsky MJ, Fahimi HD, et al. An ultrastructural study of glomerular permeability using catalase and peroxidase as tracer proteins. JExp Med 1970; 132:1153–1167.

14. Brenner BM, Hostetter TH, Humes HD. Glomerular permselectivity: barrier function based on discrimination of molecular size and charge. Am J Physiol 1978; 234: F455–F460.

15. Ruotsalainen V, Ljungberg P, Wartiovaara J, et al. Nephrin is specifically located at the slit diaphragm of glomerular podocytes. Proc Natl Acad Sci U S A 1999; 96:7962–7967.

16. Tryggvason K, Ruotsalainen V, Wartiovaara J. Discovery of the congenital nephrotic syndrome gene discloses the structure of the mysterious molecular sieve of the kidney. Int J Dev Biol 1999; 43:445–451.

17. Maddox DA, Deen WM, Brenner BM. Dynamics of glomerular filtration. VI. Studies in the primate. Kidney Int 1974; 5:271–278.

18. Brenner BM, Troy JL, Daugherty TM, et al. Dynamics of glomerular ultrafiltration in the rat. II. Plasma flow dependence of GFR. Am J Physiol 1972; 223:1184–1190.

19. Deen WM, Troy JL, Robertson CR, et al. Dynamics of glomerular filtration in the rat. IV. Determination of the ultrafiltration coefficient. J Clin Invest 1973; 52:1500–1508.

20. Navar LG, Bell PD, White RW, et al. Evaluation of the single nephron glomerular filtration coefficient in the dog. Kidney Int 1977; 12:137–149.

21. Ausiello DA, Kreisberg JJ, Roy C, et al. Contraction of cultured rat glomerular mesangial cells after stimulation with angiotensin II and arginine vasopressin. J Clin Invest 1980; 65:754–760.

22. Burg MB, Orloff J. Electrical potential difference across proximal convoluted tubules. Am J Physiol 1970; 219: 1714–1716.

23. Brant SR, Yun CH, Donowitz M, et al. Cloning, tissue distribution, and functional analysis of the human Na$^+$/H$^+$ exchanger isoform, NHE3. Am J Physiol 1995; 269: C198–C206.

24. Burg MB, Green N. Bicarbonate transport by isolated perfused rabbit proximal convoluted tubules. Am J Physiol 1977; 233:F307–F314.

25. Kokko J. Proximal tubule potential difference. Dependence on glucose, HCO$_3$ and amino acids. J Clin Invest 1973; 52:1362–1367.

26. Martino JA, Earley LE. Relationship between intrarenal hydrostatic pressure and hemodynamically induced changes in sodium excretion. Circ Res 1968; 23:371–386.

27. Spitzer A, Windhager E. Effect of peritubular oncotic pressure changes on proximal tubular fluid reabsorption. Am J Physiol 1970; 218:1188–1193.

28. Berry CA, Cogan MG. Influence of peritubular protein on solute reabsorption in the rabbit proximal tubule. J Clin Invest 1981; 68:506–516.

29. Mackenzie B, Loo DD, Panayotova-Heiermann M, et al. Biophysical characteristics of the pig kidney Na+/glucose cotransporter SGLT2 reveal a common mechanism for SGLT1 and SGLT2. J Biol Chem 1996; 271:32678–32683.

30. Wright EM, Martin MG, Turk E. Familial glucose–galactose malabsorption and hereditary renal glycosuria. In: Scriver CR, Beaudet AL, Sly WS, et al., eds. The Metabolic and Molecular Bases of Inherited Disease. 8th ed. New York: McGraw-Hill, 2001:4891–4908.

31. Silbernagl S. The renal handling of amino acids and oligopeptides. Physiol Rev 1988; 68:911–1007.

32. Palacín M, Estevez R, Bertran J, et al. Molecular biology of mammalian plasma membrane amino acid transporters. Physiol Rev 1998; 78:969–1054.

33. Palacín M, Goodyer P, Nunes V, et al. Cystinuria. In: Scriver CR, Beaudet AL, Sly WS, et al., eds. The Metabolic and Molecular Bases of Inherited Disease. 8th ed. New York: McGraw-Hill, 2001:4909–4932.

34. Waldmann TA, Strober W, Mogielnicki BP. The renal handling of low molecular weight proteins. II. Disorders of serum protein catabolism in patients with tubular proteinuria, the nephrotic syndrome, or uremia. J Clin Invest 1972; 51:2162–2174.

35. Park CH, Maack T. Albumin absorption and catabolism by isolated perfused proximal convoluted tubules of the rabbit. J Clin Invest 1984; 73:767–777.

36. de Wardener HF. The control of sodium excretion. In: Orloff J, Berliner RW, eds. Handbook of Physiology. Washington, DC: American Physiological Society, 1973:677–720.

37. Ichikawa I, Hoyer JR, Seiler MW, et al. Mechanism of glomerulotubular balance in the setting of heterogeneous glomerular injury. Preservation of a close functional linkage between individual nephrons and surrounding microvasculature. J Clin Invest 1982; 69:185–198.

38. Wright FS, Briggs P. Feedback regulation of glomerular filtration rate. Am J Physiol 1977; 233:F1–F7.

39. Schnermann J, Ploth DW, Hermle M. Activation of tubuloglomerular feedback by chloride transport. Pflügers Arch Eur J Physiol 1976; 362:229–240.

40. Brezis M, Rosen S, Silva P, et al. Selective vulnerability of the medullary thick ascending limb to anoxia in the isolated perfused rat kidney. J Clin Invest 1984; 73:182–190.

41. Strauss MB, Lamdin E, Smith WP, et al. Surfeit and deficit of sodium: a kinetic concept of sodium excretion. Arch Intern Med 1958; 102:527–536.

42. Epstein M. Cardiovascular and renal effects of head-out water immersion in man. Circ Res 1976; 39:619–628.

43. Epstein FH, Post RS, McDowell M. Effects of an arteriovenous fistula on renal hemodynamics and electrolyte excretion. J Clin Invest 1953; 32:233–241.

44. Martino JA, Earley LE. Demonstration of the role of physical factors as determinants of natriuretic response to volume expansion. J Clin Invest 1967; 46:1963–1978.

45. Lindheimer MD, Lalone RC, Levinsky NG. Evidence that an acute increase in glomerular filtration rate has little effect on sodium excretion in the dog unless extracellular volume is expanded. J Clin Invest 1967; 46:256–265.

46. Howards SS, Davis BB, Knox FB, et al. Depression of fractional sodium reabsorption by the proximal tubule of the dog without sodium diuresis. J Clin Invest 1968; 47:1561–1572.

47. Arendshorst WJ, Navar LG. Renal circulation and glomerular hemodynamics. In: Schrier RW, Gottschalk CW, eds. Diseases of the Kidney. Boston: Little, Brown & Co., 1993:75.

48. Moss NG. Renal function and renal afferent and efferent nerve activity. Am J Physiol 1982; 243:F425–F433.

49. Young DB, Guyton AC. Steady state aldosterone dose–response relationships. Circ Res 1977; 40:138–142.

50. de Wardener HE, Mills IH, Clapham WF, et al. Studies on the efferent mechanism of the sodium diuresis which follows the administration of intravenous saline in the dog. Clin Sci 1961; 21:249–258.

51. Flynn TG, Davies PL. The biochemistry and molecular biology of atrial natriuretic factor. Biochem J 1985; 232:313–321.

52. Brenner BM, Ballermann BJ, Gunning ME, et al. Diverse biological actions of atrial natriuretic peptide. Physiol Rev 1990; 70:665–699.

53. McGrath MF, de Bold ML, de Bold AJ. The endocrine function of the heart. Trends Endocrinol Metab 2005; 16:469–477.

54. de Bold AJ. Cardiac natriuretic peptides: gaining further insights into structure–function relationships. J Am Coll Cardiol 2009; 54:1033–1034.

55. Rubattu S, Sciarretta S, Valenti V, et al. Natriuretic peptides: an update on bioactivity, potential therapeutic use, and implication in cardiovascular diseases. Am J Hypertens 2008; 21:733–741.

56. Simon DB, Karet FE, Hamdan JM, et al. Bartter's syndrome, hypokalemic alkalosis with hypercalciuria, is caused by mutations in the Na–K–2Cl transporter NKCC2. Nat Genet 1996; 13:183–188.

57. Simon DB, Karet FE, Rodriguez-Soriano J, et al. Genetic heterogeneity of Bartter's syndrome revealed by mutations in the K$^+$ channel, ROMK. Nat Genet 1996; 14:152–156.

58. Simon DB, Bindra RS, Mansfield TA, et al. Mutations in the chloride channel gene, CLCNKB, cause Bartter's syndrome type III. Nat Genet 1997; 17:171–178.

59. Simon DB, Nelson-Williams C, Johnson Bia M. Gitelman's variant of Bartter's syndrome, inherited hypokalaemic alkalosis, is caused by mutations in the thiazide-sensitive Na-Cl cotransporter. Nat Genet 1996; 12:24–30.

60. Shimkets RA, Warnock DG, Bositis CM, et al. Liddle's syndrome: heritable human hypertension caused by mutations in the beta subunit of the epithelial sodium channel. Cell 1994; 79:407–414.

61. Chang SS, Grunder S, Hanukoglu A, et al. Mutations in subunits of the epithelial sodium channel cause salt wasting with hyperkalaemic acidosis, pseudohypoaldosteronism type 1. Nat Genet 1996; 12:248–253.

62. Rossier BC, Palmer LG. Mechanism of aldosterone action on sodium and potassium transport. In: Seldin DW, Giebisch G, eds. The Kidney, Physiology and Pathophysiology. New York: Raven Press, 1992:1373–1409.

63. Feldman D, Funder JW, Edelman IS. Subcellular mechanisms in the action of adrenal steroids. Am J Med 1972; 53:545–560.

64. Gottschalk CW, Lassiter WE, Mylle M. Localisation of urine adicification in the mammalian kidney. Am J Physiol 1960; 198:581–585.

65. Rodriguez Soriano J, Boichis H, Stark H, et al. Proximal renal tubular acidosis. A defect in bicarbonate reabsorption with normal urinary acidification. Pediatr Res 1967; 1:81–98.

66. Brenes LG, Brenes JN, Hernandez MM. Familial proximal renal tubular acidosis: a distinct clinical entity. Am J Med 1977; 63:244–252.

67. Hutcheon RA, Kaplan BS, Drummond KS. Distal renal tubular acidosis in children with chronic hydronephrosis. J Pediatr 1976; 89:372–376.

68. Schwartz WB, Cohen JJ. The nature of the renal response to chronic disorders of acid–base equilibrium. Am J Med 1978; 64:417–428.

69. Lassiter WE, Gottschalk CW, Myolle M. Micropuncture study of renal tubular reabsorption of calcium in normal rodents. Am J Physiol 1963; 205:771–775.

70. Burg MB, Stoner L, Cardinal J, et al. Furosemide effect on isolated perfused tubules. Am J Physiol 1973; 225:119–124.

71. Gesek FA, Friedman PA. Mechanism of calcium transport stimulated by chlorothiazide in mouse distal convoluted tubule cells. J Clin Invest 1992; 90:429–438.

72. Brodehl J, Krause A, Hoyer PF. Assessment of maximal tubular phosphate reabsorption: comparison of direct measurement with the nomogram of Bijvoet. Pediatr Nephrol 1988; 2:183–189.

73. Yu X, White KE. FGF23 and disorders of phosphate homeostasis. Cytokine Growth Factor Rev 2005; 16:221–232.

74. Shimada T, Mizutani S, Muto T, et al. Cloning and characterization of FGF23 as a causative factor of tumor-induced osteomalacia. Proc Natl Acad Sci U S A 2001; 98:6500–6505.

75. White KE, Evans WE, O'Riordan JLH, et al. Autosomal dominant hypophosphataemic rickets is associated with mutations in FGF23. Nat Genet 2000; 26:345–348.

76. Beck L, Soumounou Y, Martel J, et al. Pex/PEX tissue distribution and evidence for a deletion in the 3′ region of the Pex gene in X-linked hypophosphatemic mice. J Clin Invest 1997; 99:1200–1209.

77. Feng JQ, Ward LM, Liu S, et al. Loss of DMP1 causes rickets and osteomalacia and identifies a role for osteocytes in mineral metabolism. Nat Genet 2006; 38:1310–1315.

78. Kurosu H, Kuro-o M. The Klotho gene family as a regulator of endocrine fibroblast growth factors. Mol Cell Endocrinol 2009; 299:72–78.

79. DeLuca HF, Schnoes HK. Metabolism and actions of vitamin D. Annu Rev Biochem 1976; 45:631–666.

80. Stumpf WE, Sar M, Reid FA, et al. Target cells for 1, 25-dihydroxyvitamin D. Science 1979; 206:1188–1190.

81. Gottschalk CW, Mylle M. Micropuncture study of the mammalian urinary concentrating mechanism: evidence for the countercurrent hypothesis. Am J Physiol 1959; 196:927–936.

82. Stephenson JL, Kriz W, Jamison RL, et al. Symposium on the renal concentrating mechanism. Federation Proc 1983; 42:2377–2405.

83. Scholander PF. The wonderful net. Sci Am 1957; 196:96–107.

84. Schrier RW, Bichet DG. Osmotic and nonosmotic control of vasopressin release and the pathogenesis of impaired water excretion in adrenal, thyroid and edematous disorders. J Lab Clin Med 1981; 98:1–15.

85. Dunn FL, Brennan TJ, Nelson AE, et al. The role of blood osmolality and volume in regulating vasopressin secretion in the rat. J Clin Invest 1973; 52:3212–3219.

86. Knoers N, van den Ouweland A, Dreesen J, et al. Nephrogenic diabetes insipidus: identification of the genetic defect. Pediatr Nephrol 1993; 7:685–688.

87. Feldman BJ, Rosenthal SM, Vargas GA, et al. Nephrogenic syndrome of inappropriate antidiuresis. N Engl J Med 2005; 352:1884–1890.

88. Marcialis MA, Faa V, Fanos V, et al. Neonatal onset of nephrogenic syndrome of inappropriate antidiuresis. Pediatr Nephrol 2008; 23:2267–2271.

89. van Lieburg AF, Verdijk MA, Knoers VV, et al. Patients with autosomal nephrogenic diabetes insipidus homozygous for mutations in the aquaporin 2 water-channel gene. Am J Hum Genet 1994; 55:648–652.

6

Principles of Radiological Imaging of the Urinary Tract

Uday Patel
St George's Hospital and Medical School, London, U.K.

Miles Walkden
University College Hospital, London, U.K.

INTRODUCTION

This chapter provides an overview of the main modalities used in urological imaging and the physics behind them (except nuclear medicine which is covered elsewhere). The mention of the word physics may concern many, but this is after all a book about basic sciences. As with most things in medicine, basic concepts allow the reader a deeper understanding. The history of the various techniques, which includes contributions from urologists in the development of iodinated contrast media (CM), is also discussed.

Until fairly recently, radiology was only really involved in producing anatomical information. Functional information, such as perfusion or filtration rates, was only measurable with nuclear scintigraphy. Even then the spatial resolution (how readily two adjacent structures can be seen as separate) was poor. Improvements in technology such as multislice computed tomography (CT) scanning and faster MRI sequences have not only allowed improved spatial and contrast resolution but also started to open the door to functional imaging by increasing temporal resolution (how quickly a scan can be obtained). This means that physiological information can be obtained about a tissue. This is particularly so with prostate imaging, where the possibility of diagnosing, grading, and staging cancer with MRI is becoming a distinct possibility. This could allow more focused prostate biopsy in the future.

CREATING AN IMAGE

To make an image, a body tissue–energy interaction must be created, precisely located and measured. The different radiological modalities, X ray, MRI, and ultrasound, simply utilize different energies to create that body tissue–energy interaction. The ability to see a structure within the patient rest on three main factors.

1. *Spatial resolution*: The ability to identify two adjacent structures as separate entities.
2. *Contrast resolution*: The ability to identify adjacent tissues as texturally distinct, depending on differences in the transmission of whatever energy source is being used.
3. *Signal to noise ratio (SNR)*: This is the amount of useful energy coming from the patient that can be used to make the image, compared with the degree of useless energy (quantum mottle and scatter) that contains no meaningful information and merely degrades the image.

Further intrinsic and extrinsic parameters also affect an image. Intrinsic parameters cannot be changed and are factors inherent to the tissue being imaged such as tissue density. Extrinsic parameters are those that can be manipulated or changed such as the current or voltage used in plain film radiography. It is by manipulating these extrinsic factors that an image is created.

PLAIN AND CONTRAST RADIOGRAPHY

Plain Radiography

Plain radiography as well as CT uses the X ray to create an image. X rays are part of the electromagnetic spectrum with a very short wavelength of around 10^{-10} m. They have large amounts of energy, which when absorbed in body tissues can cause ionization and tissue damage. X rays are therefore a type of ionizing radiation, whereas other energies used in radiology such as radiowaves in MRI have insufficient energy for ionization.

In the late 19th century, many people were experimenting with cathode tubes. It was however Wilhelm Röntgen, a German physics professor, who first wrote about X rays in a paper titled "On a new kind of Rays," a preliminary communication, in December 1895 (1). The discovery was a serendipitous finding while he was experimenting with electricity. His cathode tube made a nearby barium platinocyanide screen fluoresce. Intrigued, he named his newly discovered rays "X" rays, as this is the scientific denomination for an unknown quantity. He concentrated his research on this ray and went to produce the first human radiograph when he X-rayed his wife's hand. On seeing the plate, she is said to have exclaimed "I have seen my death"; but its medical potential was immediately obvious. Indeed, by May 1896 the first dedicated radiology journal was published (Archives of Clinical Skiagraphy described as "illustrating applications of the new photography to Medicine and Surgery" and the predecessor of the present *British Journal of Radiology*) and Röntgen became the first Nobel laureate of Physics in 1901. Yet, he died nearly bankrupt of cancer of the intestines in 1923. His death was not felt to be radiation induced, but soon after the more harmful effects of X-radiation became known, and are discussed below. The medical evaluation of the plain radiograph was undertaken in many countries, and even now, after over a century of clinical use and although increasingly challenged, it remains the workhorse modality in radiology.

Urology was one of the first areas to exploit the use of X rays for the assessment of the renal tract. James Adams, a Glasgow surgeon, was the first to x-ray a renal stone in 1896. He later removed the stone as proof. The first complete retrograde pyelogram was produced by Voelcher and von Lichtenberg in 1906 (2).

X-Ray Production

An X-ray tube is shown in Figure 1. It consists of a negative electrode (cathode), a heating filament, and a positive electrode (anode), all made from tungsten and housed within a vacuum tube. The tungsten filament is heated to incandescence and emits electrons by thermionic emission. These negatively charged electrons are repelled by the negative cathode and attracted toward the positive anode at speeds of up to 1000 m/sec. On impact with the positive anode, they suddenly decelerate, and the lost kinetic energy is converted into X rays (1%) and heat (99%).

Once directed at the human body, X rays are differentially attenuated by body tissues, proportionate to that tissues atomic number, density, and thickness. The attenuation occurs as either absorption or scatter. Scatter introduces noise and degrades the image while the emergent beam carries information on the thickness and composition of the intervening body tissue. This "information" is translated into a visible image when the X ray falls on a detector. In the case of analogue plain film, this is a photographic plate made of silver haloid. X rays convert the silver ions into stable, dense, and visible silver atoms.

Five basic radiographic densities can be differentiated on plain film—air, fat, soft tissue, bone, and contrast agents. Density is the main determining factor. Air only minimally attenuates and therefore appears black. In comparison, calcium-containing structures are substantially attenuating, and therefore a renal stone will appear white. How well the stone can be seen depends on its calcium content (or rather its density): the more the calcium, the denser it is, and hence whiter and more apparent. Thick structures also attenuate more than thin structures of the same

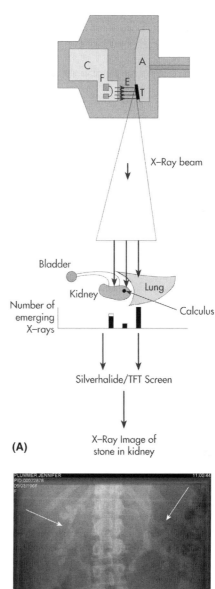

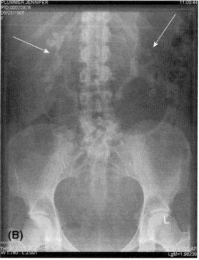

Figure 1 (**A**) A typical X-ray tube in cross section. *Abbreviations*: C, cathode; F, filament within the cathode; A, rotating anode; T, target on the anode where the electrons hit; E, electron beam. Body tissues attenuate the beam by variable amounts, depending on tissue density, tissue thickness, and atomic number (as illustrated by the bar chart—lungs being less dense allow more X rays to pass through). The emergent X-ray beam carrying this (mainly density related) information is then detected by a TFT screen and converted into a digital radiograph. The radiograph (**B**) Bilateral staghorn calculi (*white arrows*), seen as white (or relatively unexposed) areas as they are dense.

composition, which is why you can clearly see the bulky psoas muscle, as opposed to the thinner anterior abdominal muscles.

An anatomical structure will only be seen on a plain radiograph if it is outlined by tissue of a substantially different density. The kidneys (soft-tissue density) can only be seen as separate from the remaining retroperitoneal structures (also of soft-tissue density) because they are separated by the perinephric fat. Structures within the kidney cannot be differentiated as their X-ray attenuation is similar. The collecting system becomes visible only once filled by the much denser iodine-containing CM.

Table 1 (with details of film interpretation in Tables 2 and 3) shows the current uses of the plain film in urology, but a further deficiency of the plain film is the superimposition of structures on one another. Plain film tomography can partly overcome this, as it allows a "slice" of the patient to be obtained. The X-ray tube and film are simultaneously moved around a pivot point centered in the plane of interest. The structures above and below the focal plane are blurred out by motion of the tube and film, whereas structures within the focal plane are seen clearly (Fig. 2). This technique is used during excretion urography to obtain better detail of the renal collecting system.

Fluoroscopic equipment is based on the same principles of X-ray imaging except that the X rays fall onto a fluoroscopy screen. The light from this is amplified electronically by an image intensifier and displayed on a monitor. This allows real-time radiographic visualization of moving structures. Fluoroscopic images are of lower radiating dose to the

Table 1 Current Uses of Plain Films in Urology

KUB

Good for following known radio-opaque stones during treatment or as a screening tool for diagnosis of stones. However, in this respect it has probably been largely replaced by CT KUB.

IVU

IVUs were still used. However, with the introduction of multislice CT urography is starting to replace the IVU as it can assess not only the urothelium, but all the components of the renal tract as well as other intra abdominal organs.

Table 2 How to Interpret a KUB

1. Check the name, date, and side-markers on the film.
2. Look for calcification. Inspiratory and expiratory films may help as a renal stone should move on respiration.
    i. Kidneys—ensure both are present and of a normal size and outline.
    ii. Ureters—not normally seen on plain film but their course should be followed looking particularly at the PUJ, Pelvic brim and VUJ.
    iii. Bladder—can normally just be made out in the pelvis.
3. Assess the soft tissues.
    i. Look for the psoas shadows, their absence may indicate renal pathology.
    ii. Inspect other organs, such as the liver and spleen.
    iii. Asses the bowel to make sure there is no obvious bowel obstruction.
4. Assess the bones for any evidence of metastasis.

Table 3 How to Interpret an IVU

1. Check the name date and side-marker on the film.
2. Control film—check all the same points as for a KUB.
3. Immediate film.
    a. This should show bilateral symmetrical nephrograms.
    b. Assess the renal outline for any masses or scarring.
4. 5- and 10-min films of the kidney.
    a. Assess the calyceal anatomy.
    b. Ensure that all calyceals have been identified.
    c. Look for any filling defects.
5. Full-length release film.
    a. Ensure both ureters have been well opacified.
    b. Assess the bladder; looking for any filling defects.
    c. Postmicturition film.
    d. Assess adequate bladder emptying and also drainage of the upper tracts.

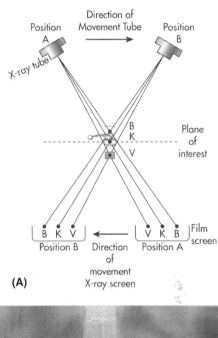

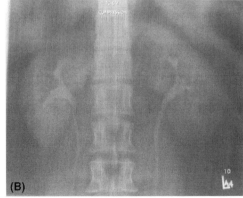

Figure 2 The principles of linear tomography. (**A**) The plane of interest is set for the kidneys (K). Structures outside the plane of interest such as the bowel (B) and the vertebral body (V) are blurred as their position on the film moves whereas structures in the plane of interest are projected in the same position and therefore appear sharp. (**B**) A tomogram through the kidneys during an IVU series. The plane of interest is set at 10 cm, which is the average depth for most kidneys. The calyceal system can be clearly seen whereas overlying structures have been blurred out.

patient; however, spatial resolution is poorer compared with the plain film.

Digital Radiography and PACS

The plain radiograph is being increasingly replaced by digital radiography (DR), where the image is acquired electronically. A thin-film transistor (TFT) screen replaces the photographic plate and converts the X ray into an electronic signal to create an image, composed of a matrix of individual cells or pixels (picture elements). Each pixel has an assigned value that is related to the intensity of X rays that falls onto it. Pixel size determines the spatial resolution—smaller pixels have better spatial resolution. The spatial resolution of digital images is currently poorer than conventional radiographs. Plain film is able to resolve 10 line pairs/mm, compared with the DR's 5.5 line pairs/mm. So, fine structure such as renal calcification is more readily apparent on conventional radiographs. Digital films do, however, have the advantage that they have superior contrast resolution, employing a wider grayscale, which can be further manipulated to the observer's satisfaction. This partly compensates for its modest spatial resolution. But most importantly, DR, being electronic, is easier to store and transmit, allowing PACS (picture archiving and communication systems) to be used.

PACS is revolutionizing radiology departments, with film-less departments that can rapidly transmit images through electronic links. Multimodality images can be instantly recalled from memory banks and displayed on a single monitor with image incorporation for surgical planning. Departments are becoming digital at a rapid pace as unit costs decline and the necessary cultural changes take place, such that radiologists and clinicians feel comfortable using monitors alone to view films. The promise is not necessarily cost saving, but promises more efficient patient management—lost films have become a thing of the past, and a complete imaging history is instantly available at any point inside or even outside the hospital, day or night.

Before the 1980s, it was impossible for anyone other than the manufacturer of a specific imaging machine to decode their images. With the increasing use of digital images and the need to be able to view these images around the hospital and indeed around the country/ world, it was realized that a standard format for viewing, storing, and transmitting medical images was required. In 1983, the American College of Radiologists (ACR) and the National Electrical Manufacturers Association (NEMA) formed a joint committee and in 1985 produced the ACR-NEMA standard. This was revised in 1993 and renamed Digital Imaging and Communications in Medicine (DICOM) (3). This standard is now updated yearly. DICOM enables the integration of scanners, servers, workstations, printers, and network hardware from multiple manufacturers into a PAC system. DICOM differs from other data formats in that it groups information into data sets. This means that a file of a KUB X ray, for example, actually contains the patient ID within the file, so that the image can never be separated from this information by mistake.

Contrast Media

One way to alter and improve the contrast resolution of a tissue is to use radio-opaque CM to outline it. CM can either be positive, such that it has a higher attenuation density than the surrounding tissues (and appearing white on the image), or it can be negative with a lower attenuation density (e.g., air) that absorbs less radiation and so appears black on the final image. Positive-contrast agents are substances with high atomic numbers. The three main categories in use in radiology currently are iodine-based, gadolinium-containing, and barium-based. Barium-based preparations are used only for the alimentary tract and are thus not readily encountered in urology, and gadolinium agents are used in magnetic resonance imaging (MRI).

Currently, the commonest intravenous contrast agent used is iodine (atomic weight 127)-containing compounds. The idea of using iodine-based compounds as an intravenous contrast agent came from the discovery that the urinary bladder could be visualized on radiographs of patients who had taken large doses of sodium iodine for the treatment of syphilis (4). Unfortunately, the collecting system was only poorly seen and the sodium iodine was found to be too toxic for clinical radiological use. In 1925, two Germans, Bruz and Rath, managed to produce less toxic iodine–containing compounds based on the pyridine ring that were initially used to treat coccal infections. In 1928 an American urology intern, Moses Swick, working with some of these drugs realized that they may be of use in visualizing the renal tract and the intravenous urogram was born (5).

All soft tissues in the body enhance with iodinated CM, but none as much as the kidneys. This is because they are the principle source of excretion (99%) with a half-life of two hours. Renal excretion is by free glomerular filtration without tubular reabsorption: this means that CT contrast–enhanced perfusion studies can be used to calculate GFR.

Adverse Effects of Contrast Media and Current Recommendations

A limitation of current CM agents is their toxicity with two broad types of adverse reaction—anaphylactoid and chemotoxic. The exact mechanism of either reaction is unclear and they can occur either early (within one hour of administration) or be delayed (one hour to one week following administration).

Anaphylactoid reactions occur unpredictably and independently of the dose or concentration of the agent. They are believed at least in part to be because of the ionic makeup of the CM, as many of the earlier ionic agents caused severe anaphylactoid reactions. With the introduction of nonionic CM, these reactions have become less frequent. Chemotoxic effects are related to the total dose, molecular toxicity, and physiological characteristics (such as osmolality)

Table 4 Prevention of Adverse Reactions Because of CM

1.	In all CM studies, the dose of CM should be kept as low as possible.	

2.	Nonrenal adverse reactions.	a. Identify patients at increased risk of reaction.
		  i. Previous moderate/severe acute reaction
		  ii. Asthma
		  iii. Allergy requiring medical treatment
		b. If increased risk detected then do the following:
		  i. Reassess the clinical indications, if still necessary.
		  ii. Use nonionic CM under careful monitoring.
		  iii. Keep the patient in the department for 30 min post administration.
		  iv. Premedication prophylaxis such as 12-hr 30-mg prednisolone and 2-hr pre-CM administration is no longer recommended.

3.	Renal adverse reactions	a. Identify patients with an increased risk of developing CM-induced nephropathy.
		  i. Raised serum creatinine particularly secondary to diabetic nephropathy.
		  ii. Dehydration.
		  iii. Congestive heart failure.
		  iv. Age >70.
		  v. Concurrent administration of nephrotoxic drugs such as NSAIDs.
		  vi. Non-insulin-dependent patient with diabetes taking metformin. Metformin is excreted unchanged in the urine. In the presence of renal failure such as can be induced by CM, metformin may accumulate in sufficient amounts to cause lactic acidosis.
		b. If increased risk then do the following:
		  i. If taking metformin, stop a time of administration of CM, check creatinine at 48 hr and if unchanged then restart metformin.
		  ii. Stop nephrotoxic drugs 24 hr prior to CM administration.
		  iii. Give IV hydration 6 hr prior to administration and for up to 24 hr after the study
		  iv. Use low or iso-osmolar CM

Special situations are as follows:

Pregnancy and lactation: No teratogenic effects of CM have been described. The free iodine does, however, have the potential to depress fetal/neonatal thyroid function. If CM is given during pregnancy, the neonatal thyroid function should be checked within the first week. Such tiny amounts of iodine enter the breast milk that there is no contraindication to breast feeding.

Thyroid disease: As CM contains small amounts of free iodine, it may cause thyrotoxic crisis in patients with Graves' disease. These patients can still receive CM but should be closely followed. The free iodine can also interfere with diagnostic and therapeutic nuclear medicine procedure for up to two months.

Phaeochromocytoma: Crises can be precipitated by CM. Patients with known phaeochromocytoma should have A and B blockade prior to the administration of CM.

Extracted from ESUR guidelines version 6.

of each agent. These are the ones thought to be responsible for nephrotoxicity. As well as being nonionic, modern CM is of low or iso-osmolality compared with plasma, and of lower chemotoxicity.

CM nephropathy is a diagnosis of exclusion, defined as an increase in serum creatinine by more than 25% or 44 nm/L occurring within three days of the use of IV CM with no alternative explanation (6). There are no characteristic or diagnostic, biochemical or histological abnormalities. It is the third highest cause of hospital-acquired acute renal failure (ARF) accounting for 12% of the cases (7). The patients with the highest risk for developing contrast-induced ARF are those with preexisting renal impairment or risk factors for renal impairment (e.g., diabetes mellitus, etc.) (8,9). The degree of renal impairment present also determines the severity of CM nephropathy. At least two risk scores for the prediction of CM-induced nephropathy have been developed (10,11) but these are not widely used, and in most radiology departments a creatinine cutoff of 200 ng/mL is used, above which intravenous CM is not used unless deemed clinically justified.

A number of preventative measures can be taken to reduce CM nephrotoxicity. These include intravenous hydration (which is probably the only intervention that has some evidence to support it), vasodilators, and antioxidants such as *N*-acetylecysteine and ascorbic acid (12). Currently, the European Society of Urogenital Radiology (ESUR) guidelines do not recommend any pharmacological manipulation for routine use in prevention of CM-induced nephropathy (13) (Table 4).

The Hazards of Ionizing Radiation

Soon after Röntgen's discovery of the X ray, their harmful effects became increasingly evident. In 1896, the first case of radiation dermatitis and hair loss were reported (14), followed soon after by cases of radiation-induced malignancy. Their frequency was sufficiently alarming for the Röntgen Society (formed in 1896) to set up a committee in 1898 to investigate radiation-induced side effects, followed in 1915 by a code of practice document with recommendations for radiation protection.

Ionization of tissues by absorption of radiation energy is the cause, and the most vulnerable molecules are proteins and deoxyribonucleic acid (DNA). Damage occurs either directly by rupture of the

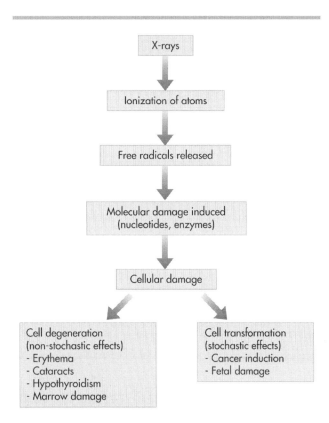

Figure 3 The damaging ionizing action of X rays has cellular and genetic consequences (see text for further explanation of stochastic and nonstochastic effects).

covalent bond or indirectly by free-radical production. Indirect free-radical production is the most commonly occurring reaction (Fig. 3). Terminologically, there are two broad groups of ionizing hazards: stochastic effects and deterministic effects (nonstochastic).

Stochastic effects means they arise by chance and have no threshold dose. The risk of an effect occurring increases with the dose, but the severity of the effect does not. Stochastic effects result in cell transformation and cancer induction. Deterministic effects have a value below which they will not occur, that is, there is a threshold dose, and include effects such as erythema and cataract formation. Once the threshold dose is exceeded, the likelihood of that effect increases rapidly up to a level, beyond which it becomes inevitable. Deterministic effects are rate dependent because the body is able to repair the damage (except in the eye, where the dose is cumulative and particular care should be taken to protect it from radiation).

Doses in diagnostic radiology on the whole do not reach deterministic threshold levels, except in interventional radiology (IR) and cumulative CT doses on the lens of the eye. Stochastic effects, however, are a risk with all X-ray imaging, no matter how small the dose. Typical doses in urological imaging are given in Table 5. It should be remembered that normal background radiation also has a risk of inducing a cancer. The quoted risk of inducing a cancer is 1:15,000/mSv. In the United Kingdom, it is estimated

Table 5 Effective Radiation Dose for Patients Undergoing Radiological Investigations

	Effective dose (mSv)	Approximate natural-background radiation
Chest X ray	0.02	3 days
Lumbar spine X ray	1.3	7 mo
IVU	2.5	14 mo
Bone scan	4.0	1.8 yr
CT		
Head	2.3	1 yr
Abdomen	10	4.5 yr
(Renal stone protocol)	(4.7)	
(CT urogram)	(10–15)	
Renal scan		
DTPA	1.0	6 mo
Mag 3	1.0	6 mo
Barium enema	7.0	3.2 yr

Average effective dose in the United Kingdom: 2.2 (87% natural sources; 13% from artificial sources of which 11% is medical sources).
Source: From Ref. 15.

that diagnostic X ray causes approximately 700 cancers a year (16). Normal background radiation for a person in this country is approximately 2.2 mSv/yr (15), unless you happen to live in Cornwall where radon gas increases this total to approximately 6 mSv/yr. Imaging accounts for approximately 14% (17) of this background radiation but is increasing. One of the main contributors to this increase is CT, which currently accounts for 10% of all radiological investigations and 40% of all radiation (18). We, therefore, need to keep the radiation dose as low as possible. Radiating radiological investigations should always have a clinical justification and, whenever possible, a substitute safer alternative should be chosen (e.g., ultrasound or MRI).

CROSS-SECTIONAL IMAGING

Plain and contrast radiography is limited to a two-dimensional (2D) format with no depth perception. However, if the source of the body tissue/energy interaction can be precisely located in the three perpendicular planes, this digitized information can be used to build a slice-by-slice sectional image. Cross-sectional imaging has made possible the noninvasive imaging of those internal tissues and organs beyond resolution by conventional radiography. CT, ultrasound, and MRI are all examples. CT uses X-radiation while ultrasound and MRI exploit novel energies and tissue/energy interactions.

Computed Tomography

CT was first developed by Sir Godfrey Hounsfield in 1973, working at the Atkinson Morley Hospital in London (19). At the time he was working with the music company EMI, who had many other nonmusic interests as well and who had recently signed the Beatles. Some of the substantial revenue that the Beatles generated for EMI made possible the investment in the development of the CT scanner. It has

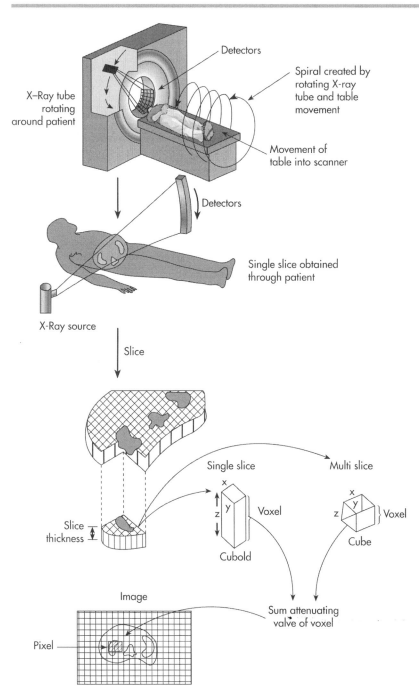

Figure 4 Principles of CT. The X-ray source does a 360° rotation around the patient to obtain a slice. This slice is divided up into a matrix made up of voxels. Each voxel is a cuboid with *x*, *y*, and *z* values. The *z*-value (or slice thickness was traditionally larger than the *x* and *y* values and thus reformats in planes other than the one of acquisition, that is, axial resulted in a loss of resolution). The sum attenuating value from the voxel is then taken and converted into a linear density scale (as Hounsfield units), which are displayed as pixels in shades of gray on the final image. Multislice machines simply acquire multiple slices per rotation, allowing the slice thickness to be significantly reduced and an isotropic voxel obtained, which allows accurate reformatting of the image in any plane.

therefore been said by some that the development of the CT scan was at least partly down to the success of the Beatles.

CT also uses X rays, and the fundamental physics of X ray/tissue interaction, as described earlier, still apply. For CT, the X-ray beam is generated as a precise pencil-thin beam, which is detected by a bank of detectors positioned diametrically opposite to the source. As the beam rotates around the body, the detectors convert the transmitted beam intensity into a cross-sectional image of between 0.6 and 10 mm thick. The image itself is composed of numerous

picture elements (pixels) (Fig. 4). As structures are no longer superimposed on one another, a far superior contrast resolution is possible compared with the plain radiograph, with at least a 10-fold improvement. Each pixel is assigned a grayscale value according to the sum attenuating power of the tissue in its corresponding volume (or voxel). The sum attenuating power is known as the CT or Hounsfield unit, and Figure 5 gives some typical values for normal body tissue. By convention, water was assigned a neutral density at zero and all other values are measured relative to water. Air is −1000, fat −100, and bone

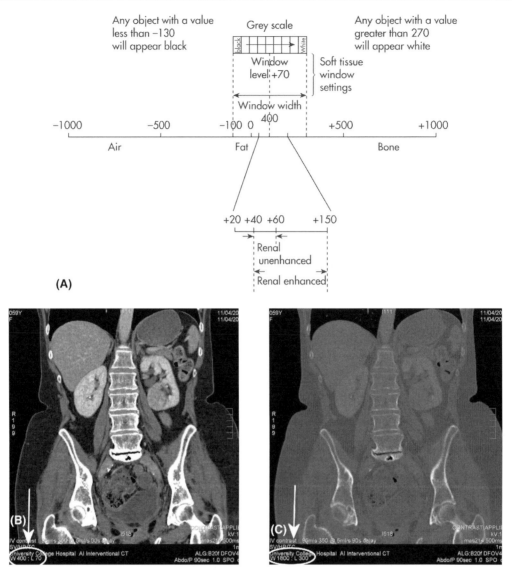

(A)

Figure 5 (**A**) A scale showing the CT (or Hounsfield) numbers of various body tissues. Water is conventionally graded as zero, air as −1000, renal stones as >200 and soft tissue such as kidney as +40 to +60 units unenhanced and +40 to +150 enhanced. The figure also demonstrates the concept of windowing to allow better contrast resolution. For soft-tissue windows the window level is set at +200. The window width 200 units either side, that is, 0 to +400. Any structure lying within this range will be seen as a shade of gray. Any structure with a value higher or lower than the window width will appear white or black, respectively, and will not be separable from other structures outside the window width. The windows are set according to the structure being scrutinized. For the majority of urological imaging, soft-tissue windows are employed. (**B**) A coronal image of the abdomen on soft-tissue windows (*white arrow* shows the window level has been set at 70 and the window width at 400). The RCC in the left lower pole is well seen. (**C**) The same coronal image on bony windows (*white arrow* shows the window level at 300 and the window width at 1800); now good bony detail is seen but the left RCC is less well seen.

above +200. The kidneys are in the soft-tissue range of +40 to +60, rising to around 150 units after intravenous contrast. Renal calculi are near the bone range and are readily identified. Structures that have a high positive value appear as white, for example, bone/renal calculi, and structures with a high negative value appear as black, for example, air.

The Hounsfield value is converted to a grayscale value for display. There are a wide range of Hounsfield values ranging from −1000 to +3000. The human eye is only able to distinguish approximately 60 shades of gray. It is, therefore, necessary to focus in on levels of interest (Fig. 5) by "windowing." A window level is set depending on the structure of interest; for example, for the kidneys as they lie in the soft-tissue range, the level is set at +20. A window width of approximately 200 Hounsfield units is then set on either side of this value. Any structure with a value inside the window width will be assigned a shade of gray, and it will be possible to differentiate it. Any structure with a value greater than $+200$ will be white and any structure less than -200 will appear black.

Spiral and Multidetector CT

The first CT scans obtained data one slice at a time, in between which the table had to be moved. This resulted in long scan times, misregistration between slices, and movement artifact. Helical scanning was then developed in which the patient is moved through the scanner at a constant speed while the X-ray tube continuously rotates around the patient. A continuous volume of data was thus obtained. Scan times were shorter and reconstruction of overlapping slices could be undertaken to improve visualization of small lesions. However, spiral CT only obtained one slice per rotation and the calculated voxels were still large (or cuboid) with the length of the Z-axis (i.e., the sliced thickness) still considerably larger than the X and Y axes (Fig. 4). This meant that image quality was good in the plane of acquisition, that is, the axial plane, but poor when attempts were made to reformat the data into other planes or three-dimensional (3D) volume images.

The advent of multidetector CT (the acquisition of multiple slices during each spiral rotation) changed this. Now instead of a single slice, 64 or even 128 slices can be obtained with one rotation of the gantry. Scan times have now plummeted with thinner slices possible, so that isotropic voxels (cubes rather than cuboids) could be obtained (Fig. 4). Isotropic voxels allow for more accurate, true 3D imaging: no matter how the data set is projected, there is no significant loss of resolution. Diagnostic quality images can be obtained in any plane. Table 6 lists the current uses of CT in urology.

Multiplanar Reformat and 3D Volume Rendering

As data are acquired as a volume with near isotropic voxels, it is possible to postprocess this information to create images in different planes and in 3D. These images do not contain any more information than the axial data, but they offer a more rapid appreciation of spatial information and anatomical relationships. This can be particularly useful in surgical planning (Fig. 6).

Multiplanar Reformats

The sagittal and coronal planes are the most commonly used and easiest to orientate. In urology the coronal

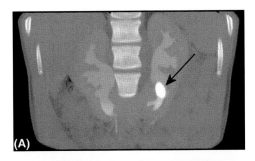

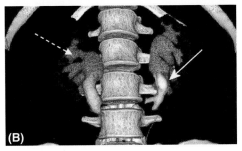

Figure 6 (**A**) Maximum-intensity projection (MIP) image of the kidneys. Note that high-density contrast in the collecting systems is well seen as is the stone in the lower pole of the left kidney (*black arrow*), but the low attenuation renal parenchyma and surrounding soft tissue is not well seen. (**B**) A 3D volume-rendered image of the same kidneys as in A. This was obtained prior to PCNL to allow delineation of the stone (*white arrow*) and its relationship to the collecting system (*dashed arrow*), which is filled with contrast. The 3D anatomical information provided by modern imaging has the potential to aid presurgical planning and navigation.

plane is excellent for visualizing the kidneys, ureters and bladder in a single view. Oblique reformats can also be made and are useful for viewing the hepatic and pancreatic regions. Curved reformats allow tortuous tubular structures such as blood vessels to be seen in one view.

Maximum- and Minimum-Intensity Projections

In maximum-intensity projection viewing, rays are traced from the viewer through the object to the display, and only the relative maximum value detected along each ray path is retained to create the image. This means that high attenuation structures such as bone and contrast are well seen and lower attenuation structures are not well visualized. This method is utilized in vascular imaging. Minimum-intensity projection involves detecting the minimum value along each ray path.

Volume Rendering

Rendering is the process of mapping a 3D data set onto a 2D screen for display. In volume rendering the CT numbers that make up the image are assigned to be either visible or invisible and can be displayed with varying colors and varying opacity levels (20). 3D volume–rendered images have proved particularly

Table 6 Current Uses of CT in Urology

1.	CT KUB	Gold standard for the investigation of renal colic. Sensitivities and specificities approach 100%. Also has the advantage of detecting other pathology in up to a third of cases.
2.	CT of kidneys	For evaluation of renal masses, renal infections, etc.
3.	CT angiography	For suspected renal artery stenosis.
4.	CT urography	For the investigation of upper tract causes of hematuria.

useful in preoperative planning for partial nephrectomy where tumor relationship to the collecting system and renal vasculature can be seen (21).

It is from using prospective rendering techniques that so-called virtual endoscopy images can be created, which are starting to be used for virtual cystography (22).

Multiphase CT Imaging

With the fast imaging capability of multidetector CT, the different phases in the handling of the contrast by the kidneys can be identified and different pathologies can be evaluated (Fig. 7).

1. *Noncontrast*: This is used for detecting stones and also is a baseline for enhancement of renal masses (Table 7).
2. *Arterial phase*: This occurs at about 15 seconds post injection. This allows high-quality multiplane images of the renal arteries to be obtained.
3. *Cortical phase*: This occurs 30 to 40 seconds post injection. Contrast filters into the proximal convoluted tubule. It permits corticomedullary differentiation. Scars are best seen and it helps differentiate renal pseudotumor (normal renal tissue) from pathology. This phase has, however, been shown to hinder mass detection in some cases and a nephrographic phase tends to be preferred.
4. *Nephrographic phase*: This phase occurs 90 to 120 seconds post injection. Contrast enters the collecting tubules. A homogenous nephrogram is obtained in which corticomedullay differentiation is lost. The detection of true renal masses is easiest in this phase.
5. *Excretory phase*: Occurs typically 10 minutes following injection. Contrast enters the pelvicalyceal system (PC), ureters, and bladder. This is the CT equivalent of the IVU. This allowed detection of filling defects within the collecting system, such as TCC, blood clot, stone, and vascular impression. As these data are obtained as a volume, it can be processed to give virtual endoscopic views.
6. *Functional imaging*: A modern 64-slice CT scanner can obtain multiple data acquisition some two or three times per second. Its ability to acquire data at such speed allows contrast-enhancing agents to be used as tracer substances, similar to many of the dynamic nuclear medicine investigations. CT number versus time curves can be constructed, which give information on parameters such as perfusion and also GFR.

If all these phases were obtained in a single scan, the radiation dose would be unacceptably high. It is therefore necessary to tailor the phases obtained to the clinical question being asked. Accurate clinical information facilitates focused imaging.

Ultrasound

Ultrasound employs sound waves that occur at a frequency above the upper limit of human hearing,

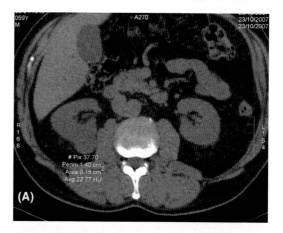

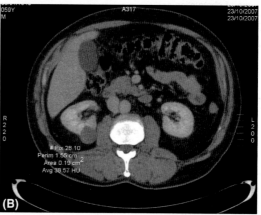

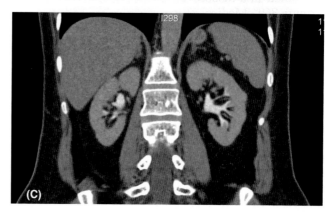

Figure 7 (**A**) Unenhanced image of the kidney shows an exophytic renal mass. It has HU above 15 and is therefore not a cyst. (**B**) Nephrographic phase obtained 100 seconds post injection of CM. The mass is seen to enhance compared with the precontrast image but not as much as the surrounding renal parenchyma. This is typical for a renal cell cancer. (**C**) Excretory phase coronal image shows contrast outlining the pelvicalyceal system. This is the CT equivalent of the IVU.

typically above 20 kHz, which are inaudible to the human ear. Ultrasound was first developed toward the end of the war in the form of SONAR (sound navigation and ranging) to detect submarines. Medical ultrasound started to be used in the 1940s as a therapeutic modality rather than a diagnostic one,

Table 7 How to Interpret a Low-Dose CT KUB

1. Look at the kidneys—assess size, cortical thickness and any evidence of stones or hydronephrosis.
2. Follow the course of the ureter—follow antegradely from the kidneys to the pelvic brim, then retrogradely from the VUJ up to the pelvic brim. Assess for any stones, thickening or stranding. Three common areas for stones to be found are at the PUJ, pelvic brim and VUJ.
3. The bladder—assess for stones and masses.
4. Assess the other organs, particularly paying attention to the appendix, pancreas, gallbladder, sigmoid colon, and in females the uterus and ovaries.

Differentiating a stone from a phlebolith: Phleboliths have comet tail of soft tissue (the tail sign), tend to be more rounded, and have a central lucency. Calculi demonstrate a rim sign (a rim of surrounding soft tissue).

Signs of obstruction: The signs include renal enlargement, calyceal dilatation, and perinephric stranding. There is a relationship between the signs of obstruction and the duration of the pain. If the patient is imaged within two hours of pain commencing, many of these signs of obstruction will not be present.

Source: From Refs. 23 and 24.

Table 8 Current Uses of Ultrasound in Urology

Renal	Hematuria
	Loin pain
	Suspected hydronephrosis
	Renal impairment
	Renal calculi
Bladder	Bladder outflow obstruction
	Hematuria
	Pelvic pain
	Lower urinary tract symptoms
	Bladder emptying
Scrotum	Testicular masses
	Testicular pain
	Suspected torsion
	Infertility
Prostate	Lower urinary tract symptoms
	Prostate size estimation
	Suspected prostate cancer
Penis	Peyronie's disease
	Erectile dysfunction

utilizing its heating and tissue disrupting effects. William Fry first used ultrasound to destroy parts of the basal ganglia in patients with Parkinson's disease (25). It was not until the 1950s that reproducible diagnostic ultrasound pictures were obtained by Holmes and Howry in America (26). One of the earliest produced was of a normal human neck and was obtained by submerging a volunteer in water (contained in a disused B29gun turret!) and scanning through 360°. Medical ultrasound can be used for both therapeutic (250 kHz to 2000 kHz) and diagnostic (3–20 MHz) purposes, the difference being the frequency of the sound wave and thus the amount of energy that is deposited in the tissue.

Diagnostic Ultrasound

This provides the cornerstone of urological imaging from which much important information on the renal tract can be obtained and of such importance that many urologists have begun to use the technique in their clinics. Diagnostic ultrasound is the safest, cheapest, and most versatile of the cross-sectional modalities and Table 8 lists its current uses in urology. The sound waves are nonionizing and so far no serious tissue consequences have been proven. It does, however, cause some minor tissue heating but normal tissue perfusion dissipates this. The ultrasound probe or transducer is both a transmitter and a receiver and continuously switches from one to the other. Within the probe is a piezoelectric disk. When a current is applied to the disk, it expands and once the current is reversed, the disk contracts emitting a sound wave proportional to the applied current. In its receiver mode, the disk is compressed by the retuning echo, producing a current proportional to the pressure.

Sound waves in the diagnostic range (3–20 MHz) will transmit through the body, but are altered in many ways by the intervening tissues and tissue-tissue interfaces. Of the numerous alterations, only three are commonly exploited for imaging—the absorption of sound by tissue, the reflection of sound at tissue-tissue interfaces, and the apparent change in frequency of sound at moving interfaces (the Doppler effect). The first two are used to build the familiar "grayscale" ultrasound image, and the last allows "vascular sonography" or duplex/color Doppler.

Grayscale Ultrasound

The amount of sound absorbed by a given tissue is calculated by analysis of the reflected echo and this is used to assign a value on a "grayscale." The factors that influence absorption and reflection are given in Figure 8. The weaker the reflection, the more "gray" or darker is the pixel value. Varying shades of grays from different points in an organ are used to build an image that can be viewed on a television monitor. As water is a good sound transmitter and poor reflector, a renal cyst is seen as black; while fat, a good reflector, is seen as white. Bone and calcium are highly sound attenuating and reflective, and demonstrate a sharp interface with a shadow beyond (Fig. 9). Unlike the other cross-sectional modalities, this is a real-time, interactive method and ideally suited for biopsy and percutaneous intervention of soft tissues.

The Doppler Effect

Christian Doppler described the change in perceived frequency of sound emitted by a moving source in 1843, and an everyday example is the crescendo/decrescendo sound of the moving train whistle, as heard by the observer on the platform. Medical ultrasound is also subject to this Doppler shift effect, and the frequency change can be recalculated to give the velocity of the moving interface—the equation for this Doppler effect is given in Figure 10. The common

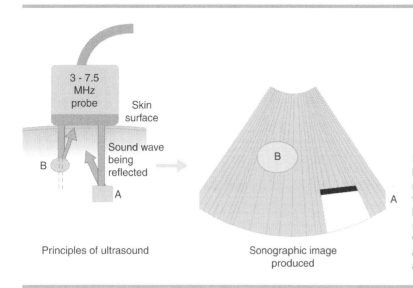

Principles of ultrasound

Sonographic image produced

Figure 8 Principles of medical ultrasound. Spatial localization is calculated from the time delay before sound is received back. Sound from deeper structures takes longer. The composition of a structure is calculated by the percentage of sound waves that are reflected back. A renal calculus reflects more sound waves than a renal cyst. The stone, therefore, appears white (hyperechoic) on ultrasound whereas a cyst appears black (hypoechoic).

moving interface in human tissues is the red blood cell and blood flow and tissue hemodynamics can be studied. Calculated velocities can be presented quantitatively as a continuous, time-framed trace of true velocity (the "Doppler or spectral waveform") or semiquantitatively/qualitatively as a "color Doppler" image.

Spectral or Duplex Doppler

Spectral Doppler represents the full spectrum of recorded velocities in a given time period. It can be used to diagnose and to grade arterial stenosis using the velocity gradient across a narrowing. This is of some value in the assessment of renal artery stenosis. As well as velocity information, the shape of a spectral waveform encodes further qualitative or semiquantitative data about tissue character. The peripheral resistance (PR) or "stiffness" of the tissue bed alters the waveform. Increased PR, as seen immediately after acute ureteric obstruction, restricts flow during diastole with reduced diastolic velocities. Waveform changes can be quantified by calculating so-called waveform indices, for example, the resistive index (RI) (Fig. 10). RI analysis is of some value in evaluation of renal dilatation. However, the diagnostic specificity of RI is modest, as adaptive physiological responses after obstruction counteract the elevated PR. Conversely, tumors have a low RI and elevated diastolic flows—because of intratumoral arteriovenous shunts and the lack of a complete smooth muscle wall in tumoral neovessels—and are seen on color Doppler as areas of hypervascularity (Fig. 11). This improves the diagnostic specificity in tumor diagnosis.

Color Doppler

With color Doppler, the peak velocity in a given time frame is assigned a value on a color scale, and this is superimposed on the grayscale image. Conventionally,

red represents flow toward the probe and blue away. Conveniently, renal arterial flow is usually toward and venous flow away from the probe, and so the "gray" and "color Doppler" findings are easily assimilated by the observer. Sonographic evaluation of the morphology of soft tissues as well as its vascularity can be carried out simultaneously, adding a qualitative or functional element to the grayscale ultrasound image. Most disease processes have some alteration of the blood flow, either increased or decreased, and color Doppler assists diagnostic evaluation. Tumors, such as renal cell carcinoma or angiomyolipoma, are seen as "hypervascular" because of the increased vessel density, as well as the higher mean velocity within tumor microvessels because of the reduced PR in the tumor.

Ultrasound Contrast Media

As with radiographic CM, certain injected agents can be used to enhance the ultrasound signal/noise. Essentially, these agents are stabilized microbubbles (2–10 μ range), which are sonovisible (27). Only intravascular agents are available at the moment with no soft-tissue distribution, but they are useful for vascular studies as they improve the strength of the Doppler effect and allow more detailed vascular analysis. They can also, under some circumstances, return signal of a specific frequency (or harmonic) that can be individually isolated and analyzed. Such harmonic imaging is currently being evaluated, and with the development of more refined agents with a tissue distribution, harmonic imaging of soft-tissue abnormalities may expand the diagnostic range of grayscale ultrasound.

Many of the recent developments in medical ultrasound are to do with improved transducer design and postprocessing. This has improved the quality of the ultrasound, but some disease processes remain frustratingly beyond current visibility. Prostate cancer is a germane example—although the prostate gland is

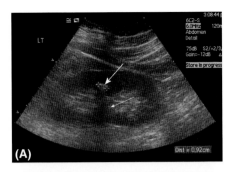

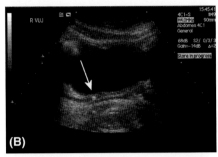

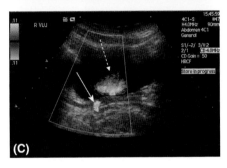

Figure 9 (**A**) Ultrasound image of a renal stone (being measured with callipers) showing it to be hyperechoic because of the increased reflection of sound waves (*thick arrow*). It also casts a hypoechoic shadow (*thin arrow*) as no sound waves can penetrate through it. Not all renal stones show this characteristic shadowing, for example, small stones may not cast a shadow. (**B**) A small hyperechoic lesion is seen in the lower ureter (*white arrow*) but it does not cast an acoustic shadow. Is it a stone? (**C**) With the color Doppler switched on, the lesion demonstrates twinkle artifact (*white arrow*), suggesting that it represents a stone. Ureteric jets can also be seen in the bladder (*dashed arrow*), suggesting that the ureter is not obstructed.

ideally suited for ultrasound examination, as with a high frequency transrectal probe, it is very close to the probe surface, with few intervening tissues to degrade the sound; yet many biopsy-proven prostate cancers are not visible. This highlights the limitation of current grayscale ultrasound. Even the most modern probes poorly resolve early or small-volume disease in the prostate gland or elsewhere. To overcome this limitation, other fundamental properties of tissue-sound interaction are being investigated for sonography. These include the imaging of harmonic frequencies (as above) and tissue sonoelasticity. Elastography

exploits the difference in stiffness of tissues. A tumor is normally significantly stiffer than the background soft tissue. When a mechanical compression such as an ultrasound wave is applied, the tumor deforms less than the surrounding tissue and this can be detected. Sonoelasticity has been explored in the prostate gland but has not yet proven useful (28,29).

Therapeutic Ultrasound

After over 30 years of constant use, there has not been even one reported case of harm attributable to the use of diagnostic ultrasound, although there are theoretical risks because of local heating or microcavitation in tissues. Theraputic ultrasound exploits these tissue-heating effects. High-intensity focused ultrasound (HIFU) is being explored as a minimally invasive treatment for solid cancers. This uses low frequency sound waves and focuses them in a small target area. The high concentration of energy at the focus point causes a dramatic rise in temperature to >55°C in a matter of seconds. This causes coagulation necrosis of the targeted tissue. The volume of destructed tissue is small—1 to 3 mm in width and 5 to 20 mm in height (30,31). The probe, therefore, has to be moved sequentially to allow a larger treatment area. The tissue outside the targeted area is not heated to cytotoxic levels; therefore, HIFU provides a trackless method of delivering ablative energy. HIFU has been used in urology to treat renal (32) and testicular cancers (33), but it is in the treatment of prostate cancer that it has gained most acceptance (34–36). It can treat those who are not candidates for standard radical therapy, as well as a salvage treatment in patients who have local recurrence following external beam radiotherapy (37). A future promising area is the use of ultrasound beams to destabilize injected microbubbles to release therapeutic agents precisely within the organ of disease (38).

MAGNETIC RESONANCE IMAGING

The nuclear magnetic resonance (NMR) phenomenon was first described in 1937 by Professor Rabi of Columbia University in the United States (39). However, it is only in the last 25 to 30 years that the medical applications of NMR have been realized.

The physics of NMR is often viewed as complex. However, the essence of the technique may be understood by reviewing extracts from quantum mechanical and classical models.

In brief, the steps in the production of an image are as follows:

- The patient is placed in a powerful magnetic field. (Typically in most hospitals this is a 1.5-Tesla magnet. This is some 30,000 times stronger than the earth's magnetic field.)
- This magnetic field aligns hydrogen nuclei within the body, creating a net magnetization.
- Radiowaves alter the alignment of the net magnetization.

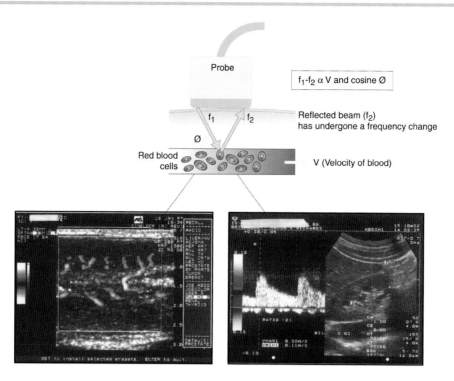

Figure 10 Principles of Doppler ultrasound. The Doppler effect is used to calculate the velocity of a moving substance, such as blood. The velocity can be presented as a continuous Doppler or spectral waveform or can be superimposed on the grayscale ultrasound image as a "color Doppler" image—as shown on the right with intrarenal arteries clearly demonstrated. The left-hand image is a power Doppler image showing the fine details of the penile vasculature. The right-hand image is a montage showing a color and spectral Doppler image—a waveform has been measured with an RI of 0.63, indicating normal PR in this nonobstructed kidney.

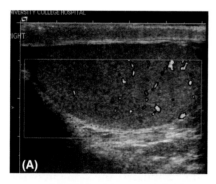

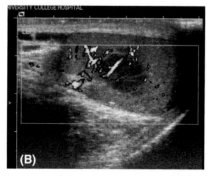

Figure 11 (**A**) Ultrasound of a patient with histologically proven seminoma of the left testicle shows the homogenously hypoechoic tumor that displays increased vascularity on color Doppler. (**B**) The patient's normal right testicle with its normal vascular pattern.

- After the radiowave is switched off, the net magnetization realigns to its original position and in doing so emits a weak radio signal.
- The frequencies contained within the radio signal can be manipulated and thereby encode spatial information.
- The signal generates a current within a coil of wire and this current is converted into an image.

To understand this process in more depth, a number of fundamental principles need to be appreciated (Fig. 12).

Useful MR Nuclei

A nucleus of an atom contains protons and neutrons that are normally spinning. Nuclei, which have an odd number of constituents, have a net charge and, because they are spinning by the law of electromagnetic induction, must generate a small magnetic field. These nuclei are the MR active nuclei and include hydrogen. The hydrogen nucleus (consisting of a single proton only) is the one used in clinical MRI because of its natural abundance within the body. Each hydrogen nucleus is in essence an extremely weak bar magnet. Luckily, the human body is not normally magnetized as these "mini magnets" are randomly aligned and the magnetic fields cancel each other out.

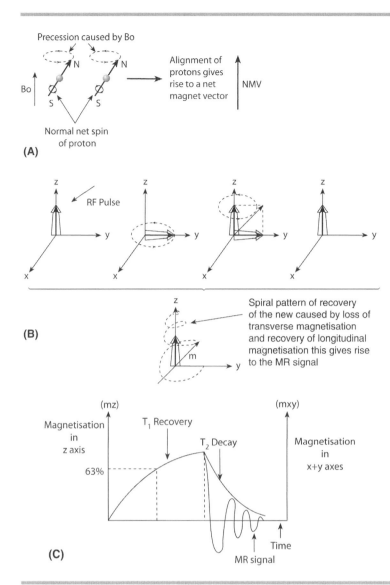

Figure 12 Principles of MRI. (**A**) Protons have a net spin that makes them act like mini bar magnets. When placed in a strong magnet field, they develop a special type of spin called precession and they align to give an NMV. (**B**) Under the influence of an externally applied radiowave, the NMV flips into the transverse plane. Once the radiowave is switched off the NMV decays in the transverse plane and recovers in the longitudinal plane. This happens in a spiral motion giving rise to the MR signal. (**C**) T_1 is the time for the longitudinal magnetization to recover to 63% of its maximum value. T_2 is the time for the MR signal to fall to 37% of its maximum value.

The Effect of an External Magnet

When the body is placed in a strong external magnetic field (B_0), two things happen.

1. Hydrogen nuclei within the body now adopt one of two distinct energy levels (high or low). Individual hydrogen nuclei constantly flip between these two levels. But at any given time, there are more nuclei in the low-energy state. Summed together, these additional low-energy hydrogen nuclei create a small net magnetic field parallel to the direction of the external magnetic field. It is the existence of this net magnetic vector (NMV), which makes MR possible.
2. The hydrogen nuclei begin to precess as well as continue to spin. The motion of precession can be described by analogy to a spinning top. As a spinning top spins on its own axis, it begins to tilt. As it tilts the top of the highest point of the spinning top starts moving in a circular orbit (precesses) while the spinning top continues to spin on its own axis. Continuing with the top

analogy, the speed of precession depends on the strength of gravity, and a top would precess far slower on the moon than on Earth. For hydrogen nuclei, the speed of precession depends on, and is in fact proportional to, the strength of the external magnetic field B_0.

Resonance

All materials have a natural frequency at which they find it easiest to vibrate, which is termed as *resonant frequency*. If a periodical force is applied at the same frequency as an object's natural frequency, the object will tend to absorb the applied energy. As this energy builds, the amplitude of its oscillations will continue to increase. The object will then either change its dynamic properties, which then alter its resonant frequency, or it loses the energy in some form. If it does not lose the energy, then the object can break apart. An example of this occurred in World War II when soldiers marching in step across a bridge caused it to collapse as they were marching at the resonant frequency of the bridge. To this day soldiers still break step when crossing bridges.

It so happens that the resonant frequency of hydrogen nuclei lies in the radiowave bandwidth.

Application of Radiofrequency Radiation (Pulse)

Why then do "resonance" and "nuclear magnetism" come together to give the term "nuclear magnetic resonance?" Recall that in an external magnetic field a NMV is set up by the alignment of the hydrogen nuclei and that this NMV lies parallel to the external magnetic field. In this equilibrium state this magnetism cannot be detected. However, when the body is exposed to radiowaves at the *resonant frequency* of the hydrogen nuclei, energy can be transferred from the radiowaves to the hydrogen nuclei.

This has two effects on the nuclei.

1. More nuclei gain enough energy to enter the high-energy state, so that the total number of "excess" nuclei in the low-energy state at any given time is reduced. This has the result of decreasing the NMV. If the radiofrequency pulse is applied for a sufficient time, then the NMV in the direction of the external magnetic field can be made to reduce to zero, and this is termed a "90°" radiofrequency pulse.
2. Another very useful property of a radiofrequency pulse is that it reforms the NMV in the plane perpendicular to the external magnetic field. It is because of this "transverse" magnetic vector that NMR signal can be detected.

    When the radiowave is stopped, the hydrogen nuclei start to lose energy and more and more nuclei once again enter the low-energy state until equilibrium is reached. Furthermore, the transverse magnetic vector begins to precess. As it precesses it generates an oscillating magnetic field, which induces an alternating current in the receiver coil. By application of a series of magnetic field gradients, the current frequencies can be varied in a controlled fashion to allow spatial encoding. This multifrequency current is then amplified and mathematically converted to an onscreen MR image.

The contrast in every MR image is dependent on three factors.

(1) The rate at which the hydrogen nuclei return from the high- to low-energy state (T_1)
(2) How quickly the transverse magnetization disperses (T_2)
(3) The density of protons within a particular area (ρ)

The greater the proton density, the higher the signal from a tissue and the brighter the MR image. The contribution of T_1 and T_2 to an image can be altered by manipulation of the imaging program (radiowaves and magnetic field gradients applied to the body to generate an image) and is completely under user control. For proton density to predominate, the T_1 and T_2 effects must be diminished.

Different body tissues may have different T_1, T_2 times and also vary in proton density, thus generating a contrast between them. If two tissues differ in T_2 times, then producing a T_2-weighted image will show a difference in contrast between these two tissues and this can sometimes be useful in differentiating tumor from normal tissue (i.e., prostate carcinoma—low T_2 signal intensity; from normal peripheral zone—high T_2 signal intensity). If T_1-weighted images were acquired from the peripheral zone of the prostate with tumor, then the tumor may be masked as the T_1 times of both tissues are similar. The multiparameter-dependent contrast of an MRI is a distinct advantage over CT where contrast is simply related to density of material.

In general, T_1 images show fluid as low signal (dark) and fat as high signal (bright). They are generally good for anatomy. They can also allow the detection of blood (at certain stages in its breakdown) such as that caused by prostate biopsy, which appears as high signal. T_2 images show fluid as high signal (bright) and tend to be more useful for distinguishing between normal and pathological tissues (Fig. 13). Heavily T_2-weighted images are used to craft MR urographic studies (Fig. 14).

A typical MRI examination consists of a selection of images of different contrasts (T_1, T_2, etc.) acquired in differing anatomical planes (saggital, coronal, axial, etc.). Exactly which planes and contrasts are used depends on the information that is required about the subject tissue (Fig. 15). Table 9 shows the current uses of MRI in urology.

Improving Signal to Noise Ratio

Improving the SNR has been a major goal in MRI. It can be achieved in many ways, but often these result in either increased scan time or loss of spatial resolution, and achieving the optimum image is a trade-off between SNR, scan time, and spatial resolution.

A simple (but rather expensive) way of getting more signal is to use a stronger magnet to generate a larger external magnetic field. Increasing the magnet strength from 1.5 to 3 Tesla should improve the SNR by a factor of 2, and 3-Tesla MRI machines are now commercially available. This "extra" signal can be traded, if required, for faster imaging or higher spatial resolutions.

Another method of improving SNR is to place the coil used to pick up the signal as close as possible to the tissue generating the signal. In urology, using an endorectal coil has been shown to improve spatial and contrast resolution for prostate imaging. Initially, there was little evidence to suggest that this dramatically improved staging accuracy, but now increasingly improved sensitivity, specificity and accuracy are being reported (40).

Contrast Media

MRI-specific CM are also available. These are paramagnetic or supaparamagnetic metal ions that affect

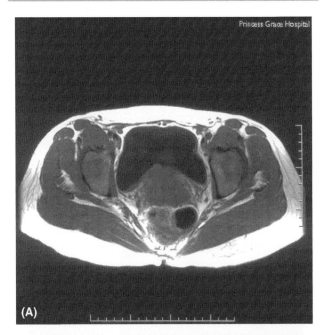

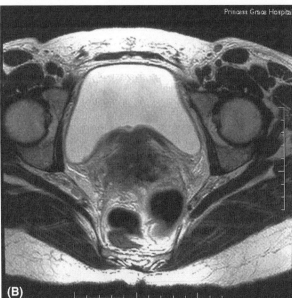

Figure 13 Magnetic resonance images of the bladder and pelvic anatomy. (**A**) T_1 image. Note that the urine is of low signal. (**B**) T_2 image, where fluid (urine) is always of high signal.

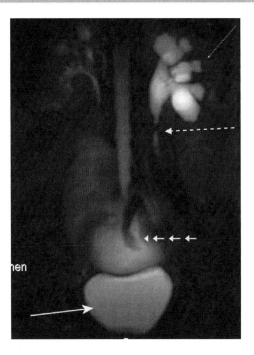

Figure 14 MR urography. A heavily T_2-weighted image shows fluid as high signal as seen here in an MR urography. A hydronephrotic left kidney is seen (*thin solid arrow*) caused by an upper ureteric stone (*dashed arrow*), which appears as a signal void. The bladder is well seen (*thick solid arrow*). The patient is also pregnant and the fetus can be seen in the uterus (*multiple white arrows*). The ability to assess the kidneys in pregnant women is a major advantage of MR urography.

the MR signal properties of surrounding tissues. Like other radiological CM they can be used to improve the SNR. Two main types exist—nonspecific extracellular agents and organ-specific agents. The organ-specific contrast agents are mainly iron oxide based, used for liver imaging, and therefore are not that relevant to urological imaging. They are, however, currently undergoing investigation for detection of lymph node metastases (41), which could have a significant effect on the accurate staging of pelvic tumors.

Gadolinium chelates are the most widely used extracellular, nonspecific contrast agents. They are strongly paramagnetic and shorten both T_1 and T_2 times of the hydrogen nuclei. Gadolinium chelates in general clinical use short-lived intravascular agents that leak into the extravascular spaces but remain extracellular. They are excreted by the kidneys by glomerular filtration without tubular secretion or reabsorption. Gadolinium-based CM can cause similar adverse reactions to iodinated CM, but much less frequently. They are quoted to occur in approximately 1% of all patients and are normally mild and transient. The prevalence of anaphylactoid reactions has been reported as between 1/100,000 and 1/500,000 (42). Contrast-induced nephropathy is not a clinical concern, but recently a link between certain gadolinium-based agents, renal failure, and nephrogenic fibrosing dermopathy has been established (43). The ESUR has published guidelines suggesting that gadolinium contrast agents should not be used in patients with a GFR <30 mL/min (44).

Dynamic Contrast–Enhanced MRI

Cancers excite neovascularity and abnormal perfusion compared with normal tissue. DCE MRI is able to detect such aberrant perfusion by obtaining a rapid series of images over a short period, following a bolus administration of gadolinium. Signal intensity–time

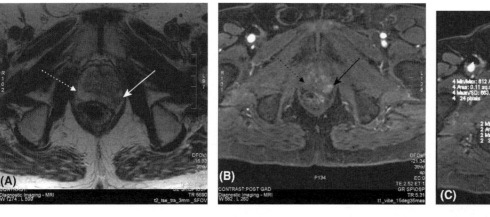
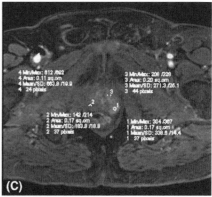
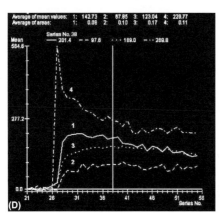
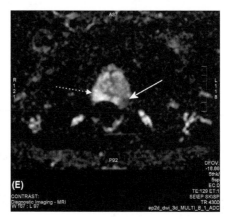

Figure 15 MRI series from a man with histological proven prostate cancer. (**A**) The peripheral zone normally displays high T_2 signal (*dashed arrow*). The low signal in the left peripheral zone (PZ, *white arrow*) is typical for tumor. (**B**) An image from a dynamic contrast-enhanced series shows the tumor to enhance early (*black arrow*) compared with the normal PZ (*dashed arrow*). (**C, D**) Signal intensity curves drawn from four regions of interest. 1 on the tumor nodule shows the tumor to have a characteristic type I curve with early enhancement and washout compared with 2, which represents normal PZ. 3 is placed in the central gland, and 4, on the femoral artery. (**E**) An ADC map shows the tumor to have restricted diffusion seen as low signal (*solid arrow*) compared with the normal PZ which has normal diffusion seen as high signal (*dashed arrow*). If a lesion demonstrates all these findings, then a confident diagnosis of cancer can be made.

Table 9 Current Use of MRI in Urology

Prostate imaging	Prostate cancer staging is probably the most common use of MRI in urology. With standard T_1 and T_2 sequences alone sensitivity and specificity are approximately 80% and 60%, respectively. The use of the newer sequences such as HMRS and diffusion-weighted images may increase this.
Renal imaging	Faster sequences have allowed improved imaging of the kidneys and MRI is often used in renal mass evaluation its improved contrast resolution being a distinct advantage over CT.
MR urography	Particularly in pregnant women where radiation is an issue.
Penile imaging	To stage penile cancer. It is also useful in the assessment of corporal fibrosis and priapism assessment.

curves can be created (Fig. 15), and these data can be assessed qualitatively or quantitatively (45). Qualitative assessment is based on the shape of the curve or descriptors, such as time to maximum enhancement, gradient of curve, or maximum signal intensity, and is relatively easy to obtain. Quantitative information involves creating concentration-time curves from pharmacokinetic models and requires special software programs (46). Currently, it is not known if the quantitative data provide more accurate information. It has been shown that prostate cancer in the peripheral zone demonstrates early nodular enhancement, before normal parenchyma and early washout (47). This pattern of enhancement, while highly suggestive of tumor, is not pathognomonic with other processes, most notably prostatitis, having a similar curve. Nevertheless, DCE is felt to improve specificity and is currently undergoing clinical evaluation.

Hydrogen Magnetic Resonance Spectroscopy

Hydrogen magnetic resonance spectroscopy (HMRS) provides metabolic information about the tissue being investigated by displaying the relative concentrations of chemical metabolites within a voxel. Cancers can have a different metabolic makeup compared with their normal surrounding tissue, because of the enhancement of the phospholipid cell membrane turnover associated with tumor cell proliferation, increased cellularity, and growth. For example, prostate cancer has a decreased level of citrate and an increased level of choline when compared with normal prostatic tissue (48) and RCC has been shown to demonstrate a decrease in free cholesterol and unsaturated fatty acids compared with normal renal parenchyma (49). HMRS has been shown to improve prostate cancer localization in the peripheral zone and provides an indication of tumor grade (50). It may also be particularly useful in detecting cancer in the previously treated prostate gland (51,52). HMRS will benefit from the use of 3T magnets as it will allow smaller voxels to be obtained, reducing volume averaging and improving the separation of the metabolite peaks (53).

Diffusion-Weighted Imaging

Diffusion is the process by which particles intermingle as the result of spontaneous movement caused by thermal agitation. MRI can be used to examine the microscopic diffusion of water molecules within tissues. Unlike free water, tissue water is limited in its movement by cellular barriers. An increase in the restriction of water diffusion has been seen in pathological tissues such as tumor and is thought to be related in part to increased cellular density. Diffusion-weighted images are able to detect and quantify this change in diffusion. Areas of restricted diffusion appear of increased signal (bright) on diffusion-weighted images and are correspondingly dark on quantitative diffusion maps (Fig. 15).

ACKNOWLEDGMENT

We would like to thank Dr Shonit Punwani for his help with the physics of MRI.

REFERENCES

1. Mould RF. Invited review: Rontgen and the discovery of X-rays. Br J Radiol 1995; 68(815):1145–1176.
2. Voeleker F, von Lichtenburg A. Pyelography (Rontgenographie des Nierenbeckens nach kullargolfullung). Munchener Med Wochenschr 1906; 53:105–106.
3. Digital Imaging and Communication in Medicine. Strategic document version 4.0. June, 2005. Available at: http://medical.nema.org.
4. Osbourne ED, Sutherland CG, Scholl AJ, Jr., et al. Roentgenology of the urinary track during excretion of sodium iodide. J Am Med Assoc 1923; 80:368–373.
5. Swick M. Darstellung der Niete und Harnwege in Roentgenbild durch intravenöse Einbringung eines neuen kontraststoffes:des uroselectans. Klin Wochenschr 1923; 8:2087–2089.
6. Morcos SK, Thomsen HS, Webb JA. Contrast-media-induced nephrotoxicity: a consensus report. Contrast media safety committee, European Society of Urogenital Radiology (ESUR). Eur Radiol 1999; 9(8):1602–1613.
7. Nash K, Hafeez A, Hou S. Hospital-acquired renal insufficiency. Am J Kidney Dis 2002; 39(5):930–936.
8. Parfrey PS, Griffiths SM, Barrett BJ, et al. Contrast material-induced renal failure in patients with diabetes mellitus, renal insufficiency, or both. A prospective controlled study. N Engl J Med 1989; 320(3):143–149.
9. Rudnick MR, Goldfarb S, Wexler L, et al. Nephrotoxicity of ionic and nonionic contrast media in 1196 patients: a randomized trial. The Iohexol Cooperative Study. Kidney Int 1995; 47(1):254–261.
10. Bartholomew BA, Harjai KJ, Dukkipati S, et al. Impact of nephropathy after percutaneous coronary intervention and a method for risk stratification. Am J Cardiol 2004; 93(12):1515–1519.
11. Mehran R, Aymong ED, Nikolsky E, et al. A simple risk score for prediction of contrast-induced nephropathy after percutaneous coronary intervention: development and initial validation. J Am Coll Cardiol 2004; 44(7):1393–1399.
12. Pannu N, Wiebe N, Tonelli M Prophylaxis strategies for contrast-induced nephropathy. JAMA 2006; 295(23):2765–2779.
13. Thomsen HS. European Society of Urogenital Radiology (ESUR) guidelines on the safe use of iodinated contrast media. Eur J Radiol 2006; 60(3):307–313.
14. Cipollaro VA. Radiation dermatitis today. J Eur Acad Dermatol Venereol 2001; 15(4):300–301.
15. The Royal College of Radiologists. Making the Best Use of Clinical Radiology Services: Referral Guidelines. London: The Royal College of Radiologists, 2007.
16. Berrington de Gonzalez A, Darby S. Risk of cancer from diagnostic X-rays: estimates for the UK and 14 other countries. Lancet 2004; 363(9406):345–351.
17. United Nations Scientific Committee on the Effects of Atomic Radiation. Sources and effects of ionising radiation. New York: United Nations, 2000.
18. Shrimpton P, Jones DG, Hillier MC, et al. Survey of CT practice in the UK. Part 2: dosimetric aspects. NRPB Report R249. Oxfordshire: National Radiological Protection Board, 1991.
19. Ambrose J, Hounsfield G. Computerized transverse axial tomography. Br J Radiol 1973; 46(542):148–149.
20. Cody DD. AAPM/RSNA physics tutorial for residents: topics in CT. Image processing in CT. Radiographics 2002; 22(5):1255–1268.
21. Coll DM, Herts BR, Davros WJ, et al. Preoperative use of 3D volume rendering to demonstrate renal tumors and renal anatomy. Radiographics 2000; 20(2):431–438.
22. Browne RF, Murphy SM, Grainger R, et al. CT cystography and virtual cystoscopy in the assessment of new and recurrent bladder neoplasms. Eur J Radiol 2005; 53(1):147–153.
23. Boridy IC, Nikolaidis P, Kawashima A, et al. Ureterolithiasis: value of the tail sign in differentiating phleboliths from ureteral calculi at nonenhanced helical CT. Radiology 1999; 211(3):619–621.
24. Varanelli MJ, Coll DM, Levine JA, et al. Relationship between duration of pain and secondary signs of obstruction of the urinary tract on unenhanced helical CT. AJR Am J Roentgenol 2001; 177(2):325–330.
25. Fry WJ, Mosberg WH Jr., Barnard JW, et al. Production of focal destructive lesions in the central nervous system with ultrasound. J Neurosurg 1954; 11(5):471–478.

26. Holmes JH, Howry DH, Posakony GJ, et al. The ultrasonic visualization of soft tissue structures in the human body. Trans Am Clin Climatol Assoc 1954; 66:208–225.

27. Cosgrove D. Ultrasound contrast agents: an overview. Eur J Radiol 2006; 60(3):324–330.

28. Linden RA, Halpern EJ. Advances in transrectal ultrasound imaging of the prostate. Semin Ultrasound CT MR 2007; 28(4):249–257.

29. Pallwein L, Aigner F, Faschingbauer R, et al. Prostate cancer diagnosis: value of real-time elastography. Abdom Imaging 2008; 33(6):729–735.

30. Watkin NA, ter Haar GR, Rivens I. The intensity dependence of the site of maximal energy deposition in focused ultrasound surgery. Ultrasound Med Biol 1996; 22(4):483–491.

31. Chapelon JY, Margonari J, Theillère Y, et al. Effects of high-energy focused ultrasound on kidney tissue in the rat and the dog. Eur Urol 1992; 22(2):147–152.

32. Wu F, Wang ZB, Chen WZ, et al. Preliminary experience using high intensity focused ultrasound for the treatment of patients with advanced stage renal malignancy. J Urol 2003; 170(6 pt 1):2237–2240.

33. Kratzik C, Schatzl G, Lackner J, et al. Transcutaneous high-intensity focused ultrasonography can cure testicular cancer in solitary testis. Urology 2006; 67(6):1269–1273.

34. Blana A, Murat FJ, Walter B, et al. First analysis of the long-term results with transrectal HIFU in patients with localised prostate cancer. Eur Urol 2008; 53(6):1194–1201.

35. Muto S, Yoshii T, Saito K, et al. Focal therapy with high-intensity-focused ultrasound in the treatment of localized prostate cancer. Jpn J Clin Oncol 2008; 38(3):192–199.

36. Illing RO, Leslie TA, Kennedy JE, et al. Visually directed high-intensity focused ultrasound for organ-confined prostate cancer: a proposed standard for the conduct of therapy. BJU Int 2006; 98(6):1187–1192.

37. Gelet A, Chapelon JY, Poissonnier L, et al. Local recurrence of prostate cancer after external beam radiotherapy: early experience of salvage therapy using high-intensity focused ultrasonography. Urology 2004; 63(4):625–629.

38. Postema M, Gilja OH. Ultrasound-directed drug delivery. Curr Pharm Biotechnol 2007; 8(6):355–361.

39. Rabi II, Zacharias JR, Millman S, et al. A new method of measuring nuclear magnetic moment. Phys Rev 1938; 53:318.

40. Futterer JJ. MR imaging in local staging of prostate cancer. Eur J Radiol 2007; 63(3):328–334.

41. Harisinghani MG, Barentsz J, Hahn PF, et al. Noninvasive detection of clinically occult lymph-node metastases in prostate cancer. N Engl J Med 2003; 348(25):2491–2499.

42. Shellock FG, Kanal E. Safety of magnetic resonance imaging contrast agents. J Magn Reson Imaging 1999; 10(3):477–484.

43. Grobner T. Gadolinium—a specific trigger for the development of nephrogenic fibrosing dermopathy and nephrogenic systemic fibrosis? Nephrol Dial Transplant 2006; 21: 1104–1108.

44. Thomsen HS. ESUR guideline: gadolinium-based contrast media and nephrogenic systemic fibrosis. Eur Radiol 2007; 17(10):2692–2696.

45. Alonzi R, Padhani AR, Allen C. Dynamic contrast enhanced MRI in prostate cancer. Eur J Radiol 2007; 63(3):335–350.

46. Tofts PS, Brix G, Buckley DL, et al. Estimating kinetic parameters from dynamic contrast-enhanced T(1)-weighted MRI of a diffusable tracer: standardized quantities and symbols. J Magn Reson Imaging 1999; 10(3):223–232.

47. Turnbull LW, Buckley DL, Turnbull LS, et al. Differentiation of prostatic carcinoma and benign prostatic hyperplasia: correlation between dynamic Gd-DTPA-enhanced MR imaging and histopathology. J Magn Reson Imaging 1999; 9(2):311–316.

48. Heerschap A, Jager GJ, van der Graaf M, et al. In vivo proton MR spectroscopy reveals altered metabolite content in malignant prostate tissue. Anticancer Res 1997; 17(3A):1455–1460.

49. Katz-Brull R, Rofsky NM, Morrin MM, et al. Decreases in free cholesterol and fatty acid unsaturation in renal cell carcinoma demonstrated by breath-hold magnetic resonance spectroscopy. Am J Physiol Renal Physiol 2005; 288(4):F637—F641.

50. Coakley FV, Qayyum A, Kurhanewicz J. Magnetic resonance imaging and spectroscopic imaging of prostate cancer. J Urol 2003; 170(6 pt 2):S69–S75; discussion S75—S76.

51. Parivar F, Hricak H, Shinohara K, et al. Detection of locally recurrent prostate cancer after cryosurgery: evaluation by transrectal ultrasound, magnetic resonance imaging, and three-dimensional proton magnetic resonance spectroscopy. Urology 1996; 48(4):594–599.

52. Pucar D, Shukla-Dave A, Hricak H, et al. Prostate cancer: correlation of MR imaging and MR spectroscopy with pathologic findings after radiation therapy-initial experience. Radiology 2005; 236(2):545–553.

53. Futterer JJ, Scheenen TW, Huisman HJ, et al. Initial experience of 3 tesla endorectal coil magnetic resonance imaging and 1H-spectroscopic imaging of the prostate. Invest Radiol 2004; 39(11):671–680.

FURTHER READING

Westbrook C, Kaut Roth C, Talbot J. MRI in Practice. 3rd ed. Oxford: Blackwell Publishing, 2005.

Allisy-Roberts P, Williams J. Farr's Physics for Medical Imaging. 2nd ed. London: WB Saunders, 2008.

Silverman SG, Cohan R. CT Urography: An Atlas. Philadelphia: Lippincott Williams & Wilkins, 2007.

7

Upper Urinary Tract Obstruction

Neil G. Docherty

The Conway Institute, University College Dublin, Ireland

John M. Fitzpatrick

Mater Misericordiae Hospital and University College Dublin, Ireland

ETIOLOGY

Upper urinary tract obstruction can result from a variety of both congenital and acquired conditions, impeding urinary flow from the renal pelvis to the bladder. Implicit in this statement is the fact that the structure affected is either the kidney (renal pelvis) or the ureter. Albeit that bilateral hydronephrosis resulting from bladder outlet obstruction shares many features of more proximal obstruction, we will restrict our discussion in this chapter to obstruction of the upper urinary tract.

The nature of ureteric obstruction (UO) can be further delineated according to whether the obstruction is intraluminal or extrinsic. The degree of obstruction can also vary from partial, to progressively occluding to acutely presenting complete obstruction. Commonly, UO is unilateral (UUO) and may involve obstruction of proximal or distal segments.

A major concern following obstruction is its effect on the proximal kidney, an effect which will depend on the site (renal pelvis, proximal or distal ureter), degree (partial, complete) and duration (acute or chronic). The combination of these considerations will determine the incidence of obstructive nephropathy in the affected kidney and in cases of UUO in individuals with a solitary kidney, the severity of acute renal failure encountered. A summary of the causes of upper urinary tract obstruction is found in Table 1.

INCIDENCE

Upper urinary tract obstruction is a frequently encountered diagnosis in urology. However, because of the fact its etiology is varied, reliable cumulative incidence rates do not exist.

Starting with neonatal obstruction, the criteria for diagnosis requires that hydronephrosis is present, with the fetal kidney producing isoosmolar urine within the first trimester of pregnancy. Antenatally hydronephrosis id detectable via ultrasonography and its incidence is reported to be around 1% (1).

The major cause of upper urinary tract obstruction in adult urology is intrinsic, intraluminal nephro-lithiasis and urolithiasis. Calcium oxalate and calcium phosphate stone disease predominates, accounting for 80% of cases, with hypercalciuria a major risk factor, underpinned by both genetic and lifestyle factors. The lifetime incidence for men is reported at 12% versus 6% in women (2).

CLINICAL PRESENTATION

Presentation of upper urinary tract obstruction is not homogeneous, reflecting differences in etiology and degree of obstruction.

Antenatal obstruction presents during routine imaging. In postnatal (inc. adult) obstruction, clinical presentation depends on the whether the obstruction is unilateral or bilateral, acute or chronic and partial or complete. Colicky flank pain is characteristic of acute UUO, with the presence of fever suggestive of infection.

DIAGNOSIS AND TREATMENT

Management of Neonatal Obstruction

Neonatal hydronephrosis secondary to obstruction frequently has its origin in antenatal uretero-pelvic junction (UPJ) obstruction or uretero-vesicular junction (UVJ) obstruction, (primary megaureter) which can be visualized on antenatal ultrasound.

Intrauterine management of obstruction is limited to close observation of the obstruction to decide the course of action in the neonate. While evidence of hydronephrosis per se does not exclude the possibility of meaningful renal function postnatally, evidence of renal hypoplasty and dysplasty predicts a poor outcome in the neonate, and reflects obstructive injury of first-trimester origin.

Postnatal ultrasound revealing dilatation should lead to the ordering of a voiding cystourethrogram (VCUG) and/or diuretic renography. Sustained deterioration of split renal function indicates pyeloplastic surgical intervention in cases of UPJ obstruction. In cases of megaureter, if adequate ureteral drainage is observed a conservative approach of antibiotic theapy throughout the first year of life is indicated. However

Table 1 Causes of Congenital and Acquired Upper Tract Obstruction

Congenital		Acquired	
Intraluminal	Extraluminal	Intraluminal	Extraluminal
PUJ obstruction	Ureterocoele (ectopic, orthotopic)	Calcus	Malignancy (pelvic: prostate, colorectal, ovarian, uterine, cervical; petroperitoneal: lymphoma, sarcoma, mesothelioma, metastases)
Ureteric actresia	Bladder diverticulum	Stricture	Gastrointestinal (pancreatitis, appendicitis, diverticulitis, Crohn's disease)
Ureteric valve	Vascular (retrocaval ureter, retroiliac ureter, lower pole renal vessels, persistent umbilical artery)	Urothelial tumor	Vascular (abdominal aortic aneurysm, Iliac artery aneurysm)
Ureteric folds		Blood clot	Pregnancy
Congenital stricture		Sloughed papilla	Gynaecological (fibrosis, endometriosis)
Vesicoureteric reflux		Benign Polyp	Retrperitoneal fibrosis
Primary megaureter		Foreign body (stent)	
VUJ obstruction		Fungal ball	

The major causes of upper urinary tract obstruction are presented and subdivided, firstly, according to cause (congenital vs. acquired) and, secondly, according to site (intraluminal vs. extraluminal).

recurrent UTI's and/or renal dysfunction indicate surgical straightening and tapering of the ureter to restore urinary flow.

Adult Obstruction

Further to history and physical examination, imaging techniques are required to make a conclusive diagnosis. These may include intravenous or retrograde pyelography and kidney-ureter-bladder CT scanning. If urosepsis is suspected, the presence of infection can be confirmed via culture and quantification of white cell counts and erythrocyte sedimentation rates. With urosepsis, percutaneous nephrostomy is indicated immediately with provision of parenteral gram-negative targeted antibiotic therapy.

In the absence of the requirement for nephrostomy, ultrasound may assist in the diagnosis of the grade of associated hydronephrosis. Immediate symptomatic relief is generally provided using oral diclofenac (50 mg) t.i.d.

An examination of the renal effects may be established using serum and urine biochemistry, with isotope renography also useful to assess split renal function, though rarely used in first-line diagnostics.

Once a diagnosis of obstruction has been established and the presence or absence of sepsis determined, a decision on management of obstruction can be made.

Nephrolithiasis

In the case of calculi contained within the renal pelvis, extracorporal shock wave lithotripsy (ESWL) is preferred for small to medium sized stones (<2cm), with some indication that its effectiveness is more limited in lower pole nephrolithiasis due to gravitational effects. Percutaneous nephrolithotomy (PNL) is preferred for larger or more numerous stones such as large pelvic staghorn calculi. Open surgery for renal calculi is rapidly disappearing but its use continues in cases where open pyelolithotomy or nephrectomy is the indicated course of action (3).

Urolithiasis

Obstruction of the ureter may require surgery if the cause is extrinsic or the result of ureteric stricturing.

When ureteric calculi are the cause, the clinical decision is based on whether spontaneous expulsion of the stone is possible. The criteria for determining this are the size and position of the calculus with small distally located calculi most amenable to spontaneous expulsion. Duration of symptoms and degree of hydronephrosis have also been shown to be predictive of spontaneous passage, possibly related to the effect of these parameters on ureteric peristalsis. Promising pharmacological promotion of spontaneous passage of distally located calculi has been demonstrated using the combination of an α-adrenergic blocker with a corticosteroid (e.g., prednisolone + tamsulosin) (4,5). The beneficial effect of medical expulsive therapy in distally located calculi is likely to be a result of the preferential expression of α1d-adrenergic receptors and adrenergic transmission in the distal versus proximal ureteric muscularis (6).

When spontaneous passage is discounted, ESWL and ureteroscopy constitute the major therapeutic modalities.

THE EFFECT OF URETERIC OBSTRUCTION ON URETERIC FUNCTION

Normal Pyelourteric Peristalsis

The peristaltic propulsion of a urine bolus from the renal pelvis to the bladder depends on coordinated contractions of the renal pelvis and ureter. In times of low urine output, renal pelvic contractions outnumber ureteric contraction. During diuresis however, contractility in the renal pelvis is increased to a point where it instigates myogenic transfer of action potentials to the ureteric muscularis, leading to coordinated pelvic/ureteric contractions, which have the combined effect of propelling urine to the bladder. Despite existence of evidence of both sympathetic and parasympathetic input and receptor expression in the renal pelvis and proximal ureter, central integrative control of ureteric peristalsis remains poorly understood. It is currently believed that the primary oscillator of ureteric peristalsis is renal pelvic urine volume and its effect on pyeloureteric pacemaker activity (7).

As mentioned above, peristalsis in the distal ureter is more dependent on adrenergic control of peristalsis making medically expulsive therapy an exciting emerging field in the treatment of distally located calculi.

Pacemaker coordination of pyelouteric peristalsis has been suggested to depend primarily on the activity of atypical smooth muscle cells and interstitial cells of Cajal-like cells which predominate in the renal pelvis, have a low depolarization threshold and act to drive depolarization (and peristalsis) in naturally more refractory typical smooth muscle cells (8).

The tonic effect of urothelium-derived factors on contractility remains an interesting area. Diclofenac is effective in preventing obstruction-associated colic and is a nonspecific inhibitor of prostaglandin producing cycloxygenase enzymes, which are localized to the urothelium. No consensus has been reached on the effect of individual prostaglandin species on ureteric contractility (7).

Acute Changes in Peristaltic Activity Following Obstruction

The frequency and amplitude of pelvic and ureteric contraction changes dramatically in response to obstruction. Graded elongation of the human and sheep intrarenal and extrarenal pelvis and distal ureter in vitro demonstrates that stretch increases both the basal and active tension (amplitude) in all segments but only increases spontaneous frequency of contraction in the pelvic segments (9).

Lennon et al. (1993) examined the effect of both complete and partial UUO of one month in duration on pelvic and ureteric contractility in vivo in dogs (10). In the case of complete obstruction baseline pelvic pressure was 1.9 mmHg, with a frequency of 9.2/min and an amplitude of 2.5 mmHg. Ureteric baseline pressure was 2.1 mmHg with a frequency of single spike contractions of 8.9/min and an amplitude of 36.2 mmHg. Following one month of obstruction both the pelvis and ureter were aperistaltic with raised baseline pressures of 15 mmHg and 16.3 mmHg, respectively. This aperistaltic effect is likely related to changes in the length/active tension relationship of the ureteric and pelvic muscularis caused by sustained urinary pooling.

A different picture was observed following one month of partial obstruction. Both pelvis and ureter remained contractile with a 50% and 66% reduction in contraction frequency, respectively. This was due to a change in contraction type to a multiphasic response with increased refractory periods between spikes. Interestingly a fivefold increase in pelvic amplitudes and a twofold increase in ureteric amplitudes were observed.

Urosepsis has also been shown to perhaps play a role in decreased contraction frequency in vitro. Urothelial application of live gram-negative species has been shown to reversibly inhibit ureteric contractility (11).

Postobstructive Ureteric Function

In the same key paper by Lennon et al. (2003) described above, measurements of ureteric function were made eight weeks after relief of both complete and partial obstruction in dogs (10). No statisitical difference versus original baseline measures was observed in ureteric contractile frequency or amplitude in the pelvis or ureter from animals with complete obstruction although baseline pressure remained twofold higher in the ureter. Baseline ureteric pressure was also increased in the partial obstruction group, however these animals retained twofold higher amplitude rates in both the pelvis and ureter and continued to show a mixed single/multphasic waveform.

OBSTRUCTIVE NEPHROPATHY

Obstructive Nephropathy Following UUO in Animal Models

The above description of the changes in ureteric function in obstructive injury has important implications for the upstream kidney.

To explain the pathophysiology of obstructive nephropathy, it is best to examine the findings of acute UUO in adult animals, which approximates most accurately to acute and complete stone mediated obstruction of the ureter in the adult human. While doing so, it is imperative to keep in mind that the results of such studies may have important differences to obstruction in divergent clinical settings (e.g., partial obstruction, bilateral affectation, neonatal vs. adult).

Overview of Macroscopic and Microscopic Changes in Acute, Complete UUO

With complete obstruction comes associated urinary pooling which, in combination with changes in ureteric contractility, gives rise to retrograde pressure transfer to the proximal kidney and hydronephrosis. These events set in motion the major gross morphological and microanatomical changes observed in renal structure. With increasing time post obstruction, the kidney becomes swollen because of pooling of urine proximal to the site of obstruction. As the renal pelvis expands, the renal parenchyma becomes affected. Flattening of the renal papilla and back filling of the collecting system occurs. This leads to compression of the renal cortex causing the characteristic cortical thinning observed in obstruction. When obstruction is sustained, tubular swelling extends to the more proximal portions of the nephron where flattening of the tubular epithelium can be observed. These mechanical changes are associated with renal tubular cell stress, which is associated with increased oxidative stress (12), the induction of cell death by apoptosis, and the initiation of both proinflammatory and profibrotic signaling (13) (Fig. 1). The result of sustained UUO is therefore progressive tubular atrophy accompanied by the development of tubulointerstitial fibrosis.

Following UUO there is relative preservation of renal microvascular structure and glomerulosclerosis

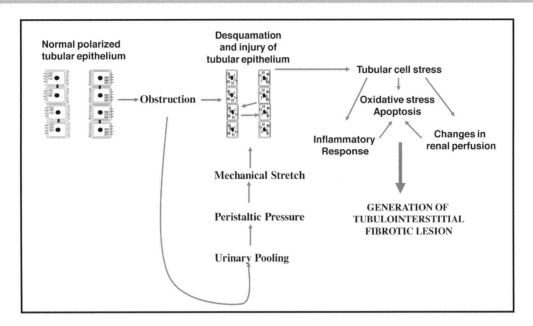

Figure 1 Mechanical stretch as a primer of obstructive nephropathy. Changes in both the frequency and amplitude of pyeloureteral contractions combined with sustained urinary pooling proximal to the site of obstruction contribute to mechanical stretch injury of the renal tubular epithelium. Apoptotic, inflammatory and haemodynamic changes thereafter give rise to the characteristic features of acute obstructive renal injury which can progress to fibrotic deterioration of the kidney.

is only a feature of the late stages of long-term chronically sustained obstruction.

The contralateral kidney undergoes adaptive changes in renal blood flow, glomerular filtration rate (GFR) and single nephron function and with sustained obstruction undergoes compensatory hypertrophy (14,15).

LINK BETWEEN CHANGES IN RENAL PELVIC PRESSURE AND BLOOD FLOW POST UUO

A well-defined phasic response to UUO is known to occur. In the first phase (0–90 minutes) there is an increase in intrapelvic pressure from values of 6 to 7 to 50 to 70 mmHg (16). Initial elevations in ipsilateral renal pelvic pressure induce a reno-renal reflex characterized by substance P release from renal sensory neurons that leads to decreased efferent sympathetic output (17,18). This neural adaptation underpins the contralateral diuresis observed in UUO. In chronic UUO in rats, artificial elevation of ipsilateral intrapelvic pressure fails to induce a further reno-renal reflex (18).

Accompanying these phasic pressure changes are nitric oxide/prostaglandin mediated decreases in afferent arteriolar resistance, which in turn raise glomerular capillary pressure to the extent that glomerular filtration rate (GFR) is maintained at around 80% of normal values despite large increases in intratubular pressure (19).

In the second phase, occurring approximately between 90 minutes and four hours after obstruction, elevated intratubular pressure is sustained but renal blood flow decreases secondary to afferent and efferent arteriolar vasoconstriction in response to vasoconstrictory substances including thromboxane A2 and endothelin (20,21). GFR is thus reduced to approximately 20% of control levels (22). Phasic changes in glomerular haemodynamics in acute UUO are presented in Figure 2.

After the initial 24 hours of obstruction, collecting system pressure is reduced, but remains around 50% elevated versus normal levels (23). The continued pooling of urine in the renal pelvis is likely to contribute to the sustained dilatation of particularly the distal tubular segments (24).

As obstruction persists, adaptive dilatation of the efferent renal lymphatics occurs secondary to increased venous pressure (25). This limits the urinary pooling effect, helps to maintain glomerular filtration by reducing intratubular pressure and ultimately limits renal damage.

Ureteric compliance also increases with sustained obstruction and the retrograde peristaltic effect is lessened as the ureter takes on a "baggy" appearance.

MECHANOSENSATION IN RENAL TUBULAR CELLS

As outlined in the above section, phasic changes in renal pelvic pressure/ureteric contraction and urinary pooling constitute a significant stress stimulus to the proximal kidney. The mechanism of mechanosensation and the subsequent responses invoked provide a link

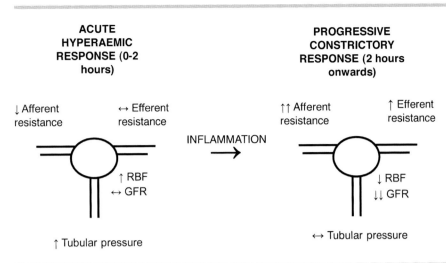

Figure 2 Changes in glomerular arteriolar tone in UUO. Early after complete UUO, vasodilatory mediators such as nitric oxide and prostaglandin E_2 cause afferent arteriolar dilatation which acts to maintain renal blood and glomerular ultrafiltration coefficient in spite of rises in intratubular hydrostatic pressure. As obstruction proceeds and an inflammatory response is established, increased release of vasoconstrictory substances (e.g., thromboxane A_2 and endothelin-1) lead to constriction of both afferent and efferent arteriolae, leading to reduced renal blood flow and a decrease in GFR.

between the biophysical stress stimuli in UUO and the apparition of renal injury. Mechanical deformation of cultured renal tubular epithelial cells elicits a wide variety of changes in cell signaling and gene expression which coordinates a set of responses which in many aspects recapitulate early tubular cell responses in UUO in vivo (26). For example, in vitro cyclic mechanical stretch of tubular epithelial cells leads to increases in transforming growth factor β-1 (TGF-β1) expression, which compliments similar finding in postobstructed renal tissue in man (27,28).

Sensing of Stretch

There are a number of mechanisms by which epithelia can sense mechanical perturbations. Firstly, epithelial adhesion to the basement membrane is mediated via the association of heterodimeric proteins called integrins to specific arginine-glycine-aspartic acid motifs on extracellular matrix (ECM) proteins such as fibronectin (29). Intracellularly the integrin heteromdimers are linked to the actin cytoskeleton at focal adhesions, sites at which the initating components of various cell signaling pathways are condensed. Mechanical stretching of cells or tissues leads to mechanosensation via this ECM-integrin-cytoskeleton complex (30). Such responses are dependent on elevations in intracellular calcium derived both from internal stores and from influx from the extracellular compartment (31).

Transient Receptor Potential Cationic Channel-1 (TRPC-1) has been identified as the putative stretch-activated calcium channel in man and is expressed in the renal tubular epithelium (32,33).

Additionally, the apical membrane of tubular cells has the capacity for mechanosensation. It is known that the renal epithelium has apically located nonmotile cilia with TRPC-1 channels residing in their base (34). Deformation of these cilia by pressure transfer leads to activation of inward calcium currents. Microvilli of the proximal tubular brush border are also known to be mechanically sensitive and respond adaptively to changes in GFR, and proximal tubular flow

rate by altering the activity of the sodium-hydrogen exchanger (35).

EFFECT OF MECHANICAL INSULT ON TUBULAR CELLS

The set of responses induced in cells mechanically stressed cells are pivotal in generating the pathophysiological changes observed in obstructive nephropathy.

The Early Epithelial Stress Response

The epithelial stress response leads to oxidative stress in affected cells. An increase in superoxide radical prodiction and a reduction in hydrogen peroxide metabolizing catalase enzyme expression has been observed both in rodent models of obstruction and during in vitro mechanical stretch (36). Such changes destabilize the mitochondria and promote the release of cytochrome C, which subsequently activates the cysteine aspartate specific protease (Caspase) mediated pathway of apoptosis. Release of cytochrome C following obstruction is also promoted by a decrease in the expression of the mitochondrial transition pore guardian Bcl-2 (37). The production of tumor necrosis factor α (TNF-α) and TGF-β1, Fas and Fas ligand also provide a means for the autocrine/paracrine induction of apoptosis early after obstruction (13).

Establishment of Renal Inflammation in UUO

However, the induction of tubular cell apoptosis following UUO in rats only attains pathological significance after all the early initial pressure and haemodynamic changes are complete (>1 day). This coincides with the establishment of a profound inflammatory infiltrate in the kidney. Early activation of the renal vascular endothelium occurs characterized by increases in adhesion molecule expression (e.g., VCAM-1 and ICAM-1) (38). The infiltrate is

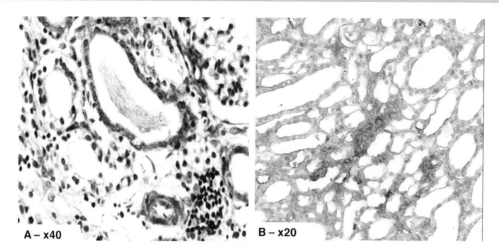

Figure 3 Fibrosis in sustained UUO in the rat. Panel A shows mature fibrillar collagen (*green*) in tubulointerstitial areas of the rat kidney 10 days post UUO. Panel B demonstrates the presence of α smooth muscle actin positive interstitial cells in the same animals, reflecting the proliferation of a matrix producing myofibroblast population.

initially composed of suppressor T-lymphocytes and macrophages, the latter possibly reflecting the fact that mechanically stretched cells(39) secrete large amounts of monocyte chemotactic protein following obstruction (40,41). Activated macrophages are a rich source of proapoptotic and profibrotic cytokines such as TNF-α and TGF-β1, leading to an exacerbation of renal injury (42).

Development of Renal Fibrosis

Sustained obstruction compounded by a progressive renal hypoxia leads to the continued production of the various growth factors and cytokines (33). In particular, TGF-β1 and its associated signaling pathways are crucial in the development of tubulointerstitial fibrosis (TIF) in the affected kidney.

Mature fibrillar collagen is laid down in the interstitium, particulary in the medullary interstitium. In addition, there is a net increase both in matrix degrading metalloproteinase expression and the expression of corresponding matrix metalloproteinase inhibitors the balance of which coordinates pathological remodeling. The fibrotic phenomenon is associated with the increased presence of fiber producing interstitial α smooth muscle actin positive myofibroblasts (Fig. 3).

INTRAOBSTRUCTIVE TUBULAR DYSFUNCTION

Associated with the development of renal injury as described above, and in addition to changes in renal haemodynamics and GFR, are a number of specific defects in tubular function that are characteristic of obstructive nephropathy. Despite the negligible GFR in the obstructed kidney, a significant amount of urine continues to pool, indicating that major changes in the systems coordinating renal reabsorption of filtered electrolytes and water is impaired in UUO.

Sodium and Potassium Handling

The opposing active transport of sodium and potassium at the basolateral membrane of the proximal tubule, the ascending limb of the loop of Henle and distal tubule is crucial to the fine tuning of renal control of extracellular fluid volume. Sodium reabsorption is coupled to luminal secretion of potassium and linked to osmotic movement of water back to the blood.

Aside from the energetic limitations on active transport imposed by progressive hypoxia. Decreased expression of apical sodium antiporters and catalytic units of the basolateral Na-K-ATPase has been described in UUO (43). Loss of sodium reabsorption interrupts the maintenance of the corticomedullary gradient and inhibits normal function of the renal countercurrent multiplier. In UUO, a reduced GFR also contributes to reductions in potassium excretion, however in the presence of a competent contralateral renal function, hyperkalemia does not ensue (44).

Evidence in a rat model of UUO shows that there is also a lesser but significant reduction in sodium transporter expression in the contralateral kidney, which contributes to early natriuresis (45).

It is interesting to note that these changes in sodium handling occur in spite of the fact that activation of the intrarenal renin angiotensin system (RAS) occurs in the obstructed kidney. Key amongst the variety of pressor effects of RAS activation are stimulation of renal sodium reabsorption, both via increases in aldosterone secretion and directly via induction of sodium transporter subunits. However, in UUO, these RAS system effects seem limited and more is

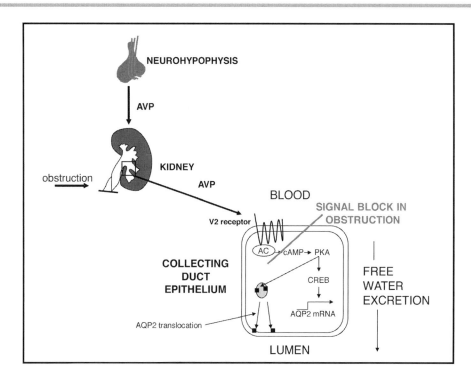

Figure 4 Defective AVP-collecting duct axis in UUO. The figure illustrates the defect in transmission of the AVP signal in the collecting duct during/after obstructive injury. The failure of AVP to stimulate cAMP induced PKA activation prevents adaptive AQP2 membrane translocation and CREB mediated AQP2 upregulation. The net result is a failure to appropriately reabsorb water from the filtrate leading to dilution of the urine (AVP-arginine vasopressin, AQP2-aquaporin 2, cAMP-cyclic adenosine monophosphate, PKA-protein kinase A CREB-cyclic adenosine monophosphate responsive element binding protein).

known regardingits role in pathophysiological changes including apoptosis, inflammation and fibrosis (46).

Distal Tubular Acidification and Collecting Duct Function

The addition of hydrogen ions to the filtrate is dependent on activity of the apical sodium coupled antiport, particulary at the level of the distal tubule. As both the expression of the antiport and general sodium reabsorptive mechanisms are impaired in the Obstructed kidney, an associated alkalization of urine is observed during and following release of obstruction (47).

The collecting duct normally receives hypotonic filtrate from the distal tubule and acts to vary the concentration of the final urine by modifying free water reabsorption. This system is tightly controlled by changes in baroreceptor and osmoreceptor firing in response to changes in blood pressure and osmololality. A decreased circulatory volume or increased plasma osmolality excites magnocellular and parvocellular neurosecretory cells of the hypothalamus to release arginine vasopressin (AVP) into the circulation from their axon terminals in the neuro-hypophysis. Interaction of AVP with V2 receptors in the collecting duct leads to cyclic adenosine-monophosphate (cAMP) generation, protein kinase A activation and the stimulation of both the expression and apical membrane localization of aquaporin-2 (AQP2) water channels.

Experimental studies in rats have demonstrated impairement of this axis in the collecting duct of kidneys with obstruction (Fig. 4) (48).

A further impairment in collecting duct function in UUO centers on the failure to correctly reabsorb urea from the filtrate. Reabsorption of urea is reliant on appropriate expression of A and B type urea transporters. Expression of these transporters is downregulated in the obstructed kidney (49). Impaired urea reabsorption has an impact on interstitial osmolality, as urea accounts for 50% of interstitial osmolality. The net result is to collapse the corticomedullary gradient required for correct functioning of the countercurrent multiplier.

The above description of changes in renal sodium, urea, and water handling explain how sustained urinary pooling can occur during obstruction in spite of such marked reductions in GFR and increases in lymphatic drainage of urine.

POSTOBSTRUCTIVE RENAL FUNCTION

Predicting Functional Recovery

Degree and duration of obstruction are clearly parameters that can affect recoverability of ipsilateral renal function in UUO, both of which are factors that are difficult to control for outwith the experimental field. Recuperation of GFR post obstruction has been noted to bear an inverse relationship to the length of prior obstruction in rats (50).

In an attempt to increase the ability to predict the outcome of obstruction in the clinical setting, a recent prospective study was made of 91 adult patients with UUO and a normally functioning contralateral kidney (51). This demonstrated that on multivariate analysis, only preoperative renographic clearance and perfusion of the obstructed kidney predicted recoverability of function. Kidneys with a renographic GFR of less than 10 mL/min/1.73 m^2 were subsequently found to be irreversibly damaged.

Postobstructive Tubular Function

The postobstructed kidney initially produces hypotonic urine. However, this is generally insignificant in individuals with intact contralateral function and only becomes clinically relevant in cases of BUO or solitary kidney UUO.

The recovery of a normal urinary osmolality and pH has been shown to take up to one month to stabilize in rats subjected to a reversible UUO of 24 hours duration reflecting the time required to reestablish correct epithelial polarity and vectorial transport (52).

Recovery of renal tubular structure concomitant with reversal has been observed in adult mice following the release of UUO of 10 days duration (53).

Effect of Nephrogenic Stage in Neonatal Obstruction

Completion of nephrogenesis is delayed postnatally in the rat, it serves as a good model to compare recovery following transient complete neonatal obstruction at different time points versus temporary and complete obstruction in adult animals. Study of animals three months subsequent to unilateral obstruction during the early postnatal phase (days 1–5, 10% of nephrons formed) revealed a relatively attenuated injury versus the results obtained in animals obstructed at two weeks of age when nephron number has peaked (54). Such studies may offer important insights into debate regarding the best time to operate on the obstructed neonate.

Evidence of Long-Term Renal Injury in UUO

Despite acute recovery of renal function in terms of the measurable GFR and renal blood flow, recent studies in rats indicate that complete obstruction of three days duration causes a progressive histological renal injury following relief (55). The authors in this study equate this progression to the establishment of an irreversible fibrotic lesion in the kidney.

EMERGING THERAPIES IN OBSTRUCTIVE NEPHROPATHY

The model of UUO in rodents is extensively used by those with a broader interest in the prevention of renal injury both in terms of the acute tubular apoptosis and chronic fibrotic progression. Administration and/or neutralization of a number of growth factors and cytokines show a beneficial effect in reducing renal injury intraobstructively (13). Chief among the growth factors which have been shown to have a positive effect intraobstructively in vivo are the administration of bone-morphogenic protein-7 (BMP-7), an epithelial growth factor downregulated in renal injury, epidermal growth factor (EGF) therapy, which provides an antiapoptotic proproliferatory stimulus to the renal epithelium, and hepatocyte growth factor (HGF) administration, which has been shown to work chiefly through the inhibition of TGF-β1 signaling (56–58). Separately, neutralizing anti-TGF-β1 antibody has been demonstrated to ameliorate tubular apoptosis following UUO in rats (59).

While the results of these studies are both interesting and useful, they are limited by two factors. Firstly, many of the demonstrations of efficacy are based on prophylactic deployment at the initiation of obstruction, a scenario irreplicable clinically and secondly, the use of recombinant proteins may in many cases prove economically unviable.

A number of studies have centered on the effectiveness of established pharmaceutical agents on injury in UUO. Angiotensin type 1 receptor antagonists and angiotensin converting enzyme inhibitors are particularly attractive agents given the involvement of the RAS in all aspects of renal injury following obstruction (13). These have been shown to particularly effective in preventing the glomerular vasoconstriction in UUO. Enalapril and Losartan have also been shown to prevent fibrosis following UUO in rats (60). This effect has been related to preservation of renal nitric oxide synthesis (61). In the same article, provision of the nitric oxide substrate L-arginine had a similar protective effect.

One recent study used the generic, tested and inexpensive anti-inflammatory sulfasalazine as an anti-inflammatory strategy implemented three days after induction of UUO in rats (62). Treated animals showed much reduced indices of renal injury in terms of inflammation and fibrosis. Results with this delayed approach to therapy have been replicated in the case of HGF in adult obstruction in rats and EGF in neonatal obstruction in mice (63,64).

The HMG-CoA reductase inhibitors simvastatin, fluvastatin and pravastatin have also shown promising antioxidative, anti-inflammatory and antifibrotic effects in UUO in rodents (65–67).

However, particular clinical relevance should be attached to studies in which therapies have been initiated in the postobstructive phase. A good example is a study in which provision of the nitric oxide synthase substrate L-arginine *ad libitum* to rats after the relief of a three-day UUO, significantly reduced tubular apoptosis, macrophage infiltration and interstitial fibrosis in the absence of any beneficial effect on GFR and renal plasma flow (68).

CONCLUSIONS

Upper urinary tract obstruction can occur secondary to a diverse range of aetiologies. Primary considerations are the type of obstruction, its location and the relevant medical and surgical approaches required to relieve obstruction. Obstructive nephropathy as a consequence of upper urinary tract obstruction as a pathology of particular importance in urology. This chapter has placed an emphasis on describing how upper urinary tract obstruction translates into changes in ureteric function and renal damage via the key primary stimulus of retrograde pressure transfer and mechanical stretch. The subsequent changes in renal haemodynamics and establishment of renal inflammation and fibrosis lead us to the characteristic features of obstructive nephropathy. The wealth of information in the literature regarding the pathophysiology of obstructive nephropathy and its treatment, combined with advances in the relief of obstruction, (particularly medical expulsive therapy) hold promise for the future minimization of obstruction induced renal injury.

REFERENCES

1. Shi Y, Pedersen M, Li C, et al. Early release of neonatal ureteral obstruction preserves renal function. Am J Physiol 2004; 286(6):F1087–F1099.
2. Coe FL, Evan A, Worcester E. Kidney stone disease. J Clin Invest 2005; 115(10):2598–2608.
3. Galvin DJ, Pearle MS. The contemporary management of renal and ureteric calculi. BJU Int 2006; 98(6):1283–1288.
4. Dellabella M, Milanese G, Muzzonigro G. Medical-expulsive therapy for distal ureterolithiasis: randomized prospective study on role of corticosteroids used in combination with tamsulosin-simplified treatment regimen and health-related quality of life. Urology 2005; 66(4):712–715.
5. Nakada SY. Tamsulosin: ureteric motility. BJU Int 2008; 101(9):1061–1062.
6. Itoh Y, Kojima Y, Yasui T, et al. Examination of alpha 1 adrenoceptor subtypes in the human ureter. Int J Urol 2007; 14(8):749–753.
7. Lang RJ, Davidson ME, Exintaris B. Pyeloureteral motility and ureteral peristalsis: essential role of sensory nerves and endogenous prostaglandins. Exp Physiol 2002; 87(2):129–146.
8. Lang RJ, Tonta MA, Zoltkowski BZ, et al. Pyeloureteric peristalsis: role of a typical smooth muscle cells and interstitial cells of Cajal-like cells as pacemakers. J Physiol 2006; 576(pt 3):695–705.
9. Thulesius O, Angelo-Khattar M, Sabha M. The effect of ureteral distension on peristalsis. Studies on human and sheep ureters. Urol Res 1989; 17(6):385–388.
10. Lennon GM, Ryan PC, Fitzpatrick JM. Recovery of ureteric motility following complete and partial ureteric obstruction. Br J Urol 1993; 72(5 pt 2):702–707.
11. Lennon GM, Ryan PC, Fitzpatrick JM. The ureter in vitro: normal motility and response to urinary pathogens. Br J Urol 1993; 72(3):284–290.
12. Kawada N, Moriyama T, Ando A, et al. Increased oxidative stress in mouse kidneys with unilateral ureteral obstruction. Kidney Int 1999; 56(3):1004–1013.
13. Docherty NG, O'Sullivan OE, Healy DA, et al. Evidence that inhibition of tubular cell apoptosis protects against renal damage and development of fibrosis following ureteric obstruction. Am J Physiol 2006; 290(1):F4–F13.
14. Paulson DF, Fraley EE. Compensatory renal growth after unilateral ureteral obstruction. Kidney Int 1973; 4(1):22–27.
15. Boberg U, Wahlberg J, Persson AE. Tubuloglomerular feedback response in the contralateral kidney after 24-hour unilateral ureteral obstruction. Ups J Med Sci 1985; 90(2):193–199.
16. Michaelson G. Percutaneous puncture of the renal pelvis, intrapelvic pressure and the concentrating capacity of the kidney in hydronephrosis. Acta Med Scand Suppl 1974; 559:1–26.
17. Kopp UC, Cicha MZ. PGE2 increases substance P release from renal pelvic sensory nerves via activation of N-type calcium channels. Am J Physiol 1999; 276(5 pt 2): R1241–R1248.
18. Ma MC, Huang HS, Chen CF. Impaired renal sensory responses after unilateral ureteral obstruction in the rat. J Am Soc Nephrol 2002; 13(4):1008–1016.
19. Gaudio KM, Siegel NJ, Hayslett JP, et al. Renal perfusion and intratubular pressure during ureteral occlusion in the rat. Am J Physiol 1980; 238(3):F205–F209.
20. Whinnery MA, Shaw JO, Beck N. Thromboxane B2 and prostaglandin E2 in the rat kidney with unilateral ureteral obstruction. Am J Physiol 1982; 242(3):F220–F225.
21. Hegarty NJ, Young LS, O'Neill AJ, et al. Endothelin in unilateral ureteral obstruction: vascular and cellular effects. J Urol 2003; 169(2):740–744.
22. Yarger WE, Griffith LD. Intrarenal hemodynamics following chronic unilateral ureteral obstruction in the dog. Am J Physiol 1974; 227(4):816–826.
23. Hsu CH, Kurtz TW, Rosenzweig J, et al. Intrarenal hemodynamics and ureteral pressure during ureteral obstruction. Invest Urol 1977; 14(6):442–445.
24. Kinn AC, Bohman SO. Renal structural and functional changes after unilateral ureteral obstruction in rabbits. Scand J Urol Nephrol 1983; 17(2):223–234.
25. Naber KG, Madsen PO. Renal function during acute total ureteral occlusion and the role of the lymphatics: an experimental study in dogs. J Urol 1973; 109(3):330–338.
26. Quinlan MR, Docherty NG, Watson RW, et al. Exploring mechanisms involved in renal tubular sensing of mechanical stretch following ureteric obstruction. Am J Physiol Renal Physiol 2008; 295(1):F1–F11.
27. Kaneto H, Ohtani H, Fukuzaki A, et al. Increased expression of TGF-beta1 but not of its receptors contributes to human obstructive nephropathy. Kidney Int 1999; 56(6): 2137–2146.
28. Sato M, Muragaki Y, Saika S, et al. Targeted disruption of TGF-beta1/Smad3 signaling protects against renal tubulointerstitial fibrosis induced by unilateral ureteral obstruction. J Clin Invest 2003; 112(10):1486–1494.
29. Pytela R, Pierschbacher MD, Ruoslahti E. Identification and isolation of a 140 kd cell surface glycoprotein with properties expected of a fibronectin receptor. Cell 1985; 40(1):191–198.
30. Matthews BD, Overby DR, Mannix R, et al. Cellular adaptation to mechanical stress: role of integrins, Rho, cytoskeletal tension and mechanosensitive ion channels. J Cell Sci 2006; 119(pt 3):508–518.
31. Glogauer M, Arora P, Chou D, et al. The role of actin-binding protein 280 in integrin-dependent mechanoprotection. J Biol Chem 1998; 273(3):1689–1698.
32. Goel M, Sinkins WG, Zuo CD, et al. Identification and localization of TRPC channels in the rat kidney. Am J Physiol 2006; 290(5):F1241–F1252.
33. Maroto R, Raso A, Wood TG, et al. TRPC1 forms the stretch-activated cation channel in vertebrate cells. Nat Cell Biol 2005; 7(2):179–185.
34. Raychowdhury MK, McLaughlin M, Ramos AJ, et al. Characterization of single channel currents from primary cilia of renal epithelial cells. J Biol Chem 2005; 280(41): 34718–34722.

35. Du Z, Yan Q, Duan Y, et al. Axial flow modulates proximal tubule NHE3 and H-ATPase activities by changing microvillus bending moments. Am J Physiol 2006; 290(2):F289–F296.

36. Sunami R, Sugiyama H, Wang DH, et al. Acatalasemia sensitizes renal tubular epithelial cells to apoptosis and exacerbates renal fibrosis after unilateral ureteral obstruction. Am J Physiol 2004; 286(6):F1030–F1038.

37. Zhang G, Oldroyd SD, Huang LH, et al. Role of apoptosis and Bcl-2/Bax in the development of tubulointerstitial fibrosis during experimental obstructive nephropathy. Exp Nephrol 2001; 9(2):71–80.

38. Ricardo SD, Levinson ME, DeJoseph MR, et al. Expression of adhesion molecules in rat renal cortex during experimental hydronephrosis. Kidney Int 1996; 50(6):2002–2010.

39. Higgins DF, Kimura K, Bernhardt WM, et al. Hypoxia promotes fibrogenesis in vivo via HIF-1 stimulation of epithelial-to-mesenchymal transition. J Clin Invest 2007; 117(12):3810–3820.

40. Crisman JM, Richards LL, Valach DP, et al. Chemokine expression in the obstructed kidney. Exp Nephrol 2001; 9(4):241–248.

41. Schreiner GF, Harris KP, Purkerson ML, et al. Immunological aspects of acute ureteral obstruction: immune cell infiltrate in the kidney. Kidney Int 1988; 34(4):487–493.

42. Diamond JR, Kees-Folts D, Ding G, et al. Macrophages, monocyte chemoattractant peptide-1, and TGF-beta 1 in experimental hydronephrosis. Am J Physiol 1994; 266(6 pt 2): F926–F933.

43. Kim SW, Lee J, Jung K, et al. Diminished expression of sodium transporters in the ureteral obstructed kidney in rats. Nephron Exp Nephrol 2004; 96(3):e67–e76.

44. Buerkert J, Martin D, Head M. Effect of acute ureteral obstruction on terminal collecting duct function in the weanling rat. Am J Physiol 1979; 236(3):F260–F267.

45. Li C, Wang W, Kwon TH, et al. Altered expression of major renal Na transporters in rats with unilateral ureteral obstruction. Am J Physiol 2003; 284(1):F155–F166.

46. Chevalier RL, Thornhill BA, Wolstenholme JT. Renal cellular response to ureteral obstruction: role of maturation and angiotensin II. Am J Physiol 1999; 277(1 pt 2):F41–F47.

47. Ribeiro C, Suki WN. Acidification in the medullary collecting duct following ureteral obstruction. Kidney Int 1986; 29(6):1167–1171.

48. Frokiaer J, Christensen BM, Marples D, et al. Downregulation of aquaporin-2 parallels changes in renal water excretion in unilateral ureteral obstruction. Am J Physiol 1997; 273(2 pt 2):F213–F223.

49. Li C, Klein JD, Wang W, et al. Altered expression of urea transporters in response to ureteral obstruction. Am J Physiol 2004; 286(6):F1154–F1162.

50. Harris RH, Yarger WE. Renal function after release of unilateral ureteral obstruction in rats. Am J Physiol 1974; 227(4):806–815.

51. Khalaf IM, Shokeir AA, El-Gyoushi FI, et al. Recoverability of renal function after treatment of adult patients with unilateral obstructive uropathy and normal contralateral kidney: a prospective study. Urology 2004; 64(4):664–668.

52. Valles P, Merlo V, Beron W, et al. Recovery of distal nephron enzyme activity after release of unilateral ureteral obstruction. J Urol 1999; 161(2):641–648.

53. Cochrane AL, Kett MM, Samuel CS, et al. Renal structural and functional repair in a mouse model of reversal of ureteral obstruction. J Am Soc Nephrol 2005; 16(12): 3623–3630.

54. Chevalier RL, Thornhill BA, Chang AY, et al. Recovery from release of ureteral obstruction in the rat: relationship to nephrogenesis. Kidney Int 2002; 61(6):2033–2043.

55. Ito K, Chen J, El Chaar M, et al. Renal damage progresses despite improvement of renal function after relief of unilateral ureteral obstruction in adult rats. Am J Physiol 2004; 287(6):F1283–F1293.

56. Mizuno S, Matsumoto K, Nakamura T. Hepatocyte growth factor suppresses interstitial fibrosis in a mouse model of obstructive nephropathy. Kidney Int 2001; 59(4):1304–1314.

57. Hruska KA, Guo G, Wozniak M, et al. Osteogenic protein-1 prevents renal fibrogenesis associated with ureteral obstruction. Am J Physiol 2000; 279(1):F130–F143.

58. Kennedy WA 2nd, Buttyan R, Garcia-Montes E, et al. Epidermal growth factor suppresses renal tubular apoptosis following ureteral obstruction. Urology 1997; 49(6): 973–980.

59. Miyajima A, Chen J, Lawrence C, et al. Antibody to transforming growth factor-beta ameliorates tubular apoptosis in unilateral ureteral obstruction. Kidney Int 2000; 58(6): 2301–2313.

60. Jones EA, Shahed A, Shoskes DA. Modulation of apoptotic and inflammatory genes by bioflavonoids and angiotensin II inhibition in ureteral obstruction. Urology 2000; 56(2):346–351.

61. Morrissey JJ, Ishidoya S, McCracken R, et al. Nitric oxide generation ameliorates the tubulointerstitial fibrosis of obstructive nephropathy. J Am Soc Nephrol 1996; 7(10):2202–2212.

62. Demirbilek S, Emre MH, Aydin EN, et al. Sulfasalazine reduces inflammatory renal injury in unilateral ureteral obstruction. Pediatr Nephrol 2007; 22(6):804–812.

63. Yang J, Liu Y. Delayed administration of hepatocyte growth factor reduces renal fibrosis in obstructive nephropathy. Am J Physiol 2003; 284(2):F349–F357.

64. Chevalier RL, Goyal S, Thornhill BA. EGF improves recovery following relief of unilateral ureteral obstruction in the neonatal rat. J Urol 1999; 162(4):1532–1536.

65. Vieira JM Jr, Mantovani E, Rodrigues LT, et al. Simvastatin attenuates renal inflammation, tubular transdifferentiation and interstitial fibrosis in rats with unilateral ureteral obstruction. Nephrol Dial Transplant 2005; 20(8):1582–1591.

66. Mizuguchi Y, Miyajima A, Kosaka T, et al. Atorvastatin ameliorates renal tissue damage in unilateral ureteral obstruction. J Urol 2004; 172(6 pt 1):2456–2459.

67. Moriyama T, Kawada N, Nagatoya K, et al. Fluvastatin suppresses oxidative stress and fibrosis in the interstitium of mouse kidneys with unilateral ureteral obstruction. Kidney Int 2001; 59(6):2095–2103.

68. Ito K, Chen J, Seshan SV, et al. Dietary arginine supplementation attenuates renal damage after relief of unilateral ureteral obstruction in rats. Kidney Int 2005; 68(2):515–528.

8

Interactive Obstructive Uropathy: Observations and Conclusions from Studies on Humans

Nicholas J. R. George

Department of Urology, Withington Hospital, University Hospitals of South Manchester, Manchester, U.K.

INTRODUCTION

It has been known for many years that dysfunctional abnormalities of the lower urinary tract may affect the performance of the upper urinary tract in several respects. Typical examples of such bladder dysfunction include those associated with benign prostatic hypertrophy and the changes that are observed after neurologic damage to the spinal cord—the neuropathic bladder. It is recognized that the renal damage caused by such interaction between the lower and upper tract may be severe, silent, and progressive, leading to terminal renal failure if the abnormalities are not recognized and corrected.

In this chapter, the basis of our physiologic understanding of the mechanisms involved in the interactive urinary tract dysfunctional states will be explored. Animal studies of such abnormalities have been few, partially because of the difficulties with complex animal experimentation and partly because natural models of lower/upper tract dysfunction do not exist. This account therefore deals with human subjects found to have a particular form of bladder dysfunction (high-pressure chronic retention) that is particularly appropriate to demonstrate the physiologic changes that occur synchronously within the lower and upper tract. Naturally, all subjects gave informed consent for the procedures, which, being undertaken without any form of anesthesia, benefited additionally from the ability of the patient to speak and comment throughout on the test procedures. Before I describe the observations and discuss the conclusions of these studies, it is pertinent to review the historical perspective relating to interactive dysfunction; such an appreciation explains previous misunderstandings and lays a more secure foundation for a rational understanding of the interactive disorder.

HISTORICAL PERSPECTIVE

In the 1840s dissections by Guthrie in Britain and Civiale in France identified a number of abnormalities in the region of the bladder neck (Fig. 1). Clearly visible in many cases were large lateral lobes of the prostate with a bladder showing trabeculation and sacculation. However, in a number of cases, there was equivalent detrusor hypertrophy, trabeculation, etc., but little to be seen in the way of prostatic hypertrophy, a thickened median bar at the bladder neck being the only possible source of obstruction (Fig. 1B). A short while later, again in Paris at the Necker hospital, Professor Guyon described a third type of dysfunctional bladder that was essentially thin-walled yet still associated with typical "prostatic" symptoms. He called this entity "prostatisme vesicale." At the time, the relationship between these three apparently discrete forms of bladder dysfunction was far from clear, and the situation was not assisted by the very high prevalence of lower urinary tract stones and infection (urgency, frequency, and incontinence) in both middle-aged and older men.

A hypothesis was however formed, which in the next 70 to 100 years became known as "the three-stage theory of prostatism" (Fig. 2). In this theory, the bladder first becomes trabeculated and hypertrophied because of outflow tract obstruction, usually as a result of an easily palpable and enlarged prostate. As obstruction develops, sacculation and diverticulum formation take place, and with "increased pressure" the ureters and subsequently upper tracts dilate, leading to hydronephrosis and eventual renal failure. In the third phase of the classically described course of events, the bladder becomes decompensated—flaccid, large, and overdistended. Overflow incontinence was said to occur.

The three-stage theory of prostatism was widely accepted in the latter part of the 19th century and first half of the 20th century, and typical accounts are to be found in urologic texts published as late as the 1980s. Examination of the theory, however, revealed inconsistencies, which were impossible to explain on a rational basis. In particular, it was not clear why a detrusor muscle, which in stage two had developed hypertrophy, trabeculation, and sacculation, should suddenly give way into a thin-walled atonic bag associated with overflow incontinence and upper tract hydronephrosis.

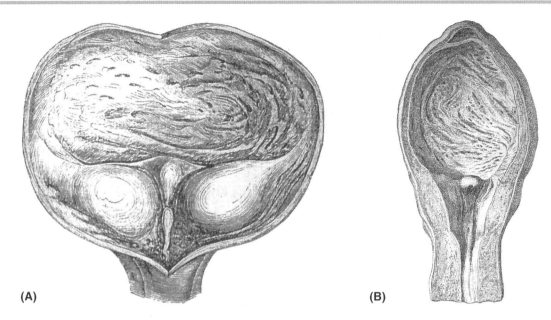

(A)   (B)

Figure 1 Drawings of original dissections by early investigators.

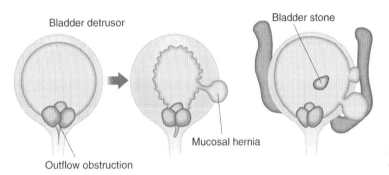

Figure 2 The classically described "three-stage theory of prostatism."

In fact, an explanation of this dilemma had been offered by some careful observational studies undertaken after World War II. In 1948, Badenoch studied 26 patients with bladder neck obstruction (Fig. 1B) whose mean age was 43, 16 of the patients being under 50 years. He noted no prostatic enlargement in these cases but made the highly significant observation that 25 of the 26 cases had diverticulum formation and bilateral hydroureter with hydronephrosis in the majority. In 1951, Wallace complemented this study. He looked at the association between lateral lobe enlargement, median lobe enlargement, and normal and dilated upper tracts. He found that 89% of patients with large prostatic lateral lobes had no upper tract dilatation, but 72% of patients with bladder neck hypertrophy alone demonstrated clear hydronephrosis with hydroureter.

These studies showed clearly that while upper tract dilatation was indeed related to obstruction, this relatively rarely involved the expected prostatic hypertrophy but was much more strongly correlated with pure bladder neck obstruction. These and other studies eventually led to the conclusion that the

unifying three-stage theory of prostatism was unlikely to be correct, and that individual or discrete disorders of the lower urinary tract (i.e., bladder neck obstruction or primary atonic/thin-walled bladder) offered a more plausible explanation for the observed clinical symptom complexes. The particular group of patients with upper tract dilatation associated with bladder neck hypertrophy originally described and clarified by Badenoch were subsequently investigated in greater detail, and the advent of sophisticated urodynamic measuring equipment enabled precise recordings of this dysfunctional state—high-pressure chronic retention—to be made for the first time. Simultaneous advances in uroradiology and nephrostomy placement, in particular, finally made possible for sophisticated simultaneous urodynamic and radiologic studies of both upper and lower urinary tracts. This chapter, therefore, describes and illustrates the physiologic interactive changes in both lower and upper tract, using records obtained by the author and colleagues from such studies on patients with uncomplicated (sterile urine) high-pressure chronic retention.

| 70 kg |
| 1.86 m |
| Temperate climate |
| 1 ml min^{-1} |
| 1500–1800 ml/24 h |

| Day/night = 450 ml × 4/0 ml | Each void approx. 1 min |

Fill phase	23 h 56 min	99.7%		
Void phase	0.3%	Worst possible case 5/60 min	8%	

Figure 3 Volumes and events during the micturition cycle.

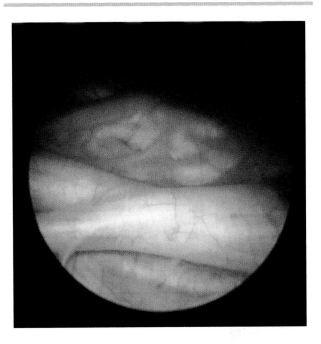

Figure 4 Endoscopic appearance in high-pressure chronic retention.

THE MICTURITION CYCLE

It is important to consider the bladder in terms of the micturition cycle. Traditionally, the terms "obstruction" and "blockage" have been associated with difficulty in passing urine, and the idea of blockage has somehow become extended to the upper tracts—rather as in the three-stage theory of prostatism. However, a moment's consideration of the micturition cycle (Fig. 3) shows that the bladder spends very little time indeed on micturition and that the vast percentage of its functional existence is spent in storage mode. A normal 70-kg adult will micturate four times in 24 hours passing approximately 1500 mL of urine. Assuming that each micturition takes approximately 1 minute to complete, it is clear that the bladder is contracting for only 0.3% of 24 hours; more emphatically, the bladder is in storage phase for 23 hours and 56 minutes of the day. Even in a case severe enough to cause the patient to spend five minutes micturating every hour, the bladder still spends 92% of its time in the filling phase.

These simple calculations show that if there is to be any effect of the lower tract on the upper tract, any abnormality thought to be responsible must act chiefly during the filling phase. An abnormality during the micturition phase—however severe—would not have sufficient time to act and lead to permanent change in the ureters or renal pelvis. Hence, the state of the bladder during filling is of critical importance to a concept of interactive urinary tract dysfunction, and in this respect the mechanical and physical properties of the bladder wall (bladder compliance) require detailed consideration.

THE BLADDER WALL IN HIGH-PRESSURE RETENTION

The bladder wall in patients with high-pressure chronic retention is characteristically thick with massive detrusor hypertrophy. Endoscopically, bars of trabecular muscle stand out, often described as a cathedral roof appearance (Fig. 4). Histologic examination and analysis of sections taken from such trabecular bars (Fig. 5A, B) show degeneration of the

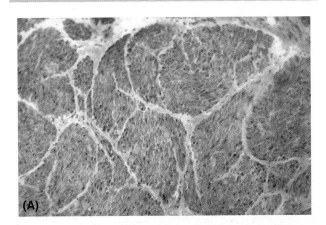

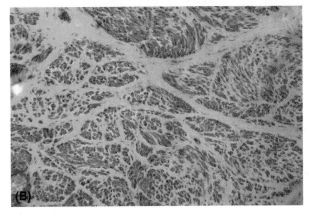

Figure 5 Histologic appearances of detrusor muscle in high-pressure chronic retention. Muscle hypertrophy (**A**) may degenerate (**B**) with collagen infiltration (*green stain*).

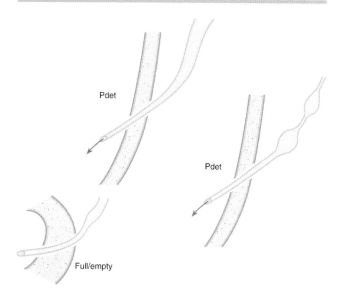

Figure 6 Ureteric passage through thickened detrusor wall. Normal (*right*), loss of peristalsis (*center*), and increasing wall thickness after micturition (*left*).

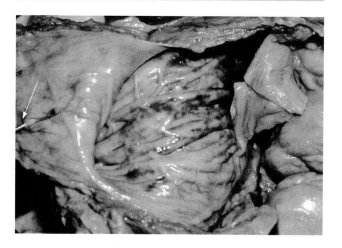

Figure 7 Whole mount bladder from case of high-pressure retention. Note the wire in the ureteric orifice (*arrow*).

smooth muscle bundles into collagen, as illustrated with the Masson trichrome stain. It is not difficult to imagine that the course of the ureter to the vesicoureteric junction (VUJ) through the wall of such a bladder may well become obstructed. The normal coapting process of ureteric peristalsis may be lost (Fig. 6, top); indeed, obstruction at the VUJ may become worse as the bladder empties (Fig. 6, bottom left). The situation is well illustrated by occasional whole mounts of such bladders (Fig. 7). Massive trabeculation and hypertrophy may well cause intramural obstruction to the

ureter, as seen in Figure 7, with a wire probe emerging from the ureteric orifice.

EFFECT OF BLADDER WALL HYPERTROPHY

As might be expected, the increase in detrusor muscle mass together with the collagen infiltration illustrated above fundamentally alters the urodynamic characteristics of the bladder as a storage organ. Normal bladders with normal compliance exhibit little or no intrinsic pressure rise during filling to capacity. By contrast, in high-pressure chronic retention, intrinsic detrusor pressure (related to abnormal sensation as discussed below) remains within the bladder after micturition has been completed, and accurate recording of this "end void" pressure is critical with regard to the analysis of associated renal dysfunction. It is not known at the present time (and it is extremely difficult to determine by experimental means) whether the upper tract dilatation develops as a result of the bladder wall hypertrophy illustrated in Figure 6 or as a result of the intrinsic detrusor postvoid pressure remaining within the bladder after micturition. This is perhaps a slightly academic point, as regardless of whether pressure precedes hypertrophy or vice versa, the end result—progressive upper tract dilatation—remains the same.

MEASUREMENT OF END VOID PRESSURE

As noted above, the accurate recording of end void pressure is an important measurement, which correlates with renal dysfunction. Figure 8 illustrates such a measurement taking place. The typical patient with high-pressure retention (painless protuberant bladder) micturates in an entirely normal fashion in private and without any Valsalva maneuver (artificial pushing). Following the void, the patient lies on the table, and under local anesthetic a small needle is placed suprapubically through the abdominal and bladder wall. Fluid rises up the tube as illustrated, clearly demonstrating the end void intrinsic detrusor pressure remaining within the bladder—this can easily be measured with reference to the pubic bone, as is standard practice, and is responsible for the "high pressure" name applied to this form of chronic retention.

This simple procedure is important because it is undertaken during the patient's natural state without stimulation of urethral or sphincteric sensory receptors. On occasion, investigators have attempted to obtain such measures following conventional urodynamic investigation of the bladder, during which the organ, after drainage of the residual, has almost invariably been filled at supranormal rates. Such abnormal filling rates significantly disrupt the functional performance of high-pressure bladders, and false recordings are obtained (see below). The measurement of end void pressure as described above is the simplest and the best method of obtaining the critical pressure that relates to renal dysfunction.

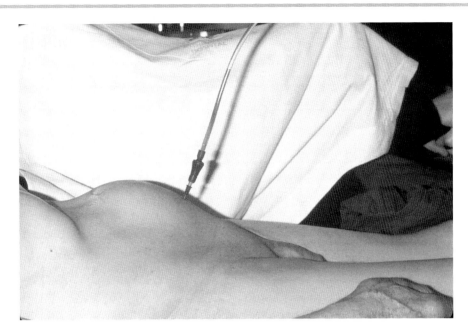

Figure 8 Direct measurement by suprapubic puncture of intrinsic detrusor pressure after void.

SUMMARY OF URODYNAMIC DATA RELATING TO BLADDERS WITH HIGH-PRESSURE RETENTION

Figure 9A illustrates in cartoon format the important concept of the "pressure cycle" that occurs within the bladder of patients with high-pressure chronic retention. Following micturition (EVP, end void point), the pressure within the bladder rises as filling takes place from the upper tracts. Eventually, the end fill pressure (EFP) is reached, at which point the patient is experiencing the normal desire to void. A detrusor contraction takes place (over and above the intrinsic pressure within the bladder), and urine is expelled in the usual fashion. At the end of micturition, the pressure returns once again to the EVP, thus completing the pressure "loop."

It can thus be seen that in the state of high-pressure chronic retention the bladder fills and empties in cyclical fashion at an abnormally raised pressure throughout the 24 hours. Micturition may occur with apparent normality, but at no time are the upper tracts able freely to empty into the bladder storage organ. Thus, it might be predicted that within the upper tracts a similar cycle might be observed—reduced pressure when urine was able to drain easily into the bladder but rising pressure as the bladder filled and passage of urine distally through the vesicoureteric junction became more difficult. This hypothesis is tested by the experiment described below.

Patients with high-pressure retention never drain their bladder below the EVP unless urine is removed artificially. Evidence from cases observed at intervals (years) before initiation of treatment suggest that the EVP gradually rises with time, and as the range of pressure within the bladder cycles—fill/void/fill/void, etc., slowly elevates it becomes progressively more difficult for the ureter to empty into the storage organ. This change is initially observed radiologically as a "snake's head" at the lower end followed by a gradually filling hydroureter to a full hydroureteronephrosis (Fig. 12A) when the intrinsic detrusor pressure at EVP becomes significantly elevated. If a catheter is placed in the bladder and urine drained (Fig. 9A, dashed line), pressure will drop toward zero, and, of course, the suprapubic mass will disappear. As already noted, subsequent measurements taken under these circumstances are highly misleading and do not give useful prognostic information regarding renal function.

Fill-Void Observations

The broad categories of filling phase abnormality that may be seen in the human bladder are noted in Figure 9B. Patients with normal (normal compliance) inflow phases have a pressure rise to the physiologic bladder capacity (approximately 500 mL) of less than 5 cm water. Cases of poor compliance are those in which the bladder pressure rises to a greater degree during filling. This mechanical process can be easily understood when the bladder wall has been replaced by fibrous tissue such as occurs in interstitial cystitis or tuberculosis, or after radiation therapy. By contrast, in high-pressure retention, the reduced compliance during filling is related to a pathophysiologic abnormality of smooth muscle—detrusor hypertrophy and associated collagen formation, as discussed earlier. In any one case the proportion of compliance loss because of muscle hypertrophy (ameliorated to a degree by stress relaxation) or collagen (essentially unable to relax) cannot be known with certainty; however, there is little doubt that those bladders

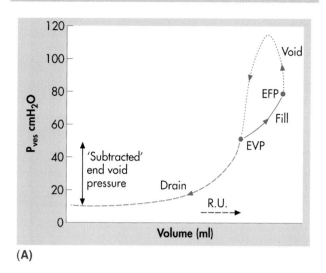

(A)

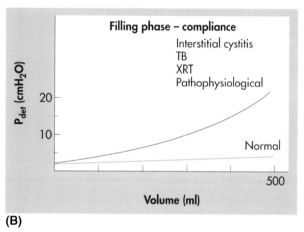

(B)

Figure 9 (**A**) Pressure-volume relationship in high-pressure chronic retention. (**B**) Types of abnormal bladder compliance. *Abbreviations*: EFP, end fill pressure; EVP, end void pressure; RU, residual urine.

with a higher proportion of collagen replacement are more injurious to the upper tract and renal function, as is seen in the significant therapeutic challenge offered by the pediatric "valve bladder."

By definition, storage organs with abnormal compliance will be variably sensitive to filling rates, whether by ureter or urodynamic catheter. Figure 10 panels A and B are from an ambulatory (natural fill) study on a 61-year-old man with relatively early HPCR visualized radiologically as retention with snake's head lower ureters but minimal hydronephrosis. By comparison, a medium-fill (60 mL/min) videocystometric inflow study is shown from a patient with a similar condition (Fig. 10C). In the latter the familiar smooth curve (to 45 cm H_2O) of poor compliance is seen, whereas under conditions of ureteric filling (Fig. 10A) such traces are in reality shown to be made up of a series of contractions gradually rising from EVP 9 cm H_2O to maximum 46 cm H_2O prior to the void. The patient remains completely unaware of filling until, in this case, a sensory threshold

of about 35 cm H_2O is breached. The filling rate is thus responsible for the appearance of the urodynamic trace.

The reason for the development of the high-pressure characteristic remains unknown. Undoubtedly, this detrusor reaction to obstruction may occur with any form of distal urethral lesion, such as dense phimosis, urethral stricture or, in children, urethral valves (the final common pathway). Such pathologic or embryologic abnormalies (or iatrogenic damage such as catheter damage to the urethra) carry a significant risk of silent and irreversible renal damage. By contrast, obstruction that involves the prostate rarely seems to lead to the high-pressure filling type of change (as noted in the historical series). The "typical" prostate (lateral lobe) obstruction characterized by high-pressure/low-flow voiding seldom develops filling phase abnormalities other than phasic overactive waves against a background of near-normal compliance (Fig. 9B). This may perhaps be related to the irritation caused by prostatic obstruction, such as detrusor overactivity protecting against the development of painless retention.

Abnormal sensation appears to be the critical factor in the development of this condition. Urethral sensation, as judged during catheterization, remains normal to touch, thermal stimuli, and pain as classically described and illustrated. Likewise, sensation from periurethral and external urethral sphincter regions appears normal as a catheter passes into the bladder. The sensation of bladder filling, however, is lost until some point toward the end of filling when gradually the patient becomes aware of the impending need to void. At the EFP a perfectly synergic voiding episode takes place with detrusor contraction and synchronous urethral relaxation, no Valsalva maneuver being required (Fig. 10B). Subsequently, all sensation is lost as the pressure settles back to the EVP prior to the start of a new cycle. Whether this loss relates to receptor failure, pelvic nerve dysfunction, or spinal long tract disorder remains unknown at the present time.

RADIOLOGIC ASSESSMENT OF HIGH-PRESSURE BLADDERS

Reflux cystograms (Fig. 11) show, as might be expected, a trabeculated, sacculated picture entirely consistent with the cystoscopic appearance. It might also be expected that reflux would not be seen when one considers the oblique path of the ureter through the massively hypertrophied bladder wall (Fig. 7). Naturally, for the purpose of these human studies into interactive dysfunction, all patients received cystograms to exclude the possibility of reflux, which would be expected to lead to unrelated and entirely different changes within the upper tracts. In the patients studied, urine was always sterile and reflux never present.

Intravenous urography demonstrates the typical picture of well-preserved renal parenchyma with general distension of the collecting system from the

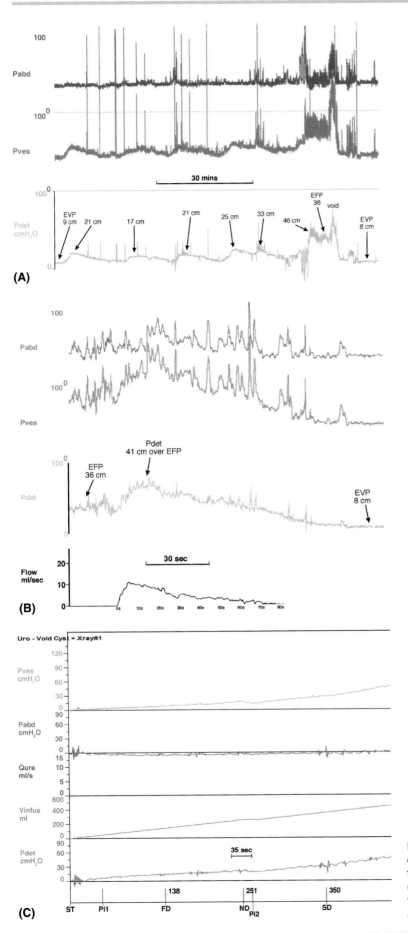

Figure 10 HPCR. (**A**) Ambulatory (*natural fill*) record of one "cycle" lasting 1 hour and 40 minutes taken from filling phase. (**B**) Ambulatory record from above expanded to illustrate voiding characteristics. (**C**) Conventional medium fill (60mL/mn) urodynamics in HPCR after bladder residual drained.

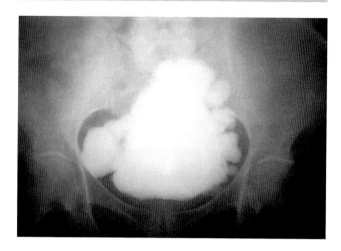

Figure 11 Reflex cystogram in high-pressure retention, demonstrating competent vesicoureteric junction.

calyces to the vesicoureteric junction (Fig. 12). Figure 12A particularly well illustrates the typical snake's head appearance of high-pressure retention at the lower end of the left ureter—a near-certain sign of raised intravesical pressure and a warning, if not otherwise suspected, that renal function might be at risk. Such appearances allow a relatively easy target for a skilled nephrostomist, and the placement of such a tube at last allows the synchronous measurement of upper and lower urinary tract pressures to be contemplated.

INTERACTIVE PRESSURE RECORDINGS IN PATIENTS WITH HIGH-PRESSURE CHRONIC RETENTION AND HYDROURETER/ HYDRONEPHROSIS

Following careful screening to exclude default conditions such as prostate cancer or urinary tract infection, consenting patients underwent the investigation protocol illustrated in Figure 13. A nephrostomy tube was placed in the renal pelvis (via the renal substance to avoid leakage) and connected to standard Whitaker

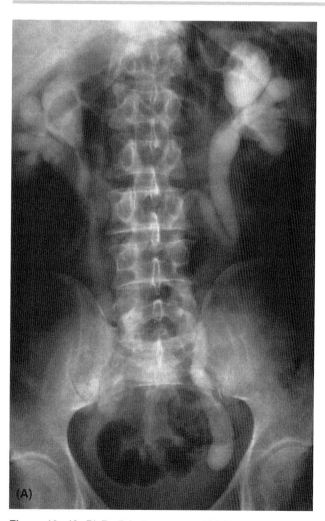

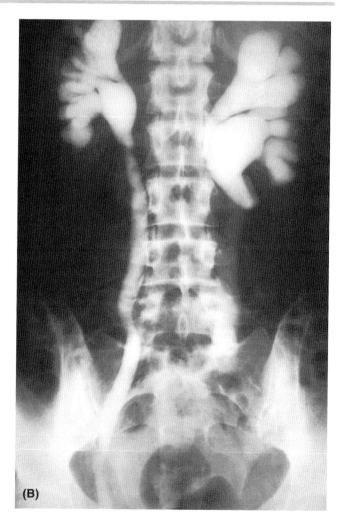

Figure 12 (**A**, **B**) Radiologic aspects of high-pressure retention.

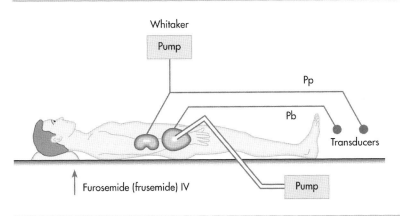

Figure 13 Experimental protocol for bladder and renal pressure measurement.

pump/measurement apparatus. A suprapubic pressure line was inserted, and finally a urethral catheter allowed bladder volume to be increased or decreased at will. The patient was made warm and comfortable on the investigation table, as the studies took an extended period of time. Patients rarely experienced any discomfort during the tests and commonly fell asleep during measurements.

States of Hydration

Three differing states of hydration were identified. Baseline hydration determined that the patient was comfortable—enough water had been drunk to satisfy thirst. Water drinking determined that patients were asked to drink 1 to 1.5 L of water fairly rapidly, a load well in excess of what they would normally ingest. A third level of fluid loading was attained by administration of furosemide (frusemide) 0.5 mg/kg IV. These three forms of hydration were used to "front-end load" the urinary tract—that is present differing diuretic loads to the drainage system of the renal mass.

In addition to fluid loads presented to the kidney, it was possible to vary the rate with which the fluid passed through the vesicoureteric junction. This was performed by filling and emptying the bladder through the urethral catheter, the resultant pressure being recorded by the suprapubic pressure line. As will be evident from Figure 9, such artificial filling and emptying of the bladder results in marked swings of intrinsic detrusor pressure, which may be expected to affect vesicoureteric transport.

Experimental Observations

The results of these experiments are illustrated in Figures 14 to 20. During prolonged baseline recordings (Fig. 14), in which the patient was resting comfortably and simply hydrated, there was no identifiable correlation or connection between bladder and pelvic pressure measurements. Occasional pelvic pressure waves were seen, as were occasional detrusor contractions (unstable waves), but these bore no temporal relationship to each other. Subsequently

(Fig. 15), the bladder was filled at a rate of 60 mL/min and the effect on bladder and pelvic pressure noted. As expected from the pressure–volume characteristic of high-pressure bladders, the bladder pressure rose rapidly, but at the same time pelvic pressure was also seen to rise, albeit much more slowly. When 100 mL of water was removed from the bladder (Fig. 16),

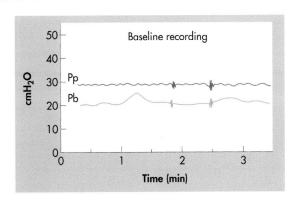

Figure 14 Baseline recordings of renal pelvic (P_p) and bladder (P_b) pressures.

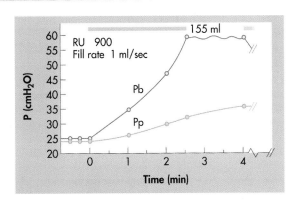

Figure 15 Subsequent pressure variations.

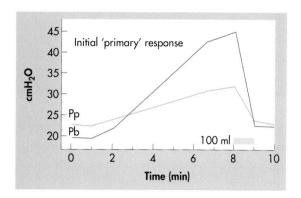

Figure 16 Effect of bladder pressure variation.

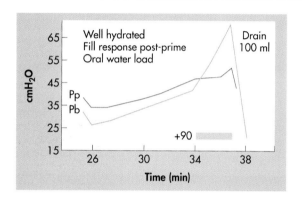

Figure 17 Further pressure variations with water loading and an additional 90 mL in the bladder.

bladder pressure dropped rapidly, as again would be expected, but pelvic pressure also dropped following the slow initial rise, demonstrating that the artificial "cycling" of bladder pressure (see above) had induced a form of artificial cycling of the upper tract pressure.

The cycling linkage continued but was more precisely interlinked when oral water loading increased the perfusion pressure at the proximal end of the urinary tract (Fig. 17). Natural diuresis and subsequent bladder drainage produced sharp swings in bladder and pelvic pressure measurements, although, as might be expected, bladder pressure swings were more acute than those seen in the renal pelvis.

Subsequently, under maximal "front-end loading" caused by furosemide IV, bladder pressure cycling via the urethral catheter led to similar sharp swings of pressure being recorded from the renal pelvis. Occasionally, small reductions in pelvic pressure were observed that were not related to any variation of bladder volume; these were thought to represent periods of ureteric "creep," during which smooth muscle of the upper urinary tract dilated marginally, thus reducing pressure and accommodating a greater volume. This is the mechanism thought experimentally to account for the development of hydroureter and hydronephrosis over the long term (Fig. 19).

The interactive pressure experiments are summarized in Figure 20. During baseline periods, bladder and renal pressures are dissociated, and variation of bladder pressure in particular has no effect on upper tract distension. However, prolonged increase of bladder pressure (unlikely to be tolerated by the patient) or increased fluid loading/diuretic therapy (a reasonably common occurrence) might well "prime" the upper tracts, and thereafter pressures within the pelvis may mimic precisely pressures within the bladder. It is very important to appreciate that this synchronous pressure state occurs in the absence of the vesicoureteric reflux. The pressure measured within the pelvis is not a reflection of bladder pressure "passing backward" up the ureter; it is a pressure required to be exerted by the upper tract if profusion through the vesicoureteric junction is to occur.

It is proposed therefore that these experiments give some insight into the development of hydronephrosis in the simple, uncomplicated (uninfected)

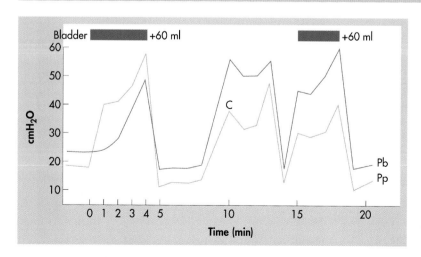

Figure 18 Coordinated pressure movements within bladder and renal pelvis. Drainage volumes not shown. C: Possible time of ureteric "creep."

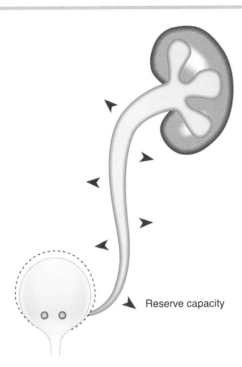

Figure 19 Schematic diagram of ureteric "creep"—gradual dilatation under stress.

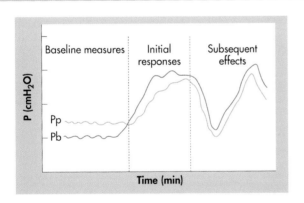

Figure 20 Summary of interactive pressure-volume effects.

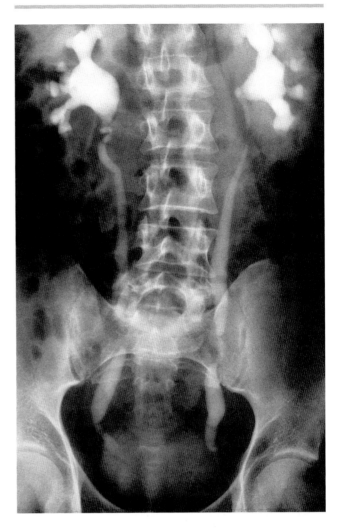

Figure 21 Urographic changes in early high-pressure retention.

case of high-pressure retention. It is now possible to consider what might be the consequences of such changes for renal function. By the same experimental model, it is possible to examine both renographic and biochemical aspects of renal function, and the technique and results of these studies will be briefly described.

EXCRETORY FUNCTION MEASURED BY GAMMA CAMERA RENOGRAPHY

It has already been noted that the lack of coapting peristaltic waves would be likely fundamentally to

affect drainage function from the upper urinary tract. The ureter, previously divided into segments, becomes an open column of fluid as hydronephrosis supervenes, and such an open column is capable of exerting forces very dissimilar to those acting in the normal state. It might be hypothesized, for example, that such an open hydroureter would, under certain critical circumstances, exert pressures on the vesicoureteric junction in the vertical position that would not be present in the horizontal position. Clearly, in this respect, the pressure on the other side of the vesicoureteric junction (i.e., within the bladder) would be critical, but there might be defined circumstances where significant differences in drainage from the upper tracts would be seen when the patient was in the erect rather than the horizontal position.

Such patients can be identified, and one such is illustrated in Figures 21 to 23. The IVP of this 41-year-old man is not, at first glance, overtly hydronephrotic, but an open hydroureter can be seen on both sides, most marked on the left, and the typical snake's head at the lower end of the ureter typical of high-pressure

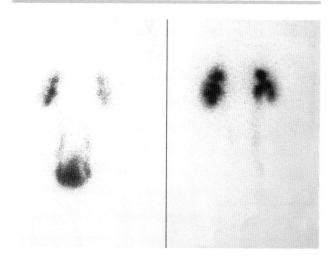

Figure 22 Erect and supine renographic images.

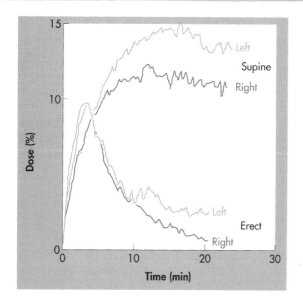

Figure 23 Erect and supine renographic curves.

position. This simple study in a young man with early high-pressure retention demonstrates conclusively that drainage through the vesicoureteric junction can be affected by postural conditions; loss of the normal coapting mechanism might well be responsible for the observations.

GRAVITATIONAL THEORY OF DRAINAGE

This gravitational theory of the open hydroureter may be tested with the human high-pressure retention model (Fig. 24). In these studies, men with sterile high-pressure retention have a suprapubic line and catheter inserted under local anesthetic. Thus, the volume and hence pressure within the bladder may be varied at will while the patient is seated or lying in front of a gamma camera.

The results of various studies are depicted in Figures 25 to 28. In the first experiment, a man underwent ^{123}I gamma camera renography in the sitting position. He was comfortably hydrated but had been asked not to void prior to the examination. It was thus envisaged that his bladder pressure would be relatively advanced up the pressure–volume curve illustrated in Figure 9A. Injection of the isotope was given, and the curves elaborated are shown. At 25 minutes, 120 mL of urine was withdrawn through the suprapubic catheter, and the effect on renal clearance of the isotope observed. The acute reduction in intravesical volume and thus pressure allowed vesicoureteric transport to take place, urine from the previously

retention can be seen. The relatively small but high-pressure bladder fails to opacify. [123]I gamma camera renography was performed in erect and supine positions under identical circumstances a few days apart. Figure 22 shows accumulated frames between 10 and 15 minutes. The panel showing the erect study clearly demonstrates upper tract drainage, particularly from the left, and bladder filling, while the panel relating to the supine study shows near-total stasis within the renal pelvis and calyces and no image whatever of the bladder. Graphical analysis (Fig. 23) shows equally good uptake for either test but little excretion in the supine position as compared with near-normal excretion (renal area of interest demonstrated) in the erect

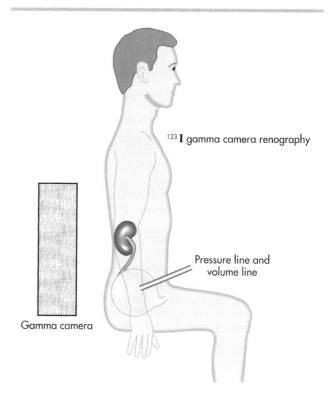

Figure 24 Experimental protocol for drainage experiments.

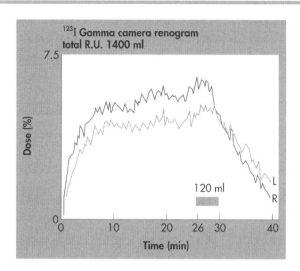

Figure 25 Effect of bladder drainage.

obstructed kidney passing rapidly onward and down the hydroureter. In Figure 26, the same experiment is repeated, but the intravesical pressure is recorded on the same time base as that for the renogram curves. Under these conditions, little isotope escaped the renal substance until the reduction of the bladder volume once again caused a sharp drop of bladder pressure, following which rapid reduction in isotope counts from the kidney took place. These experiments demonstrate an important hydrodynamic aspect of high-pressure retention. A vertical line drawn at the moment isotope counts begin to reduce (urine leaving the kidney) bisects the intravesical pressure recording

at approximately 25 cm of water. Thus, when the intravesical pressure is above this level, little or no drainage occurs from the upper tract. As the pressure falls through 25 cm, rapid drainage starts to commence, suggesting that the figure of 25 cm is particularly important for the maintenance of upper tract function.

The robust and resilient nature of the lower tract changes are illustrated in Figure 27. In these experiments, bladder pressure was recorded as before during gamma camera renography. However, to stimulate to the maximum the upper tract—and thus, if possible, to force perfusion into the bladder—an injection of furosemide was given 15 minutes after the isotope injection. As can be seen, despite this front-end loading, the renographic counts do not diminish and the renographic curves do not deflect until, once again, bladder pressure has been significantly reduced by removing fluid from within. Lower tract intrinsic pressure and dynamics appear to dominate renal function, and such an effect may still be seen in relatively advanced obstructive renal failure (Fig. 28). In this case, relatively poor uptake during gamma camera renography signifies relatively high serum creatinine, but, on draining the bladder, there is still an effect seen in the erect position that is not identified if the renography is carried out supine.

In conclusion, therefore, it is possible to advance a hypothesis on high-pressure chronic retention to account for the variation seen in upper and lower tract pressures. It is postulated that an open hydroureter (approximate length in the adult, 25 cm) (Fig. 29) may maintain profusion through the vesicoureteric junction as long as the cyclic intrinsic detrusor pressure remains under 25 cm for the

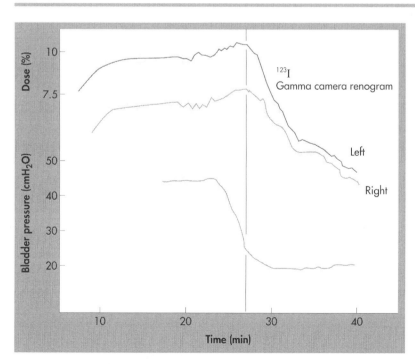

Figure 26 Bladder pressure and renal drainage compared.

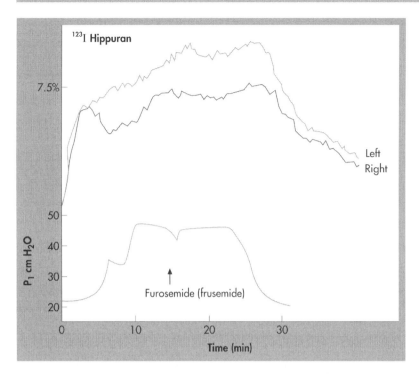

Figure 27 Lack of furosemide (frusemide) effect until bladder drained. See text for details.

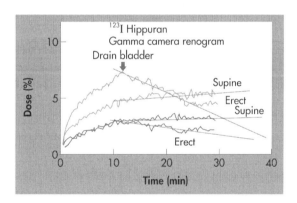

Figure 28 Bladder effect in advanced renal failure.

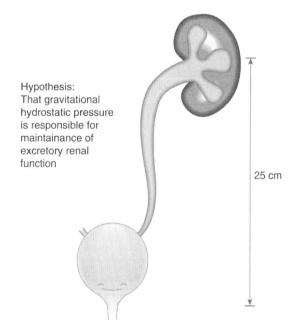

Figure 29 Hypothesis for gravitational theory in open hydroureter.

majority of the cycle. If the intrinsic detrusor pressure rises above 25 cm for the majority of the filling phase, ureteric stasis should supervene and obstructed renal failure would follow. This hypothesis was explored in the original report describing high-pressure retention where a graph of intrinsic detrusor pressure against serum creatinine (Fig. 30) appeared to show that above 25 cm of water there was indeed a steep rise in creatinine, as would be expected from the experimental evidence. Although there were few patients with significantly raised creatinine levels in this series, other results from workers have tended to support the importance of the 25- to 30-cm water pressure range with respect to maintenance of renal profusion and function.

APPLICATION TO RECONSTRUCTIVE SURGERY

The urodynamic observations on HPCR patients may assist those considering orthotopic or neobladder techniques for patients requiring radical pelvic surgery. Naturally, bladder walls constructed from other

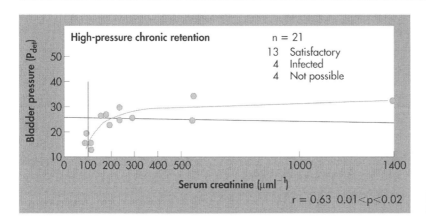

Figure 30 Intrinsic detrusor pressure related to serum creatinine.

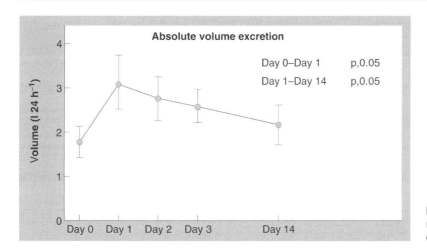

Figure 31 Volume excretion before and after relief of obstruction. Day 0: prior to relief of obstruction by bladder catheterization.

than the original detrusor muscle will be neurologically independent of the patient micturition reflex, so sensory/motor and compliance abnormalities might be anticipated following such surgery.

Filling phase pressure within the reconstructed storage organ will clearly be critical for successful outcome with regard to incontinence, enuresis, and upper tract function. Physiologic wall characteristics, detubularization techniques, and other refinements of design should enable low-pressure storage, ideally less than 25 cm of water but certainly no greater than 35 cm of water for the majority of the "micturition cycle." Failure to attain these objectives will inevitably lead to complications as predicted by the high-pressure model.

BIOCHEMICAL STUDIES BEFORE AND AFTER THE RELIEF OF OBSTRUCTION

This subject has been extensively studied in the literature and in our own department during the last few years by Jones and coworkers. An understanding of the abnormalities of tubular function that may occur

under such circumstances is important for the practicing urologist, who not infrequently has to manage a patient with postobstructive diuresis on the urology ward. Absolute volumes (Fig. 31) and electrolyte excretion (Fig. 32) are maximal within 24 hours and usually stabilize by 14 days. Synchronous studies of glomerular filtration rate by various mechanisms (Fig. 33) illustrate that most of the early improvement is related to tubular recovery, although a late glomerular recovery phase can be identified. Precisely similar urodynamic, renographic, and biochemical changes may be seen in children as well as adults—infants and children with urethral valves have a near-identical syndrome to high-pressure retention (the valve bladder), and in those cases that are not associated with reflux, similar patterns of obstructive renal failure take place. Unfortunately, the destructive nature of the severe obstruction on the detrusor muscle frequently leads to marked collagen infiltration and fibrotic damage, resulting in very poor compliance. By contrast, in the adult, long-term studies both from our own unit and others suggest that the majority of patients recover well, both as regards bladder and renal function.

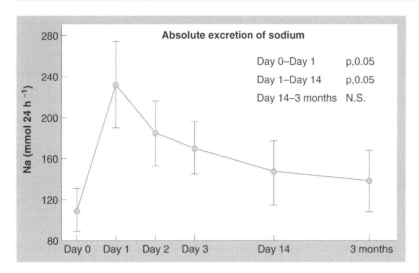

Figure 32 Sodium excretion before and after release of obstruction. Day 0: as in Figure 31.

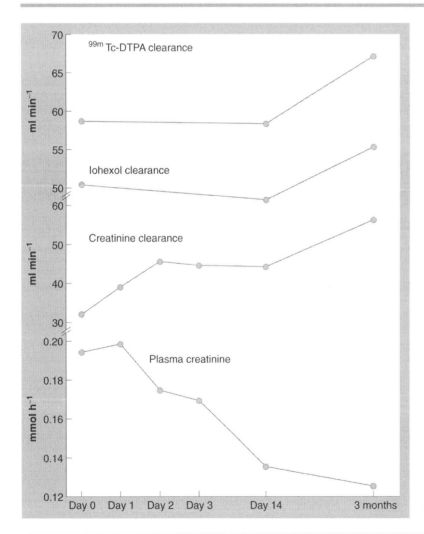

Figure 33 Summary of glomerular and tubular changes in obstructive uropathy before and after the release of obstruction.

The observations recorded above have, of course, been made in a particular group of patients studied with a particular form of bladder dysfunction. It might be argued that patients with neurogenic bladder dysfunction—acknowledged to be chiefly at risk because of obstructive renal problems—could not be linked urodynamically or therapeutically with the high-pressure retention group. There is no doubt that neurogenic bladders may demonstrate a profile of much more aggressive hyperreflexic contractions than that seen in high-pressure retention cases (although, in the latter, moderate overactivity may be seen on ambulatory studies), and it is possible that the hyperreflexic contractions themselves may be responsible for the obstructive renal failure. Nevertheless, there are enough signs in common (clinical, radiologic, renographic, and biochemical) to consider that the conditions may be associated at least in part; therapeutic and reconstructive lessons learned in one group may well be applicable to the other.

CLINICAL ADDENDUM

The classical high-pressure presentation of a tense, painless bladder, late onset enuresis, hypertension, and progressive renal impairment associated with bilateral hydroureteronephrosis is comparatively uncommon, occurring in 10% or less of patients attending "lower urinary tract" clinics. Patients whose urine remains sterile do *not* complain of "prostatic symptoms" such as hesitancy or poor stream and are often astonished when the distended bladder is pointed out to them.

Unfortunately, the combination of suboptimal diagnostic skills and the many reasons for abnormal renal function in the elderly male have led to overdiagnosis of the condition with subsequent illogical treatment of a postobstructive diuresis, which is usually no more than resolving acute on chronic (low pressure) retention or residual urine associated with underactive detrusor function. By association, the real threat posed by a marked diuresis in a genuine case may pass unnoticed until postural hypotension supervenes. Informed history taking, accurate fluid chart records, appropriate radiology and familiarity with renal function in the elderly can help reduce these errors of clinical judgment.

FURTHER READING

1. Badenoch AW. Congenital obstruction of the bladder neck. Ann R Coll Surg Engl 1949; 4:295–307.
2. George NJR, O'Reilly PH, Barnard RJ, et al. High-pressure chronic retention. BMJ 1983; 286:1780–1783.
3. George NJR, O'Reilly PH, Barnard RJ, et al. Practical management of patients with dilated upper tracts and chronic retention of urine. Br J Urol 1984; 56:9–12.
4. George NJR, Feneley RC, Roberts JBM. Identification of the poor risk patient with "prostatism" and detrusor failure. Br J Urol 1986; 58:290–295.
5. Ghose RR. Prolonged recovery of renal function after prostatectomy for prostatic outflow obstruction. BMJ 1990; 300:1376–1377.
6. Holden D, George NJR, Rickards D, et al. Renal pelvic pressures in human chronic obstructive uropathy. Br J Urol 1984; 56:565–570.
7. Jones DA, George NJR, O'Reilly PH, et al. Reversible hypertension associated with unrecognised high-pressure chronic retention of urine. Lancet 1987; 11:1052–1054.
8. Jones DA, George NJR, O'Reilly PH. Post-obstructive renal function. Semin Urol 1987; 5:176–190.
9. Jones DA, George NJR, O'Reilly PH, et al. The biphasic nature of renal functional recovery following relief of chronic obstructive uropathy. Br J Urol 1988; 61:192–197.
10. Jones DA, Holden D, George NJR. Mechanism of upper tract dilatation in patients with thick walled bladders, chronic retention of urine and associated hydroureteronephrosis. J Urol 1988; 140:326–329.
11. Jones DA, Lupton EW, George NJR. Effect of bladder filling on upper tract urodynamics in man. Br J Urol 1990; 65:492–496.
12. Jones DA, Atherton JC, O'Reilly PH, et al. Assessment of the nephron segments involved in post-obstructive diuresis in man, using lithium clearance. Br J Urol 1989; 64:559–563.
13. Jones DA, Gilpin SA, Holden D, et al. Relationship between bladder morphology and long-term outcome of treatment in patients with high pressure chronic retention of urine. Br J Urol 1991; 67:265–285.
14. Sacks SH, Aparicio SAJR, Bevan A, et al. Late renal failure due to prostatic outflow obstruction: a preventable disease. BMJ 1989; 298:156–159.
15. Styles RA, Neal DE, Ramsden PD. Chronic retention of urine. The relationship between upper tract dilatation and bladder pressure. Br J Urol 1986; 58:647–651.
16. Styles RA, Neal De, Griffiths CJ, et al. Long term monitoring of bladder pressure in chronic retention of urine: the relationship between detrusor activity and upper tract dilatation. J Urol 1988; 140:330–334.
17. Wallace DM. The bladder neck in urinary obstruction. Proc R Soc Med 1951; 44:434–437.

9

Urinary Tract Infection

Nicholas J. R. George

Department of Urology, Withington Hospital, University Hospitals of South Manchester, Manchester, U.K.

INTRODUCTION

The infectious process encompasses a highly complex series of events that surround the relationship between the defending host and the offending parasite. Virulence factors available to the microorganism will be combated by a wide range of specific and nonspecific defense mechanisms, and the result of this encounter, "the microbiological battleground," will determine whether infectious disease is established.

Conventionally, accounts of infection of the urinary tract concentrate on the response of the urothelium to bacterial invasion. However, a continuing and perhaps increasing tendency to open surgery in certain groups of patients determines that a basic understanding of the broader concepts of the infectious process is likely to be advantageous for the practicing urological surgeon. Therefore, in this account of urinary tract infection (UTI), before dealing with specific issues relating to organisms and the urothelium, a general description will be made of the host-parasite relationship as it applies to the urogenital system both in health and disease. Some important fundamental definitions are noted in Table 1. Such general microbiological points may be considered under the following headings.

1. Colonizing microorganisms in health
2. General defense mechanisms
3. General modifying factors
4. Properties of commensal organisms

Colonizing Microorganisms in Health

Table 2 lists common colonizing microorganisms by site in healthy humans. The widespread presence of staphylococci and streptococci on the skin and surrounding the lower genitourinary tract will be appreciated, as will the occurrence of *Candida* and lactobacilli within vaginal flora. The colon contains enormous numbers of bacteria—up to 10^{11} organisms per gram. The majority of these organisms are obligate anaerobes, although aerobic and facultative anaerobic organisms, such as enterobacteriaceae and *Enterococcus* spp., are present in significant numbers (approximately $10^8/g$ of colonic contents), these species being the most common source of uropathogens.

The normally balanced environment of the bowel flora is significantly affected by antimicrobial agents. Antibiotic therapy results in normally sensitive *Escherichia coli* strains as well as anaerobic species being replaced by more resistant strains and organisms such as *Pseudomonas aeruginosa* (1). Cessation of broad-spectrum therapy allows recolonization by resident flora, but slower-growing anaerobic organisms may initially be displaced by faster-growing enterobacteriaceae. Hence, injudicious broad-spectrum

Table 1 Essential Definitions of Basic Microbiological Terms

Term	Definition
Pathogenicity	Ability to cause disease
Opportunistic infection	Weakened defenses predispose to infection, often by nonpathogens
Virulence	Degree of pathogenicity

Table 2 Organisms by Site in Health (Normal Flora): Commensal Organisms That Exist in Symbiotic Relationship with the Host Protecting Against Uropathogens

Skin
  Staphylococci (*Staphylococcus aureus* and *Staphylococcus epidermidis*)
  Corynebacterium spp.
  Candida spp.
Lower genitourinary tract
  Staphylococci
  Streptococci
  Anaerobic cocci
    Corynebacterium spp.
    Lactobacilli (vagina)
Large intestine
  Anaerobes
    Bacteroides spp.
    Clostridium spp.
    Fusobacterium spp.
  Aerobes/facultative anaerobes
    Escherichia coli
    Klebsiella spp.
    Streptococci Enterococci (*Streptococcus faecalis*)
    Yeasts

Table 3 General Nonspecific (Constitute) Host Defense Mechanisms

Surface	Compromised	Subsurface	Compromised	Cellular	Compromised
Commensal flora	Antibiotics	Lysozyme			Alcholism
Mechanical integrity	Surgery	Lactoferrin		Phagocytosis	Advanced cancer
Acidity	Cannulae	Acute-phase	Drugs	Polymorphonuclear	Renal disease
		response	Corticosteroids	Mononuclear	Liver disease
			Immunosuppression		HIV
			Infections		
Secretions		Inflammatory			
Lysozyme		response			
Lactoferrin					
IgA					
Flow	Surgery	Complement			
Peristalsis	Obstruction	Fibronectin			
Irritation					

These are conveniently described in terms of the degree to which the organism penetrate the surface. General factors that may compromise these defenses are noted.

therapy may increase the size of the colonic reservoir from which uropathogens are normally drawn (2); as noted above, these organisms usually account for only 0.1% of total colonic flora. The presence of a large volume of potential uropathogens may clearly be an ascending threat to the lower urinary tract, particularly in the presence of any abnormality such as outflow tract obstruction or congenital anomalies.

General Defense Mechanisms

Nonspecific host defense mechanisms are outlined in Table 3. General resistance to invasion may be described in terms of events at the surface of the host, events at a deeper level, and mechanisms that depend on cellular function.

The role of commensal flora is further explored below. The mechanical integrity of skin and mucous membranes may clearly be breached in a number of ways. The breakdown of lipids into fatty acids (approximate pH 5–6) by skin flora constitutes a mildly hostile environment for pathogens. Lysozyme, found in every mucosal secretion, splits the muramic acid linkage in cell walls of gram-positive organisms in particular. The iron-binding properties of lactoferrin disrupt the normal metabolism of the microorganism. IgA secretion may prevent attachment of organisms to host cells.

Penetration of the initial line of defense leads to more substantial but nonspecific reactions such as the acute-phase response and the inflammatory response. Humoral and cellular components, such as protease inhibitors and adherence proteins, are delivered to the site, and the classical inflammatory reaction supervenes. Activation of the complement cascade by the alternative pathway may lead to bacterial lysis as well as enhancement of phagocytosis. The antiadherence properties of the glycoprotein fibronectin may prevent attachment of pathogenic organisms. Increased phagocytosis by various cells, including neutrophil polymorphs, mononuclear phagocytes, and natural-killer cells, is stimulated by a complex series of events, which may vary according to the nature of the microbiological challenge.

General Modifying Factors

A number of generalized factors may affect the standard host defense mechanisms. Patients at the extremes of life are vulnerable to infections. Postmenopausal hormonal changes in the lower urinary tract are of particular interest to urologists.

Poor nutrition or overt malnutrition, particularly in the elderly, may weaken defenses in a number of ways relating to protein synthesis and vitamin deficiency. Generalized disorders, such as diabetes mellitus, alcoholism, and renal failure, may markedly increase susceptibility to disease, as may overwhelming infection and certain types of drug therapy as well as the general debility related to advanced malignancy. Pathological conditions, which further expose the individual to risk of infection, such as stone disease or obstruction, will be considered below.

Properties of Commensal Organisms

Commensal organisms have an important role to play in the protection of the host by resisting the growth of more pathogenic organisms. The mechanisms by which they attain this objective are listed in Table 4. Competition for a limited supply of nutrients acts to restrict the growth of pathogens, while the ability of the commensal organisms to occupy certain cell surface receptors (tropism) limits the adherence possibilities for the invader. Bacterial products known as bacteriocins may be toxic to other organisms, often of the same species. As noted above, fatty acid production by sebum and lipids results in a hostile microenvironment. Low-level but continued stimulation of the immune system, as well as the stimulation of cross-reacting "natural" antibodies (such antibodies

Table 4 Mechanisms of Protection by Commensal Flora

Competition for nutrients (interference)
Competition for receptors (tropism)
Bacteriocin production
Fatty acid production
Stimulation of immune system
Stimulation of natural antibodies

are raised against organisms, which the host has not encountered because of antigenic cross-reaction with organisms that have been experienced), further enhances resistance to pathogenic bacteria. Apart from antibiotic therapy, the normal commensal flora may be significantly affected by general factors such as diet, hygienic habits, and underlying disease.

The described general mechanisms are, under the normal circumstances of health, remarkably effective at excluding pathogenic invasion. For a more complete account of the highly complex processes involved, the reader is referred to standard bacteriological texts. The remainder of this chapter will address, first, specific microbiological aspects of UTI in humans and, second, a clinical account of the more important forms of inflammatory disease.

HOST DEFENSE MECHANISMS: LOWER URINARY TRACT

Apart from the broad concepts outlined above, the lower urinary tract has a number of specific defense mechanisms, which allow it to counter the threat posed by the reservoir of potential pathogens, which is located chiefly in the lower bowel and on the perineal skin. Naturally, the anatomy of the male and in particular the length of the urethra determine that ascending infection is extremely uncommon when compared with the female. However, the lower urogenital tract, while clearly offering a bacteriological threat to the female urothelium, does offer some defense mechanisms against ascending infection by pathogenic bacteria.

Commensal Organisms

An outline of the advantages of commensal flora has been described above. During the reproductive years, circulating estrogens affect the vaginal epithelium, which stores increased amounts of glycogen within the cells (Fig. 1). The glycogen is metabolized by

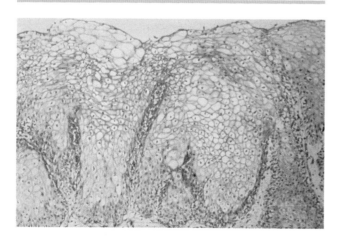

Figure 1 Vaginal epithelial cells stuffed with glycogen. Produced in response to estrogens, the glycogen is broken down by *Lactobacillus acidophillus*, thus increasing local vaginal acidity.

Lactobacillus acidophilus into lactic acid, and the resultant drop in pH produces an unfavorable microenvironment for the majority of pathogenic bacteria attempting to ascend into the bladder (see also discussion of adhesion theory). Lactobacilli and other gram-positive rods are collectively known as Döderlein's bacilli, and disruption of this vaginal flora by vaginitis or other infection leads to a rise in pH and loss of the natural defense barrier. Lactobacilli are one of the main causes of milk going sour and indeed are the active organisms in "live" yoghurt, which for this reason is frequently advocated by health magazines as a topical application that can prevent recurrent lower UTI without the need for antibiotic therapy. Naturally, such protection is not available either before or after the menopause, one fact that possibly explains the increased incidence of ascending lower UTI in elderly women, whose introital skin is oftenthin and atrophic because of lack of circulating estrogens.

Urine

Urine, normally a good culture medium, may under some circumstances be inhibitory or even bactericidal against some uropathogens. Low urinary pH levels in particular, as well as raised blood urea and high osmolarity, are inhibitory for some organisms (3).

Genital Skin

Although strictly unrelated to the urothelium, penetration of the natural barrier afforded by genital skin can have serious consequences for the patient (Fig. 2A, B). Any perforation of penile skin may be followed by infection, but this is particularly the case when the patient is diabetic; such patients are commonly exposed to increased risk during self-administration of vasoactive substances for erectile dysfunction.

Urine Flow

Urine flow from the kidney by ureteric peristalsis and from the bladder by periodic detrusor contraction constitutes the main defense mechanism of the urinary tract against ascending infection (4). Loss of competence at the vesicoureteric junction for any reason may lead under certain circumstances to significant renal damage; additionally, reflux prevents efficient bladder emptying, thus compromising the flushing mechanism of micturition, which is similarly impeded by any form of lower urinary tract obstruction.

Bladder Surface Mucin

In a series of experiments on rabbit bladders, Parsons et al. (5–7) proposed that a bladder surface mucin layer consisting of a glycosaminoglycan (GAG) was secreted by transitional cells and acted as an "anti-adherence factor" by inhibiting bacterial attachment to bladder mucosa, thereby facilitating removal of bacteria by the voiding process. These workers demonstrated that removal of the GAG layer by acid

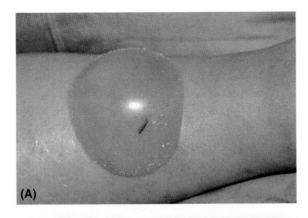

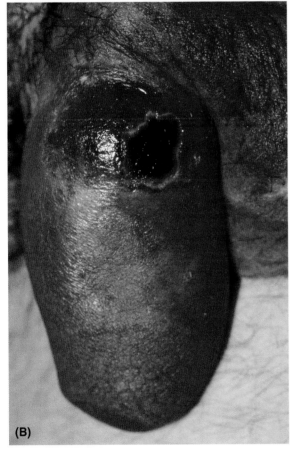

Figure 2 The importance of skin epithelial integrity. **(A)** Large blister on forearm—no infection within perfect subblister culture medium because of integrity of ultrathin residual epithelial covering. **(B)** Puncture site of intracavernosal therapy in diabetic—despite full precautions, serious widespread inflammation has taken place.

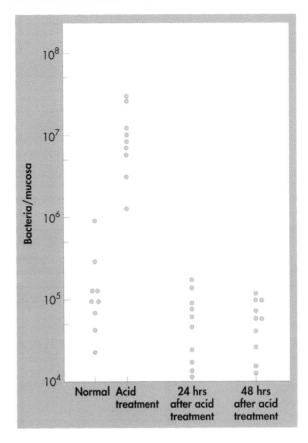

Figure 3 Effect of bladder surface mucin. Binding of 14C-labelled *Escherichia coli* to normal bladder mucosa and acid-treated mucosa. Acid treatment removes the mucin layer, and bacterial adhesion to the bladder mucosa increases significantly. Twenty-four hours after acid treatment, the mucin layer has recovered sufficiently to prevent epithelial attachment (rabbit bladder). *Source*: From Ref. 8.

markedly increased adhesion to the urothelium (Fig. 3) and, furthermore, that instillation of heparin (a synthetic GAG) into bladders previously denuded of their GAG layer by acid resulted in restoration of the antimucosal adherence properties. Pretreatment of the bacteria with heparin had no effect on adherence, and the authors concluded that the surface mucin provided a protective barrier for the urothelium, thus preventing bacterial adherence to the uroepithelial cells. Subsequently, the bacteria trapped in the GAG layer are expelled by urination (5–7).

Tamm-Horsfall Protein

Tamm-Horsfall protein is secreted by the cells of the ascending loop of Henle and is the most common mucoprotein of renal origin in urine. Also known as uromucoid, Tamm-Horsfall protein was originally noted to react with influenza virus (9), but subsequently, it was established that the protein was capable of binding strongly to *E. coli* expressing type 1 mannose-sensitive fimbriae (10), probably because of mannose-containing side chains within the mucoprotein. After entrapment, it is proposed that the uromucoid/coliform complex is mechanically cleared from the urinary tract by urination. Recent studies confirm that in these circumstances the mannose-binding properties of type I pili are critically related to the FimH tip adhesin (see below) (11).

Mucosal Shedding

Attachment to uroepithelial cells by pathogenic bacteria offers both defense and attack possibilities for host and invading organism alike. Exfoliation rates for bladder mucosal cells under normal conditions of sterile urine are approximately four weeks (12); following infection, greatly increased rates are observed within hours of inoculation, a process apparently linked to FimH adhesion and the apoptotic pathway involving caspases and epithelial cell DNA fragmentation (13,14).

Exfoliation of cells with adherent bacteria (Fig. 4) by bulk flow of urine is likely to be of benefit to the host, although the consequent exposure of less mature epithelial cells may provide an opportunity for colonization and invasion by other uropathogenic organisms. It has been suggested that such sequestration of organisms within deeper layers of the bladder wall might explain problems related to persistent infection in some cases of cystitis (17).

Local Immune Response

The role of immunity in the defense of the urinary tract remains poorly understood. Although considerable

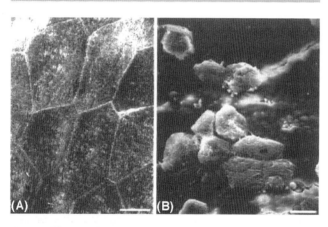

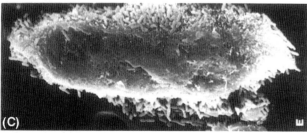

Figure 4 Mucosal shedding of epithelial cells in response to *Escherichia coli* infection. (**A**) Scanning electron micrograph of superficial epithelial cells of uninfected mouse bladder. (**B**) Following infection with type 1 pilated *E. coli*, superficial cells exfoliate, exposing deeper less mature cells. Scale bars 50 μm. (**C**) Magnified view of exfoliated mouse epithelial cell showing vesical surface coated with *E. coli* while the recently separated inferior surface is devoid of organisms (× 440). *Source*: From Refs. 15 and 16.

humoral and cellular response may be observed in upper UTI, serum production of urinary antibody in bladder infection is characteristically difficult to detect, perhaps reflecting the relative superficiality of the infection.

VIRULENCE MECHANISMS

Virulence mechanisms are those properties of the parasite that enable it first to colonize and then flourish within the host. Such mechanisms may be directed against external agents administered to eradicate the organism or against the host itself, including natural host defenses that have developed over time to counter the invading microorganism (Table 5).

Virulence Against External Agents: Antimicrobial Resistance

Before World War II there were few agents with reliable antimicrobial properties, and the virulence capability of organisms was almost entirely directed against the natural properties of the host. After the discovery and clinical usage of penicillin, organisms learnt rapidly to develop systems for evasion of the toxic effects of antibiotics, and the consequent emergence of resistant strains today constitutes a significant threat, particularly for certain groups of the population such as hospital inpatients. *Staphylococcus aureus*, once almost entirely penicillin sensitive, is now approximately 90% resistant to the agent. *Neisseria gonorrheae* remained penicillin sensitive for many years, but its acquisition of β-lactamase activity has resulted in high levels of penicillin resistance. Hospital-based doctors will be well aware of the extremely serious threat posed by methicillin-resistant *S. aureus* (MRSA) infections, which may spread rapidly throughout whole wards and effectively be untreatable. These examples underscore the extreme flexibility and adaptability of the invading microorganism, which, through evolutionary processes, has managed to match and subsequently often overcome the best efforts of scientific antibiotic endeavor.

Types of Resistance

Organisms may acquire antimicrobial resistance by two basic mechanisms. *Intrinsic resistance* means that the organism may naturally resist antibiotics by the production of natural enzymes, such as β-lactamases; or because the usual antibiotic target within the cell is lacking; or by the presence of an impenetrable cell wall. *Acquired resistance* develops as a result of the evolution of new or altered genetic material, which may occur through either mutations or gene transfer.

Table 5 General Classification of Virulence Mechanisms

Against external agents	Antimicrobial resistance
Against the host	Toxin production
	General mechanisms
	Adherence
	mechanisms

Table 6 Target Sites of Common Antimicrobial Drugs

Drug	Target/mechanism
β-Lactams (penicillin, cephalosporin)	Cell wall: disruption of peptidoglycan X-linkage
Aminoglycosides	Ribosomal interference: misreading mRNA
Erythromycin	Translocation interference
Tetracyclines	RNA-binding interference
Trimethoprim	Nucleic acid interference: dihydrofolate reductase inhibition
Fluoroquinolones (ciprofloxacin)	Inhibit DNA gyrase

It is convenient to consider the action of the antibiotic as it relates to bacterial cell structure—cell wall, cytoplasmic membrane, ribosomal function, and nucleic acid synthesis.

Such mutations and transfers result in a number of well-described mechanisms by which the organism may evade the action of the antibiotic.

Enzyme inactivation. β-Lactamase production is the most important resistance mechanism against the penicillins and cepha losporins. The enzyme hydrolyzes the β-lactam bond in the antibiotic structure, rendering it inactive. β-Lactamase production is commonly found in *S. aureus, N. gonorrhea*, and enterobacteria.

Altered permeability. Various alterations in receptor activity and transport mechanisms may prevent access of the antibiotic to the microorganism. Aminoglycosides and tetracyclines are actively taken up into organisms, and resistance may occur either by inactivation of the transport mechanism or by development of additional systems, allowing increased expulsion of the drug from the cell.

Alteration of binding site. Antibiotics may bind to specific targets within the cell. Genetic variation may alter or delete the antibiotic target, thus leading to resistance to the drug. The site of action of the more commonly used antibiotics is summarized in Table 6. The complex nature of antimicrobial resistance determines that a detailed account is beyond the scope of this text; for a comprehensive overview, the reader is referred to definitive studies of resistance mechanisms (18).

VIRULENCE AGAINST THE HOST ITSELF

Toxin Production

Toxins are proteins that are able to harm the cells or tissues of the host. Many organisms elaborate toxins that may either assist with the process of local invasion or be themselves responsible for the characteristics of disease. Important examples of such virulent toxins are those that produce the clinical manifestations of diphtheria, tetanus, and botulism.

A number of organisms, including *E. coli*, exhibit hemolysin activity, which may damage erythrocytes in a variety of ways, including phospholipase C activity (cell-membrane damage) and osmotic lysis. *E. coli* strains commonly associated with UTI (01, 02, 04, 06, 07, 016, 018, and 075) frequently elaborate hemolysins, and such strains may be disproportionately promoted from the colonic reservoir (19,20). Cytotoxic necrotizing factor 1 is another toxin elaborated by pathogenic coliforms to facilitate colonization of the host (21). Despite the strong association of such strains with the ability to cause ascending UTI, the

precise mechanism of enhanced virulence remains unknown.

General Mechanisms

Apart from toxin production, there are a number of general mechanisms that facilitate the organism's attempt to enter and multiply within the host.

1. Penetration
2. Antihumoral activity
3. Evasion of phagocytosis
4. Competition for nutrients

Penetration

In general, organisms are unable to penetrate the intact epithelium of the host unless prior damage (Fig. 2B) has taken place. However, certain parasites may do so, the best example in the urinary tract being the fork-tailed cercariae of *Schistosoma haematobium*, which are able to penetrate unbroken skin for a few hours after being shed by the intermediate snail host (Fig. 5A).

Antihumoral Activity

As noted above, antibodies such as secretory IgA may be active against organisms before mucosal invasion occurs. Organisms such as *N. gonorrheae* and *Proteus mirabilis* elaborate anti-IgA proteases that inactivate this defense mechanism. A further antihumoral virulence factor is exhibited by certain isolates of *N. gonorrheae* that are able to resist the lytic effects of complement. Such strains are thus able to multiply and enter the host bloodstream, whereas those isolates that lack this virulence factor are unable to invade and so remain localized on the surface of the genital tract (22). Resistance to the bactericidal effect of serum/complement has been linked to the integrity of the lipolysaccharide cell wall (O-antigen). Additionally, loss of capsular polysaccharide (K antigen) has been associated with lack of resistance to compliment mediated lysis (23).

Evasion of Phagocytosis

A number of bacteria have developed mechanisms for resisting phagocytic attack by the host. Variation in surface antigens and the properties of some polysaccharide capsules may constitute a successful defense mechanism by preventing interaction between the phagocytic cell and the invading organism (22).

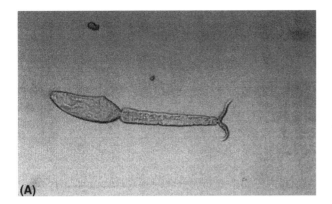

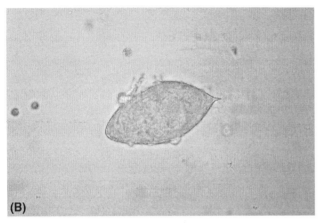

Figure 5 *Schistosoma haematobium*. (**A**) The fork-tailed cercariae have a free-swimming existence of 24 to 28 hours. Intact skin or mucosa may be penetrated, the fork-tailed structure being lost in the process, allowing the organism (now known as a schistosomulum) to reach the subcutaneous tissues. (**B**) The spike-like projection at the end of the egg identifies the organism, in contrast to the projections of *Schist. mansoni*, which are located in the equatorial region. The eggs sequester within the wall of the urinary tract and are shed to the exterior in the urine. Typical egg dimensions of *S. haematobium*: 112/170 × 40/70 μm. *Source*: Courtesy of Dr Allan Curry, UHSM.

Competition for Nutrients

To be successful, any invading microorganism will require an adequate supply of nutrients. In particular, free iron is required for metabolism and multiplication of *E. coli*, iron uptake being facilitated by the siderophore aerobactin and enterobactin (21). The ability to produce these agents thus confirms an advantage on strains invading the urinary tract, and an association has been observed between aerobactin production and the expression of P fimbriae (see below) in patients with symptomatic UTI (24).

Adherence Mechanisms

The adherence of a cell to another structure is an extremely important biological characteristic that can be observed widely throughout nature. Early reports of this phenomenon (25) were slightly misleading, as the particular mechanisms of attachment were not

Table 7   Recognized Adhesion Mechanisms

Afimbrial adhesions
Adherence pedestals
Fimbriae

fully understood at that time. General observations of bacteria and algae adhering to inert plastic or rocks in streams were brought together with other observations of various bacteria adhering in vivo to a number of epithelial surfaces. It is now possible to distinguish the individual mechanisms by which adhesion takes place in each of these specialized circumstances (Table 7). Although fimbriae are of overriding importance in UTI, it is helpful briefly to describe and contrast other methods of adhesion. Adherence is defined as the initial interaction of a microorganism with the host. An adhesin is a microbiological molecule that leads to bacterial adhesion to cells or tissues. Adhesins predominantly react with specific receptors on the host cell surface, although nonspecific adhesion (as by surface charge) may occur (26).

Types of Adhesins

Afimbrial Adhesions

Afimbrial adhesins consist of polymers, polysaccharides, lipoteichoic acid, and other proteins associated with the cell wall of the organism. Collectively, these are known as a "glycocalix," and together they serve to attach the organism to the target cell. The classical studies into glycocalix formation involved *Streptococcus mutans*, an organism that colonizes human teeth, leading to decay. Enzymatic activity at the cell surface degrades sucrose, providing fructose for ongoing nutrition, but it also polymerizes glucose into polysaccharide chains used to construct the glycocalix. Thus, the organism attaches itself to its target, at the same time protecting itself against attack and concentrating its nutrients by wrapping itself within the glycocalix—also known as a "biofilm" (27).

Helicobacter pylori

Helicobacter pylori provides a typical example of an organism that attaches itself via small cellular projections known as adherence pedestals. This organism, with its unmistakable flagella (approximately three times the size of fimbriae; see below), attaches itself to cells within the gastric epithelium, leading to ulceration and perhaps gastric carcinoma (Fig. 6A). Presumably, the flagella drive the organism downward into the mucosa, following which adhesion to the target cells takes place (Fig. 6B).

Fimbriae

Fimbriae (also known as pili) are very important virulence structures that mediate attachment to host tissues and are particularly important in the pathogenesis of *E. coli* UTI. A typical organism may have 100 to 500 appendages, each approximately 5 to 10 nm

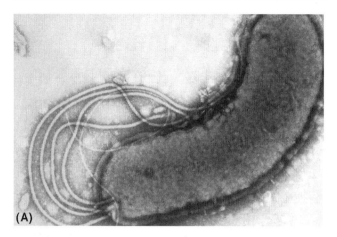

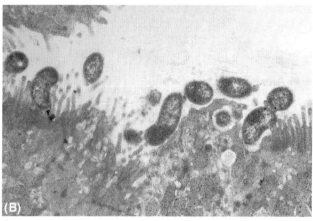

Figure 6 *Helicobacter pylori*. (**A**) The flagella of the organism are easily identified (significantly larger than fimbriae). (**B**) Flagella used to propel organism into gastric mucosa where adhesins provide attachment. *Source*: Courtesy of Dr Alan Curry, UHSM.

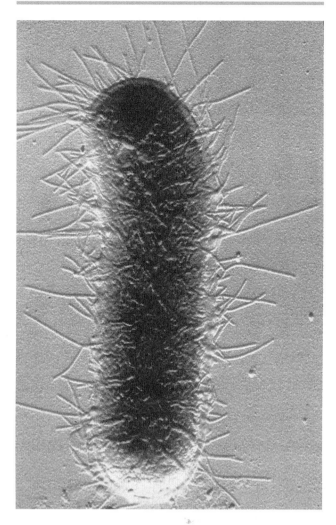

Figure 7 *Escherichia coli*, showing fimbriae. *Source*: Courtesy of Dr Pauline Handley, University of Manchester.

in diameter and 2 μm in length (Fig. 7). Isolates of *E. coli* may produce a number of antigenically distinct fimbriae, although some strains produce no fimbriae at all.

Supramolecular Adhesins Associated with Pathogenic Strains of *Escherichia coli*

Early distinction between types of fimbriae was made by the ability of mannose, respectively, to inhibit (mannose sensitive) or not to inhibit (mannose resistant) the agglutination of guinea pig erythrocytes. For some years, it had been known that type I pili were specifically bound to Tamm-Horsfall protein (10) and foreign bodies such as catheters and prosthetic implants (28). More recently, a variety of techniques, including hemagglutination, electron microscopy, X-ray crystallography, and molecular methodologies, have enabled a more precise identification of a number of specific adhesion organelles that are recognized as critically important virulence factors for uropathological *E. coli* (UPEC) (Table 8).

Type I Fimbriae

These structures are the most common adhesion organelles found on pathogenic coliforms isolated from the urinary tract (32). They are of variable length (1–2 μm) and approximately 7 nm thick, being of helical construction (Fig. 8). The FimH terminal adhesin is a two-domain protein approximately 3 nm in width to which mannose-containing glycoprotein receptors can attach (33,34). Uroplakin (UP1a) is a complex glycoprotein that covers the internal surface of the bladder in a form of membrane or plaque (35). This and other related compounds (UP1b, UPII and UPIII) are the primary receptors (docking sites) for the type I pilus of pathogenic bacteria (34) (Table 8). The defensive role of Tamm-Horsfall protein, which preferentially binds type I pili, has been mentioned above (11).

Initiation of the Infective Process

Traditionally, pathogenic coliforms were considered to exert their influence by epithelial adherence and

Table 8 Adhesin and Receptor Characteristics Identified in Pathogenic Coliform Infections

Organelle	Guinea pig hemaglutination characteristic	Adhesin		Host receptors	Host cells	Clinical disease
Type I fimbriae	Inhibited by mannose (mannose sensitive)	Fim H		Uroplakin 1a (mannosylated glyco protein), Tamm-Horsfall protein (uromucoid), collagen types I, IV, laminin, fibronectin	Bladder:kidney: buccal epithelial cells, erythrocytes, neutrophils, foreign bodies (i.e., catheters)	Cystitis Sepsis
Type P fimbriae	Not inhibited by mannose (mannose resistant)	PapG Epitope Class	I	Globo**tria**osylceramide	Kidney epithelial cells	Not in human Pyronephritis
			II	Globo**tetra**ceramide (globoside)		
			III	Globo**penta**ceramide (Forssmann antigen)	Human P blood group antigen	Cystitis
S/F1C fimbriae		Sfas SfaA/FocH		α-sialyl-2,3-β-galactoside Plasminogen Lactosylceramide	Bladder/kidney Epithelial cells Erythrocytes	Ascending UTI Sepsis Meningitis
Dr adhesins		Various		Type IV collagen α5β, integrin	Bladder/kidney Epithelial cells	Cystitis Diarrhea Sepsis

The description of the organelle, the characteristic of the tip adhesin and specific host receptor "docking port" on particular host cells are tabulated. The critical chemical structure of the PapG receptor has been emphasized by bold underlined text. For further details concerning the site of the disaccharide Gal-Gal core receptor, see Ref. 29. Globo A is similar but not identical to the Forssmann antigen and has been investigated as part of comparative receptor studies.
Source: From Refs. 15, 21, 30, and 31.

subsequent metabolic disruption as a result of factors expressed from the epithelial locus. Recent work suggests that under certain circumstances coliform organisms may become opportunistic intracellular pathogens. Using human bladder epithelial cells, Martinez and coworkers observed cellular invasion by organisms expressing type I pili, but not by those with type G pili (36). The process required FimH-activated submembranous actin organization, phosphoinositide 3-kinase activation and tyrosine phosphorylation (Fig. 9A). Such internalization might allow (assuming no shedding) the organisms to replicate in the relative shelter (vacuole) of the uroepithelial cell, thus propagating the infective process. Similar observations have been made relating to bacterial survival within host macrophages (37). Recent studies (38) have shown the sophistication of such intracellular bacterial communities (IBCs) wherein UPEC are able to adjust virulence systems including iron acquisition mechanisms and various adhesins that may be up- or downregulated presumably to give the organism a survival advantage on release (Fig. 9B). *Klebsiella pneumoniae* may also form IBCs though expression of type I pili is minimal as compared with UPEC (39) (see below).

Expression of Type I Pili

Expression of adhesins can be markedly affected by a wide variety of factors, including environmental cues, adhesin "cross-talk" and the adherence environment in which the organism is placed; coliforms in liquid culture (no adherence required) may fail to develop any adhesion organelles at all.

Schwan and coworkers varied growth conditions and found that fewer type I pili were expressed in a low-pH/high-osmolarity environment (40). Other cues include temperature change, oxygen tension, and nutrient availability. Transcription of type I fimbrial genes is controlled by a promoter located on an invertible element; during UTI, the orientation of the element ("on") that allows the expression of type I pili was maximal at 24 hours, suggesting that the switch (phase variation) was a significant virulence mechanism in the early stages of an infection (41). Expression of organelles is also significantly affected by other adhesins that may be present on the bacterium. PapB, a regulator of type P pilus expression, may modulate type I expression, increasing the "off" phase noted above (42). Such interpilus variations may enable the organism to adapt and change targets; for example, such a mechanism would be advantageous for a PapP pathogenic organism trying to reach the upper tracts via the epithelial barrier of the bladder.

Further studies have explored the complex relationship between type I pilus expression and motility as related to flagellum expression. The presence of type I pili significantly reduced flagella expression and motility while loss of type I surprisingly did not result in increased motility (43).

Type P Fimbriae

P fimbriae are particularly important in disease of the upper urinary tract, and their clinical significance is discussed below. It has already been noted that some pathogenic organisms may variably express both type I

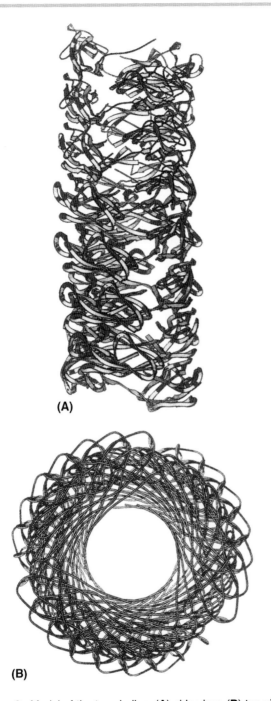

Figure 8 Model of the type I pilus. (**A**) side view; (**B**) top view. External diameter approximately 70 Å. FimH tip adhesin; rod predominantly FimA subunits. *Source*: Courtesy of Ref. 33.

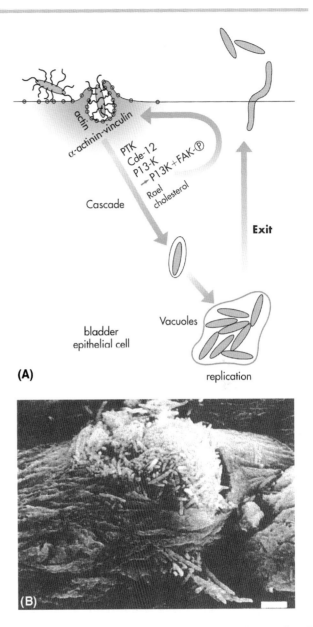

Figure 9 (**A**) Possible mechanism of type I pilus-mediated invasion of bladder epithelial cells. FimH adhesion to cell surface triggers envelopment followed by activation of a cascade involving protein tyrosine kinases, PI-3 kinases and Cdc 42. The transduction cascade facilitates the internalization of the organism within membrane-bound vacuoles that protect it from host defense mechanisms. The organisms replicate within the intracellular environment, effectively converting the epithelial cell into a "bacterial factory." (**B**) Finally, the organisms burst out and are released from the surface of the epithelial cell. Note smaller rupture at base of cell with emerging rod-like organisms. Bar 5 μm. *Source*: Courtesy of Refs. 15, 17, and 36.

and P pili (44), a factor that may complicate attempts to identify virulence factors by in vitro bacterial studies.

Structure and Ultrastructure of P Fimbriae

Advances in molecular biology have enabled the structure of P fimbriae to be elucidated (Fig. 10). The Pap pili (*p*ili *a*ssociated with *p*yelonephritis) essentially consist of four proteins, PapA, PapE, PapF and PapG, constructed and assembled on a platform of PapC protein, the fiber being 7 nm wide. PapG is chiefly responsible for binding to the receptor, while protein PapA constitutes the bulk of the "stem" of the pilus,

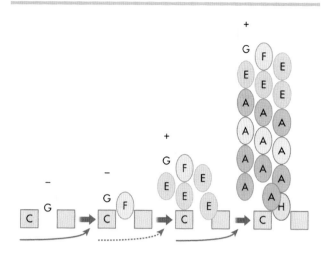

Figure 10 Pilus assembly and structure. The Pap pilus is constructed and assembled on a platform of PapC protein. The adhesion characteristics are chiefly determined by the terminal PapG protein, which must be some distance from the platform before it is able to function (−, no adhesion; +, able to adhere). The PapA subunits are formed in an helical fashion into the stem of the pilus, the entire structure being approximately 1000 subunits long. *Source*: From Ref. 45.

approximately 1000 subunits being arranged in a helical fashion between the surface of the organism and the active tip proteins (21). Experimental observations suggest that the adhesion characteristics are maintained by the GFE tip proteins even in the absence of the helical structure of PapA stem subunits. It has been suggested that the reason for the seemingly dispensable fiber structure is that this length places the adhesin outside the lipopolysaccharide cell surface structure of *E. coli* (see below), thus maintaining the integrity of the individual virulence mechanisms (45).

Recent advances in the understanding of the receptor structure for the G tip protein are leading to significant advances in knowledge concerning the mechanisms of UTI. Table 8 annotates the globoseries glycolipid isoreceptor types, each of which contains the disaccharide α-GAL-1-4-β-GAL (known colloquially as GAL-GAL), and their association with disease. Different positioning of the disaccharide within the molecule in each of the isoreceptors determines the adherence capability of the G tip proteins. Organisms with class I tip proteins do not adhere and do not cause disease in man because of the absence of the globo isoreceptor. Those with class II are strongly associated with pyelonephritis, while class III adhesins are commonly found in patients with cystitis (29). Hence, the structure of the globo isoreceptor determines the outcome between invading organism and host—patients with infections from coliforms expressing class II adhesins are unlikely to suffer from cystitis, globoside being the major isoreceptor in the human kidney (46). Similarly, the association of class III adhesion with cystitis suggests a predominance of Forssman receptors on the urothelium of the lower

urinary tract. Further studies of receptor expression by means of differential blood group analysis (30) have demonstrated that minor differences in receptor core structure profoundly affect disease patterns, and emphasize the importance of precise "fitness" if bacteria are to persist and multiply within the lower urinary tract (31). However, the complexity of the relationship between PapG adhesins and their receptors on target cells has recently been reemphasized. Most *E. coli* express a single fimbrial type at any one time while loss may promote another, a form of compensatory virulence. The multiple renal putative targets for Pap pili are mentioned below; this and the variable surface adhesion expression of experimental coliforms make specific conclusions as to the etiology of infectious disease problematical (47,48). Nevertheless, despite the complexity of adhesin/receptor interactions, the importance played by nonspecific mechanisms, such as electrostatic and hydrophobic attractive forces, should not be overlooked (46).

Historical Relevance of Fimbrinated Status

Long before the mechanisms of adherence were fully understood, observational studies had indicated a connection between the macroscopically observed bacterial adherence and severity of UTI. This phenomenon was first reported in *The Lancet* in 1976 by Catharina Svanborg Eden and colleagues from the Department of Immunology in Göteborg, Sweden, a department that has continued at the forefront of adherence research. Uroepithelial cells from freshly voided morning urine samples were added to bacterial cells, and the mixture was incubated during rotation for 60 minutes. Adherent bacteria (Fig. 11) were counted under direct light microscopy. The results (Fig. 12) demonstrated convincingly that pyelonephritic strains were more adherent than strains from other disorders of the lower urinary tract (49). This effect was negated when the organisms were incubated with antibodies against the strain tested. Two years later the same laboratory described hairlike appendages (Fig. 7), which might have been responsible for the effect (50). These observations were extended by Fowler and Stamey, who studied adherence to vaginal cells from controls and from women susceptible to lower UTI (Fig. 13). Significant adherence was demonstrated, suggesting the possibility that general cellular characteristics might be involved in the adherence process (51). This concept was taken further by Schaeffer and coworkers, who confirmed the findings on vaginal cells and then showed that the same phenomenon could be observed on buccal cells (Fig. 14). These observations clearly indicated that there might be a widespread alteration in the surface characteristics of mucosal epithelial cells in particular susceptible individuals (52).

Previously, Sellwood and coworkers at the Veterinary Agricultural Research Council had noted that *E. coli* strains expressing K-88 surface antigen caused neonatal diarrhea when administered to some piglets, but not others. This phenomenon was observed to be because of K-88 adherence to intestinal cell brush

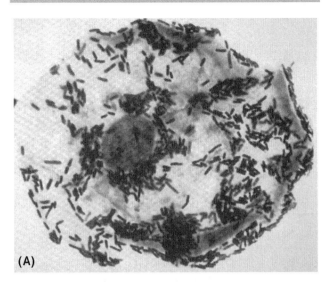

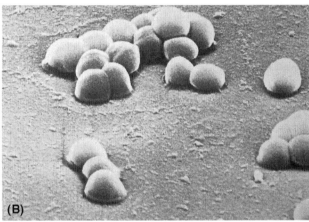

Figure 11 Examples of bacterial adherence. (**A**) Adherence of *Escherichia coli* to epithelial cell. (**B**) Adhesion of colonies to the surface of a urinary catheter. Such adhesion is thought to be mediated by type 1 fimbriae. *Source*: From Ref. 28.

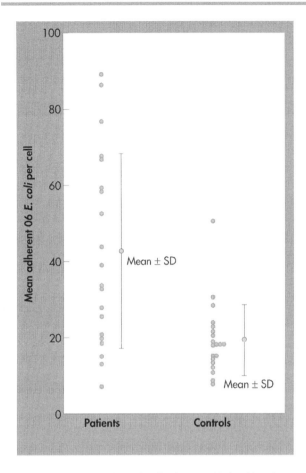

Figure 12 *Escherichia coli* adhering to 40 healthy, human, urinary tract epithelial cells. Organisms from patients with ABU adhered minimally when compared with those from cases of pyelonephritis. *Source*: From Ref. 49.

borders in piglets that developed diarrhea, while those that remained well did not show this phenomenon (53,54). Subsequently, it was found that "adhesive" and "nonadhesive" piglets inherited these intestinal cellular characteristics in a simple Mendelian manner, and these findings have since been acknowledged as the first report of a genetic basis for resistance to enteric disease (55). Schaeffer, quoting this work, noted that it might explain in part why some patients' resistance to infectious disease could correlate with their blood groups (56).

Subsequent ability to identify P-fimbriated varieties of *E. coli* allowed further investigation into the mechanisms of UTI. Källenius et al. (57) examined 97 children with UTI and compared them with 82 healthy controls. P-fimbriated forms were found in 33/35 (91%) of urinary strains causing acute pyelonephritis, but in only 19% of patients with cystitis and 14% of cases with asymptomatic bacteriuria (ABU). By contrast, only 7% of fecal isolates from healthy controls carried such fimbriae. Further evidence of the importance of P fimbriation was observed by Johnson et al. (58), who investigated host conditions that might be associated with increased frequency of P fimbriae or other virulence factors. These studies clearly showed that, while P-fimbriated forms remained relatively common in the presence of anatomical urinary tract abnormality or after instrumentation, the fimbriated form was absolutely essential if infection was to occur when none of these predisposing abnormalities were present. In summary, coliform strains with a variety of characteristics are capable of causing upper UTI in the presence of (i.e., with the help of) obstruction or other abnormalities; however, for infection to supervene in a completely normal upper urinary tract, the presence of the P-fimbriated form of *E. coli* is almost essential. Nevertheless, other adhesins have been mapped to other "docking" molecules at various sites within the human kidney (Fig. 15), underscoring the complexity of ascending UPEC infection in the urinary tract.

Recently, in an elegant experiment, Wullt and coworkers examined the ability of P fimbriae to

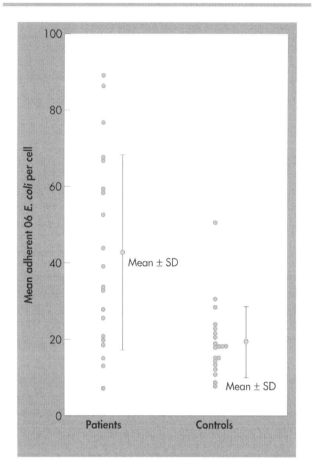

Figure 13 In vitro adherence of *Escherichia coli* to vaginal epithelial cells in patients susceptible to recurrent UTI compared with controls. *Source*: From Ref. 51.

induce inflammation in the human urinary tract, and at the same time they sought to satisfy Koch's "molecular" postulates linking P pilus expression to the host inflammatory response. Koch's postulates state that, from diseased tissue, isolates should be recoverable, be reproducible in culture and, on reintroduction to a susceptible host, be the cause of further recognizable disease. At molecular level, the same postulates can be examined with respect to various factors such as the putative virulence mechanisms of the coliform bacillus.

It has already been noted that P fimbriation is associated with pyelonephritis in approximately 90% of cases, but in 20% of patients with ABU (57,60,61). Nevertheless, other adhesins—type I, type S, and Dr adhesins—may also be isolated from patients with upper tract infection, and the question arises as to which of these characteristics is the preeminent cause of disease. However, other lines of evidence (the ability to enter the bloodstream, to enhance experimental infection and to promote a cytokine response) suggest strongly that P fimbriae are indeed the significant independent virulence factors. To resolve this problem, 17 human volunteers received intravesical inoculation of either a nonfimbriated ABU coliform strain or Pap transformants of the same strain, the former acting as control to negate the possibility of nonspecific adhesin formation linked to DNA sequences carried by the ABU strain. The result (Fig. 16) demonstrated that the presence of the Pap transformants invariably caused higher neutrophil and cytokine responses; furthermore, loss of Pap expression was linked to a reduction in background inflammatory levels. Control strains did not cause a significant host response. Taken as a whole, the results provided convincing evidence that P fimbriation per se converted a low- into a high-virulence strain, suggesting in turn that Koch's molecular postulates were indeed fulfilled (62).

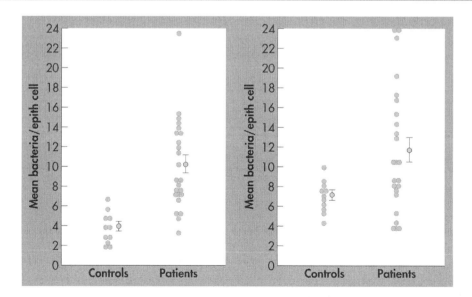

Figure 14 In vitro adherence of *Escherichia coli* to vaginal cells (*left panel*) and buccal cells (*right panel*) from patients with recurrent UTIs as compared with controls. *Source*: From Ref. 52.

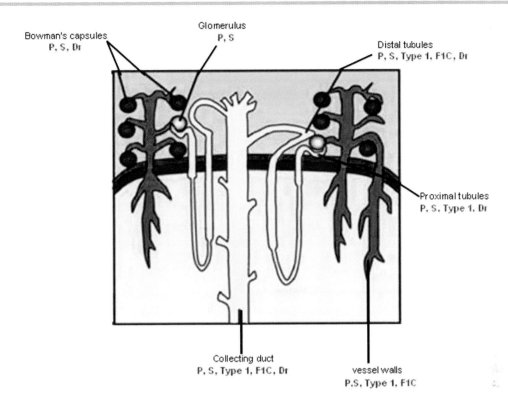

Figure 15 Binding sites of various *Escherichia coli* adhesins in the human kidney. The complexity of variable adhesin expression on uropathogenic *E. coli* and the possible relationship to pyelonephritis can be appreciated. Adhesins in red. *Source*: Courtesy of Ref. 59.

Type S Pili

Less well defined than the preceding types of pili, S types nevertheless share a similar structure of Sfa A subunits, with the Sfa S subunit localized to the tip and interacting with sialic acid receptors on renal vascular and epithelial cells. The fimbriae may facilitate bacterial dissemination, and the type has been associated with pathogenic strains that are associated with sepsis and meningitis as well as ascending UTI (63). FIC pili are homologous with type S and may be present on approximately 14% of pathogenic coliforms.

Dr Adhesin Family

The family includes both pilus-like adhesin Dr and nonfimbrial adhesion molecules. Their function remains open to question, but they can be isolated in a high proportion of children with UTI and one-third of pregnant women with pyelonephritis. They may be responsible for long-term bacterial persistence within the upper tract (64).

Clinical Aspects of Adhesion Theory

The ability to adhere and thus to persist within the host is an advantage to the microorganism in a number of circumstances; it helps the pathogen to remain within its source (reservoir), survive during the journey to the target tissue, and establish and replicate on

arrival within the lower urinary tract. Receptors for P fimbriae have been identified within the colon, and this attachment mechanism has been proposed to explain persistence of pathogenic organisms within the reservoir (65). Such strains expressing Pap established themselves more rapidly in children susceptible to UTI than organisms without the adhesin (61). Recent studies of cystitis in young schoolgirls (66), chosen (by age) to exclude the effect of sexual intercourse, observed that the clones of organisms responsible for the infection were P fimbriated, whereas those forms were not usually found on the perineum—where clones exhibiting type I fimbriae and other virulence factors predominated. These observations, when summarized, indicate that both type I and type P fimbriae are commonly found in the fecal reservoir, as well as the periurethral zone, and may variously facilitate the initial move toward the lower urinary tract. Clearly, phase variation, cross-talk, and an altered microenvironment (the effect of *L. acidophyllus* is noted above) may significantly alter fimbrial expression (Fig. 17), both to evade host defenses and maintain optimal pathogenicity en route to the target cells. Needless to mention, this ability rapidly to vary expression makes the study of virulence factors particularly difficult for microbiological researchers. Hence, it is not entirely clear which virulence factors are responsible for colonization and development of clinical disease in the lower urinary tract. Certainly, the variability mentioned above means that it is difficult at this time to

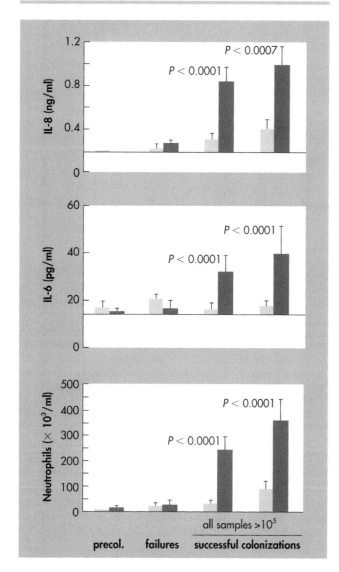

Figure 16 Neutrophil, IL-6 and IL-8 responses to intravesical inoculation with ABU *Escherichia coli* 83972 nonfimbriated strain (*gray bars*) and the same *E. coli* 83972 strain transformed with recombinant plasmids encoding class II or class III P fimbriae (*black bars*). Responses identified in urine; see text for details. *Abbreviation*: Precol, precolonization. *Source*: From Ref. 62.

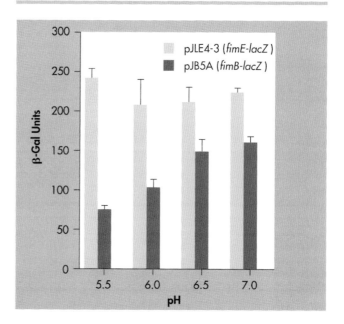

Figure 17 Microenvironment and pathogenicity. Effect of altered pH in human urine on pilus expression. With a sodium phosphate buffer, the expression of FimB almost doubles at pH 7.0, whereas FimE levels remain constant throughout. *Source*: From Ref. 40.

renal pelvis and calyces, a fact that might explain the observed lack of systemic response. Both type I and Pap III/Forsmann antigen mechanisms have been implicated in cystitis, but the interaction remains obscure, as do the various forms of inflammatory responses initiated during infection (37,67). Transmission of the organism and subsequent establishment of clinical disease are clearly highly complex microbiological processes that remain minimally understood at the present time.

Therapeutic Implications

The observations noted above might assist treatment of affected individuals in a number of ways. Variation in adhesion potential might identify at-risk groups. Fimbriae would appear to be a rational target for antimicrobial therapy and vaccine development. In the veterinary piglets experiment referred to above, effective vaccines based initially on the K-88 antigen were developed and successfully prevented neonatal diarrhea in the susceptible groups. Immunization with purified P fimbriae has been attempted in a number of animal models, with variable success. In a primate setting, vaccination with a FimH adhesin–chaperone complex protected three of four treated monkeys while all control animals developed cystitis, suggesting that such techniques might have application in humans with chronic lower UTI (68). As might be expected, phase variation and other types of antigen variability might be expected to cause problems in this type of therapeutic approach.

predict infection on the basis of adhesin analysis of introital or periurethral organisms (66).

Finally, it should be noted that the identification of certain forms of an organism associated with particular tissues does not per se prove a relationship with clinical disease—hence the need to test Koch's postulates. In particular, type I fimbriae are found in a majority of enterobacteria, on both nonpathogenic as well as pathogenic *E. coli*. In the experiments of Wullt and coworkers mentioned above, it was acknowledged that the inflammatory responses induced in urine were not observed systemically, where all patients remained well (62). This, however, was an experiment on the bladder of humans, and not on the acknowledged target of Pap pili, the urothelium of the

Virulence Factors in Other Uropathogens

Not surprisingly, studies of other species involved in UTI have demonstrated the presence of adherence mechanisms. *P. mirabilis* and *Klebsiella* spp. have been found to express fimbriae in animal experiments (69,70), although the fimbrial expression of type I pili is considerably less than that of UPEC, which might explain why *Klebsiella* is a less prevalent agent for UTI than the former organism (39). *Staphylococcus saprophyticus* is known to be able to adhere avidly to uroepithelial cells, probably by nonspecific adherence mechanisms.

Summary of Virulence Factors in Urinary Tract Infections

It is appropriate to bring together those factors that are thought to be important with respect to the virulence of gram-negative bacteria in general and *E. coli* in particular (Fig. 18 and Table 9).

The antigenic structure of the bacterial surface is classically described in terms of three classes of antigens. O-Antigens represent the polysaccharide side chains of the lipopolysaccharide structure found in all gram-negative bacteria. The polysaccharide is anchored to the outer membrane by lipid A (Fig. 18),

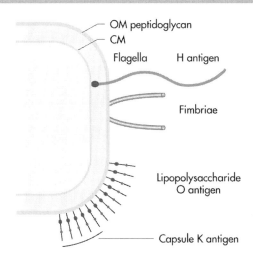

Figure 18 Schematic diagram of cell-wall gram-negative bacteria and associated structures. *Abbreviations*: CM, cytoplasmic membrane; OM, outer membrane. Note differential size of flagella and fimbriae. Lipid A (see text) is on the innermost aspect of the lipopolysaccharide O antigen, next to the outer membrane (see also Fig. 28).

Table 9 Virulence Factors Associated with *Escherichia coli*

Specific O serotypes
K capsular antigen
Adherence mechanisms
Resistance to serum bactericidal activity
Hemolysin production
Aerobactin production
Colicin V

the agent thought to be responsible for endotoxic shock, as described below. O-antigens are heat stable and classically certain serogroups (01, 02, 04, 06, 07, 016, 018, and 075) responsible for urinary infections, such strains being responsible for up to 80% of cases of pyelonephritis. Modern theory suggests that the O-antigen is not itself specifically responsible for pathogenicity; rather, the identified serogroups represent clones of organisms with a selection or panel of various virulence properties that enable successful colonization of the urinary tract. Other serogroups and hence other combinations of virulence factors may enable successful colonization of other areas such as the gastrointestinal tract. K capsular antigen is partially heat stable and may, on occasion, partially obscure the O-antigen (Fig. 18). K capsular polysaccharide antigen has been strongly associated with pyelonephritis for many years, both in adults (71) and in children (72). Some 70% of strains from children with pyelonephritis were associated with K1, K2, K3, K12, and K13 antigens, of which K1 is acknowledged to be the most frequently associated strain with pyelonephritic disease. Interestingly, K1 strains have also been associated with 80% of *E. coli* strains causing neonatal meningitis (72).

Adherence mechanisms have been fully described above, and the relationship between type 1 fimbriae and P fimbriae and their ability to cause UTI have been noted. Typically, *E. coli* may be killed by serum bactericidal activity relating to both the classical and alternative pathway of complement. Cell wall lipopolysaccharide (O-antigen) is thought to provide a degree of resistance against complement-mediated digestion, and, recently, Leying and associates have suggested that the K1 polysaccharide antigen may also confer significant levels of serum resistance on the organism (23). The advantages conferred on those organisms expressing hemolysin and aerobactin have been noted above. Colicin V is another virulence factor that has selectively been found to be present in isolates from urine, but not from isolates in the fecal reservoir. Colicin V is assumed to interfere with host defense mechanisms (19,20).

ORGANISMS RESPONSIBLE FOR URINARY TRACT INFECTION

The great majority of UTIs are caused by single bacterial species; among these, *E. coli* is by far the most common, accounting for approximately 85% of general or community-based infections at the present time. Previous studies (Table 10) have emphasized the differences between general practice and hospital practice, where *E. coli* accounts for only approximately 50% of the isolates. *Proteus*, *Klebsiella*, enterococci, and *Pseudomonas* are all more frequently isolated from hospital patients, especially if an in-dwelling catheter is present (73,74). Remaining organisms include *Enterobacter*, *Citrobacter*, and *Serratia*; fungal infections are rarely encountered outside hospital practice. These classical studies, though dated, serve to emphasize the differing bacteriological environments between

Table 10 Organisms Causing Urinary Tract Infection in Community and Hospital Practice

	General practice		Hospital practice	
	1976	1971	1971	1978
Escherichia coli	72	78.5	55.4	50.7
Proteus mirabilis	9	9.2	11.4	10.6
Staphylococci	6	5.1	3.3	2.7
Streptococcus faecalis	3.3	2.3	4.0	4.3
Klebsiella spp.	2.7	2.3	16.8	21.6
Pseudomonas	–	–	2.7	2.8
Remainder	7.0	2.6	6.4	7.3

Although the proportions of organisms have remained relatively similar, it is accepted that in the 1990s approximately 80% to 85% of community UTI was related to *E. coli*. The comparable figure for hospital-based infections has remained steady at approximately 50%. *Source*: Data from Refs. 73 and 74.

hospital and community that has only partially been affected by the publicity surrounding the "superbug" threats of MRSA and *Clostridium difficile*.

The presence of abnormalities in the urinary tract, as may be found in congenital abnormality or obstruction, often leads to infection by noncoliform organisms, such as *Proteus and Klebsiella*, and, under these circumstances, mixed infections are also frequently encountered. Naturally, obstruction related to stone formation is often associated with *P. mirabilis*. *S. saprophyticus* has been identified, particularly in the United States of America, as a cause of acute cystitis in young, sexually active females (75). Anaerobic organisms are rarely pathogens in the urinary tract. Maskell et al. supported the concept that slow-growing CO_2-dependent, gram-positive bacteria might be responsible for the "urethral syndrome" (76), although these suggestions that "fastidious" organisms could be responsible for the symptom complex were strongly denied by other workers (77). Apart from lactobacilli, *Gardinerella vaginalis* and *Ureaplasma urealyticum* are not infrequently isolated, but their role in infection of the lower urinary tract remains unproven.

Routes of Infection

Organisms may enter the urinary tract via the ascending route, the hematogenous route, or the lymphatic route.

Ascending Route

The difference in the incidence of lower UTI between men and women strongly suggests that the ascending urethral route is the most common pathway for infection; in the female, organisms have been isolated from the bladder after both urethral massage (78) and sexual intercourse (79). One insertion of a urinary catheter into the bladder has been observed to result in lower UTI in 1% to 2% of patients (80). It is widely agreed that the presence of a urethral catheter for more than 36/48 hours almost invariably results in bladder bacteriuria. Recent studies suggest that spermicidal agents encourage the colonization of the introital region with uropathogenic bacteria (81). The

relationship between the introital flora and lower UTI is further considered below.

The question of ascent into the upper tract from the bladder in the absence of reflux appears problematical. Presumably, various virulence factors must aid progression through the vesicoureteric junction; perhaps mucosal edema caused by local inflammation disrupts the valvular mechanisms and allows passage of organisms, which then successfully colonize the upper tracts by means of the appropriate fimbriated structures. Diuresis and loss of the usual coapting ureteral mechanisms have also been suggested as a mechanism whereby organisms may gain entry into the upper tract.

Hematogenous Route

Blood-borne infection of the kidney is a well-described, though uncommon, mechanism of renal infection in individuals who are otherwise normal. Staphylococcal spread from dental abscesses may occur, and these and other organisms may originate from sites such as diseased heart valves. Hematogenous spread of *Candida albicans* has been observed in experimental circumstances, although this fungus is not usually observed unless a chronic in-dwelling catheter is present. Interestingly, if one ureter is tied and bacteria are introduced into the bladder during experimentation on animals, infection supervenes in the nonobstructed kidney, but not on the hydronephrotic side (82). This convincingly demonstrates the overriding importance of the ascending route and the relative resistance to hematological spread, even in the presence of severe obstruction—conditions under which it is acknowledged that hematogenous infection should easily supervene.

Lymphatic Route

Theoretically, infection could spread via lymphatics into various parts of the urinary tract, but, in practice, there is little clinical evidence for such a mode of infection. Occasional experimental reports have failed to convince that the lymphatic route is other than of academic interest.

CLINICAL ASPECTS OF URINARY TRACT INFECTION

The Significance of "Significance"

Historically, there have always been difficulties distinguishing between true bacteriuria, defined as actual residence of bacteria within the urinary tract, and contamination, defined as the adventitious entry of bacteria into the urine during the collection of the specimen. This problem was most notably tackled in the mid-1950s by Edward H. Kass from Boston, who performed a number of studies on women with various disorders of the lower urinary tract in both the normal and pregnant state. In his most important study, the urine of female patients attending as outpatients was studied, specimens being obtained by catheterization and cultured promptly thereafter (83). He found (Fig. 19) that the patients could broadly be divided into two groups. In the first group were patients with bacterial counts between 0 and 100,000/mL of urine; of these, only approximately 15% had a past history of UTI, instrumentation, or catheterization of the urinary tract. He noted that the bacteria obtained in this group were usually the common saprophytes of the urinary tract, and his contention that these were contaminated specimens was further supported by the fact that second samples obtained from the same group usually demonstrated dissimilar organisms and counts.

By contrast, in the second group with more than 100,000 bacteria/mL, 55% had a past history of UTIs, and repeat sampling in these patients revealed similarly high counts, both specimens yielding commonly accepted pathogens of the urinary tract. These simple yet ground-breaking observations define the level of "bacterial significance" widely used to this day—10^5 organisms or colony-forming units (CFU) per milliliter from midstream urine.

For a quarter of a century, the scientific distinction between patients with contaminants and patients with true infection was broadly welcomed. Gradually, however, it became clear that there were a significant number of women with dysuria and frequent urination whose midstream urines did not contain "significant" bacteriuria, and to these women the label "acute urethral syndrome" was applied. In an important study, Stamm et al. investigated 59 women with acute urethral syndrome, from whom bladder urine was obtained either by suprapubic aspiration or clean urethral catheterization. Forty-two patients had abnormal pyuria, and 37 of these were infected with coliforms, *S. Saprophyticus, or Chlamydia trachomatis.* Patients without pyuria had little demonstrable infection. Stamm et al. concluded that the classic Kass criteria of 10^5 CFU/mL was an insensitive diagnostic criterion when applied to symptomatic lower UTI in this group of relatively young, sexually active women (84).

This and other similar studies (85) provoked a flurry of editorial comment (86,87). Doubt was cast over the suggestion that 10^2 CFU/mL organisms could reliably discriminate between patients with infected and uninfected lower urinary tracts. Additionally, it was noted that many midstream urine cultures were mixed—ignoring the conventional wisdom that true pathogens are usually found in pure culture. Nevertheless, it was acknowledged that most of Stamm's bacteriuric patients (10^2, 10^5) had pyuria, suggesting that this was indeed a true infection (60). Stamm himself made further comment and reviewed the situation in 1984 (87). He pointed out that the essence of Kass's original work (often forgotten) concerned patients with pyelonephritis, not women with acute frequency/dysuria lower tract symptoms. He made a plea for closer communication between clinicians and laboratory so as to obtain better information from the more flexible approach to quantitative bacteriological sampling. There is little doubt that urologists should be aware that "no significant growth" may mean different things according to definitions in different bacteriological laboratories. It is the responsibility of each clinician to determine whether such a report refers to 10^5 CFU/mL or 10^2 CFU/mL—as usual, optimum results result only from close cooperation between clinical and laboratory service.

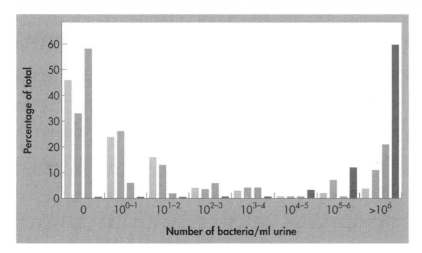

Figure 19 Bacterial counts in urine of various population groups. Kass noted that most of the patients with low counts did not have a history of UTI, and in these cases reculture frequently demonstrated different organisms. However, patients with >105 organisms frequently had pure cultures associated with significant clinical infections (pyelonephritis). *Source*: From Ref. 83.

The Introital Question

Another major microbiological debate concerns the means whereby pathogenic organisms pass from the (presumed) fecal reservoir to the lower urinary tract. In particular, the importance of organisms that colonize the vaginal introitus and periurethral region has been discussed at great length, and the debate continues to the present day.

There seems little doubt that *E. coli*—pathogenic or otherwise—may obtain a foothold in the introital area, and, in this respect, it has been noted above that mannose-sensitive type 1 pili adhere powerfully to vaginal epithelial cells (52), vaginal mucus (88) and uromucoid (10). It has also been emphasized that type 1 fimbriae are to be found on nonpathogenic as well as pathogenic enterobacteria.

Three essential questions may be asked.

1. Do women at risk of UTIs carry pathogenic organisms in the introital and periurethral area?
2. If so, are these organisms responsible for the symptomatic bladder or pyelonephritic infection?
3. In such cases, what is the state of the introital and periurethral area between overt symptomatic clinical infections?

A number of workers support the concept that abnormal periurethral flora are to be found in women with recurrent infections. Hinman's group (89) studied 43 patients and found that the flora contained a higher percentage of pathogenic microorganisms than that of female subjects without urological disease. In a general practice study from London, Grüneberg observed that the infecting strain of *E. coli* was isolated from rectal, vaginal, and periurethral flora in nearly all cases. Furthermore, he noted that chemotherapy eradicated the organism from the urine but not necessarily from the introital/urethral area (90). Stamey studied cultures from 20 premenopausal controls compared with cultures from nine women with recurrent urinary infections (91). He observed that not only was introital colonization significantly higher in the patients, but also enterobacteria persist after the infectious episode, and he postulated that the introital mucosa in women with infection was biologically different from the same area in women who never suffer from lower UTI. This postulate was supported some years later by Pfau and Sacks (92), who had previously shown that the predominant bacterial flora of the introital and periurethral area consisted of lactobacilli

and staphylococci, gram-negative bacteria being infrequent and transitory. These workers found *E. coli* to be the predominant microorganism recovered from 68% of introital, 60% of vaginal, and 42% of urethral cultures.

Despite these apparently conclusive results by American researchers, a number of British workers failed to confirm the findings (93–96). Nevertheless, although an absolute association between periurethral flora and lower UTI could not be demonstrated, it was acknowledged that the presence of *E. coli* in the introital area might constitute a "permissive factor" for the subsequent development of overt infection (93). Similarly, O'Grady et al. could find no difference in the carriage rate between normal women and women with symptoms suggestive of UTI, although, again, these workers acknowledged that introital bacteria were more commonly recovered in patients when symptomatic (34%) than when symptom free (19%)(94). In a further development, Brumfitt and coworkers observed that women with recurrent urinary infections were susceptible to perineal and periurethral colonization with gram-negative bacteria, but they noted that the infection need not be with the colonizing enterobacteria (95). Kunin, in an editorial comment, attempted to reconcile these positions (92) by suggesting that most workers could agree that infections were indeed preceded by colonization of the periurethral area with gram-negative bacteria, but he considered that the evidence for colonization of this area between infections was less convincing. It may be argued that the presence or absence of organisms is not so critical as the ability of any organisms that may be present—that is, the virulence mechanism carried on those organisms—to ascend and invade the lower urinary tract. In summary, colonization is important, but the critical factor relates to the presence or absence of essential virulence mechanisms.

Urinary Tract Infection: Variation by Age and Sex

It is appropriate at this point to review the changes that may occur in the urinary tract of either sex as a result of invasion by microorganisms. Table 11 records the prevalence of bacteriuria by age in either sex as determined by studies in the literature. It is immediately apparent that bacteriuria is more common in females at all times of life, with the single exception of babies under three months old, among whom boys are more than twice as likely to have clinical infection than girls.

Table 11 Prevalence of Bacteriuria by Age (%)

	$<1/12$	$<3/12$	<5	School age	Young men	Nonpregnant females	Pregnant females	Pregnant females (previous bacteriuria)	65–70	>80
Male	0.075	Circumcised, 0.07 Noncircumcised, 0.77	0.5	0.03	<0.1	–	–	–	2–3	>20
Female	0.077	0.3	4.5	1.2	–	1.3	4–7	35	20	>20
Reference	73	73	77	78–82	–	83	82, 71, 85	80, 81	86	86

The identified groups of patients are fully discussed in the text.

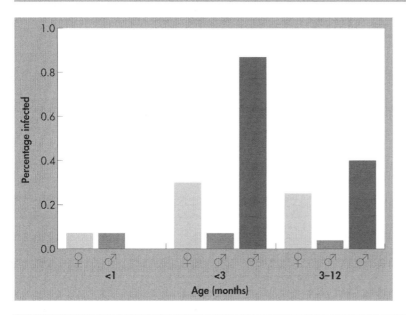

Figure 20 Urinary tract infection in infants under one year. The incidence of infection between sexes is approximately similar under one month, but thereafter girls have more infections than boys unless the boys have not been circumcised. ▨ Circumcised; ▬ uncircumcised. *Source*: From Ref. 97.

Infants

In the first month of life, there is a virtually identical incidence of UTI in girls and boys (97). Interestingly, in infants under three months old, the infection rate in males depends on whether circumcision has been performed. For those who have had the operation, the incidence of infection is significantly less than that of girls of the same age. For uncircumcised infants, however, the risk is considerably greater, and it is clear that the presence of the foreskin is linked to an increased incidence of lower UTI. These observations were made in a remarkable study of 422,328 children born to members of the U.S. services over a 10-year period. Precision military record keeping allowed the result of circumcision to be accurately documented (Fig. 20). A surprising 80% of the male population underwent circumcision, but the 20% who did not suffered 70% of the male UTIs (97). The authors later proved their point by noting that a subsequent decline in the circumcision rate was associated with an increased incidence of male infant infection (98).

Preschool Children

Urinary tract infection is important in children of this age group, as most pediatricians consider renal development to be most at risk at this time. Both symptomatic and asymptomatic infections are more common in girls, although the line between the two is difficult to draw—careful history taking in children with "asymptomatic bacteriuria" often reveals symptoms strongly suggestive of UTI (99). From the first year onward, infections become increasingly uncommon in male infants; indeed, the presence of such an infection may indicate significant disease or other abnormality of the urinary tract. Infections in girls may be troublesome and, as noted above, permanent damage relating to the reflux of

infected urine may occur by mechanisms such as those described by Ransley (100). It is difficult to avoid the conclusion that bacteriuria is a very important finding in this group of children (101).

Bacteriuria in Schoolchildren

As can be seen from Table 11, the problem of bacteriuria in schoolchildren relates almost entirely to girls. There is an impressive body of evidence concerning the nature and outcome of such infections. In Charlottesville, Virginia, an area with a stable local population, Kunin prospectively studied the characteristics and natural history of UTI in schoolgirls between 1959 and 1968. It was observed that bacteriuria was common in schoolgirls and symptoms were often absent; recurrence frequently occurred (102). Approximately one-third of the girls had symptoms of the infection at the time of detection. In the United Kingdom, Meadow et al. reported broadly similar findings in Birmingham schoolchildren. Infection in schoolboys was essentially undetectable, but 1% of girls had significant ABU (103). In another important prospective study, the Cardiff/Oxford bacteriuria study group followed 208 girls from 5 to 12 years of age who had been identified as suffering from bacteriuria. The girls were followed for four years, and the authors noted that treatment had little effect on the emergence of symptoms, the clearance of vesicoureteric reflux, renal growth, or the progression of renal scars. These observations seemed to suggest that renal damage had occurred before five years of age, as noted above (104).

Effect of bacteriuria on subsequent pregnancy. Both Kunin's group and the Oxford/Cardiff group continued to follow their young women as they grew up and eventually became pregnant. These irreplaceable studies have emphasized the importance of vigilance with respect to young bacteriuric schoolgirls.

Gillenwater reported the U.S. results in 1979. Sixty schoolgirls with bacteriuria and 38 matched controls had been followed for periods ranging up to 18 years. Renal scars and/or caliectasis were observed to occur only in the bacteriuric group, but renal function and blood pressure were not affected. The study group had 10 times as many bacteriuric episodes as did controls, and infections were particularly common during subsequent pregnancy. Most interestingly, seven children of the bacteriuric mothers, but none of the controls themselves, showed UTIs (105).

The Oxford/Cardiff group studied 52 pregnancies in 34 women who had been found to have bacteriuria in childhood. At the first antenatal visit, the prevalence of bacteriuria in the study group was significantly greater (35%) than that in the control group (5%). During pregnancy, pyelonephritis developed in 10% of the study group and in 4% of controls. The data suggested that previously bacteriuric women known to have renal scars were at increased risk of hypertension and preeclampsia of pregnancy, findings that have not been universally accepted. No comment was made about the children resulting from these pregnancies and their susceptibility or otherwise to UTI (106).

In summary, therefore, these observations show that ABU in schoolgirls persists over long periods. Subsequently, such young women are at greater risk of infection during pregnancy, and if renal damage has occurred in earlier life, the pregnancy may perhaps be complicated by hypertension or preeclampsia. The children of such women appear to inherit an ongoing susceptibility to bacteriuria and infection.

Young, Nonpregnant Females

It is generally accepted that the prevalence of bacteriuria in this group is approximately 1% per decade. To investigate the assumption that these cases were largely intercourse-related, Kunin's group compared the prevalence of significant bacteriuria in nuns and married women. As expected, they found that celibacy was associated with a lower frequency of infection, but young nuns still had a higher frequency of urinary infection than young males. He commented later that it was not clear from this study whether there was a subpopulation of women who were inherently susceptible to urinary infection that was not the result of sexual intercourse (107).

Bacteriuria During Pregnancy

There is general agreement that 4% to 7% of pregnant women have bacteriuria (108,109), and of these 20% to 40% will develop symptomatic infection later in the pregnancy, usually in the third trimester. Bacteriuria in the lower urinary tract more commonly leads to pyelonephritis in pregnant than nonpregnant women, presumably because of the various changes that occur in the upper tracts as a result of the pregnancy. The prevalence of bacteriuria during pregnancy rises with parity, sexual activity, age, diabetes mellitus, and sickle-cell trait. It has already been mentioned that

pregnant women who were bacteriuric as schoolgirls carry a significantly greater risk of UTI during pregnancy (104,105).

Urinary Tract Infection in Young Adult Men

As previously emphasized, UTI in otherwise healthy adult men is very uncommon. Presumably, the large difference in prevalence between men and women is related to the length of the urethra and the difficulties that face uropathogens attempting to reach the urethral meatus from the fecal reservoir. The antibacterial nature of prostatic fluid is noted below. Presumably, most infections that occur arise because of sexual intercourse with an infected female partner, or, in the case of homosexuality, direct contamination from the fecal reservoir.

Older Patients

The bias in favor of female patients that operates throughout most of life begins to reverse in old age. Presumably because of prostatic obstruction, residual urine, and other problems in the lower urinary tract of older men, the incidence of bacteriuria rises steeply to significant levels, particularly after the age of 70 (Table 11). It has been observed that the place of residence has an important influence on the presence or otherwise of bacteriuria. Older men living at home have a lesser incidence of bacteriuria than those living in nursing homes, where the prevalence in both sexes is approximately 20%. Figures for those resident in hospital inpatient facilities are even higher (110).

Uncomplicated Cystitis in Females

Approximately 20% of women experience an episode of simple cystitis during their lifetime. Most of these settle rapidly, but 2% to 3% suffer from repeat infections. In a Danish study, nonpregnant women 16 to 65 years of age were referred to the medical outpatient clinic, where a placebo study of patients with acute symptomatic lower UTI was undertaken. Fifty-three female patients were given placebo and were followed for longer than 12 months following the initial infection; 43 of these (81%) spontaneously cleared their urine within 5 months (111). Unfortunately, nearly half these patients became reinfected within a year, and similar observations were found in the antibiotic-treated group. The author concluded that host defense and eradication mechanisms could be very effective, but to keep recurrence of bacteriuria to a minimum, it would be necessary to recheck urine samples for at least six months after the initial elimination of bacteriuria.

Typically, uncomplicated lower UTI is caused by *E. coli* in 80% of domicillary cases. *S. saprophyticus* may be implicated in up to 5% of cases, this organism being particularly noted in the literature from North America. The causes of the acute urethral syndrome, as reported by Stamm et al., have already been noted (84). It seems reasonable that a pure growth of organism at concentrations between 10^2 and 10^5 accompanied by pyuria, should be accepted as a case of true cystitis. The case of bladder urine with mixed organisms and equivocal pyuria is much more debatable; these may perhaps be better described as equivocal cystitis, in contradistinction to the true urethral syndrome described below in which the symptoms of urethral irritation are accompanied neither by organisms nor by pyuria—the female equivalent of "prostatodynia."

The Urethral Syndrome

A critical definition of the female urethral syndrome refers to the symptoms of frequency and dysuria in the absence of bacteriuria and pyuria in both initial [voided bladder 1 (VB1)] and midstream (VB2) urine when analysis is made on several separate occasions. This definition assumes that such female patients have been thoroughly screened to exclude vesical motor dysfunction (bladder overactivity) as well as systemic and local (such as trauma, tumor and irradiation injury) disease (112).

A number of workers have stressed the importance of pyuria in patients with such urethral symptomatology. O'Grady et al. (113) proposed that pyuria was significant even when tests failed to identify bacteriuria. In their studies, if cultures were performed over extended periods, bacteria were eventually identified; thus, this patient group was designated as being "between infections" (113). *C. trachomatis* was identified in 10 of 16 patients with pyuria, but in only one of 16 patients without white cells in the urine (57). The controversy surrounding more fastidious carbon dioxide–dependent organisms—chiefly lactobacilli—has also been noted (76). In summary, although considerable effort may be required, the presence of pyuria may often give a clue as to the true bacteriological cause of the frequency dysuria syndrome. Those who have neither bacteriuria nor pyuria constitute the essential core of those who are said to suffer from the true urethral syndrome.

Pyelonephritis

The clinical, radiographic, and therapeutic aspects of acute and chronic pyelonephritis are beyond the remit of this work. The important virulence factors that enable colonization of the upper tract have been noted, as have those factors in childhood that later predispose to pyelonephritis of pregnancy. It is generally agreed that uncomplicated pyelonephritis in adults—as opposed to infants under five years—rarely leads to permanent and progressive renal damage with scarring. Renal function usually remains stable.

Stones and Infection

Most urinary infections are caused by *E. coli*, but a substantial minority—around 10%—may be because of *P. mirabilis*, which is also found in the normal fecal flora. Most patients with simple *Proteus* infections do not form stones, but stone formation is a risk, this being particularly high when stones are already present. Urease-producing bacteria, of which *Proteus* is the most notable genus, may split urea into ammonia and carbon dioxide, with alkalization of the urine and

precipitation of crystals of magnesium, ammonia, and calcium phosphate, "triple phosphate," leading to stone formation. Such struvite stones may grow rapidly in infected urine, and a vicious circle ensues whereby the organisms themselves are trapped within the stone safe from the action of antibiotics and the natural host defense mechanisms. Urine cultures at these times may show pyuria but, misleadingly, no bacterial growth. Hence, removal of the stone is an essential part of the treatment of patients with *Proteus* and other urea-splitting UTIs.

Infections of the Male Genital Tract

Prostatitis

Until relatively recently, considerable confusion surrounded the symptom complex of men thought to have "prostatitis." In no small part, this was related to problems of terminology—various authorities were describing aspects of prostatitis in the literature but calling these symptom complexes by different names such as "pelvic floor tension myalgia." As a result, no one was sure exactly who was investigating which group of patients.

This situation was clarified by Drach et al., who suggested a classification in a letter to the Journal of Urology (114), which was accepted by most workers in the field. Subsequently, this suggestion was in large part taken up by an NIH consensus classification in 1998 as illustrated in Table 12.

These four conditions have many symptoms in common, but they are also distinguished by specific clinical and microbiological features. Successful treatment in each group depends on meticulous attention to diagnostic detail, without which failure is inevitable.

Organisms responsible for acute bacterial and chronic bacterial prostatitis are generally similar and resemble those organisms responsible for lower UTI. The majority are grown in pure culture; most often, *E. coli* is isolated, while institutionalized patients may harbor more virulent organisms such as *Pseudomonas* or *Streptococcus faecalis*. It has been suggested that the (rare) episodes of cystitis that occur in young men are all secondary to infection of the prostatic ducts.

Etiological factors thought to be important in acute or chronic bacterial prostatitis include ascending urethral infection and reflux of infected urine into ejaculatory and prostatic ducts. Blacklock (115) noted

Table 12 The Classification of Drach et al. and Subsequent Adjustments by the NIH Consensus Committee (1998)

Drach et al.	Clinical descriptor	NIH Consensus
1	Acute bacterial prostatis	I
2	Chronic bacaterial prostatis	II
3	Nonbacterial prostatitis	III
	Inflammatory[a]	IIIA
4	Prostatodynia[b] noninflammatory	IIIB
	Asymptomatic inflammatory	IV

[a]WBC semen > 10^6/mL, WBC EPS > 5p hpf, WBC VB3 > 10p hpf.
[b]Drach defined as literally "prostatic pain" without evidence of inflammation.
Source: From Ref. 114.

that patients with chronic bacterial prostatitis frequently had the same pathogens as identified in vaginal cultures of their sexual partners. Kirby et al. injected carbon particles into the bladders of men about to undergo transurethral resection and found the particles within the prostate on later histological examination, thus proving that significant intraprostatic reflux had taken place (116).

Localization of Infection

It is evident that with a unified genitourinary tract emerging at the urethral meatus, specimens obtained there may relate to urethral, prostatic, or bladder infections. To overcome this difficulty, specific techniques have been developed for localization of infection (117). A possible scheme for carrying out such studies is illustrated in Fig. 21. The localization tests are not difficult, but they do require attention to detail and a state of preparedness—failure to attend to such detail usually results in negative findings and a disappointed tertiary referral.

Following arrival in the clinic, the patient passes a VB1 specimen (10 mL—voided bladder 1). This is a "washout" specimen and relates to urethral disease. After passage of a further 100 to 200 mL, the patient collects a standard specimen of midstream urine (VB2). Following this, the prostate is massaged in the usual fashion, and prostatic secretion is collected for analysis, as described below. Subsequently, the next voided 10 mL is collected for further examination (VB3), and, within this specimen, organisms of prostatic origin may be cultured. Hence, by comparison of specimens obtained from urethral urine, bladder urine, and postmassage urine, it is generally possible to localize the source of the patient's infection. As is evident, diagnostic and analytical care is required to make an exact diagnosis by Drach/NIH criteria. The schema illustrated (Fig. 21) are still necessary to isolate conventional bacteriological organisms, but modern point of care tests based on molecular techniques have largely replaced standard culture methodologies for *C. trachomatis*, as described in chapter 36. The prevalence of this organism is discussed below.

Examination of Prostatic Fluid

Examination of material obtained after prostatic massage is an important step in the diagnosis of genital infection. In general, cases of prostatic inflammation are found to have more than 15 white cells per high-powered field when such microscopy is performed; as noted above, it is important to check that urethral and bladder specimens do not have similar levels of pyuria. A number of biochemical examinations may be made of expressed prostatic fluid (Fig. 22). The pH of the fluid, normally around 6.5, becomes alkaline as a result of decreased levels of citric acid (119). Zinc levels also reduce significantly (118), this element having previously been known as prostatic antibacterial factor because of its potent bactericidal action on most bacteria capable of causing UTI. It is not clear, however, whether these changes are the cause or the result of bacterial infection of the prostate gland.

Nonbacterial Prostatitis

The cause of nonbacterial prostatitis is essentially unknown. Meticulous investigations may reveal pyuria, but no positive cultures will be obtained by the selective methodology described above. It is not clear whether the symptom complex—which is

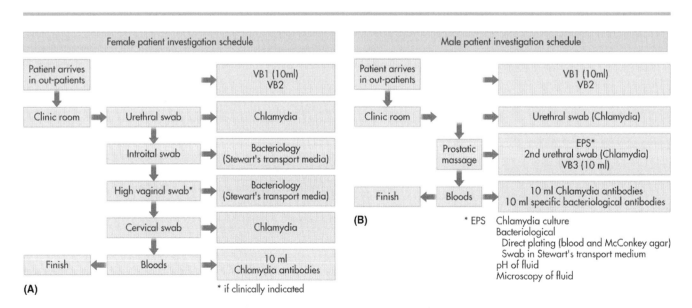

Figure 21 Possible investigation schedule for female (**A**) and male (**B**) patients with possible urogenital infection. The tests are time intensive and require meticulous planning—see text for details.

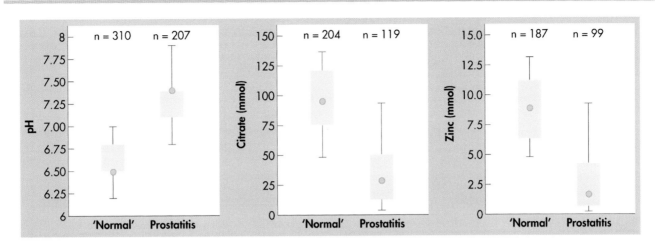

Figure 22 Differences in expressed prostatic secretion composition (EPS) between "normal" samples and men with prostatitis. Circles: median values; boxes: central 50% of samples. Error bars 10th/90th percentile. All differences significant ($P < 0.001$). Infection causes a rise in pH but a decrease in citrate and zinc concentration. See text for details. *Source*: From Ref. 118.

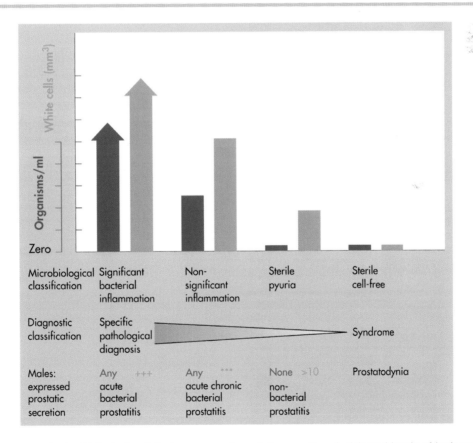

Figure 23 The spectrum of microbiological activity in expressed prostatic secretion. Anticipated levels of both organisms and white cells in the various clinical groups as classified by Drach and NIH criteria (see text). The major clinical problems relate to patients with nonbacterial prostatitis and prostatodynia.

similar to chronic bacterial prostatitis—is related to infectious disease by an unidentified pathogen or is a noninfectious inflammatory process (Fig. 23). A number of causes of nonbacterial prostatitis have been discussed in the literature, including previous antibiotic therapy, viral infection (herpes), *U. urealyticum*, chemical inflammatory processes, and autoimmune disease. The role of *C. trachomatis* is controversial.

Mardh et al. studied 53 patients with nonbacterial prostatitis and found only one positive chlamydial isolate (120), and most other investigators have been similarly unsuccessful in identifying this organism in prostatic fluid or even in prostatic aspirates obtained by direct transrectal ultrasound-guided needle puncture of the gland (121). Nevertheless, identification of this agent as the causative organism of epididymitis in younger men (Figs. 24 and 25) raises questions as to how the infection reaches the epididymis. In this study, a tender, swollen epididymis was associated with chlamydial infection in 19 of 23 patients (83%) 15 to 25 years of age, and these findings were consolidated by the observation that 9 of 12 consorts were also positive for this infection (122). Presumably, these observations are reconciled by assuming that the

organism may pass from urethra to epididymis, but the biological environment within the prostate ducts themselves is hostile to this agent. Further defined studies using the new diagnostic techniques noted below should resolve this question.

Prevalence and Diagnois of Chlamydia trachomatis

Infection rates with *C. trachomatis* have markedly increased in recent years. Younger sexually active males (18–29 years) and females (16–24 years) are, as expected, the main source of the infection (see Fig.10 of chapter 36, page 554), 2% to 6% of the population under the age of 25 being infected by the organism (123,124). The alarming increase in prevalence has prompted the U.K. Department of Health to institute a National *Chlamydia* Screening Programme (NCSP) within the United Kingdom as described in chapter 36. In part, the increase in prevalence might be because of better health awareness, increased sporadic screening, or more sensitive diagnostic tests (125). The new rapid point of care tests in particular are expected to make a significant impact on both immediate treatment and contact tracing (126).

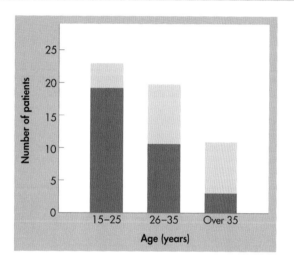

Figure 24 Age distribution of patients with epididymitis according to recovered organism. ▨ negative for *Chlamydia trachomatis*, ■ positive for *C. trachomatis*. *Source*: From Ref. 97.

Antibiotic Penetration in Prostatitis

The specific physicochemical characteristics of the prostate and prostatic fluid govern the penetration of antibiotics into the organ. To penetrate the lipid membrane of the prostatic epithelium, a drug must be lipid soluble; furthermore, the acid-base characteristic of the drug will determine the concentration of the antibiotic in the fluid. Experiments on normal dog prostates (secretion pH 6.4) demonstrate that only bases are able to penetrate successfully into prostatic fluid. However, as noted above, during infection of the human prostate, pH becomes more alkaline and the dissociation gradient may reverse. Nevertheless, fat-soluble bases, such as erythromycin and trimethoprim, are effective in acute or chronic bacterial prostatitis despite experimental evidence, which suggests that concentration of the drug should deteriorate as the pH of the expressed prostatic fluid becomes more alkaline.

Tuberculosis

Tuberculosis remains an important disease worldwide with an estimated 8 to 10 million new cases per annum. The incidence of the disease in its pulmonary form is increasing steadily, particularly in certain ethnic groups and geographical locations. A national survey in England and Wales in 1998 identified an annual rate of 10.9 per 100,000 population, representing increases of 11% and 21%, respectively, over similar surveys undertaken in 1993 and 1988 (127).

However, these figures mask a more complex picture; there has been relatively little change in most regions, but a 71% increase in London and other major urban areas with significant ethnic population. The per 100,000 rate among the whole population

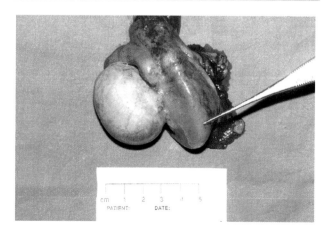

Figure 25 Tuberculous epididymitis removed from 38-year-old white patient; histology revealed florid tuberculous changes within the descending genital tract.

Table 13 Annual Number of Patients with Tuberculosis and Rate of Disease in England and Wales by Ethnic Group

	Annual number cases/rate per 100,000		
Ethnic group	1988	1993	1998
White	2504/5.36	2267/4.78	2108/4.38
Indian subcontinent	1784/132	2101/128	2141/121
Black African	77/64.4	355/151	743/210
Black Caribbean	137/29.4	104/21.6	125/26.4
Chinese	48/36.2	41/30.7	103/77.3

Note the relatively stable data in whites and patients from the Indian subcontinent but marked increases within the Chinese and Black African groups, especially those recently arrived from their native countries.
Source: From Ref. 127.

(4.4) was many times lower than that of immigrants from the Indian subcontinent (121), while significant increases were recorded for groups of black Africans (210) and Chinese (77.3) origin (Table 13). As expected, recent immigrants had a higher incidence of the disease than those who had arrived more than five years previously (127), and the demographic profile of the disease shows wide variation between ethnic groups (Fig. 26). Nonpulmonary disease in developed countries presents chiefly as lymph adenopthy or genitourinary disease (128), the latter

accounting for approximately 25% of cases surveyed in North America and the United Kingdom. Paradoxically, in these populations, genitourinary tuberculosis is less common in ethnic minority groups (approximately 5%) than in white Europeans (27%), although these observations might be related to age differences at diagnosis (129). Approximately 3% of all adults with pulmonary or nonpulmonary disease are coinfected with HIV (130).

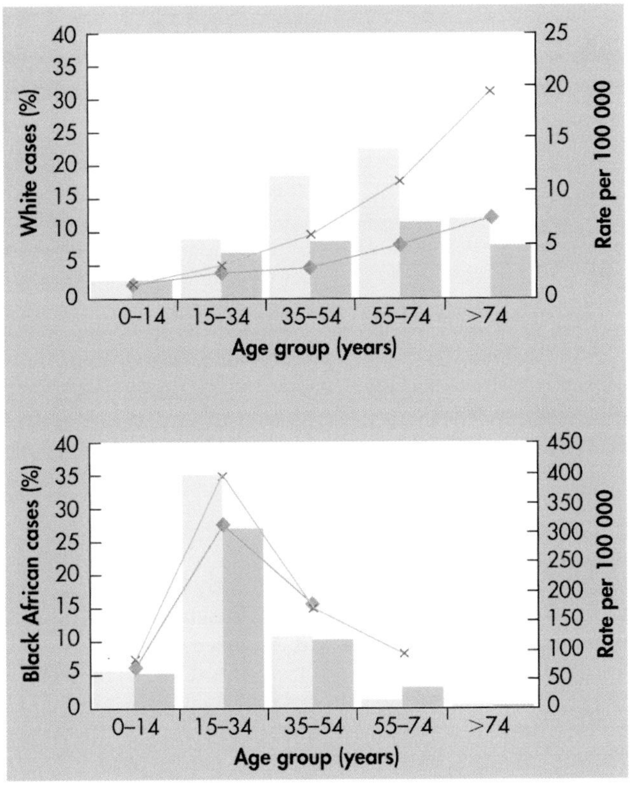

Clinical Features

Descriptions of the classical presentation of genitourinary tuberculosis are to be found in clinical textbooks; some, however, are worthy of note to urologists. Disseminated disease may affect patients with renal or other types of organ transplantation, a situation further complicated by therapeutic immunosuppression (131). Prophylactic chemotherapy (isoniazid) has been demonstrated to be of benefit in such high-risk renal transplant situations. In one study, 6 of 27 patients without prophylaxis developed disease while no treated patients became infected (132). Length of treatment prophylaxis is probably best linked to the necessary duration of immunosuppression. Rarely, patients with chronic renal failure may develop genitourinary tuberculosis and hypercalcaemia (133). Usually, raised calcitriol levels are more commonly found in patients with disseminated but nongenitourinary disease, probably because of active synthesis of vitamin D by activated macrophages within granulomas.

Laboratory Diagnosis

The great majority of cases are infected by the human tubercle bacillus, *Mycobacterium tuberculosis*. *M. bovis* is now rarely (1%) a cause of disease although it may be isolated in reactivated dormant disease or that associated with HIV infection. Bacillus Calmette-Guérin vaccine strain-associated lesions are now regularly encountered by laboratories in those centers where intravesical immunotherapy of superficial bladder cancer is widely practiced.

Classically, the diagnosis of genitourinary tuberculosis was made by culture on solid Lowenstein-Jensen median, the process taking up to six weeks. In cases with a high index of clinical suspicion, modern liquid culture systems may deliver a diagnosis

Figure 26 Age and sex distribution of proportion of patients with tuberculosis, comparing (*top*) ethnic white population with (*bottom*) black African patients. Note very different age distribution and rate per 100,000 population. ■: male; □: female; ×: male rate; ♦: female rate. *Source*: From Ref. 127.

in half this time. In recent years, polymerase chain reaction (PCR) amplification techniques have been investigated for the diagnosis of both pulmonary and genitourinary tuberculosis and have been found to deliver good sensitivity and specificity (135,136). Other workers have attempted to use the technique to diagnose active pulmonary tuberculosis in HIV patients by means of urine analysis (134). It was concluded that PCR diagnostics may provide much faster confirmation of disease (24–48 hours), although the intermittent excretory nature of M. tuberculosis may lead to false-negative results, and urine concentration techniques may be required to reduce this error (135).

To an extent, this diagnostic divide is a good example of the difference between an efficacy trial (what works in perfect conditions) and an effectiveness trial (what works in the real world) (136). It is well known that techniques that function satisfactorily with dedicated researchers and refined techniques perform poorly when applied to mass populations and routine laboratories. PCR diagnostics are suspect at organism concentrations of 10^3 CFU/mL (roughly the lower detectable limit for light microscopy), and for most situations a high index of clinical suspicion, effective communication, and modern culture systems leads to optimal outcomes in the search for M. tuberculosis in the genitourinary tract.

Bacteraemia and Septic Shock

Septic shock is a relatively common and extremely serious complication of infection, usually of gram-negative origin. In urological practice, the complication is most often encountered in the management of stones, usually complex in nature and located in the upper tract. Septicemic shock, however, may occur after apparently simple and uncomplicated instrumentation of the urinary tract.

Figure 27 illustrates organisms isolated from blood cultures, and the surgical procedures involved are taken from a typically busy stone service. The endotoxin, which may be encased within the stone (137), may not always respond to appropriate antibiotic prophylaxis (138). The toxin lies between the outer membrane and the core oligosaccharide that makes up the O-serotype antigen common to gram-negative bacteria (Fig. 28). Known as lipid A, this lipopolysaccharide may trigger release of large amounts of cytokines, such as tumor necrosis factor and the interleukins, which participate in the classically described cascade illustrated in Fig. 29. A full description of the sepsis syndrome is beyond the scope of this text, but urologists will be aware of the urgent need to maintain adequate tissue profusion by volume replacement at the same time as instituting appropriate antimicrobial therapy as judged by repeated blood cultures if necessary.

Papilloma Viruses and Cancer

Human papilloma viruses (HPV) are a group of DNA-containing viruses numbering over 100 types, which stimulate rapid cell division. External genital warts

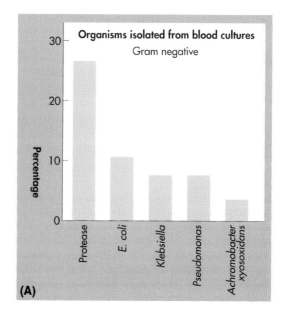

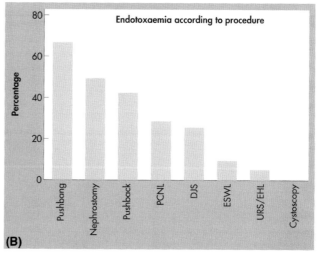

Figure 27 Organisms (**A**) recovered from blood cultures following procedures (**B**) carried out in a busy interventional stone center. Unfortunately, septic shock occurs in a significant number of these cases.

are most frequently caused by HPV types 6 and 11 (Fig. 30). Other HPV types (mainly 16 and 18, less often 31 and 33) are frequently present in the anogenital region and have been associated with the development of high-grade, premalignant cervical lesions [cervical intraepithelial neoplasia (CIN) III] as well as anogenital cancer, principally of the anus and vulva. Types 16 and 18 are thought to cause over 70% of squamous cell cancers while type 18 may be responsible in 50% adenocarcinomas from the endocervix. DNA sequences from such HPVs are detectable in the majority of cervical and anal tumors; PCR studies of apparently normal cervical smears showed increased levels of sequences from "high-risk virus types," and subsequent colposcopy confirmed the

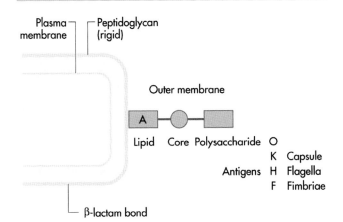

Figure 28 Detailed structure of the O polysaccharide antigen associated with *Escherichia coli*. Lipid adjacent to the outer membrane (lipid A) is thought to be responsible for the manifestations of endotoxic shock.

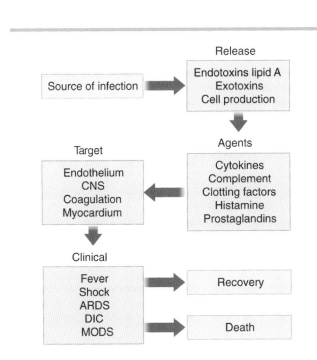

Figure 29 The classical cascade described in endotoxic septicemic shock. *Abbreviations*: ARDS, adult respiratory distress syndrome; DIC, disseminated intravascular coagulation; MODS, multiple organ dysfunction syndrome.

presence of underlying high-grade CIN III (139). Not all women infected with high-risk HPV types develop cancer, and the reason for this discrepancy remains unclear at the present time.

Recombinant vaccines have been developed against the higher risk type 16 and 18 viruses based on L1 protein shell particles; however, at least 15 oncogenic types have been identified, which lead to neoplastic transformation under certain circumstances, and hence routine cervical screening will continue

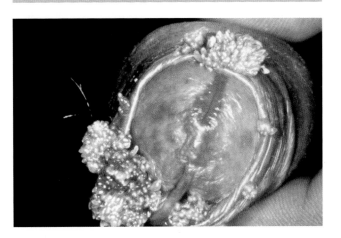

Figure 30 Exophytic papilloma virus, usually caused by type 6 or type 11 infection.

to be important. Early reports suggested high efficacy in women not previously exposed to virus (preintercourse) although later studies were less clear-cut, generating considerable controversy (140,141).

The vaccines (Gardasil, MSD, Cervarix GSK) naturally are not active against existing HPV infection or established cervical neoplasia; Gardasil alone, however, is active against the genital wart types 6 and 11. The cost, marketing, and ethics—where vaccination has to be given to girls not yet exposed to virus (sexually inactive, target 12–13 years)—continue to generate comment on both sides of the Atlantic (142,143).

Early surveys involving PCR assays for HPV DNA in squamous cell carcinoma of the penis have been reported. About half of patients with Basaloid and warty squamous cell carcinomas were found to be associated with HPV 16 and 18. The role of vaccines in such disease has yet to be determined (144).

Localization Studies in the Urinary Tract

It is pertinent to summarize the various localization studies that may be employed to identify the site of infection of any particular organism. When efficiently and accurately performed, such studies can be of great help to the urologist attempting to identify the source of organisms within the urinary tract.

Studies on prostatic fluid described by Meares and Stamey (117) have already been noted. Stamey has also refined localization studies designed to determine the source of bacteriuria emanating from the upper urinary tract. Essentially, this test involves ureteric catheterization of the appropriate unit in question after meticulous steps to eradicate bacteria from the bladder that would otherwise contaminate the ureteric sample. Such techniques have been equally useful when attempting to determine the source of cells with abnormal cytological features. Earlier methods for differentiating kidney from bladder infections (Fairley bladder washout test) have fallen into disuse, although such studies can, on occasion, be clinically helpful.

Summary of Definitions

Adherence	Initial interaction of microorganism with host
Adhesin	Microbiological molecule that leads to adhesion to cells or tissues
Bacteriuria	The residence of bacteria within the urinary tract
Contamination	Adventitious entry of bacteria during urine collection
Fitness	The ability of bacteria to establish and maintain a population in a specific ecological habit
GAL-GAL	Essential core of disaccharide receptor for P fimbriae
Pathogenicity	The ability to cause disease
Phase variation	Variation of virulence antigens, often to protect organism
Tropism	The restriction of commercials and pathogens to certain host tissues and cell types
Virulence	The degree of pathogenicity

REFERENCES

1. Lincoln K, Lidin-Janson G, Winberg J. Resistant urinary infections resulting from changes in resistance pattern of faecal flora induced by sulphonamide and hospital environment. BMJ 1970; 3:305–309.
2. Finegold SM, Mathisen GE, George WL. Changes in human intestinal flora related to administration of antimicrobial agents. In: Hentges DJ, ed. Human Intestinal Microflora in Health and Disease. New York: Academic Press, 1983:355–446.
3. Kaye D. Antibacterial activity of human urine. J Clin Invest 1968; 47:2374–2390.
4. Cox CE, Hinman F, Jr. Experiments with induced bacteriuria, vesical emptying and bacterial growth on a mechanism of bladder defence to infection. J Urol 1961; 86:739–748.
5. Parsons CL, Greenspan C, Mulholland SG. The primary antibacterial defence mechanism of the bladder. Invest Urol 1975; 13:72–76.
6. Parsons LC, Shrom SH, Hanno PM, et al. Bladder surface mucin—examination of possible mechanisms for its antibacterial effect. Invest Urol 1978; 60:196–200.
7. Parsons CL, Mulholland SG, Anwar H. Antibacterial activity of bladder surface mucin duplication by exogenous glycosaminoglycan (heparin). Infect Immun 1979; 24:552–557.
8. Parsons CL, Greenspan C, Moore SW, et al. Role of surface mucin in primary antibacterial defense of bladder. Urology 1977; 9:48–52.
9. Tamm I, Horsfall FL. A mucoprotein derived from human urine which reacts with influenza, mumps and Newcastle disease viruses. J Exp Med 1952; 95:71–97.
10. Orskov I, Ferencz A, Orskov F. Tamm–Horsfall protein or uro-mucoid is the normal urinary slime that traps type I fimbriated Escherichia coli. Lancet 1980; 1:887.
11. Pak J, Pu Y, Xhang ZT, et al. Tamm–Horsfall protein binds to type I fimbriated E. coli and prevents E. coli from binding to uroplakin 1a and 1b receptors. J Biol Chem 2001; 276:9924–9930.
12. Jost SP. Cell cycle of normal bladder urothelium in developing and adult mice. Virchows Arch B Cell Pathol Incl Mol Pathol 1989; 57:27–36.
13. Mulvey MA, Lopez-Boado YS, Wilson CL, et al. Induction and evasion of host defences by type I pilated uropathological E. coli. Science 1998; 282:1494–1497.
14. Klump DJ, Weiser AC, Sangupta S, et al. Uropathogenic E. coli potentiates type I pilus induced apoptosis by suppressing NF-kappaB. Infect Immun 2001; 69:6689–6695.
15. Mulvey MA. Adhesion and entry of uropathogenic Escherichia coli. Cell Microbiol 2002; 4:257–271.
16. Gunther NW, Lockatelle V, Johnson DE, et al. In vivo dynamics of type I fimbria regulation in uropathogenic Escherichia coli during experimental urinary tract infection. Infect Immun 2001; 69:2838–2853.
17. Mulvey MA, Schilling JD, Hultgren SJ. Establishment of a persistent E. coli reservoir during the acute phase of bladder infection. Infect Immun 2001; 69:4572–4579.
18. Mayer KH, Opal SM, Mederios AA. Mechanisms of antibiotic resistance. In: Mandell GL, Douglas, Benett JE, et al., eds. Principles and Practice of Infectious Diseases. Edinburgh: Churchill Livingstone, 1995:212–224.
19. Cooke EM, Ewins SP. Properties of strains of Escherichia coli isolated from a variety of sources. J Med Microbiol 1975; 8:107–111.
20. Minshew BH, Jorgenson J, Swanstrum M. Some characteristics of E. coli strains isolated from extra-intestinal infections of humans. J Infect Dis 1978; 137:648–654.
21. Johnson JR. Virulence factors in E. coli urinary tract infection. Clin Microbiol Rev 1991; 4:80–128.
22. Mayer TF. Pathogenic neisseriae—a model of bacterial virulence and genetic flexibility. Int J Microbiol 1990; 274:135–154.
23. Leying H, Suerbaum S, Kroll H P, et al. The capsular polysaccharide is a major determinant of serum resistance in K-1 positive blood culture isolates of Escherichia coli. Infect Immun 1990; 58:222–227.
24. Jacobson SH, Hammarlind M, Lidefeldt KJ, et al. Incidence of aerobactin-positive Escherichia coli strains in patients with symptomatic urinary tract infection. Eur J Clin Microbiol Infect Dis 1988; 7:630–634.
25. Costerton JW, Geesey GG, Cheng K J. How bacteria stick. Sci Am 1978; 238:86–95.
26. van Oss CJ, Good RJ, Chaudhury MK. The role of Van de Waals forces and hydrogen bonds in hydrophobic interactions between biopolymers and low energy surfaces. J Colloid Interface Sci 1986; 3:378–384.
27. Gibbons RJ, van-Houte J. Bacterial adherence in oral microbial ecology. Ann Rev Microbiol 1975; 29:19–41.
28. Mobley HLT, Chippendale GR, Tenney JH, et al. Expression of type I fimbriae may be required for persistence of Escherichia coli in the catheterised urinary tract. J Clin Microbiol 1987; 25:2253–2257.
29. Roberts JA. Tropism in bacterial infections: urinary tract infections. J Urol 1996; 156:1552–1559.
30. Senior D, Baker N, Cedergren B, et al. Globo-A—a new receptor specificity for attaching Escherichia coli. FEBS Lett 1988; 237:123–127.
31. Lindstedt R, Larson G, Falk P, et al. The receptor repertoire defines the host range for attaching Escherichia coli strains that recognise Globo-A. Infect Immun 1991; 59:1086–1092.
32. Langermann S, Palaszynski S, Barnhart M, et al. Prevention of mucosal E. coli infection by FimH adhesin based systemic vaccination. Science 1997; 276:607–611.
33. Choudhury D, Thompson A, Stojanoff V, et al. X-ray structure of the FimC–FimH chaperone–adhesin complex from uropathogenic E. coli. Science 1999; 285:1061–1066.
34. Zhou G, Mo WJ, Sebbel P, et al. Uroplakin is the urothelial receptor for uropathogenic E. coli: evidence from in vitro FimH binding. J Cell Sci 2001; 114:4095–4103.

35. Sunn TT, Zhao H, Provet J, et al. Formation of asymmetric unit membrane during urothelial differentiation. Mol Biol Rep 1996; 23:3–11.

36. Martinez TS, Mulvey MA, Schilling JD. Type I pilus mediated bacterial invasion of bladder epithelial cells. EMBO J 2000; 19:2803–2812.

37. Baorto DM, Gao Z, Malaviya R, et al. Survival of FimH expressing enterobacteria in macrophages relies on glycolipid traffic. Nature 1997; 389:636–639.

38. Berry RE, Klumpp DJ, Schaeffer AJ. Urothelial cultures support intracellular bacterial community formation by uropathogenic *E. coli*. *Infect Immun* 2009; 77:2762–2772.

39. Rosen DA, Pinkner JS, Jones JM, et al. Utilization of an intracellular bacterial community pathway in *Klebsiella pneumoniae* UTI and the effects of FimK on type I pilus expression. Infect Immun 2008; 76:3337–3345.

40. Schwan WR, Lee JL, Lenard FA, et al. Osmolarity and pH growth conditions regulate fim gene transcription and type I pilus expression in uropathogenic *E. coli*. Infect Immun 2002; 70:1391–1402.

41. Gunther WW, Synder JA, Lockatell V, et al. Assessment of virulence of uropathogenic *E. coli* type I fimbrial mutants in which the invertible element is phase locked on or off. Infect Immun 2002; 70:3344–3354.

42. Xia Y, Gally D, Forsman-Sembk, et al. Regulatory cross talk between adhesin operant in *E. coli*: inhibition of fimbriae expression by the PapB protein. EMBO J 2000; 19:1450–1457.

43. Lane MC, Simms AN, Mobley HLT. Complex interplay between Type I Fimbrial Expression and Flagellum mediated motility of uropathogenic *E. coli*. J Bacteriol 2007; 189:5523–5533.

44. Eisenstein BI. Phase variation of type I fimbriae in *Escherichia coli* is under transcriptional control. Science 1981; 214: 337–339.

45. Lindberg F, Lund B, Johansson L, et al. Localisation of the receptor-binding protein adhesin at the tip of the bacterial pilus. Nature 1987; 328:84–87.

46. Roberts JA, Kaack MB, Baskin G, et al. Epitotes of the P-fimbrial adhesin of *E. coli* cause different urinary tract infections. J Urol 1997; 158:1610–1613.

47. Lane MC, Mobley HLT. Role of P-fimbrial-mediated adherence in pyelonephritis and persistence of uropathogenic *E. coli* (UPEC) in mammalian kidney. Kidney Int 2007; 72:19–25.

48. Holden NJ, Gally DL. Switches, cross-talk and memory in *E. coli* adherence. J Med Microbiol 2004; 53:585–593.

49. Svanborg, Edén C, Hanson LC5, Jodal U, et al. Variable adherence to normal human urinary tract epithelial cells of *Escherichia coli* strains associated with various forms of urinary tract infection. Lancet 1976; 2:490–492.

50. Edén CS, Hansson HA. *E. coli* pili as possible mediators of attachment to human urinary tract epithelial cells. Infect Immun 1978; 21:229–237.

51. Fowler JE, Stamey TA. Studies of introital colonisation in women with recurrent urinary tract infections—role of bacterial adherence. J Urol 1977; 177:472–476.

52. Schaeffer AJ, Jones JM, Dunn JK. Association of in vitro *Escherichia coli* adherence to vaginal and buccal epithelial cells with susceptibility of women to recurrent urinary tract infections. N Engl J Med 1981; 304:1062–1066.

53. Sellwood R, Gibbons RA, Jones GW, et al. A possible basis for the breeding of pigs relatively resistant to neonatal diarrhoea. Vet Rec 1974; 95:574–575.

54. Sellwood R, Gibbons RA, Jones GW, et al. Adhesion of enteropathogenic *Escherichia coli* to pig intestinal brush borders: the existence of two pig phenotypes. J Med Microbiol 1975; 8:405–411.

55. Rutter JM, Burrows MR, Sellwood R, et al. A genetic basis for resistance to enteric disease caused by *E. coli*. Nature 1975; 257:135–136.

56. Buckwalter JA, Naifeh GS, Auer JE. Rheumatic fever and the blood groups. BMJ 1962; 2:1023–1027.

57. Källenius G, Möllby R, Svenson SB, et al. Occurrence of P-fimbriated *Escherichia coli* in urinary tract infections. Lancet 1981; 2:1369–1372.

58. Johnson JR, Roberts PL, Stamm WE. P-fimbriae and other virulence factors in *Escherichia coli* urosepsis: association with patients' characteristics. J Infect Dis 1987; 156: 225–228.

59. Virkola R, Westerlund B, Holthöfer H, et al. Binding characteristics of E. Coli adhesins in human urinary bladder. Infect Immun 1988; 56:2615–2622.

60. Leffler H, Svanborg-Edén C. Glycolipid receptors for uropathogenic *E. coli* on human erythrocytes and uroepithelial cells. Infect Immun 1981; 34:920–929.

61. Plos K, Carter T, Hull S, et al. Intestinal carriage of P fimbriated *E. coli* and the susceptibility to urinary tract infection in young children. J Infect Dis 1995; 171: 625–631.

62. Wullt B, Bergsten G, Connell H, et al. P-fimbriae trigger mucosal responses to *E. coli* in the human urinary tract. Cell Microbiol 2001; 3:255–264.

63. Hacker J, Kestler H, Hoschntzky H, et al. Cloning and characterisation of the S fimbrial adhesin II complex of *E. coli* 018 K1 meningitis isolate. Infect Immun 1993; 61: 544–550.

64. Nowicki B, Selvarangan R, Nowick S. Family of *E. coli* Dr adhesins: delay-accelerating factor receptor recognition and invasiveness. J Infect Dis 2001; 183:S24–S27.

65. Wold A, Thorssén M, Hull S, Svenborg-Edén C. Attachment of *E. coli* via mannose or Gal-Gal containing receptors to human colonic epithelial cells. Infect Immun 1988; 56:2531–2537.

66. Schlager TA, Whittam TS, Hendley JO, et al. Comparison of expression of virulence factors by *Escherichia coli* causing cystitis and *E. coli* colonising the peri-urethra of healthy girls. J Infect Dis 1995; 172:772–778.

67. Hedlund M, Svensson M, Wilsson A, et al. Role of the ceramide-signalling pathway in cytokine responses to P fimbriated *E. coli*. J Exp Med 1996; 183:1037–1044.

68. Langermann S, Mollby R, Burlein JE, et al. Vaccination with Fim H adhesin protects cynomolgus monkey from colonisation and infection by uropathogenic *E. coli*. J Infect Dis 2000; 181:774–778.

69. Silverblatt FS. Host–parasite interaction in the rat renal pelvis: a possible role of pili in the pathogenesis of pyelonephritis. J Exp Med 1974; 140:1696–1699.

70. Fader RC, Davis CP. Effect of pilation on *Klebsiella pneumoniae* infection in rat bladders. Infect Immun 1980; 30:554–561.

71. Glynn AA, Brumfitt W, Howard CJ. K antigens of *Escherichia coli* and renal involvement in urinary tract infections. Lancet 1971; 1:514–516.

72. Kaijser B, Hanson LA, Jodal U, et al. Frequency of *E. coli* K antigens in urinary tract infections in children. Lancet 1977; 2:663–664.

73. Crump J, Pead L, Maskell R. Urinary infections in general practice. Lancet 1976; 1:1184

74. Grüneberg RN. Antibiotic sensitivies of urinary pathogens, 1971–1978. J Clin Pathol 1980; 33:853–856.

75. Jordan PA, Iravani A, Richard GA. Urinary tract infection caused by *Staphylococcus saprophyticus*. J Infect Dis 1980; 142:510–515.

76. Maskell R, Pead L, Allen J. The puzzle of ''urethral syndrome:'' a possible answer? Lancet 1979; 1:1058–1059.

77. Brumfitt W, Hamilton-Miller JMT, Ludlam H, et al. Lactobacilli do not cause frequency and dysuria syndrome. Lancet 1981; 2:393–394.

78. Bran JL, Levison ME, Kaye D. Entrance of bacteria into the female urinary bladder. N Engl J Med 1972; 286:626–629.

79. Buckley RM, McGuckin M, MacGregor RR. Urine bacterial counts following sexual intercourse. N Engl J Med 1978; 298:321–324.

80. Hinman F, Jr. Mechanisms for the entry of bacteria and the establishment of urinary infection in female children. J Urol 1966; 96:546–550.

81. Hooton TM, Hillier S, Johnson C. *Escherichia coli* bacteriuria and contraceptive method. JAMA 1991; 265:64–69.

82. Vivaldi E, Cotran R, Zangwill DP. Ascending infection as a mechanism in pathogenesis of experimental non-obstructive pyelonephritis. Proc Soc Exp Biol Med 1959; 102:242–247.

83. Kass EH. Bacteriuria and the diagnosis of infections of the urinary tract. AMA Arch Intern Med 1957; 100:709–714.

84. Stamm WE, Wagner KF, Amsell R, et al. Causes of the acute urethral syndrome in women. N Engl J Med 1980; 303:409–415.

85. Stamm WE, Counts GW, Running KR, et al. Diagnosis of coliform infection in acutely dysuric women. N Engl J Med 1982; 307:463–468.

86. Editorial. Can Kasstigation beat the truth out of the urethral syndrome? Lancet 1982; 2:694–695.

87. Stamm WE. Quantitative urine cultures revisited. Editorial. Eur J Clin Microbiol 1984; 3:279–281.

88. Venegas MF, Navas EL, Gaffney RA, et al. Binding of type I pilated *Escherichia coli* to vaginal mucous. Infect Immun 1995; 73:416–421.

89. Cox CE, Lacy SS, Hinman F, Jr. The urethra and its relationship to urinary tract infection. II. The urethral flora of the female with recurrent urinary infection. J Urol 1968; 99:632–638.

90. Grüneberg RN. Relationship of infecting urinary organism to the faecal flora in patients with symptomatic urinary infection. Lancet 1969; 2:766–768.

91. Stamey TA, Sexton CC. The role of vaginal colonisation with enterobacteriaceae in recurrent urinary infections. J Urol 1975; 113:214–217.

92. Pfau A, Sacks T. The bacterial flora of the vaginal vestibule, urethra and vagina in premenopausal women with recurrent urinary tract infections. J Urol 1981; 126:630–634.

93. Marsh FP, Murray M, Panchamia P. The relationship between bacterial cultures of the vaginal introitus and urinary infection. Br J Urol 1972; 44:368–375.

94. O'Grady FW, Richards B, McSherry MA, et al. Introital enterobacteria, urinary infection and the urethral syndrome. Lancet 1970; 2:1208–1210.

95. Brumfitt W, Grogan RA, Hamilton-Miller JMT. Periurethral enterobacterial carriage preceding urinary infection. Lancet 1987; 1:824–826.

96. Cattell WR, McSherry MA, Northeast A, et al. Periurethral enterobacterial carriage in the pathogenesis of recurrent urinary infection. BMJ 1974; 4:136–139.

97. Wiswell TE, Roscelli JD. Corroborative evidence for the decreased incidence of urinary tract infections in circumcised male infants. Paediatrics 1986; 78:96–99.

98. Wiswell TE, Enzenauer RW, Holton ME, et al. Declining frequency of circumcision: implications for changes in the absolute incidence and male to female sex ratio of urinary tract infections in early infancy. Paediatrics 1987; 79: 338–342.

99. Feld L, Greenfield S, Ogra P. Urinary tract infections in infants and children. Paediatr Rev 1989; 11:71–77.

100. Ransley PG, Risdon RA. The pathogenesis of reflux nephropathy. Contrib Nephrol 1979; 16:90–98.

101. Siegel S, Siegel B, Sokoloff B. Urinary infection in infants and preschool children. Am J Dis Child 1980; 134:369–372.

102. Kunin CM. A ten year study of bacteriuria in schoolgirls: final report of bacteriologic, urologic, and epidemiologic findings. J Infect Dis 1970; 122:382–393.

103. Meadow RS, White RHR, Johnston NM. Prevalence of symptomless urinary tract disease in Birmingham schoolchildren. I. Pyuria and bacteriuria. BMJ 1969; 3:81–84.

104. Cardiff/Oxford Bacteriuria Study Group. Sequelae of covert bacteriuria in schoolgirls. A four-year follow-up study. Lancet 1978; 1:889–894.

105. Gillenwater JY, Harrison RB, Kunin CM. Natural history of bacteriuria in schoolgirls. N Engl J Med 1979; 301:396–399.

106. Sacks SH, Verrier Jones K, Roberts R, et al. The effect of symptomless bacteriuria in childhood on subsequent pregnancy. Lancet 1987; 2:991–994.

107. Kunin CM. Sexual intercourse and urinary infections. N Engl J Med 1978; 298:336–337.

108. Norden CW, Kass EH. Bacteriuria of pregnancy: a critical appraisal. Annu Rev Med 1968; 19:431–437.

109. Kass EH. Bacteriuria and pyelonephritis of pregnancy. AMA Arch Intern Med 1960; 105:194–198.

110. Brocklehurst JC, Dillane JB, Griffiths L. The prevalence and symptomatology of urinary infection in an aged population. Gerontol Clin 1968; 10:242–253.

111. Mabeck CE. Treatment of uncomplicated urinary tract infection in non-pregnant women. Postgrad Med J 1972; 48:69–75.

112. George NJR. Urethral syndrome—clinical features. In: George NJR, Gosling JA, eds. Sensory Disorders of the Bladder and Urethra. New York: Springer-Verlag, 1986:91–102.

113. O'Grady FW, Charlton CAC, Fry IK, et al. Natural history of intractable "cystitis" in women referred to a special clinic. In: Brumfitt W, Ascher AW, eds. Urinary Tract Infection. Oxford: Oxford University Press, 1973:81–91.

114. Drach GW, Fair WR, Meares EM, Stamey TA. Classification of benign diseases associated with prostatic pain: prostatitis or prostatodynia? J Urol 1978; 120:226.

115. Blacklock NJ. Anatomical factors in prostatitis. Br J Urol 1974; 46:47–50.

116. Kirby RS, Lowe D, Bultitude MI. Intraprostatic urinary reflux: an aetiological factor in abacterial prostatitis. Br J Urol 1982; 54:729–731.

117. Meares EM, Jr, Stamey TA. Bacteriologic localisation patterns in bacterial prostatitis and urethritis. Invest Urol 1968; 5:492–518.

118. Kavanagh JP, Darby C, Costello CB. Differences in expressed prostatic secretion composition (EPS) between "normal" samples and from men with prostatitis. Int J Androl 1982; 5:487–496.

119. Blacklock NJ, Beavis JP. Response of prostatic fluid pH in inflammation. Br J Urol 1974; 46:537–542.

120. Mardh PH, Ripa KT, Colleen S, et al. Role of *Chlamydia trachomatis* in non-acute prostatitis. Br J Vener Dis 1978; 54:330–334.

121. Doble A, Thomas BJ, Walker MM. The role of *Chlamydia trachomatis* in chronic abacterial prostatitis: a study using ultrasound guided biopsy. J Urol 1989; 141:332–335.

122. Grant JBF, Costello CB, Sequeira PJL, et al. The role of *Chlamydia trachomatis* in epididymitis. Br J Urol 1987; 60:355–359.

123. Anderson B, Olesen F, Moller JK, et al. Population based strategies for outreach screening of urogenital *Chlamydia trachomatis* infections: a randomised controlled trial. J Infect Dis 2002; 185:252–258.

124. Fenton KA, Korovessis C, Johnson AM, et al. Sexual behaviour in Britain: reported sexually transmitted infections

and prevalent genital *Chlamydia trachomatis* infection. Lancet 2001; 358:1851–1854.

125. Macleod J, Salisbury C, Low N, et al. Coverage and uptake of systemic postal screening for genital *Chlamydia trachomatis* and prevalence of infection in the United Kingdom general population: cross-sectional study. BMJ 2005; 230:940–943.

126. Mahilum-Tapay L, Laitila V, Wawrzyniak JJ, et al. New point of care *Chlamydia* rapid test—bridging the gap between diagnosis and treatment: performance evaluation study. BMJ 2007; 335:1190–1194.

127. Rose AMC, Watson JM, Graham C, et al. Tuberculosis at the end of the 20th century in England and Wales: the results of a national survey in 1998. Thorax 2001; 56: 173–179.

128. Garcia-Rodriguez JA, Garcia-Sanchez JE, Munoz Bellido JL, et al. Genitourinary TB in Spain: a review of 81 cases. Clin Infect Dis 1994; 18:557–561.

129. Grange JM, Yates MD, Ormerod LP, et al. Factors determining ethnic differences in the incidence of bacteriologically confirmed genitourinary tuberculosis in south east Engl J Infect 1995; 30:37–40.

130. Churchill D, Hannan M, Miller R, et al. HIV associated culture proved tuberculosis has increased in north central London from 1990–1996. Sex Transm Infect 2002; 76:43–45.

131. Gwoeltje KF, Matthew A, Rothstein M, et al. Tuberculosis infection and anergy in haemodialysis patients. Am J Kidney Dis 1998; 31:848–852.

132. Higgins RM, Cahn AP, Porter D, et al. Microbacterial infections after renal transplantation. Q J Med 1991; 78:145–153.

133. Paces R, de la Torre M, Alcazar F, et al. Genitourinary tuberculosis as the cause of unexplained hypercalcaemia in a patient with pre-end stage renal failure. Nephrol Dial Transplant 1998; 13:488–490.

134. Romano L, Sanquinetti, Posteraro B, et al. Early detection of negative BACTEC MCIT 960 cultures by PCR-reverse cross blot hybridization assay. J Clin Microbiol 2002; 40:3499–3501.

135. Van Vollenhoven P, Heynes CF, de Beer PM, et al. PCR in the diagnosis of urinary tract tuberculosis. Urol Res 1996; 24:107–111.

136. When to act on evidence? Editorial. BMJ 2002; 325:7371.

137. Mc Aleer IM, Kaplan GW, Bradley JS, et al. Endotoxin content in renal calculi. J Urol 2003; 169:1813–1814.

138. Mariappen P, Smith G, Mousssa SA, et al. One week of ciprofloxacin before percutaneous nephrolithotomy significantly reduces upper tract infection and urosepsis: a prospective controlled study. BJU Int 2006; 98:1075–1079.

139. Cuziack J, Szarewski A, Terry G. Human papilloma virus testing in primary cervical screening. Lancet 1995; 345: 1533–1536.

140. The Future II study group: quadrivalent vaccine against human papilloma virus to prevent high-grade cervical lesions. N Engl J Med 2007; 356:1915–1927.

141. Haug C. Human papilloma virus vaccination—reason for caution. N Engl J Med 2008; 359:861–862.

142. Editorial. Cheaper HPV vaccines needed. Lancet 2008; 371:1638.

143. Rothman SM, Rothman DJ. Marketing HPV vaccine. JAMA 2009; 302:781–786.

144. Miralies-Guri C, Bruni L, Cubilla A. HPV prevalence and type destribution in penile carcinoma. J Clin Pathol 2009; 62:870–878.

10

The Scientific Basis of Urinary Stone Formation

William G. Robertson

Physiology Department, Royal Free and University College Medical School, London, U.K.

INTRODUCTION

Urolithiasis is a disorder that has cut across all historical, geographical, demographic and social boundaries. From the days of the predynastic Egyptians until the present time, kidney stones have perplexed patients and physicians alike and, although during that time the methods for removing stones have advanced from the crudely barbaric to the highly sophisticated, the problem of how successfully to prevent their recurrence in a given patient continues to challenge urologists and nephrologists.

If patients are not provided with proper preventative management, the risk of recurrence is traditionally high—40% within 3 years rising to 74% at 10 years and to 98% at 25 years in the days when open surgery and transurethral basket or loop extraction were the main techniques for removing stones (1). In the era of extracorporeal shock wave lithotripsy (ESWL) and percutaneous nephrolithotomy (PCNL), the recurrence rate became even higher (Fig. 1), a fact which is not surprising since both techniques, particularly ESWL, often leave particles behind in the kidney that provide ideal nuclei for further stone formation (2). However, with the recent advent of flexible ureterorenoscopy (FURS), a procedure which promises to be more efficient with respect to the removal of stones and their fragments, it may be that recurrence rates may decrease to those experienced in the days of open surgery. Unfortunately, the relative success of ESWL, PCNL and FURS in the disintegration and removal of stones has lulled many into the belief that the problem can be managed solely by these means, a trend that has been increased by opportune cost-cutting by many Health Authorities, for although these minimally invasive techniques may be the procedures of choice for the removal of stones, they do not treat the underlying cause(s) of stone formation. Without biochemical screening and appropriate dietary and/or medical management, the patient will generally return for further stone removal in the future.

Not only is the failure to provide proper prophylactic treatment for the patient bad clinical management, in the long term it is economically more expensive (3). Financial analysis has shown that the projected cost of treating stone patients solely by removing their stones by minimally invasive technologies every time they form them is considerably more expensive than removing their initial stones and then screening the patients thoroughly to identify their risk factors to provide them with appropriate prophylactic management (4).

During the six millennia since the formation of the earliest recorded stones, the pattern of urolithiasis has changed in many respects, particularly within the past century. In Western countries before 1900, for example, stones occurred commonly in children, particularly boys, and were formed mainly in the bladder. These stones usually consisted of ammonium urate and/or calcium oxalate and were caused by poor nutrition. Although this form of the disorder is still found today in rural areas within the "endemic stone belt" stretching from Jordan, through Iraq, Iran and the Indian subcontinent to the furthest extremities of South-East Asia, it is rapidly disappearing with improving standards of nutrition, as it did in most developed countries about 100 years ago (5).

As the incidence of bladder stones in children has decreased, however, the prevalence of upper urinary tract stones in adults has increased. Within this general increase in stone occurrence, there have been peaks and troughs in incidence that coincide with periods of economic prosperity and recession, respectively (Fig. 2). Kidney stones occur more frequently in the more industrially developed nations and are less common in those countries whose economies are more dependent on agriculture. Overall, the incidence of upper tract stone disease increases in parallel with the level of affluence, presumably through the effect of the latter on diet and lifestyle (6).

Other changes in the pattern of stone formation have also been noted during this time. Although stones generally occur more frequently in men than in women (male: female ratio about 2.5:1), recent studies have shown that, within the past 25 years, there has been a progressive decrease in the age at onset of stone formation in both males (Fig. 3A) and females (Fig. 3B), particularly females (7). Within the population of stone formers as a whole, the male: female ratio among patients who formed their first stone before the age of 20 is now 1.5:1 (cf. 3.0:1 in 1975). In those patients currently aged under 20, the

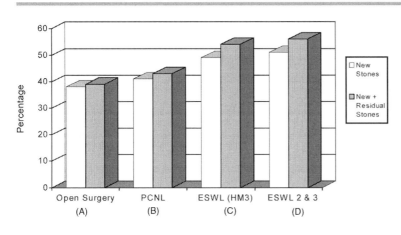

Figure 1 The percentage of patients with new stones or with new + residual stones within three years of the (A) open surgery, (B) percutaneous nephrolithotomy (PCNL), (C) extracorporeal shock wave lithotripsy using a Dornier HM3 lithotripter [ESWL (HM3)], or (D) extracorporeal shock wave lithotripsy using 2nd or 3rd generation lithotripters [ESWL (2,3)].

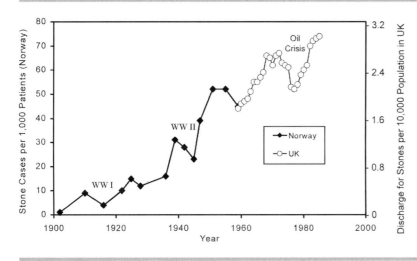

Figure 2 The number of stone cases per 1000 patients attending hospital in Norway and in the United Kingdom during the past 100 years. Oil Crisis refers to the Middle East Oil crisis in the early 1970s. Abbreviation: WW, World War.

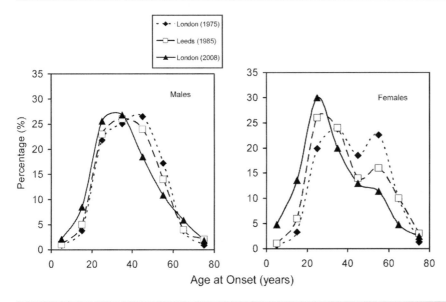

Figure 3 The decrease in age at onset of stone formation in males and females in the UK during the past 25 years.

ratio has fallen to 1.15:1 (cf 1.6:1 in 1975). The main changes have taken place in the teenage years and may be attributed to alterations in diet and lifestyle in that group during the past 33 years. The combination of an earlier age at onset and an increasing life expectancy means that more young first-time stone formers will have a longer span of life over which they are likely to experience recurrence of the disorder. This will add to the burden on urological resources required to manage the stone problem in the future.

STONE COMPOSITION

The vast majority (75–80%) of urinary calculi consist predominantly of calcium oxalate (Fig. 4), either on its own or mixed with calcium phosphate or, increasingly more frequently, mixed with uric acid (8). In about 90% of these cases, there is no obvious metabolic cause for their stones (idiopathic stone formers). In the remainder, stones form secondarily to some disorder of calcium metabolism, oxalate metabolism or acid-base balance (see section on calcium stone disease).

"Infection stones" composed of magnesium ammonium phosphate, usually in conjunction with calcium phosphate, constitute between 4% and 12% of all calculi. They are caused by urinary tract infections involving a urea-splitting organism and occur more commonly in women than in men (9). They may also occur secondarily to the formation of most types of sterile stone. The relative incidence of infection stones has decreased over the past 25 years in most Western countries, presumably as a result of better clinical diagnosis and earlier treatment of urinary tract infections.

Uric acid calculi constitute between 4% and 15% of all stones and generally depend on the relative consumption of animal and vegetable protein in the population concerned. Over the past two decades, there has been an increase in the occurrence of uric acid–containing stones in many Western countries which has been attributed to the increase in the prevalence of "metabolic syndrome," a disorder associated with obesity, hypertension and type 2 diabetes (10) (see later). "Pure" uric acid stones are rare in developing countries and are most common in the oil-rich states of the Arabian Gulf (Fig. 4) and other affluent populations, or in countries where there is a cheap local source of animal protein (8). Most uric acid stones are idiopathic in origin; a small number form secondarily to some disorder of purine metabolism or to some condition in which there is a high tissue turnover.

In all stone series, 1% to 3% of stones consist of one of a range of "rare" constituents derived either from some hereditary or congenital inborn error of metabolism, such as cystinuria, xanthinuria or 2,8-dihydroxyadeninuria, or from a prescribed drug or one of its metabolites that is relatively insoluble in urine, such as silica, sulfonamides (such as sulfadiazine), indinavir or triamterene.

All stones contain a small percentage by weight of mucoproteinaceous matrix. A few consist almost entirely of mucoprotein ("matrix calculi") and usually result from inflammation of the urinary tract in patients whose urine is not sufficiently supersaturated with calcium salts to mineralize the organic matrix (11). Apart from these rare entities, the role of the organic matrix in the formation of stones is unclear. By analogy with organized mineralized tissues such as bones and teeth, where the matrix plays a major role not only in the laying down of the mineral phase but also in defining the structure and architecture of the completed tissue, some researchers believe that the matrix of stones plays an equally important role in their initiation and growth (12–14). Others, however, maintain that it is present merely as an adventitious inclusion, as a consequence of the calcium-binding properties of certain glycoproteins in the matrix material (8).

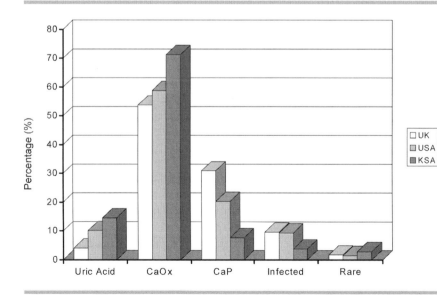

Figure 4 The percentage of urinary stones classified according to the predominant mineral in the United Kingdom (UK), United States of America (USA), and Kingdom of Saudi Arabia (KSA). *Abbreviations:* CaOx, calcium oxalate; CaP, calcium phosphate.

THEORIES OF STONE FORMATION

The essential features of a complete theory of stone formation are that it should account for the formation and retention within the urinary system of some critical nucleus, which then enlarges by the processes of crystal growth and agglomeration until it produces the clinical symptoms associated with the disorder, namely, renal colic, dysuria and hematuria. To understand the current theories on how stones begin to form, it is necessary to appreciate some simple chemical principles involved in the stone-forming process.

CHEMICAL PRINCIPLES OF URINARY STONE FORMATION

Supersaturation

The overriding factor that is common to all types of stone is the relative insolubility of their respective mineral component(s) in urine. When a substance is allowed to dissolve in water, dissolution proceeds until the rate of return of the dissolved material to the solid phase equals the rate at which the solid phase goes into solution. The concentration of the substance in solution at this equilibrium point is known as the substance's solubility under the conditions of temperature and ionic strength concerned. Examples of the solubilities in water at 37°C and at pH 6 of various salts and acids present in urine are shown in Table 1. Clearly, the substances that turn up in kidney stones have much lower solubilities than those that do not. For a sparingly soluble substance, it is usual to express this equilibrium value as a product of the concentrations (or more correctly activities) of the constituent ions rather than as the absolute solubility of the substance in mass per unit volume. This equilibrium activity product is known as the thermodynamic solubility product of the substance concerned and is a constant at a given temperature.

In the absence of crystals of a particular substance, it is possible to add the ionic constituents of that substance to water and reach an activity product in the ensuing solution that is considerably above the solubility product of the substance without crystal nucleation occurring (8). Such a solution is said to be in a state of metastable supersaturation, and it may survive in this state without *de novo* crystals forming

Table 1 Solubilities of Various Possible Urinary Salts and Acids in Water at 37°C and pH 6

Salt	Solubility (g/l)	Properties
Calcium oxalate	0.0071	
Calcium phosphate	0.08	
Uric acid	0.08	
Cystine	0.17	All occur in kidney stones.
Magnesium ammonium phosphate	0.36	
Calcium sulfate	2.1	
Calcium citrate	2.2	
Magnesium sulfate	293	Never occur in kidney stones.
Calcium chloride	560	

for several hours. There is, however, an upper limit to this region of metastability, known as the "formation product" of the substance. This is not a true thermodynamic constant, like the solubility product, but covers a band of supersaturation values within which de novo crystal nucleation may take place within a relatively short interval of time. Nucleation is dependent on the time of incubation and on the concentration of heterogeneous nuclei (that is, particles consisting of materials other than the substance under consideration) in the system. The upper limit of this band of formation products, beyond which the solution becomes completely unstable, corresponds to the level at which homogeneous nucleation takes place (8).

From these general considerations of solubility, it is evident that urine may fall into one of three zones of relative supersaturation with respect to each of the stone-forming minerals (Fig. 5). Urines lying below the solubility product of a given mineral are said to be undersaturated with respect to that mineral; in this region, no new crystals can form and any existing crystals will dissolve. There is no risk of forming stones in undersaturated urine. Urines lying between the solubility product and the formation product band are in a state of metastable supersaturation; in this region, urines can exist for quite long time periods without new crystals forming, but any existing crystals of the mineral concerned would be expected to grow [subject to the presence of possible inhibitors of crystallization (see below)]. Urines lying above the formation product band are said to be labile or unstable. Since urine is never a pure solution but usually contains particles of cell debris, polymerized glycoproteins, or even crystals of another salt, it is extremely unlikely that the point of homogeneous nucleation will ever be attained, since these particles will most likely have caused spontaneous heterogeneous nucleation to take place long before reaching this level of supersaturation (8).

No simple method exists for measuring supersaturation directly in urine, and this has to be obtained indirectly by computational techniques. To calculate the relative supersaturation of urine with respect to every stone-forming salt and acid requires the measurement of the concentrations of 15 different urinary constituents (15,16). These are fed into a computer that calculates the concentrations of all the soluble complexes formed between these constituents, the ionic strength of the urine and the activity coefficients of all the ions in solution. From this information, the activity products of each of the stone-forming substances are calculated and compared with the relevant solubility products. The ratio of activity product to solubility product is termed the relative supersaturation of urine with respect to the substance concerned. Values of 1 indicate that the urine is at the solubility product of the substance; values below 1 indicate that the urine is undersaturated with respect to the substance, and values greater than 1 indicate that the urine is supersaturated with that substance (16).

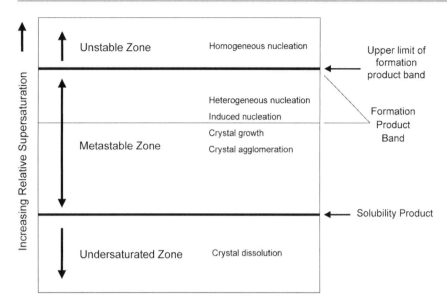

Figure 5 Diagram showing the three main regions of relative supersaturation of urine with respect to a sparingly soluble mineral and the crystallization processes that may occur in each region.

Whether or not supersaturation is the only factor responsible for the formation of stones is still open to debate. Broadly, there are two main schools of thought regarding the initiation of stones. Proponents of the "free-particle" model of urolithiasis believe that stones are initiated when urine becomes so excessively supersaturated with one of the salts or acids that turn up in kidney stones that crystals of that constituent spontaneously precipitate in urine (17,18). If this happens frequently and if the crystals grow or aggregate sufficiently within the transit time of urine through the kidney, the risk increases that one of these particles will become trapped at some narrow point in the urinary tract and form the focus around which a stone may form (19). Alternatively, blockage may occur through a "log-jamming" mechanism in a urinary stream overcrowded with crystals (Fig. 6) (8).

An alternative theory claims that the formation of a critical particle by such a free-particle mechanism cannot take place within the transit time of urine through the kidney and that the only way that a stone can be initiated is through chemical "fixation" of a crystal or aggregate of crystals to the renal epithelial lining (Fig. 6). In this "fixed-particle" theory, formation is postulated to occur either through damage to the cell walls (caused either by the crystals themselves or by viruses or bacteria) and/or through the participation of some "gluing" material present in the urine of stone formers (but absent from the urine of non–stone formers) that causes crystals to adhere to these sites and there act as foci for stone formation (20–26). Recently, a variant of the fixed-particle model has been proposed which postulates that stone formation is initiated by so-called "Randall's plaques," subepithelial flecks of calcium phosphate that are more frequently found in the renal papillae of stone formers than in those of individuals who do not have a history of urolithiasis (27,28). The plaques, originally described by Randall in 1937 (29), are considered to

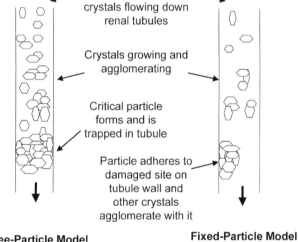

Free-Particle Model of Stone Initiation   **Fixed-Particle Model of Stone Initiation**

Figure 6 Diagrammatic representation of how stones are initiated according to the "free-particle" and "fixed-particle" models of stone formation.

form as a result of high supersaturation of tubular fluid with respect to calcium phosphate in the descending limb of the Loop of Henle (27,28). If these plaques erupt through the papillary epithelium, they may be exposed to urine supersaturated with respect to calcium oxalate and/or other stone-forming salts and acids in the renal calyces, thereby leading to the nucleation of a stone at the tip of renal papilla concerned. All the above theories require urine to be supersaturated to some degree with respect to the stone-forming salt or acid concerned, sufficient to cause crystals to be formed by spontaneous or heterogeneous nucleation.

Processes of Crystallization

Nucleation, as described above, is the first step in the process of crystallization. This causes a fall in the supersaturation of urine as new crystals are formed but does not usually reduce the level of supersaturation immediately down to the solubility product. There is then a period during which the initially formed nuclei grow in the remaining metastable urine, and in the moving stream of urine, the growing crystals may impact with each other and aggregate to form larger particles. This process is called agglomeration and is the stage in the crystallization process during which the particle size increases most rapidly (18,19,30). In the free-particle theory, crystal agglomeration is essential to create a particle that is large enough to be retained in the collecting tubule before the urine is expelled through the ducts of Bellini (18,19,31,32). Crystal growth per se is normally too slow a process to allow this to happen within the transit time of urine through the renal tubule.

Agglomeration may be less important in the fixed-particle model, since the initial particle that causes the stone to form round it is considered, by definition, to be glued to the renal tubular epithelial wall or formed round an exposed Randall's plaque. Once the initial entrapment (free-particle model) or fixation step (fixed-particle model) has taken place, both theories require the immobilized particle to increase in size through further crystal growth and agglomeration until it becomes a "stone" that causes problems for the patient (17–20,29,31,32).

Modifiers of Crystallization

One factor that may affect the kinetics of the processes involved in both theories is the presence or absence in urine of so-called modifiers of crystallization (8). These are claimed to be of particular importance in the formation of calcium-containing stones. Indeed, no specific, naturally occurring modifier has been reported to have any effect on the crystallization of cystine, uric acid or magnesium ammonium phosphate. One group of crystallization modifiers is claimed to retard the rate of growth and/or aggregation of crystals of calcium salts and/or the binding of calcium-containing crystals to cell walls. These are known as inhibitors of crystallization and include magnesium (33), citrate (34), pyro-phosphate (35,36), adenosine diphosphate (37), adenosine triphosphate (37), at least two phosphopeptides (38), various glycosaminoglycans (39,40), nonpolymerised Tamm-Horsfall protein (also known as uromodulin) (41,42), nephrocalcin (43–46), calgranulin (47), various plasma proteins (12), osteopontin (also known as uropontin) (48,49), α-1-microglobulin (13), β-2-microglobulin (50), urinary prothrombin fragment 1 (51,52) and inter-α-trypsin inhibitor (bikunin light chain) (53,54).

The second group of modifiers is claimed to stimulate one or more of the processes involved in the crystallization of calcium salts. These are known as promoters of stone formation and include matrix substance A (13), various uncharacterized urinary proteins and glycoproteins (55–57) and the polymerized form of Tamm-Horsfall protein (uromucoid) (58–60).

Unquestionably, urine does possess a certain ability to modify the rate of crystal growth and/or agglomeration of calcium oxalate crystals and may also contain factors that influence the binding of these crystals to renal epithelial cells. Currently, it would seem, however, that the "crystallization-modifying activity" is unlikely to be attributable to one single magic factor X but is probably due to the net effect of all the above promoters and inhibitors (and probably others not yet identified). None of the above factors appears to dominate the kinetics of crystal nucleation, growth, aggregation and binding to cells, and none has yet been accepted as being uniquely different, either quantitatively or qualitatively, between stone formers and normal subjects. Therefore, the assertion that a deficiency in one particular inhibitor or an excess of one particular promoter is the cause of stone formation is open to question (61).

In the final analysis, stone formation is probably due to an abnormal combination of factors that affect both the thermodynamic driving force (supersaturation) and the kinetic (rate-controlling) processes involved in the crystallization of the various stone-forming minerals. For some types of stone formation (cystine, xanthine, 2,8-dihydroxyadenine, uric acid and probably magnesium ammonium phosphate), the thermodynamic factors appear to predominate; in others (calcium-containing stones), both sets of factors may be involved (8).

Crystalluria

Whatever the detailed mechanism of stone initiation, an individual's propensity to produce crystals of one of the stone-forming constituents is an important prerequisite for stone formation, either because the crystals lead directly to the initiation of stones (as postulated in the free-particle model) or because their production is a signal that urine is so supersaturated with respect to that constituent that heterogeneous nucleation and crystal growth are likely to occur at one of the critical sites postulated in the fixed-particle model. Crystalluria occurs more frequently and more abundantly in the urine of stone formers than in that of controls, and, in patients with calcium stone disease, the crystals are larger and more agglomerated (18–19). The severity of the disorder, as defined by the stone episode rate in a given patient is proportional to the percentage of large crystals and aggregates in the patient's urine (Fig. 7). It would appear that particle size is a vital factor in the stone-forming process.

CYSTINE STONE FORMATION

Cystinuria is a congenital disorder characterized by a defect in the renal tubular reabsorption of cystine, lysine, ornithine and arginine, but the lesion also affects the intestine (62,63). As a consequence, the urinary excretion of these amino acids is greatly

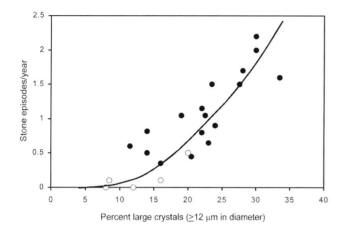

Figure 7 The relationship between the severity of stone formation (as defined by the stone episode rate) in recurrent calcium oxalate stone formers and the proportion of large calcium oxalate crystals and aggregates in their freshly voided urine: •, untreated patients; o, patients on orthophosphate supplements.

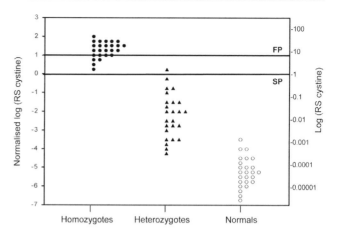

Figure 8 The relative supersaturation (RS) of urine with respect to cystine in homozygous cystinurics, heterozygous cystinurics and normal subjects. The data are plotted on a log scale (*right axis*), where the solubility product (SP) has a value of 1, and on a normalized log scale (*left axis*) such that the SP has a value of 0 and the upper limit of the formation product band (FP) has a value of 1.

increased. Lysine, ornithine and arginine are all fairly soluble in urine, but cystine is relatively insoluble and, as a result, these patients tend to have cystine crystalluria and to form cystine stones (64,65).

The sole risk factor for cystine stone formation is the supersaturation of urine with respect to cystine, as defined by the urinary concentration of cystine and urine pH (Fig. 8). Within the normal pH range of urine (5–7), the supersaturation is defined by the concentration of cystine. In normal urine, this is generally low (10–100 μmol/l), at which concentrations urine is well undersaturated with respect to cystine; therefore, cystine crystalluria is never found in normal urine. In heterozygous cystinurics, whose urinary cystine concentrations are in the range 20 to 1000 μmol/l, the supersaturation values are higher but still below the solubility of cystine in urine. As a rule, these patients do not have cystine crystalluria in fresh urine and do not form cystine stones (66). Homozygous cystinurics, however, have much higher urinary concentrations of cystine (1400–4200 μmol/l), above the solubility of

cystine in saline at 37° (1250 μmol/l), and so their urines are considerably supersaturated with respect to cystine (Fig. 8). These patients often pass large cystine crystals in their urine and form cystine stones (64,65). This form of stone formation is therefore readily explained in terms of excessive excretion → excessive supersaturation → abnormal crystalluria → stones. The complete risk factor model of cystine stone formation is outlined in Figure 9.

Prevention of cystine stones requires the supersaturation of urine to be substantially reduced to prevent continued crystalluria (Fig. 10). Although cystine is more soluble in alkaline urine than under acidic or neutral conditions, alkali therapy is not always practicable, as large doses of sodium bicarbonate are required to maintain urinary pH above 7.6 (67). Less alkali may be required if the patient is also put on a high fluid intake (>3 l/day) (68). Alternatively, reduction in cystine concentration may be achieved

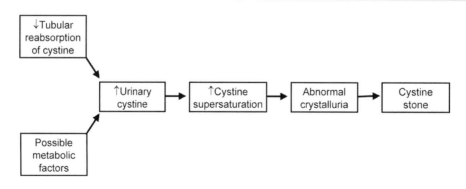

Figure 9 A risk factor model of cystine stone formation.

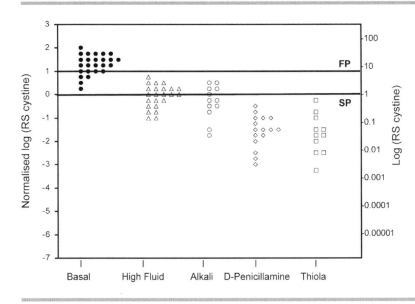

Figure 10 The effect of various treatments on the relative supersaturation (RS) of urine with respect to cystine in cystinuric stone formers. The data are plotted on a log scale (*right axis*), where the solubility product (SP) has a value of 1, and on a normalized log scale (*left axis*) such that the SP has a value of 0 and the upper limit of the formation product band (FP) has a value of 1.

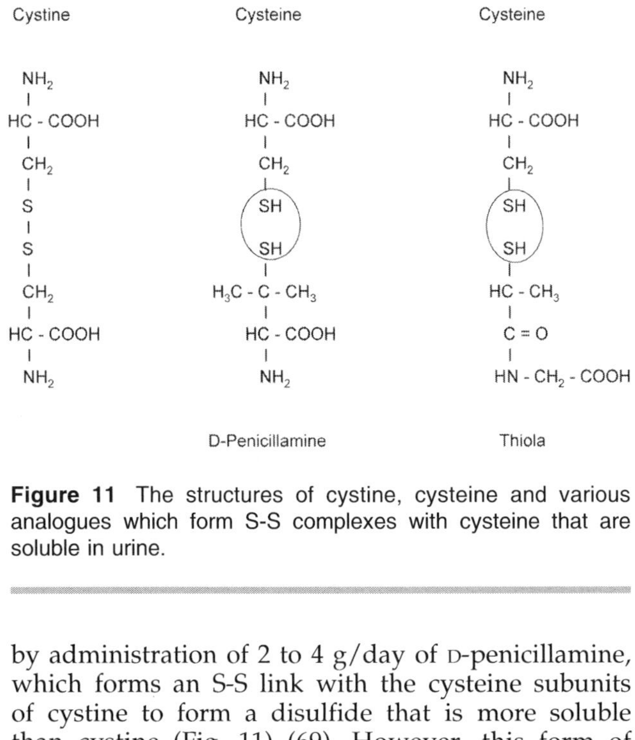

Figure 11 The structures of cystine, cysteine and various analogues which form S-S complexes with cysteine that are soluble in urine.

by administration of 2 to 4 g/day of D-penicillamine, which forms an S-S link with the cysteine subunits of cystine to form a disulfide that is more soluble than cystine (Fig. 11) (69). However, this form of therapy has a high risk of side-effects, including rashes, neutropenia, thrombo penia, nephrotic syndrome and fever. Severe proteinuria is experienced in about 10% to 15% of patients (65). A number of analogues, such as N-acetyl-D-penicillamine and α-mercaptopropionylglycine, have been tried with some degree of success as less toxic alternatives (70–72). If the above forms of therapy are pursued tenaciously, the supersaturation of urine with respect to cystine can be reduced (Fig. 10) and with it the risk of stone recurrence (65,73,74).

It is also possible to explain the formation of the other rare stones (such as 2,8-dihydroxyadenine,

xanthine and silica) simply on the basis of their insolubility in urine. These stones form purely from the excessive excretion in urine of the particular substance concerned, either as a result of some metabolic defect or from the administration of a drug that is itself insoluble (or one of its metabolites is insoluble) in urine. Urine becomes excessively supersaturated with the substance concerned, resulting in abnormal crystalluria and stone formation (8).

URIC ACID STONE FORMATION

Uric acid is the end-product of purine metabolism and is normally excreted in urine in the range 2 to 5 mmol/day (75,76). Patients with urinary excretions above this range are prone to form uric acid stones, but hyperuricosuria per se is not the sole cause or even the most important factor in uric acid lithiasis (77). Dehydration is as important as hyperuricosuria, and a low urine pH is more critical than both of these factors (78,79). The main causes of hyperuricosuria are listed in Table 2. The most recent addition to this list is fructose, which has been shown to increase the urinary excretion of uric acid following the breakdown of fructose by fructokinase (80).

Table 2 Causes of Hyperuricosuria

Primary gout
Increased purine intake
Increased fructose intake
Glycogen storage disease—glucose-6-phosphatase deficiency
Increased phosphoribosyl pyrophosphate synthetase activity
Hypoxanthine—guanine phosphoribosyltransferase deficiency
  (Lesch-Nyhan syndrome)
Neoplastic disease
Secondary polycythaemia
Anaemia and haemoglobinopathy
Psoriasis
Cystinuria

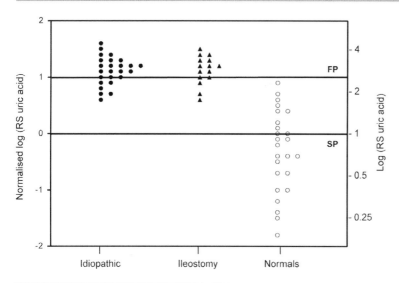

Figure 12 The relative supersaturation (RS) of urine with respect to uric acid in idiopathic uric acid stone formers, patients with an ileostomy and uric acid stones and normal subjects. The data are plotted on a log scale (*right axis*), where the solubility product (SP) has a value of 1, and on a normalized log scale (*left axis*) such that the SP has a value of 0 and the upper limit of the formation product band (FP) has a value of 1.

As with the formation of rare stones, uric acid stone formation can be completely explained in terms of excessive supersaturation of urine with respect to uric acid (8). Chemically, the two factors that determine the risk of uric acid crystalluria are the concentration of uric acid and the pH of urine. The pKa of uric acid is 5.46, so that any urine with a pH of less than this figure will contain more of the relatively insoluble, undissociated form of the acid. Uric acid crystalluria becomes increasingly more likely as urine pH drops below 5.3 (81). Normal urine, on the other hand, generally lies in the metastable or undersaturated region with respect to uric acid (8) with little or no risk of forming uric acid crystals (Fig. 12).

The causes of an acid urine are listed in Table 3. These include a high acid-ash diet containing large amounts of meat, fish and poultry (82). As this type of diet is also high in purines, these patients usually have hyperuricosuria in conjunction with their acid urine, and so the risk of uric acid stone formation is compounded (8). In the idiopathic uric acid stone formers, the tendency to pass an acid urine has been attributed to a low rate of ammonia synthesis;(78,83) ammonia is normally synthesized in the kidney to buffer hydrogen ions. Impaired renal ammoniagenesis leading to the passage of a more acidic urine than expected from the potential renal acid load, is probably the defect which leads to the formation of uric acid–containing stones in patients with metabolic syndrome, through the effects of insulin-resistance on both

Table 3 Possible Causes of Acid Urine

Dehydration
Oliguria
Diarrhoea
Permanent ileostomy
Colostomy
Low rate of renal production of ammonia
Increased titratable acidity
High acid ash diet (as in a high intake of animal protein)
"Metabolic syndrome"

phosphate-dependent and phosphate-independent ammonia production in the renal tubules (84,85). Patients with a permanent ileostomy also pass urine that is highly supersaturated with respect to uric acid (86). As a result their urine is highly concentrated and very acidic as a result of losing water and bicarbonate through their ileostomy. The risk factor model of uric acid stone formation is shown in Figure 13.

Treatment is designed to lower the supersaturation of urine with respect to uric acid (Fig. 14). This can be achieved relatively cheaply by increasing urinary pH to above 6.2 (but not higher than 6.5 to avoid formation of calcium phosphate stones) with oral sodium bicarbonate or potassium citrate and maintaining the urine volume above 2.5 l/day with a high fluid intake (78,79,87). Allopurinol, which inhibits the metabolic production of uric acid from xanthine by blocking the enzyme xanthine oxidase, may be necessary for patients who cannot tolerate alkali (88,89). Allopurinol has few side-effects, but care has to be taken with patients with enzyme defects that lead to a very high production of uric acid (such as Lesch-Nyhan syndrome or neoplastic disease), since allopurinol administration may result in xanthinuria and xanthine stones (90,91).

INFECTED STONE FORMATION

Urinary tract infections involving urea-splitting organisms often lead to the formation of stones that consist of calcium phosphate often mixed with magnesium ammonium phosphate (92). Chemically, the process involves the breakdown of urea by the enzyme urease to form ammonium, bicarbonate and hydroxyl ions (Fig. 15) with an accompanying marked alkalinization of urine (pH > 7.2). Under these conditions, the supersaturation of urine with respect to both calcium phosphate and magnesium ammonium phosphate reaches values that cause spontaneous precipitation of these salts and massive crystalluria

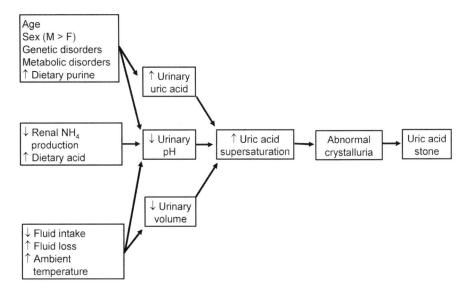

Figure 13 A risk factor model for uric acid stone formation.

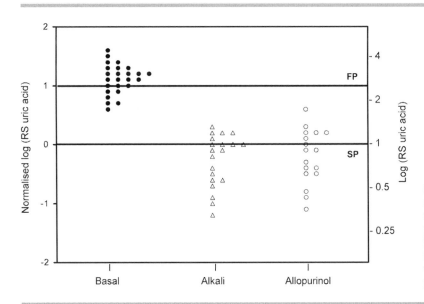

Figure 14 The effect of various treatments on the relative supersaturation (RS) of urine with respect to uric acid in uric acid stone formers. The data are plotted on a log scale (*right axis*), where the solubility product (SP) has a value of 1, and on a normalized log scale (*left axis*) such that the SP has a value of 0 and the upper limit of the formation product band (FP) has a value of 1.

$$3H_2O + \underset{H_2N}{\overset{H_2N}{\diagdown}}C=O \xrightarrow{\text{Urease}} 2NH_4 + HCO_3^- + OH^-$$

Figure 15 The breakdown of urea by urease to form ammonium ions and alkali.

(Fig. 16) (92,93). In addition, two of the known inhibitors of calcium phosphate crystal growth, pyrophosphate and citrate, are often low in the urines of patients with urinary tract infections, and this may allow the formation of larger than normal crystals and aggregates of calcium phosphate, thereby increasing the risk of stone formation (8). A list of the organisms causing urinary tract infection and their ability to produce urease is contained in Table 4. The risk factor model of infected stone formation is shown in Figure 17.

Treatment of infected stone patients usually involves the combined efforts of the surgeon and the physician. The first important stage is to remove the stone completely and, if possible, to correct any anatomical obstruction that might have caused the underlying infection. Medical management is necessary

Table 4 The Relative Prevalence of Organisms Causing Urinary Tract Infection and Their Ability to Produce Urease

Organisms causing urinary tract infection	Patients with infection (%)		Ability to produce urease	
	In hospital	At home	Frequently	Occasionally
Escherichia	5	0	0	1
Proteus	16	5	1	0
Klebsiella	9	2	0	1
Streptococcus	7	0	0	0
Staphylococcus	5	3	1	0
Pseudomonas	3	0	0	1
Ureaplasma urealyticum	1	0	1	0

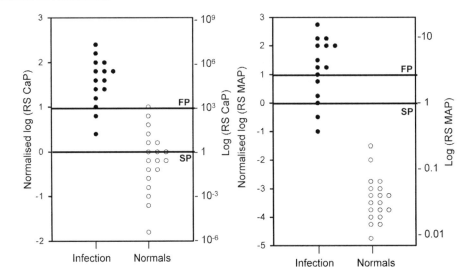

Figure 16 The relative supersaturation (RS) of urine with respect to calcium phosphate (CaP) (*left panel*) and magnesium ammonium phosphate (MAP) (*right panel*) in infected stone formers and normal subjects. The data are plotted on a log scale (*right axis of each panel*), where the solubility product (SP) has a value of 1, and on a normalized log scale (*left axis of each panel*) such that the SP has a value of 0 and the upper limit of the formation product band (FP) has a value of 1.

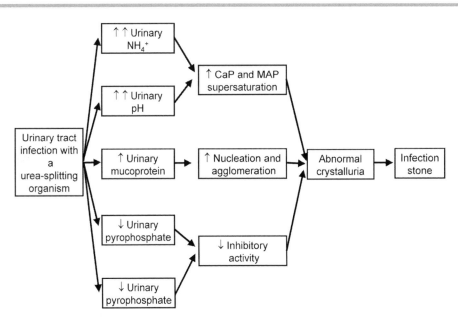

Figure 17 A risk factor model of infected stone formation.

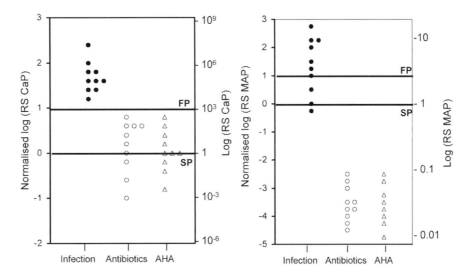

Figure 18 The effect of various treatments on the relative supersaturation (RS) of urine with respect to calcium phosphate (CaP) (*left panel*) and magnesium ammonium phosphate (MAP) (*right panel*) in infected stone formers. The data are plotted on a log scale (*right axis of each panel*), where the solubility product (SP) has a value of 1, and on a normalized log scale (*left axis of each panel*) such that the SP has a value of 0 and the upper limit of the formation product band (FP) has a value of 1. *Abbreviation:* AHA, acetohydroxamic acid.

before and after stone removal to sterilize the urine (94). This may not always be easy to achieve since the infecting organism may be resistant to several anti-biotics (95,96). In this situation, urease-inhibiting drugs, such as acetohydroxamic acid or one of its analogues, may be helpful (97–99), although there may be side-effects (Fig. 18) (97). A high fluid intake is necessary in all patients, and some acidification may be required to lower the urine pH to around 6. Drinking cranberry juice may be beneficial in this respect (100). It should be noted that cranberry juice is the only fruit juice known to acidify urine; all other fruit juices including those which are acidic to the taste, alkalinise urine.

CALCIUM STONE DISEASE

Stones consisting of calcium oxalate, often mixed with calcium phosphate, are the most common types of calculi in most series (8). Pure calcium phosphate stones are quite rare, suggesting that calcium oxalate is the main problem behind the formation of calcium-containing stones. The reason for this is the very poor solubility of calcium oxalate in aqueous media (Table 1). Whereas urine can often be undersaturated with respect to all other constituents of urinary calculi, particularly in non–stone formers, in the case of calcium oxalate urine is always supersaturated to some degree with the salt, even in normal subjects (Fig. 19). This means, firstly, that urine is relatively close to the formation product of calcium oxalate in most individuals and, secondly, that once calcium oxalate deposits form and become lodged in the kidney, they can never dissolve spontaneously. Stones containing calcium

oxalate can be disintegrated by ESWL and other methods and the fragments (probably) passed, but they cannot be easily redissolved, even with aggressive irrigation techniques.

The vast majority of calcium stone formers are said to be idiopathic, since they exhibit no obvious metabolic cause for their stones. About 10% to 12% of patients are found to have a metabolic cause, such as primary hyperparathyroidism, distal renal tubular acidosis or primary or enteric hyperoxaluria (8). The complete list of conditions and lifestyle practices that lead to secondary calcium stones is contained in Table 5.

Unlike most other types of stone formation, calcium lithiasis does not appear to be attributable to a single urinary abnormality or even to a simple combination of abnormalities. It is a truly multifactorial disorder in which various combinations of (often) small increases or decreases in certain urinary factors may compound the risk of forming stones (8). These include a low urine volume (<1.3 l/day) (101,102), a raised urinary pH (>6.3) (8,103). hypercalciuria (>6 mmol/day) (104–108), mild hyperoxaluria (>0.45 mmol/day) (29,109,110), hypocitraturia (<2 mmol/day) (111–113), hyperurico-suria (>4.5 mmol/day) (82) and a low urinary magnesium excretion (<3.2 mmol/day) (114). All of these factors have been found to be different between stone formers and normals, although in each case there is a considerable overlap between the data in the two groups (115,116). All the abnormalities described are known to increase the supersaturation of urine with respect to calcium oxalate and/or calcium phosphate, although they are not all equally important in this respect. In addition to their ability to influence supersaturation, citrate and magnesium are mild inhibitors of crystallization of calcium salts (33,34), and uric acid is a mild

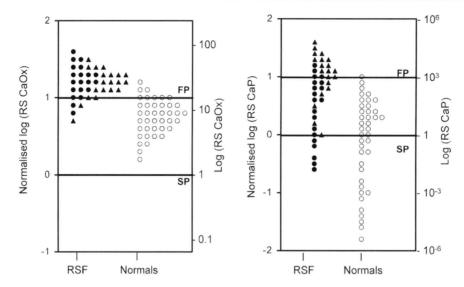

Figure 19 The relative supersaturation (RS) of urine with respect to calcium oxalate (CaOx) (*left panel*) and calcium phosphate (CaP) (*right panel*) in recurrent idiopathic calcium stone formers (RSF) and normal subjects. The RSF are divided into those with "pure" CaOx stones (•) and those with "mixed" CaOx/CaP stones (▲). The data are plotted on a log scale (*right axis of each panel*), where the solubility product (SP) has a value of 1, and on a normalized log scale (*left axis of each panel*) such that the SP has a value of 0 and the upper limit of the formation product band (FP) has a value of 1.

Table 5 List of Medical Conditions and Lifestyle Practices That May Lead to Secondary Calcium Stone Formation

Primary hyperparathyroidism
Distal renal tubular acidosis (type I)
Hereditary hyperoxaluria
Enteric hyperoxaluria
Pancreatitis
Medullary sponge kidney
Cushing's disease and steroid treatment
Sarcoidosis
Immobilization
Milk-alkali syndrome
Vitamin D intoxication
Bariatric surgery
Betel nut chewing
Laxative abuse
Antacid abuse (with calcium carbonate–containing preparations)
Stress
Tropical holidays
Strenuous exercise (without sufficient rehydration)

promoter of calcium stone formation (117,118). Risk factor analysis has shown that, taking all their properties into account, the overall order of importance of the above seven factors in determining the risk of forming calcium-containing stones is as follows: low urine volume > mild hyperoxaluria > raised urinary pH > hypercalciuria > hypocitraturia > hyperuricosuria > hypomagnesiuria (116).

The risk factor model of calcium stone formation makes use of these seven measurements to generate a number of algorithms that represent an estimate (P_{SF}) of the overall biochemical risk of forming various types of calcium-containing stones (115,116). The model has recently been extended to include uric acid-containing stones so that predictions can be made from an analysis of two 24-hour urines on the likelihood of forming all combinations of stone types involving uric acid, calcium oxalate and calcium phosphate (116). The values of P_{SF}, which are calculated on a probability scale from 0 to 1, are higher in stone formers than in non–stone formers. In recurrent stone formers, the values are generally over 0.5, whereas in normal subjects they are usually under 0.5. This function therefore provides quite a good discriminator between the two groups (Fig. 20). Furthermore, within the group of recurrent stone formers, the severity of the disorder (as defined by the stone recurrence rate of the patient) is related to the patient's average P_{SF} value. This method of combining risk factors is a useful means of assessing the risk of forming stones in a given individual and for following the efficacy of the particular form of prophylaxis prescribed for the patient. A summary of the urinary risk factors involved in all types of stone formation is given in Table 6.

Epidemiological Factors in the Formation of Urinary Stones

There are three groups of epidemiological factors that have been found to be of importance in the formation of urinary stones—demographic, environmental and pathophysiological. Each of these groups contains a number of categories. These are summarized in Table 7. Each has been shown to increase the risk of stone formation through its effect on the balance between supersaturation, inhibitors and promoters of crystallization in urine (8). For calcium stone formation, the most common form of the disorder, the

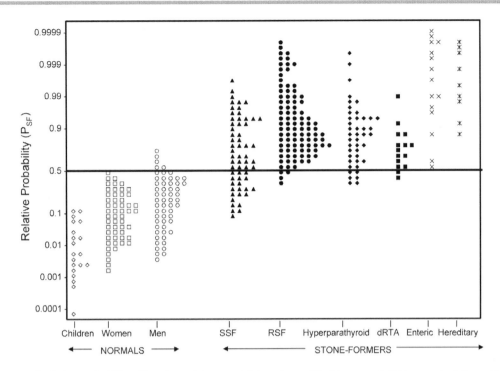

Figure 20   The overall relative probability of forming calcium-containing stones (P_{SF}) in normal children and adults and in single episode (SSF) and recurrent episode (RSF) idiopathic calcium stone formers. Also shown are the P_{SF} values in various groups of patients at risk of forming secondary calcium stones: hyperparathyroid, patients with primary hyperparathyroidism; dRTA, distal renal tubular acidosis; enteric, patients with enteric hyperoxaluria; hereditary, patients with hereditary hyperoxaluria.

Table 6   Summary of the Urinary Risk Factors for the Various Types of Stone Formation and Their Effects on the Parameters of Crystallization

Stone type	Urinary risk factor	Chemical effect
Rare stones	↑ Cystine, ↑ xanthine, ↑ 2,8-dihydroxyadenine, ↑ silica, ↑ indinavir, ↑ triamterene, etc.	↑ Supersaturation with respect to corresponding stone constituent
Cystine stones	Cystine	↑ Cystine supersaturation
Uric acid stones	↓ pH ↑ Uric acid ↓ Volume	↑ Uric acid supersaturation
Infection stones	↑ pH ↑ Ammonium ions ↑ Mucosubstances	↑ Magnesium ammonium phosphate and ↑ calcium phosphate supersaturation ↑ Agglomeration of crystals
Calcium stones	↓ Volume ↑ Oxalate ↑ Calcium ↑ pH ↓ Citrate ↓ Magnesium	↑ Calcium oxalate and/or calcium phosphate supersaturation
	↓ Macromolecular inhibitors	↓ Crystallization-inhibitory activity
	↑ Uric acid ↑ Macromolecular promoters	↑ Crystallization-promotive activity

main epidemiological factors are age (8), gender (8), season (119,120), climate (121,122), stress (123,124), occupation (122,125,126), affluence (127–129), diet (including fluid intake) (8,130–134), genetic/metabolic (135–137) and lifestyle factors (8).

The role of diet, in particular, has been studied in detail, and it appears to explain much of the changing pattern of stone incidence over the past 100 years (8,132,138), As the composition of the diet becomes "richer" in a given population (owing to an increased

Table 7 The Epidemiological Factors Involved in Uric Acid and Calcium Stone Formation and Their Effects on Urinary Risk Factors

Epidemiological factor	Urinary risk factors
Age and sex	↑ Calcium, ↑ oxalate, ↑ uric acid, ↑ pH, ↓ volume, ↓ citrate, ↓ magnesium, ↓ macromolecular inhibitors, ↑ promoters
Climate and season	↓ Volume, ↑ calcium, ↑ oxalate, ↓ pH
Stress	↑ Calcium, ↑ oxalate, ↑ uric acid, ↓ magnesium
Low fluid intake or strenuous exercise	↓ Volume, ↓ pH
Affluence and diet	↑ Calcium, ↑ oxalate, ↑ uric acid, ↓ citrate, ↓ pH
Metabolic and lifestyle disorders	
Gout	↑ Uric acid
Glycogen storage disease	↑ Uric acid
Lesch-Nyhan syndrome	↑ Uric acid
Neoplastic disease	↑ Uric acid
Ileostomy	↓↓ Volume, ↓↓ pH
"Metabolic syndrome"	↑ Uric acid, ↓↓ pH
Primary hyperparathyroidism	↑↑ Calcium, ↑ pH
Distal renal tubular acidosis	↑ pH, ↑ calcium, ↓ citrate
Hereditary hyperoxaluria	↑↑ oxalate
Enteric hyperoxaluria	↑ Oxalate, ↓ pH, ↓ citrate, ↓ magnesium
Medullary sponge kidney	↑ Calcium
Cushing's disease	↑ Calcium, ↑ pH
Vitamin D intoxication	↑↑ Calcium
Milk-alkali syndrome	↑ Calcium, ↑ pH
Bariatric surgery	↑ Oxalate
Topiramate	↑ Calcium, ↑ pH, ↓ citrate
Sarcoidosis	↑↑ Calcium
Immobilization	↑ Calcium, ↑↑ pH (from urinary tract infection)
Betel-nut chewing	↑ Calcium, ↑ pH
Antacid abuse	↑↑ Calcium, ↑ pH
Tropical holidays	↓ Volume, ↑ calcium

consumption of protein, particularly animal protein, fat, refined sugars and salt (the so-called "bad Western diet"), the incidence of stones increases (132,138) (Fig. 21). This often follows periods of economic expansion (Fig. 2). During periods of recession, on the other hand, the incidence of stones has been noted to decrease in parallel with a return to a more healthy form of diet containing more fiber and fewer energy-rich foods (8,138). The risk factor model for calcium stone formation, incorporating all of these factors, is shown in Figure 22.

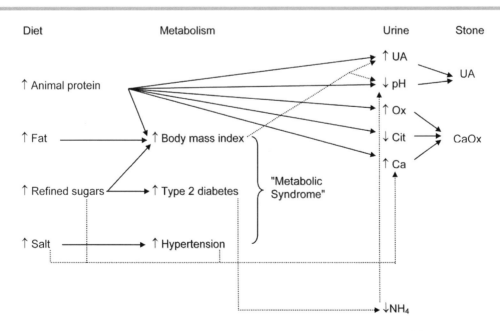

Figure 21 The effects of the "bad Western diet" on the risk of forming calcium oxalate and uric acid stones.

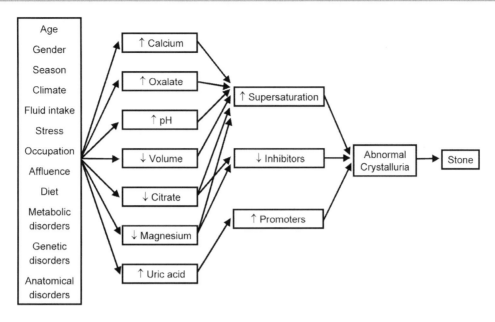

Figure 22   A risk factor model for calcium stone formation.

Prevention of Stone Recurrence

The main aim in the prevention of stone recurrence is to decrease the likelihood of crystals forming in the urinary tract by reducing the supersaturation of urine with respect to the particular constituent(s) that occur in the patients' stones (139–141). A summary of the available dietary and medical treatments for the various types of urinary calculi is shown in Table 8.

Although most of these are effective in reducing the risk of stone recurrence, the main problem in the long-term management of stone patients is compliance (142). Generally, stone formers feel well for most of the time, except when they are experiencing an attack of renal colic. It is often difficult, therefore, to maintain their cooperation and motivation to adhere to their preventative treatment over a long period after their

Table 8   Medical Methods for Prevention of Urinary Stone Disease

Stone type	Treatment
2,8-Dihydroxyadenine	Very high fluid intake (>3 l/day) + allopurinol (300 mg/day)
Silica	Discontinue magnesium trisilicate antacids
Xanthine	Hereditary form: high fluid intake + oral alkali (urine pH >7.4) Iatrogenic form: withdraw allopurinol
Cystine	Very high fluid intake (>3 l/day) + oral alkali (urine pH >7.5) or D-penicillamine (2–4 g/day) or α-mercaptopropionylglycine
Uric acid	High fluid intake (>2.5 l/day) + oral alkali (urine pH >6.2) or allopurinol (300 mg/day) or reduce purine intake
Infected	High fluid intake + antibiotics + oral acid (pH < 6.2)
Calcium	
Idiopathic	High fluid intake + dietary advice or thiazide diuretics (bendrofluazide 10 mg/day) or magnesium supplements (500 mg mg/day) or potassium citrate (20 mequiv t.d.s.)
Hyperparathyroid	Parathyroidectomy or, if contraindicated, high fluids + oral acid
Hereditary hyperoxaluric	High fluid intake (>3 l/day) + pyridoxine (300 mg/day)
Enteric hyperoxaluric	High fluid intake + low oxalate/high calcium diet or potassium citrate
Renal tubular acidotic	High fluid intake + thiazides or potassium citrate
Medullary sponge kidney	Treat as for idiopathic
Corticosteroid induced	Discontinue corticosteroids: treat as for idiopathic
Sarcoidosis	High fluid intake
Milk-alkali syndrome	Discontinue alkali and moderate calcium intake + high fluid intake
Vitamin D intoxication	Discontinue high vitamin D intake + high fluid intake
Betel nut chewing	Discontinue practice
Immobilization	High fluid intake; remobilize as far as possible; treat any urinary tract infection with antibiotics
Iatrogenic	Discontinue drug concerned as far as possible and replace with alternative therapy + high fluid intake
Antacid abuse	Discontinue calcium-containing antacids; change to proton pump inhibitors
Tropical holidays	Protect skin from UV radiation + increase fluid intake (not alcohol) while on holiday

stone episode. If they do not have a recurrence of their problem within a few months of their episode, most stone formers will regress to their original abnormal pattern of urine biochemistry within three to six months and will eventually produce another stone (143). Once they have had several episodes of renal colic, it is usually easier to motivate them on a more continuous basis. It is important to review the patient regularly as an outpatient and to repeat the 24-hour urine analysis, preferably annually but at least biennially, to ensure that they are adhering to the prophylaxis prescribed and to check that their biochemical risk of stones remains low (116,142).

REFERENCES

1. Williams RE. Long-term survey of 538 patients with upper urinary tract stone. B J Urol 1963; 35:416–437.
2. Pearl MS, Clayman RV. Outcomes and selection of surgical therapies of stones in the kidney and ureter. In: Coe FL, Favus MJ, Pak CYC, et al., eds. Kidney Stones—Medical and Surgical Management. Philadelphia: Lippincott-Raven, 1996:709–755.
3. Robertson WG. The economic case for the biochemical screening of stone patients. In: Rodgers AL, Hibbert BE, Hess B, et al., eds. Urolithiasis 2000. Cape Town: University of Cape Town, 2000:403–405.
4. Parks JH, Coe FL. The financial effects of kidney stone prevention. Kidney Int 1996; 50:1706–1712.
5. Andersen DA. Environmental factors in the aetiology of urolithiasis. In: Cifuentes Delatte L, Rapado A, Hodgkinson A, eds. Urinary Calculi. Basel: Karger, 1973:130–144.
6. Robertson WG, Peacock M, Heyburn PJ, et al. The risk of calcium stone-formation in relation to affluence and dietary animal protein. In: Brockis JG, Finlayson B, eds. Urinary Calculus. Littleton, MA: PSG Publishing, 1981:3–12.
7. Robertson WG, Whitfield HN, Unwin RJ, et al. Possible causes of the changing pattern of the age of onset of urinary stone disease in the UK. In: Rodgers AL, Hibbert BE, Hess B, et al., eds. Urolithiasis 2000. Cape Town: University of Cape Town, 2000:366–368.
8. Robertson WG. Urinary tract calculi. In: Nordin BEC, Need AG, Morris HA, eds. Metabolic Bone and Stone Disease. 3rd ed. Edinburgh: Churchill Livingstone, 1993:249–311.
9. Griffith DP, Osborne CA. Infection (urease) stones. Miner Electrolyte Metab 1987; 13:278–285.
10. Maalouf NM, Cameron MA, Moe OW, et al. Low urine pH: a novel feature of the metabolic syndrome. Clin J Am Soc Nephrol 2007; 2:883–888.
11. Wickham JEA. Matrix and the infective renal calculus. Br J Urol 1976; 47:727–732.
12. Boyce WH, King JS. Present concepts concerning the origin of matrix and stones. Ann N Y Acad Sci 1963; 104:563–578.
13. Morse RM, Resnick MI. A new approach to the study of urinary macromolecules as a participant in calcium oxalate crystallization. J Urol 1988; 139:869–873.
14. Morse RM, Resnick MI. A study of the incorporation of urinary macromolecules onto crystals of different mineral compositions. J Urol 1989; 141:641–644.
15. Robertson WG. Measurement of ionized calcium in biological fluids. Clin Chim Acta 1969; 24:149–157.
16. Werness P, Brown C, Smith LH, et al. EQUIL2: a BASIC computer program for the calculation of urinary saturation. J Urol 1985; 134:1242–1244.
17. Vermeulen CW, Ellis JE, Hsu TC. Experimental observations on the pathogenesis of urinary calculi. J Urol 1966; 95:681–690.
18. Robertson WG, Peacock M, Nordin BEC. Calcium crystalluria in recurrent renal stone-formers. Lancet 1969; 2:21–24.
19. Kok DJ, Papapoulos SE, Bijvoet OLM. Crystal agglomeration is a major element in calcium oxalate urinary stone-formation. Kidney Int 1990; 37:51–56.
20. Finlayson B, Reid F. The expectation of free and fixed particles in urinary stone disease. Invest Urol 1978; 15:442–448.
21. Kumar S, Sigmon D, Miller T, et al. A new model of nephrolithiasis involving tubular dysfunction/injury. J Urol 1991; 146:1384–1389.
22. Bigelow MW, Wiessner JH, Kleinman JG, et al. Calcium oxalate crystal attachment to cultured kidney epithelial cell lines. J Urol 1998; 160:1528–1532.
23. Verkoelen CF, van der Boom BG, Houtsmuller AB, et al. Increased calcium oxalate monohydrate crystal binding to injured tubular epithelial cells in culture. Am J Physiol 1998; 274:F958–F965.
24. Scheid C, Koul H, Hill WA, et al. Oxalate toxicity in LLC-PK$_1$ cells: role of free radicals. Kidney Int 1996; 49:413–419.
25. Lieske JC, Leonard R, Swift HS, et al. Adhesion of calcium oxalate monohydrate crystals to anionic sites of renal epithelial cells. Am J Physiol 1996; 270:F192–F199.
26. Koul H, Menon M, Koul S, et al. Effect of oxalate on calcium oxalate crystal adherence to renal epithelial cells in culture. In: Rodgers AL, Hibbert BE, Hess B, et al, eds. Urolithiasis 2000. Cape Town: University of Cape Town, 2000:267–269.
27. Matlaga BR, Williams JC, Kim SC, et al. Endoscopic evidence of calculus attachment to Randall's plaque. J Urol 2006; 175:1720–1724.
28. Matlaga BR, Coe FL, Evan AP, et al. The role of Randall's plaques in the pathogenesis of calcium stones. J Urol 2007; 177:31–38.
29. Robertson WG, Peacock M, Nordin BEC. Calcium oxalate crystalluria and urine saturation in recurrent renal stone-formers. Clin Sci 1971; 40:365–374.
30. Randall A. The origin and growth of renal calculi. Ann Surg 1937; 105:1009–1027.
31. Kok DJ, Khan SR. Calcium oxalate nephrolithiasis, a free or fixed particle disease? J Urol 1994; 46:847–854.
32. Robertson WG. Kidney models of calcium oxalate stone-formation. Nephron Physiol 2004; 98:21–30.
33. Borden TA, Lyon ES. The effects of magnesium and pH on experimental calcium oxalate stone disease. Invest Urol 1969; 6:412–422.
34. Meyer JL, Smith LH. Growth of calcium oxalate crystals. II. Inhibition by natural urinary crystal growth inhibitors. Invest Urol 1975; 13:36–39.
35. Fleisch H, Bisaz S. Isolation from urine of pyrophosphate, a calcification inhibitor. Am J Physiol 1962; 203:671–675.
36. Fleisch H, Bisaz S. The inhibitory effect of pyrophosphate on calcium oxalate precipitation and its relation to urolithiasis. Experientia 1964; 20:276–277.
37. Meyer JL, McCall JT, Smith LH. Inhibition of calcium phosphate crystallization by nucleoside phosphates. Calcif Tissue Res 1974; 15:289–293.
38. Howard JE, Thomas WC, Barker LM, et al. The recognition and isolation from urine and serum of a peptide inhibitor to calcification. Johns Hopkins Med J 1967; 120:119–136.
39. Robertson WG, Peacock M, Nordin BEC. Inhibitors of the growth and aggregation of calcium oxalate crystals in vitro. Clin Chim Acta 1973; 43:31–37.

40. Ryall RL, Harnett RM, Marshall VR. The effect of urine, pyrophosphate, citrate, magnesium and glycosaminoglycans on the growth and aggregation of calcium oxalate crystals in vitro. Clin Chim Acta 1981; 112:349–356.

41. Robertson WG, Scurr DS, Bridge CM. Factors influencing the crystallization of calcium oxalate in urine – a critique. J Cryst Growth 1981; 53:182–194.

42. Worcester EM, Nakagawa Y, Coe FL. Glycoprotein calcium oxalate crystal growth inhibitor in urine. Miner Electrolyte Metab 1987; 13:267–272.

43. Worcester EM, Nakagawa Y, Wabner CL, et al. Crystal adsorption and growth slowing by nephrocalcin, albumin and Tamm-Horsfall protein. Am J Physiol 1988; 255: F1197–F1205.

44. Nakagawa Y, Ahmed MA, Hall SL, et al. Isolation from human calcium oxalate stones of nephrocalcin, a glycoprotein inhibitor of calcium oxalate crystal growth. Evidence that nephrocalcin from patients with calcium oxalate nephrolithiasis is deficient in gamma-carboxyglutamic acid. J Clin Invest 1987; 79:1782–1787.

45. Hess B, Nakagawa Y, Coe FL. Inhibition of calcium oxalate monohydrate crystal aggregation by urine proteins. Am J Physiol 1989; 257:F99–F106.

46. Coe FL, Parks JH. Defenses of an unstable compromise: crystallization inhibitors and the kidney's role in mineral regulation. Kidney Int 1990; 38:625–631.

47. Pillay SN, Asplin JR, Coe FL. Evidence that calgranulin is produced by kidney cells and is an inhibitor of calcium oxalate crystallization. Am J Physiol 1998; 275: F255–F261.

48. Shiraga H, Min W, Van Dusen WJ, et al. Inhibition of calcium oxalate crystal growth in vitro by uropontin: another member of the aspartic acid-rich protein superfamily. Proc Natl Acad Sci USA 1992; 89:426–430.

49. Tsuji H, Tohru U, Hirotsugu U, et al. Urinary concentration of osteopontin and association with urinary supersaturation and crystal formation. Int J Urol 2007; 14:630–634.

50. Dussol B, Geider S, Lilova A, et al. Analysis of the soluble matrix of five morphologically different kidney stones. Urol Res 1995; 23:45–51.

51. Stapleton AMF, Dawson CJ, Grover PK, et al. Further evidence linking urolithiasis and blood coagulation: urinary prothrombin fragment 1 is present in stone matrix. Kidney Int 1996; 49:880–888.

52. Grover PK, Ryall RL. Inhibition of calcium oxalate crystal growth and aggregation by prothrombin and its fragments in vitro: relationship between protein structure and inhibitory activity. Eur J Biochem 1999; 263:50–56.

53. Dawson CJ, Grover PK, Ryall RL. Inter-alpha-inhibitor in urine and calcium oxalate urinary crystals. Br J Urol 1998; 81:20–26.

54. Evan AP, Bledsoe S, Worcester EM, et al. Renal inter-alpha-trypsin inhibitor heavy chain 3 increases in calcium oxalate stone-forming patients. Kidney Int 2007; 72: 1503–1511.

55. Spector AR, Gray A, Prien EL. Kidney stone matrix. Differences in acidic protein composition. Invest Urol 1976; 13:387–389.

56. Lian JB, Prien EL, Glimcher MJ, et al. The presence of protein-bound c-carboxyglutamic acid in calcium-containing renal calculi. J Clin Invest 1977; 59:1151–1157.

57. Jones WT, Resnick MI. The characterization of soluble matrix proteins in selected human renal calculi using two-dimensional polyacrylamide gel electrophoresis. J Urol 1990; 144:1010–1014.

58. Rose GA, Sulaiman S. Tamm-Horsfall mucoproteins promote calcium oxalate crystal formation in urine: quantitative studies. J Urol 1982; 127:177–179.

59. Scurr DS, Robertson WG. Modifiers of calcium oxalate crystallization found in urine. III. Studies on the role of Tamm-Horsfall mucoprotein and of ionic strength. J Urol 1986; 136:505–507.

60. Grover PK, Ryall RL, Marshall VR. Does Tamm-Horsfall mucoprotein inhibit or promote calcium oxalate crystallization in human urine? Clin Chim Acta 1990; 190:223–238.

61. Robertson WG. 'Take-home message' on the epidemiology and basic science of stone-formation. In: Rodgers AL, Hibbert BE, Hess B, et al., eds. Urolithiasis 2000. Cape Town: University of Cape Town, 2000:841–849.

62. Dent CE, Senior B, Walshe JM. The pathogenesis of cystinuria. II. Polarographic studies of the metabolism of sulphur-containing amino acids. J Clin Invest 1954; 33:1216–1226.

63. Milne MD, Asatoor AM, Edwards KDG, et al. The intestinal absorption defect in cystinuria. Gut 1961; 2:323–337.

64. Ettinger B, Kolb FO. Factors involved in crystal formation in cystinuria. In vivo and in vitro crystallization dynamics and a simple colorimetric assay for cystine. J Urol 1971; 106:106–110.

65. Dahlberg PJ, Van den Berg CJ, Kurtz SB, et al. Clinical features and management of cystinuria. Mayo Clin Proc 1977; 52:533–542.

66. Crawhall JC, Purkiss P, Watts RWE, et al. The excretion of amino acids by cystinuric patients and their relatives. Ann Hum Genet 1969; 33:149–169.

67. Dent CE, Friedman M, Green H, et al. Treatment of cystinuria. Br Med J 1965; 1:403–407.

68. Dent CE, Senior B. Studies on the treatment of cystinuria. Br J Urol 1955; 27:317–332.

69. Crawhall JC, Scowen EF, Watts RWE. Effect of penicillamine on cystinuria. Br Med J 1963; 1:588–590.

70. Stokes GS, Potts JT, Lotz M, et al. New agent in the treatment of cystinuria: N-acetyl-D-penicillamine. BMJ 1968; 1:284–288.

71. Remien A, Kallistratos G, Burchardt P. Treatment of cystinuria with thiola (α-mercapto-propionyl glycine). Eur Urol 1975; 1:227–228.

72. Pak CYC, Fuller C, Sakhaee K, et al. Management of cystine nephrolithiasis with mercaptopropionylglycine. J Urol 1986; 136:1003–1008.

73. Frimpter GW. Medical management of cystinuria. Am J Med Sci 1968; 255:348–357.

74. Koide Y, Kinoshita K, Takemoto M, et al. Conservative treatment of cystine calculi: effect of oral alpha-mercaptopropionylglycine on cystine stone dissolution and on prevention of stone recurrence. J Urol 1982; 128:513–516.

75. Gutman AB, YFC TF. Uric acid nephrolithiasis. Am J Med 1968; 45:657–779.

76. Seegmiller JE, Grayzel AI, Laster L, et al. Uric acid production in gout. J Clin Invest 1961; 40:1304–1314.

77. Atsmon A, De Vries A, Frank M. Uric Acid Lithiasis. Amsterdam: Elsevier, 1963.

78. Metcalfe-Gibson A, MacCallum FM, Morrison RBI, et al. Urinary excretion of hydrogen ion in patients with uric acid calculi. Clin Sci 1965; 28:325–345.

79. Kursh ED, Resnick MI. Dissolution of uric acid calculi with system alkalinization. J Urol 1984; 132:286–287.

80. Johnson RJ, Segaj MS, Sautin Y, et al. Potential role of sugar (fructose) in the epidemic of hypertension, obesity and the metabolic syndrome, diabetes, kidney damage and cardiovascular disease. Am J Clin Nutr 2007; 86: 899–906.

81. Cifuentes Delatte L, Rapado A, Abehsera A, et al. Uric acid lithiasis and gout. In: Cifuentes Delatte L, Rapado A, Hodgkinson A, eds. Urinary Calculi. Basel: Karger, 1973:115–118.

82. Coe FL, Moran E, Kavalich AG. The contribution of dietary purine over-consumption to hyperuricosuria on calcium oxalate stone-formers. J Chron Dis 1976; 29: 793–800.

83. Henneman PH, Wallach S, Dempsey EF. The metabolic defect responsible for uric acid stone-formation. J Clin Invest 1962; 41:537–542.

84. Maalouf NM, Sakhaee K, Parks JH, et al. Kidney Int 2004; 65:1422–1425.

85. Robertson WG, Nair D, Lang C, et al. The role of "Metabolic Syndrome" in the formation of uric-acid-containing stones. Urol Res 2010 (in press).

86. Bambach CP, Robertson WG, Peacock M, et al. Effect of intestinal surgery on the risk of urinary stone formation. Gut 1981; 22:257–263.

87. Pak CYC, Sakhaee K, Fuller C. Successful management of uric acid nephrolithiasis with potassium citrate. Kidney Int 1986; 30:422–428.

88. Rundles WR, Wyngaarden JB, Hitchings GH, et al. Effect of xanthine oxidase inhibitor on thiopurine metabolism, hyperuricaemia and gout. Trans Assoc Am Physicians 1963; 76:126–140.

89. Godfrey RG, Rankin TJ. Uric acid renal lithiasis: management by allopurinol. J Urol 1969; 101:643–647.

90. Greene ML, Fujimoto WY, Seegmiller JE. Urinary xanthine stones – a rare complication of allopurinol therapy. N Engl J Med 1969; 280:426–427.

91. Band PR, Silverberg DS, Henderson JF, et al. Xanthine nephropathy in a patient with lymphosarcoma treated with allopurinol. N Engl J Med 1970; 283:354–357.

92. Griffith DP, Musher DM, Itin C. Urease. The primary cause of infection-induced urinary stones. Invest Urol 1976; 13:346–350.

93. Robertson WG, Peacock M, Nordin BEC. Activity products in stone-forming and non-stone-forming urine. Clin Sci 1968; 32:579–594.

94. Lerner SP, Gleeson MJ, Griffith DP. Infection stones. J Urol 1989; 141:753–758.

95. Cox CE. Urinary tract infection and renal lithiasis. Urol Clin N Am 1974; 1:279–297.

96. Chinn RH, Maskell R, Mead JE, et al. Renal stone and urinary infection: a study of antibiotic treatment. BMJ 1976; 2:1411–1413.

97. Griffith DP, Gibson JR, Clinton CW, et al. Acetohydroxamic acid: clinical studies of a urease inhibitor in patients with staghorn renal calculi. J Urol 1978; 119:9–15.

98. Martelli A, Buli P, Cortecchia V. Urease inhibitor therapy in infected renal stones. Eur Urol 1981; 7:291–293.

99. Griffith DP, Gleeson MJ, Lee H, et al. Randomized, double-blind trial of Lithostat (acetohydroxamic acid) in the palliative treatment of infection-induced urinary calculi. Euro Urol 1991; 20:243–247.

100. Kinney AB, Blount M. Effect of cranberry juice on urinary pH. Nurs Res 1979; 28:287–290.

101. Pak CYC, Sakhaee K, Crowther C, et al. Evidence justifying a high fluid intake in treatment of nephrolithiasis. Ann Intern Med 1980; 93:36–39.

102. Jaeger P, Portmann L, Jacquet AF, et al. Drinking water for stone-formers: is the calcium content relevant? Eur Urol 1984; 10:53–54.

103. Marshall RW, Cochran M, Robertson WG, et al. The relation between urine saturation and stone composition in patients with calcium-containing renal stones. Clin Sci 1972; 43:433–441.

104. Albright F, Henneman P, Benedict PH, et al. Idiopathic hypercalciuria. Proc R Soc Med 1953; 46:1077–1081.

105. Hodgkinson A, Pyrah LN. The urinary excretion of calcium and inorganic phosphate in 344 patients with calcium stone of renal origin. Br J Surg 1958; 46:10–18.

106. Pak CYC, Kaplan RA, Bone H, et al. A simple test for the diagnosis of absorptive, resorptive and renal hypercalciurias. N Engl J Med 1975; 292:497–500.

107. Coe FL, Favus MJ. Idiopathic hypercalciuria in calcium nephrolithiasis. Disease-a-Month 1980; 26:1–36.

108. Halabé A, Sutton RAL. Primary hyperparathyroidism and idiopathic hypercalciuria. Miner Electrolyte Metab 1987; 13:235–241.

109. Robertson WG, Peacock M. The cause of idiopathic calcium stone disease: hypercalciuria or hyper oxaluria? Nephron 1980; 26:105–110.

110. Rose GA. Current trends in urolithiasis research. In: Rous SN, ed. Stone Disease: Diagnosis and Management. Orlando, FL: Grune & Stratton, 1987:383–416.

111. Rudman D, Kutner MH, Redd SC, et al. Hypocitraturia in calcium nephrolithiasis. J Clin Endocrinol Metab 1982; 55(6):1052–1057.

112. Nicar MJ, Skurla C, Sakhaee K, et al. Low urinary citrate excretion in nephrolithiasis. Urology 1983; 21:8–14.

113. Hosking DH, Wilson JW, Liedtke RR, et al. Urinary citrate excretion in normal persons and patients with idiopathic calcium urolithiasis. J Lab Clin Med 1985; 106:682–689.

114. Tiselius H G, Almgård LE, Larsson L, et al. A biochemical basis for grouping of patients with urolithiasis. Eur Urol 1978; 4:241–249.

115. Robertson WG, Peacock M, Heyburn PJ, et al. Risk factors in calcium stone disease of the urinary tract. Br J Urol 1978; 50:449–454.

116. Robertson WG. A risk factor model of stone-formation. Front Biosci 2003; 8:1330–1338.

117. Coe FL, Kavalich AG. Hypercalciuria and hyperuricosuria in patients with calcium nephrolithiasis. N Engl J Med 1974; 291:1344–1350.

118. Grover PK, Ryall RL. Urate and calcium oxalate stones: from repute to rhetoric to reality. Miner Electrolyte Metab 1994; 20:361–370.

119. Prince CL, Scardino PL, Wolan CT. The effect of temperature, humidity and dehydration on the formation of renal calculi. J Urol 1956; 75:209–215.

120. Robertson WG, Peacock M, Marshall RW, et al. Seasonal variations in the composition of urine in relation to calcium stone-formation. Clin Sci Mol Med 1975; 49:597–602.

121. Pierce LW, Bloom B. Observations on urolithiasis among American troops in a desert area. J Urol 1945; 54:466–470.

122. Blacklock NJ. The pattern of urolithiasis in the Royal Navy. In: Hodgkinson A, Nordin BEC, eds. Proceedings of the Renal Stone Research Symposium. London: Churchill, 1969:33–47.

123. Brundig P, Berg W, Schneider HJ. Stress und Harnsteinbildungsrisiko. I. Einfluss von Stress auf lithogene Harnsubstanz. Urol Int 1981; 36:199–207.

124. Diniz DHMP, Schor N, Blay SL. Stressful life events and painful recurrent colic of renal lithiasis. J Urol 2006; 176:2483–2487.

125. Larsen JF, Phillip J. Studies on the incidence of urolithiasis. Urol Int 1962; 13:53–54.

126. Clark JY. Renal calculi in army aviators. Aviat Space Environ Med 1990; 61:744–747.

127. Robertson WG, Peacock M, Hodgkinson A. Dietary changes and the incidence of urinary calculi in the UK between 1958 and 1976. J Chron Dis 1979; 32:469–476.

128. Robertson WG, Peacock M, Baker M, et al. Studies on the prevalence and epidemiology of urinary stone disease in men in Leeds. Br J Urol 1983; 55:595–598.

129. Power C, Barker DJP, Blacklock NJ. Incidence of renal stones in 18 British towns. Br J Urol 1987; 59:105–110.

130. Robertson WG, Peacock M, Heyburn PJ, et al. Should recurrent calcium oxalate stone-formers become vegetarians? Br J Urol 1979; 51:427–443.

131. Robertson WG, Peacock M, Marshall DH. Prevalence of urinary stone disease in vegetarians. Eur Urol 1982; 8:334–339.

132. Robertson WG. Diet and calcium stones. Miner Electrolyte Metab 1987; 13:228–234.

133. Iguchi M, Umekawa IT, Ishikawa T, et al. Dietary intake and habits of Japanese renal stone patients. J Urol 1990; 143:1093–1095.

134. Curhan GC, Willett WC, Rimm EB, et al. A prospective study of dietary calcium and other nutrients and the risk of symptomatic kidney stones. N Engl J Med 1993; 328:833–838.

135. Resnick MI, Pridgen DB, Goodman HO. Genetic predisposition to formation of calcium oxalate renal calculi. N Engl J Med 1968; 278:1313–1318.

136. Coe FL, Parks JH, Moore ES. Familial idiopathic hypercalciuria. N Engl J Med 1979; 300:337–340.

137. Aladjem M, Modan M, Lusky A, et al. Idiopathic hypercalciuria: a familial generalized renal hyper excretory state. Kidney Int 1983; 24:549–554.

138. Blacklock NJ. Epidemiology of renal lithiasis. In: Wickham JEA, ed. Urinary Calculous Disease. Edinburgh: Churchill Livingstone, 1979:21–39.

139. Coe FL, Parks JH, Asplin JR. The pathogenesis and treatment of kidney stones – medical progress. N Engl J Med 1992; 327:1142–1152.

140. Fine JK, Pak CYC, Preminger GM. Effect of medical management and residual fragments on recurrent stone formation following shock wave lithotripsy. J Urol 1995; 153:27–33.

141. Pak CYC. Kidney stones. Lancet 1998; 351:1797–1801.

142. Robertson WG. Is it possible to motivate patients with recurrent stones to adhere to their treatment regimen?In: Rodgers AL, Hibbert BE, Hess B, et al., eds. Urolithiasis 2000. Cape Town: University of Cape Town, 2000:624–627.

143. Norman RW, Bath SS, Robertson WG, et al. When should patients with symptomatic stone disease be evaluated metabolically? J Urol 1984; 132:1137–1139.

11

Pathophysiology and Management of Shock

Iain M. J. Mackenzie

*Department of Anaesthesia and Critical Care, University Hospital Birmingham NHS
Foundation Trust, Edgbaston, Birmingham, U.K.*

> The manifestation of a rude unhinging of the machinery of life.
> *Dr Samuel D. Gross*
>
> A momentary pause in the act of death.
> *Dr R. Adams Cowley*

WHAT IS SHOCK?

The war of the Spanish Succession was eventually concluded by the treaty of Utrecht on the April 11, 1713, after two grueling battles on the Franco-Belgian border, which left staggering numbers of dead and wounded in their wake: about 37,000 at the Battle of Malplaquet in 1709 and a further 23,000 at the Battle of Denain in 1712. Even compared with earlier battles of the campaign, such as the Battles of Blenheim (1704) and Ramillies (1706), these casualty figures were alarmingly high. Besides the change in military tactics that had occurred since the Thirty Years' War almost a half century earlier, the other major contributor was the replacement of the infantryman's pike for the flintlock musket. Tending to the wounded in Louis XIV's army was the young military surgeon Henri Le Dran (1685–1770), who was later appointed as a surgeon at La Charité in Paris (1724), and eventually became the Chief Surgeon to the French army. Drawing on his extensive experience, Le Dran published in 1737 a monograph on the management of gun-shot wounds (1) in which he undoubtedly described both hemorrhagic and septic shock, although contrary to some accounts he never used the word "choc" himself. Six years later, in 1743, the English translation of Le Dran's now famous treatise was published in London, and it is in the translation that the first use of the word "shock" is made as a mistranslation of the French "secousse."

Although subsequent military conflicts, such as the Crimean War[a] (1853–1856), the American Civil War[b] (1861–1865), and the Spanish-American War[c] (1898), contributed a number of theories to the etiology of "wound shock," a proper understanding of this complex phenomenon required hemodynamic measurements that only became available during the course of the 20th century (2).

In clinical terms shock describes a constellation of signs and symptoms that reflect widespread organ dysfunction caused by cellular metabolic failure. This may arise from an intracellular failure of substrate utilization, but is often driven, or at least accompanied by, a failure of substrate delivery, either locally or systemically (Fig. 1). More formally the definition of shock varies depending on the clinical context (Tables 1 and 2). By the time that the clinical features attract attention, hypotension, relative or absolute, is a common finding, accompanied by one or more features of organ dysfunction such as confusion or oliguria—with the conspicuousness of the clinical presentation arising from the interplay between severity and duration. Both the severity and duration of the initiating insult determine the extent and reversibility of cellular/organ dysfunction, exacerbated by stress signals from other sites.

The number of patients admitted to an intensive care unit (ICU) with shock has risen steadily since 1997 (Fig. 2), although the overall proportion of patients admitted in shock has remained much the same. As the Intensive Care National Audit and Research Centre (ICNARC) only collects data from England[d], one can extrapolate this figure on a population basis to estimate an incidence of over 31,300 cases per year for the United Kingdom as a whole. Of note, the proportion of patients admitted in shock with an underlying genitourinary problem has almost doubled in the same period, now accounting for just under 7% of all cases of shock admitted to ICU (Fig. 3). The proportion by pathophysiological cause is hard to

---

[a]Shock identified as a distinct entity from haemorrhage.
[b]George Crile.
[c]Shock identified with infection.

[d]By the 2001 census 94% of the UK population lived in England.

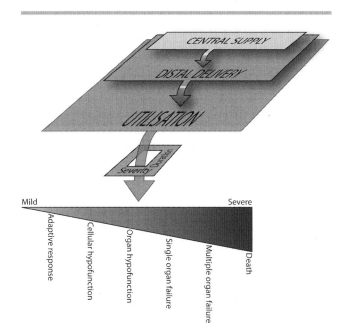

Figure 1 Schematic overview of the pathophysiological cascade of dependencies leading to shock. The top half of the diagram illustrates the cascade of dependencies, where tissue substrate utilization depends on the regional (distal) delivery of substrate via arterioles and capillaries, which in turn is dependent on the central supply of this substrate from the heart and major arteries. The bottom half of the diagram illustrates the interplay between the severity and duration of metabolic failure that then result in a spectrum of abnormalities from an adaptive response at one end of the spectrum to death at the other.

determine, but in a consecutive series of patients admitted to ICU with shock, 53% had septic shock, 28% cardiogenic shock, and 19% hypovolemic shock (7). However, this data is from a small series and was performed in a surgical ICU, explaining the absence of the many other, nonsurgical, causes of shock.

Nevertheless, it is likely that these three forms of shock account for up to 75% or 80% of cases. The hospital mortality of these patients increases with the severity of shock and the number of failed organs, but overall varies from around 33% in patients with septic shock (8), 41.6% in patients with cardiogenic shock (9), and up to 54% in patients with hemorrhagic shock (10).

HEMODYNAMIC PATHOPHYSIOLOGY

Traditionally, shock has been divided into four etiological categories, namely hypovolemic, cardiogenic, obstructive, and distributive (11), with the later addition of "endocrine shock" as a fifth category. This classification implies a single underlying hemodynamic problem in each category, which is almost invariably not the case. The schema shown in Figure 1 illustrates the cascade of dependencies, with tissue substrate utilization requiring adequate peripheral delivery, which itself requires an adequate central supply.

Central Supply

The central supply of substrate is generated by the cardiac output, which is the product of stroke volume and heart rate.

$$\text{Cardiac output (CO)} = \text{stroke volume (SV)} \times \text{heart rate (HR)} \tag{1}$$

Stroke Volume

There are three factors that determine the stroke volume: preload, contractility, and afterload (Fig. 4). The factors that influence each of these is discussed below.

Preload. The maximum force that a strip of cardiac muscle can exert is an intrinsic property of its precontraction length and determined by the degree of overlap between the thick (myosin-bearing) and thin (actin-bearing) myofilaments (Fig. 5). The three-dimensional corollary of this two-dimensional

Table 1 Formal Definitions of Septic and Cardiogenic Shock

	Septic[a]	Cardiogenic[b]
Blood pressure	SBP < 90 mmHg	SBP < 80 mmHg
	or	*or*
	↓SBP > 40 mmHg	↓MAP ≥ 30%
	or	
	MAP < 60 mmHg	
	and	*and*
Intravascular volume	Adequate volume resuscitation	LVEDP > 18 mmHg
		or
		RVEDP > 10 mmHg
	and	*and*
Other criteria 1	Other organ dysfunction[c]	CI < 1.8 L/min[1]/m² without support
		or
		CI < 2.2 L/min[1]/m² with support
	and	
Other criteria 2	Sepsis[a]	

[a]Data taken from Ref. 3
[b]Data taken from Ref. 4
[c]Data taken from Ref. 5
Abbreviations: CI, cardiac index; LEVDP, left ventricular end-diastolic pressure; MAP, mean arterial pressure; REVDP, right ventricular end-diastolic pressure; SBP, systolic blood pressure.

Table 2 Classification of Hypovolemic Shock

	Class I	Class II	Class III	Class IV
Volume loss (%)	<15%	15–30%	31–40%	>40%
Pulse (beats/min)	<100	100–120	121–140	>140
Blood pressure	Normal	Decreased	Decreased	Decreased
Respiratory rate (breaths/min)	14–20	21–30	31–40	>35
Urine output (mL/hr)	>30	20–30	5–19	<5
Neurology	Normal	Anxious	Confused	Obtunded

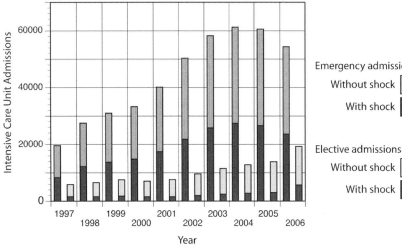

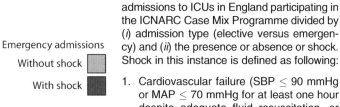

Figure 2 Annual incidence of shock. Annual admissions to ICUs in England participating in the ICNARC Case Mix Programme divided by (*i*) admission type (elective versus emergency) and (*ii*) the presence or absence or shock. Shock in this instance is defined as following:

1. Cardiovascular failure (SBP ≤ 90 mmHg or MAP ≤ 70 mmHg for at least one hour despite adequate fluid resuscitation, or the use of vasopressors)
2. Failure of at least one other organ system by the PROWESS criteria (data taken from Ref. 6)

Data courtesy of Case Mix Programme Database, ICNARC (Intensive Care National Audit and Research Centre), Tavistock House, Tavistock Square, London WC1H 9HR.

phenomenon is that stroke volume is determined by the precontraction ventricular volume, which is itself determined by the rate and duration of ventricular filling. Ventricular filling has three phases: early, mid-, and end diastolic (13).

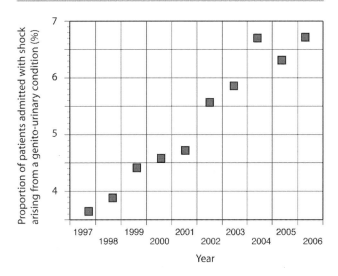

Figure 3 Annual proportion of shock cases arising from a genitourinary condition. Data courtesy of Case Mix Programme Database, ICNARC (Intensive Care National Audit and Research Centre), Tavistock House, Tavistock Square, London WC1H 9HR.

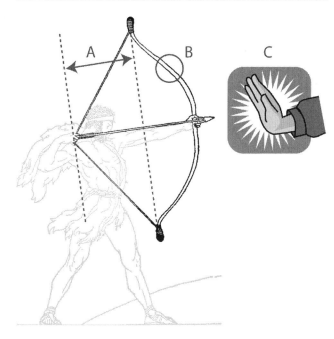

Figure 4 Conceptual analogy for the relationship between preload, contractility, and afterload in determining stroke volume. Using the analogy of an arrow being fired into a target, it becomes intuitively obvious that the depth of penetration (stroke volume) is determined by the draw of the bowstring [(**A**) preload], the stiffness of the bow [(**B**) contractility], and the resistance of the target [(**C**) afterload].

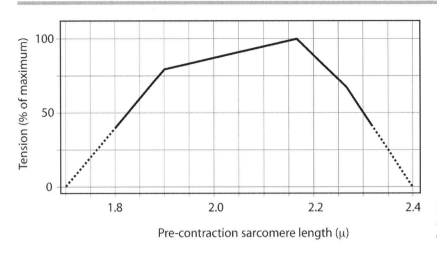

Figure 5 Relationship between precontraction sarcomere length and tension generated on contraction. *Source*: Adapted from Ref. 12.

Early diastolic ventricular filling is augmented by the elastic recoil of the ventricle that springs back to its resting volume at the beginning of diastole, "sucking" blood into the ventricle as it does so.

Mid-diastolic ventricular filling, which under normal circumstances is the principle determinant of the end-diastolic ventricular volume, occurs at a rate determined by (i) the veno-ventricular pressure gradient, more commonly referred to as the "filling pressure," and (ii) ventricular stiffness (Fig. 6). It is worth emphasizing three points that are the source of common misconceptions. First, "preload" is defined by the ventricular end-diastolic volume, and not, as is widely believed, simply the filling pressure (often measured clinically as the central venous pressure [CVP]). This is illustrated in Figure 6 as a normal stroke volume arising from the combination of either a low filling pressure and a compliant ventricle (panel A), or a high filling pressure and a stiff ventricle (panel D). Second, filling pressure arises from the combined effects of circulating volume (also referred to as blood volume or intravascular volume) and venous tone, not just circulating volume alone. This is illustrated in Figure 7 where it can be seen that a normal circulating volume can generate a high (Panel A), normal (Panel C), or low (Panel E) filling pressure depending on whether the venous tone is high, normal, or low, respectively. Conversely, a normal filling pressure can arise with a low (Panel B), normal (Panel C), or high (Panel D) circulating volume if the venous tone is high, normal, or low, respectively. Third, body weight cannot be used to estimate circulating volume in patients who may have leaky capillaries and interstitial edema (Fig. 8). Stiffness, properly termed elastance, describes the relationship between pressure (*y*-axis) and volume (*x*-axis), and for a simple elastic body, for example, a rubber balloon, plots an upward curve (Fig. 9). Passive ventricular stiffness is determined by the viscoelastic properties and mass of the ventricle, and is increased in conditions that result in either myocardial fibrosis, or ventricular wall thickening, displacing the elastance curve upward (Fig. 9A).

Unlike a rubber balloon, however, the ventricle is encased in a pericardial sac that is not only considerably stiffer, but whose limited volume has to be shared with the other cardiac chambers. Therefore, at low/normal diastolic volumes ventricular elastance is determined by the ventricle alone (Fig. 10A, B, C), but at a critical diastolic volume pericardial elastance becomes superimposed on the ventricular elastance and, being much greater, becomes dominant (Fig. 10D). Although pericardial elastance itself can increase even further as a result of pericardial fibrosis or calcification, the impact of the pericardium's increased stiffness becomes much more significant if the critical diastolic volume is reduced. This may occur if any of the other cardiac chambers are enlarged, or if there is fluid within the pericardial sac (Fig. 10B). The second difference from a simple elastic body is that the ventricle is composed of cardiac muscle. Total ventricular elastance is therefore composed of a passive component, described above, and an active component that is determined by the extent of ventricular relaxation in diastole. In molecular terms relaxation is a process in which the myofibrillar myosin heads disengage from the actin filaments as a result of energy-dependent calcium sequestration into the sarcoplasmic reticulum. Being energy-dependent, relaxation is impaired in ischemic myocardium.

Finally, ventricular volume is given a presystolic "boost" by atrial contraction. This effect is lost in patients with atrial fibrillation or flutter, but this is of little consequence in patients with well-preserved ventricular function. However, in patients with significant impairment of left ventricular function, the loss of the atrial boost is much more noticeable, and may precipitate or exacerbate symptoms of heart failure such as exercise intolerance, dyspnea, and fluid retention.

In the absence of changes in contractility, or afterload, increases in preload result in an increase in the force generated by myofibril contraction (Fig. 5) and stroke volume (Fig. 10) up to the point of optimal preload. Thereafter, further increases in preload cause

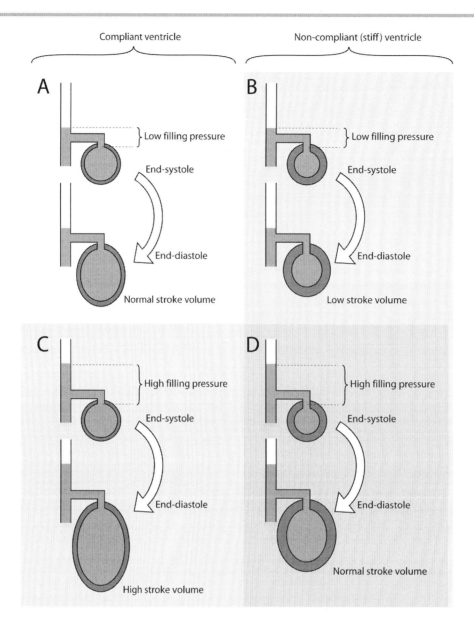

Figure 6 Effect of filling pressure and ventricular elastance (stiffness) on end-diastolic ventricular volume. Preload is defined by the ventricular end-diastolic volume (LVEDV) and may result in a normal stroke volume (**A** and **D**) with a low filling pressure and a compliant ventricle (**A**), or a high filling pressure and a stiff ventricle (**D**). A low filling pressure and stiff ventricle (**B**) results in a low LVEDV and a low stroke volume, while a high filling pressure and compliant ventricle (**C**) results in a high LVEDV and a high stroke volume.

a decrease in both the force generated by myofibril contraction (Fig. 5) and stroke volume (Fig. 11). Factors affecting preload are shown in Table 3.

Contractility. Changes in myocardial contractility account for changes in stroke volume under similar conditions of preload and afterload (Fig. 11) and may be effected physiologically, pharmacologically, or pathologically (Table 2). In practical terms, the commonest causes of depressed contractility in patients with shock are myocardial ischemia or infarction, or sepsis. Clinically contractility is optimized by correcting any relevant electrolyte disturbances, and avoid-

ing or minimizing the use of pharmacological agents that reduce contractility (negative inotropes). Finally, contractility can be directly augmented by drugs that increase the effect of myocyte cytosolic calcium on troponin, either by increasing the myocyte calcium content, or by sensitizing the tropinin to the effects of calcium (Table 4).

Afterload. Constant blood flow through vital organs is achieved by maintaining a constant perfusion pressure by the regulation of afferent and efferent vasomotor tone. Increases in mean arterial pressure (MAP) are regulated by afferent arteriolar

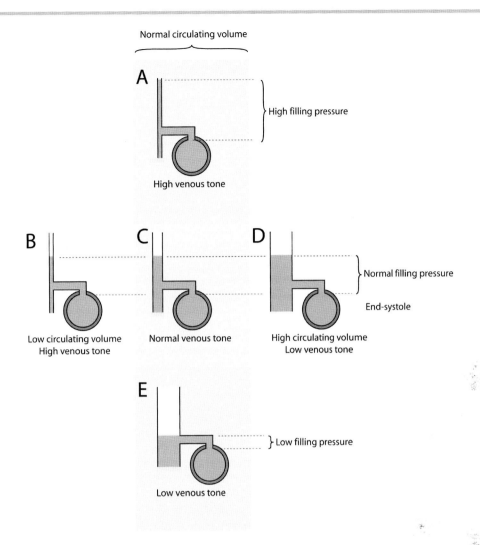

Figure 7 Effect of intravascular volume and venous tone on filling pressure. Filling pressure arises from the combined effects of circulating volume and venous tone. Thus, a normal circulating volume can generate a high (**A**), normal (**C**), or low (**E**) filling pressure depending on whether the venous tone is high, normal, or low, respectively. Conversely, a normal filling pressure can arise with a low (**B**), normal (**C**), or high (**D**) circulating volume if the venous tone is high, normal, or low, respectively.

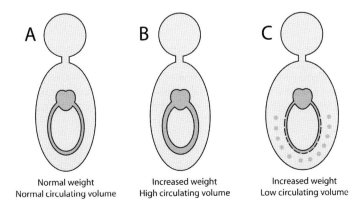

Figure 8 Body weight and circulating volume. In the absence of capillary leak and "third space" losses body weight provides a reasonable estimate of intravascular volume (**A** and **B**). However, in the context of systemic inflammation (**C**), which is invariably associated with capillary leak, body weight and intravascular volume are not related.

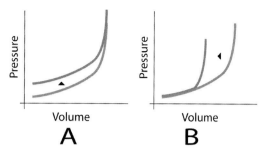

Figure 9 Increases in ventricular elastance (stiffness). An increase in ventricular elastance as a consequence of either increased ventricular muscle mass (pressure overload of the ventricle, e.g., hypertension or stenosis of the ventricular exit valve) or ventricular fibrosis (ischemic heart disease) causes the elastance curve to be displaced upward (**A**). A reduction in the ventricular volume at which pericardial elastance becomes dominant (**B**) arises when the available pericardial volume is reduced, either by the overdistension of any of the other cardiac chambers, or by the presence of pericardial fluid (pericardial effusion or hemopericardium) resulting in pericardial "tamponade."

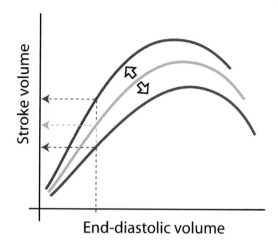

Figure 11 Effect of changes in contractility on the relationship between end-diastolic volume (preload) and stroke volume. The green curve represents the normal relationship between stroke volume and end-diastolic volume. The red curve shows the effect of an increase in contractility, while the blue curve shows the effect of a decrease in contractility. At the same end-diastolic volume, an increase in contractility results in an increase in stroke volume, while a decrease in contractility has the opposite effect.

vasoconstriction, while decreases in MAP are accommodated initially by afferent arteriolar vasodilatation. However, when arteriolar vasodilatation is maximal, perfusion pressure is maintained by efferent vasoconstriction, which inevitably reduces flow. This means that the perfusion of these vital organs is compro-

mised by reductions in MAP. If the amount of cardiac work per unit time (cardiac power) is held constant then the MAP is proportional to systemic vascular resistance [SVR, eq. (2)], which is a measure of cardiac

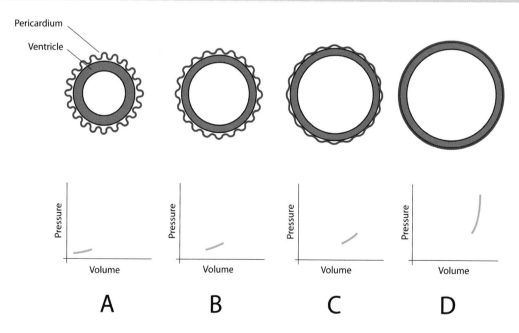

Figure 10 Ventricular elastance curves. In each of the panels the cartoon above the graph represents the ventricle (*brown*) surrounded by the pericardium (*blue*). In panels A, B, and C ventricular volume can be seen to trace a smooth upward curve in relation to ventricular pressure, and as the ventricular volume increases progressively more of the pericardial "slack" is taken up. At a critical volume, represented by panel D, the pericardial slack is completely taken up by the expanding ventricle. Ventricular elastance is now principally determined by the pericardium, and as the latter is considerably stiffer than the ventricle, the gradient of the pressure/volume curve (the elastance) becomes markedly steeper.

Table 3 Factors Affecting Preload

	Increased preload	Decreased preload

Physiological	• Increased intravascular volume
	  Renal retention of salt and water
	  (↑ ADH, ↑ angiotensin II,
	  ↑ cortisol, ↓ ANP)
	  ↑ Fluid intake (thirst)
	• Increased venous tone
	  ↑ Sympathetic drive
		• Decreased intravascular volume
		  Renal diuresis (↓ ADH, ↓ angiotensin II, ↓ cortisol, ↑ ANP)
		  ↓ Fluid intake
		• Decreased venous tone
		  ↑ Parasympathetic drive

Pharmacological	• Intravenous fluids	• Decreased intravascular volume
		  Diuretics
		• Decreased venous tone
		  Diuretics
		  Opiates

Pathological	• Fluid retention
	  Renal failure
	  Cardiac failure
	  Liver failure
		• Decreased intravascular volume
		  Hemorrhage
		  Inappropriate renal diuresis (polyuric ATN, diabetes insipidus, diabetes mellitus, hypocortisolism)
		  Fluid loss from GI tract (vomiting, diarrhea) or impaired fluid reabsorption from GI tract (ileus)
		  Increased insensible losses (fever, burns)
		  Capillary leak (systemic inflammation, anaphylaxis)
		• Decreased venous tone
		  ↑ Parasympathetic drive
		• Increased intrathoracic pressure
		  Tension pneumothorax
		  Positive pressure ventilation
		  Continuous positive airway pressure (CPAP)
		• Reduced diastolic ventricular compliance
		  Pericardial effusion
		  Ventricular hypertrophy or infiltration
		  Ventricular dilatation (Bernheim effect)

Table 4 Factors Affecting Cardiac Contractility

	Increased contractility	Decreased contractility
Physiological	• Cardiac sympathetic nerve stimulation (sympathetic nerves → noradrenaline → cardiac β1-adrenoreceptors) • Adrenomedullary drive (adrenaline release → cardiac α1-adrenoreceptors) • Hypercalcemia	• ↑ Parasympathetic drive

Pharmacological	• ↑ Myocyte calcium load
	  ↑ cAMP synthesis
	  ~ β1-adrenergic receptor agonists (adrenaline, dopamine, dobutamine, dopexamine, noradrenaline)
	  ~ Glucagon receptor
	  ↓ cAMP degradation
	  Phosphodiesterase inhibitors (milrinone, amrinone)
	  ↑ Na^+/Ca^{2+} exchange
	  ~ Cardiac glycosides (digoxin)
	  ↑ Extracellular calcium concentration (calcium)
	• ↑ Myocyte calcium sensitivity (levosimendan)
		• β-Blockers
		• Calcium channel blockers (verapamil, nicardipine)
		• Amiodarone
		• Volatile anesthetic agents

Pathological	• Hyperthyroidism (early)	• Ischemia/hypoxia
		• Infarction
		• Sepsis
		• Electrolyte disturbance
		  Hypocalcemia
		  Hyperkalemia
		  Hypokalemia
		• Hypothermia
		• Acidemia
		• Cardiomyopathy
		• Myocarditis

Table 5 Factors Affecting Afterload

	Increased LV afterload	Decreased LV afterload
Physiological	• Arteriolar vasoconstriction Cold Pain Fear	• Arteriolar vasodilatation Exercise Hypercapnia Pyrexia

Pharmacological	• Arteriolar vasoconstrictors
	 α-Adrenergic agonists
	  (noradrenaline, metaraminol)
	 β-Adrenergic antagonists
		• Arteriolar vasodilators
		 α-Adrenergic antagonists (phentolamine, phenoxybenzamine,
		  doxasozin)
		 β-Adrenergic agonists (dobutamine, dopexamine, dopamine)
		 ↑ Smooth muscle cGMP (nitrates)
		 Smooth muscle Ca^{2+} channel blockers (nifedipine, verapamil)
		 ↓ Angiotensin II (angiotensin converting enzyme inhibitors,
		  angiotensin II receptor antagonists)
		 Smooth muscle relaxant (hydralazine, prostacyclin)

Pathological	• ↑Sympathetic drive (hypovolemia) • 1° or 2° hypertension (LV) • Aortic valve stenosis • Aortic coarctation	• Arteriolar vasodilatation Sepsis Anaphylaxis • Systemic AV shunts • Loss of sympathetic tone Thoracic epidural or high spinal Cervical or thoracic spinal cord damage
	Increased RV afterload	Decreased RV afterload
Physiological	• Low partial pressure of inspired gas (high altitude, hypoxic gas mixture, upper airway obstruction) • Very low (pneumothorax) or very high lung volumes	• Pulmonary AV shunts
Pharmacological		• Inhaled nitric oxide
Pathological	• Acute or chronic pulmonary thromboembolism • Pulmonary hypertension • Pulmonary valve stenosis • Mitral valve stenosis	• Pulmonary AV shunts

afterload, and the MAP is inversely proportional to the cardiac output [eq. (3)].

$$SVR \propto MAP \qquad (2)$$

$$\frac{1}{SVR} \propto \text{cardiac output} \qquad (3)$$

What these equations tell us is that under conditions of constant cardiac power output, a reduction in afterload allows the cardiac output to rise, whereas an increase in afterload (MAP) causes the cardiac output to fall. In this latter situation, achieving the minimum MAP required to maintain vital organ perfusion may only be possible with an increase in afterload that then reduces total blood flow to less than that required by the vital organs. Taken together, this tells us that the perfusion of vital organs requires the central supply of both pressure and flow.

Clinically, cardiac power output is only ever fixed when a patient is operating at the upper limit of their heart's capacity. This occurs when there is an imbalance between the demand being placed on the heart, and the heart's capacity, which may entail an increase in demand, a decrease in capacity, or both. Factors affecting afterload are presented in Table 5.

Heart Rate

By virtue of the relationship between cardiac output and heart rate defined above, cardiac output declines linearly as the heart rate falls, providing that the stroke volume remains constant. Under normal circumstances the decline in cardiac output is mitigated by a protective reflex mediated by sympathetic drive that increases the stroke volume. This mechanism is limited by a maximum stroke volume, beyond which further reductions in heart rate result in a steep decline in cardiac output. Where the falling heart rate is being driven by parasympathetic (vagal) drive, or in patients who cannot mount an adequate sympathetic response (sympathetic outflow blocked by a thoracic epidural or high spinal block, α adrenergic blockade, Table 6), this protective reflex is severely compromised and the cardiac output declines more precipitously. As the cardiac output falls below the critical perfusion thresholds for brain and heart, the patient starts to lose consciousness and cardiac function is further compromised by ischemia. Commonly, this sequence of events occurs over a minute or two and, in the absence of intervention, culminates in cardiorespiratory arrest. While some patients will be found to be asystolic, others develop a degenerative rhythm under these conditions such as

Table 6 Factors Affecting Cardiac Output

Increased cardiac output	Decreased cardiac output

• Optimized preload
• Increased contractility
• Decreased afterload
• Increased heart rate (within normal range)
	• Suboptimal or supraoptimal preload
	• Decreased contractility
	• Increased afterload
	• Bradycardia
	  ↑ Parasympathetic drive
	  ~ Reflex (pneumoperitoneum, mesenteric traction, pain, nausea, inferior MI)
	  ~ Opiates
	  ~ Volatile anesthetic agents
	  ↓ Sympathetic drive
	  ↓ Sinus node automaticity
	  Atrioventricular conduction defect
	• Tachycardia

ventricular fibrillation or torsades de pointes. In rapidly progressive bradycardia this sequence of events can be aborted providing (i) appropriate monitoring is in place to provide both visual and auditory warning of the impending disaster, (ii) intravenous access is immediately available, and (iii) appropriate rescue therapy, such as atropine (0.5–1 mg) or ephedrine (6–12 mg), is administered quickly enough. In urological practice, where spinal anesthesia is commonly employed in the frail and elderly undergoing transurethral procedures, rapidly progressive bradycardia is a trap for the unwary that may spring immediately following the completion of surgery. At this time, the combination of (i) sympathetic blockade from a high spinal anesthetic, (ii) hypovolemia from preoperative fasting, vasodilatation, and intraoperative blood loss, and (iii) nausea secondary to hypotension, all synergize to produce vagal drive and hypotension precipitated by removing the patient's legs from the lithotomy stirrups. Not uncommonly, the anesthetist will already have removed the monitoring equipment in anticipation of transferring the patient into the recovery area, and with the distraction of theater staff preparing for the next case, the patient's loss of consciousness may not be immediately appreciated.

Although it may seem obvious that an increase in heart rate would de facto result in an increase in cardiac output, this is not, in fact, the case. This is explained by the observation that as the heart rate increases there is progressively less time during diastole for the left ventricle to fill with blood, resulting in a paradoxical decrease in stroke volume. Under most circumstances, however, increases in heart rate are driven by stimuli, which also increase the stroke volume, for example, endogenous or exogenous catecholamines. In the absence of an extracardiac stimulus for an increased heart rate, a symptomatic tachycardia is usually driven by an atrial or ventricular dysrhythmia. The urgency of intervention is determined by the degree of circulatory failure and, where the patient is symptomatically hypotensive, or shocked, requires immediate recognition and synchronized DC cardioversion.

ASSOCIATED PATHOPHYSIOLOGY

Although shock is primarily defined by the characteristic hemodynamic disturbance that leads to the failure of substrate delivery, the shocked state is inextricably linked to associated abnormalities in other organ systems that this failure of substrate delivery provokes.

Hypotension and Organ Ischemia

The loss or reduction of normal organ perfusion will have consequences that will depend not only on the extent and duration of hypoperfusion, but also on the presence of coexisting abnormalities, such as ischemic heart disease, peripheral vascular disease, or hypertension. In susceptible patients, therefore, shock can precipitate ischemia or infarction of the heart, gut, kidneys, liver, or brain. Myocardial ischemia or infarction has immediate hemodynamic consequences, either by reducing myocardial contractility or by precipitating abnormalities of rhythm or conduction, thus complicating the hemodynamic picture. The consequences of gut, kidney, liver, or brain damage may be less immediately damaging, but are no less important in terms of their impact on morbidity and mortality. Gastrointestinal ischemia can lead to bacterial translocation, discussed below, as well as precipitating gastric or duodenal stress ulceration and GI hemorrhage, ileus, or even GI perforation. Hepatic ischemia is rather more subtle in its manifestations, which may range from an elevation of hepatic enzymes and hypoabuminemia, which are very common, to a failure of hepatic function with prolongation of the prothrombin time, worsening lactic acidemia and intractable hypoglycemia, which are less common. Renal function is almost always disturbed in patients with shock, although oliguria may not be present if in fact it is a failure of renal concentrating ability, which is responsible for, or contributing to, the hypovolemia. Although renal function is readily supported by hemofiltration, renal failure remains an independent risk factor for mortality, the reason for which remains unclear. Finally, neurological

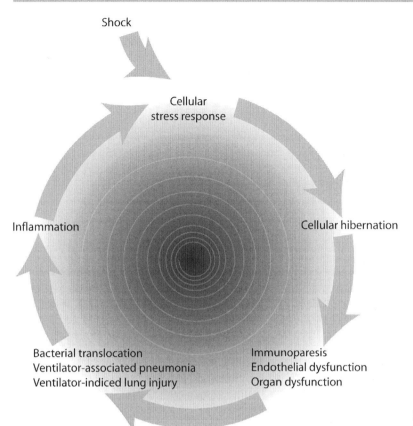

Figure 12 Positive feedback cycle connecting shock, cellular dysfunction, and inflammation.

disturbances are commonly seen in the acute phase of shock, but persisting "brain failure" in the form of delirium is commonly seen in patients during the recovery phase of critical illness.

Systemic Inflammation

Although a systemic inflammatory response may result in shock, for example, as a result of sepsis, anaphylaxis, or pancreatitis, shock can itself provoke a systemic inflammatory response by exposing the tissues to an ischemic insult. For example, pure hemorrhagic shock has been shown to cause significantly increased plasma concentrations of the inflammatory cytokines interleukin-1 (IL-1), IL-6, and tumor necrosis factor α (TNFα)(14), and in patients with trauma particular cytokine profiles have been associated with outcome (15). Disseminated activation of the innate immune system has a number of consequences. Within the circulation endothelial cell activation leads to the expression of cell surface receptors, promoting the margination and vascular emigration of activated leukocytes. Activationt of the vascular endothelium leads to a profound relaxation of the interendothelial cell junctions, resulting in fluid extravasation, and increased endothelial expression of tissue factor resulting in intravascular activation of the coagulation cascade and the deposition of microthrombi in the capillaries. A number of inflammatory mediators,

which include TNFα and nitric oxide, have also been implicated in the loss of smooth muscle and myocardial contractility. Thus, the hypovolemia precipitated by the capillary leak is then compounded by both arteriolar and venous vasodilatation as well as by reduced myocardial contractility, creating a positive feedback loop for hemodynamic deterioration. Within the splanchnic circulation, ischemia and circulating inflammatory mediators also impair the barrier function of the intestinal epithelium, allowing the ingress of bacteria and bacterial toxins such as endotoxin. These agents are themselves potent activators of the innate immune system and there is a growing body of circumstantial and animal data to suggest that this process of "bacterial translocation" plays a role in driving the pathophysiology of multiple organ failure (16) (Fig. 12).

In septic patients with an elevated cardiac output but evidence of tissue hypoxia (lactic acidosis) and organ dysfunction, it was originally believed that the problem was caused by regional ischemia, with flow being diverted away from the tissues by arteriovenous shunts or intracapillary microthrombi. While this has certainly been seen to occur in some tissue beds (17), elevated tissue oxygen tensions have been documented in both septic animals (18) and man (19). These observations, and others, have led to the identification of a phenomenon referred to as cytopathic dysoxia (20), a condition in which cellular dysfunction arises from a failure of substrate utilization rather than delivery. Although more typically associated with primary systemic inflammation, especially sepsis, rather than shock-induced "secondary" systemic inflammation, it is likely to be a feature of both conditions, and may represent a cellular stress response in which mitochondrial function is downregulated rather than actually driving the observed abnormalities in cellular function. This is discussed further below.

MANAGEMENT OF SHOCK

The range of clinical conditions associated with the presence of cellular metabolic failure (i.e., shock) can vary from cardiac arrest, at one end of the spectrum, to subtle biochemical abnormalities in a patient who otherwise gives no cause for concern, at the other end of the spectrum. However, the same logical and methodical approach to the assessment and management for all these patients ensures that the former are treated effectively, and shock in the latter is not overlooked.

The assessment begins with an evaluation of respiratory function and, in particular, the quality of the airway and breathing. Four broad situations can usually be recognized by (*i*) respiratory arrest, (*ii*) agonal respiration, (*iii*) abnormal breathing, and (*iv*) normal breathing. Tachypnea is an early and useful sign of clinical deterioration (21) and, in patients with shock, may reflect acidosis (tissue hypoperfusion, renal dysfunction) or increased carbon dioxide production associated with the hypermetabolism of sepsis. More recently, it has been shown that sepsis (22) induces early contractile failure in the diaphragm, a fact that may explain ventilatory failure in patients with an extrapulmonary source of sepsis. In adults, respiratory arrest is almost always secondary to cardiac arrest, the management of which is beyond the scope of this chapter. Agonal respiration is usually easily recognized as intermittent stertorous and labored respiration accompanied by marked impairment of neurological function. Assessment using the Glasgow scale is likely to reveal a patient whose eyes open to pain (2) or not at all (1), who is able to make incomprehensible sounds (2), and who either localizes (5) or withdraws from a painful stimulus. This peri-arrest situation requires immediate attention, with urgent tracheal intubation and mechanical ventilation by members of the ICU team. In the meantime, having established vascular access and initiated fluid resuscitation, further examination of the patient is likely to provide clues as to the underlying problem. Warm peripheries with a brisk capillary refill are typical of systemic inflammation, and in some patients gentle pressure on the nail-bed elicits the capillary pulsation of Quincke's sign. Otherwise, cool peripheries with a prolonged capillary would be expected. Most patients in shock are likely to have a tachycardia up to 150/min, with a bounding pulse being typical of systemic inflammation, and a weak thready pulse indicating other types of shock.

Pulse rates higher than this may simply reflect profound hemodynamic disturbance, but may in fact indicate a tachydysrhythmia. If this is confirmed on electrocardiography, and the rhythm is causing symptomatic hypotension, consideration should be given to immediate DC cardioversion. If time allows, blood gas analysis may reveal hypokalemia, which ought to be corrected before, or as soon as possible after, cardioversion. Bradycardia or a normal pulse rate would be highly unusual in most cases of shock, unless the bradycardia itself was driving the hemodynamic condition, for example, in patients with significant parasympathetic drive. Finally, in most cases of overt shock one would expect hypotension. Serious hypotension (systolic blood pressure <70 mmHg) that does not appear to be responding to fluid therapy deserves a little pharmacological support. In tachycardic patients increments of 1 mg of metaraminol, a potent α-agonist, are usually very effective in preventing any further deteriorations in the blood pressure, amd may be accompanied by a modest fall in the heart rate. In bradycardic patients incremental doses of 3 to 6 mg of ephedrine may be effective in increasing both the heart rate and blood pressure, as would small doses (0.5–1 mL) of adrenaline 1:10,000. In the seriously compromised patient additional hemodynamic monitoring is required to clarify the hemodynamics and guide therapy.

Assessment and Optimization of Preload

Clinical assessment of the jugular venous pressure can only serve as a very rough guide to right ventricular preload, which is best measured by the placement of a central venous catheter. Even then, the CVP is itself a relatively poor indicator of left ventricular preload and makes the following assumptions:

1. Left ventricular end-diastolic pressure (LVEDP) $\propto$ Left ventricular end-diastolic volume (assumes constant and normal LV compliance)
2. Left atrial pressure (LAP) $\propto$ LVEDP (assumes normal mitral valve)
3. Pulmonary artery pressure (PAP) $\propto$ LAP (assumes constant and normal pulmonary resistance)
4. Right ventricular end-diastolic volume (RVEDV) $\propto$ PAP (assumes normal pulmonary valve)
5. Right ventricular end-diastolic pressure (RVEDP) $\propto$ RVEDV (assumes constant and normal RV compliance)
6. Right atrial pressure (RAP) $\propto$ RVEDP (assumes normal tricuspid valve)
7. CVP $\propto$ RAP

However, providing ventricular compliance and pulmonary resistance remain constant, changes in CVP will reflect changes in ventricular preload within an individual. Between individuals there is too much variation in these factors to detect any relationship even between pulmonary artery occlusion pressure (PAOP) and LVEDV (Fig. 13). Nevertheless, it is worth noting that it is almost impossible for a correctly measured CVP to underestimate ventricular preload,

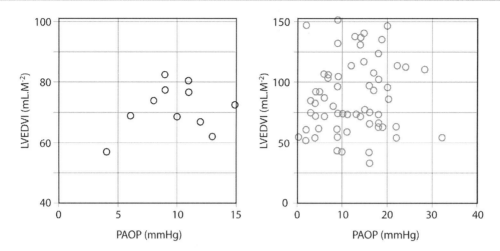

Figure 13 Relationship of the left ventricular end-diastolic index (LVEDVI) to the PAOP. Data from 12 normal subjects (*left*). Data from 61 patients with acute respiratory distress syndrome (ARDS) (*right*). *Source*: From Refs. 23 and 24.

and therefore an abnormally low CVP almost certainly reflects functional hypovolemia.

The pulmonary artery catheter (PAC) eliminates some of the assumptions inherent in the CVP and allows direct measurement of the PAP, which is very helpful in patients with right ventricular dysfunction or raised PAPs (pulmonary thromboembolism or pulmonary hypertension). In unselected patients use of the PAC has not been shown in either of two large prospective trials to be associated with any benefit (25,26), and its use is falling out of favor. In place of the PAC some centers are now using other techniques for hemodynamic assessment such as esophageal Doppler or pulse-contour analysis. These techniques are not only less invasive, but also provide continuous measurement of stroke volume, cardiac output, and SVR. This is particularly helpful in allowing dynamic assessment of the patient's response to fluid loading. Where there is doubt of the patient's preload status, this is an effective technique and involves challenging the patients with repeated boluses of fluid (sufficient to cause an elevation of CVP or PAOP of >3 mmHg) until there is no further improvement in cardiac output.

Transthoracic echocardiography is a rapid, noninvasive, and useful method of assessing the hemodynamics, if somewhat underutilized. Echocardiography not only provides information about contractility and preload, but also eliminates valve failure, pericardial effusion/tamponade, and pulmonary embolism as causes for shock.

There is currently no evidence to favor isotonic crystalloids over colloids although large volume fluid resuscitation with 0.9% sodium chloride risks hyperchloremic acidosis and may be associated with a number of other adverse effects. In cases of hemorrhage these fluids must be accompanied by packed red blood cells. Current recommendations (27) are to give fresh frozen plasma (10–15 mL/kg) if the prothrombin time is $\geq$ 1.5 times normal, with cryopreci-

pitate if the plasma fibrinogen concentration falls below 1 g/L and platelet concentrate to maintain the count above 50,000 cells/mm^3. Overt blood loss, such as hemorrhage from an open wound, is impossible to overlook, but equally significant blood loss can occur covertly, such as that associated with pelvic and long bone fractures, gastrointestinal bleeding, or even following transurethral resection of the prostate. In the young or fit patient significant hypovolemia can be obscured by highly effective reflex mechanisms that are capable of maintaining an almost normal blood pressure and heart rate. In these patients hemodynamic decompensation is a late and precipitous event, and there may be other signs of "covert" shock such as metabolic acidosis[e] or elevated plasma lactate concentration. Thus, in patients with septic shock, for example, the addition of a mixed venous saturation greater than 70% as a therapeutic end point for resuscitation was associated with a 16% reduction of hospital mortality (28). Although some patients respond to volume resuscitation alone, most will also require pharmacological support of either contractility, or afterload, or both.

Management of Contractility and Afterload

The effect of vasopressor and inotropic agents is most commonly determined by their activity at endogenous receptors of the adrenergic (α and β) and dopaminergic families, although there are agents that work in other ways (Table 4). This knowledge combined with an understanding of the effects of receptor activation on preload, contractility, and afterload allows clinicians to estimate which agent, or combination of agents, is most likely to produce the desired effects (Table 7). However, the actual effects produced in

---

[e]Indicated by a fall in pH or an elevated base deficit.

Table 7 Agents Used to Manipulate Preload, Contractility, and Afterload

	Preload	CO	SVR	MAP	HR	SBF
Adrenaline	+	+++	++	↑	↑	↓
Dobutamine	−	++	−−	↓	↑	↑
Dopamine (<5 µg/kg/min)	±	+	±	↑	(↑)	↑
Dopamine (5–10 µg/kg/min)	+	+	+	↑	(↑)	?
Dopamine (>10 µg/kg/min)	+	+	++	↑	(↑)	↓
Dopexamine	−	+	−	↓	↑	↑
Nitrates	−−	NC	−	↓	↑	?
Isoprenaline	−	+	−	↓	↑	?
Milrinone	−	++	−−	↓	↑	?
Noradrenaline	+	++	+++	↑	↓	↑ or ↓
Phentolamine	−	NC	−−	↓	↑	↑

Abbreviations: CO, cardiac output (a clinical surrogate for contractility but is strongly influenced by afterload); SVR, systemic vascular resistance (a good reflection of afterload); MAP, mean arterial pressure; HR, heart rate; SBF, splanchnic blood flow; ?, unknown or unpredictable; NC, no change.

vivo may differ from those expected because of the effects of adrenoreceptor up- and downregulation during critical illness (29), the effect of polymorphisms in the adrenoreceptor genes (30), and alterations to adrenoreceptor activation[f] caused by free radicals (31). In practice, therefore, the desired effect may require a therapeutic trial of more than one agent, or the use of a combination of agents. Unfortunately, the quality of evidence on which to base the choice, or combination, of agents, is generally low (32) and largely based on animal data, small studies in patients, and expert opinion. Currently, either norepinephrine or dopamine is recommended as first-line agents (33) for the treatment of septic shock. For norepinephrine this represents the culmination of two decades of rehabilitation, having originally been believed to increase blood pressure at the expense of tissue (especially splanchnic) perfusion. Norepinephrine increases the blood pressure more rapidly and reliably than dopamine (34) and improves renal function, but only produces a modest rise in cardiac output. Its effects on the liver and gastrointestinal mucosa are unpredictable. Dopamine, on the other hand, despite increasing splanchnic blood flow at low doses does produce increased gut oxygen consumption or improvements in hepatic function. Moreover discomfort is growing about a range of negative effects attributable to dopamine, including the reduction of gut motility, hypoprolactinemia-mediated immunosuppression, reduced anabolism related to a fall in the production of growth hormone and dehydroepiandrosterone, and impaired thyroid function (35). In a recent observational study involving 198 centers in 24 European countries, the use of dopamine in the subset of patients with sepsis (*n* = 1058) was associated with an increased risk of hospital death (36) (relative risk 1.19, 95% confidence interval 1.04–1.36). Epinephrine is now rarely used as a single agent, if at all, as it causes a fall in splanchnic perfusion and, in some patients, a lactic acidosis.

---

[f]See also: Inactivation of catecholamines by superoxide gives new insights on the pathogenesis of septic shock. Proc Natl Acad Sci U S A. 2000 Aug 15;97(17):9753-8.

CELLULAR RESPONSES TO SHOCK: THE MOLECULAR BASIS OF MULTIPLE ORGAN FAILURE

Adaptation to adverse conditions is the foundation of evolution and has been the driving force behind the cumulative complexity and sophistication of metazoan organisms. This applies not only to the acquisition and inheritance of traits that enhance survival in the face of long-term changes in conditions, such as changes in the availability of food sources, but also to the acquisition of defensive mechanisms against unfavorable conditions arising in the short term. In other words, one of evolution's end points is the acquisition of adaptability itself. Within the confines of the "normal" variation of environmental conditions, this adaptability has resulted in mechanisms that maintain homeostasis at every level of the organism, including mechanisms to deal with tissue injury and attack from other organisms, large or small. Clinicians are most familiar with these "stress responses" at the level of entire organs and organ systems, and indeed this has formed the basis of this chapter so far. However, stress responses also exist at a cellular level, and indeed are quite specific to the various cellular components.

Cytosolic Response to Stress

The existence of an organized response to cellular stress was uncovered entirely by accident. In the early 1960s Ferrucio Ritossa was trying to identify the type of nucleic acid synthesized in the chromosomal puffs of salivary gland cells of *Drosophila* when a colleague inadvertently increased the temperature of the incubator. The following morning Ritossa was struck by the different puffing pattern of the chromosomes and had the foresight to wonder whether this was connected to the change in temperature (37). Not surprisingly this change in gene expression was subsequently referred to as the "heat shock response," and the protein products of these genes, identified in 1974 (38), became known as the "heat shock proteins" (Hsp). It has since emerged that Hsp are among the most phylogenetically conserved proteins identified, having been found in all three kingdoms of life,[g] and that their expression can be induced by a host of stressors besides heat, including oxidant stress, ischemia/reperfusion, hypoxia, and sepsis (39). Even under basal conditions Hsp are normal constituents of the cell's "housekeeping" armamentarium, where they act as molecular chaperones. In this role they are responsible for ensuring the successful attainment and maintenance of correct protein tertiary (folding) and quaternary (subunit assembly) structure, transmembranous protein transport for secretion or entry into cellular organelles, and finally the identification and disposal of denatured or abnormal proteins. By convention, the Hsp in vertebrates are categorized into families on the basis of molecular size, for example, Hsp70, Hsp90 or Hsp110, although the discovery that previously identified proteins have a role in the stress response, for example, heme oxygenase (Hsp32), ubiquitin, or inhibitor of κB (iκBα), means that the convention is not water tight. Increased gene expression is mediated by a small family of transcription factors with a helix-turn-helix DNA-binding domain called the "heat shock factors" (HSF), of which three have been identified in man, HSF1, HSF2 and HSF4.[h] HSF1 is a 57 kD protein coded on the long arm of chromosome 8 that is constitutively present in a monomeric form in the cytosol, where it is sequestered by forming complexes with the chaperone Hsp90. An excess of chaperone demand over supply distracts the HSF1-anchoring Hsp90, liberating the naked HSF1 monomers to homotrimerize, whereupon DNA-binding activity is acquired. The HSF1 trimers then migrate to the nucleus where they bind recognition sequences, known as "heat shock elements" (HSE), in the promoter regions of the Hsp. Although DNA binding is an essential step in gene regulation, binding alone is not sufficient for regulatory activity that requires modification of HSF-1 by phosphorylation, sumoylation, or the activity of coregulatory factors such as DAXX (40). A genome-wide search of functional HSE in human cells (HeLa) under conditions of heat shock identified 46 and 26 genes that were up- and downregulated, respectively, by HSF1 (41). Upregulated genes included those coding for Hsp, for example, Hsp70 and Hsp90, thus redressing the imbalance between the supply and demand for molecular chaperones, as well as genes involved in oxidant defense, immune function, gut epithelial permeability, and antiapoptotic proteins. Downregulated genes include those that code for IL-1β, TNFα, and genes induced by FOS. Mice lacking a functional HSF-1 allele are less likely to survive to birth, with survivors showing a number of phenotypic abnormalities including growth-retardation, female infertility, and a significantly reduced survival following endotoxin challenge (42).

Endoplasmic Reticulum Stress Responses

While ATP might be the currency of life and DNA the "secret of life,"[i] proteins are the fabric of life. Proteins that are destined for secretion (hormones, cytokines, neurotransmitters) or expression on the cell surface (receptors, adhesion molecules) are guided through aqueous pores by the Sec61 complex into the lumen of the endoplasmic reticulum (ER) as they are translated by cytosolic ribosomes. In contrast to any other cellular compartment, the ER maintains an oxidizing environment necessary for the formation of disulfide bonds and glycosylation, processes vital to the stabilization of a functional tertiary conformation following protein folding. The correct execution of these post-translational events are mediated and monitored by a repertoire of molecular chaperones that are able to detect misfolded or aggregated proteins, which are then exported to the cytosol for proteasomal degradation. When the capacity for ER processing cannot meet demand, for example, as a consequence of increased protein synthesis or degradation of the ER's processing capacity (hypoxia, hypoglycemia, oxidative stress), the ER chaperone Grp78 (BiP) is distracted from the lumenal aspect of the ER membrane where it anchors the N-terminal transmembranous portion of three molecules that are then freed to generate the "unfolded protein response" (UPR) (43).

The first of these, IRE1 (inositol-requiring transmembrane kinase and endonuclease), migrates in the plane of the membrane to form oligomers that transactivate each other by phosphorylation. Phosphorylated IRE1 is then able to initiate two separate pathways. On the one hand, its carboxy terminus acquires endonuclease activity, which removes a 26-nucleotide intron from native XBP-1 mRNA. This generates a frameshift that translates a 371 amino acid protein from the edited mRNA instead of a 267 amino acid protein from the native mRNA. Unlike the product of the native mRNA, the translation product of the edited XBP-1 mRNA is a transcription factor of the basic leucine zipper family (bZIP) responsible for the upregulation of a number of genes that code for ER chaperones (44). On the other, the phosphorylated IRE1 forms a scaffold for the attachment of TRAF2 (TNF receptor-associated factor 2), which can then bind and activate the ASK1/JNK kinase cascade. This pathway not only cross talks with the cytosolic version of the UPR by upregulating the transcription of HSF-1 but also promotes insulin resistance and gluconeogenesis by phosphorylating IRS1 (insulin receptor substrate 1) (45) at serine 307 and activating glucose-6-phosphatase, respectively. Finally, this pathway also promotes autophagy, although intermediaries in this process remain to be identified (46).

The second, ATF6 (activating transcription factor 6), is a bZIP transcription factor that on release of its BiP anchor migrates to the Golgi where the N-terminal intramembranous domain is cleaved by the S1P and S2P serine proteases. This frees the carboxy terminus

[g]Archaea, Bacteria and Eukaria.
[h]Hsf-3 appears to be uniquely avian.

[i]See Watson J. DNA. The Secret of Life. London: Random House; 2003. Page 53.

moiety to translocate to the nucleus and engage in transcriptional regulation, where it induces increased expression of genes coding for ER chaperones.

The third, PERK (PKR-like ER kinase), is a serine/threonine kinase that, like IRE1, oligomerizes on release of its BiP anchor and autoactivates by transphosphorylation. Its substrate is the eukaryotic translation initiation factor 2α (eIF2α), which in its naked form binds eIF2B to exchange GDP for GTP to become active. Activated eIF2a can then load tRNA-Met on to the 40S ribosome to initiate protein translation. Phosphorylation of eIF2a on serine 51 prevents it from interacting with eIF2B, thus shutting down general protein translation. However, protected translation from ATF4 (activating transcription factor 4) is enhanced following phosphorylation of eIF2α, because of the presence of an alternative open reading frame 5' upstream in the ATF4 mRNA. As with both XBP-1 and ATF6, ATF4 increases the production of molecular chaperones and antioxidant systems, as well as being important in gluconeogenesis (47).

Nuclear Responses to Stress

The physiological circumstances that induce the cytosolic and ER UPR increase the generation of DNA damage such as nucleotide depurination or deamination, oxidative damage, single- and double-strand breaks, and the generation of nonsense mRNA. DNA damage is recognized by, and activates, a family of phosphoinositide-3-kinase-related protein kinases, including ataxia telangiectasia and Rad-3 related, ataxia telangiectasia mutated, DNA-dependent protein kinase, and SMG1, that not only effect DNA repair,[j] which is important in its own right, but also all converge on the activation of the transcription factor p53. Although more commonly viewed as a tumor suppressor because of its key role in precipitating cell cycle arrest, p53 also exerts pressure on other cellular processes where, for example, it suppresses translation,[k] increases antioxidant defenses (48), and enhances anaerobic metabolism by activation of AMP-dependent protein kinase (49) (AMPK). In persistently unfavorable circumstances p53 enhances autophagy, a highly conserved mechanism for autocannibalizing and recycling old or damaged organelles (see below). This mechanism is invoked under these circumstances in a "last-ditch" bid to source cellular substrate for continued cell function, and is driven by p53 both through the downregulation of mTOR and the upregulation of damage-regulated autophagy modulator (50). Finally, where the situation is deemed irrecoverable, p53 invokes a dignified apoptotic cell death both through transrepression of BCL-2 (an inhibitor of apoptosis) as well as upregulation of PUMA, BAX, BIDD, and PIDD. However, in situations where the genetic damage is extensive, overwhelming activation of the enzyme poly-ADP ribose polymer-

ase-1 leads to the rapid cellular depletion of both NAD^+ and ATP, culminating in cellular necrosis (51).

Energy Depletion, Hypoxic Stress, and the Mitochondrial Responses to Stress

Oxygen was entirely absent from the Earth's early atmosphere but was produced as a by-product of the photosynthetic activity of marine cyanobacteria. Although there is evidence that cyanobacteria (and eucaria) were present at least 2700 million years ago (MYA) (52), oxygen did not begin to accumulate for a further 250 million years and only reached present day concentrations a further 1850 to 1900 million years later (550–600 MYA).[l] The oxygenation of earth's atmosphere appears to have been permissive for metazoan life-forms, and within a geologically short time resulted in the appearance of a multitude of these organisms in the fossil record recognized as the "Cambrian explosion," which started 540 MYA. Today, the vast majority of metazoan organisms rely on oxygen and oxidative phosphorylation to generate their cellular energy. But in the absence of any means of storing this component of the energy supply chain (unlike other substrates), metazoan cells had to develop mechanisms to cope with temporary interruptions to its supply.

A fall in the supply of oxygen is detected in three ways. First, the rate at which the mitochondrial F1F0ATPase (complex V) can generate ATP falls, and in the absence of attenuated consumption this immediately results in a fall in the intracellular ratio of ATP to AMP, activating the cytosolic AMPK. Second, as the supply of oxygen continues to fall, mitochondrial generation of reactive oxygen species (ROS) increases (53). Third, the fall in oxygen tension induces the expression of the transcription factor HIF-1 (hypoxia-induced factor-1).

AMPK is a heterotrimeric protein kinase composed of a catalytic α subunit (α1 or α2) and two regulatory subunits (β1 or β2 and γ1, γ2 or γ3) that is only susceptible to activation (phosphorylation) when AMP is bound to the γ subunit. In addition, AMP allosterically activates AMPK and renders the activated kinase less susceptible to the action of deactivating phosphatases. The action of adenylate kinase in maintaining the ADP:ATP ratio in equilibrium by converting ADP into ATP and AMP acts as a "gearing ratio" between ATP and AMP. This, together with AMP's activating influence, makes AMPK activation exquisitely sensitive to energy deprivation. Not surprisingly, therefore, AMPK activity aims to redress the balance between energy consumption and energy production. Energy consumption is reduced in a number of ways. First, phosphorylation of tuberous sclerosis complex 2 promotes the conversion of GTP to

---

[j]Nucleotide excision repair (NER), base excision repair (BER) and nonsense mutation.

[k]Via the TSC2 → mTOR → S6 kinase and 4EBP1 pathways.

[l]For further information on this fascinating subject see: (1) Knoll AH. *Life on a Young Planet.* Princeton: Princeton University Press, 2003, and (2) Lane N. *Oxygen. The Molecule That Made the World.* Oxford: Oxford University Press, 2002.

GDP on RHEB, inactivating mTOR and shutting down protein translation. Second, cell division is arrested both directly, through activation of a cyclin-dependent kinase inhibitor, and indirectly by upregulation of signaling through the family of forkhead transcription factors (54). Energy synthesis, on the other hand, is enhanced through both glycolysis and β-oxidation. Cellular glucose uptake is enhanced by the translocation of GLUT1 and GLUT4 to the plasma membrane, while glycolytic flux is promoted by the inhibition of glycogen synthase. Insulin signaling is inhibited by phosphorylation of IRS-1 at Ser794 and oxidative phosphorylation is downregulated by AMPK-mediated increased transcription of pyruvate dehydrogenase kinase 4, an enzyme that inactivates the pyruvate dehydrogenase complex, thus preventing the entry of pyruvate into the Krebs cycle. β-Oxidation is enhanced by AMPK-mediated inhibition of acetyl-coA carboxylase. This prevents the synthesis of malonyl-CoA, removing the latter's allosteric inhibition of long-chain acyl-CoA transport into mitochondria by carnitine palmitoyltransferase-1.

HIF-1 is another phylogenetically conserved molecule. This heterodimer is made up of a constitutively expressed HIF-1β subunit and an HIF-1α subunit that is hydroxylated in the presence of oxygen, ascorbate, Fe(II), and α-ketoglutarate. The stable HIF-1αβ heterodimer is therefore only formed under hypoxic conditions when it translocates into the nucleus to regulate the expression of a range of glycolytic enzymes, including lactate dehydrogenase, that promote anaerobic glycolysis. HIF-1 also increases the transcription of genes involved in angiogenesis, erythropoeisis, and the maintenance of blood pressure (endothelin 1, tyrosine hydroxylase). Another important role for HIF-1 appears to involve the suppression of mitochondrial function during hypoxia. Under hypoxic conditions there is a paradoxical increase in the mitochondrial generation of ROS from complex III of the electron transport chain (55), which can then lead to mitochondrial depolarization, the release of cytochrome C from the inner mitochondrial membrane, and triggering of apoptosis. To prevent this, HIF-1 shuts down oxidative phosphorylation by activating pyruvate dehydrogenase kinase 1, which in turn phosphorylates and inactivates the pyruvate dehydrogenase complex, thus preventing pyruvate from entering the Krebs cycle. Furthermore, HIF-1 appears to reduce mitochondrial biogenesis, mitochondrial respiration, and the generation of ROS by inhibiting MYC-regulated activation of PPAR-γ coactivator 1β (56) (PGC-1β), as well as promoting the dismantling (autophagy) of mitochondria to provide raw materials (57).

Autophagy, Apoptosis, and Necrosis

In the normal course of cellular activity intracellular components become damaged or redundant. These components are then biochemically "tagged" and then incorporated into double-membrane vesicles, which then fuse with lysosomes. The contents of these autophagosomes are then digested, and the metabolic building blocks reexported to the cytoplasm for recycling. As described above, this highly selective process, known as "autophagy," may become nonselective when cell survival is at risk (58). Ultimately, under circumstances where the supply of essential substrates continues to fall short of the requirement for cellular survival, a decision has to be made to either struggle on, and risk a necrotic cell death, or to abandon the fight gracefully, and activate a highly ordered form of cell death referred to as apoptosis. The apoptotic pathway involves two distinct phases. The first phase, commitment, is believed to be integrated by endogenous signals arriving at the mitochondria that provide information on cellular "well-being" and culminates in an irreversible increase in mitochondrial membrane permeability. The molecular details of this decision phase remain to be elucidated in detail. In contrast the second phase, execution, is more clearly understood and involves the activation of a cascade of enzymes, known as caspases, that culminate in the orderly dismantling of the cellular contents, including the nucleus, which are then packaged into vesicles for phagocytosis by neighboring cells (59). In marked contrast, cellular necrosis occurs when the integrity of the cell membrane can no longer be maintained. Membrane rupture results in the release of intracellular content and provokes a local inflammatory reaction. This increases the metabolic demands of the local environment, which, in the context of a local shortage of substrate supply, may then jeopardize the survival of neighboring cells.

Multiple Organ Dysfunction

The cellular outcomes from the pathways described above are limited, varying along the continuum between normal function and a threshold of dysfunction that then triggers a commitment to cellular senescence, apoptosis, or necrosis (Fig. 14). As our understanding of the cellular mechanisms of stress improves, it is becoming apparent that the pathways identified may vary between different species, different tissues types, or indeed between different experimental situations between transformed or native cells in vitro, or whole tissues in vivo. Furthermore, the ultimate outcome for any given cell will depend on the integration of a complex interplay between multiple pathways, some of which undoubtedly remain to be described, as well as the influence of particular genotypes. However, common end points clearly emerge from the stress pathways described above, which include the minimization of free-radical damage (enhanced antioxidant defenses, reduced oxidative phosphorylation), enhanced anaerobic glycolysis, the recycling of endogenous substrate by autophagy, and the conservation of energy by reduced protein translation. Ultimately, where survival appears impossible, energy is expended in an apoptotic cell death in an altruistic effort to minimize damage to neighboring cells (Fig. 15). At the organ level, where each constituent cell is subjected to particular conditions of substrate supply and extracellular signals, the

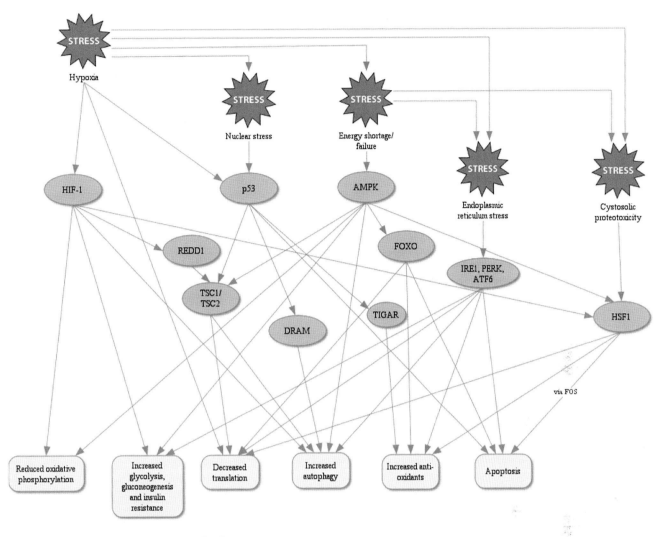

Figure 14 The spectrum of cellular end points.

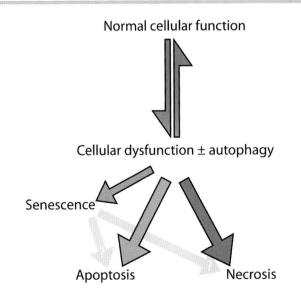

Figure 15 Molecular pathways mediating multiple organ dysfunction.

outcome can be very heterogeneous, with the function of the whole organ reflecting the sum of all the different outcomes for each constituent cell. Significant organ dysfunction (Table 8), sufficient to contribute to a patient's death, can be present with only modest cellular evidence of apoptosis (60). Survival in this condition for days or weeks is an entirely artificial situation made possible by modern medicine, and the cellular stress response, akin to hibernation, in the context of modern intensive care and organ support, establishes a vicious cycle (Fig. 12). While there has been strong evolutionary pressure to develop mechanisms to cope with, and survive, short periods of acute severe illness, this is not the case for prolonged critical illness (Fig. 16). An excellent example of this phenomenon is stress hyperglycemia. This particular response to stress is highly phylogenetically conserved and is seen not only in mammals, but even in fish (61), crustacea (62), and insects (63). This trait must, therefore, confer a survival benefit. In man, however, stress hyperglycemia has been associated with a poorer outcome in patients following stroke (64), acute myocardial infarction (65), and admission

Table 8 Clinical Manifestations of Cell Stress and Cell Death

	Clinical manifestations of cell stress (± cell senescence)	Clinical manifestations of cell death
Nervous system	Impaired arousal (stupor, coma) Impaired content (confusion, delirium) Motor and/or sensory neuropathy	Irreversible neurological deficits
Respiratory system	Failure to synthesize surfactant Failure to repopulate alveoli with type I pneumocytes Failure of gas exchange (hypoxia and hypercapnia) Contractile failure of respiratory muscles Persistent pulmonary inflammation	
Heart	Depressed contractility Rhythm disturbances	Raised plasma concentration of cardiac enzymes ECG changes
Kidneys	Impaired handling of water and solutes	Anuric renal failure
Liver	Impaired synthetic function Impaired drug and metabolite clearance	Raised plasma concentration of hepatic enzymes
Gut	Impaired gastric acid buffering/protection leading to gastric erosions Impaired enterocyte production leading to delayed healing Impairment of gut barrier function leading to bacterial translocation Impaired motility (ileus and constipation)	
Skeletal muscle	Atrophy Impaired contractility	Rhabdomyolysis
Immune system	Failure to clear infection	Lymphocytopenia Neutropenia
Bone marrow	Anemia Neutropenia Thrombocytopenia	
Connective tissue	Poor and slow wound healing	
Metabolism	Insulin resistance Impaired glucose tolerance	

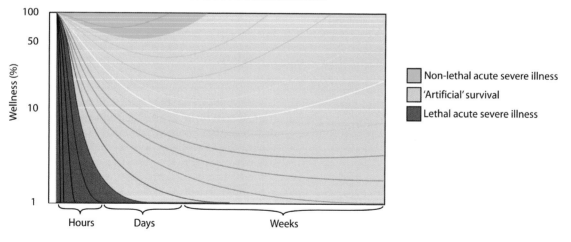

Figure 16 Time course of acute severe illness in man. The red zone represents the course of acute severe illnesses that are, and always have been, fatal. The green zone represents the course of acute severe illnesses that men, in some cases, have been able to survive. The responses to these conditions have therefore been under evolutionary selective pressure. The gray zone represents the course of acute severe illness that, in the absence of medical developments introduced in the past 50 years, would have been fatal. This zone represents a biological condition for which there has been no evolutionary precedent.

to intensive care (66). Furthermore, tight control of blood glucose with intravenous insulin has been shown to reduce morbidity and mortality in critically ill adults in both a historical cohort comparison (67) and two large prospective randomized trials (68,69). For this reason teleological and phylogenetic arguments that the stress response "must serve some purpose" cannot be applied in the context of patients whose acute severe illness and multiple organ failure have been "artificially" prolonged by modern intensive care.

REFERENCES

1. Le Dran H. Traite Ou Reflexions Tirées De La Pratique Sur Les Playes D'armes À Feux. Paris: Charles Osmont, 1737.
2. Mackenzie IMJ. The haemodynamics of human septic shock. Anaesthesia 2001; 56:130–144.
3. Levy MM, Fink MP, Marshall JC, et al. 2001 SCCM/ ESICM/ACCP/ATS/SIS International Sepsis Definitions Conference. Crit Care Med 2003; 31(4):1250–1256.
4. Reynolds HR, Hochman JS. Cardiogenic shock: current concepts and improving outcomes. Circulation 2008; 117 (5):686–697.
5. Ferreira FL, Bota DP, Bross A, et al. Serial evaluation of the SOFA score to predict outcome in critically ill patients. JAMA 2001; 286(14):1754–1758.
6. Bernard GR, Vincent JL, Laterre PF, et al. Efficacy and safety of recombinant human activated protein C for severe sepsis. N Engl J Med 2001; 344:699–709.
7. Caille V, Chiche JD, Nciri N, et al. Histocompatibility leukocyte antigen-D related expression is specifically altered and predicts mortality in septic shock but not in other causes of shock. Shock 2004; 22(6):521–526.
8. Sprung CL, Annane D, Keh D, et al. Hydrocortisone therapy for patients with septic shock. N Engl J Med 2008; 358(2):111–124.
9. Zeymer U, Vogt A, Zahn R, et al. Predictors of in-hospital mortality in 1333 patients with acute myocardial infarction complicated by cardiogenic shock treated with primary percutaneous coronary intervention (PCI): results of the primary PCI registry of the Arbeitsgemeinschaft Leitende Kardiologische Krankenhausarzte (ALKK). Eur Heart J 2004; 25(4):322–328.
10. Heckbert SR, Vedder NB, Hoffman W, et al. Outcome after hemorrhagic shock in trauma patients. J Trauma 1998; 45(3):545–549.
11. Weil MH, Shubin H. Proposed reclassification of shock states with special reference to distributive defects. Adv Exp Med Biol 1971; 23(0):13–23.
12. Sonnenblick EH, Skelton CL. Reconsideration of the ultrastructural basis of cardiac length-tension relations. Circ Res 1974; 35:517–526.
13. Gilbert JC, Glantz SA. Determinants of left ventricular filling and of the diastolic pressure-volume relation. Circ Res 1989; 64(5):827–852.
14. Kentner R, Rollwagen FM, Prueckner S, et al. Effects of mild hypothermia on survival and serum cytokines in uncontrolled hemorrhagic shock in rats. Shock 2002; 17(6):521–526.
15. Lausevic Z, Lausevic M, Trbojevic-Stankovic J, et al. Predicting multiple organ failure in patients with severe trauma. Can J Surg 2008; 51(2):97–102.
16. Clark JA, Coopersmith CM. Intestinal crosstalk: a new paradigm for understanding the gut as the "motor" of critical illness. Shock 2007; 28(4):384–393.
17. Spronk PE, Zandstra DF, Ince C. Bench-to-bedside review: sepsis is a disease of the microcirculation. Crit Care 2004; 8(6):462–468.
18. VanderMeer TJ, Wang H, Fink MP. Endotoxemia causes ileal mucosal acidosis in the absence of mucosal hypoxia in a normodynamic porcine model of septic shock. Crit Care Med 1995; 23(7):1217–1226.
19. Boekstegers P, Weidenhofer S, Pilz G, et al. Peripheral oxygen availability within skeletal muscle in sepsis and

20. Fink MP. Bench-to-bedside review: cytopathic hypoxia. Crit Care Dec 2002; 6(6):491–499.
21. Fieselmann JF, Hendryx MS, Helms CM, et al. Respiratory rate predicts cardiopulmonary arrest for internal medicine inpatients. J Gen Intern Med 1993; 8(7):354–360.
22. Lanone S, Taille C, Boczkowski J, et al. Diaphragmatic fatigue during sepsis and septic shock. Intensive Care Med Dec 2005; 31(12):1611–1617.
23. Kumar A, Anel R, Bunnell E, et al. Pulmonary artery occlusion pressure and central venous pressure fail to predict ventricular filling volume, cardiac performance, or the response to volume infusion in normal subjects. Crit Care Med 2004; 32(3):691–699.
24. Raper R, Sibbald WJ. Misled by the wedge? The Swan-Ganz catheter and left-ventricular pre-load. Chest 1986; 89(3):427–434.
25. Harvey S, Harrison DA, Singer M, et al. Assessment of the clinical effectiveness of pulmonary artery catheters in management of patients in intensive care (PAC-Man): a randomised controlled trial. Lancet 2005; 366(9484):472–477.
26. Wheeler AP, Bernard GR, Thompson BT, et al. Pulmonary-artery versus central venous catheter to guide treatment of acute lung injury. N Engl J Med 2006; 354(21):2213–2224.
27. Spahn DR, Cerny V, Coats TJ, et al. Management of bleeding following major trauma: a European guideline. Crit Care 2007; 11(1):R17.
28. Rivers E, Nguyen B, Havstad S, et al. Early goal-directed therapy in the treatment of severe sepsis and septic shock. N Engl J Med 2001; 345(19):1368–1377.
29. Bucher M, Kees F, Taeger K, et al. Cytokines downregulate alpha1-adrenergic receptor expression during endotoxemia. Crit Care Med 2003; 31(2):566–571.
30. Schaak S, Mialet-Perez J, Flordellis C, et al. Genetic variation of human adrenergic receptors: from molecular and functional properties to clinical and pharmacogenetic implications. Curr Top Med Chem 2007; 7(2):217–231.
31. Takakura K, Taniguchi T, Muramatsu I, et al. Modification of alpha1-adrenoceptors by peroxynitrite as a possible mechanism of systemic hypotension in sepsis. Crit Care Med 2002; 30(4):894–899.
32. Mullner M, Urbanek B, Havel C, et al. Vasopressors for shock. Cochrane Database Syst Rev 2004(3):CD003709.
33. Beale RJ, Hollenberg SM, Vincent JL, et al. Vasopressor and inotropic support in septic shock: an evidence-based review. Crit Care Med 2004; 32(11 suppl):S455–S465.
34. Martin C, Papazian L, Perrin G, et al. Norepinephrine or dopamine for the treatment of hyperdynamic septic shock? Chest 1993; 103(6):1826–1831.
35. Debaveye YA, Van den Berghe GH. Is there still a place for dopamine in the modern intensive care unit? Anesth Analg 2004; 98(2):461–468.
36. Sakr Y, Reinhart K, Vincent JL, et al. Does dopamine administration in shock influence outcome? Results of the Sepsis Occurrence in Acutely Ill Patients (SOAP) Study. Crit Care Med 2006; 34(3):589–597.
37. Ritossa F. A new puffing pattern induced by temperature shock and DNP in *Drosophila*. Experientia 1962; 18 (12):571–573.
38. Tissieres A, Mitchell HK, Tracy UM. Protein synthesis in salivary glands of *Drosophila melanogaster*: relation to chromosome puffs. J Mol Biol 1974; 84(3):389–398.
39. Ryan AJ, Flanagan SW, Moseley PL, et al. Acute heat stress protects rats against endotoxin shock. J Appl Physiol 1992; 73(4):1517–1522.
40. Boellmann F, Guettouche T, Guo Y, et al. DAXX interacts with heat shock factor 1 during stress activation and

enhances its transcriptional activity. Proc Natl Acad Sci U S A 2004; 101(12):4100–4105.

41. Page TJ, Sikder D, Yang L, et al. Genome-wide analysis of human HSF1 signaling reveals a transcriptional program linked to cellular adaptation and survival. Mol Biosyst 2006; 2(12):627–639.

42. Xiao X, Zuo X, Davis AA, et al. HSF1 is required for extra-embryonic development, postnatal growth and protection during inflammatory responses in mice. EMBO J 1999; 18(21):5943–5952.

43. Marciniak SJ, Ron D. Endoplasmic reticulum stress signaling in disease. Physiol Rev 2006; 86(4):1133–1149.

44. Lee AH, Iwakoshi NN, Glimcher LH. XBP-1 regulates a subset of endoplasmic reticulum resident chaperone genes in the unfolded protein response. Mol Cell Biol 2003; 23(21):7448–7459.

45. Ozcan U, Cao Q, Yilmaz E, et al. Endoplasmic reticulum stress links obesity, insulin action, and type 2 diabetes. Science 2004; 306(5695):457–461.

46. Ogata M, Hino S, Saito A, et al. Autophagy is activated for cell survival after endoplasmic reticulum stress. Mol Cell Biol 2006; 26(24):9220–9231.

47. Scheuner D, Song B, McEwen E, et al. Translational control is required for the unfolded protein response and in vivo glucose homeostasis. Mol Cell 2001; 7(6):1165–1176.

48. Bensaad K, Tsuruta A, Selak MA, et al. TIGAR, a p53-inducible regulator of glycolysis and apoptosis. Cell 2006; 126(1):107–120.

49. Feng Z, Hu W, de Stanchina E, et al. The regulation of AMPK beta1, TSC2, and PTEN expression by p53: stress, cell and tissue specificity, and the role of these gene products in modulating the IGF-1-AKT-mTOR pathways. Cancer Res 2007; 67(7):3043–3053.

50. Crighton D, Wilkinson S, O'Prey J, et al. DRAM, a p53-induced modulator of autophagy, is critical for apoptosis. Cell 2006; 126(1):121–134.

51. Virag L, Szabo C. The therapeutic potential of poly(ADP-ribose) polymerase inhibitors. Pharmacol Rev 2002; 54(3):375–429.

52. Brocks JJ, Logan GA, Buick R, et al. Archean molecular fossils and the early rise of eukaryotes. Science 1999; 285(5430):1033–1036.

53. Clanton TL. Hypoxia-induced reactive oxygen species formation in skeletal muscle. J Appl Physiol 2007; 102(6):2379–2388.

54. Greer EL, Oskoui PR, Banko MR, et al. The energy sensor AMP-activated protein kinase directly regulates the mammalian FOXO3 transcription factor. J Biol Chem 2007; 282(41):30107–30119.

55. Guzy RD, Schumacker PT. Oxygen sensing by mitochondria at complex III: the paradox of increased reactive oxygen species during hypoxia. Exp Physiol 2006; 91(5):807–819.

56. Zhang H, Gao P, Fukuda R, et al. HIF-1 inhibits mitochondrial biogenesis and cellular respiration in VHL-deficient renal cell carcinoma by repression of C-MYC activity. Cancer Cell 2007; 11(5):407–420.

57. Zhang H, Bosch-Marce M, Shimoda LA, et al. Mitochondrial autophagy is an HIF-1-dependent adaptive metabolic response to hypoxia. J Biol Chem 2008; 283(16):10892–10903.

58. Kundu M, Thompson CB. Autophagy: basic principles and relevance to disease. Annu Rev Pathol 2008; 3:427–455.

59. Kroemer G, Galluzzi L, Brenner C. Mitochondrial membrane permeabilization in cell death. Physiol Rev 2007; 87(1):99–163.

60. Hotchkiss RS, Swanson PE, Freeman BD, et al. Apoptotic cell death in patients with sepsis, shock, and multiple organ dysfunction. Crit Care Med 1999; 27(7):1230–1251.

61. Suski CD, Cooke SJ, Danylchuk AJ, et al. Physiological disturbance and recovery dynamics of bonefish (*Albula vulpes*), a tropical marine fish, in response to variable exercise and exposure to air. Comp Biochem Physiol A Mol Integr Physiol 2007; 148(3):664–673.

62. Telford M. The effects of stress on blood sugar composition of the lobster, *Homarus americanus*. Can J Zool 1968; 46(5):819–826.

63. Schilder RJ, Marden JH. Metabolic syndrome and obesity in an insect. Proc Natl Acad Sci U S A 2006; 103(49):18805–18809.

64. Capes SE, Hunt D, Malmberg K, et al. Stress hyperglycaemia and prognosis of stroke in nondiabetic and diabetic patients: a systematic overview. Stroke 2001; 32:2426–2432.

65. Capes SE, Hunt D, Malmberg K, et al. Stress hyperglycaemia and increased risk of death after myocardial infarction in patients with and without diabetes: a systematic overview. Lancet 2000; 355(9206):773–778.

66. Krinsley JS. Association between hyperglycaemia and increased hospital mortality in a heterogeneous population of critically ill patients. Mayo Clin Proc 2003; 78:1471–1478.

67. Krinsley JS. Effect of an intensive glucose management protocol on the mortality of critically ill adult patients. Mayo Clin Proc 2004; 79(8):992–1000.

68. Van den Berghe G, Wouters P, Weekers F, et al. Intensive insulin therapy in critically ill patients. N Engl J Med 2001; 345(19):1359–1367.

69. Van den Berghe G, Wilmer A, Hermans G, et al. Intensive insulin therapy in the medical ICU. N Engl J Med 2006; 354(5):449–461.

12

Acute Renal Failure

Rona Smith and John R. Bradley
Cambridge University Hospitals NHS Foundation Trust, Cambridge, U.K.

INTRODUCTION

Until recently more than 30 definitions for acute renal failure have been used in the literature. The majority mention a rapid deterioration in renal function, with the accumulation of nitrogenous wastes in the body, often associated with oliguria or anuria. However, there was no agreed definition. The huge variation not only caused confusion but also made comparisons between studies very difficult. As a consequence, a group of experts, the acute dialysis quality initiative (ADQI), developed the RIFLE criteria as a consensus definition for acute kidney injury (AKI), an alternative term now commonly used and which henceforth will be used in this chapter (1). The RIFLE criteria divides renal dysfunction into five categories—risk, injury, failure, loss, and end stage kidney disease (ESKD)—on the basis of glomerular filtration rate (GFR) and urine output criteria, which are illustrated in Figure 1.

AKI is common, although the incidence depends on the definition used. In a United Kingdom–based community study, the incidence of severe AKI (creatinine >500 mmol/L) was 172 cases/million adults/yr, with 22 cases/million adults/yr requiring dialysis (2). AKI complicates 5% to 20% of hospital admissions and approximately 30% of admissions to the intensive care unit. Rates of survival are dependent on cause. However, mortality is high (40–80%) in patients with multiple organ failure, with death being likely if AKI is associated with failure of more than three other organ systems. In patients acquiring AKI in the community, mortality is much lower (10–30%) (3).

The potential causes of AKI can be divided into three categories: prerenal failure (approximately 55% of cases) due to inadequate perfusion of blood through the kidney, often termed physiological prerenal failure, which resolves when the underlying hypovolaemia is corrected, and pathological prerenal failure due to an interruption of blood flow to the kidney when there is an anatomical cause for disturbed renal blood flow, such as an aortic dissection; renal failure as a consequence of intrinsic injury to the kidney (about 40% of cases); and postrenal failure (less than 5% of AKI cases) due to the obstruction of urine outflow (Fig. 2). However, in 50% of cases of hospital acquired AKI, the cause is multifactorial, with hypotension, sepsis, and nephrotoxic drugs commonly being involved (4).

PRESENTATION

Presenting symptoms are usually dominated by those of the underlying etiology, especially in cases of prerenal AKI. Often symptoms are those of hypovolaemia, namely thirst, dizziness, decreased urine output, and postural hypotension. Conversely, patients may present in a state of fluid overload, with peripheral edema and shortness of breath. Symptoms of uremia are nonspecific, but include anorexia, nausea, vomiting, lethargy, weakness, myoclonic jerks, seizures, confusion, and coma.

INVESTIGATIONS

On any sick patient, a number of investigations are performed. It may only be at this point that a diagnosis of AKI is made, when elevated serum urea and creatinine levels are identified on blood tests. Once the diagnosis is made, further tests are required to determine the severity and urgency of any treatment required, such as dialysis, and also the etiology of the renal failure. The key tests required are listed below.

Blood Tests

Biochemical tests identify high urea and creatinine levels. Other features of AKI include high serum potassium and phosphate levels due to reduced renal excretion, and typically a low calcium level. A high serum calcium level would make one suspicious of multiple myeloma, which would be confirmed by performing serum protein electrophoresis, and the presence of a monoclonal immunoglobulin band. Elevated creatinine kinase (CK) levels are seen in rhabdomyolysis. Serum levels of any potential nephrotoxins (vancomycin, gentamicin, cyclosporine, and tacrolimus) should be determined.

Hematological investigations include a full blood count and coagulation screen. Anemia is a feature of chronic renal failure due to a number of factors, but predominantly decreased erythropoietin levels. Thrombocytopaenia is suggestive of sepsis or systemic lupus erythematosus (SLE) or thrombotic thrombocytopaenic purpura (TTP). A blood film may be useful if hemolysis is suspected as in hemolytic uremic syndrome (HUS). Clotting may be deranged if severe sepsis or liver disease is present

	GFR criteria	Urine output (UO) criteria
Risk	Increased creatinine × 1.5 or GFR decrease >25%	UO < 0.5mL/kg/hr × 6 hr
Injury	Increased creatinine × 2 or GFR decrease >50%	UO < 0.5mL/kg/hr × 12 hr
Failure	Increase creatinine × 3 or GFR decrease >75%	UO < 0.3mL/kg/hr × 24 hr or anuria × 12 hr
Loss	Persistent AKI = complete loss of kidney function >4 wk	
ESKD	End-stage kidney disease (>3 mo)	

Figure 1 RIFLE criteria for acute renal dysfunction.

Prerenal

Volume depletion	GI losses (diarrhoea and vomiting) Renal losses (diuretics) Hemorrhage
Decreased cardiac output	Pulmonary embolus Heart failure/myocardial infarction/ severe valvular disease Abdominal compartment syndrome
Systemic vasodilatation	Sepsis/anaphylaxis
Afferent arteriolar constriction	Hypercalcaemia Drugs—calcineurin inhibitors, NSAIDS, radio contrast agents Hepatorenal syndrome
Efferent arteriolar constriction	ACE inhibitors or angiotensin receptor blockers

Intrinsic

Acute tubular injury	Ischaemic Cytotoxic—heme pigment (rhabdomyolosis), crystals, drugs, for example, gentamicin
Glomerulonephritis	Antiglomerular basement membrane disease ANCA associated, for example, Wegner's granulomatosis, MPA Immune complex GN—lupus, post infective, cryoglobulinaemia
Tubulointerstitial nephritis	Drugs, for example, NSAIDS, penicillin Infection Systemic disease—for example, sarcoid
Acute vascular nephropathy	Renal artery obstruction Renal vein obstruction Microangiopathy Atheroembolic disease

Postrenal

Ureteric obstruction	Intrinisic (stones), extrinsic (retroperitoneal fibrosis, lymph nodes)
Bladder neck obstruction	Prostate carcinoma, benign prostatic hypertrophy, bladder tumours, hemorrhage/clot

Figure 2 Causes of acute renal failure.

but must be performed if a biopsy is contemplated. Elevated erythrocyte sedimentation rate (ESR) is seen in vasculitis and multiple myeloma.

Serological investigations are performed if glomerular pathology is suspected. Key tests are antinuclear antibody (ANA) and double-stranded DNA levels, which are positive in SLE; antineutrophil cytoplasmic antibodies (ANCA), which are divided into proteinase PR3 positive in Wegner's granulomatosis; and myeloperoxidase (MPO) positive; and anti-GBM (glomerular basement membrane) antibody is found in Goodpasture's disease. Complement levels, namely C3 and C4, should be measured and cryoglobulins tested in patients with unexplained glomerular disease. Serum complement levels tend to be low in immune-mediated renal conditions because of consumption within the kidney. Cryoglobulins are immunoglobulin proteins that precipitate in the cold and can be deposited in the kidney where they are associated with immune inflammation. They may be idiopathic or associated with autoimmune disease, hematological disease, or infection, including hepatitis C.

Urine Testing

Dipstick testing identifies hematuria and proteinuria, which are suggestive of glomerular pathology as a cause of intrinsic renal failure. In cases of prerenal failure, ATN, and obstruction, the urine should be bland. Leukocytes and nitrites may also be identified and if that is the case a urine culture should be performed.

Microscopy looks for red cells or white cells, or cellular casts, in which red or white cells adhere to proteins excreted by tubules. Red cells are seen in bleeding from anywhere in the renal tract, but red cell casts usually indicate glomerular bleeding. White cell casts imply tubular inflammation.

Osmolality and urinary sodium concentrations can help distinguish prerenal failure from established ATN. Prerenal failure is characterised by a urine sodium <20 mmol/L and an urine/plasma urea ratio >8, because the tubules are working normally and reabsorbing salt and water maximally. Once ischemic damage occurs to the tubules and ATN is established, the tubules can no longer reabsorb sodium or concentrate the urine and so the urine sodium concentration is typically high at >40 mmol/L and the urine/plasma urea ratio low at <3. Sometimes this information is presented as a fractional excretion of sodium (FeNa), which is calculated using the following formula.

$$FeNa = (urine\ Na/plasma\ Na)/(urine\ creatinine/plasma\ creatinine)$$

A FeNa <1% is suggestive of prerenal AKI, while a FeNa >1% indicates tubular damage and ATN (5). However, in the following situations, the FeNa may be <1%, but the cause of renal impairment is not prerenal—urinary tract obstruction, hepatorenal syndrome, renal allograft rejection, contrast induced ATN, rhabdomyolysis, and acute glomerulonephritis.

Imaging

Chest radiography is performed on a routine basis to look for evidence of pulmonary edema and fluid overload. It is also important to look for pulmonary infiltrates, which can be seen in pulmonary renal syndromes, such as Wegner's granulomatosis and Goodpasture's syndrome.

Renal ultrasound looks at the size, shape, and texture of the kidneys. In AKI, kidneys are often normal sized or larger than normal and may show increased echogenicity. However, in chronic renal failure, the kidneys are not only smaller than expected, but also show increased echogenicity, probably because of fibrosis. Ultrasound can also identify signs of hydronephrosis, such as a dilated pelvicalyceal system, although it must be remembered that a normal ultrasound does not completely exclude obstruction.

Renal Biopsy

Renal biopsies are an invasive procedure and should therefore be reserved for evaluation of cases of AKI when the cause is uncertain. They are particularly useful when a glomerular pathology is suspected not only for confirming the diagnosis but also for guiding treatment decisions and indicating prognosis.

MANAGEMENT OF ACUTE KIDNEY INJURY

While investigation into the cause of AKI progresses, early medical intervention to reverse any potential underlying cause, such as hypovolaemia, and prevent further iatrogenic injury, for example, by the administration of nephrotoxic drugs, is key. Attention must be focused on optimal fluid balance, whether that is aggressive rehydration with intravenous fluids if dry or attempts at inducing a diuresis with various agents if the converse is true. If lower urinary tract obstruction is suspected, a urinary catheter should be inserted. Its placement will also help with accurate fluid balance measurement, but it is a potential source of infection, and urinary catheter placement is not obligatory to manage fluid balance closely.

Patients with nonoliguric AKI have decreased mortality rates, and improved renal recovery rates (6). Therefore, in the past diuretics were often used in an attempt to convert oliguric AKI into nonoliguric AKI. However, randomised double-blind controlled trials have failed to show any benefit (7), and now diuretics are only used in fluid overloaded patients to promote a diuresis in an attempt to avoid the need for dialysis. Furosemide is the most commonly used agent. Very high doses, up to 250 mg intravenously may be required to have an effect when renal function is poor, but carry a risk of ototoxicity.

There is also often confusion regarding the role of low-dose dopamine, generally considered to be a dose less than 2.5 µg/kg/min, in AKI. Dopamine is a potent vasodilator acting via DA1 receptors, and also inhibits active sodium transport in the proximal tubule leading to a naturesis and diuresis. At moderate doses it has β-adrenergic effects increasing cardiac output and renal blood flow and perfusion. A meta-analysis by Kellum (8) and a randomised controlled trial by Bellomo et al. (9), have both shown that low-dose dopamine may increase urine output, but has no beneficial effect in terms of decreased mortality or the need for renal replacement therapy (RRT). Documented side effects include depression of respiratory drive, cardiac arrhythmias, and tissue necrosis and digital gangrene (10). Therefore, at present, the use of dopamine in AKI, whether it be prophylactically or therapeutically, is not advised.

COMPLICATIONS OF ACUTE KIDNEY INJURY

Hyperkalemia

Hyperkalaemia is a medical emergency. In AKI serum potassium levels rise for several reasons including decreased GFR, reduced tubular secretion, a catabolic state and a metabolic acidosis. It is particularly marked in situations where endogenous potassium production is high, such as in rhabdomyolysis or tumor lysis syndrome. Often the patient will not have any specific symptoms, but the ECG may show typical changes including tented T waves, broadening of the QRS complex, flattening of P waves and prolongation of the PR interval. If the K+ >7 mmol, then treat immediately. Most people would advocate treating a K+ level greater than 6.5 mmol if ECG changes are present. Initially 10 mL 10% calcium gluconate should be given intravenously to stabilize the myocardium. It does not lower the potassium level. This is achieved by administering 50 mL 50% dextrose with 10 units of actrapid insulin intravenously over 20 to 30 minutes to drive potassium intracellularly. 5 mg nebulized salbutamol can be given as an adjunct to drive potassium into cells, as can intravenous sodium bicarbonate. Calcium resonium, 15g orally, four times a day, reduces absorption of dietary potassium from the gut, but works over many hours. Drugs that raise serum potassium levels, such as ACE inhibitors, angiotensin receptor blockers and potassium sparing diuretics must be stopped. Ultimately, if hyperkalaemia proves refractory to the above treatments, then dialysis will be required.

Fluid Overload

Patients with AKI may present with fluid overload because of salt and water retention and a decrease in GFR. It also commonly occurs after oliguric/anuric patients are given intravenous fluids by medical staff in an attempt to improve urine output. Clinically, patients complain of feeling short of breath, and on physical examination signs of fluid overload include a raised jugular venous pressure, peripheral edema, a gallop rhythm, and bibasal crepitations on auscultation of the chest.

Bleeding Tendency

Patients with severe renal failure have an increased likelihood of bleeding, which may occur even though their platelet counts and clotting are normal. This is thought to occur because platelets do not adhere normally to the endothelium and stop bleeding. Experimental work in rats has suggested that nitric oxide is the mediator of bleeding tendency in uremia. Rats that have extensive surgical ablation of renal tissue develop renal failure because of progressive glomerulosclerosis. Like uremic humans, these rats have a prolonged bleeding time. Administration of L-NMMA, a specific inhibitor of nitric oxide normalized the bleeding time in uremic rats. This effect was completely reversed by giving the animals the NO precursor L-arginine (11).

Infection

Infections develop in 30% to 70% of patients with ATN, probably because of a combination of factors including impaired defences due to uremia, excessive use of antibiotics and multiple invasive procedures.

DIALYSIS

Indications for urgent dialysis or RRT are as follows:

1. Persistent hyperkalaemia (K+ >7 mmol).
2. Fluid overload refractory to diuretic therapy.
3. Acidosis (pH <7.1, or bicarbonate <12 mmol).
4. Symptomatic uremia (tremor, cognitive impairment, fits, coma or pericarditis). This usually occurs when urea >45 mmol.

Three principle methods for RRT exist, namely intermittent hemodialysis, peritoneal dialysis and continuous venovenous haemofiltration (CVVH). Each method has its advantages and disadvantages. Intermittent hemodialysis is probably the most widely available technique, and it is very efficient at removing volume from the intravascular compartment. However, its use is often complicated by

hypotension, and it is in this situation that CVVH may be more appropriate. Peritoneal dialysis can be used in the acute setting, but this is certainly more unusual, and it is more difficult to remove large fluid volumes.

ACUTE TUBULAR NECROSIS

Pathogenesis of Acute Tubular Necrosis

The commonest form of intrinsic AKI is acute tubular necrosis (ATN) secondary to ischemic and, or nephrotoxic injury. It is often the result of multiple insults, rather than a single event, and multiple mechanisms contribute to the final outcome of reduced urine output. The key processes involved are illustrated in Figure 3. The clinical course of ATN can be divided into three phases: initiation, maintenance and recovery. Figure 4 illustrates the key features of each phase. Research into the pathogenesis of ATN aims to develop strategies to prevent it developing initially, and the secondly to discover interventions that might accelerate recovery.

ATN is characterised pathologically by varying degrees of tubular cell damage and cell death. In biopsy specimens regenerating cells are often found together with freshly damaged cells, suggesting multiple cycles of injury and repair. The histological sequence of events is as follows:

*   Patchy loss of tubular epithelial cells, leading to gaps and exposure of a denuded basement membrane
*   Loss of proximal tubular brush border
*   Patchy necrosis of tubules most commonly in the outer medulla
*   Tubular dilatation and formation of intraluminal casts
*   Cellular regeneration

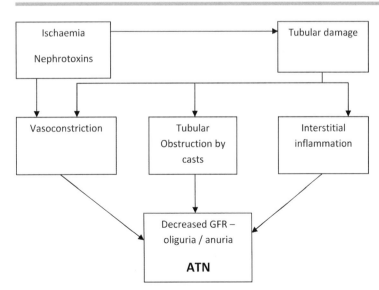

Figure 3 Key process involved in acute tubular necrosis.

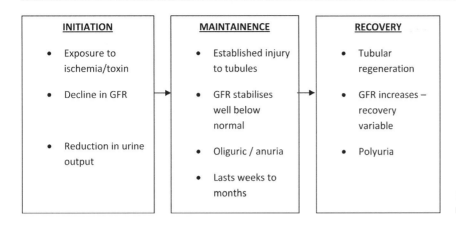

INITIATION	MAINTAINENCE	RECOVERY
• Exposure to ischemia/toxin	• Established injury to tubules	• Tubular regeneration
• Decline in GFR	• GFR stabilises well below normal	• GFR increases – recovery variable
• Reduction in urine output	• Oliguric / anuria	• Polyuria
	• Lasts weeks to months	

Figure 4 The clinical course of acute tubular necrosis.

In almost all experimental models of ATN and in clinical experience of patients with AKI, volume loading with saline and the establishment of natriuresis, will minimize or even prevent ATN developing. Conversely, volume depletion increases the risk of ATN. Therefore, alterations in renal haemodynamics and tubular function are two key factors in the pathogenesis of ATN.

Alterations in Renal Hemodynamics

The kidneys (less than 0.5% of total body mass) have one of the highest blood flow rates per unit tissue mass in the body, receiving approximately 20% of cardiac output. This is mainly to filter the blood, with only a small percentage being required for their metabolism. If cardiac output, or effective intravascular volume decreases, compensatory mechanisms such as afferent arteriolar dilatation (as a result of myogenic responses and prostaglandins) and efferent arteriolar constriction (via angiotensin II) attempt to maintain renal perfusion. However, if prolonged, decompensation occurs. Excessive stimulation of the renin angiotensin system and the sympathetic nervous system, leads to profound renal vasoconstriction and tubular hypoxia and damage. Drugs that interfere with these compensatory mechanisms, such as NSAIDS inhibiting prostaglandin synthesis, calcineurin inhibitors (e.g., cyclosporine and tacrolimus), which are potent vasoconstrictors, and ACE inhibitors accelerate the process.

Blood flow in the outer cortex is approximately six fold greater than the outer medulla and twenty fold greater than the inner medulla. The limited blood flow in the medulla prevents wash out of the gradients of solute formed by the loops of Henle, which are important for normal urine concentration. Therefore, even under normal conditions the medulla is relatively hypoxic, with a partial pressure of oxygen being 10 to 20 mmHg, compared with 50 mmHg in the cortex. So, tubules in the medulla are particularly vulnerable to ischemic damage when renal perfusion is reduced (12). Although reduction in renal blood flow is thought to be the dominant cause of ATN, it cannot be the sole factor, as restoration of adequate blood flow by volume expansion or vasodilatation does not correct GFR.

Mediators such as endothelin-1, adenosine and angiotensin II, all potent vasoconstrictors and reduced levels of vasodilators such as nitric oxide and prostaglandins are thought to lead to prolonged medullary vasoconstriction and hypoxic damage to tubules. It is not understood why this occurs. During periods of ischemia and reperfusion, the ET-1 gene is upregulated (13) and elevated levels of endothelin-1 have been demonstrated in experimental models of AKI, and endothelin-1 receptor antagonists shown to improve renal function and renal histological features of ischemic injury (14,15). Adenosine is thought to play a role in contrast nephropathy. Pretreatment with adenosine receptor antagonists, such as theophylline, prior to the administration of contrast have been shown to limit the reduction in GFR, but have no effect in established ATN (16). The role of angiotensin II is somewhat unclear. Expansion of the juxtaglomerular apparatus and an increase in plasma rennin levels have been shown in experimental cases of ATN, but inhibition of angiotensin II, rather than ameliorate AKI has been shown to precipitate renal failure in patients with reduced blood volume.

A deficiency of vasodilators, such as endothelium-derived nitric oxide and prostaglandins may play a role in the initiation of ATN, but no evidence exists that administration of either molecule alters the course of established ATN. As a consequence of the initial severe vasospasm occurring in an attempt to maintain renal perfusion, focal and segmental necrosis of the media in resistance arterioles is found. Endothelial cells swell, and platelets and leukocytes adhere to sites of endothelial cell injury, obstructing the lumens of capillaries. Activated adherent neutrophils inactivate endothelium-derived nitric oxide, promoting further vasoconstriction and renal hypoperfusion and further leukocyte adhesion, probably via up-regulation of adhesion molecules, such as ICAM-1 (Intercellular adhesion molecule-1). Administration of monoclonal antibodies to ICAM-1, protected rats against AKI (18), and ICAM-1 deficient mice are protected against ischemic renal injury (18).

There is a rationale for giving vasodilators in ATN. However, nitric oxide donors such as nitroprusside, do not improve the course of ischemic ATN (19). The lack of effect may not be due to a failure in vasodilatation, but due to the paradoxical toxic effect of nitric oxide on the proximal tubules, by the generation of oxygen free radicals. The cell swelling seen after ischemic damage in ATN, not only obstructs the tubular lumens, but together with interstitial edema obstructs the ascending vessels impairing venous return from the medulla, further exacerbating tubular ischemia.

Alterations in Tubular Function

Tubular obstruction due to the exfoliation of mainly viable rather than necrotic tubular cells into the lumen, contributes to reduction in GFR. It also leaves behind an exposed basement membrane, and the loss of tight junctions between the proximal tubule cells results in tubular back leak of various substances in the ultrafiltrate. The sloughed cells in the lumen exacerbate this by increasing intratubular pressure.

Tubular obstruction is especially relevant in certain causes of AKI. In myeloma, haemoglobulinuria, myoglobinuria and crystalluria, casts contribute to tubular obstruction in addition to denuded tubular cells. In these situations, establishing a diuresis and alkalinizing the urine are strategies to minimize the risk of tubular obstruction.

Activation of tubuloglomerular feedback also contributes to the reduction in GFR. As well as losing their tight junctions, proximal tubule cells lose their polarity, by the relocation of the Na^+/K^+ adenosine triphosphate (ATP)ase from the basolateral to the apical membrane. This impairs sodium and water transport, and consequently the loss of chloride reabsorption in the thick ascending limb of the loop of Henle activates the feedback mechanism at the macula densa because of increased chloride delivery. This leads to afferent arteriolar constriction via the adenosine A1 receptor (A1AR) in the glomerulus and a decrease in the GFR. Therefore, it may be expected that knockout of the A1AR may limit the decline in GFR. However, paradoxically the reverse is true (20). Activation of A1AR is actually protective, probably by limiting delivery of ions and solutes to the damaged cells of the proximal tubule, thereby reducing the demand for ATP dependent reabsorption. An alternative explanation may be that adenosine has differential effects in the cortex and medulla. In the cortical circulation it is a potent vasoconstrictor via A1 receptors, but in the medulla it is a vasodilator acting via A2 receptors.

Oxygen deprivation, as occurs with renal hypoperfusion, leads to the catabolism of ATP to adenosine diphosphate (ADP) and adenosine monophosphate (AMP). Prolonged ischemia results in the breakdown of adenine nucleotides to adenosine and hypoxanthine. Consequently, ATP dependent transport mechanisms are inhibited. One effect is a rise in intracellular free calcium, as ATP is required to pump calcium out of cells or sequester it in the endoplasmic reticulum. High calcium levels activate proteases and phospholipases, cause mitochondrial damage, generate oxygen free radicals and disrupt the cell cytoskeleton. Calcium channel blockers have been show to limit ischemic renal injury in animal models, although the exact mechanism is unclear (21). Possible effects include membrane stabilization of tubular epithelial cells, or antagonism of calmodulin, or improved renal haemodynamics in addition to preventing calcium overloading of cells. Calcium channel blockers have been shown to ameliorate ATN in humans. The best evidence comes from the transplant population, where administration of calcium channel blockers to recipients reduces the prevalence of ATN (22,23). In addition, there is some evidence that administration of calcium channel blocking agents prior to radiocontrast materials offers some protection to their nephrotoxicity (21).

Recovery from Acute Tubular Necrosis

Once renal perfusion has been reestablished, the majority of individuals with ATN recover most of their renal function. For recovery to occur, tubular cell polarity and the integrity of tight junctions need to be restored in viable cells. In addition, dead cells must be removed by apoptosis, and lost tubular epithelial cells must regenerate. Following reperfusion, there is marked up-regulation of a number of genes involved in cell proliferation, including insulin-like growth factor 1 (IGF-1) (24), fibroblast growth factor (FGF), hepatocyte growth factor (HGF) (25) and epidermal growth factor (EGF) (26). In animal models of AKI, administration of these various growth factors accelerated renal recovery. However, when IGF-1 was given to human subjects with AKI, no benefit was demonstrated. In addition to the above factors, heat shock proteins (HSP) are likely to play a key role in tubular regeneration. Both HSP-70 and HSP-25 have been shown to be over expressed in renal tubular cells following ischemia and reperfusion in animal models (27,28). Their role in humans is yet to be determined.

CONCLUSIONS

Treatment of patients with AKI is still largely supportive. Of course strategies to prevent the development of AKI, such as volume expansion prior to administration of radiocontrast materials is important, but most research has focused on interventions to accelerate regeneration and recovery of the tubular epithelium following an episode of ATN. Much of this work is still very experimental, and although successes have been seen in animal models, translating such work into human subjects remains difficult. It is likely that as the cause of most cases of ATN is multifactorial, and the development of ATN requires a number of pathological processes, that any single drug therapy will be the cure, and multiple agents will be required to promote a rapid recovery.

REFERENCES

1. Bellomo R, Kellum JA, Ronco C. Defining and classifying acute renal failure: from advocacy to consensus and validation of the RIFLE criteria. Intensive Care Med 2007; 33 (3):409–413.
2. Lameire N Van Biesen W, Vanholder R. Acute renal failure. Lancet 2005; 365(9457):417–430.
3. Chertow GM, Christionsen CL, Cleary PD, et al. Prognostic stratification in critically ill patients with AKI requiring dialysis. Arch Intern Med 1995; 155(14):1505–1511.
4. Kalra PA. Early management and prevention of acute renal failure. EDTNA ERCA J. 2002(suppl 2):34–38, 42.
5. Miller TR, Anderson RJ, Linas SL, et al. Urinary diagnostic indices in acute renal failure: a prospective failure. Ann Intern Med 1978; 89:47–50.
6. Anderson RJ, Linas SL, Berns AS, et al. Nonoliguric acute renal failure. N Engl J Med 1977; 296:1134–1138.
7. Shilliday I, Quinn K, Allison M. Loop diuretics in the management of acute renal failure: a prospective, double-blind, placebo-controlled, randomized study. Nephrol Dial Transplant 1997; 12(12):2592–2596.
8. Kellum JA, Decker J. Use of dopamine in acute renal failure: a meta-analysis. Crit Care Med 2001; 29(8):1526–1531.
9. Bellomo R, Chapman M, Finfer S, et al. Low-dose dopamine in patients with early renal dysfunction: a placebo-controlled randomised trial. Lancet 2000; 356:2139–2143.
10. Debaveye YA, Van de Berghe GH. Is there still a place for dopamine in the modern intensive care unit? Anesth Analg 2004; 98:461–468.
11. Remuzzi G, Perico N, Zoja C, et al. Role of endothelium-derived nitric oxide in the bleeding tendency of uremia. J Clin Invest 1990; 86(5):1768–1771.
12. Heyman SN, Fuchs S, Brezis M. The role of medullary ischemia in acute renal failure. New Horiz 1995; 3(5): 597–607.
13. Wilhelm SM, Simonson MS, Robinson AV, et al. Endothelin up-regulation and localization following renal ischemia and reperfusion. Kidney Int 1999; 55:1011–1018.
14. Gellai M, Jugus M, Fletcher T, et al. Nonpeptide endothelin receptor antagonists. V. Prevention and reversal of acute renal failure in the rat by SB 209670. J Pharmacol Exp Ther 1995; 275:200–206.
15. Gellai M, Jugus M, Fletcher T, et al. Reversal of postischemic acute renal failure with a selective endothelin$_A$ receptor antagonist in the rat. J Clin Invest 1994; 93:900–906.
16. Ix JH, McCulloch CE, Chertow GM. Theophylline for the prevention of radiocontrast nephropathy: a meta-analysis. Nephrol Dial Transplant 2004; 19(11):2747–2753.
17. Kelly KJ, Williams WW Jr., Colvin RB, et al. Antibody to intercellular adhesion molecule 1 protects the kidney against ischemic injury. Proc Natl Acad Sci USA 1994; 91: 812–816.
18. Kelly KJ, Williams JJ, Colvin RB, et al. Intracellular adhesion molecule-I deficient mice are protected against renal ischemia. J Clin Invest 1996; 97:1056–1063.
19. Lopez-Neblina F, Toledo-Pereyra LH, Mirmiran R, et al. Time dependence of Na-nitroprusside administration in the prevention of neutrophil infiltration in the rat ischaemic kidney. Transplantation 1996; 61(2):179–183.
20. Lee HT, Xu H, Nasr SH, et al. A1 adenosine receptor knockout mice exhibit increased renal injury following ischemia and reperfusion. Am J Physiol Renal Physiol 2004; 286:F298–F306.
21. Michael U, Lee SM. The role of calcium antagonists in nephrotoxic models of renal failure. In: Epstein M, Loutzenheimer R, eds. Calcium Antagonists and the Kidney. Philadelphia: Hanley and Belfus, 1990:187–201.
22. Neumayer HH, Kunzendorf U, Schreiber M. Protective effects of calcium antagonists in human renal transplantation. Kidney Int 1992; 41:S87–S93.
23. Alcaraz A, Oppenheimer F, Talbot-Wright R, et al. Effect of diltiazem in the prevention of acute tubular necrosis, acute rejection, and cyclosporine levels. Transplant Proc 1991; 23(5):2383–2384.
24. Miller SB, Martin DR, Kissane J, et al. Insulin-like growth factor I accelerates recovery from ischaemic acute tubular necrosis in the rat. Proc Natl Acad Sci 1992; 89(24): 11876–11880.
25. Miller SB, Martin DR, Kissane J, et al. Hepatocyte growth factor accelerates recovery from acute ischaemic renal injury in rats. Am J Physiol Renal Physiol 1994; 266:F129–F134.
26. Humes HD, Cieslinski DA, Coimbra TM, et al. Epidermal growth factor enhances renal tubule cell regeneration and repair and accelerates the recovery of renal function in postischemic acute renal failure. J Clin Invest 1989; 84: 1757–1761.
27. Aufricht C. Heat-shock protein 70: molecular supertool? Pediatr Nephrol 2005; 20:707–713.
28. Kelly KJ. Heat shock (stress response) proteins and renal ischemia/reperfusion injury. Contrib Nephrol 2005; 148: 86–106.

13

Chronic Renal Failure

Sanjay Ojha and John R. Bradley
Cambridge University Hospitals NHS Foundation Trust, Cambridge, U.K.

DEFINITION

The kidneys perform a number of roles, which include regulation of water and inorganic ion balance, removal of metabolic waste products from the blood, and secretion of certain hormones. Chronic renal failure is a state in which there has been irreversible loss of these functions, sufficient to cause an impact on an individual's health. Given that there is a significant amount of "renal reserve," this only occurs when more than 50% of renal excretory capacity has been lost; for example, removal of a single kidney from a healthy person (e.g., living kidney donors) does not cause any long-term sequelae.

Traditionally, serum creatinine has been used as a marker of renal function. This has always posed two problems. First, creatinine is affected by a number of variables apart from glomerular filtration rate (GFR), such as age, gender, race and body mass. Second, serum creatinine tends not to rise outside the normal range until around 50% of GFR has been lost. As a consequence certain groups of patients with renal disease—the frail and the elderly—tend to be detected late.

Estimated GFR (eGFR) is now being used to provide a more accurate assessment of kidney function. This utilizes the four-variable modification of diet in renal disease (MDRD) equation, which takes into account age, gender, and race as well as serum creatinine, to give a measure of renal function.

The U.S. Kidney Disease Outcomes Quality Initiative (K/DOQI) has introduced the term chronic kidney disease (CKD) to replace chronic renal failure. This classifies renal impairment into five stages on the basis of eGFR (Table 1) (1).

All stages are associated with hypertension as well as an increased risk of cardiovascular disease. From stage 3 onward complications of renal failure such as renal anemia and renal bone disease start to develop. Stage 4 tends to be the point at which uremic symptoms occur. Stage 5 should prompt consideration of initiating renal replacement therapy (RRT), unless a conservative management plan has been agreed.

The chief advantage to this classification is that it allows early identification of those patients who are at risk of progressive renal impairment (i.e., stages 1 and 2). In addition, it provides a standardized nomenclature worldwide for severity of chronic renal disease.

EPIDEMIOLOGY

CKD is a common condition. Extrapolating data from the third National Health and Nutrition Examination Survey (NHANES III) in the United States indicates a prevalence of 11% in the adult population (2). However, only a small proportion of these patients require RRT. The majority of patients with CKD fall into stages 1 to 3 and will not progress to more severe renal failure. They often require no specific interventions, apart from addressing cardiovascular risk factors.

Accurate data for the incidence and prevalence of end-stage renal failure (ESRF) exist, thanks to the establishment of various national renal registries (Table 2) (3–5). In 2006, 113 patients per million population were accepted onto dialysis programs in the United Kingdom. This is approximately double the number compared with 20 years ago, and although this increase is in part because of improved provision of RRT, there has undoubtedly been a real increase in the incidence of ESRF. A number of elements have contributed to this. Diabetes and obesity, both of which predispose to CKD, are now far commoner. In addition, there is a larger elderly population to care for, and it is well recognized that the incidence of ESRF rises exponentially with age. The median age of patients starting dialysis in the United Kingdom was 65 years in 2006, with the highest acceptance rate in the 75- to 79-year age group (3).

CKD is also commoner in ethnic populations. Afro-Caribbeans and Asians are two to four times more likely to start RRT than the white (Caucasian) population (4). To an extent this is explained by the predisposition of these groups to develop type 2 diabetes. Furthermore, hypertension is particularly common among people of Afro-Caribbean background. However, this is not the full story. Other genetic and environmental factors contribute to the tendency of these populations to develop ESRF. For example, conditions such as lupus nephritis and focal segmental glomerulosclerosis are also overrepresented in the ethnic communities. In addition to the greater

Table 1 Staging of CKD

CKD stage	GFR (mL/min/1.73 m^2)	Description
1	>90	Normal renal function but other evidence of kidney damage[a]
2	60–89	Mild reduction in renal function, with other evidence of kidney damage[a]
3	30–59	Moderately reduced GFR
4	15–29	Severely reduced GFR
5	<15	End-stage renal failure or on dialysis

[a]Evidence of kidney damage is suggested by abnormal urinalysis for blood and/or protein, structural abnormalities (e.g., abnormal renal imaging), or known inherited renal disease (e.g., ADPKD).
Abbreviations: CKD, chronic kidney disease; GFR, glomerular filtration rate.

Table 2 Incidence and Prevalence of End-Stage Renal Failure

	United Kingdom (2006)	United States of America (2006)	Australia (2006)
Incidence (pmp/yr)	113	347	115
Prevalence (pmp)	725	1569	778

frequency of renal diseases in these two populations, it has been noted that there is a faster decline in GFR in Afro-Caribbeans and Asians with nephropathy compared with Caucasians. This may partly explain the overrepresentation of these groups on dialysis programs.

There is a disparity between the genders with a male to female ratio of 1.5:1 in both the U.S. and the U.K. dialysis cohorts (3,4). This may be related to the fact that diseases such as atherosclerosis and hypertension are commoner in men. In addition, there is evidence that many renal diseases (including diabetic nephropathy, ADPKD, IgA nephropathy, and membranous nephropathy) progress more quickly in males than females (6).

There continues to be a steady increase in the number of patients initiating dialysis at a rate of 5% to 7% per year, and it seems likely that a steady state will not be reached for at least another 10 years.

ETIOLOGY

There are a number of causes for renal failure. Their frequency will vary according to the population that is evaluated. For example, in the United States, diabetes is responsible for 45% of all new patients commencing dialysis (4). In contrast, glomerulonephritis and hypertension together account for over 90% of new cases of ESRF in sub-Saharan Africa (7). This geographical discrepancy largely reflects differences in diet, lifestyle, and environmental factors that exist between Western and developing countries.

Table 3 shows the common diseases that result in ESRF in the U.K. population. In most cases, there is a chronic underlying process. However, 16% of patients who have severe acute renal failure do not recover renal function and remain on long-term dialysis (8).

Table 3 Common Causes of ESRF in the United Kingdom

Cause of ESRF	Percentage of all patients
Diabetes	22.2
Glomerulonephritis	10.4
Pyelonephritis/interstitial nephritis	7.2
Polycystic kidney disease	6.7
Hypertension	5.4
Renovascular disease	6.8
Etiology uncertain[a]	26.2
Others	15.3

[a]In many cases the cause is presumed to be glomerulonephritis, but this is not biopsy proven.
Abbreviation: ESRF, end-stage renal failure.

The underlying diagnosis changes depending on the age group that is considered. In children, congenital urinary system anomalies and reflux nephropathy constitute the commonest causes of ESRF. In the elderly, renal vascular disease and hypertension are more prevalent. In the U.K. dialysis population, renal vascular disease is five times more common in those aged over 65 compared with patients under 65.

CLINICAL PRESENTATION

The commonest presentation of CKD is the finding of an elevated urea and creatinine on blood tests in an otherwise asymptomatic individual. It is well recognized that the symptoms of renal failure are nonspecific and occur late—usually when 80% to 90% of renal function has been lost. Consequently, it is now recommended that renal function should be measured at least annually in adult patients who are at high risk of silent development of CKD (Table 4) (9).

Table 4 Indications for Annual Measurement of Renal Function

Diseases associated with high risk of silent development of CKD
- Hypertension
- Diabetes
- Heart failure
- Atherosclerotic disease (coronary/cerebral/peripheral vascular)

Diseases associated with high risk of obstructive nephropathy
- Urinary stone disease
- Urinary diversion surgery
- Known or suspected bladder outflow obstruction
- Neurogenic bladder

Diseases requiring long-term treatment with potentially nephrotoxic drugs
- ACE inhibitors and angiotensin receptor blockers
- Nonsteroidal anti-inflammatory drugs
- Lithium
- Calcineurin inhibitors

Multisystem conditions that may involve the kidney
- Systemic lupus erythematosus
- Vasculitis
- Rheumatoid arthritis

Previously diagnosed CKD

Abbreviation: CKD, chronic kidney disease.

Identifying these patients early is important as it allows measures to be instituted to preserve kidney function, as well as ensuring that the complications of renal failure can be prevented or ameliorated in a timely fashion.

Despite this targeted screening process, many patients with CKD are detected late. Twenty-three percent of patients who commence dialysis will have seen a nephrologist for the first time less than 90 days prior to starting RRT (3).

The typical early symptoms of renal failure are lethargy, malaise, fatigue, and dyspnea, which are predominantly a consequence of renal anemia. Later symptoms include pruritus, anorexia, nausea and vomiting, headache, difficulty in concentrating, unintentional weight loss, peripheral edema, and restless legs.

It is less common now for ESRF to present as a uremic emergency, but in these situations, symptoms of encephalopathy will often be present. Patients will have a reduced conscious level and evidence of neuromuscular irritability such as asterixis. In addition, they have an increased bleeding tendency; there may be evidence of skin bruising or gastrointestinal bleeding. Uremic pericarditis (characterized by a pericardial friction rub) or pulmonary edema can also occur. The presence of any of these features is an indication to commence dialysis urgently.

CLINICAL APPROACH TO CKD

When faced by an individual with impaired renal function, there are four key aspects to be considered in the initial assessment (Table 5):

Is the Renal Failure Acute or Chronic?

Determining chronicity is vital as it provides prognostic information and alters patient management. The best way of distinguishing between acute and chronic renal failure is to find out what the patient's renal function has been in the past. Looking through old notes and laboratory records or phoning the patient's

GP are simple tasks, which can yield important information.

In the absence of old blood results, ultrasonography of the kidneys may be helpful. The finding of two shrunken kidneys with increased echogenicity can allow a diagnosis of chronic renal failure to be made with confidence.

What Is the Underlying Diagnosis?

It is vital to make a diagnosis where possible as some causes of CKD are treatable. In addition, if the condition is inherited there are implications for family members.

The diagnosis may sometimes be obvious from the history and exam; a patient with longstanding diabetes and evidence of retinopathy is almost certain to have diabetic nephropathy. Older gentlemen with longstanding urinary symptoms and a palpable bladder on abdominal examination are likely to have obstructive uropathy because of prostatic pathology.

An ultrasound scan is a mandatory investigation in all patients with CKD. It not only looks for evidence of obstruction, but also allows diagnoses such as ADPKD to become apparent. Furthermore, in patients with evidence of atherosclerotic disease, the finding of asymmetric kidneys on ultrasound should raise the possibility of renovascular disease, which can be further investigated with either magnetic resonance angiogram or formal invasive angiography.

Urine dipstick is the other obligatory test; the presence of blood and protein on urinalysis should raise the possibility of a chronic glomerulonephritis. In these circumstances, it would be reasonable to check immunological blood tests to assess for an underlying autoimmune condition.

If the initial assessment fails to elucidate the etiology, consideration should be given to performing a renal biopsy. This should not be undertaken, however, if the kidneys are small. A biopsy is unlikely to provide useful information and the risk of bleeding is significant in this situation.

Are There Any Reversible Factors That Can Be Addressed?

Even when renal failure is confirmed to be chronic, there are a number of factors that can cause an acute decline in GFR (termed "acute-on-chronic" renal failure). Hypovolemia, use of nephrotoxins, urinary tract sepsis, and urinary tract obstruction should all be actively looked for and excluded.

Have Any Complications of Renal Failure Arisen?

Questioning should be directed at determining whether there are symptoms of uremia or fluid overload. The examination should also focus on these, looking for evidence of hypertension, peripheral or pulmonary edema, and excoriations, which would suggest pruritus.

Table 5 Clinical Approach to Chronic Kidney Disease

Acute vs. chronic	Historical values for renal function
	Ultrasound of kidneys
Underlying diagnosis	History and examination
	Ultrasound
	Immunology
	Renal biopsy
Reversible factors	Hypovolemia
	Nephrotoxins
	Obstruction
	Urinary tract infection
Complications	Fluid overload
	Hypertension
	Hyperkalemia
	Acidosis
	Anemia
	Calcium/phosphate imbalance
	Renal osteodystrophy

A number of blood tests assessing for electrolyte disturbances, acidosis, anemia, and hyperparathyroidism should be checked.

The complications of renal failure will be dealt with in more detail later in the chapter.

PATHOPHYSIOLOGY

This section will deal with the mechanisms that lead to the development and progression of CKD. It will then address the interventions that may be undertaken to prevent deterioration of renal function in patients with established CKD.

Mechanisms of Progression of Renal Disease

The first step in the development of renal failure is an insult, which results in loss of functioning nephrons. This may be acute, for example, hemodynamic compromise leading to renal ischemia, or chronic such as in the case of a persistent glomerulonephritis. Not all insults lead to progressive kidney disease; for example, patients with renal impairment secondary to urinary tract obstruction can maintain stable renal function in the long-term once the obstruction has been relieved.

However, once a threshold has been passed—usually when 60% to 70% of renal function has been lost, CKD tends to become progressive. This is the consequence of pathogenic processes, which lead to glomerulosclerosis and tubulointerstitial fibrosis.

Glomerulosclerosis

Glomerular scarring can arise because of ongoing damage from the primary disease process (glomerulonephritis and diabetes being the main culprits here). However, it also occurs because of maladaptive responses, which attempt to compensate for the loss of functioning renal mass. The evidence for this comes from an animal model in which rats underwent subtotal nephrectomy (10). In the remnant kidney, hemodynamic changes were noted, specifically preferential vasodilatation of afferent glomerular arterioles, together with increases in glomerular transcapillary hydraulic pressure and filtration fraction. This functional change—so-called hyperfiltration—is an attempt by the remaining nephrons to maintain GFR.

Unfortunately, hyperfiltration contributes to the progressive destruction of remaining glomeruli; over a period of weeks, these rats developed structural lesions within the remaining kidney tissue, including mesangial expansion and focal segmental glomerulosclerosis. This was associated with progressive hypertension, proteinuria, and renal insufficiency, eventually leading to the death of the animals.

The mechanism by which hyperfiltration causes renal scarring is thought to relate to increased glomerular capillary pressure, which in turn causes stretch of these capillaries and initiates endothelial cell damage. As a result of this, an inflammatory response ensues with release of proinflammatory and profibrotic cytokines, as well as growth factors (such as PDGF). This leads to mesangial cell proliferation and extracellular matrix deposition. Combined with the platelet aggregation and fibrin deposition that also occur following endothelial injury, the end point is glomerulosclerosis.

In addition to this process, glomerular hypertension with consequent endothelial and epithelial cell stress leads to proteinuria, which also plays a pathogenic role in progression of kidney disease (see below).

Tubulointerstitial Scarring

The extent of tubular and interstitial damage seen within a kidney often correlates better with long-term renal prognosis than the degree of glomerular injury.

As with glomerulosclerosis, tubulointerstitial inflammation and fibrosis may arise as a consequence of a primary disease process (Table 6).

However, it can also be a secondary effect of glomerular pathology and this is thought to be largely mediated by proteinuria. There are a number of mechanisms that have been implicated. Tubular cell injury can occur either because of the direct toxic effects of filtered proteins, or as a consequence of complement activation within the tubules (11). This in turn leads to release of proinflammatory cytokines with the development of an inflammatory infiltrate within the interstitium. Resolution of this is by fibrosis.

Increased deposition of extracellular matrix in the interstitium is driven by a number of profibrotic factors within the filtrate, which have the effect of activating renal fibroblasts, as well as increasing their number by causing tubular cells to change phenotype.

The outcome of tubulointerstitial damage is chronic ischemia within this part of the kidney. This arises because of loss of peritubular capillaries, causing impaired blood flow to the interstitium. In addition, there is reduced oxygen diffusion because of the interstitial fibrosis. As a consequence of the hypoxia, further tubular damage occurs, and so a

Table 6 Primary Causes of Tubulointerstitial Nephritis

Drugs	Metabolic
NSAIDs	Hyperuricemia
Calcineurin inhibitors	Hyperoxaluria
Lithium	Chronic hypokalemia
Cystic diseases	Obstructive
ADPKD	Obstructive uropathy
Medullary sponge kidney	Reflux nephropathy
Medullary cystic disease	
Infection	Sickle cell nephropathy
Pyelonephritis	
Heavy metals	Immunological
Lead	Sjogrens
Cadmium	Sarcoidosis

Table 7 Risk Factors for Progression of Chronic Kidney Disease

Modifiable	Nonmodifiable
Hypertension	Age
Proteinuria	Gender
Hyperglycemia	Race
Dyslipidemia	Genetics
Obesity	Underlying renal disease
Smoking	

vicious cycle of self-perpetuating renal damage emerges (12).

Slowing Progression of Renal Disease

The majority of patients with CKD will not progress to a point where they require RRT. Death from cardiovascular disease is a far more likely outcome. However, a significant proportion of patients do progress to ESRF and there are a number of factors that predispose to this (Table 7).

The strategy for slowing progression of renal disease entails three approaches.

1. *Diagnosis and treatment of the underlying disease*: Not all diseases are treatable; polycystic kidney disease tends to have a relentless progression. However, many causes of chronic renal failure are amenable to treatment, which is why a diagnosis should always be sought. For example, relieving urinary tract obstruction is often a straightforward procedure that can yield satisfying results. More complex cases such as glomerulonephritis and vasculitis may entail interventions such as immunosuppression, which can address the underlying pathogenic process and preserve renal function.
2. *Avoidance of nephrotoxins and other insults to the kidney*: Kidneys that are already damaged are more vulnerable to new insults, which can cause further, sometimes irreversible, decline in GFR. This can be avoided through simple measures; patients should be told to steer clear of NSAIDs. Radiocontrast and aminoglycoside antibiotics should be used with caution. Urinary tract infections and episodes of hypovolemia need to be treated promptly.
3. *Modulating factors that promote progression*: The importance of this cannot be overstated, for all of these influences are recognized as risk factors for cardiovascular disease. Hence controlling them will provide a dual health benefit. These will be dealt with in detail.

Hypertension

Given the kidney's central role in the control of blood pressure, it is not surprising that hypertension is a finding in most patients with CKD. It arises because of salt and water retention with subsequent expansion of the extracellular space. Furthermore, the renin-angiotensin-aldosterone system (RAAS) is upregulated in renal disease. This contributes to salt and water retention through increased production of aldosterone, as well as promoting arteriolar vasoconstriction and sympathetic nervous system activation via the effects of angiotensin II.

Systemic hypertension promotes renal damage, as it exacerbates glomerular capillary hypertension and thus induces increased glomerular filtration and proteinuria.

There is a clear association between elevated blood pressure and a faster rate of progression of CKD, although this relationship is modulated by the amount of proteinuria that is also present. The MDRD trial demonstrated that a lower blood pressure target (125/75 vs. 140/90) in patients with more than 1 g proteinuria per day was associated with a slower decline in GFR (13). A more recent meta-analysis showed that in nondiabetic patients with CKD, the lowest risk of progression was in those who achieved a systolic blood pressure between 110 and 129 (14).

Current guidelines state that all patients with CKD should have a target blood pressure of less than 130/80 (15). In cases where there is significant proteinuria (>1 g/day) tighter blood pressure control is desirable with a target of less than 125/75.

Treatment of hypertension needs to closely involve the patient; restricting dietary sodium load is a vital aspect of management, as is ensuring compliance with any medications that are prescribed. It often requires three or more agents to achieve the appropriate blood pressure target. The choice of antihypertensive medication is determined by several variables. In general, ACE inhibitors and angiotensin II receptor blockers (ARBs) are first line as they have antiproteinuric as well as antihypertensive effects (see below). Furthermore, in patients with concomitant diabetes or cardiovascular disease, they are recognized to reduce morbidity and mortality. However, this has to be tempered by the fact that they often exacerbate hyperkalemia, which is a familiar complication of CKD. Their use can also be limited by a decline in renal function that is seen in some cases soon after these drugs are started. The commonest situation in which this is observed is silent renovascular disease. In this setting, angiotensin II plays a vital role in maintaining renal perfusion pressure by preferentially vasoconstricting the efferent arteriole. When this is blocked the adverse effect on renal hemodynamics causes an acute drop in GFR. It is imperative that all patients commenced on an ACE inhibitor or ARB have their renal function checked within seven days. If there is a fall in eGFR of >20%, these drugs should be stopped, and consideration given regarding investigation for renovascular disease (9).

Diuretics are useful second-line antihypertensives, especially in the context of fluid overload. However, in more advanced CKD (stages 4 and 5) thiazide diuretics tend to be ineffective. Calcium channel blockers, α-blockers, β-blockers, and centrally acting antihypertensive drugs can all be used thereafter.

Proteinuria

Proteinuria is a powerful risk factor for the progression of renal disease, via mechanisms that have been explained above. It is widely accepted that in proteinuric renal disease, the aim should be to achieve less than 1 g/day proteinuria. The rationale for this comes from the observation that the greater the degree of proteinuria, the more rapidly patients will progress to ESRF. A seminal study from 1996 looked at renal survival in patients with a variety of proteinuric kidney disease; in the group that had <1 g/day proteinuria, less than 10% had progressed to ESRF after two years. Conversely, nearly 25% of the group with >3 g/day proteinuria had reached this end point by 18 months (16). A number of other studies have confirmed this relationship between proteinuria and poorer renal outcomes (9).

Indeed, on the basis of the strength of this link, reduction in proteinuria is now accepted as a good surrogate marker for assessing whether an intervention has a role in slowing kidney damage.

A number of antiproteinuric interventions in CKD have been evaluated. The largest body of evidence exists for blockade of the RAAS. Overactivation of this system leads to increased production of angiotensin II, which drives renal efferent arteriolar vasoconstriction. This causes increased glomerular capillary pressure and hence hyperfiltration and proteinuria.

In both diabetic and nondiabetic patients with renal impairment, ACE inhibitors and ARBs have been shown to reduce protein leak and progression of nephropathy (17–21). Each of these drugs targets a different step in the RAAS pathway, and there are theoretical reasons why individually they cannot provide complete blockade of this system. For example, angiotensin I can be converted to angiotensin II by enzymes that are not affected by ACE inhibitors (e.g., chymase). Conversely, ARBs cause elevated angiotensin II levels. Normally, angiotensin II inhibits renin secretion via a negative feedback mechanism mediated by the angiotensin receptor (AT1). When this is blocked, the subsequent rise in renin and angiotensin II levels can antagonize the therapeutic effects of the ARB.

With this rationale in mind, there has been a focus on using dual blockade therapy, especially in those patients who have persistent proteinuria of more than 1 g/day despite monotherapy. The COOPERATE study assessed the efficacy of combined ACE inhibitor (trandolapril) and ARB (losartan) treatment in nondiabetic patients with chronic proteinuric nephropathy (22). Patients who received dual therapy had a 50% reduction in their relative risk of doubling their serum creatinine or developing ESRF compared with patients on monotherapy.

In type 2 diabetic patients, the CALM study has also provided evidence that combination treatment with ACE inhibitor (lisinopril) and ARB (candesartan) produces better reductions in blood pressure and microalbuminuria compared with using these drugs in isolation (23).

The main concern with using these drugs together is the risk of severe hyperkalemia. Given that nondihydropyridine calcium channel blockers (ditiazem and verapamil) have also been shown to reduce proteinuria and progression of renal disease, a safer option is to add in one of these medicines to achieve satisfactory control of proteinuria.

Rather more controversial than RAAS blockade, is the role for dietary protein restriction as an antiproteinuric intervention. Analysis of the MDRD study showed that in those patients with severe renal impairment (GFR 13–24 mL/min), reduction in dietary protein intake by 0.2 g/kg/day slowed decline in GFR by 1.15 mL/min/yr (13).

A meta-analysis of data from 1413 nondiabetic patients confirmed that dietary protein restriction effectively slows the progression of renal disease (24). Nonetheless, many physicians will avoid this strategy because of concerns that it may result in malnutrition. It is recognized that a significant proportion of patients with CKD have an inadequate calorie intake and this could be made worse if dietary restrictions are imposed.

Hyperglycemia

Diabetes is the commonest cause of ESRF in the Western world. Therefore, it is imperative that this disease is optimally managed to reduce the incidence of renal complications. Data from the Diabetes Control and Complications Trial (DCCT) showed that tight glycemic control in type 1 diabetics prevented the development of microalbuminuria by 34%, and reduced progression of microalbuminuria to frank diabetic nephropathy by 56% (25). In type 2 diabetics, the United Kingdom Prospective Diabetes Study (UKPDS) showed that maintaining HbA1C levels at 7% as compared with 7.9% also reduced the development of microalbuminuria (26). What remains to be seen, however, is whether attaining tighter glycemic control has any impact on the rate of progression of established diabetic renal disease.

Obesity

There is a growing body of evidence linking obesity to the development of CKD. One study has shown that patients with a BMI of over 30 are more likely to develop proteinuria and renal insufficiency following nephrectomy compared with nonobese patients (27). The pathophysiology underlying this is not clear.

Many patients with obesity will have associated hypertension, impaired glucose tolerance, and dyslipidemia. This is known as the metabolic syndrome and is associated with hyperfiltration.

It is also postulated that deposition of excessive adipose tissue in the renal viscera can cause compression of the loop of Henle, resulting in sluggish tubular flow. Consequently, there is increased sodium reabsorption and so reduced delivery of sodium to the macula densa. The outcome is vasodilatation of the afferent arteriole and hence glomerular hyperfiltration (28).

Smoking

Smoking should be discouraged in all patients with CKD, not only to preserve renal function, but also to reduce the risk of cardiovascular disease and cancer. It is well recognized that smoking increases the risk of ESRF, though the precise mechanisms for this remain unclear (29–31) It is postulated that cigarette smoke causes renal injury through adverse effects on renal hemodynamics. More recently, it had been shown that nicotine promotes mesangial cell proliferation and production of extracellular matrix. This could accelerate glomerulosclerosis (32).

Dyslipidemia

Dyslipidemia is common in patients with CKD. Both experimental and clinical studies show that it is associated with faster progression of renal disease. Hyperlipidemia can cause both increased glomerular permeability, which can progress to glomerulosclerosis, as well as tubulointerstitial injury (33). In the MDRD study a low serum HDL was an independent risk factor for more rapid decline in GFR (13).

However, it remains unclear as to whether lipid-lowering therapy is beneficial in retarding progression of CKD. A meta-analysis of 13 small trials suggests that treatment of hyperlipidemia does preserve GFR and reduce proteinuria in patients with renal disease (34). Further evidence is awaited though. The Study of Heart and Renal Protection (SHARP) trial is currently ongoing and aims to give a definitive answer as to whether lipid-lowering drugs improve outcomes in patients with CKD.

HMG CoA reductase inhibitors do carry an increased risk of side effects in patients with CKD, notably myositis and rhabdomyolysis. Hence, current recommendations are that they should only be used to address cardiovascular risk, rather than as a therapy to protect renal function.

CONSEQUENCES OF ADVANCED CKD

Having considered the ways in which GFR can be preserved, we now need to reflect on the consequences of advanced CKD and how to manage the complications that arise when there is insufficient renal function to maintain health.

Table 8 shows the functions that the kidneys perform. The effect of loss of each of these functions will be considered individually.

Table 8 Functions of the Kidney

Regulation of sodium and water balance
Regulation of inorganic ion balance
Regulation of acid-base balance
Removal of metabolic waste products
Secretion of hormones
- Renin
- Erythropoietin
- 1,25-Dihydroxycholecalciferol
Gluconeogenesis

Salt and Water

In healthy individuals the kidneys are able to maintain sodium and water homeostasis despite wide variations in the intake of these substances. Salt intake may be up to 20 g/day in a Western diet, while water intake may fluctuate hugely on a day-to-day basis. Nonetheless, renal mechanisms ensure that serum sodium is tightly regulated between 135 and 145 mmol/L and serum osmolality is kept between 280 and 300 mOsm.

Sodium

Sodium balance is managed because of the ability of the tubules to vary the fractional excretion of filtered sodium from less than 1% normally, up to 30% in advanced CKD. However, once GFR falls to <10 mL/min, the kidneys can no longer cope with sodium loads. The consequence of this is salt and water retention, which manifests itself as hypertension and tissue edema.

To prevent this, patients should be advised to limit their salt intake to <4 g/day. When hypertension and fluid overload are present, diuretics should be used to promote natriuresis. Loop diuretics are the most effective, but their action can be potentiated by addition of a thiazide diuretic. Caution needs to be taken when using these drugs as they can precipitate dehydration and hypotension, which can worsen renal failure.

Water

The kidneys control water balance through their capacity to produce very dilute or concentrated urine. This is mediated by variations in water reabsorption from the collecting duct from <1% (for a water-loaded individual) to >24% (for a dehydrated person).

In renal failure, the kidneys lose the ability to produce concentrated urine. This is because of a number of mechanisms.

- Hyperfiltration leads to an increased solute load in each nephron, thus promoting a diuresis.
- Tubulointerstitial scarring diminishes the high interstitial osmolality that drives water reabsorption from the collecting ducts.
- Tubular damage causes the collecting ducts to become resistant to antidiuretic hormone.

As a consequence patients tend to develop polyuria, nocturia, and then thirst. They are prone to dehydration if they cannot maintain satisfactory oral fluid intake.

Hyperkalemia

Extracellular potassium ion concentration needs to be tightly regulated; otherwise, life-threatening cardiac dysrhythmias occur. Potassium excretion by the kidneys is predominantly controlled by the effect of

Table 9 Causes of Hyperkalemia in Chronic Kidney Disease

High potassium intake
Hyporeninemic hypoaldosteronism
- Diabetes
- Interstitial nephritis

Medications
- ACE inhibitors/angiotensin II receptor blockers
- Aldosterone antagonists (spironolactone)
- NSAIDs
- β-Blockers

Acidosis

aldosterone, which increases potassium secretion by the principal cells of the distal tubules.

Hyperkalemia does not tend to be a problem until GFR falls to <10 mL/min as the kidneys retain the ability to excrete potassium normally till this stage. There are some exceptions to this rule: diseases in which there is reduced production of aldosterone (e. g., diabetes) or cases where the distal tubule becomes less responsive to aldosterone (obstructive uropathy, chronic pyelonephritis) can cause hyperkalemia despite a much higher GFR.

In CKD a number of other factors can promote hyperkalemia (Table 9). The management of hyperkalemia relies mainly on restriction of dietary intake of potassium. In a normal diet an individual will consume around 100 mmol potassium each day. A low-potassium diet will contain half this amount.

Other measures that should be taken are correction of acidosis and stopping medications that promote hyperkalemia. If the serum potassium remains elevated despite these measures, it is an indication to start dialysis.

Acidosis

The kidneys regulate acid-base balance through excretion of hydrogen ions, as well as reabsorption of bicarbonate. Acidosis only occurs once GFR has fallen to <20 mL/min.

This has multiple detrimental consequences on health (Table 10). The respiratory system attempts to compensate for metabolic acidosis through hyperventilation. Consequently, patients describe symptoms of breathlessness and exhaustion. Acidosis also exacerbates hyperkalemia by stimulating movement of potassium ions from the intracellular to the extracellular compartment, in exchange for hydrogen ions.

Bone attempts to buffer the acidosis, but this leads to calcium loss from bone as well as impaired mineralization, hence contributing to renal osteodystrophy. Finally, acidosis increases skeletal muscle

Table 10 Consequences of Acidosis

Hyperventilation
Hyperkalemia
Exacerbation of renal bone disease
Skeletal muscle breakdown
Reduced cardiac output

Table 11 Effects of Uremic Toxins

Chronic inflammation
Accelerated atherogenesis
Sensorimotor peripheral neuropathy
Autonomic neuropathy
Defective immune system
Impaired platelet function

catabolism, contributing to loss of body mass and general weakness.

To avoid these complications, acidosis should be treated with oral sodium bicarbonate once the serum bicarbonate concentration is <20 mmol/L. Unfortunately, this therapy contributes to salt and water retention and can worsen hypertension.

Uremia

One of the principal functions of the kidneys is the excretion of organic waste products. These include breakdown products of protein metabolism, such as urea and creatinine, as well as metabolites of various hormones. Although urea and creatinine are used as measures of renal function, they are not themselves harmful (35). However, when their levels are elevated it reflects the accumulation of a number of small (<500 Da) and middle (500–5000 Da) molecules, which are normally excreted by healthy kidneys. These molecules are termed uremic toxins and they exert several deleterious effects on the body (Table 11).

Over 90 such compounds have been recognized, which include free water-soluble solutes such as guanidines, protein-bound solutes such as phenol, and middle molecules including β_2 microglobulin, complement factor D, and multiple cytokines (36). Many other uremic toxins remain unidentified.

These molecules are responsible for many of the symptoms that are observed in advanced CKD, including anorexia, nausea and vomiting, the features of neuropathy and encephalopathy, and pericarditis. If any of these symptoms develop, dialysis should be commenced.

Anemia

Anemia is a common complication of CKD and can occur early—once GFR has fallen to <50 mL/min. Typically, it is normochromic and normocytic. There are a number of factors that contribute to its development; the primary mechanism is reduced renal production of the peptide hormone erythropoietin (EPO). This hormone is secreted by peritubular cells in the interstitium, in response to a reduction in the partial pressure of oxygen in the kidneys. It stimulates erythroid lines within the bone marrow to proliferate and mature, hence increasing production of red blood cells.

Other explanations for anemia include reduced intake of iron and folic acid because of anorexia, impaired intestinal absorption of iron as a consequence of uremia, gastrointestinal blood loss because of bleeding tendency, and shortened red cell survival.

Anemia has a significant impact on the quality of life in patients with CKD. They suffer from fatigue, reduced exercise tolerance, slowing of cognitive function, and reduced libido. In patients with ESRF, there is also evidence that anemia contributes to increased morbidity and mortality. This is thought to be secondary to increased left ventricular hypertrophy.

Correction of anemia is therefore a priority in the management of CKD patients. Iron stores must be assessed first. If they are deficient, they can be restored through the use of oral or intravenous iron. Once patients are iron replete, recombinant EPO can be administered.

There has been much debate over what hemoglobin target to aim for. Until recently, it was mistakenly thought that a normal hemoglobin target would improve clinical outcomes. However, the publication of two trials—CREATE (cardiovascular risk reduction by early anemia treatment with epoetin β) (37) and CHOIR (correction of hemoglobin and outcomes in renal insufficiency) (38)—has exploded this myth. In these trials, patients with a GFR of between 15 and 50 mL/min were found to derive no benefit from achieving a higher ("normal") hemoglobin target. Indeed, the CHOIR study found that patients with CKD-related anemia were at higher risk of death from cardiovascular events when the target hemoglobin level was 13.5 g/dL rather than 11.3 g/dL.

Consequently, current guidelines state that all patients with CKD should aim to achieve target hemoglobin between 10.5 g/dL and 12.5 g/dL.

Renal Bone Disease

Renal bone disease is a complex entity that starts to develop early in the course of progressive renal disease. It is characterized by a spectrum of metabolic bone disorders, all of which have the effect of reducing bone strength and hence predisposing to fractures. The main pathologies are as follows:

- *Osteitis fibrosa cystica* ("high turnover bone disease"): This occurs because of secondary hyperparathyroidism (SHPT) with increased osteoblast and osteoclast activity, leading to rapid bone formation and resorption. The outcome is weakened bone structure.
- *Adynamic bone disease* ("low turnover bone disease"): This is characterized by reduced bone formation and resorption. Parathyroid hormone (PTH) levels are suppressed in this case, either as a consequence of excessive use of vitamin D analogues, or because the patient has undergone parathyroidectomy.
- *Osteomalacia*: This normally arises as a result of low 1,25-dihydroxycholecalciferol levels, as well as metabolic acidosis. Both lead to impaired bone mineralization. Osteomalacia commonly coexists with adynamic bone disease.

- *Mixed renal osteodystrophy*: This has features of osteitis fibrosa, adynamic bone disease, and osteomalacia.

The interplay between a number of factors is involved in the evolution of renal osteodystrophy. The two main mechanisms are SHPT and 1,25-dihydroxycholecalciferol deficiency.

Secondary Hyperparathyroidism

SHPT is driven by three processes. Hyperphosphatemia arises in renal failure because of the reduction in filtered phosphate load that occurs once GFR falls below 40 mL/min. It promotes SHPT through a direct effect on the parathyroid glands, as well as by precipitating a fall in serum calcium levels.

Loss of functioning renal mass leads to reduced 1α-hydroxylase activity. This enzyme is produced by renal tubular cells and is required for the production of active vitamin D (1,25-dihydroxycholecalciferol). CKD thus results in low 1,25-dihydroxycholecalciferol levels, which then stimulate release of PTH.

Both the mechanisms mentioned above cause hypocalcemia. This is detected by the calcium-sensing receptor on the parathyroid glands and acts as the strongest driver for PTH release.

The effects of elevated PTH are diverse, with an overall aim of attempting to maintain calcium-phosphate homeostasis. PTH increases urinary excretion of phosphate as well as stimulating 1α-hydroxylase in an effort to increase active vitamin D levels. It also tries to correct hypocalcemia through increased resorption of calcium from bone. This effect is responsible for causing high turnover bone disease.

Prolonged hyperparathyroidism can have other detrimental consequences. These include left ventricular hypertrophy and cardiac fibrosis, as well as EPO-resistant anemia.

1,25-Dihydroxycholecalciferol Deficiency

Active vitamin D plays a number of roles in bone metabolism. Low levels prevent mineralization of bone and hence predispose to osteomalacia, which is characterized by bone fragility and proximal muscle weakness.

It is well recognized that the abnormal mineral metabolism that occurs in CKD can also have extra-skeletal effects; disturbances of calcium and phosphate homeostasis lead to their deposition in soft tissues. Blood vessels are a prime target for the ensuing calcification and this leads to arterial stiffening as well as accelerated atherosclerosis. Calcification of heart valves (usually the mitral valve annulus or aortic valve leaflets) plays a role in the development of left ventricular dysfunction. Both of these factors contribute to cardiovascular morbidity and mortality in patients with CKD.

Treatment of renal bone disease requires a multipronged approach. Control of hyperphosphatemia is the primary objective. There is evidence showing that hyperphosphatemia is an independent risk factor for all-cause and cardiovascular mortality in hemodialysis patients (39). This is in part because it promotes vascular calcification. Current guidelines suggest phosphate targets of 0.9 to 1.5 mmol/L in stages 3 and 4 CKD, and 1.1 to 1.8 mmol/L in stage 5 CKD. Achieving this requires a combination of dietary phosphate restriction, as well as the use of oral phosphate binders, which are taken with meals.

There are a number of phosphate binders currently available, which fall into two categories: calcium-based binders (calcium acetate and calcium carbonate) and non-calcium-based binders (sevelamer hydrochloride and lanthanum carbonate). Use of the calcium-based preparations is limited by the fact that patients with CKD should not take in more than 2 g of elemental calcium per day, as this may again promote vascular calcification.

Correction of SHPT is the other key target in the treatment of renal osteodystrophy. A certain degree of SHPT is desirable to maintain bone health, so a careful balancing act needs to be achieved. For patients with ESRF, PTH levels should ideally be maintained between 150 and 300 pg/mL. This is based on the observation that these levels are associated with normal bone turnover as monitored by bone histology.

Therapy for SHPT involves the use of active forms of vitamin D. These can cause hypercalcemia, in which case second-line agents such as vitamin D analogues (e.g., paracalcitol) or calcimimetic agents (cinacalcet) should be prescribed. In cases of refractory hyperparathyroidism, surgical removal of the parathyroid glands may be needed.

Cardiovascular Complications of CKD

The commonest cause of death in patients with CKD is cardiovascular disease. Individuals at each stage of CKD are more likely to die from a cardiovascular event than progress to ESRF. The outlook is worst for those patients who require dialysis; they have an annual mortality rate of 10% to 15% and cardiovascular disease accounts for 55% of all deaths in ESRF (40). The explanation given for this is that they have accelerated atherogenesis. It is certain that these patients have a preponderance of the so-called classical risk factors for atherosclerosis including hypertension, dyslipidemia, glucose intolerance, and hyperinsulinemia. As described above these factors also promote accelerated loss of GFR. Hence, close attention needs to be paid to addressing these problems.

Controversy remains as to how effective statins are in reducing cardiovascular risk in CKD. No randomized controlled studies thus far have shown them to be of benefit in dialysis patients.

This is probably attributable to a number of pathogenetic factors, which are not modifiable by statins. The uremic milieu promotes a state of inflammation and oxidative stress that encourages the formation of atherosclerotic plaques. Furthermore, hyperhomocysteinemia is a common finding in ESRF, and this is also believed to accelerate atherogenesis.

It is not only atherosclerosis that causes cardiovascular mortality. Left ventricular hypertrophy and dysfunction, which predispose to sudden cardiac death are highly prevalent in CKD. These arise as a consequence of hypertension, volume overload, anemia, and loss of arterial elasticity because of vascular calcification.

The combination of all these factors creates a significant challenge for physicians who care for the CKD population.

RENAL REPLACEMENT THERAPY

Commencement of RRT should be considered once patients have an eGFR of less than 15 mL/min. This is not a precise cut-off and the decision regarding initiation of dialysis has to take into account the patient's overall well-being. Some individuals do not feel unwell despite this low level of renal function, and are reluctant to start a treatment that will involve major disruption to their lives. Conversely, if symptoms of uremia develop, RRT should not be delayed.

There are three modalities of RRT available: renal transplantation, hemodialysis, and peritoneal dialysis. For those patients fit enough to withstand the operation and subsequent immunosuppression, the transplant option is best. It provides better quality of life as well as increased longevity compared with dialysis.

The majority of patients who commence RRT will start out on dialysis though. Ideally, these patients should have been under the care of a nephrologist well in advance so that they can be prepared physically (in terms of dialysis access and vaccination against hepatitis B) as well as psychologically for the rigors of dialysis.

Not all patients are suitable for dialysis; the frail elderly patient with multiple comorbidities may not tolerate this treatment. In cases such as this, good conservative care aimed at managing the complications and relieving the symptoms of ESRF is likely to be a kinder option.

REFERENCES

1. National Kidney Foundation. Kidney disease outcome quality initiative. Am J Kidney Dis 2002; 39(suppl 1): S1–S266.
2. Coresh J, Astor BC, Greene T, et al. Prevalence of chronic kidney disease and decreased kidney function in the adult US population: Third National Health and Nutrition Examination Survey. Am J Kidney Dis 2003; 41:1–12.
3. The UK Renal Registry. The Tenth Annual Report. December 2007.
4. US Renal Data System: USRDS Annual Data Report. 2007.
5. ANZDATA Registry. The 30th Annual Report. 2007.
6. Locatelli F, Del Vecchio L. Natural history and factors affecting the progression of chronic renal failure. In: El Nahas AM, Anderson S, Harris KPG, eds. Mechanisms and Management of Progressive Renal Failure. London: Oxford University Press, 2000:20–79.
7. Naicker S. End-stage renal diseases in sub-Saharan and South Africa. Kidney Int 2003; 63:S119–S122.
8. Bhandari S, Turney JH. Survivors of acute renal failure who do not recover renal function. Q J Med 1996; 89: 415–421.

9. Joint Specialty Committee on Renal Medicine of the Royal College of Physicians and the Renal Association, and the Royal College of General Practitioners. Chronic Kidney Disease in Adults: UK Guidelines for Identification, Management and Referral. London: Royal College of Physicians, 2006.

10. Hostetter TH, Olson JH, Rennke HG, et al. Hyperfiltration in remnant nephrons: a potentially adverse response to renal ablation. Am J Physiol 1981; 241:F85–F93.

11. Hong SI, Couser WG. Chronic progression of tubulointerstitial damage in proteinuric renal disease is mediated by complement activation: a therapeutic role for complement inhibitors? J Am Soc Nephrol 2003; 14(7 suppl 2):S186–S191.

12. Nangaku M. Chronic hypoxia and tubulointerstitial injury: a final common pathway to end-stage renal failure. J Am Soc Nephrol 2006; 17:17–25.

13. Klahr S, Levey AS, Beck GJ, et al. The effects of dietary protein restriction and blood-pressure control on the progression of chronic renal disease. N Engl J Med 1994; 330: 877–884.

14. Jafar TH, Stark PC, Schmid CH, et al. Progression of chronic kidney disease: the role of blood pressure control, proteinuria, and angiotensin-converting enzyme inhibition: a patient-level meta-analysis. Ann Intern Med 2003; 139:244–252.

15. Li PK, Weening JJ, Dirks JA, et al. A report with consensus statements of the International Society of Nephrology 2004 consensus workshop on prevention of progression of renal disease, Hong Kong, June 29, 2004. Kidney Int Suppl 2005; 94:S2–S7.

16. Locatelli F, Marcelli D, Comelli M, et al. Proteinuria and blood pressure as causal components of progression to end-stage renal failure. Nephrol Dial Transplant 1996; 11:461–467.

17. Lewis EJ, Hunsicker LG, Bain RP, et al.; For the Collaborative Study Group. The effect of angiotensin-converting enzyme inhibition on diabetic nephropathy. N Engl J Med 1993; 329:1456–1462.

18. The GISEN group. Randomized placebo-controlled trial of effect of ramipril on decline in glomerular filtration rate and risk of terminal renal failure in proteinuric non-diabetic nephropathy. Lancet 1997; 349:1857–1863.

19. Lewis EJ, Hunsicker LG, Clarke WR, et al. Renoprotective effect of the angiotensin-receptor antagonist irbesartan in patients with nephropathy due to type 2 diabetes. N Engl J Med 2001; 345:851–860.

20. Brenner BM, Cooper ME, de Zeeuw D, et al. For the RENAAL study investigators. Effects of losartan on renal and cardiovascular outcomes in patients with type 2 diabetes and nephropathy. N Engl J Med 2001; 345:861–869.

21. Parving HH, Lehnert H, Brochner-Mortensen J, et al. The effect of irbesartan on the development of diabetic nephropathy in patients with type 2 diabetes. N Engl J Med 2001; 345:870–878.

22. Nakao N, Yoshimura A, Morita H, et al. Combination treatment of angiotensin-II receptor blocker and angiotensin-converting-enzyme inhibitor in non-diabetic renal disease (COOPERATE): a randomized controlled trial. Lancet 2003; 361:117–124.

23. Morgensen CE, Neldam S, Tikkanen I, et al. Randomised controlled trial of dual blockade of renin–angiotensin system in patients with hypertension, microalbuminuria and non-insulin dependent diabetes: the candesartan and lisinopril microalbuminuria (CALM) study. BMJ 2000; 321: 1440–1444.

24. Pedrini MT, Levey AS, Lau J, et al. The effect of dietary protein restriction on the progression of diabetic and nondiabetic renal diseases: a meta-analysis. Ann Intern Med 1996; 124(7):627–632.

25. The effect of intensive treatment of diabetes on the development and progression of long-term complications in insulin-dependent diabetes mellitus. The Diabetes Control and Complications Trial Research Group. N Engl J Med 1993; 329:977–986.

26. Intensive blood-glucose control with sulphonylureas or insulin compared with conventional treatment and risk of complications in patients with type 2 diabetes (UKPDS 33). UK Prospective Diabetes Study (UKPDS) Group. Lancet 1998; 352:837–853.

27. Praga M, Hernandez E, Herrero JC, et al. Influence of obesity on the appearance of proteinuria and renal insufficiency after unilateral nephrectomy. Kidney Int 2000; 58:2111–2118.

28. Hall JE. Mechanisms of obesity-associated cardiovascular and renal disease. Am J Med Sci 2002; 324:127–137.

29. Gonzalez E, Gutierrez E, Morales E, et al. Factors influencing the progression of renal damage in patients with unilateral renal agenesis and remnant kidney. Kidney Int 2005; 68(1):263–270.

30. Orth SR, Stockmann A, Conradt C, et al. Smoking as a risk factor for end-stage renal failure in men with primary renal disease. Kidney Int 1998; 54:926–931.

31. Schiffl H, Lang SM, Fischer R. Stopping smoking slows accelerated progression of renal failure in primary renal disease. J Nephrol 2002; 15:270–274.

32. Jaimes EA, Tian RX, Raij L. Nicotine: the link between cigarette smoking and the progression of renal injury? Am J Physiol Heart Circ Physiol 2007; 292:76–82.

33. Moorhead JF, Chan MK, El-Nahas M, Varghese Z. Lipid nephrotoxicity in chronic progressive glomerular and tubulo-interstitial disease. Lancet 1982; 2(8311):1309–1311.

34. Fried LF, Orchard TJ, Kasiske BL. Effect of lipid reduction on the progression of renal disease: a meta-analysis. Kidney Int 2001; 59:260–269.

35. Johnson WJ, Hagge WW, Wagoner RD, et al. Effects of urea loading in patients with far-advanced renal failure. Mayo Clin Proc 1972; 47:21–29.

36. Vanholder R, De Smet R, Glorieux G, et al. Review on uremic toxins: classification, concentration, and interindividual variability. Kidney Int 2003; 63:1934–1943.

37. Drueke TB, Locatelli F, Clyne N, et al. Normalization of hemoglobin level in patients with chronic kidney disease and anaemia. N Eng J Med 2006; 355:2071–2084.

38. Singh AK, Szczech L, Tang KL, et al. Correction of anemia with epoetin alfa in chronic kidney disease. N Eng J Med 2006; 355:2085–2098.

39. Block GA, Hulbert-Shearon TE, Levi NW, et al. Association of serum phosphorus and calcium × phosphate product with mortality risk in chronic haemodialysis patients: a national study. Am J Kidney Dis 1998; 31:607–617.

40. Baber U, Toto RD, de Lemos JA. Statins and cardiovascular risk reduction in patients with chronic kidney disease and end-stage renal failure. Am Heart J 2007; 153:471–477.

Structure and Function of the Lower Urinary Tract

Anthony R. Mundy

Institute of Urology, University College Hospital, London, U.K.

INTRODUCTION

Before starting, the reader should be aware of certain problems in discussing the subject.

First of all, a great deal is known (relatively speaking) about the structure of the bladder, urethra and pelvic floor, but as one works back proximally through the innervation of the lower urinary tract to the spinal cord and up to the brain, and as one turns more from structure to function, so knowledge of the subject becomes exponentially less.

Secondly, much of the published research on the lower urinary tract has been done on animals other than humans and there are considerable species differences that make interpretation of such work very difficult.

Thirdly, in the same vein, many of the experimental studies have been done after neuronal ablation or otherwise in circumstances that are very far from physiological. Extrapolation from ablative pathophysiology in experimental animals to normal physiology in humans is also problematic.

Fourthly, many experimental studies have been based on the identification of receptors for neurotransmitters, or on the demonstration by radioimmunoassay of the presence of neurotransmitters themselves or have attempted to infer the presence of a physiologically significant mechanism from the presence of one component of a presumed "reflex arc." Two examples will show the fallacy of such an extrapolation. Firstly, one of the most significant medical advances in recent years has been in the development of β-adrenergic receptor-active drugs for the treatment of bronchospasm, but there is no significant β sympathetic innervation to the human lung. Receptors are present that may be therapeutically manipulated, but they have no apparent physiological significance. Secondly, and more obviously, "receptors" can be identified in human platelets but no one imagines that platelets have an innervation.

Finally, it should be appreciated that just because a reflex mechanism exists does not mean that that mechanism is active, let alone important in normal circumstances. Thus, a reflex may be present or elicitable or evident in disease, but it does not necessarily mean that it is active or important in health.

These various points should be borne in mind when reading about studies of the structure and function of the lower urinary tract. Equally, it is hoped that the reader will forgive the author for the speculation that will creep in to provide a reasonably smooth narrative when substance is lacking.

The discussion begins distally in the bladder and urethra and then moves proximally, considering structure first and function second but integrating both as far as possible.

THE STRUCTURE OF THE BLADDER AND URETHRA

The bladder and urethra have three layers to which is added, in the male, the additional component of the prostate. The prostate is considered in detail in chapter 19 and is not considered further here. These three layers are, from the outside in, the adventitial layer, the muscular layer and the epithelial layer.

The Adventitial Layer

The bladder and proximal urethra lie in the pelvis, covered over the dome of the bladder with peritoneum. Deep to the peritoneum the bladder is held in place by an adventitial layer consisting of two fascial layers—the first on the anterior and lateral aspect of the bladder and the second on the dome and posterior aspect of the bladder—the two fusing together anteriorly and laterally to form what Uhlenhuth (1) described as the superior hypogastric wing (Fig. 1), which runs laterally to the external iliac vessels and anteriorly onto the anterior abdominal wall, ensheathing the medial umbilical ligaments and the urachus. The same two layers form the anterior layer of the sheath around the ureters and the superior and inferior vesical vessels posterolaterally in what Uhlenhuth described as the inferior hypogastric wing (Fig. 2). Posteriorly, the sheet of fascia that covers the dome and posterolateral aspect of the bladder sweeps back onto the posterolateral pelvic side wall and to ensheath the rectum as Uhlenhuth's presacral fascia (Fig. 3). These fascial layers and the neurovascular structures that they ensheath hold the bladder in place, as does the urethra, and the prostate in males,

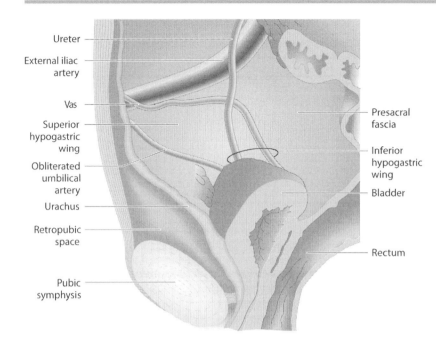

Ureter

External iliac
artery

Vas

Superior
hypogastric
wing

Obliterated
umbilical
artery

Urachus

Retropubic
space

Pubic
symphysis

Presacral
fascia

Inferior
hypogastric
wing

Bladder

Rectum

Figure 1 Diagram of the distribution of pelvic fascia to show the superior hypogastric wing. *Source*: From Ref. 2.

with which the bladder is continuous. The urethra and prostate have their attachments too, notably the endopelvic fascia, which tethers them to the pelvic side wall and the periurethral component of the levator ani muscle in males (it is vestigial in females) and the anterior vaginal wall in females, to which the female urethra is intimately related (Fig. 4).

There are other supporting structures that are thought to be important in lower urinary tract function, particularly in the female.

First and foremost, in the female, are the pubourethral ligaments, which sling the full length of the urethra but particularly the proximal urethra from the inferior pubic area (Fig. 5). These have been particularly studied by Zacharin (5), and his findings have since been confirmed by others, and all of these authors have sought somehow to link a deficiency in these ligaments to the genesis of stress incontinence.

The homologous structures in the male are the puboprostatic ligaments, which have become of particular interest since the development by Walsh (6) of his technique of radical retropubic prostatectomy.

One supporting structure identified in the anatomical and more traditional urological literature, the existence of which is now disputed, is the so-called urogenital diaphragm. Described as the layer on which the prostate sits, (7) it has proved elusive to others (8) and probably does not exist as a separate entity.

THE MUSCULAR LAYER

The smooth muscle of the bladder, which accounts for the most component of the bladder wall, is called the detrusor. There have been various attempts to identify specific bundles of muscle within the bladder wall, (9)

largely to substantiate a hypothetical mechanism to account for the opening of the bladder neck at the initiation of voiding, but there is no good evidence that such layering exists (10). The bladder should be considered as a single homogeneous layer of relatively large muscle bundles in a relatively small amount of connective tissue. These muscle bundles have no particular orientation (Fig. 6). As one approaches the bladder base from above down, there is the triangular region of the trigone between the two ureters and the internal urinary meatus, where there is a flimsy additional superficial layer of smooth muscle quite separate from the underlying smooth muscle, which is typical detrusor. This additional trigonal layer is derived from the ureters and shows several distinct characteristics. The muscle fibers form bundles that are much smaller with a higher connective tissue component and a fairly dense adrenergic innervation (11) (Fig. 7). The trigonal muscle was once thought also to have a role in opening the bladder neck, but this too has not been substantiated. As one approaches closer to the bladder neck, the disposition and orientation of the detrusor change uniformly around it. The muscle bundles get smaller, there is a relatively greater amount of connective tissue, and the orientation of the muscle bundles becomes more uniform, to loop obliquely around the bladder neck (Fig. 8).

Below the bladder neck in both sexes, the muscle bundles continue to be relatively small in size and interspersed with a relatively larger connective tissue component and they continue to show an oblique looping arrangement around the urethra. The vascular component of the wall increases by comparison with the bladder, particularly in females (12). In the male, the prostate forms an additional component at this level, and at the upper part, where the prostate and

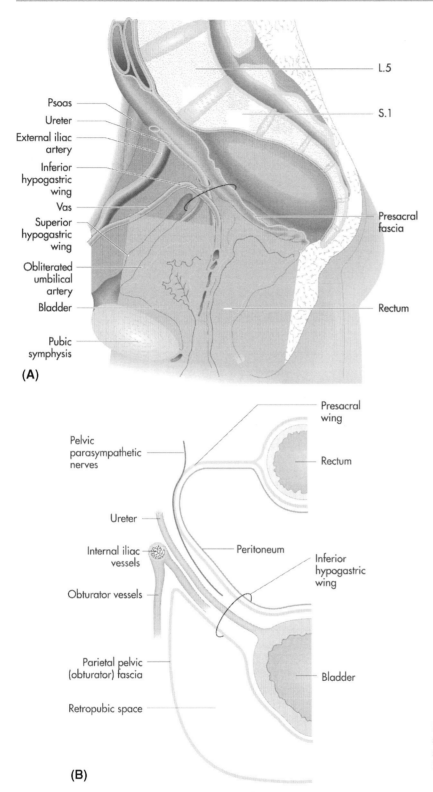

Figure 2 (**A**) Diagram of the pelvic fascia to show the inferior hypogastric wing. (**B**) Cross-section of the inferior hypogastric wing to show its structure, origin, disposition and contents. *Source*: From Ref. 2.

the bladder neck merge, there is the preprostatic sphincter in which adrenergically innervated smooth muscle bundles form a distinct sphincter around the urethra to prevent retrograde ejaculation (Fig. 9) (11). It should be emphasized that this adrenergically innervated smooth muscle component—the preprostatic sphincter—which is present in males but not in females, is a genital sphincter and not the bladder neck urinary sphincter mechanism in the strict sense, which is presumably the same in both sexes.

The preprostatic sphincter and the trigone are the only areas to show a distinct adrenergic innervation;

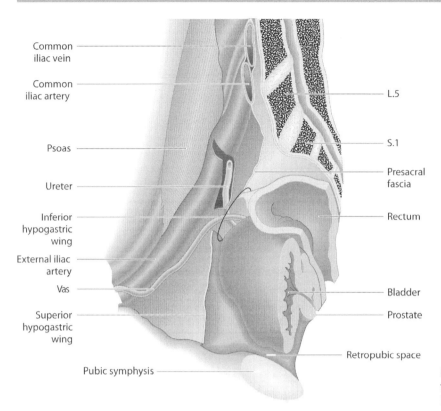

Common iliac vein

Common iliac artery

Psoas

Ureter

Inferior hypogastric wing

External iliac artery

Vas

Superior hypogastric wing

Pubic symphysis

L.5

S.1

Presacral fascia

Rectum

Bladder

Prostate

Retropubic space

Figure 3 Diagram of the pelvic fascia to show the distribution of the presacral fascia. *Source*: From Ref. 2.

otherwise the only adrenergic neurons in the bladder are those that supply the blood vessels (11). This is not to say that there are not adrenergic receptors present; indeed, there are α receptors in the bladder base and β receptors elsewhere in the bladder dome, (13) but there is no evidence that there is a functionally important innervation to these receptors in the normal individual. Further down the urethra at the apex of the prostate in males and in the mid-urethra in females, there is the urethral sphincter mechanism, sometimes called the "distal sphincter mechanism" to distinguish it from the proximal sphincter mechanism, which is the other name for the bladder neck. Whereas there is a readily identifiable sphincter mechanism in the "sphincter-active" area of the urethra in both sexes, there is no anatomically identifiable sphincter mechanism at the bladder neck in either sex (using the term "bladder neck" in its strictest sense—as distinct from the preprostatic sphincter). The urethral sphincter mechanism has three components (Fig. 10). The innermost is the urethral smooth muscle and the middle layer is the striated muscle component within the urethral wall. These two components within the urethral wall itself are separated from the third component, which is the periurethral component of the levator ani, or pubourethral sling, which is slung around the urethra in much the same way as the puborectal sling is disposed round the rectum (4). These two sling components, the pubourethral and the puborectal slings, are distinct from and below the diaphragmatic layer of the levator ani (Fig. 11) (14). They both form substantial components of their respective sphincter mechanisms and they share several common features.

THE URETHRAL SPHINCTER MECHANISM

Of the three layers of the urethral sphincter mechanism, two are relatively quickly dealt with. The outermost layer—the pubourethral sling—is the levator ani component most closely related to the urethra; (4) it is typical striated muscle; it has typical striated muscle innervation; it is relatively insignificant in the female compared with the male because of the presence of the vagina; and it is activated along with the rest of the levator ani under "stress conditions," acting specifically on the urethra at such times to augment urethral occlusion pressure.

The urethral smooth muscle is dealt with relatively quickly for an entirely different reason: we know very little about its function. The innervation is more complicated than the detrusor with both excitatory and inhibitory innervation. Small ganglia, smaller than in and around the bladder, are present, and both acetylcholine and noradrenaline (norepinephrine) mediate contraction. The sympathetic innervation involves a distinct subtype of the α1 adrenoceptor in the male, particularly in the prostatic urethra, which has particular implications for the treatment of bladder outflow obstruction due to benign prostatic hyperplasia as described in chapter 19.

When the striated muscle of the urethral sphincter mechanism is paralyzed, the urethral smooth muscle

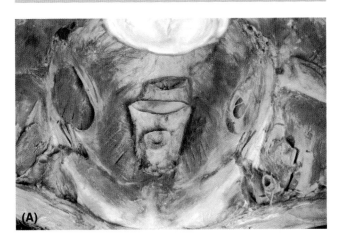

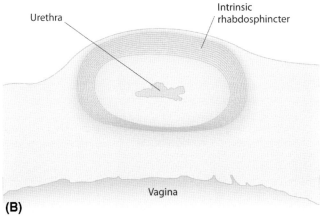

Figure 4 (**A**) The relationship of the urethra to the anterior vaginal wall. (**B**) Cross-section to show the integration of the urethra, below the bladder neck within the anterior vaginal wall. *Source*: From Refs. 2 and 3.

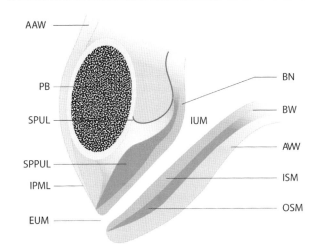

Figure 5 The orientation of the pubourethral ligaments. *Abbreviations*: AAW, anterior abdominal wall; PB, pubic bone; BN, bladder neck; BW, bladder wall; AVW, anterior vaginal wall; ISM, inner smooth muscle; OSM, outer striated muscle; IUM, internal urinary meatus; EUM, external urinary meatus; SPUL, superior pubourethral ligament; SPPUL, subpubic pubourethral ligament; IPML, inferior pubomeatal ligament. *Source*: From Ref. 4.

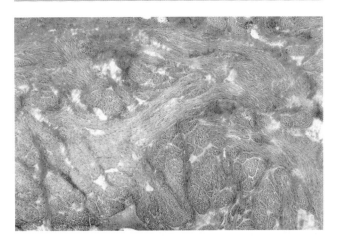

Figure 6 Low-power microscopy of the detrusor stained with Masson's trichrome to show the orientation of the smooth muscle bundles. *Source*: From Ref. 3.

continues to produce a high-pressure zone, which suggests that it is tonically active (14)—whereas the bladder smooth muscle is phasically active—and recent experimental studies suggest that this tonic smooth muscle contraction may be relaxed by nitric oxide (15–17). Indeed, there are both ganglia and nerves innervating the urethral smooth muscle, which contain nitric oxide synthase. The current opinion is that this nitric oxide-related relaxant mechanism in this area of the urethra and bladder neck is responsible for the opening of the bladder neck and the relaxation of the urethra that occurs when the bladder contracts at the onset of voiding (17).

It appears that it is the striated muscle component within the urethral wall that is the most important component for continence. It is sometimes called the intrinsic rhabdosphincter (11). This striated muscle is unusual in a number of ways (11). It is orientated predominantly anteriorly in both the vertical and horizontal planes and is relatively deficient posteriorly, giving it, overall, a signet ring distribution (Fig. 12). This is clearly seen microscopically in both sexes (Fig. 13). The reason for this is not clear, but it is common experience that the easiest way of stopping

water flowing through a hosepipe is to kink it rather than to squeeze it circumferentially. It may be that the distribution of the fibers of the intrinsic striated muscle of the urethra produces a kinking rather than a circumferential compression when it contracts, for this sort of reason, but this is entirely conjectural. This intrinsic striated muscle sphincter is composed of relatively very small muscle fibers when compared with typical striated muscle; the fibers themselves are disposed in small muscle bundles within a very much greater connective tissue component than is seen in typical striated muscle (Fig. 14); the muscle fibers themselves are stuffed with mitochondria; there are

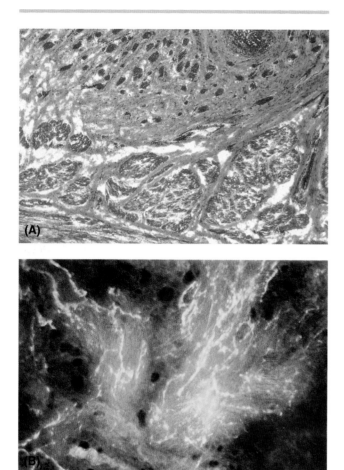

Figure 7 (**A**) Low-power microscopy of the detrusor stained with Masson's trichrome to show the distribution of the smooth muscle bundles in relation to the trigone superficially, compared with the detrusor proper, more deeply. (**B**) Immunofluorescent microscopy study to show the presence of adrenergic nerves in the trigone. *Source*: From Ref. 3.

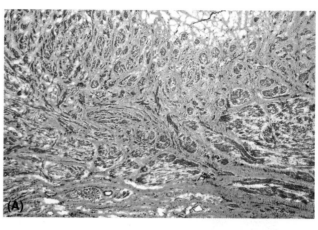

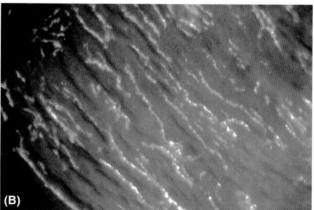

Figure 8 (**A**) Low-power microscopy of the detrusor stained with Masson's trichrome to show the distribution of the smooth muscle bundles at the bladder neck. (**B**) Immunofluorescent microscopy to show the presence of adrenergic nerve fibers in the bladder neck. *Source*: From Ref. 3.

no muscle spindles; and there are several distinct histochemical staining characteristics of these muscle fibers, most notably a uniform staining with acid-stable myosin adenosine triphosphatase (ATPase) (Fig. 15) (18). By contrast, the typical striated muscle of the pubourethral sling that is immediately adjacent to the intrinsic rhabdosphincter shows larger muscle fibers in larger muscle bundles, with little connective tissue, fewer mitochondria, muscle spindles present and a mixed pattern of staining for acid-stable myosin ATPase (Fig. 16). Furthermore, whereas the nerve supply to the levator ani originates in typical cell bodies in the motor cell nuclei of the anterior horn of the sacral spinal cord, the cell bodies of the fibers that innervate the intrinsic rhabdosphincter appear to arise in a nucleus more medially situated in the sacral anterior horn, as do the fibers innervating the anal sphincter mechanism, and this spinal cord nucleus is known as spinal nucleus X, sometimes called Onuf's nucleus (Fig. 17) (19). The fibers from Onuf's nucleus to the intrinsic rhabdosphincter run out of the anterior

primary rami and the nerve fibers run initially with the nervi erigentes, which are the preganglionic parasympathetic neurons. They run with these fibers through the pelvic plexuses and down with the postganglionic parasympathetic neurons into the urethra (8).

Whether this is the sole innervation of the intrinsic rhabdosphincter or whether there is a separate component arising from the pudendal nerve is not clear, (20) but after pudendal neurectomy or pudendal nerve blockade, the urethral sphincter mechanism is intact so there is clearly a source other than the pudendal nerve.

These characteristics of the intrinsic rhabdosphincter are very unusual but not unique; the intrinsic laryngeal muscles are very similar in structure and in the nature of their innervation.

The Epithelial Layer

The urothelial layer of the bladder is a multilayered transitional epithelium that is continuous with the ureters above and the prostatic urethra below. Under the light microscope, the urothelium is similar

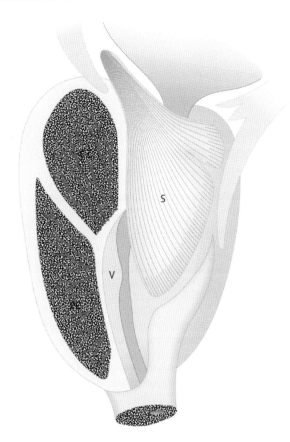

Figure 9 A diagram to show the preprostatic sphincter. *Abbreviations*: CZ, central zone; PZ, peripheral zone; S, preprostatic sphincter; V, verumontanum.

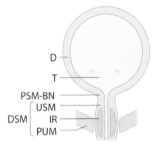

Figure 10 Diagrammatic representation of the components of the urethral sphincter mechanism. *Abbreviations*: D, detrusor; T, trigone; PSM-BN, proximal sphincter mechanism bladder neck; DSM, distal sphincter mechanism; USM, urethral smooth muscle; IR, intrinsic rhabdosphincter; PUM, periurethral musculature.

in the bladder and the prostatic urethra, but there are differences on scanning electron microscopy that become more marked the further one proceeds down the urethra toward the bulbar segment where it changes to a columnar epithelium and changes again toward the meatus to a squamous epithelium. The urothelium has numerous so-called tight junctions (chap. 1), which make it impermeable to fluids and solutes. This relative impermeability should not

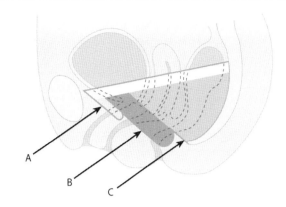

Figure 11 Illustration of the various components of levator ani showing separate sling and diaphragmatic components. *Abbreviations*: A, pubourethral sling; B, puborectal sling; C, levator diaphragm.

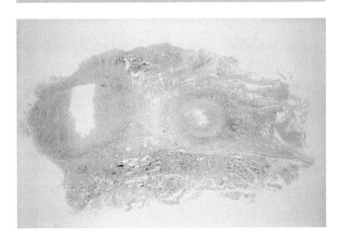

Figure 12 Low-power microscopy of a transverse section of the male sphincter-active urethra to show the "signet ring" distribution of the intrinsic rhabdosphincter (anterior to the right of the figure).

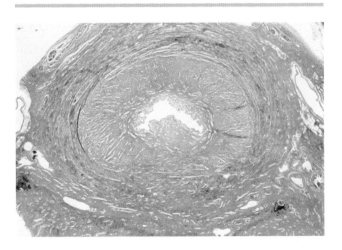

Figure 13 Low-power microscopy of a transverse section of the female sphincter-active urethra to show the "signet ring" distribution of the intrinsic rhabdosphincter (anterior to the top of the figure).

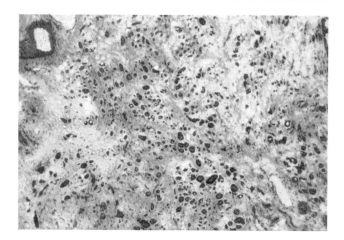

Figure 14 Low-power microscopy of the intrinsic rhabdosphincter to show the relative distribution of muscle bundles and connective tissue. *Source*: From Ref. 3.

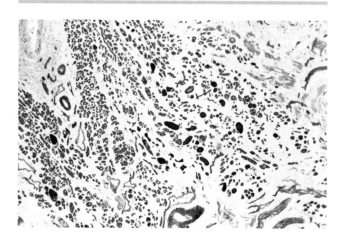

Figure 15 Low-power histochemistry of the intrinsic rhabdosphincter to show the distribution of acid-stable myosin ATPase. *Source*: From Ref. 3.

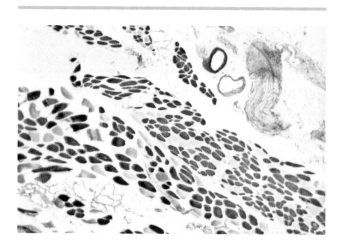

Figure 16 Low-power histochemistry of the typical striated muscle, in this case the pubourethral sling, to show the distribution of acid-stable myosin ATPase. *Source*: From Ref. 3.

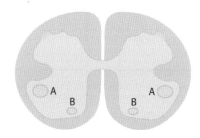

Figure 17 Diagram to show the separate origin of the innervation of the intrinsic rhabdosphincter from Onuf's nucleus as distinct from the site of origin of typical striated muscle from anterior horn cells. *Abbreviations*: A, a motor neuron group; B, Onuf's nucleus.

be taken to mean that the urothelium is inert. Indeed, various drugs can be absorbed from the bladder and instilled intravesically. In addition, the urothelium has a sensory role. Various sensory nerves have been recognized in the epithelium and subepithelium, which have been presumed to act as touch receptors and chemoreceptors. There are also cells in the epithelium sensitive to hydrostatic pressure, which appear to have an important role in continence and voiding.

Deep to the basal lamina of the epithelial layer, in the lamina propria, is a thin layer of muscle cells, formerly called interstitial cells and now more commonly known as myofibroblasts (21). Although only a thin layer, these cells are closely connected to each other by numerous gap junctions facilitating electrical coupling (22). They are also closely connected to the overlying epithelium by numerous fine nerves, some of which are related to the cells, receptors and nerves mentioned in the last paragraph. Together these three components—epithelium, myofibroblasts and the interconnecting network of nerves—are thought to act as a sort of "unitary stretch receptor" responsible for sensing bladder filling (23,24). This is discussed further below.

THE INNERVATION OF THE BLADDER AND URETHRA

Four separate neuronal pathways to the lower urinary tract have been alluded to (Fig. 18). The principal one is derived from cell bodies in the intermediolateral column of the second, third and fourth sacral segments of the spinal cord. These are preganglionic parasympathetic fibers that run out of the anterior primary rami of S2, S3, and S4 and then separate out from the somatic component, which runs to the sacral plexus, to run as the nervi erigentes to the pelvic plexuses. These preganglionic parasympathetic neurons end by synapsing in ganglia on the cell bodies of the postganglionic parasympathetic nerves, which then run to the bladder and to the urethra (and more proximally to the rectum and the genital structures). In humans, 50% of the ganglia of the pelvic plexus are in the adventitial tissue around the base and posterolateral aspects of the bladder and 50% are

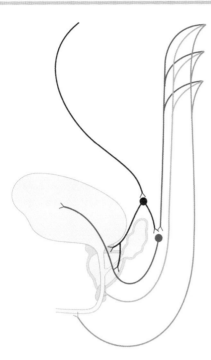

Figure 18 Diagram to show the four components of innervation of the lower urinary tract. —, sympathetic; —, parasympathetic; —, somatic innervation of intrinsic rhabdosphincter; —, pudendal nerve. *Source*: From Ref. 3.

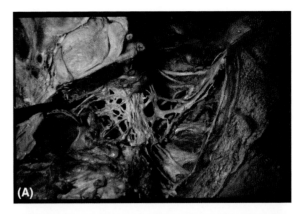

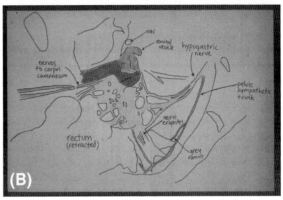

Figure 19 (**A**) Cadaveric dissection of the right half of the pelvis to show the pelvic plexus and its origins and distribution on that side, and its anatomical relationships. (**B**) Diagram of the dissection identifying the structures demonstrated. *Source*: From Ref. 25.

within the bladder wall itself (11). For this reason it is, strictly speaking, technically impossible to denervate the bladder because the 50% within the bladder wall itself will still remain and there will therefore still be reflex activity, even if this is not physiologically significant. A more semantically correct term would therefore be "decentralization" rather than "denervation" when discussing the stripping of the nerves from around the outside of the bladder.

The somatic nerve fibers that arise from Onuf's nucleus and that travel with the otherwise autonomic parasympathetic nerve fibers of the nervi erigentes and pass ultimately to the intrinsic rhabdosphincter have already been mentioned.

The third component is the sympathetic nerve component that arises from the intermediatolateral column of the 10th, 11th and 12th thoracic and the 1st and 2nd lumbar segments of the spinal cord. These preganglionic sympathetic fibers and their postganglionic sympathetic derivatives travel as the hypogastric nerves, which innervate the trigone, the blood vessels of the bladder and the smooth muscle of the prostate in males, including the preprostatic sphincter. They also have postganglionic branches that end in the parasympathetic ganglia, (11) where they exert an inhibitory effect that is described in detail below.

Finally, there is the pudendal nerve component, also arising from S2, S3, and S4, in this instance from typical anterior horn motor neuron cell bodies, which innervates the urethra and the pelvic floor musculature and provides afferent innervation to the urethra.

By comparison with typical anatomical "nerves" such as the obturator nerve, the femoral nerve and even the sciatic nerve, the total mass of the autonomic nerves in the pelvis is large. The autonomic nerves are not as discrete and easily identifiable as the somatic nerves referred to, disposed as they are as a sheet within the fascial layers that invest the rectum, the genital structures and the lower urinary tract, but if the nerve fibers are dissected out and considered as a whole, their volume is considerable (Fig. 19). It is this sheer mass that protects pelvic autonomic function from extensive damage during pelvic surgery such as hysterectomy or rectal resection, but they are nonetheless vulnerable to traction injuries during such procedures (26), as of course they are in females during childbirth.

FUNCTIONAL ASPECTS OF THE INNERVATION OF THE BLADDER AND URETHRA

Cholinergic nerves cannot be stained directly for microscopical study—only indirectly by staining for acetylcholinesterase, the enzyme that breaks down acetylcholine at the neuromuscular junction. Staining for acetylcholinesterase shows a dense "presumptive cholinergic" innervation of the detrusor smooth

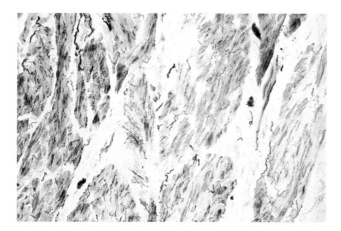

Figure 20 Low-power microscopy of the muscle wall after staining with acetylcholinesterase to show the distribution of presumptive cholinergic nerves in the bladder wall. *Source*: From Ref. 3.

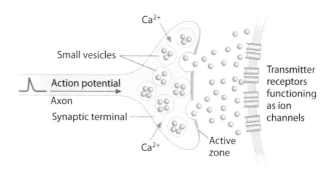

Figure 22 Diagram of a nerve ending and neuromuscular junction to show the release of "fast" neurotransmitters into the neuromuscular junction. *Source*: From Ref. 29.

muscle (Fig. 20) with a nerve to muscle cell ratio of about 1:1, and a less dense cholinergic innervation of the urethral smooth muscle (11). Under the electron microscope, the terminal branches of the parasympathetic neurons within the bladder wall are seen to contain varicosities (Fig. 21). These varicosities are there because of the presence of numerous vesicles within the terminal neuron at that point and these vesicles contain neurotransmitter substances. Alongside the varicosity is the specialized area of the smooth muscle cell membrane that constitutes the receptor site, although this is not very specialized by comparison with the receptor site—the neuromuscular junction—in striated muscle. Adjacent smooth muscle cells are connected by so-called "regions of close approach," like gap junctions in effect, which could, at least theoretically, allow electrotonic spread of activity from one smooth muscle cell to the next and

which thereby confer so-called "cable properties" on the smooth muscle fibers. This would supplement the spreading neuronal stimulus as a sort of "parallel pathway," and help to ensure a uniform simultaneous contraction of all the bladder smooth muscle cells at the time of voiding.

Vesicles are of two main types (28): small clear vesicles and larger vesicles with a dense core. The small clear vesicles are thought to contain so-called "fast" neurotransmitter substances, which are released directly into the area between the neuron and the adjacent neuron across a synapse, or the adjacent smooth muscle cell across a neuromuscular junction (Fig. 22) to open ligand-gated ion channels on the receptor site that will initiate an action potential—so-called "electromechanical coupling." Outside the central nervous system, the commonest neurotransmitter to be found in these small clear vesicles is acetylcholine and the commonest receptor is the nicotinic acetylcholine receptor, although acetylcholine does not exclusively act as a fast neurotransmitter to open ligand-gated ion channels in this way, nor is the nicotinic receptor the only type of acetylcholine receptor (see below). In the central nervous system, γ-aminobutyric acid (GABA) is also found in small clear vesicles (28).

Large, dense-cored vesicles contain so-called "slow" neurotransmitters (30), which are called slow because they are released nonspecifically from around the area of the varicosity (Fig. 23) rather than specifically into the receptor site; and because they generally act by binding to G protein–linked receptors (chap. 1) and initiating smooth muscle contraction through second messengers systems. This is so-called "pharmacomechanical" coupling of the neuronal stimulus to smooth muscle contraction, as distinct from the "electromechanical" coupling initiated by the binding of ligand-gated ion channels by fast neurotransmitters.

A single nerve impulse will empty about half the vesicles in a varicosity, each of which will release about 5000 molecules of acetylcholine as a quantum. These vesicles empty their contents in response to a rise in cytosolic calcium within the varicosity as a result of the opening of membrane calcium channels induced by the neuronal electrical impulse (voltage-gated calcium

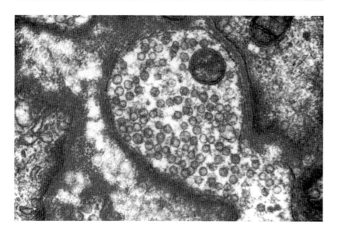

Figure 21 Electron microscopy of a terminal neuron within the detrusor smooth muscle layer to show a varicosity containing small clear vesicles containing acetylcholine. *Source*: From Ref. 27.

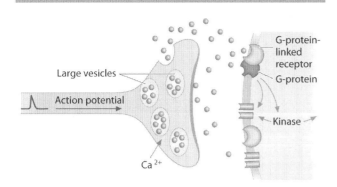

Figure 23 Diagram of a nerve ending and neuromuscular junction to show the release of "slow" neurotransmitters from around the neuromuscular junction. *Source*: From Ref. 29.

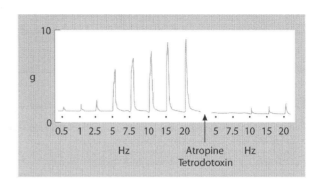

Figure 25 A frequency-response curve before and after Tetrodotoxin showing a very small residual contraction that is not nerve mediated and due to direct smooth muscle stimulation. *Source*: From Ref. 31.

channels), causing an influx of extracellular calcium (30).

There are other ways of demonstrating the primacy of parasympathetic cholinergic activity in the excitatory innervation of the bladder other than by showing the density of staining of acetylcholinesterase on light microscopy and the vesicles on electron microscopy. The most convincing way is by the physiological study of strips of detrusor smooth muscle in an organ bath (Fig. 24). The organ bath keeps the muscle strip at the right temperature, sufficiently oxygenated and in the right fluid medium to keep it viable sufficiently long for adequate study. The excitatory nerve supply to the muscle fibers within the muscle strip is stimulated by using an electrical impulse. If the strength and amplitude are optimized and the frequency of the electrical stimulus is then varied, a frequency-response curve is produced between about 0.5 Hz and 20 Hz, above which the response rate plateaus until the electrical impulse is of sufficiently high frequency to cause damage (Fig. 25). This response can be abolished by the application of tetrodotoxin, which is a sodium channel blocker which, therefore, blocks nerve conduction (32). (Tetrodotoxin is extracted from the liver of the puffer fish—called fugu in Japan—and will be known as such to James Bond aficionados.) If a frequency-response curve is plotted after the application of tetrodotoxin, there will be a very small response at higher frequencies that is not nerve mediated but due to direct stimulation of the smooth muscle cell membrane itself. If the frequency-response curve is performed after the application of atropine at a sufficient dose to give complete cholinergic blockade, then the

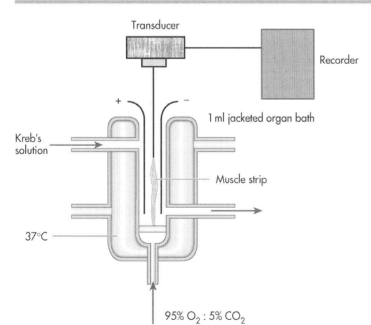

Figure 24 Diagrammatic representation of an organ bath experiment. *Source*: From Ref. 31.

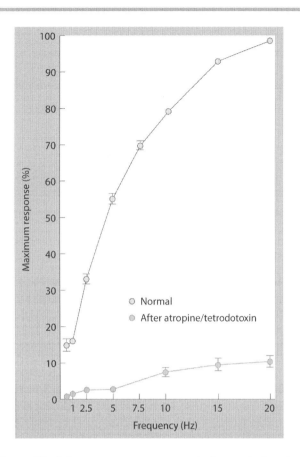

Figure 26 A frequency-response curve before and after atropine in a human showing a very small residual response. In this case it is a graphical representation of the percentage response. *Source*: From Ref. 31.

only response left will be the same as that after tetrodotoxin (Fig. 26). In other words, in the normal human specimen (stressing both adjectives), there is no excitatory component left after atropine blockade and there is no "atropine-resistant" component to excitatory neurotransmission. Normal excitatory neurotransmission in the human bladder is therefore exclusively muscarinic cholinergic (33–35). In other mammals, it is a completely different story. In some small mammals, there may be as much as 30% of the frequency-response curve that is atropine resistant. This is thought to be due to the presence of an alternative excitatory neurotransmitter that, in most animal species showing this type of excitatory neurotransmission, is thought to be adenosine triphosphate (ATP) (30). This is thought to give rise to the type of bladder contraction responsible for the excretion of a small amount of urine for the purposes of territorial marking. In those animals that exhibit territorial marking, it seems likely that a normal voiding detrusor contraction is cholinergic in origin, whereas the small-volume "squirt" of urine excreted for territorial marking is under so-called purinergic (ATP-mediated) innervation.

This is not to say that ATP cannot be made to cause contraction of human detrusor smooth muscle.

It has indeed been shown to do so (32), but it does not appear to be a component of normal human voiding. It may, however, be a cause of abnormal detrusor function in detrusor instability.

OTHER NEUROTRANSMITTERS

To qualify as a neurotransmitter, a potential candidate must satisfy certain stringent criteria. In the last 20 years or so, numerous compounds have been identified as potential neurotransmitters, many of which fail to satisfy these criteria but nonetheless appear to be involved in the process of neurotransmission, either as neurotransmitters or as neuromodulators (30).

A further observation is that many of these compounds seem to be related to nerves that show the characteristics of cholinergic or adrenergic neurons. In other words, the putative neurotransmitter or neuromodulator appears to be "colocalized" with a known "classical" transmitter or with another putative neurotransmitter (26).

Several of these putative neurotransmitters are peptides, which have been grouped together as neuropeptides. This group includes substance P (36,37) vasoactive intestinal polypeptide (38,39) and neuropeptide Y, to name but a few. Substance P is thought to be involved in afferent neurotransmission (36). Vasoactive intestinal polypeptide relaxes detrusor smooth muscle (39) and has been shown in some studies to be coreleased with acetylcholine. Similarly, neuropeptide Y has been colocalized in adrenergic neurons. This concept of colocalization, corelease and cotransmission is interesting as it provides a means of modifying the effects of neural activity either temporally or spatially. Thus, the same nerves could produce two transmitters with different effects, both being simultaneously released but with one predominating in one area and the other in the other area. For example, an excitatory and an inhibitory transmitter, if coreleased, might cause bladder contraction if the former predominated in the bladder and relaxation of the bladder neck if the latter predominated at that site. This is indeed what is thought to happen with acetylcholine and nitric oxide, colocated in and coreleased from the parasympathetic nerves that supply this area (17,40). This type of neuromodulatory activity could have other effects, which would less dramatically act to "fine tune" the actions of the lower urinary tract.

RECEPTORS

The acetylcholine released from the varicosities at the ends of parasympathetic nerves has a variety of different actions depending on exactly where it is released and particularly on the nature of the receptors present. As a general rule, the same applies to all transmitters and all nerves. Many transmitters are associated with several different types of receptors and each type of receptor has several subtypes, each with different effects. When acetylcholine is released from preganglionic nerve fibers in the parasympathetic ganglia of the pelvic plexus and in the bladder wall its principal targets are the receptors on the cell bodies of the postganglionic nerves. These receptors are nicotinic in type, which are ligand-gated ion channels.

At the neuromuscular junctions in the detrusor smooth muscle itself, the most important excitatory receptors are muscarinic—the other main type of cholinergic receptor—and specifically of the M3 subtype (41,42). These are not the only muscarinic receptors present—there are muscarinic receptors on the nerve terminals from which the acetylcholine is released which can enhance (M1 subtype) or suppress (M4 subtype) transmitter release depending on the intensity of the nerve impulse (43) There are also M2 receptors on the bladder smooth muscle cells themselves as a separate population of muscarinic receptors whose function is not clear. M2 receptors have various actions, both as ligand-gated ion channels and as G protein–linked receptors; M3 receptors are G protein–linked receptors.

Muscarinic receptors are not restricted to the ganglia and the neuromuscular junctions; they are also found in the urothelim and in the suburothelial lamina propria, in relation to myofibroblasts, where have a role in bladder sensation and probably also in normal motor function. Acetylcholine is not the only transmitter released by parasympathetic nerves and muscarinic receptors are not the only receptors to be found in the bladder and urethra. Nitric oxide is released by parasympathetic nerves, particularly in the bladder neck and urethra (17,40); there are purinergic receptors of various different types (41), and there are of course a few sympathetic nerves with various associated types and subtypes of receptors, mainly associated—outside the prostate—with vasomotor function.

Because ATP was first identified in experimental animals as the factor responsible for atropine resistance in detrusor contraction most attention until recently was concentrated on its contractile properties. ATP acts through two types of purinergic receptor: the P2X receptor (with seven subtypes), which is an ion channel, and the P2Y receptor (with eight subtypes), which is a G protein–linked receptor (41). The contractile response to ATP is mediated through the P2X receptor subtypes; the sensory role of ATP is mediated by P2Y receptor subtypes.

Mechanisms of Contraction and Relaxation of the Bladder and Urethral Smooth Muscle in Health and Disease

This is described in detail in the next chapter.

THE AFFERENT INNERVATION OF THE BLADDER

So far, we have mainly concentrated on the efferent innervation of the bladder. The afferent innervation is equally important, but is less well understood. Afferent impulses arise from the nerve plexus in the lamina propria associated with the myofibroblasts immediately deep to the urothelium, from within the muscle layer itself, and, presumably, from the adventitia. Afferent nerve endings have been identified, but their nature is poorly understood (44). Substance P and ATP are thought to be sensory neurotransmitters and there is good evidence to support this view, but again the mechanism is not well understood. Other presumptive sensory nerves have been shown to contain calcitonin gene-related peptide (CGRP) and other transmitters, including neurokinin A (45).

The emerging explanation for the sensation of bladder filling centers on the layer of myofibroblasts in the lamina propria, referred to above as forming a sort of "unitary stretch receptor" with the epithelium and the interconnecting network of nerves between the two (21–24). Thus, although there are stretch receptors (in the traditional physiological sense) throughout the bladder wall, current opinion is that the bulk of afferent activity originates in this functional syncitium forming the unitary "stretch receptor;" the receptors involved in this system are many and varied but principally muscarinic and purinergic; and that onward transmission of the afferent impulse in the pelvic and other afferent nerves is largely purinergic.

Importantly it is now thought likely that the activity in these receptors in the lamina propria might be a better explanation for bladder overactivity states and for the clinical response to anticholinergic medication in such states than the activity in the receptors in the detrusor layer (46,47).

The majority of the afferents from the bladder run in the pelvic nerves (48). Only a small, albeit important, percent run in the sympathetic and somatic nerves. Pelvic nerve afferents consist of myelinated A-δ and unmyelinated C axons. The A-δ myelinated axons arise from tension receptors in the smooth muscle of the bladder and respond to increasing muscle wall tension during bladder filling. These are the afferent neurons responsible for eliciting the so-called micturition reflex in normal healthy individuals. Most of the C-fiber unmyelinated axons arise from receptors in the suburothelial layer, although some nociceptors sensitive to overdistension may also be found in the muscle and adventitia. Some of the suburothelial receptors respond to stretching of the mucosa and thus act as bladder volume sensors. The remainder are insensitive to normal bladder distension and are referred to as "silent afferents" (49). These afferents are thought to become mechanosensitive when irritated or inflamed, thereby lowering the threshold of bladder contraction in such situations. It is thought that this may be due to the release of neurokinin A, which then acts on its own specialist receptor binding sites and sensory nerve endings in the suburothelial layer (50).

What is clear, from the work of Nathan (51), is that there are three types of sensation arising from the bladder (Fig. 27). The first and most general sensation of bladder filling arises from receptors throughout the bladder. The afferent fibers run with the parasympathetic nerves back to the sacral cord, where there is some local synapsing on preganglionic parasympathetic cell bodies in the intermediolateral column of the sacral cord, but the majority of afferent neurons run in the ascending tracts of the spinal cord and up to the pons, where they synapse with preganglionic neurons in the

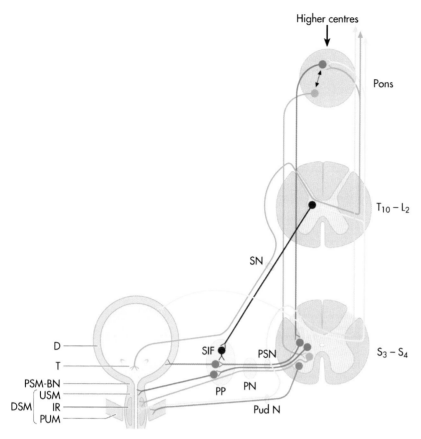

Figure 27 The nervous pathways concerned with the three different types of sensation from the lower urinary tract. ——, from the bladder; ——, from the trigone; ——, from the urethra and pelvic floor. *Source*: From Ref. 31.

nucleus locus coeruleus in the rostral pons. Other fibers pass up to the cerebral cortex to give rise to sensory awareness. This type of afferent stimulus gives rise to a volume-related awareness of bladder filling that is easily suppressed.

Less easily suppressed is the next type of bladder sensation, which is stimulated by definite fullness of the bladder. This is a stimulus that arises in the trigonal area and the afferent impulses are transmitted in neurons that run with the sympathetic nerves up to the thoracolumbar cord. Once again, there are local relays in the cord, but most fibers run up in the ascending tracts to the pons and to the cerebral cortex to give awareness.

Finally, there is the feeling of severe urgency and the sense that voiding is imminent. This sensation cannot be overlooked. It arises in the urethra and the afferent fibers run with the pudendal nerve, again giving rise to local relays in the sacral cord, but with most fibers running in the ascending tracts to the pons and to the cerebral cortex.

Within the spinal cord, the ascending and descending fibers all run in an equatorial plane through the spinal canal, as also shown by Nathan (Fig. 28) (52). The medial tracts are visceral efferent, the intermediate tracts are somatic efferent to the intrinsic rhabdosphincter and the pelvic floor, and the most lateral fibers lying at the periphery of the cord between the corticospinal and the spinothalamic tracts are visceral afferent. The location of these tracts

in relation to the urinary tract was found by postmortem studies of patients who had undergone the neurosurgical procedure of percutaneous cordotomy during life for relief for severe visceral pain, usually malignant in origin.

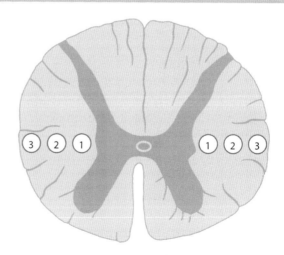

Figure 28 The orientation within the spinal cord of the pathways related to lower urinary tract function. *Abbreviations*: 1, autonomic efferent; 2, somatic efferent; 3, afferent. *Source*: From Ref. 31.

The nature of the neurotransmitters in both the afferent and efferent pathways of the spinal cord (53) is still largely unknown (54). Glutamic acid is thought to be the principal excitatory transmitter of both the ascending and descending limbs of the micurition reflex pathway as well as in the reflex pathway controlling sphincter function at both the spinal and supraspinal levels. Likewise, GABA and the opioid peptides (enkephalins) are the most important inhibitory modulators. It is clear that several other substances may exert significant modulatory influences, including supraspinal cholinergic and dopaminergic influences at the supraspinal level and adrenergic influences at the spinal level. All of these transmitters have variable effects according to their site of action within the neuraxis and the type of receptor activated.

CEREBRAL CONTROL OF VOIDING

Within the brain, there are five areas that are concerned with continence and voiding (Fig. 29). The first has already been alluded to the nucleus locus coeruleus in the rostral pons where afferent nerves synapse on the cell bodies of efferent nerve fibers. There are two connections of importance at this site. The first is the synapse, by which means an adequate afferent impulse gives rise to an efferent impulse that will generate a detrusor contraction that is sufficient in amplitude and duration to cause complete bladder emptying. The second connection that occurs at this site coordinates this contraction with relaxation of the bladder outflow to given unobstructed voiding. The details of these two mechanisms and their coordination are unclear; it is, however, quite clear that this is the site where both these actions—generation of a normal voiding contraction and reciprocal relaxation

of the sphincter mechanism—occur and are coordinated. If there is such a thing as a "micturition center," then this is it (55).

This view of a unitary "pontine micturition center" has been revised in recent years largely by the work of Blok and Holstege (56). They have shown experimentally that micturition and continence are independently organized in the brain, and this has since been confirmed by PET scanning in humans (55). Their experimental studies in the cat have shown that the pontine micturition center is exactly where Barrington said it was in the medial part of the dorsolateral pons (55,56) (Fig. 30). This they call the M-region. Neurons from the M-region project downward to the

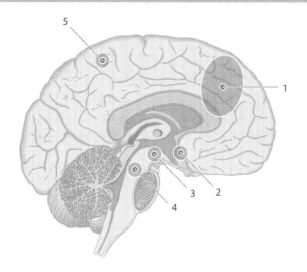

Figure 29 Five areas of the brain concerned with lower urinary tract function. *Abbreviations*: 1, medial aspect of frontal lobe; 2, septal and preoptic nuclei; 3, hypothalamus; 4, nucleus locus coeruleus (Barrington's pontine micturition center); 5, paracentral lobule. *Source*: From Ref. 31.

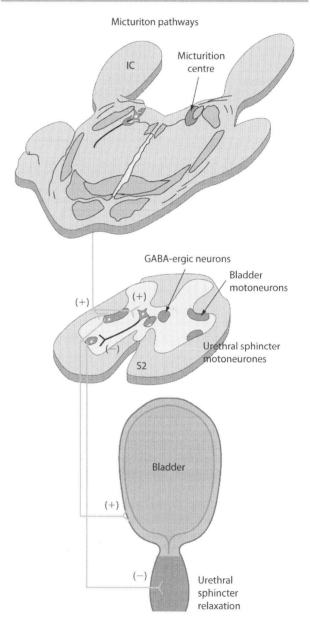

Figure 30 Schematic diagram of the spinal and supraspinal structures and their pathways involved in micturition. Pathways are indicated on one side only. *Abbreviations*: IC, inferior cellulus; S2, second sacral segment.

sacral intermediolateral gray column. There are also projections to the sacral intermediomedial cell column, which is also known as the dorsal gray commissure (DGC). Thus, impulses from the M-region simultaneously excite the preganglionic parasympathetic neurons in the sacral intermediolateral gray column to cause bladder contraction and excite GABA-ergic interneurons in the DGC in the same area of the spinal cord, which inhibit the urethral sphincter motor neurons and thereby cause relaxation of the sphincter. The presence of the M-region has been shown in exactly the same area in humans by PET.

It has also been shown that afferent impulses do not project directly to the pontine micturition center (M-region) but to a relay center in the mesencephalic periaqueductal gray matter (PAG). This is an important relay center between the pontine micturition center and a number of higher centers in the brain, which seems to act as an interface between the afferent and efferent components of bladder control and specifically in registering the degree of bladder filling both with the pontine micturition center and with the higher centers responsible for conscious awareness (57).

Ventral and lateral to the pontine micturition center of M-region is another group of neurons responsible for the storage of urine during continence. This is known as the pontine storage center (PSC) or L-region (Fig. 31). Neurons project from the L-region to the urethral sphincter motor neurons in Onuf's nucleus, reducing tonic urethral sphincter contraction. The presence of this center in humans has also been shown on PET scanning but with less certainty than the M-region.

Clearly, as this is largely an autonomic event, parasympathetically mediated, the hypothalamus is important, and this is the second of the five centers. The third is the paracentral lobule of the cerebral cortex, which is responsible for the control of the pelvic floor musculature. The importance of this center becomes manifest in spastic conditions such as congenital cerebral palsy, in which failure of relaxation can cause quite severe voiding difficulties. The normal physiological role of other related areas of the brain, such as the basal ganglia, is not clear, although diseases that affect these areas, such as Parkinson's disease and multiple system atrophy, have obvious adverse effects.

At the junction of the diencephalon and telencephalon are the septal and preoptic nuclei where the "associated acts" of both micturition and defecation (and, for that matter, coition) are coordinated (58). In some animals, such as the cat, these associated acts of voiding are quite elaborate, but in the human being they are restricted to fixation of the diaphragm and anterior abdominal wall musculature.

Finally, there is the area in the medial aspect of the frontal lobe—specifically the right inferior frontal gyrus (57)—that, although described initially as an inhibitory area (59), seems to facilitate or inhibit voiding according to circumstances. Thus, it would appear, this area of the frontal lobe can facilitate the

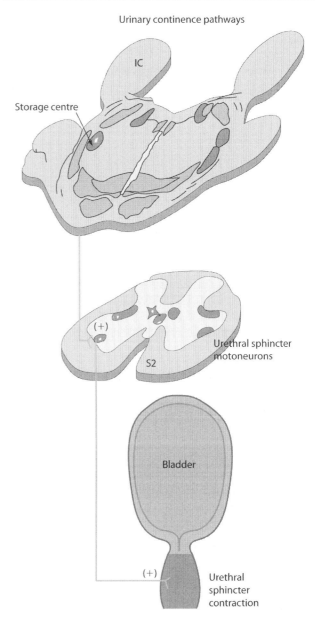

Urinary continence pathways

IC

Storage centre

(+)

S2

Urethral sphincter motoneurons

Bladder

(+)

Urethral sphincter contraction

Figure 31 Schematic diagram of the spinal and supraspinal structure and their pathways involved in bladder control problems.

nucleus locus coeruleus to cause voiding when the bladder is only partially full and afferent activity is therefore subthreshold. This is the way in which the bladder can be emptied before going to bed or before undertaking a long journey to avoid, perhaps, the need to void during the night or the journey. Equally, if afferent activity has reached a threshold level but there is a good program on the television, then this area of the frontal lobe can suppress the need to void until a more appropriate time.

The details of our understanding of the spinal cord mechanisms involved in voiding are sparse—in the brain, our knowledge of the mechanisms involved in continence and voiding is scant indeed.

THE NORMAL BLADDER FILLING-VOIDING CYCLE

So far, a summary has been given of our anatomical and physiological knowledge peripherally in the bladder and urethra themselves and then centrally within the nervous system. It has been seen that the most important reflex arcs are mediated through the nucleus locus coeruleus in the rostral pons; that excitatory neurotransmission in the normal human is exclusively cholinergic, and specifically muscarinic in origin; that relaxation of the bladder neck and urethral smooth muscle is probably mediated through the action of nitric oxide; and that the intrinsic rhabdosphincter is the most important component of the sphincter mechanism for continence and must be reciprocally relaxed through a coordinating mechanism in the rostral pons for normal voiding to occur. However, these issues and the other matters discussed do not explain all that we need to know about normal continence and voiding.

It is apparent during the normal filling and voiding cycle of a cystometrogram, with synchronous measurement of pressure within the sphincter-active urethra (Fig. 32), that bladder pressure stays almost completely unchanged throughout filling to a normal capacity despite an increasing afferent stimulus. Indeed, in health, the bladder is quiescent for over 99.5% of the day. There is, however, a small but definite rise in intraurethral pressure that is volume related. Then, just before or synchronous with the onset of voiding, there is a drop in intraurethral pressure, matched by a cessation of the electromyographic activity of the intrinsic rhabdosphincter, after which or synchronous with which detrusor pressure starts to rise (14). This rise in pressure is then sustained until the bladder is empty, by which time detrusor pressure has returned to normal and urethral resistance has risen back to normal. The cycle then starts over again.

WHAT KEEPS THE BLADDER PRESSURE LOW DURING FILLING?

This ability of the bladder to keep its pressure almost unchanging irrespective of bladder volume and afferent stimulation is known as compliance. The bladder is highly compliant: it shows very little change in pressure for a substantial change in volume. A steady rise in pressure during filling, which is sometimes seen when the bladder wall is "stiff" because of disease, is known as low compliance or poor compliance.

The exact nature of normal bladder compliance is not clear, but it can be observed to be present in the bladder post-mortem, at least up to a certain filling volume (60). This has been explained on the basis of the physical characteristics of the protein fibers that constitute the cellular and connective tissue structures of the bladder wall. They can be imagined as being coiled in the collapsed bladder and filling simply uncoils them, at least until 100 to 200 mL of filling has occurred (Fig. 33). Detrusor smooth muscle cells have a striking ability to change their length without

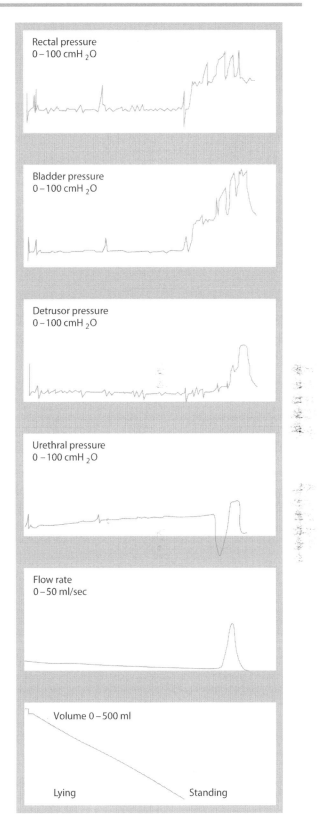

Figure 32 Synchronous urethral and bladder pressure studies to show the urethra pressurized during bladder filling and pressure fall before the onset of detrusor contraction. *Source*: From Ref. 31.

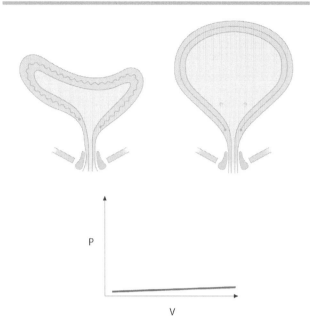

Figure 33 The contribution of passive properties of the bladder wall to normal bladder compliance. *Source*: From Ref. 31.

any change in tension. They may lengthen as much as fourfold during bladder filling, in a linear relationship with increasing bladder radius.

Our understanding of what happens over and beyond this elastic component and a certain "visco-elastic" property of the bladder is due to the work of de Groat and his coworkers, who have studied this mechanism in great detail in the cat (61). In a series of elegant experiments, de Groat has shown that there is a "gating" mechanism in the parasympathetic ganglia of the pelvic plexuses, which means that subthreshold activity in the preganglionic neurons is not transmitted to postganglionic efferent neurons (Fig. 34). There is also an inhibitory interneuron mechanism within the spinal cord that helps to keep afferent impulses from being transmitted onward until they reach a critical level. At low levels of afferent activity, the inhibitory

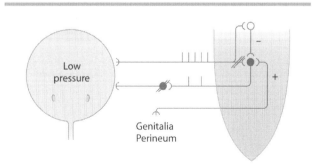

Figure 34 The "gating" mechanism by which, with minor degrees of activity in the afferent and preganglionic efferent nerves, there is no transmission to postganglionic efferent nerves.

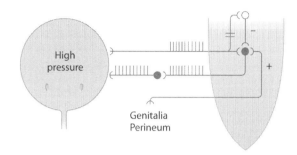

Figure 35 The "gating" mechanism showing that, with threshold afferent and preganglionic efferent activity, efferent activity is transmitted to postganglionic neurons.

interneurons prevent the transmission of impulses from the afferent nerves to the preganglionic efferent nerves. As afferent activity builds up, the inhibitory interneurons are progressively inhibited and impulses start to appear in the preganglionic efferent neurons, but the gating mechanism prevents these from being transmitted to the postganglionic efferent neurons until preganglionic efferent activity has reached a critical "threshold" level. When this level is reached, a barrage of impulses is then transmitted down the postganglionic efferent neuron to the bladder, which therefore contracts (Fig. 35).

In addition, there are the inhibitory effects of the sympathetic neurons that have postganglionic branches ending on parasympathetic ganglion cells, as mentioned earlier in the chapter. The afferent fibers are presumably those that arise in the trigone, conveying fullness of the bladder and running up to the thoracolumbar cord, where the local relay gives rise to efferent sympathetic activity that tends to inhibit neurotransmission across the parasympathetic ganglia of the pelvic plexuses, thereby enhancing de Groat's gating mechanism (Fig. 36).

WHAT CAUSES THE RISE IN URETHRAL PRESSURE DURING BLADDER FILLING?

This appears to be due to local reflex activity within the sacral cord by which afferent impulses from the bladder cause a local reflex rise in efferent activity to the urethral smooth muscle. It is thought to be spinal because it persists after complete spinal cord transection above the level of the sacral segments. Other than that, the mechanism is unclear.

WHAT CAUSES THE FALL IN URETHRAL PRESSURE AT THE ONSET OF VOIDING?

The mechanism of this is not clear either, but it has regularly been observed that intraurethral pressure drops to a degree that indicates that both the smooth and the striated components of the urethral sphincter mechanism are relaxed (14). Cessation of rhabdosphincter electromyogram activity synchronous with

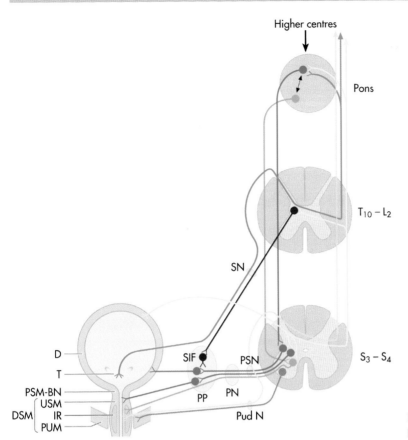

Figure 36 The action of sympathetic fibers. ─, on parasympathetic ganglia. *Source*: From Ref. 31.

the fall in urethral pressure has also been observed to support this conclusion. This possibly explains why the most urgent sense of a very full bladder is more a urethral than a bladder sensation, transmitted through the pudendal nerve. It seems, in fact, that the urethral sphincter mechanism is reflexly opening, and only voluntary contraction of the pelvic floor and suppression of the micturition reflex can stop it occurring. It seems, therefore, that at this point there has been threshold activation of the efferent cell bodies in the nucleus locus coeruleus and only positive intervention by higher centers to suppress the process can prevent the urethra from relaxing and stop reflex detrusor contraction from following.

HOW DOES THE BLADDER NECK OPEN?

There have been several theories to account for this. It used to be thought that there was a reciprocal innervation of the bladder by the parasympathetic system and of the bladder neck by the sympathetic system and that when the one caused contraction the other caused relaxation (Fig. 37) (62), but that was discounted when the role of the sympathetic system in the lower urinary tract was effectively ruled out, as discussed above. With the recent discovery of the role of nitric oxide, however, this reciprocal innervation theory has been resuscitated, although not in so many words. Nitric oxide may be cotransmitted

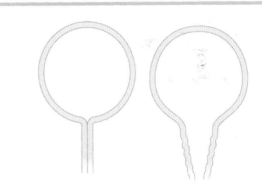

Figure 37 Diagrammatic representation of the theory of "reciprocal innervation."

with acetylcholine and it may be that the acetylcholine component causes contraction of the detrusor smooth muscle, whereas at the bladder neck and in the urethra there is a dominant nitric oxide effect released from the same type of neurons, which causes bladder neck and urethral relaxation. This does not explain the relaxation of the intrinsic rhabdosphincter, but if one presupposes that relaxation of the rhabdosphincter is a necessary precondition for detrusor contraction to occur, then bladder neck and urethral smooth muscle relaxation at the onset of detrusor contraction is all that is left to explain.

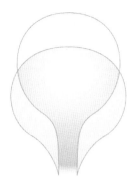

Figure 38 Diagrammatic representation of Lapides' theory of bladder neck opening.

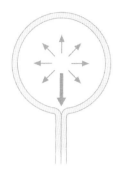

Figure 40 A simple hydrokinetic explanation of bladder neck opening.

Another explanation popularized by Lapides (63) (Fig. 38) was that the bladder neck and the urethral musculature were continuous and fixed like a system of guy ropes at the urogenital diaphragm. Contraction therefore caused shortening, which therefore caused opening of the bladder neck. This theory was never widely held and was eventually discounted by the demonstration that the urogenital diaphragm did not exist.

The next theory to explain bladder neck opening was Hutch's "base plate" theory (Fig. 39) (64). This was based on the importance of the trigonal musculature and of certain bands of detrusor smooth muscle that acted to trip open the base plate of the bladder neck, but the presence of such layers and bands has never been demonstrated convincingly by anybody else and so this theory, too, has been discounted.

There is the simple hydrokinetic observation that there is only actually one way out of the bladder and that is through the bladder neck, so that when the detrusor contracts, the force is likely to be transmitted in that direction (Fig. 40). It may well be that this simplistic point of view is at least in part correct, perhaps in conjunction with the reciprocal relaxation

theory modified to incorporate the action of nitric oxide rather than the sympathetic nervous system. In addition, it should be noted that it has been observed in spinal cord-injured patients fitted with a sacral anterior root stimulator that the bladder neck can be made to open and close separately from events in the main body of the detrusor, indicating that there may be a separate innervation to the bladder neck (Giles Brindley, personal communication). Clearly, as it can only be demonstrated in this way and then only under certain circumstances and in some patients, this innervation cannot readily be dissected out from innervation of the bladder as a whole, but again it would tend to support the reciprocal innervation theory, with the corelease of nitric oxide in the sphincter-active area to explain opening coincident with cholinergic-mediated detrusor contraction.

VESICOURETHRAL REFLEXES

As many as 12 "micturition reflexes" have been described, largely following the descriptions by Barrington earlier this century (55) and by Kuru more

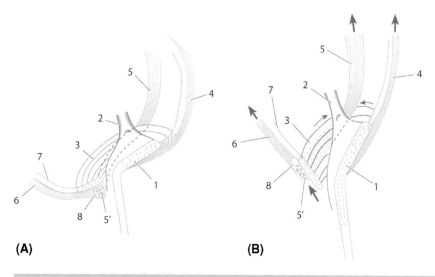

(A)   **(B)**

Figure 39 (**A, B**) Diagrammatic representation of Hutch's theory of bladder neck opening. Figures refer to hypothetical muscle bundles identified by Hutch. *Source*: From Ref. 9.

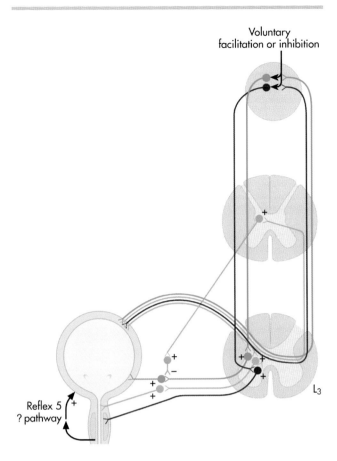

Voluntary
facilitation or inhibition

Reflex 5
? pathway

L₃

Figure 41 Diagram to show the bladder reflexes described in this chapter. ——, reflex 1; ——, reflex 2; ——, reflex 3; ——, reflex 4. *Source*: From Ref. 31.

recently (65). Some of these are only active in experimental animals subject to various neural ablation procedures and at least one of them is the genital reflex of closing off the bladder neck to ensure antegrade ejaculation. Some have been observed in animals but not in humans. So far in this chapter, reference has been made to four reflexes (Fig. 41). The first is the afferent impulse routed up to the pons to cause the parasympathetic efferent contraction of the bladder of sufficient amplitude and duration to give complete bladder emptying; and the second is that which causes reciprocal relaxation of the intrinsic rhabdosphincter to allow unobstructed voiding. The third is the local spinal reflex increase in urethral pressure during bladder filling. The fourth reflex is the one that causes sympathetic inhibition of parasympathetic ganglionic transmission in the pelvic plexuses with more advanced degrees of bladder filling.

There is, therefore, one local sacral reflex causing a rise in urethral pressure during filling, and one thoracolumbar reflex causing sympathetic inhibition of ganglionic transmission in the parasympathetic innervation to the bladder, thereby supporting de Groat's gating mechanism that keeps the bladder quiescent during filling. Then, there are the two pontine reflexes, the one to cause a bladder contraction of adequate

amplitude and duration and the second to coordinate this with reciprocal relaxation of the intrinsic rhabdosphincter.

In addition, there is a reflex facilitation that occurs during a detrusor contraction that is mediated by afferents in the pudendal nerve. The mechanism for this is unclear, but Brindley has noted that after pudendal blockade, the force of detrusor contraction is considerably reduced (66): hence, the afferent pathway can be identified as pudendal but the rest of the reflex is unclear.

This is not to say that other reflexes do not exist and particularly that other reflexes do not exist in disease, but these are the only ones that can be positively identified as being important in health.

SUMMARY

It will be apparent to the reader that there is a great deal to be learnt about the structure and even more about the function of the lower urinary tract, particularly about the spinal and supraspinal mechanisms that control it.

The fundamental features are that during bladder filling, intravesical pressure changes very little despite the bladder filling by 400 mL or more, and this "compliance" is achieved by a gating mechanism that prevents afferent neuronal activity being transmitted to postganglionic efferent activity until that afferent activity reaches a critical level. Critical afferent activity, probably originating in the myofibroblasts of the lamina propria of the bladder, is transmitted by ascending spinal pathways that synapse on cell bodies in the nucleus locus coeruleus in the rostral pons in addition to providing conscious awareness of bladder filling. When afferent activity to the nucleus locus coeruleus, subject to suprapontine facilitation or inhibition, reaches a threshold level, efferent activity is initiated, mediated through the pelvic parasympathetic nerves and muscarinic receptors. This causes a detrusor contraction of sufficient amplitude and duration to give complete bladder emptying and a synchronous coordinated reciprocal relaxation of the urethral sphincter mechanism to allow unobstructed voiding until the bladder is empty. It seems clear that excitatory neurotransmission in the normal human detrusor is exclusively cholinergic, and it is becoming increasingly clear that reciprocal relaxation of the urethral sphincter is a prerequisite for detrusor contraction, and that the synchronous relaxation of the bladder neck and urethral smooth muscle is probably mediated by nitric oxide, which is cotransmitted with acetylcholine from postganglionic parasympathetic neurons. Unfortunately, although this fundamental mechanism appears reasonably clear, a lot of the details are lacking at present.

REFERENCES

1. Uhlenhuth E, Hunter DT, Loechel WE. Problems in the Anatomy of the Pelvis. Philadelphia: Lippincott, 1953.
2. Mundy AR. Urodynamic and Reconstructive Surgery of the Lower Urinary Tract. Edinburgh: Churchill Livingstone, 1993.

3. Gosling JA, Dixon JS, Humpherson JR. The Functional Anatomy of the Urinary Tract. Edinburgh: Churchill Livingstone, 1983.

4. Chilton CP. The urethra. In: Webster G, Kirby R, King L, et al., eds. Reconstructive Urology. Cambridge: Blackwell Scientific, 1993:59–73.

5. Zacharin RF. The anatomical supports of the female urethra. Obstet Gynaecol 1968; 32:754–759.

6. Walsh PC, Partin AW. Anatomic radical retropubic prostatectomy. In: Wein AJ, Kavoussi LR, Novick AC, et al., eds. Campbell—Walsh Urology. 9th ed. Philadelphia: Saunders, 2007:2956–2978.

7. Redman JF. Anatomy of the genitourinary system. In: Gillenwater JR, Grayhack JT, Howards SS, et al., eds. Adult and Pediatric Urology. 3rd ed. Philadelphia: Mosby, 1996:3–61.

8. Kaye KW, Milne N, Creed K, et al. The urogenital diaphragm external urethral sphincter and radical prostatectomy. Aust N Z J Surg 1997; 67:40–44.

9. Hutch JA. Anatomy and Physiology of the Bladder, Trigone and Urethra. London: Butterworths, 1972.

10. Gosling J. The structure of the bladder and urethra in relation to function. Urol Clin North Am 1979; 6:31–38.

11. Dixon J, Gosling J. Structure and innervation in the human. In: Torrens M, Morrison FB, eds. The Physiology of the Lower Urinary Tract. London: Springer Verlag, 1987:3–22.

12. Raz S, Caine M, Zeigler M. The vascular component in the production of intraurethral pressure. J Urol 1972; 108:93–96.

13. Sundin T, Dahlstrom A, Norlen L, et al. The sympathetic innervation and adrenoreceptor function of the human lower urinary tract in the normal state and after parasympathetic denervation. Invest Urol 1977; 14:322–328.

14. Tanagho EA. The anatomy and physiology of micturition. Clin Obstet Gynaecol 1978; 5:3–26.

15. James MJ. Relaxation of the human detrusor. University of Nottingham, MD Thesis, 1993.

16. Bridgewater M, MacNeil HF, Brading AF. Regulation of tone in pig urethral smooth muscle. J Urol 1993; 150:223–228.

17. de Groat WC, Fraser MO, Yoshiyama M, et al. Neural control of the urethra. Scand J Urol Nephrol Suppl 2001; 207:35–43.

18. Gosling JA, Dixon JS, Critchely HOD, et al. A comparative study of the human external sphincter and periurethral levator ani muscles. Br J Urol 1981; 53:35–41.

19. Schroder HD. Onuf's nucleus X: a morphological study of a human spinal nucleus. Anat Embryol (Berl) 1981; 162:443–453.

20. Zrara P, Carrier S, Kour NW, et al. The detailed neuroanatomy of the human striated urethral sphincter. Br J Urol 1994; 74:182–187.

21. Wiseman OJ, Fowler CJ, Landon DN. The role of the human bladder lamina propria myofibroblast. BJU Int 2003; 91:89–93.

22. Sui GP, Rothery S, Dupont E, et al. Gap junctions and connexin expression in human suburothelial interstitial cells. BJU Int 2002; 90(1):118–129.

23. Wu C, Sui GP, Fry CH. Purinergic regulation of guinea pig suburothelial myofibroblasts. J Physiol 2004; 559:231–243.

24. Fowler CJ, Griffiths D, de Groat WC. The neural control of micturition. Nat Rev Neurosci 2008; 9(6):453–466.

25. Kirkham APS, Mundy AR, Heald RJ, et al. Cadaveric dissection for the rectal surgeon. Ann R Coll Surg Engl 2001; 83:89–95.

26. Mundy AR. An anatomical explanation for bladder dysfunction following rectal and uterine surgery. Br J Urol 1982; 54:501–504.

27. Gosling JA, Dixon JS. Anatomy of the bladder, urethra and pelvic floor. In: Mundy AR, Stephenson TP, Wein AJ, eds. Urodynamics—Principles, Practice and Application. Edinburgh: Churchill Livingstone, 1984.

28. Burnstock G. Autonomic innervation and transmission. Br Med Bull 1979; 35:255–262.

29. Goodman SR. Medical Cell Biology. Philadelphia: JB Lippincott, 1994.

30. Burnstock G. The changing face of autonomic transmission. Acta Physiol Scand 1986; 126:67–91.

31. Mundy AR, Thomas PJ. Clinical physiology of the bladder, urethra and pelvic floor. In: Mundy AR, Stephenson TP, Wein AJ, eds. Urodynamics—Principles, Practice and Application. 2nd ed. Edinburgh: Churchill Livingstone, 1994.

32. Brading AF. Physiology of the urinary tract smooth muscle. In: Webster G, Kirby R, King L, et al., eds. Reconstructive Urology. Cambridge: Blackwell Scientific, 1993:15–26.

33. Brindley GS, Craggs MD. The effect of atropine in the urinary bladder of the baboon and of man. J Physiol 1975; 255:55P.

34. Kinder RB, Mundy AR. Atropine blockade of nerve-mediated stimulation of the human detrusor. Br J Urol 1985; 57:418–421.

35. Sibley GA. An experimental model of detrusor instability in the obstructed pig. Br J Urol 1985; 57:292–298.

36. Alm P, Alumets J, Brodin E, et al. Peptidergic (substance P) nerves in the genito-urinary tract. Neuroscience 1978; 3:419–425.

37. Maggi CA, Barbanti G, Santicioli P, et al. Cystometric evidence that capsaicin sensitive nerves modulate the afferent branch of the micturition reflex in humans. J Urol 1989; 142:150–154.

38. Gu J, Restorick J, Blank MA, et al. Vasoactive intestinal polypeptide in the normal and unstable bladder. Br J Urol 1983; 55:645–647.

39. Alm P, Alumets J, Hakenson R, et al. Peptidergic (vasoactive intestinal peptide) nerves in the genito-urinary tract. Neuroscience 1977; 2:751–754.

40. Bennett BC, Kruse MN, Roppolo JR, et al. Neural control of urethral outlet activity in vivo: role of nitric oxide. J Urol 1995; 153:2004–2009.

41. Andersson KE, Arner A. Urinary bladder contraction and relaxation: physiology and pathophysiology. Physiol Rev 2004; 84:935–986.

42. Fetscher C, Fleichman M, Schmidt M, et al. M(3) muscarinic receptors mediate contraction of human urinary bladder. Br J Pharmacol 2002; 136:641–643.

43. Somogyi GT, Zernova GV, Yoshiyama M, et al. Frequency dependence of muscarinic facilitation of transmitter release in urinary bladder strips from nerally intact or chronic spinal cord transected rats. Br J Pharmacol 1998; 125:241–246.

44. Fergusson DR, Kennedy I, Burton TJ. ATP release from rabbit urinary bladder epithelial cells by hydrostatic pressure change – a possible sensory mechanism. J Physiol 1997; 505:503.

45. de Groat WC. Spinal cord projections and neuropeptides in visceral afferent neurons. Prog Brain Res 1986; 67:165–188.

46. Hawthorn MH, Chapple CR, Cock M, et al. Urothelium-derived inhibitory factor(s) influences on detrusor muscle contractility in vitro. Br J Pharmacol 2000; 129:416–419.

47. de Groat WC. The urothelium in overactive bladder: passive bystander or active participant? Urology 2004; (suppl 1):7–11.

48. Lincoln J, Burnstock G. Autonomic innervation of the urinary bladder and urethra. In: Maggi CA, ed. Nervous Control of the Urogenital System. London: Harwood Academic Publishers, 1993:33–68.

49. Habler HJ, Janig W, Koltzenburg M. Activation of unmyelinated afferent fibres by mechanical stimuli and inflammation of the urinary bladder in the cat. J Physiol 1990; 425:545–562.

50. Wen J, Morrison JFB. Sensitisation of pelvic afferent neurones from the rat bladder. J Auton Nerv Sys 1996; 58:187.

51. Nathan PW. Sensations associated with micturition. Br J Urol 1956; 28:126–131.

52. Nathan PW. The central nervous connections of bladder. In: Chisholm GD, Williams DI, eds. Scientific Foundation of Urology. London: Heinemann, 1976.

53. MacMahon SB, Morrison JFB. Spinal neurones with long projections activated from the abdominal viscera of the cat. J Physiol 1982; 332:1–20.

54. Sillen U. Central neurotransmitter mechanisms involved in the control of urinary bladder function. Scand J Urol Nephrol Suppl 1980; 58:1–45.

55. Barrington FJF. The effect of lesions on the hind and midbrain on micturition in the cat. Q J Exp Physiol 1915; 15:181–202.

56. Blok BFM, Holstege G. The central control of micturition and continence: implications for urology. BJU Int 1999; 83(suppl 2):1–6.

57. Kavia R, Dasgupta R, Fowler CJ. Functional imaging and central control of the bladder. J Comp Neurol 2005; 493:27–32.

58. Hess WR. The Functional Organisation of the Diencephalon. London: Grune & Stratton, 1957.

59. Andrew J, Nathan PW. Lesions of the anterior frontal lobes and disturbances of micturition and defecation. Brain 1964; 87:233–261.

60. Tang PC, Ruch TC. Non-neurogenic basis of bladder tonus. Am J Physiol 1955; 181:249–257.

61. de Groat WC. Physiology of the urinary bladder and urethra. Ann Int Med 1980; 92:312–315.

62. Denny-Brown D, Robertson EG. On the physiology of micturition. J Physiol 1933; 56:149–190.

63. Lapides J. Structure and function of the internal vesical sphincter. J Urol 1958; 80:341–353.

64. Hutch J. A new theory of the anatomy of the internal urinary sphincter and the physiology of micturition. Invest Urol 1965; 3:36–58.

65. Kuru M. Nervous control of micturition. Physiol Rev 1965; 45:425–494.

66. Brindley GS, Craggs MD. The pressure exerted by the external sphincter of the urethra when its motor nerve fibres are stimulated electrically. Br J Urol 1974; 46:453–462.

15

Physiological Properties of the Lower Urinary Tract

Christopher H. Fry

Postgraduate Medical School, University of Surrey, Guildford, U.K.

INTRODUCTION

Since the last edition of the *Scientific Basis of Urology*, there has been considerable progress in our elemental understanding of lower urinary tract (LUT) physiology. The previous edition included two chapters LUT physiology—one on detrusor physiology and the other on detrusor pathophysiology. With advancing knowledge it has become clear that it is increasingly difficult to discuss one without the other. Moreover, while detrusor smooth muscle behavior may be the "end organ," which generates measurable changes such as overactivity or incontinence, the urothelium and suburothelium appear to be at least as important as the muscle itself in determining the contractile properties of the LUT.

THE UROTHELIUM, BARRIER FUNCTIONS, AND BACTERIAL INFECTIONS

Structure of the Urothelium and Suburothelium

The urothelium is a transitional epithelium and its barrier function, to separate underlying tissues of the bladder wall from urine, has long been appreciated. The cells have a high turnover rate, therefore, if damaged, the barrier function is maintained. However, it is more than a mere passive barrier and additionally has transport as well as sensory/signaling (section "Secretory and Signaling Properties of the Urothelium/Suburothelium") functions. Figure 1 shows a cross-section of the bladder wall consisting of four layers: urothelium, suburothelium, detrusor, and serosa. For consideration of transport and barrier properties, the urothelium can be considered alone; however, when sensory/signaling properties are discussed the urothelium and suburothelium seem to form a single integrated structure. The inset in Figure 1 shows in more detail the urothelium/suburothelium layer: in the suburothelium is embedded a functional syncitium of interstitial cells observed as the cell network in the figure, as well as a capillary network and unmyelinated and myelinated nerves.

The urothelium has three layers in

1. an apical (umbrella) cell layer with a very low permeability to urine and pathogens,
2. an intermediate layer, and

3. a basal layer (lamina propria) that interacts with the extracellular matrix of the suburothelial region for structural support.

The apical cells have several important characteristics.

1. 70% to 90% of the apical surface area is covered by protein plaques separated by lipid membrane called the *hinge area*. Each plaque contains about 1000 subunits composed of an inner ring of six large, and an outer ring of six smaller particles (1). The subunits are formed from five proteins collectively called *uroplakins*, two of which have four transmembrane domains (UPIa and UPIb), while the others are type 1 transmembrane proteins (UPII, UPIIIa, and UPIIIb). UPIa associates with UPII, and UPIb associates with UPIIIa or UPIIIb.
2. Their cytoplasm has a high density of fusiform vesicles, formed by two apposing plaques joined together by hinge membrane. The vesicles and surface membrane plaques are joined by a network of cytoplasmic filaments that attach to tight junctions at the apical/lateral membrane interface, and desmosomes in the basolateral membrane (2). Their function is considered below.
3. Umbrella cells are joined by tight junctions. Solute movement across the urothelium can be through the cell (transcellular) or through the tight junction and the lateral intercellular space (paracellular) pathway. The tight junctions ensure that this urothelial layer is the major impedance for the movement of substances from urine to plasma.

Whether alterations in uroplakin expression relate to urinary tract disease is unclear. Ablation of the uroplakin-II gene in mice (3) or loss of uroplakin expression in myelomeningocele patients (4) led to hyperplastic urothelial growth and may interfere with smooth muscle development. UPIII expression is also a prognostic factor in patients with upper urinary tract urothelial carcinoma (5).

Storage Properties of the Bladder: Role of the Urothelium

Addition of cytoplasmic vesicles into the apical membrane during bladder filling and their removal during

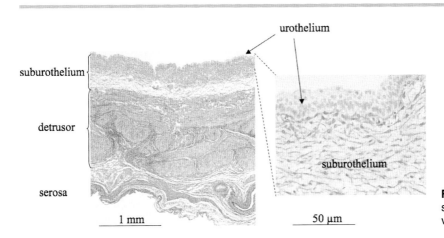

Figure 1 Cross-section of the bladder wall showing the principal layers; right is an expanded view of the suburothelial layer.

contraction (6,7) minimizes the surface to volume ratio of the bladder and hence the flux of substances over the urothelium. Recent studies have shown that stretch to either apical or basolateral membrane exerts opposite effects (8). Stretch also increases protein secretion into the urine, raises cell cAMP levels (7), and stimulates ATP release into the blood side (9) (the latter is also considered in section "Secretory and Signaling Properties of the Urothelium/Suburothelium"). Release of ATP results in its binding to purinergic (P2X) receptors on the basolateral membrane of the apical cells and stimulates an increase in the intracellular $[Ca^{2+}]$, $[Ca^{2+}]_i$, which in turn stimulates vesicle fusion (7,10). Raised $[Ca^{2+}]_i$ is also induced by capsaicin and blocked by the vanilloid receptor antagonists. The molecular basis of vesicle fusion shares many features with synaptic vesicle fusion. The apical membrane and the fusiform/discoidal vesicles contain SNAP 23 and SNARES—synaptobrevin and syntaxin. Another key component for synaptic vesicle fusion is the Rab proteins, with Rab 27b found in umbrella cells (11).

Urothelial Permeability and Transport

The urothelium is very impermeable to major ions in urine (Na^+, K^+, and Cl^-) (12), with an electrical resistance some 15,000 to 20,000 time that of the proximal tubule epithelium. Both the tight junctions and transcellular routes contribute significantly to this resistance. This low transport of ions means that urine composition does not change greatly during storage. Uroplakins may contribute to the low solute and water permeability of the urothelium. With UPIII knockout mice, water fluxes were twofold greater, although transepithelial resistance, rate of ion transport, and urea fluxes were not different (13).

It has also been proposed that a glycosaminoglycan (GAG) layer on the apical membrane represents a major permeability barrier to small electrolytes and nonelectrolytes and that derangement of the barrier contributes to bladder pathologies such as painful bladder syndrome (14). The GAG layer is a multicharged anionic polysaccharide that is supposed to trap water and hence hinder diffusion to the apical

cells. However, the evidence is not entirely convincing for the following reasons:

- There is no significant electrical resistance across the GAG layer; the Na^+ channel blocker amiloride rapidly diffuses through the GAG layer and blocks apical Na^+ channels.
- Alteration of luminal $[Na^+]$ rapidly alters membrane transport.
- Enzymatic cleavage of GAG does not alter ion transepithelial permeability (13).

The mammalian urothelium has a transepithelial potential (-20 to -120 mV, apical surface negative) (12,15), with Na^+ the predominant transported ion. Na^+ transport is blocked by the epithelial Na^+ channel (ENaC) blocker amiloride, applied to the apical face, and more slowly by ouabain on the basolateral face to block the Na pump. The rate of transepithelial Na^+ transport mirrors the permeability of the apical membrane to Na^+; amiloride decreases and aldosterone increases Na^+ permeability. The presence of Na^+ channels in the apical membrane of mammalian urothelium as well as in cytoplasmic vesicles has been confirmed by immunohistochemistry (16). The exit of intracellular Na^+ across the basolateral membrane via the Na/K ATPase raises cell $[K^+]$ to 70 to 90 mM (17,18), which subsequently leaves through K^+ channels in the same membrane (19).

In addition to the amiloride-sensitive Na^+ channel, the apical membrane contains three other channels: a stretch-activated channel (20), permeable to Na^+ and K^+ and blocked by high amiloride concentrations (>100 μM)—two degradation products of the amiloride-sensitive channel; a nonselective, amiloride-insensitive cation channel (21); and a separate nonselective ion channel. The basolateral membrane contains, in addition to the Na/K ATPase and K^+ channel, a large (64 pS) Cl^- conductance (22) that is responsible for the passive distribution of Cl^- under physiological conditions and is also permeable to HCO_3. These cells also regulate their volume during osmotic stress (23). A raised basolateral extracellular osmolality results in cell shrinkage and a decrease in basolateral membrane K^+ and Cl^- permeability and activation of Na^+/H^+ and Cl^-/HCO_3^- exchangers. The net effect, in concert with Na/K ATPase activity, increases cell $[K^+]$ and $[Cl^-]$ and hence water flux to restore cell volume. Water movement across the basolateral membrane is also facilitated by aquaporins (24).

Uropathogenic Bacteria

Uropathogenic *Escherichia coli* (UPEC) is the most common causative agent for urinary tract infections in women (5). UPEC have part of their pathogenic cycle as an intracellular phase within urothelial cells where replication and formation of bacterial communities occurs before exiting the host cell (25). Cellular invasion is facilitated by adhesive fibers—type I pili (26). Thus, UPEC can form intracellular bacterial reservoirs that persist for several weeks and may be resistant to antibiotics. Much of this work has been carried out on animal models; however, intracellular bacterial communities from exfoliated urothelial cells have also been detected in the urine of patients (27).

FUNCTIONS OF THE LOWER URINARY TRACT: TENSION AND PRESSURE

The LUT has two functions: to store and periodically void urine. To achieve these functions various regions of the LUT have different physical states.

Filling: The bladder wall is highly compliant (low wall stress), coupled to a high outflow resistance.
Voiding: The bladder wall stress is high, coupled to a low outflow resistance.

These physical properties depend in large measure on changes to the physical (biomechanical) properties of LUT tissues.

Before considering the physiological background to contraction and relaxation in the LUT, it is essential to understand the relationship between wall tension and intraluminal pressure. Muscles lining any hollow organ exhibit a state of tension, T, because of either physical stretch of the tissue (passive tension) or contraction of the muscular elements (active tension). The most important tensile component is that tangential to the wall of the organ. The manifestation of this wall tension (stress) is a pressure, P, within the lumen. However, the relationship between T and P is not linear, but depends on the radius of the organ, r, and the wall thickness, d (Laplace's law).

$$P = 2Td/r \qquad (1)$$

Thus, a large sphere generating the same unit wall tension as a smaller sphere will produce a smaller pressure change. This can lead to confusion when changes of pressure, regardless of the vessel size, are equated to changes of wall tension and muscle performance. Two situations exemplify the need to understand this interrelationship between pressure and wall tension.

1. *Changes to internal pressure by passively filling the bladder*: When pressure-volume relationships are generated during bladder filling plots are nonlinear

and crucially depend on the volumes used to fill the bladder. When normalized to wall tension versus changes to bladder radius, the plots are linearized, enabling more meaningful estimates of tissue compliance or stiffness (28).

2. *Estimation of active wall tension (muscle contractility) from internal pressure changes*: This has been attempted from urodynamic measurements to compare contractile properties of the bladder in patients with different pathologies (29,30). The approach is really only useful when the pressure is generated isovolumically (31), that is, energy is not also being used to move fluid. Figure 2A shows calculations of the change of pressure during the development of wall tension when a bladder is emptying, or remaining at constant volume. In the latter case more pressure develops as the bladder empties, because the radius is reducing as a function of time, despite contractile effort being similar in the two cases. Caution must be applied therefore in ascribing changes of luminal pressure purely to alterations of muscle contractility.

BIOMECHANICAL PROPERTIES OF THE BLADDER WALL

Passive and Active Properties

The bladder is composed of four major layers: urothelium; lamina propria; smooth muscle (detrusor) and an outer serosal layer. The biomechanical properties of the bladder wall are mainly determined by the connective tissues of the lamina propria and detrusor layers, as well as the detrusor itself. The detrusor layer, which is 60% to 70% of the thickness of the normal bladder wall, is composed of smooth muscle cells aligned in longitudinal and circumferential layers that are highly variable in cross-section, length and orientation and embedded in a collagen/elastin matrix. The passive tissue characteristics result from the viscoelastic properties of the collagen and elastin fibers in the extracellular matrices of the lamina propria and detrusor as well as the detrusor muscle cells themselves. The active properties result from contraction of the muscular structures within and surrounding the LUT and transmission of the resultant force via the extracellular and cellular tissues. Whether the high compliance of the filling bladder is merely an absence of muscular contraction or is contributed by active muscle relaxation remains a subject of debate.

Passive Forces and Bladder Compliance

The stiffness of a body is the ratio of an applied force to the resulting change of dimension; the inverse parameter is compliance and is a measure of its "distensibility." In three dimensional terms pressures and volumes are substituted for force and distension, for example, bladder compliance (C) is the ratio of change to bladder volume, V, per change to unit intravesical pressure, P, that is, $C = \Delta V/\Delta P$. In principle, it is difficult to state a standard value for bladder

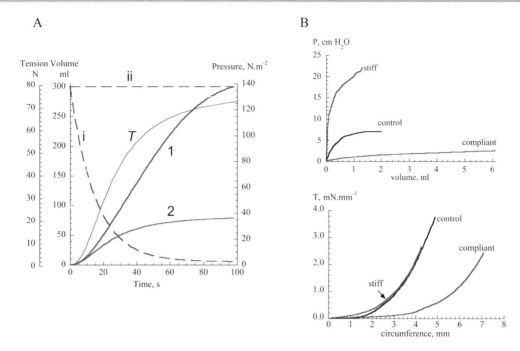

Figure 2   (**A**) Derived bladder pressure-time plots (1,2) as a result of an increase in wall tension, *T*, and calculated using Laplace's relationship for a thin-walled sphere, equation (1). The two pressure-time plots correspond either to a bladder emptying along the relationship shown in (*i*) curve 1, or at constant volume shown in (*ii*) curve 2. The *tension* and *volume* relationships are scaled by the left-hand side vertical axes and the *pressure* relationships scaled by the right-hand side verical axis. (**B**) *Upper plot*: Ex vivo experimental pressure-volume curves from three bladders, labeled "stiff," "control," and "compliant." The stiff and compliant curves were obtained from obstructed bladders and the control from an unobstructed bladder. *Lower plot*: Derived tension-length (circumference) curves from the above data using Laplace's law (see text for details); circumference was calculated from bladder volume assuming a spherical shape. *Source*: Adapted from Ref. 28.

compliance: bladder capacity increases with age whereas intravesical pressures are less variable; intravesical pressure itself is a function of bladder volume and thus compliance would vary as the bladder fills. Furthermore, compliance is a steady-state property and measurements must only be made when any stress-relaxation has fully subsided. Several approaches have been used to account for these confounding factors. Normalization factors have been introduced in urodynamic studies to correct for values obtained in different size bladders (32,33) and ex vivo, when nonlinear pressure-volume relationships have been transformed into linear stress-strain relationships (28), when more direct comparison can be made with data from tissue strips (Fig. 2B) (28,34).

Outflow tract obstruction has variable effects on bladder compliance: brief periods have little effect (35), but after longer periods compliance may either decrease (36,37) or increase (28,34,38). These different effects may result from the severity and duration of the obstruction. Decreased compliance will raise intravesical pressures for a given amount of filling and so initiate a micturition reflex at lower volumes. If maintained a significantly raised bladder pressure may cause upper tract damage (39). Conversely, if compliance is increased detrusor muscle contractions will be less effective in raising pressure and thus make voiding more difficult.

Stress Relaxation

Stress-relaxation is a viscoelastic feature of the whole bladder and isolated muscle strips and manifests as a partial reduction of stress (pressure or tension) after a rapid change of strain (volume or length). This is of benefit to the filling bladder as steady-state changes of pressure are minimized during filling. With urodynamic measurements it means that if a bladder is rapidly filled then changes to intravesical pressure may be greater than during slow-fill. Thus, rapid-fill would underestimate compliance, as it is a steady-state property. Measurement of pressure or tension should only be made when any stress-relaxation has finished. Stress-relaxation may reside from a rearrangement of the cellular and extracellular elements. In the over-compliant obstructed bladder the extent of stress-relaxation diminishes in the same proportion as steady-state stiffness (34). Because the proportion of extracellular material increases in these bladders this suggests that the phenomenon may reside in both the cellular and extracellular components.

Collagen and the Extracellular Matrix

The most significant extracellular components in determining the passive properties of LUT tissues are collagen (especially types I and III) and elastin

(40). In obstructed bladders collagen content is raised, particularly in the detrusor muscle layer, with an increased ratio of type III to type I reported in some (41–43). Collagen-I forms large fibers and predominates in tissues with high tensile strength, while collagen III, forming smaller fibers, imparts increased tissue flexibility and an ability to rearrange during bladder filling (44), which may be of importance to bladders undergoing hypertrophy. Collagen synthesis by cells is upregulated by physical stretch, which may provide the basic stimulus in bladder outflow obstruction (45). During bladder development the collagen III:I ratio shows an inverse relation to compliance (46); however, other geometrical factors, as mentioned above, will also determine compliance so that changing collagen ratio per se is only one factor, among many.

The nonenzymatic adduction (combination) of sugar to protein (glycation) is associated with diabetes and ageing and is a significant factor in damage to extracellular and cellular proteins by promoting cross-linking and aggregation. The formation of advanced glycation end-products increases tissue stiffness of (47). However, several studies have shown that bladder compliance actually increases in animal models of diabetes (48,49), so the role of glycation product formation remains unclear.

THE ACTIVE PROPERTIES OF MUSCLES IN THE LOWER URINARY TRACT

Interaction between contractile proteins in the muscle cell generates "active" tension that manifests itself as an increase of tension within the cell or a shortening of the muscle. If a muscle generates tension without shortening, this is termed an isometric contraction.

In a hollow organ, such as the bladder, such an increase of tension would be manifest as a rise of pressure (above). If the muscle shortens against a load, the contraction is termed isotonic.

Isometric Contractions and Length-Tension Relationships

All muscles exhibit a bell-shaped dependence for active force on initial resting length, that is, there is an optimum resting length, L_0, at which active force is maximal (Fig. 3A). However, this length-tension curve extends over a greater range of initial lengths for smooth compared with striated muscle and is particularly true of detrusor where passive extension much beyond L_0 does not greatly reduce force (50). Thus, large changes in bladder circumference will still permit adequate force development by individual myocytes and, when normalized to L_0, L-T relationships are similar in control and pathological organs (51).

Isotonic Contractions and Force-Velocity Relationships

In this case the muscle shortens against an opposing load, and observation shows that the heavier the load (and hence the force, F, opposing shortening) the slower is the initial velocity of shortening, v. The relationship between force and velocity was described by Hill (52) and is shown in Figure 3B:

$$(F + a) \cdot (v + b) = (F_0 + a) \cdot b \qquad (2)$$

where a and b are constants. Note that where the curve crosses the abscissa (F axis), the opposing load is so large that the muscle cannot shorten, and contraction becomes isometric. A characteristic of this curve is the

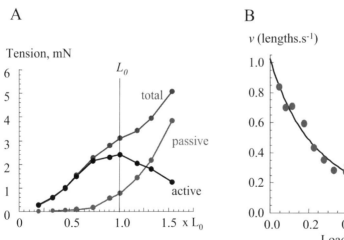
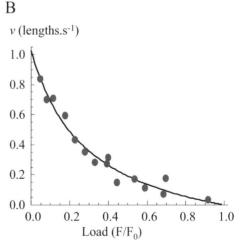

Figure 3 (**A**) Length-tension curve for a detrusor smooth muscle strip, in vitro. Active (peak twitch) force; passive, resting force and the sum of the two forces (total) are shown for contractions elicited at 16-Hz stimulation. Muscle forces are measured over a range of resting muscle lengths, normalized to the length (L_0) at which maximum active force was generated. (**B**) Force-velocity curve for a shortening smooth muscle strip subject to different loads, F. The load is normalized to the maximum load, F_0, above which shortening can no longer occur (i.e., an isometric contraction). Shortening rate is expressed in muscle lengths per second. The line is a fit of equation (2) and extrapolated to the v and F/F_0 axes.

extrapolation to a maximum velocity of shortening at zero load, V_0, as this is related to the maximum frequency of cross-bridge cycling (see below). This curve bears a resemblance, but only superficial, to the pressure-flow plots obtained in urodynamics (53) but have been used by some to estimate the contractile state of the bladder (54). However, such extrapolations should be treated with caution as the relationship between pressure-flow measurements and force-velocity determinations is not linear for the same dimensional reasons as discussed above when considering Laplace's law.

The Contractile State

There is lack of agreement whether absolute force (normalized to cross-sectional area) varies in samples from normal and pathological bladders. This is important, as it is necessary to know if conditions such as detrusor underactivity or overactivity are mirrored by changes to the contractile state of detrusor muscle. Alternatively, these conditions may be because of other causes such as alteration to the proportion of muscle in a bladder sample, the extent of functional innervation, or the physical properties of the extracellular matrix. Therefore, in this respect care must be exercised in the interpretation of experimental data, as contractile responses evoked by agents such as muscarinic receptor agonists may give different responses compared with nerve-mediated responses. Some animal models of bladder obstruction suggest contractile failure (34,55), but not in all cases (28) and it is possible that failure is a feature of later growth when a decompensated, more compliant bladder is generated by obstruction. The most obvious clinical correlate for this is the "valve" bladder—in which all the clinical manifestations expected from the above changes can be seen, and in a few patients, a progression may be demonstrable. It remains far more difficult to predict those in whom progression, or not, will occur or those in whom the diseased bladder function plateaus. With human detrusor there is little evidence that detrusor contractility is different in normal and overactive bladders (56).

Energetics of Contraction and Bladder Blood Flow

Compared with skeletal and cardiac (striated) muscle, smooth muscle exhibits high economy, as contractions can be maintained for a relatively long period with a lower ATP consumption than in the initial stages of force development. However, to perform external work (work = force × distance), smooth muscle has a lower efficiency than striated muscle. Efficiency is the work produced per unit change of free energy for the driving chemical reaction, that is, ATP hydrolysis, and is about 5 compared with 20 kJ/mol for smooth and striated muscle, respectively (57). One reason for this decreased efficiency may be that in smooth muscle ATP is needed not just for cross-bridge cycling but also to phosphorylate the myosin light chain (see below) (58).

A particular feature of smooth muscle metabolism is that oxidative metabolism and lactate production occur together and their respective rates are not correlated. In some smooth muscles, force development and O_2 consumption are closely correlated, whereas lactate production is associated with other ATP-consuming processes such as the Na pump (59). This has led to the suggestion that metabolism is functionally compartmentalized, with O_2 consumption above basal levels directed toward meeting the needs for ATP consumption associated with contraction. The relevance of this metabolic division to detrusor muscle has not been tested.

A decrease in bladder blood flow occurs during filling, and is associated with tissue hypoxia and acidosis (60,61). It is assumed that these changes occur because the bladder wall is stretched and the blood vessels occluded. In the hypertrophied bladder, angiogenesis does not keep pace with increased muscle growth so that such ischemic conditions would be exacerbated. Tissue hypoxia has complex effects on detrusor contractility, which may contribute to overactive behavior. In the short term, there is an increase of detrusor contractility before a longer-term reduction (62). The increased contractility is probably because of an intracellular acidosis that increases muscle contractility, in contrast to striated muscle (63). In the long term, the reduction of aerobic metabolism will limit the ability of the cell to regulate intracellular $[Ca^{2+}]$ and so generate the conditions for spontaneous activity.

DETRUSOR SMOOTH MUSCLE: CONTRACTILE MECHANISMS

Contractile Proteins and Intracellular Ca^{2+}

Smooth muscle cells of the bladder are spindle-shaped, single nucleated cells organized into bundles separated by connective tissue. The thin filaments are composed of α- and β-actin, which are attached to dense bodies on the cell membrane, and provide binding sites for the myosin thick filaments. There are four smooth muscle myosin isoforms (SM1A, 1B, 2A, 2B) that exhibit different contractile properties. Adult bladders are composed of nearly equal amounts of SM1B and SM2B (64). SM1 produces more force than SM2; SM-A types are more slowly contracting than SM-B. In obstruction, there is a shift to more SM1A, which results in slower and more forceful contractions to overcome increased resistance (65).

An increase in the sarcoplasmic $[Ca^{2+}]$, $[Ca^{2+}]_i$, from a basal level of 50 to 100 nM is required to initiate detrusor contraction; half maximal activation is achieved at about 1 μM (66). The source of Ca^{2+} can be extracellular, via L- and T-type Ca^{2+} channels (67,68), or from intracellular stores (69). Release from intracellular stores may be separately mediated by activation of IP_3 receptors, as it can be blocked by receptor inhibitors, or via ryanodine receptors (70). The increase in $[Ca^{2+}]_i$ is transient and Ca^{2+} are either removed from the cell via Na^+/Ca^{2+} exchange (71), or reaccumulated in intracellular stores via a SERCA

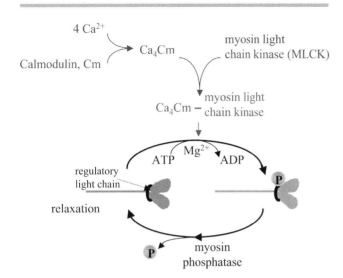

Figure 4 Schematic diagram of myosin activation (phosphorylation, P) and inactivation (dephosphorylation) by the calcium-calmodulin complex and associated kinase and phosphatase reactions.

pump; the activity of the latter is modulated by intracellular proteins, such as phospholamban (72). As with other smooth muscles, the contractile proteins are activated by phosphorylation of myosin by a myosin light chain kinase (MLCK), which in turn is activated by a Ca^{2+}_4-calmodulin complex. Relaxation will occur if the myosin light chain is dephosphorylated, by a myosin light chain phosphatase (MLCP). The sensitivity of the contractile system can therefore be altered by modulating the activities of MLCK or MLCP. A schematic diagram of contractile activation is shown in Figure 4. Intracellular messengers that can modulate the activity of these enzymes and hence contractile activity, in response to receptor activation by extracellular neurotransmitters and other signaling compounds, are described below.

MLCH activity can be decreased itself, being phosphorylated via a number of kinases including CaM kinase II, mitogen-activated protein (MAP) kinase, cAMP-dependent kinase (protein kinase A, PKA), and p21-activated kinase (73). An example of the relevance of such modulation is by consideration of the action of caffeine, application of which causes near-maximum release of Ca^{2+} from intracellular stores, but evokes little or no tension. The absence of contractile activation is probably through its actions as a phosphodiesterase (PDE) inhibitor that will enhance levels of intracellular cAMP, and hence activation of PKA.

MLCP activity can also be reduced by phosphorylation, which increases the Ca^{2+} sensitivity of the contractile system. Of significance is inhibition of MLCP activity by *rho*-associated kinase (ROK or ROCK) (74), which in turn is activated by small G proteins of the *rho*-family. In detrusor two isoforms of ROCK (I and II) have been identified (74). Inhibitors

of ROCK activity, such as Y-27632 and HA-1077, attenuate agonist-induced contractions, but do not affect depolarization-mediated [with high (KCl)] contractures (75), which suggests that the *rho*-kinase pathway plays a role in the contractile state of the bladder.

Detrusor Activation and Muscarinic Mechanisms

Acetylcholine (ACh) is released not just from parasympathetic and somatic motor nerves to smooth and skeletal muscle targets, respectively, but also from nonneuronal sources such as the urothelium. In the normal human bladder ACh is the sole neurotransmitter eliciting contraction, that is, there are no atropine-resistant contractions, while in many pathologies associated with bladder overactivity ATP is an additional activator (56,76,77). With animal bladders, except for old-world monkeys, a dual muscarinic-purinergic activation is present.

Muscarinic receptors are one of the main targets for ACh and they are expressed throughout the LUT. There are five subtypes of muscarinic receptors based on molecular (m_{1-5}) and pharmacological (M_{1-5}) characteristics. In detrusor, immunoprecipitation analyses show that m_2 and m_3 subtypes are expressed, with m_2 receptors in three- to ninefold excess (78). In normal human detrusor the minor M_3 fraction is responsible for contractile activation (79). More recently, the role of M_2 receptors has been reevaluated and it has been proposed that M_2 receptors exert a more significant role in certain pathological conditions (e.g., denervated or hypertrophied bladders), or when M_3 receptors are desensitized (80). One possibility is that M_2-dependent actions may derive from the urothelium. It has also been proposed that M_2 receptors in the normal bladder facilitate the function of other receptors, such as M_3 receptors, or counteract the relaxant effect of β-adrenoceptor agonists (81,82). However, there is little difference on overactive bladder function between the effect of more selective M_1/M_3-selective blockers and those with a less specific action, although the side effect profiles are different (83).

M_3 receptors are coupled to $G_{q/11}$ proteins, which importantly activate the enzyme phospholipase C (PLC) to convert membrane phosphoinositides to the second messengers, inositol trisphosphate (IP_3) and diacylglycerol (DAG). IP_3 in turn releases Ca^{2+} from intracellular stores, after binding to an IP_3 receptor, to activate the contractile proteins. There is a body of experimental evidence to support the relevance of this pathway in detrusor: muscarinic agonists generate a rise in $[Ca^{2+}]$ independent of membrane potential, and its release is blocked by IP_3 receptor blockers (70); the potency of the muscarinic receptor agonist carbachol is reduced by other IP_3 receptor blockers such as heparin and PLC inhibitors (84). Moreover inositol phosphate production mirrors tension generation in detrusor strips exposed to muscarinic agonists (85). However, other work suggests that this is not the exclusive pathway, in part because of the relative ineffectiveness of other PLC inhibitors to reduce carbachol-induced tension. It has been suggested that activation of the *rho*-kinase pathway and of protein kinase C by G protein activation and DAG, respectively, reduces the activity of myosin light chain phosphatase to increase the Ca^{2+} sensitivity of the contractile proteins; the rise of intracellular Ca^{2+} is explained by activation of nonspecific cation channels coupled to L-type Ca^{2+} channel activation (86). Several attempts to reconcile this controversy have been attempted, and it may be that there are considerable species differences in the relative importance of inositol phosphate and other pathways (87).

M_2 receptors are coupled to G_i protein that reduces cAMP production by its influence on adenylate cyclase activity. It has been proposed that M_2 receptor activation inhibits the effect of other agonists that increase cAMP production, such as β-receptor stimulation.

Recent reviews summarize the role of muscarinic-dependent pathways in the bladder and their relevance to contractile activation (79,88): M_3 pathways are summarized in Figure 5 and M_2 pathways in Figure 6.

Presynaptic muscarinic receptors have also been described where it is proposed that they modulate transmitter release in either a negative ($M_{2/4}$) or positive (M_1) feedback mode. Knockout experiments indicate that M_4, rather than M_2, receptors inhibit transmitter release (89).

Desensitization of muscarinic receptors results in detrusor smooth muscle being less sensitive to nerve

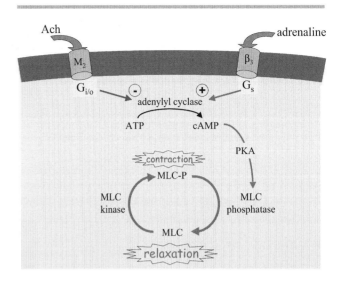

Figure 6 Schematic diagram of the intracellular signaling pathways activated after muscarinic (M_2) and adrenergic (β$_3$) receptor activation. *Abbreviations*: $G_{i/o1}$ and G_s, G proteins; camp, cyclic adenosine monophosphate; PKA, protein kinase A.

stimuli. This is mediated by phosphorylation of the muscarinic receptor by guanosine phosphate–binding G protein–coupled receptor kinase (GRK) (90); m$_2$ and m$_3$ GRK$_2$ mRNAs have been described. Protein expression of GRK$_2$ is significantly reduced in detrusor from patients with benign prostatic hyperplasia (91) and may therefore contribute to detrusor overactivity.

Purinergic Transmission

The role of ATP as an extracellular signaling molecule is now well accepted. In most mammalian species, ATP is coreleased with ACh from parasympathetic nerves, which activates purinergic receptors to initiate detrusor contraction. This is in contrast to healthy human bladders where contraction is predominately mediated by ACh. However, purinergic nerve–mediated contraction is increased in a number of bladder pathologies including hypertrophy, idiopathic overactivity, interstitial cystitis, and neurogenic damage. The increase in atropine resistance in bladder disorders may be because of increased sensitivity of detrusor cells to ATP, increased release from motor nerves, or reduced ATP hydrolysis within the neuromuscular junction. The three possibilities have been investigated using human detrusor samples from stable and overactive bladders. Only the last hypothesis was considered a possibility as ectonucleotidase (ATPase) activity in overactive human bladder samples is significantly reduced (92).

ATP binds to purinergic, P2, receptors that are in turn divided into P2X and P2Y families on the basis of pharmacological and molecular studies (93,94). P2X receptors are ionotropic ligand–gated nonspecific

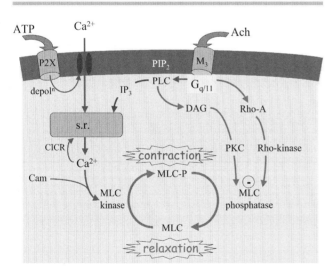

Figure 5 Schematic diagram of the intracellular signaling pathways activated after purinergic (P2X) and muscarinic (M_3) receptor activation, by adenosine triphosphate (ATP) and acetylcholine (ACh), respectively. *Abbreviations*: IP$_3$, inositol trisphosphate; PLC, phospholipase C; PIP$_2$, phosphatidylinositol 4,5-bisphosphate; $G_{q/11}$, a G protein; s.r., sarcoplasmic reticulum; DAG, diacylglycerol; PKC, protein kinase C; rho-A, Ras homologue gene family, member A—a small GTPase protein; *rho*-kinase, rho-associated, coiled-coil containing protein kinase 1 (ROCK); CICR, Ca^{2+}-induced Ca^{2+} release; Cam, calmodulin; MLC, myosin light chain (P-phosphorylated form).

cation channels, while P2Y receptors are metabotropic G protein coupled. Currently, seven P2X receptors subtypes have been cloned and characterized (P2X$_{1-7}$). P2X$_1$ labeling is present on detrusor muscle (95) and activation generates an inward, depolarizing current sufficient to activate L-type Ca^{2+} channels to generate an action potential (AP) and Ca^{2+} influx to initiate contraction (96).

There are eight subtypes of P2Y receptors (P2Y$_{1,2,4,6,11-14}$) linked either to G$_{q/11}$ (P2Y$_{1,2,6}$), G$_i$ (P2Y$_{12-14}$) or several proteins: G$_{q/11}$/G$_i$ (P2Y$_4$); G$_{q/11}$/G$_s$ (P2Y$_{11}$) (97,98). P2Y receptors, although not a specific subtype, have been implicated in relaxation of smooth muscle, possibly via cAMP-dependent PKA activity.

Metabolism of Neurotransmitters in the Neuromuscular Junction

A general principle of neuromuscular transmission is that neurotransmitter concentrations are locally high and postjunctional receptors have a relatively low affinity. Thus, the transmitter can fully activate and rapidly dissociate from its receptor. This, coupled to an efficient enzymatic removal of the transmitter, ensures that the action is transient and thus in a muscle contributes to a transient activation of contraction.

ACh is broken down by acetylcholinesterases (AChE), and the chief product, choline, is taken up by the nerve terminal to act as a substrate for further transmitter production. Several agents, such as physostigmine, attenuate AChE activity and prolong and enhance detrusor contractile activation. ATP is also broken down by extracellular endonucleotidases, and in human detrusor where ATP is functionally ineffective as an excitatory transmitter, it is assumed that it is completely hydrolyzed before it can activate the muscle cell. This is corroborated by the observation that in human detrusor samples displaying atropine-resistant contractions, endonucleotidase activity was reduced (92).

OTHER MODULATORS OF DETRUSOR CONTRACTILE FUNCTION

Adrenergic Mechanisms

There are five distinct adrenergic receptor types—α_1, α_2, β_1, β_2, and β_3—with each being further divided into subtypes. All three β-subtypes are expressed in detrusor muscle with the β_3-receptor the most highly expressed (99). Activation of β_2- and β_3-receptors can cause significant relaxation of detrusor smooth muscle (100). Thus, there is much interest in specifically targeting β_3-receptors for treatment of detrusor overactivity (101) and for producing an agent suitable for human use. The β-receptor-mediated relaxatory mechanism is thought to involve a rise in cAMP (Fig. 6) and modulation of large conductance Ca^{2+}-activated K$^+$ channels. There is a comprehensive survey of the in vitro and in vivo actions of β-receptor modulators (102).

Nitrergic Mechanisms

There are three nitric oxide synthase (NOS) isoforms, encoded by separate genes, named for the tissue from which they were first isolated from, or the order in which the genes were cloned: neuronal NOS (nNOS, NOS 1); inducible NOS from macrophage (iNOS, NOS 2); and endothelial NOS (eNOS, NOS 3); there is also a form of nNOS that is localized within mitochondria (mtNOS). Each of these enzymes can be found in every cell type of the LUT. The expression of several factors determine whether there is a relaxatory effect to nitric oxide (NO): NOS; the NO receptor, soluble guanylate cyclase (sGC); and PDE, the enzyme that degrades cGMP, the product of sGC activity. There are 11 PDE isoforms so far identified: PDE$_{1-5}$ are described to be present in the bladder (103). PDE$_5$-selective inhibitors such as sildenafil (Viagra) and vardenafil are structural analogs of cGMP and competitively inhibit PDE. NO donors have a small relaxatory effect on detrusor (104), but PDE inhibitors, such as vardenafil, relaxed precontracted detrusor (105), suggesting a relatively high endogenous PDE activity. These findings are supported by the beneficial effects of PDE$_5$ inhibitors with LUTS, when used to treat erectile dysfunction (106). The cellular pathways in relaxation that are mediated by NO are shown in Figure 7.

Nicotine and Nicotinic Receptors

Transmission at parasympathetic pelvic ganglia is mediated largely by nicotinic receptors, and these receptors may also be involved at other sites in the LUT. Nicotine can evoke ACh release from motor

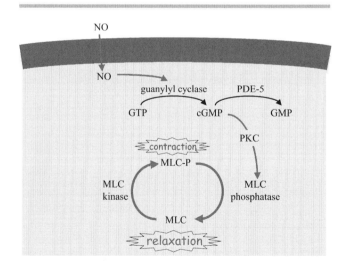

Figure 7 Schematic diagram of the intracellular signaling pathways activated after NO (nitric oxide) exposure. Pathways that cause contraction are shown by solid lines, those that cause relaxation by dotted lines. *Abbreviations*: GTP, guanosine triphosphate; cGMP, cyclic guanosne monophosphate; PDE-5, phosphodiesterase, type 5.

nerves, which itself may be upregulated by tachykinins acting via NK_2 receptors (107). This contractile effect of nicotine is blocked by the nicotine receptor antagonist hexamethonium. The nicotinic receptor is a pentamer of subunits, with 17 different subunits identified so far (α_{1-10}, β_{1-4}, γ, δ, ε). Mutation studies suggest that the α_3 and β_4 subunits are required for bladder function (108).

Adenosine Receptors

While purinergic, P2, receptors have received much attention, the pyrimidine P1 receptor family is less well studied. Four subtypes have been cloned—A_1, A_{2A}, A_{2B}, and A_3—and all are G protein–coupled receptors. $A_{1/3}$ receptors are negatively coupled to adenylyl cyclase activity, while A_2 receptors are positively coupled. Adenosine relaxes bladder preparations precontracted by carbachol through an A_2 (possibly A_{2B}) receptor mechanism (109). Adenosine also reduces nerve-mediated contractions, possibly by reducing neurotransmitter release via A_1 receptors (M Hussain, Y Ikeda, CH Fry, unpublished data). The relevance of P1-receptor activation is evidenced by the fact that adenosine is a breakdown product of ATP by the action endonucleotidases. Thus, P1-receptors exert a negative-feedback effect on the excitatory action of the neurotransmitter ATP.

Neuropeptides

Various neuropeptides, including calcitonin gene–related peptide (CGRP), substance P, neurokinin A, vasoactive intestinal polypeptide (VIP) and pituitary adenylate cyclase-activating peptide (PACAP), are released in the bladder from efferent and afferent (110) nerves and urothelial cells. These peptides may also be released by noxious stimuli and promote inflammation. CGRP inhibits spontaneous activity and relaxes ACh-induced tension. Tachykinins (substance P and neurokinin A) are prototypic of endogenous agonists of specific G protein–coupled receptors: tachykinin NK_1 and NK_2. NK_1 receptors have been found in blood vessels and the urothelium of all species thus far examined, whereas their expression in muscle cells seems restricted to only a few animal species [rats, guinea pigs (111)]. The stimulation of NK_1 receptors activates PLC, leading to inositol phosphate accumulation, and is linked to smooth muscle contraction. Substance P also stimulates detrusor smooth muscle. NK_2 receptors are localized on detrusor muscle of all mammalian species studied, including humans (112). The stimulation of NK_2 receptors is coupled to inositol phosphate accumulation and has a contractile effect on the bladder. VIP and PACAP receptors ($VPAC_{1/2}$ and PAC_1) are G protein–coupled receptors on neurons and smooth muscle. They are coupled to several signal transduction pathways, including activation of adenylate cyclase and elevation of cyclic guanylate monophosphate levels in tissues (65). VIP release evokes relaxation of detrusor and urethra smooth muscle.

Endothelin

The three isoforms of endothelin (ET-1,2,3) mediate their actions via ET_A and ET_B receptors (113): ET_A receptors have a dominant role in human detrusor, but their function is unclear. Because they initiate only a slow rise of tension, it has been proposed that they may potentiate nerve-mediated responses (114). ET_A receptors might contribute to premicturition contractions, and receptor antagonists, such as YM598, may have ameliorating effects in patients with bladder overactivity associated with obstruction (115).

SPONTANEOUS ACTIVITY

Significance of Spontaneous Activity

Nonneuronal contractions, resistant to the neurotoxins such as tetrodotoxin (TTX), occur in the detrusor and have several synonyms: intrinsic, autonomous, phasic, rhythmic, nonmicturition, spontaneous or transient activity, and micromotion. This activity was first reported by Sherrington in cats, as transient rises in bladder pressure seen during filling. Spontaneous smooth muscle contractions could also stimulate afferent fibers to generate centrally mediated reflex bladder contractions.

Investigation of the significance of phenomena, such as spontaneous activity, in human bladder function is often difficult to gauge for practical reasons and animal models can provide valuable insight. In neonatal rats, spontaneous, TTX-resistant, activity is absent at birth, increases in amplitude by week two, then changes from high-amplitude low-frequency to adult-like low-amplitude high-frequency activity by week six (116) (Fig. 8). At this time, micturition in the neonate is mediated by a somato-bladder spinal reflex pathway, activated by the mother licking the perineum. As development progresses, this primitive reflex

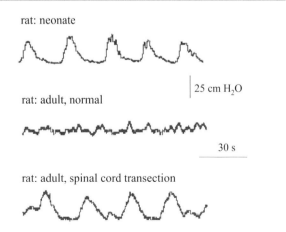

Figure 8 Pressure transients recorded ex vivo in bladders from a normal neonatal rat (*upper trace*); a normal adult rat (*middle trace*); an adult rat subjected to spinal cord transection to obtain a functional bladder outlet obstruction (*lower trace*). *Source*: From Ref. 118.

is replaced by supraspinal mechanisms that control brain-to-bladder reflexes and voluntary voiding. Thus, developmental changes in the central control of voiding occur in concert with changes in peripheral neurotransmission and the spontaneous properties of the bladder smooth muscle (117). In bladders from spinal cord–transected (SCT) rats (118) and outlet-obstructed (119) bladders, there is a reemergence of high-amplitude low-frequency spontaneous activity similar to that observed in neonatal bladders. The question therefore arises if the pattern of spontaneous activity is modulated by peripheral nervous control in the human bladder.

Origin of Spontaneous Activity

Detrusor overactivity is likely to be a multifactorial process with several possible origins.

1. *The neurogenic hypothesis*: Reduced peripheral or central inhibition increases activation of the micturition reflex and contractions associated with detrusor overactivity (120).
2. *The myogenic hypothesis*: Changes in the excitability and coupling of smooth muscle cells with other myocytes or interstitial cells leads to the generation of uninhibited contractions (121).
3. *The urotheliogenic hypothesis*: Changes in the sensitivity and coupling of the suburothelial myofibroblast network enhances spontaneous detrusor activity (122).
4. *The autonomous hypothesis*: Structures within the bladder wall coordinate to drive spontaneous contractions, which somehow become enhanced in pathology (123).
5. A leak of transmitter from motor fibers causes small local contractions or increases tone (124).

Neurogenic detrusor overactivity, explained by hypothesis 1, may pertain to a distinct subset of patients. Muscle samples taken from such bladders are similar to those from stable bladders (56).

Increased spontaneous activity is recorded from isolated muscle strips and cells obtained from other overactive (e.g., idiopathic) bladders. Contractions are resistant to neurotoxins but labile to Ca^{2+} channel blockers or K^+ channel openers (65). While upregulated activity in isolated cells may be present, this alone will not explain spontaneous activity in multicellular preparations that requires intercellular coordination of responses within and between muscle bundles. Two possibilities have been proposed for increased intercellular communication.

1. Increased intercellular coupling through gap junctions. Gap junctions are composed of the connexin (Cx) family of proteins. In human detrusor, expression of the main intermuscular connexin, Cx45, is actually less in samples from idiopathically overactive bladders, correlated with a higher gap junction resistance in such samples (125). Other groups, however, suggest that another connexin isoform, Cx43, is upregulated in overactive bladders (125).

2. Cx43 antibodies label interstitial cells in the detrusor layer, which exist between muscle bundles. These cells are also characterized by their labeling for the tyrosine kinase receptor protein *c-kit* and the generation of spontaneous and carbachol-evoked Ca^{2+} and electrical activity (126). It is postulated that rather than initiate spontaneous activity in the detrusor syncitium, interstitial cells modulate its activity (127), possibly by coordinating activity in different muscle bundles. However, these cells could form a control point for regulation of spontaneous activity; they are innervated by afferent nerves labeling for NOS (128), and they also express cGMP activity. However, the origin of spontaneous activity in muscle bundles remains unclear.

The urotheliogenic hypothesis is premised on a urothelial–myofibroblast network connected by gap junctions supporting pacemaker-driven spontaneous activity where bladder pathology, because of spinal cord transection for example, leads to an upregulation of gap junctions in the urothelium and myofibroblast network. This, in turn, leads to an increasingly functional myofibroblast syncytium with focal pacemaker activity that drives spontaneous contractions.

The autonomous hypothesis takes into account the potential role of interstitial cells within the bladder wall but does not clearly indicate a specific mechanism to generate spontaneous activity. It probably represents a qualitative description of a combined myogenic/urotheliogenic hypothesis. As with the urotheliogenic hypothesis spontaneous bladder contractions are enhanced by low-dose muscarinic stimulation, via M_3 receptors on suburothelial myofibroblasts and several agents such as ATP, substance P, nicotinic receptor agonists, noradrenaline, and NO (129).

SECRETORY AND SIGNALING PROPERTIES OF THE UROTHELIUM/SUBUROTHELIUM

Urothelium/Nerve Interactions

The urothelium releases many chemical factors, such as ATP (9), ACh (130), NO (131), and substance P (132), in several cases in response to stimuli such as stretch and changes in local osmolarity (9,133). The urothelial/suburothelial region is well supplied with sensory neurons that label for receptors to some of these releasates and suggests that these neurones interact with the urothelium to detect changes in bladder fullness. Urothelial cells also express receptors typically found on afferent nerves, such as purinergic receptors (134,135), members of the vanilloid receptor group $TRPV_{1,2,4}$ (136), $TRPA_1$ (137), $TRPM_8$ (138), $B_{1,2}$ bradykinin receptors (139), and adrenergic receptors (131,140), suggesting a complex interaction between urothelium and sensory nerves.

ATP Release

Most work has been applied to ATP release: it is hypothesized that when the urothelium is stretched

ATP is released and targets purinergic (P2X$_3$) receptors on sensory neurons. This hypothesis is inferred from data using P2X$_3$ knockout mice, which exhibited a reduced afferent firing and micturition reflex (141,142) on bladder filling. A layer of suburothelial interstitial cells (ICs, myofibroblasts—see below) is also in intimate association with these nerve endings, and ICs also generate excitatory responses to exogenous ATP through P2Y receptor activation. It has been proposed that these cells modulate the urothelium/neurone interaction (143,144). In pathologies associated with bladder overactivity and enhanced bladder sensation ATP release, IC number and neuronal P2X$_3$ labeling are increased, and the latter is decreased when overactivity is reduced, as with bladders treated with botulinum toxin (Botox-A) (145–147). Therefore, it may be further hypothesized that increased release of urothelial ATP contributes to afferent sensitization through enhanced activation of suburothelial nerves and/or ICs.

Acetylcholine Release

ACh is also released by the urothelium in response to stretch, increasing with age and estrogen status (130,148,149). Release may be through a nonvesicular mechanism (150), and thus is different from vesicular, neural release from parasympathetic nerves in stimulating bladder contraction. Urothelial-derived ACh, like ATP, may also have a role in promoting sensory activation. Hence, it is hypothesized that anticholinergics exert their effect not on detrusor muscle but on urothelial muscarinic receptors. All five subtypes of muscarinic receptors are expressed throughout the urothelial layers (151). There was specific localization of the M$_2$ subtype to the umbrella cells and M$_1$ to the basal layer, with M$_3$ receptors more generally distributed. There is some evidence that receptor subtype ratios may change (increased M$_2$:M$_3$) in detrusor overactivity but the significance of this remains unclear (152). The mechanism by which ACh modulates urothelial secretory activity is also unclear, but blockade of urothelial muscarinic receptors with atropine inhibits stretch-induced ATP release (153). Stretch-released ACh may therefore act in a feedback mechanism to induce urothelial ATP release.

Suburothelial Interstitial Cells

A network of interstitial myofibroblast-like cells (ICs) has been identified in the suburothelium; these cells have demonstrable cell markers including vimentin (an intracellular filament protein seen in cells of mesodermal origin) and *c-kit* (a cell surface marker). They are connected by gap junctions containing connexin, Cx43, and are closely apposed to unmyelinated nerve endings (154,155). ICs may mediate urothelium-derived ATP responses by generating propagating depolarizing Ca^{2+} waves across the IC network, through P2Y$_6$ activation, thus amplifying local responses to exogenous ATP (144,155). The ability of myofibroblasts to form functional networks can

involve mechanisms other than via gap junctions: if two isolated cells are pushed together, each cell demonstrates enhanced responses to ATP without the obvious formation of gap junctions. The cellular adhesion molecule, Cadherin-11, has been demonstrated on myofibroblast membranes (156) and the activation of the membranes by intercellular adhesion may offer a mechanism. This enhancement of response is abolished by the *c-kit* receptor ligand glivec.

These purinergic responses are mimicked by extracellular acidosis and attenuated by capsaicin and NO donors. The latter effect is in keeping with the demonstration of NOS/GC activity in these cells (128). The effect of extracellular acidosis and capsaicin is of significance as it proposes a mechanism for the response of the bladder wall to local ischemia—a feature of bladder filling—especially in the presence of outflow obstruction or reduced compliance (60,157,158).

Muscarinic M$_2$ and M$_3$ receptor labeling has also been localized to suburothelial ICs and is increased in samples from idiopathic overactive bladders and painful bladder syndrome (159). Isolated ICs do not respond to exogenous muscarinic receptor agonists by a rise of intracellular [Ca^{2+}], so the intracellular signaling mechanism(s) remains unknown (143). However, these observations may be significant as sensory C-fiber and Aδ-fiber afferent firing in response to bladder filling was reduced by M$_3$-selective antimuscarinics (160), or less-selective agents such as oxybutynin (161) or tolterodine (162).

Interactions Between Urothelium/Suburothelium and Detrusor

Several lines of evidence indicate that the urothelium/suburothelium directly affects detrusor function, through both inhibitory and excitatory mechanisms. With in vitro detrusor preparations the potency and maximum contractile responses to ACh, but not KCl, are reduced if the urothelium is intact. The active substance is unknown, but diffusible, and may involve activation of a β-adrenoreceptor (163,164). A similar phenomenon is present in ureter, which in this case may involve a cyclo-oxygenase product (165).

Optical imaging of transverse sections of the bladder wall shows propagating Ca^{2+} and membrane potential waves in the suburothelial layer in response to physical stretch or very low concentrations of the muscarinic agonist carbachol. After a delay these responses may spread to the detrusor layer initiating activity there (166) (Fig. 9A). Optical imaging of bladder sheets, with the urothelial surface uppermost, showed similar propagating waves of Ca^{2+} transients but only on the surface where the mucosa was intact (Fig. 9B). These waves may be initiated by stretch, muscarinic agonists, or purines such as UTP. UTP was chosen as the purine elicits excitatory responses from suburothelial ICs, but not directly from detrusor muscle. Isolated strips of detrusor generate spontaneous activity, especially if the urothelium/suburothelium is intact, and such activity is also upregulated by exogenous UTP (167). These observations are of interest as

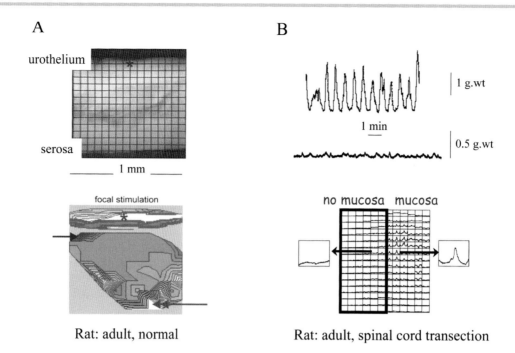

A

urothelium

serosa

_____ 1 mm _____

focal stimulation

Rat: adult, normal

B

1 g.wt

1 min

0.5 g.wt

no mucosa   mucosa

Rat: adult, spinal cord transection

Figure 9 (**A**) *Upper panel*: Photograph of a section through the bladder wall, with a superimposed grid. *Lower panel*: Isochronal maps for the spread of Ca^{2+} transients after mechanical focal stimulation of the suburothelial layer at the red star. The darker the shading the longer the isochrones after the initial evoked Ca^{2+} transient. Conduction initially occurs along the suburothial space, and only after a delay is there a limited wave in the detrusor layer (*left, single-headed arrow*). A separate activation source is also present in the detrusor layer (*bottom, double-headed arrow*). (**B**) *Upper panel*: Tension transients recorded from bladder sheets dissected from a spinal cord–transected (*top*) and normal (*bottom*) rat bladders. *Lower panel*: Ca^{2+} transients recorded from a spinal cord–transected rat bladder from which half the mucosa was removed (*solid, black box region*). Separate transients are recorded simultaneously from each grid square. An individual transient from each half of the preparation is also shown. *Source*: From Refs. 70 and 122.

they indicate that spontaneous activity could originate in the suburothelium region of the bladder wall. Furthermore, the specificity of site of action of some activators offers particular targets that may modulate such activity.

Thus, there is evidence that a suburothelial population of ICs is an intermediate stage in the sensory response to bladder wall stimuli. It acts as a variable amplifier, mediating signals between the urothelium and sensory afferents or the detrusor smooth muscle layer. Moreover, the increase in myofibroblast numbers in conditions associated with bladder overactivity (117,168) suggests that this cell layer may offer a therapeutic target to alleviate the condition. Agents that modulate IC activity, such as glivec, also reduce spontaneous activity in the bladder (169,170). These agents offer an alternative therapeutic avenue to manage detrusor overactivity.

ELECTRICAL ACTIVITY AND ACTION POTENTIALS

Cellular Activation and Propagation

Detrusor smooth muscle is an electrically excitable tissue capable of generating evoked and spontaneous APs (Fig. 10). The function of electrical activity

remains unclear in the human bladder, but could have two functions.

1. To initiate cellular events such as contractile activation
2. To propagate to adjacent regions of the tissue and so coordinate activity of a multicellular tissue

The role of APs in initiating and maintaining contractile function in detrusor muscle remains equivocal, as many excitatory neurotransmitters have significant actions that are independent of changes to the membrane potential. However, the presence of electrical activity means that APs should at least exert a modulatory role over contractile function, and may assume a greater significance during certain bladder pathologies when ionotropic neurotransmitters, such as ATP, assume a more important role.

It is unclear whether APs propagate extensively throughout detrusor tissue. In true functional syncitia, such as myocardium, APs propagate from cell to cell through gap junctions, composed of different isoforms of the protein connexin (Cx), and concentrated in intercalated disks. Gap junctions, as observed under the electron microscope, are sparser in detrusor. This has led many to conclude that APs do not freely propagate. However, electrophysiological experiments show electrical coupling between cells, and the

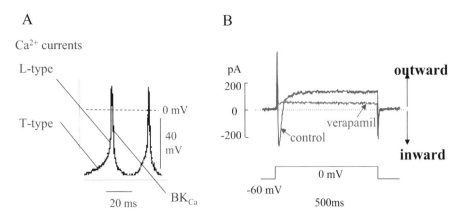

Figure 10 (**A**) APs recorded from an isolated human detrusor cell. The major currents contributing to the different phases of the AP are shown. (**B**) Voltage-clamp traces from an isolated human detrusor cell. Membrane current is recorded in response to a step depolarization from −60 to 0 mV. Inward current is carried by an influx of cations and outward current by an efflux of cations. Two traces are superimposed: in the absence and presence of the L-type Ca^{2+} channel blocker verapamil (10 μM). Note both inward current (mainly Ca^{2+} entry through L-type Ca^{2+} channels) and outward current (mainly K^+ efflux through Ca^{2+} activated BK_{Ca} channels) are attenuated by verapamil.

connexin isoform Cx45 has been identified (171). The relatively poor electrical coupling, compared with detrusor, and the failure of Cx45 to be found in intercalated disk-like structures may account for the relative difficulty in observing gap junctions in detrusor.

Ion Channels

The membrane potential is sufficiently negative (−40 to −50 mV) for regenerative APs to be initiated. The AP upstroke phase is carried by Ca^{2+} influx, predominantly through L-type Ca^{2+} channels, and repolarization is mediated by K^+ efflux through several K^+ channels (67,172). Such Ca^{2+} influx is sufficient to elicit further release from intracellular stores to sustain contractions. T-type Ca^{2+} channels have also been described in detrusor muscle and the proportion of total inward Ca^{2+} current is increased in cells from overactive bladders (173). Because T-type channels are activated at more negative membrane potentials, they may contribute to increased spontaneous activity in the overactive bladder. Several receptor modulators that alter detrusor contractility also affect the L-type Ca^{2+} current. Antimuscarinic agents such as propiverine attenuate L-type Ca^{2+} current (174), an effect probably mediated via M_3 receptors. β-agonists also attenuate Ca^{2+} current by a cAMP/ protein kinase A–dependent mechanism (175).

The most significant K^+ channel in detrusor is the Ca^{2+}-activated large conductance K^+ channel (BK_{Ca}). This channel has physiological roles in determining membrane potential, AP repolarization (176), and regulating contractile events (70): channel opening is coupled to intracellular Ca^{2+} sparks emanating from intracellular Ca stores via ryanodine receptors (176). Outward current is also modulated by Ca^{2+} current influx through L-type and T-type Ca^{2+} channels. In the former case this has been proposed as a mechanism to regulate Ca^{2+} influx into the myocyte

(70), and in the latter case as a basis for spontaneous fluctuations of membrane potential (177). Reduction in BK channel activity may contribute to myogenic bladder overactivity, as deletion of the *slo*-gene that encodes for the channel protein enhances muscle sensitivity to cholinergic and purinergic agonists (178); conversely injection of *slo*-cDNA reduced overactivity (179). BK channel activity is regulated by phosphorylation of the pore-forming α-subunit, or associated proteins (180), and affords a mechanism whereby cAMP and cGMP, through PKC, can regulate channel function. Conversely, the Ca^{2+}-dependent phosphatase, calcineurin, decreased BK_{Ca} conductance (181) so that overall Ca^{2+} exerts a complex control of channel function.

Intracellular ATP-gated K^+ channels (K_{ATP}) have also been described in detrusor smooth muscle, and channel openers hyperpolarize the cell and reduce spontaneous activity. A problem with the use of these channel modulators is that of tissue specificity, as many are as potent, if not more, in generating similar responses in vascular smooth muscle.

Stretch-activated channels could serve a dual purpose in the detrusor myocyte: to permit cation influx to depolarize the cells and thus cause contraction to counter an initial stretch; and to initiate intracellular signaling cascades that may initiate cellular reconfiguration or growth (182,183). Physical stretch of detrusor myocytes opens nonselective cation channels, depolarizes the cell, and augments Ca^{2+} influx through Ca^{2+} channels (184). However, stretch also increases K^+ channel activity (185). The net effect would be to increase spontaneous activity.

THE BLADDER BASE

The bladder base consists of the trigone, ureterovesical junction, and deep detrusor, and the anterior bladder wall may be considered to form a functional entity to provide an effective reflux mechanism as well as control urine outflow during filling and voiding (186). It is defined as the triangular region between the ureteral orifices and the bladder outlet and plays a crucial role in ureterovesical function, continence and micturition. The trigone is believed to develop, with the ureter, from an outgrowth of the mesonephric duct, with a common mesodermal origin of the vesical neck musculature, the trigone, and the ureterovesical junction. More recent studies, however, suggest that the trigone is formed predominantly from bladder muscle, and the contribution from ureteral longitudinal fibers at the lateral edges is more limited (187).

In general, the bladder base is thought to provide a rather stable structure against which the bladder dome can contract and relax during the micturition cycle. This might be the reason for the relatively high amount of connective tissue and greater spontaneous activity within individual myocytes, compared with detrusor. The spontaneous activity is mainly driven by ion fluxes through membrane L-type Ca^{2+}-channels and Ca^{2+}-actvated Cl^- channels. Extensive gap junction coupling ensures electrical propagation and coordination of function throughout the tissue (188).

The bladder base and trigone represents an area of dual sympathetic/parasympathetic innervation. Both systems significantly control contractile function (102,189), demonstrated from experiments using adrenergic and muscarinic receptor agonists and antagonists. The α_{1D}-adrenoceptor seems to be the most abundant subtype in humans; muscarinic receptor representation is similar to the in detrusor (102). It is generally agreed, through animal studies, that sympathetic activation is active during the storage phase and induces contraction of the bladder base, as well as the internal urethral smooth muscle sphincter. The role of the parasympathetic innervation is more controversial, even that there may be a relaxatory component through the generation of NO during micturition (190). However, there is considerable synergy of action between the adrenergic and muscarinic systems in the trigone, with respect to contractile activation. The two systems probably act through different cellular pathways; the adrenergic system primarily operates through Ca^{2+} sensitization of the contractile machinery, while muscarinic-dependent activation is a $[Ca^{2+}]_i$-dependent process (189,191). This synergistic mechanism may contribute to the prevention of urinary reflux into the ureter and increase outflow closure pressure, as the trigone is sited to regulate both functions.

However, during micturition the trigone may relax and cause a "funneling" effect to facilitate voiding. As in the urethra, animal experiments have shown that NO is the key relaxing factor in the bladder base (190). NO effectively relaxes isolated smooth muscle preparations from the outflow region, suggesting that it may be involved in the decrease in intraurethral pressure observed at the start of normal micturition. This NO-based relaxation provides an effective mechanism to allow the bladder base and trigone to switch from a closed to open state, especially in combination

with the adrenergic control of the Ca^{2+} sensitization of the contractile machinery.

MUSCLES OF THE URETHRA

Role of the Musculature

During voiding, relaxation of the bladder outlet precedes detrusor contraction and during filling the outlet is contracted. Several processes contribute to these functions, mediated through urethral smooth and skeletal muscle as well as the mechanical properties of the lamina propria. Smooth muscle is arranged in an outer circular and an inner longitudinal layer. Contraction of the circular muscle should maintain continence, and the longitudinal muscle may shorten during micturition. It has been proposed that the pelvic organs also provide a support for the intra-abdominal portion of the urethra, especially in women. However, up to half of total urethral pressure in women is because of smooth muscle tone (192,193). The urethra is innervated by both the sympathetic and parasympathetic systems. Activity in pelvic nerve parasympathetic fibers relaxes urethral smooth muscle, especially in the proximal portion, and therefore the outflow region; sympathetic fibers (T10-L2) generate contraction.

Urethral Smooth Muscle

Sympathetic and parasympathetic branches of the autonomic nervous system exert control over uretheral smooth muscle. Sympathetic control is mediated by α_1 receptors, mainly the $\alpha_{1A/L}$ subtype in both human and animal tissue (194,195) and about half of the urethral pressure is maintained by adrenergic receptor activation (190). Partial $\alpha_{1A/L}$ agonists, such as Ro 115-1240, have been proposed as agents that may be used to manage stress urinary incontinence (SUI) in women without significant cardiovascular side effects (196).

Urethral relaxation is believed to be because of release of NO (190) and prejunctional muscarinic receptors may also limit noradrenaline release from sympathetic fibers (197). Urethral relaxation can be mediated by β-receptor activation, predominantly the β_2 subtype. However, this mechanism is probably less important than in detrusor (102). The β_2 agonist clenbuterol also increased urethral skeletal muscle contraction, raising the possibility that it may have a role in the treatment of urinary incontinence by inhibiting detrusor contraction and augmenting external urethral sphincter activity (198). NO-mediated relaxation is because of production of cGMP and activation of cGMP-dependent protein kinase, cGK. Electrical field stimulation generates relaxations that are abolished by inhibitors of NO production and are absent in mice lacking cGK (199). CO can also exert relaxation through a rise of cGMP, which may be equivalent in magnitude to the effect of NO (200). Derangements of the NO system have been demonstrated in several disorders associated with LUT function, such as diabetes, bladder outlet obstruction, or bladder inflammation (201,202).

Sex hormones play an important role in modulating urinary tract smooth muscle function, including urethral muscle. Lack of estrogen following menopause may contribute to decreased urethral tone, urothelial integrity, and incontinence, and the earlier papers suggested that estrogen supplementation may be beneficial. However, recent clinical studies indicate that supplemental estrogen lowers collagen content in the periurethral connective tissue and decreases urethral closure pressure (203), thereby worsening the symptoms of incontinence (204).

Urethral smooth muscle exhibits spontaneous electrical and mechanical activity that contributes to the overall muscular tone. Electrical activity occurs because of bursts of spikes superimposed on a slower more rhythmic activity, and could be initiated by autonomic transmitters (205). Two types of Ca^{2+} currents—L type and T type—have been recorded in isolated myocytes. Blockade of the former type reduced the number of spikes in each burst; the frequency within bursts was attenuated by blockade of T-type current (206). However, both channels represent targets that may modulate spontaneous activity. The muscle cells are closely associated with interstitial cells that may at least modify their activity (207). The observation that interstitial cells are closely associated with NOS synthase–containing nerves suggests that they may be intermediaries between nerves and urethral smooth muscle (208).

Urethral Skeletal Muscle

Urethral skeletal muscle (rhabdosphincter) forms an incomplete ring around the urethral conduit (209). In human tissue three fiber types have been described: fast twitch fatigue sensitive, fast twitch fatigue resistant, and slow twitch, with the majority fatigue resistant (210). Muscle bulk decreases with age and with parity in women, and SUI may be associated with a loss of muscle mass (211). A decrease in motor nerve function may also contribute to SUI: In a mouse model vaginal distension reduced leak point pressures and the number of urethral nerves, without affecting muscle mass (212). The decline of sphincter, and striated muscle, function has motivated the development of myoblast implants that may improve continence (213), or the use of basic fibroblast growth factor to facilitate muscle cell generation (214). When using implants, muscle fiber cells showed improved results over the use of fibroblasts (215).

Selective inhibitors of serotonin (5-HT) and noradrenaline (NA) uptake, such as duloxetine, are potential agents for the therapeutic management of SUI because 5-HT and NA terminals are present in Onuf's nucleus that supplies the rhabdosphincter with motor nerves (216). Clinical trials suggest that the effect of duloxetine on alleviating USI is small, but significant (217)—clinical uptake of this drug has been slow.

The striated muscle of the urethral sphincter may undergo abnormal activity, resulting in urinary retention, Fowler's syndrome (218). The origin of the condition is unknown, but one hypothesis is that it is because of ephaptic (i.e., direct cross talk) electrical transmission between cells, much as can occur between nerve axons under certain conditions (219). Neuromodulation may be effective in restoring voiding activity, but there remain significant complication rates (220).

REFERENCES

1. Walz T, Häner M, Wu X R, et al. Towards the molecular architecture of the asymmetric unit membrane of the mammalian urinary bladder epithelium: a closed "twisted ribbon" structure. J Mol Biol 1995; 248:887–900.
2. Minsky BD, Chlapowski FJ. Morphometric analysis of the translocation of lumenal membrane between cytoplasm and cell surface of transitional epithelial cells during the expansion–contraction cycles of mammalian urinary bladder. J Cell Biol 1978; 77:685–697.
3. Schlager TA, Grady R, Mills SE, et al. Bladder epithelium is abnormal in patients with neurogenic bladder due to myelomeningocele. Spinal Cord 2004; 42:163–168.
4. Ohtsuka Y, Kawakami S, Fujii Y, et al. Loss of uroplakin III expression is associated with a poor prognosis in patients with urothelial carcinoma of the upper urinary tract. BJU Int 2006; 97:1322–1326.
5. Ronald A. The etiology of urinary tract infection: traditional and emerging pathogens. Dis Mon 2003; 49:71–82.
6. Lewis SA, de Moura JL. Incorporation of cytoplasmic vesicles into apical membrane of mammalian urinary bladder epithelium. Nature 1982; 297:685–688.
7. Truschel ST, Wang E, Ruiz WG, et al. Stretch-regulated exocytosis/endocytosis in bladder umbrella cells. Mol Biol Cell 2002; 13:830–846.
8. Yu W, Khandelwal P, Apodaca G. Distinct apical and basolateral membrane requirements for stretch-induced membrane traffic at the apical surface of bladder umbrella cells. Mol Biol Cell 2009; 20:282–295.
9. Ferguson DR, Kennedy I, Burton TJ. ATP is released from rabbit urinary bladder epithelial cells by hydrostatic pressure changes—a possible sensory mechanism? J Physiol 1997; 505:503–511.
10. Apodaca G. The urothelium: not just a passive barrier. Traffic 2004; 5:1–12.
11. Khandelwal P, Ruiz WG, Balestreire-Hawryluk E, et al. Rab11a-dependent exocytosis of discoidal/fusiform vesicles in bladder umbrella cells. Proc Natl Acad Sci U S A 2008; 105:15773–15778.
12. Lewis SA, Diamond J. Active sodium transport by mammalian urinary bladder. Nature 1975; 253:747–748.
13. Tzan CJ, Berg JR, Lewis SA. Mammalian urinary bladder permeability is altered by cationic proteins: modulation by divalent cations. Am J Physiol 1994; 267:C1013–C1026.
14. Parsons CL. The role of the urinary epithelium in the pathogenesis of interstitial cystitis/prostatitis/urethritis. Urology 2007; 69(4 suppl):9–16.
15. Wickham JE. Active transport of sodium ion by the mammalian bladder epithelium. Invest Urol 1964; 2:145–153.
16. Smith PR, Mackler SA, Weiser PC, et al. Expression and localization of epithelial sodium channel in mammalian urinary bladder. Am J Physiol 1998; 274:F91–F96.
17. Lewis SA, Wills NK. Apical membrane permeability and kinetic properties of the Na pump in rabbit urinary bladder. J Physiol 1983; 341:169–184.

18. Lewis SA, Wills NK, Eaton DC. Basolateral membrane potential of a tight epithelium: ionic diffusion and electrogenic pumps. J Membr Biol 1978; 41:117–148.

19. Lewis SA, Hanrahan JW. Apical and basolateral membrane ionic channels in rabbit urinary bladder epithelium. Pflugers Arch 1985; 405:S83–S88.

20. Wang EC, Lee J M, Johnson JP, et al. Hydrostatic pressure-regulated ion transport in bladder uroepithelium. Am J Physiol 2003; 285:F651–F663.

21. Lewis SA, Ifshin MS, Loo DDF, et al. Studies of sodium channels in rabbit urinary bladder by noise analysis. J Membr Biol 1984; 80:135–151.

22. Hanrahan JW, Alles WP, Lewis SA. Single anion-selective channels in basolateral membrane of a mammalian tight epithelium. Proc Natl Acad Sci U S A 1985; 82:7791–7795.

23. Donaldson P, Lewis SA. Effect of hyperosmotic challenge on basolateral membrane potential in rabbit urinary bladder. Am J Physiol 1990; 27:C248–C257.

24. Spector DA, Wade JB, Dillow R, et al. Expression, localization, and regulation of aquaporin-1 to -3 in rat urothelia. Am J Physiol 2002; 282:F1034–F1042.

25. Wright KJ, Seed PC, Hultgren SJ. Development of intracellular bacterial communities of uropathogenic *Escherichia coli* depends on type 1 pili. Cell Microbiol 2007; 9:2230–2241.

26. Anderson GG, Palermo JJ, Schilling JD, et al. Intracellular bacterial biofilm-like pods in urinary tract infections. Science 2003; 301:105–107.

27. Rosen DA, Hooton TM, Stamm WE, et al. Detection of intracellular bacterial communities in human urinary tract infection. PLoS Med 2007; 4:e329.

28. Farrugia MK, Godley ML, Woolf AS, et al. Experimental short-term fetal bladder outflow obstruction: II effects on bladder stiffness and detrusor contractility. J Paediatr Urol 2006; 2:254–260.

29. Bross S, Braun PM, Michel MS, et al. Bladder wall tension during physiological voiding and in patients with an unstable detrusor or bladder outlet obstruction. BJU Int 2003; 92:584–588.

30. Bross S, Braun PM, Michel MS, et al. Preoperatively evaluated bladder wall tension as a prognostic parameter for postoperative success after surgery for bladder outlet obstruction. Urology 2003; 61:562–566.

31. Thiruchelvam N, Godley ML, Fry CH. Comment on: bladder wall tension during physiological voiding and in patients with an unstable detrusor or bladder outlet obstruction. BJU Int 2004; 93:1117–1118.

32. Wahl EF, Lerman SE, Lahdes-Vasama TT, et al. Measurement of bladder compliance can be standardized by a dimensionless number: clinical perspective. BJU Int 2004; 94:898–900.

33. Wahl EF, Lerman SE, Lahdes-Vasama TT, et al. Measurement of bladder compliance can be standardized by a dimensionless number: theoretical perspective. BJU Int 2004; 94:895–897.

34. Thiruchelvam N, Wu C, David A, et al. Neurotransmission and viscoelasticity in the ovine fetal bladder after in utero bladder outflow obstruction. Am J Physiol 2003; 284:R1296–R1305.

35. Farrugia MK, Woolf AS, Fry CH, et al. Radiotelemetered urodynamics of obstructed ovine fetal bladders: correlations with ex vivo cystometry and renal histopathology. BJU Int 2007; 99:1517–1522.

36. Liao LM, Schaefer W. Cross-sectional and longitudinal studies on interaction between bladder compliance and outflow obstruction in men with benign prostatic hyperplasia. Asian J Androl 2007; 9:51–56.

37. Shaw MB, Herndon CD, Cain MP, et al. A porcine model of bladder outlet obstruction incorporating radio-telemetered cystometry. BJU Int 2007; 100:170–174.

38. Kohan AD, Danziger M, Vaughan ED, Jr, et al. Effect of aging on bladder function and the response to outlet obstruction in female rats. Urol Res 2000; 28:33–37.

39. Ghoniem GM, Bloom DA, McGuire EJ, et al. Bladder compliance in meningomyelocele children. J Urol 1989; 141:1404–1406.

40. Macarak EJ, Ewalt D, Baskin L, et al. The collagens and their urologic implications. Adv Exp Med Biol 1995; 385:173–177.

41. Tekgul S, Yoshino K, Bagli D, et al. Collagen types I and III localization by in situ hybridization and immunohistochemistry in the partially obstructed young rabbit bladder. J Urol 1996; 156:582–586.

42. Kim JC, Yoon JY, Seo SI, et al. Effects of partial bladder outlet obstruction and its relief on types I and III collagen and detrusor contractility in the rat. Neurourol Urodyn 2000; 19:29–42.

43. Thiruchelvam N, Nyirady P, Peebles D, et al. Urinary outflow obstruction increases apoptosis and deregulates Bcl-2 and Bax expression in the fetal ovine bladder. Am J Pathol 2003; 162:1271–1282.

44. Chang SL, Howard PS, Koo HP, et al. Role of type III collagen in bladder filling. Neurourol Urodyn 1998; 17:135–145.

45. Coplen DE, Macarak EJ, Howard PS. Matrix synthesis by bladder smooth muscle cells is modulated by stretch frequency. In Vitro Cell Dev Biol Anim 2003; 39:157–162.

46. Baskin LS, Contantinescu S, Duckett JW, et al. Type III collagen decreases in normal fetal bovine bladder development. J Urol 1994; 152:688–691.

47. Furber JD. Extracellular glycation crosslinks: prospects for removal. Rejuvenation Res 2006; 9:274–278.

48. Poladia DP, Bauer JA. Functional, structural, and neuronal alterations in urinary bladder during diabetes: investigations of a mouse model. Pharmacology 2005; 74:84–94.

49. Daneshgari F, Liu G, Imrey PB. Time dependent changes in diabetic cystopathy in rats include compensated and decompensated bladder function. J Urol 2006; 176:380–386.

50. Malmqvist U, Arner A, Uvelius B. Mechanics and Ca^{2+} sensitivity of human detrusor muscle bundles studied in vitro. Acta Physiol Scand 1991; 143:373–380.

51. Ekström J, Uvelius B. Length–tension relations of smooth muscle from normal and denervated rat urinary bladders. Acta Physiol Scand 1981; 112:443–447.

52. Hill AV. The force–velocity relation in shortening muscle. In: First and Last Experiments in Muscle Mechanics. Cambridge: Cambridge University Press, 1970:23–41.

53. Griffiths DJ. The mechanics of the urethra and of micturition. Br J Urol 1973; 45:497–507.

54. Malone-Lee J, Wahedna I. Characterisation of detrusor contractile function in relation to old age. Br J Urol 1993; 72:873–880.

55. Williams JH, Turner WH, Sainsbury GM, et al. Experimental model of bladder outflow tract obstruction in the guinea-pig. Br J Urol 1993; 71:543–554.

56. Bayliss M, Wu C, Newgreen D, et al. A quantitative study of atropine-resistant contractile responses in human detrusor smooth muscle, from stable, unstable and obstructed bladders. J Urol 1999; 162:1833–1839.

57. Paul RJ. Smooth muscle energetics. Ann Rev Physiol 1989; 51:331–349.

58. Hai CM, Murphy RA. Ca^{2+}, crossbridge phosphorylation, and contraction. Ann Rev Physiol 1989; 51:285–298.

59. Paul RJ, Bauer M, Pease W. Vascular smooth muscle: aerobic glycolysis linked to Na–K transport processes. Science 1979; 206:1414.

60. Azadzoi KM, Pontari M, Vlachiotis J, et al. Canine bladder blood flow and oxygenation: changes induced by filling,

contraction and outlet obstruction. J Urol 1996; 155: 1459–1465.

61. Bellringer JF, Ward J, Fry CH. Intramural pH changes in the anaesthetised rabbit bladder during filling. J Physiol 1994; 480:82P–83P.

62. Thomas PJ, Fry CH. The effects of cellular hypoxia on contraction and extracellular ion accumulation in isolated human detrusor smooth muscle. J Urol 1996; 155:726–731.

63. Liston TG, Palfrey EL, Raimbach SJ, et al. The effects of pH changes on human and ferret detrusor muscle function. J Physiol 1991; 432:1–21.

64. Martin AF, Bhatti S, Pyne-Geithman GJ, et al. Expression and function of COOH terminal myosin heavy chain isoforms in mouse smooth muscle. Am J Physiol Cell Physiol 2007; 293:C238–C245.

65. Andersson KE, Arner A. Urinary bladder contraction and relaxation: physiology and pathophysiology. Physiol Rev 2004; 84:935–986.

66. Wu C, Kentish JC, Fry CH. Effect of pH on myofilament Ca^{2+}-sensitivity in α-toxin permeabilized guinea-pig detrusor muscle. J Urol 1995; 154:191–194.

67. Montgomery BS, Fry CH. The action potential and net membrane currents in isolated human detrusor smooth muscle cells. J Urol 1992; 147:176–184.

68. Sui GP, Wu C, Fry CH. A description of Ca^{2+} channels in human detrusor smooth muscle. BJU Int 2003; 92:476–482.

69. Fry CH, Gallegos CRR, Montgomery BS. The actions of extracellular H^+ on the electro-physiological properties of isolated human detrusor smooth muscle cells. J Physiol 1994; 480:71–80.

70. Wu C, Sui, GP, Fry CH. The role of the L-type Ca^{2+} channel in refilling functional intracellular Ca^{2+} stores in guinea-pig detrusor smooth muscle. J Physiol 2002; 538:357–369.

71. Wu C, Fry CH. Evidence for Na^+/Ca^{2+} exchange and its role in intracellular Ca^{2+} regulation in guinea-pig detrusor smooth muscle cells. Am J Physiol Cell Physiol 2001; 280:C1090–C1096.

72. Nobe K, Sutliff RL, Kranias EG, et al. Phospholamban regulation of bladder contractility: evidence from gene-altered mouse models. J Physiol 2001; 535:867–878.

73. Yamaguchi O. Response of bladder smooth muscle cells to obstruction: signal transduction and the role of mechanosensors. Urology 2004; 63(3 suppl 1):11–16.

74. Kimura K, Ito M, Amano M, et al. Regulation of myosin phosphatase by Rho and Rho-associated kinase (Rho-kinase). Science 1996; 273:245–248.

75. Durlu-Kandilci NT, Brading AF. Involvement of Rho kinase and protein kinase C in carbachol-induced calcium sensitization in beta-escin skinned rat and guinea-pig bladders. Br J Pharmacol 2006; 148:376–384.

76. Sjögren C, Andersson KE, Husted S, et al. Atropine resistance of transmurally stimulated isolated human bladder muscle. J Urol 1982; 128:1368–1371.

77. Palea S, Artibani W, Ostardo E, et al. Evidence for purinergic neurotransmission in human urinary bladder affected by interstitial cystitis. J Urol 1993; 150:2007–2012.

78. Wang P, Luthin GR, Ruggieri MR. Muscarinic acetylcholine receptor subtypes mediating urinary bladder contractility and coupling to GTP binding proteins. J Pharmacol Exp Ther 1995; 273:959–966.

79. Hegde SS. Muscarinic receptors in the bladder: from basic research to therapeutics. Br J Pharmacol 2006; 147:S80–S87.

80. Braverman AS, Doumanian LR, Ruggieri MR, Sr. M_2 and M_3 muscarinic receptor activation of urinary bladder contractile signal transduction. II. Denervated rat bladder. J Pharmacol Exp Ther 2006; 316:875–880.

81. Ehlert FJ, Griffin MT, Abe DM, et al. The M_2 muscarinic receptor mediates contraction through indirect mechanisms in mouse urinary bladder. J Pharmacol Exp Ther 2005; 313:368–378.

82. Ehlert FJ, Ahn S, Pak KJ, et al. Neuronally released acetylcholine acts on the M_2 muscarinic receptor to oppose the relaxant effect of isoproterenol on cholinergic contractions in mouse urinary bladder. J Pharmacol Exp Ther 2007; 322:631–637.

83. Chapple CR, Khullar V, Gabriel Z, et al. The effects of antimuscarinic treatments in overactive bladder: an update of a systematic review and meta-analysis. Eur Urol 2008; 54:543–562.

84. Braverman AS, Tibb AS, Ruggieri MR Sr. M_2 and M_3 muscarinic receptor activation of urinary bladder contractile signal transduction. I. Normal rat bladder. J Pharmacol Exp Ther 2006; 316:869–874.

85. Harriss DR, Marsh KA, Birmingham AT, et al. Expression of muscarinic M3-receptors coupled to inositol phospholipid hydrolysis in human detrusor cultured smooth muscle cells. J Urol 1995; 154:1241–1245.

86. Frazier EP, Braverman AS, Peters SL, et al. Does phospholipase C mediate muscarinic receptor-induced rat urinary bladder contraction? J Pharmacol Exp Ther 2007; 322:998–1002.

87. Wuest M, Hiller N, Braeter M, et al. Contribution of Ca^{2+} influx to carbachol-induced detrusor contraction is different in human urinary bladder compared to pig and mouse. Eur J Pharmacol 2007; 565:180–189.

88. Frazier EP, Peters SL, Braverman AS, et al. Signal transduction underlying the control of urinary bladder smooth muscle tone by muscarinic receptors and beta-adrenoceptors. Naunyn Schmiedebergs Arch Pharmacol 2007; 377:449–462.

89. Zhou H, Meyer A, Starke K, et al. Heterogeneity of release-inhibiting muscarinic autoreceptors in heart atria and urinary bladder: a study with M2- and M4-receptor-deficient mice. Naunyn Schmiedebergs Arch Pharmacol 2002; 365:112–122.

90. Pals-Rylaarsdam R, Xu Y, Witt-Enderby P, et al. Desensitization and internalization of the m2 muscarinic acetylcholine receptor are directed by independent mechanisms. J Biol Chem 195; 27048:29004–29011.

91. Furuya Y, Araki I, Kamiyama M, et al. Decreased expression of G protein-coupled receptor kinases in the detrusor smooth muscle of human urinary bladder with outlet obstruction. Int J Urol 2006; 13:1226–1232.

92. Harvey RA, Skennerton DE, Newgreen D, et al. The contractile potency of adenosine triphosphate and ecto-adenosine triphosphatase activity in guinea pig detrusor and detrusor from patients with a stable, unstable or obstructed bladder. J Urol 2002; 168:1235–1239.

93. Ralevic V, Burnstock G. Receptors for purines and pyrimidines. Pharmacol Rev 1998; 50:413–492.

94. Burnstock G. Physiology and pathophysiology of purinergic neurotransmission. Physiol Rev 2007; 87:659–797.

95. Elneil S, Skepper JN, Kidd EJ, et al. Distribution of P2X$_1$ and P2X$_3$ receptors in the rat and human urinary bladder. Pharmacology 2001; 63:120–128.

96. Wu C, Bayliss M, Newgreen D, et al. A comparison of the mode of action of ATP and carbachol on isolated human detrusor smooth muscle. J Urol 1999; 162:1840–1847.

97. IUPHAR receptor database. Available at: http://www.iuphar-db.org/index_ic.jsp.

98. Abbracchio MP, Burnstock G, Boeynaems JM, et al. International Union of Pharmacology LVIII: update on the P2Y G protein-coupled nucleotide receptors: from molecular mechanisms and pathophysiology to therapy. Pharmacol Rev 2006; 58:281–341.

99. Yamaguchi O. Beta3-adrenoceptors in human detrusor muscle. Urology 2002; 59(5 suppl 1):25–29.

100. Badawi JK, Uecelehan H, Hatzinger M, et al. Relaxant effects of beta-adrenergic agonists on porcine and human detrusor muscle. Acta Physiol Scand 2005; 185:151–159.

101. Leon LA, Hoffman BE, Gardner SD, et al. Effects of the beta3-adrenergic receptor agonist CL-316243 on bladder micturition reflex in spontaneously hypertensive rats. J Pharmacol Exp Ther 2008; 326:178–185.

102. Michel MC, Vrydag W. Adrenoceptors in the lower urinary tract. Br J Pharmacol 2006; 147:S88–S119.

103. Uckert S, Stief CG, Mayer M, et al. Distribution and functional significance of phosphodiesterase isoenzymes in the human lower urinary tract. World J Urol 2005; 23:368–373.

104. Qiu Y, Kraft P, Craig EC, et al. Identification and functional study of phosphodiesterases in rat urinary bladder. Urol Res 2001; 29:388–392.

105. Filippi S, Morelli A, Sandner P, et al. Characterization and functional role of androgen-dependent PDE5 activity in the bladder. Endocrinology 2007; 148:1019–1029.

106. Mulhall JP, Guhring P, Parker M, et al. Assessment of the impact of sildenafil citrate on lower urinary tract symptoms in men with erectile dysfunction. J Sex Med 2006; 3:662–667.

107. Shinkai M, Takayanagi I. Effect of tachykinins on the acetylcholine output stimulated by nicotine from guinea-pig bladder. Regul Pept 1993; 46:399–401.

108. de Biasi M, Nigro F, Xu W. Nicotinic acetylcholine receptors in the autonomic control of bladder function. Eur J Pharmacol 2000; 393:137–140.

109. Nicholls J, Hourani SM, Kitchen I. Characterization of P1-purinoceptors on rat duodenum and urinary bladder. Br J Pharmacol 1992; 105:639–642.

110. Fahrenkrug J, Hannibal J. Pituitary adenylate cyclase activating polypeptide immunoreactivity in capsaicin-sensitive nerve fibres supplying the rat urinary tract. Neuroscience 1998; 83:1261–1272.

111. Candenas L, Lecci A, Pinto FM, et al. Tachykinins and tachykinin receptors: effects in the genitourinary tract. Life Sci 2005; 76:835–862.

112. Templeman L, Sellers DJ, Chapple CR, et al. Investigation of neurokinin-2 and -3 receptors in the human and pig bladder. BJU Int 2003; 92:787–792.

113. Davenport AP, Battistino B. Classification of endothelin receptors and antagonists in clinical development. Clin Sc (Lond) 2002; 103(suppl 48):1S–3S.

114. Donoso MV, Salas C, Sepulveda G, et al. Involvement of ETA receptors in the facilitation by endothelin-1 of non-adrenergic non-cholinergic transmission in the rat urinary bladder. Br J Pharmacol 1994; 111:473–482.

115. Ukai M, Yuyama H, Noguchi Y, et al. Participation of endogenous endothelin and ETA receptor in premicturition contractions in rats with bladder outlet obstruction. Naunyn Schmiedebergs Arch Pharmacol 2006; 373:197–203.

116. Ng YK, de Groat WC, Wu HY. Smooth muscle and neural mechanisms contributing to the downregulation of neonatal rat spontaneous bladder contractions during postnatal development. Am J Physiol Regul Integr Comp Physiol 2007; 292:R2100–R2112.

117. Szell EA, Somogyi GT, de Groat WC, et al. Developmental changes in spontaneous smooth muscle activity in the neonatal rat urinary bladder. Am J Physiol Regul Integr Comp Physiol 2003; 285:R809–R816.

118. Ikeda Y, Fry CH, Hayashi F, et al. The role of gap junctions in spontaneous activity of the rat bladder. Am J Physiol Renal Physiol 2007 293:F1018–F1025.

119. Chua WC, Liu L, Mansfield KJ, et al. Age-related changes of P2X$_1$ receptor mRNA in the bladder detrusor from men with and without bladder outlet obstruction. Exp Gerontol 2007; 42:686–692.

120. de Groat WC. A neurologic basis for the overactive bladder. Urology. 1997; 50:36–52.

121. Brading AF. A myogenic basis for the overactive bladder. Urology 1997; 50:57–67.

122. Ikeda Y, Kanai A. Urotheliogenic modulation of intrinsic activity in spinal cord transected rat bladders—the role of mucosal muscarinic receptors. Am J Physiol Renal Physiol 2008; 295:F454–F461.

123. Drake MJ, Hedlund P, Harvey IJ, et al. Partial outlet obstruction enhances modular autonomous activity in the isolated rat bladder. J Urol 2003; 170:276–279.

124. Andersson KE. Antimuscarinics for treatment of overactive bladder. Lancet Neurol 2004; 3:46–53.

125. Christ GJ, Day NS, Day M, et al. Increased connexin43-mediated intercellular communication in a rat model of bladder overactivity in vivo. Am J Physiol Regul Integr Comp Physiol 2003; 284:R1241–R1248.

126. McCloskey KD, Gurney AM. Kit positive cells in the guinea pig bladder. J Urol 2002; 168:832–836.

127. Hashitani H, Yanai Y, Suzuki H. Role of interstitial cells and gap junctions in the transmission of spontaneous Ca^{2+} signals in detrusor smooth muscles of the guinea-pig urinary bladder. J Physiol 2004; 559:567–581.

128. Smet PJ, Jonavicius J, Marshall VR, et al. Distribution of nitric oxide synthase-immuno-reactive nerves and identification of the cellular targets of nitric oxide in guinea-pig and human urinary bladder by cGMP immunohistochemistry. Neuroscience 1996; 71:337–348.

129. Gillespie JI, Drake MJ. The actions of sodium nitroprusside and the phosphodiesterase inhibitor dipyridamole on phasic activity in the isolated guinea pig bladder. BJU Int 2004; 93:851858.

130. Yoshida M, Inadome A, Maeda Y, et al. Non-neuronal cholinergic system in human bladder urothelium. Urology 2006; 67:425–430.

131. Birder LA, Apodaca G, De Groat WC, et al. Adrenergic- and capsaicin-evoked nitric oxide release from urothelium and afferent nerves in urinary bladder. Am J Physiol 1998; 275:F226–F229.

132. Marchand JE, Sant GR, Kream RM. Increased expression of substance P receptor encoding mRNA in bladder biopsies from patients with interstitial cystitis. Br J Urol 1998; 81:224–228.

133. Sun Y, Chai TC. Augmented extracellular ATP signaling in bladder urothelial cells from patients with interstitial cystitis. Am J Physiol Cell Physiol 2006; 290:C27–C34.

134. Wang EC, Lee JM, Ruiz WG, et al. ATP and purinergic receptor-dependent membrane traffic in bladder umbrella cells. J Clin Invest 2005; 115:2412–2422.

135. Birder LA, Ruan HZ, Chopra B, et al. Alterations in P2X and P2Y purinergic receptor expression in urinary bladder from normal cats and cats with interstitial cystitis. Am J Physiol Renal Physiol 2004; 287:F1084–F1091.

136. Birder LA, Kanai AJ, de Groat WC, et al. Vanilloid receptor expression suggests a sensory role for urinary bladder epithelial cells. Proc Natl Acad Sci U S A 2001; 98:13396–13401.

137. Andrade EL, Ferreira J, Andre E, et al. Contractile mechanisms coupled to TRPA1 receptor activation in rat urinary bladder. Biochem Pharmacol 2006; 72:104–114.

138. Stein RJ, Santos S, Nagatomi J, et al. Cool (TRPM8) and hot (TRPV1) receptors in the bladder and male genital tract. J Urol 2004; 172:1175–1178.

139. Chopra B, Barrick SR, Meyers S, et al. Expression and function of bradykinin B1 and B2 receptors in normal and inflamed rat urinary bladder urothelium. J Physiol 2005; 562:859–871.

140. Birder LA, Nealen ML, Kiss S, et al. Beta-adrenoceptor agonists stimulate endothelial nitric oxide synthase in rat

urinary bladder urothelial cells. J Neurosci 2002; 22: 8063–8070.

141. Cockayne DA, Hamilton SG, Zhu QM, et al. Urinary bladder hyporeflexia and reduced pain-related behaviour in P2X3-deficient mice. Nature 2000; 407:1011–1015.

142. Vlaskovska M, Kasakov L, Rong W, et al. P2X3 knock-out mice reveal a major sensory role for urothelially released ATP. J Neurosci 2001; 21:5670–5677.

143. Wu C, Sui GP, Fry CH. Purinergic regulation of guinea pig suburothelial myofibroblasts. J Physiol 2004; 559:231–243.

144. Sui GP, Wu C, Fry CH. Characterization of the purinergic receptor subtype on guinea-pig suburothelial myofibroblasts. BJU Int 2006; 97:1327–1331.

145. Sun Y, Keay S, De Deyne PG, et al. Augmented stretch activated adenosine triphosphate release from bladder uroepithelial cells in patients with interstitial cystitis. J Urol 2001; 166:1951–1956.

146. Salas NA, Somogyi GT, Gangitano DA, et al. Receptor activated bladder and spinal ATP release in neurally intact and chronic spinal cord injured rats. Neurochem Int 2007; 50:345–350.

147. Khera M, Somogyi GT, Kiss S, et al. Botulinum toxin A inhibits ATP release from bladder urothelium after chronic spinal cord injury. Neurochem Int 2004; 45:987–993.

148. Yoshida M, Miyamae K, Iwashita H, et al. Management of detrusor dysfunction in the elderly: changes in acetylcholine and adenosine triphosphate release during aging. Urology 2004; 63(3 suppl 1):17–23.

149. Yoshida M, Masunaga K, Satoji Y, et al. Basic and clinical aspects of non-neuronal acetylcholine: expression of non-neuronal acetylcholine in urothelium and its clinical significance. J Pharmacol Sci 2008; 106:193–198.

150. Hanna-Mitchell AT, Beckel JM, Barbadora S, et al. Non-neuronal acetylcholine and urinary bladder urothelium. Life Sci 2007; 80:2298–2302.

151. Zarghooni S, Wunsch J, Bodenbenner M, et al. Expression of muscarinic and nicotinic acetylcholine receptors in the mouse urothelium. Life Sci 2007; 80:2308–2313.

152. Mansfield KJ, Liu L, Moore KH, et al. Molecular characterization of M_2 and M_3 muscarinic receptor expression in bladder from women with refractory idiopathic detrusor overactivity. BJU Int 2007; 99:1433–1438.

153. Birder LA, Barrick SR, Roppolo JR, et al. Feline interstitial cystitis results in mechanical hypersensitivity and altered ATP release from bladder urothelium. Am J Physiol Renal Physiol 2003; 285:F423–F429.

154. Davidson RA, McCloskey KD. Morphology and localization of interstitial cells in the guinea pig bladder: structural relationships with smooth muscle and neurons. J Urol 2005; 173:1385–1390.

155. Sui GP, Wu C, Fry CH. Electrical characteristics of suburothelial cells isolated from the human bladder. J Urol 2004; 171:938–943.

156. Kuijpers KA, Heesakkers JP, Jansen CF, et al. Cadherin-11 is expressed in detrusor smooth muscle cells and myofibroblasts of normal human bladder. Eur Urol 2007; 52:1213–1221.

157. Greenland JE, Brading AF. The effect of bladder outflow obstruction on detrusor blood flow changes during the voiding cycle in conscious pigs. J Urol 2001; 165:245–248.

158. Kershen RT, Azadzoi KM, Siroky MB. Blood flow, pressure and compliance in the male human bladder. J Urol 2002; 168:121–125.

159. Mukerji G, Yiangou Y, Grogono J, et al. Localisation of M_2 and M_3 muscarinic receptors in human bladder disorders and their clinical correlations. J Urol 2006; 176:367–373.

160. Iijima K, de Wachter S, Wyndaele JJ. Effects of the M3 receptor selective muscarinic antagonist darifenacin on bladder afferent activity of the rat pelvic nerve. Eur Urol 2007; 52:842–849.

161. de Laet K, de Wachter S, Wyndaele JJ. Systemic oxybutynin decreases afferent activity of the pelvic nerve of the rat: new insights into the working mechanism of antimuscarinics. Neurourol Urodyn 2006; 25:156–161.

162. Hedland P, Streng T, Lee T, et al. Effects of tolterodine on afferent neuro-transmission in normal and resiniferotoxin treated conscious rats. J Urol 2007; 178:326–331.

163. Hawthorn MH, Chapple CR, Cock M, et al. Urothelium-derived inhibitory factor(s) influences on detrusor muscle contractility in vitro. Br J Pharmacol 2000; 129:416–419.

164. Murakami S, Chapple CR, Akino H, et al. The role of the urothelium in mediating bladder responses to isoprenaline. BJU Int 2007; 99:669–673.

165. Mastrangelo D, Iselin CE. Urothelium-dependent inhibition of rat ureter contractile activity. J Urol 2007; 178: 702–709.

166. Kanai A, Roppolo J, Ikeda Y, et al. Origin of spontaneous activity in neonatal and adult rat bladders and its enhancement by stretch and muscarinic agonists. Am J Physiol Renal Physiol 2007; 292:F1065–F1072.

167. Sui GP, Wu C, Roosen A, et al. Modulation of bladder myofibroblast activity: implications for bladder function. Am J Physiol 2008; 295:F688–F697.

168. Kubota Y, Hashitani H, Shirasawa N, et al. Altered distribution of interstitial cells in the guinea-pig bladder following bladder outlet obstruction. Neurourol Urodyn 2008; 27:330–340.

169. Biers SM, Reynard JM, Doore T, et al. The functional effects of a c-kit tyrosine inhibitor on guinea-pig and human detrusor. BJU Int 2006; 97:612–616.

170. Kubota Y, Biers SM, Kohri K, et al. Effects of imatinib mesylate (Glivec) as a *c-kit* tyrosine kinase inhibitor in the guinea-pig urinary bladder. Neurourol Urodyn 2006; 25:205–210.

171. Sui GP, Coppen SR, Dupont E, et al. Impedance measurements and connexin expression in human detrusor muscle from stable and unstable bladders. BJU Int 2003; 92:297–305.

172. Imaizumi Y, Torii Y, Ohi Y, et al. Ca^{2+} images and K^+ current during depolarization in smooth muscle cells of the guinea-pig vas deferens and urinary bladder. J Physiol 1998; 510:705–719.

173. Sui GP, Wu C, Severs N, et al. The association between T-type Ca^{2+}-current and outward current in isolated human detrusor cells from stable and overactive bladders. BJU International 2007; 99:436–441.

174. Zhu HL, Brain KL, Aishima M, et al. Actions of two main metabolites of propiverine (M-1 and M-2) on voltage-dependent L-type Ca^{2+} currents and Ca^{2+} transients in murine urinary bladder myocytes. J Pharmacol Exp Ther 2008; 324:118–127.

175. Kobayashi H, Miwa T, Nagao T, et al. Negative modulation of L-type Ca^{2+} channels via beta-adrenoceptor stimulation in guinea-pig detrusor smooth muscle cells. Eur J Pharmacol 2003; 470:9–15.

176. Herrera GM, Heppner TJ, Nelson MT. Voltage dependence of the coupling of Ca^{2+} sparks to BK(Ca) channels in urinary bladder smooth muscle. Am J Physiol Cell Physiol 2001; 280:C481–C490.

177. Yanai Y, Hashitani H, Kubota Y, et al. The role of Ni^{2+}-sensitive T-type Ca^{2+} channels in the regulation of spontaneous excitation in detrusor smooth muscles of the guinea-pig bladder. BJU Int 2006; 97:182–189.

178. Werner ME, Knorn AM, Meredith AL, et al. Frequency encoding of cholinergic- and purinergic-mediated signaling to mouse urinary bladder smooth muscle: modulation

by BK channels. Am J Physiol Regul Integr Comp Physiol 2007; 292:R616–R624.

179. Christ GJ, Day NS, Day M, et al. Bladder injection of "naked" hSlo/pcDNA3 ameliorates detrusor hyperactivity in obstructed rats in vivo. Am J Physiol Regul Integr Comp Physiol 2001; 281:R1699–R1709.

180. Tian L, McClafferty H, Chen L, et al. Reversible tyrosine protein phosphorylation regulates large conductance voltage- and calcium-activated potassium channels via cortactin. J Biol Chem 2008; 283:3067–3076.

181. Loane DJ, Hicks GA, Perrino BA, et al. Inhibition of BK channel activity by association with calcineurin in rat brain. Eur J Neurosci 2006; 24:4334–4341.

182. Adam RM, Eaton SH, Estrada C, et al. Mechanical stretch is a highly selective regulator of gene expression in human bladder smooth muscle cells. Physiol Genomics 2004; 20:36–44.

183. Aitken KJ, Block G, Lorenzo A, et al. Mechanotransduction of extracellular signal-regulated kinases 1 and 2 mitogen-activated protein kinase activity in smooth muscle is dependent on the extracellular matrix and regulated by matrix metalloproteinases. Am J Pathol 2006; 169:459–470.

184. Wellner MC, Isenberg G. Stretch effects on whole-cell currents of guinea-pig urinary bladder myocytes. J Physiol 1994; 480:439–448.

185. Baker SA, Hennig GW, Han J, et al. Methionine and its derivatives increase bladder excitability by inhibiting stretch-dependent K^+ channels. Br J Pharmacol 2008; 1530:1259–1271.

186. Tanagho EA. The ureterovesical junction. In: Chisholm GD, Williams DI, eds. Scientific Foundations of Urology. London: Heinemann, 1982:395–404.

187. Viana R, Batourina E, Huang H, et al. The development of the bladder trigone, the center of the anti-reflux mechanism. Development 2007; 134:3763–3769.

188. Roosen A, Wu C, Sui GP, et al. Characteristics of spontaneous activity in the bladder trigone. Eur Urol 2009 56(2):346–153.

189. Roosen A, Wu C, Sui GP, et al. Synergistic effects in neuromuscular activation and calcium-sensitisation in the bladder trigone. BJU Int 2008; 101:610–614.

190. Andersson KE, Wein AJ. Pharmacology of the lower urinary tract: basis for current and future treatments of urinary incontinence. Pharmacol Rev 2004; 56:581–631.

191. Roosen A, Sui GP, Fry CH, et al. Adreno-muscarinic synergism in the bladder trigone: calcium-dependent and -independent mechanisms. Cell Calcium 2009 45(1):11–17.

192. Tanagho EA, Meyers FH, Smith DR. Urethral resistance: its components and implications. I. Smooth muscle component. Invest Urol 1969; 7:136–149.

193. Awad SA, Downie JW. Relative contributions of smooth and striated muscles to the canine urethral pressure profile. Br J Urol 1976; 48:347–354.

194. Nishimatsu H, Moriyama N, Hamada K, et al. Contractile responses to alpha1-adrenoceptor agonists in isolated human male and female urethra. BJU Int 1999; 84:515–520.

195. Bagot K, Chess-Williams R. Alpha(1A/L)-adrenoceptors mediate contraction of the circular smooth muscle of the pig urethra. Auton Autacoid Pharmacol 2006; 26:345–353.

196. Musselman DM, Ford AP, Gennevois DJ, et al. A randomized crossover study to evaluate Ro 115-1240, a selective alpha(1A/1L)-adrenoceptor partial agonist in women with stress urinary incontinence. BJU Int 2004; 93:78–83.

197. Mattiasson A, Andersson K E, Sjögren C. Adrenoceptors and cholinoceptors controlling noradrenaline release from adrenergic nerves in the urethra of rabbit and man. J Urol 1984; 131:1190–1195.

198. Morita T, Kihara K, Nagamatsu H, et al. Effects of clenbuterol on rabbit vesicourethral muscle contractility. J Smooth Muscle Res 1995; 31:119–127.

199. Persson K, Pandita RK, Aszodi A, et al. Functional characteristics of urinary tract smooth muscles in mice lacking cGMP protein kinase type I. Am J Physiol Regul Integr Comp Physiol 2000; 279:R1112–R1120.

200. Schroder A, Hedlund P, Andersson KE. Carbon monoxide relaxes the female pig urethra as effectively as nitric oxide in the presence of YC-1. J Urol 2002; 167:1892–1896.

201. Ho MH, Bhatia NN, Khorram O. Physiologic role of nitric oxide and nitric oxide synthase in female lower urinary tract. Curr Opin Obstet Gynecol 2004; 16:423–429.

202. Yang Z, Dolber PC, Fraser MO. Diabetic urethropathy compounds the effects of diabetic cystopathy. J Urol 2007; 178:2213–2219.

203. Jackson S, James M, Abrams P. The effect of oestradiol on vaginal collagen metabolism in postmenopausal women with genuine stress incontinence. BJOG 2002; 109:339–344.

204. DuBeau CE. Estrogen treatment for urinary incontinence: never, now, or in the future? JAMA 2005; 293:998–1001.

205. Callahan SM, Creed KE. Electrical and mechanical activity of the isolated lower urinary tract of the guinea-pig. Br J Pharmacol 1981; 74:353–358.

206. Bradley JE, Anderson UA, Woolsey SM, Thornbury KD, McHale NG, Hollywood MA. Characterization of T-type calcium current and its contribution to electrical activity in rabbit urethra. Am J Physiol Cell Physiol 2004; 286:C1078–C1088.

207. McHale N, Hollywood M, Sergeant G, Thornbury K. Origin of spontaneous rhythmicity in smooth muscle. J Physiol 2006; 570:23–28.

208. Lyons AD, Gardiner TA, McCloskey KD. Kit-positive interstitial cells in the rabbit urethra: structural relationships with nerves and smooth muscle. BJU Int 2007; 99:687–694.

209. Strasser H, Ninkovic M, Hess M, et al. Anatomic and functional studies of the male and female urethral sphincter. World J Urol 2000; 18:324–329.

210. Creed KE, van der Werf BA. The innervation and properties of the urethral striated muscle. Scand J Urol Nephrol Suppl 2001; 207:8–11.

211. Strasser H, Tiefenthaler M, Steinlechner M, et al. Age dependent apoptosis and loss of rhabdosphincter cells. J Urol 2000; 164:1781–1785.

212. Lin YH, Liu G, Daneshgari F. A mouse model of simulated birth trauma induced stress urinary incontinence. Neurourol Urodyn 2008; 27:353–358.

213. Furuta A, Jankowski RJ, Honda M, et al. State of the art of where we are at using stem cells for stress urinary incontinence. Neurourol Urodyn. 2007; 26:966–971.

214. Takahashi S, Chen Q, Ogushi T, et al. Periurethral injection of sustained release basic fibroblast growth factor improves sphincteric contractility of the rat urethra denervated by botulinum-a toxin. J Urol. 2006; 176:819–823.

215. Kwon D, Kim Y, Pruchnic R, et al. Periurethral cellular injection: comparison of muscle-derived progenitor cells and fibroblasts with regard to efficacy and tissue contractility in an animal model of stress urinary incontinence. Urology 2006; 68:449–454.

216. Thor K. Serotonin and norepinephrine involvement in efferent pathways to the urethral rhabdosphincter: implication for treating stress urinary incontinence. Urology 2003; 62(suppl 4A):3–9.

217. Mariappan P, Ballantyne Z, N'Dow JM, et al. Serotonin and noradrenaline reuptake inhibitors (SNRI) for stress

urinary incontinence in adults. Cochrane Database Syst Rev 2005; 20(3):CD004742.

218. Fowler CJ, Christmas TJ, Chapple CR, et al. Abnormal electromyographic activity of the urethral sphincter, voiding dysfunction, and polycystic ovaries: a new syndrome? BMJ 1988; 297:1436–1438.

219. Sanders DB. Ephaptic transmission in hemifacial SPASM: a single-fiber EMG study. Nerve Muscle 1989; 12:690–694.

220. Datta SN, Chaliha C, Singh A, et al. Sacral neurostimulation for urinary retention: 10-year experience from one UK centre. BJU Int 2008; 101:192–196.

16

Scientific Basis of Urodynamics

Michael Craggs and Sarah Knight
London Spinal Cord Injuries Centre, Royal National Orthopaedic Hospital, Stanmore, U.K.

INTRODUCTION

The lower urinary tract comprises the bladder, urethra and striated sphincter, which act as a single functional unit under nervous control. The bladder has two principal functions; first, to be a secure low-pressure storage reservoir for the entire urine output from the kidneys and, second, to contract efficiently and empty at socially convenient times. The normal person voids on average about 300 mL completely in about 40 seconds six times a day with no leakage and little sensation of bladder filling in between. However, if these functions are ever compromised, as, for example, in patients presenting with symptoms such as incontinence, urgency, frequency or obstructed voiding, it is important that we are able to assess the operation of the lower urinary tract objectively during both the storage and voiding phases.

Such investigations form the basis of urodynamics, a study that attempts to measure and determine the relationship between bladder volume, bladder pressure (cystometry) and urine flow (flowmetry) under the best physiological conditions possible. The physiological basis and coordination of normal bladder and sphincter function are described fully elsewhere (chap. 15).

Much is said about the lack of correlation between symptoms and urodynamic measures in some patients; for example, it is not always possible to observe unstable contractions of the detrusor in the untreated patient complaining of urge incontinence. This sort of finding has made some urologists skeptical of the value of invasive urodynamics (pressure monitoring by catheter per urethra) to the extent that they believe the method is unnatural, offers little to the diagnosis of a patient's problems and introduces infection to the bladder. On the other hand, there are many clinicians who do accept urodynamics as a useful investigative tool but only as a practiced art requiring years of experience and careful evaluation.

However, there is an important scientific basis of urodynamics, which, if properly standardized and interpreted, can lead to significant findings for making a proper diagnosis of a patient's problems. An example of this is in the derived measure of "urethral resistance," where an analysis relating detrusor pressure to flow can objectively define obstructed voiding,

a condition not always accurately diagnosed from flow measurement alone (1). Therefore, to transform urodynamics from an art form to a science, we must have a full understanding of the principles of the technique, the underlying physics and mechanics, the derivation of parameters and an appreciation of the extent and limitations of urodynamics as a diagnostic tool.

PHYSICS AND MECHANICS OF THE LOWER URINARY TRACT

From an engineering point of view, the bladder and urethra act as a single functional unit, which can be modeled as a system comprising reservoir, valves and connecting tubes, with pressure, flow and volume as measured variables. To understand the working of this unit during the normal micturition cycle, it is easiest to consider storage and voiding separately, but before that we should be clear about the definition of the measures, specifically, pressure.

Pressure is defined as the force acting per unit area, and force is a vector quantity, which has a direction; however, pressure is scalar and has no direction. In urodynamics, pressure is usually quoted in the units of cmH_2O. The standard international (SI) unit is the kilopascal (kPa), which is approximately equal to $10\ cmH_2O$.

Storage Phase

Bladder filling is an essentially passive process during which the normal functional capacity of 300 to 500 mL should be reached with only a small increase in pressure and before sensations of bladder fullness are perceived. It is possible to account for the bladder as a low-pressure, high-capacity reservoir in purely physical terms.

The small pressure rise within the bladder as it fills is mainly the result of elastic forces generated within the bladder wall. If the bladder is assumed to behave as a thin-walled sphere, its pressure-volume characteristics can be described by Laplace's law ($P = 2T/R$) where P—pressure, R—radius, and T—tension per unit width of bladder wall (Fig. 1). As the bladder fills and the volume increases ($R\uparrow$), the wall tension increases ($T\uparrow$), but the ratio T/R remains constant,

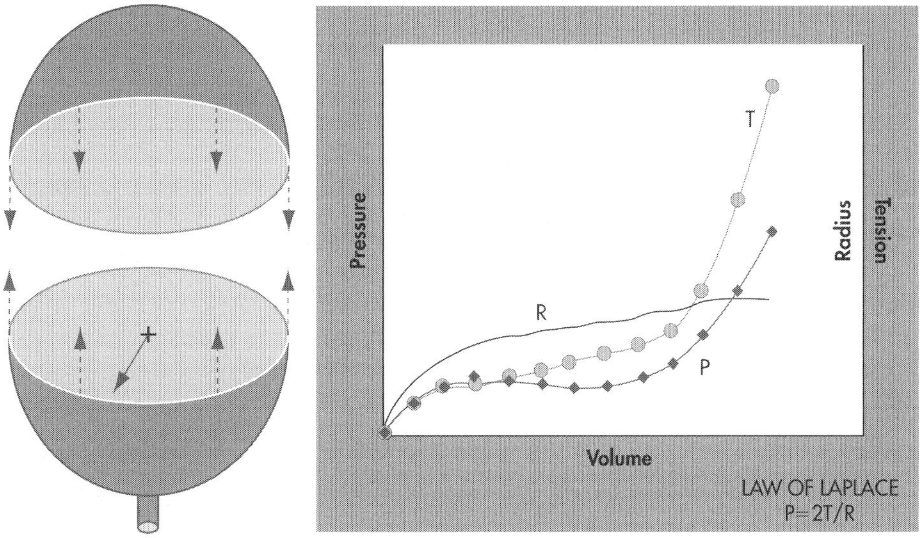

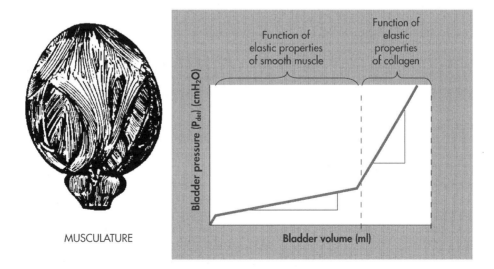

Figure 1 The physics of the bladder as a low-pressure reservoir. The bladder modeled as a thin-walled sphere obeying the law of Laplace. Relationships between volume, pressure, radius and tension in a thin-walled sphere.

resulting in little change in intravesical pressure until the bladder is almost full.

The use of Laplace's law to determine wall tension and pressure is based on the assumption that the bladder is a thin-walled sphere during the whole of the filling phase. However, the bladder actually progresses from a relatively thick-walled irregular shape when empty to a thin-walled multicurved vessel when full, but the model is a sufficient approximation for a relatively full bladder.

The property of the bladder wall that allows a large increase in volume with only a small associated pressure rise is known as compliance, which is defined as the change in volume divided by the corresponding change in pressure ($\Delta V/\Delta P$). The wall also exhibits the property of elasticity, as it can return to its normal size after voiding with no permanent deformation (plastic) changes. The bladder wall is composed of three layers: an outer covering of connective tissue (serosa), a smooth muscle layer (detrusor) and a mucous membrane (urothelium) which lines the interior of the bladder. These layers comprise collagen and elastin fibers as well as muscle. The layers in combination make the bladder very compliant until the structural capacity of the bladder is reached, and further increases in volume cause increased wall stiffness as the properties of the collagen fibers in the wall dominate and reduce compliance (Fig. 2).

Figure 2 Structure, compliance and capacity of the bladder. Bladder musculature and graph showing relationship between bladder volume and pressure with respect to structural properties.

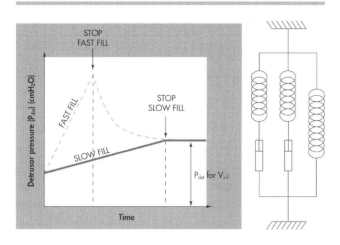

Figure 3 Viscoelastic properties of the bladder wall. The effect of bladder fill rate on measured detrusor pressure. A typical spring and dashpot model of the viscoelastic behavior of the bladder wall.

In addition to compliance and elasticity, the bladder exhibits the time-dependent property of viscoelasticity in which the bladder wall tension and extension are dependent on rate of filling. When the bladder wall is stretched rapidly, as during fast filling, it appears stiffer than when filled more slowly; however, when the filling is stopped, the wall exhibits relaxation in an exponential manner. Viscoelasticity is often modeled as a combination of spring (purely elastic) and dash-pot (purely viscous) elements (Fig. 3) (2).

These properties of the bladder wall during storage are likely to be purely passive physical mechanisms attributable to the properties of the tissues, although there may be some active neuromodulatory effects brought about by reflex contractions of the detrusor muscle.

Throughout the storage phase, the urethra must remain closed with a pressure (P_{ura}), which exceeds

that of the bladder pressure (P_{ves}) to ensure no leakage of urine ($P_{ura} > P_{ves}$). The urethral closure pressure may be divided into passive and active forces (3). Passive forces are maintained by the mucosal seal, which occurs when the urethral walls oppose each other. Active forces are exerted by the contraction of the urethral and periurethral muscles.

The urethral pressure increases as the bladder fills and during periods when the intra-abdominal pressure increases—for example, as a result of postural change or coughing and sneezing—thus maintaining continence.

Voiding Phase

Voiding is initiated voluntarily following sensation of bladder fullness and is preceded by relaxation of the urethral sphincter. The detrusor muscle contracts in response to uninhibited parasympathetic stimulation, but urine does not flow until the bladder pressure exceeds the urethral pressure ($P_{ves} > P_{ura}$). This initial detrusor contraction is isometric since there is no significant change in bladder volume and no external work done in passing urine.

As soon as the bladder pressure exceeds the urethral closure pressure, the detrusor contraction becomes isotonic, and there is shortening of the detrusor muscle, producing increased external work as the flow reaches a maximum. The isotonic contraction is sustained by reflex activation mediated by increased tension in the receptors in series with the contracting muscle fibers until it falls below a threshold as the detrusor begins to relax at the end of voiding (Fig. 4).

As with any fluid flow, the rate of urine output (Q_{ura}) is dependent on both the driving force (P_{ves}), and the resistance to flow (R_{ura}) ($Q_{ura} \propto P_{ves}/R_{ura}$). Other fluid properties, such as viscosity, are normally constant and relatively unimportant, but the use of radio-opaque substances, which can be quite viscous, for X-ray imaging of the urinary tract during urodynamics may have small effects on flow. Physiologically,

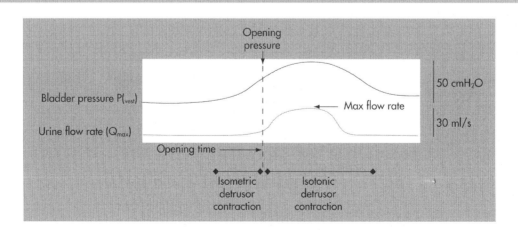

Figure 4 Pressure relationships from storage to voiding, indicating the transition from isometric to isotonic detrusor contraction.

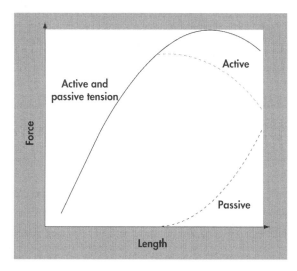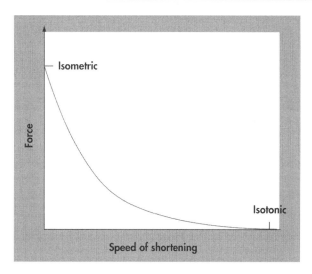

Figure 5 Force-length curve and force-velocity curve for detrusor muscle contraction.

the isometric part of the detrusor contraction should follow the standard force-length (or volume) and force-velocity curves that can be demonstrated for other muscles (Fig. 5) (4).

If the bladder is overstretched or not sufficiently full, a submaximal isometric contraction will be produced and reduced flow rate will be achieved. The optimal contraction of the detrusor will be at bladder volumes within the normal functional capacity. The isotonic contraction of the detrusor, that is, when the bladder is emptying, is related to the velocity of shortening of the detrusor muscle. As the force changes from isometric to isotonic, the maximum speed of shortening increases with decreasing load until, in the theoretical limit, no force is required when the muscle becomes unloaded. The resistance to flow is dependent on both active and passive factors in the urethra, including urethral lumen shape and length, active contraction of the sphincter, and intrinsic muscle and anatomical features. These factors may change throughout the voiding phase; therefore, a simple interpretation of urethral resistance may be difficult to evaluate, and it may be more useful to describe these changes in terms of impedance that includes a time-dependent element. Although the viscosity of urine can

be approximated as a constant, the type of urine flow is likely to alternate between laminar and turbulent, depending on changes in the urethral impedance.

Understanding these basic principles of physics and mechanics is important if we are to develop good scientific methodology for urodynamic investigations, the measurement of and relationship between pressure, flow and volume during the storage and voiding phases of bladder function.

METHODOLOGY, PRACTICE, AND PROBLEMS

The basic aim of urodynamics is to provoke the lower urinary tract in the relatively controlled environment of a clinical laboratory so as to provide an objective basis for a patient's symptoms, lead to a clear diagnosis of the dysfunction and, hopefully, give a guide to rational treatment. Perhaps the greatest failure in this endeavor is poor practice and the misinterpretation of urodynamic tests. There are a number of techniques available for the practice of urodynamics depending on whether the individual patient has a voiding or storage problem, or a combination of both, these are summarized in Table 1. In standard

Table 1 Techniques Used in Urodynamics for Measurement of Lower Urinary Tract Function

Technique	Function	Indication
Cystometry	Measurement of bladder storage and voiding function, including sensation	Incontinence and dysfunction of detrusor
Flowmetry	Measurement of voiding function	Incontinence and voiding dysfunction
Urethral pressure profilometry	Measurement of urethral closure pressures	Incontinence due to sphincter incompetence
Ambulatory urodynamics	Behavior of bladder and urethra during activities of daily living	Incontinence
Videourodynamics	Measurement of bladder storage and voiding in conjunction with imaging of bladder morphology	Multifactorial incontinence or suspected abnormalities in lower urinary tract
Neurophysiological	Neurophysiological assessment of urethral sphincter and pelvic floor function	Incontinence or dyssynergic voiding

urodynamic testing, we usually measure only pressure, flow and volume and leave other physiological measures, such as the electromyography of sphincters, too more specialized investigations. To interpret accurately the results of urodynamic tests and carry them out in a scientific and reproducible manner, free from technical artefact, it is important to have a full understanding of the physical principles of these measurements, as described in the previous section.

Pressure can be measured in a number of ways; simple manometry is based on the height of a fluid column, with the pressure proportional to the height of the column. Alternatively, the fluid column can be connected (e.g., via a fluid-filled catheter) to an external strain gauge pressure transducer in which the pressure is proportional to the electrical signal output from the transducer. This is the most commonly used pressure measurement technique in urodynamics. Microtip catheter transducers utilize a miniature pressure sensor mounted in the tip (or along the side) of a catheter, which can be inserted into the bladder.

Bladder pressure is usually expressed with reference to atmospheric pressure; therefore, the correct zeroing of transducers to atmospheric pressures is very important. In addition, the position of the catheter tip transducer within the bladder can affect the pressure recording, as the pressure measured at the top of the bladder is approximately 10 cmH$_2$O lower than that at the base because of the height of the water within the bladder itself, and the fluid-filled catheters are very dependent on relative height of external transducer and tip of catheter (Fig. 6). The standard zero reference is the level of the symphisis pubis [International Continence Society (ICS)].

Cystometry

The aim of cystometry is to investigate the pressure-volume relationship of the bladder during the filling and storage phases. To measure pressure, a catheter is introduced into the bladder either per urethra or, if access is available, suprapubically. In addition to measuring bladder pressure, it is important to measure intra-abdominal pressure, usually through a catheter placed in the rectum. In this way, the intra-abdominal pressure (P_{abd}) can be subtracted from the intravesical pressure (P_{ves}) to give a true detrusor pressure (P_{det}) free from artefacts caused by extravesical pressure increases, such as coughing or straining. However, it must be noted that in addition to abdominal pressure changes, P_{abd} will also reflect intrinsic bowel activity (Fig. 7).

During a filling cystometrogram, fluid is retrogradely instilled into the bladder in a physiological manner. In the ideal situation, this means using isotonic saline at body temperature, at a rate close to that of natural diuresis from the kidneys ($\ll$10 mL/min). However, because of constraints of time and convenience, filling rates are normally much faster (10–100 mL/min), though these rates may be too provocative for some overactive bladders, and may lead to overfilling in others that are hypoactive. As described earlier, a normal bladder shows very little change in pressure during filling (high compliance), but because of possible decreases in the viscoelastic nature of the bladder wall (e.g., in the neuropathic bladder), it may be necessary to fill much more slowly in some patients. A further matter is the position of the patient during cystometry—lying down, sitting or standing may be important if we are to replicate the conditions in which patients' symptoms are revealed, but this cannot always be practical. Most filling

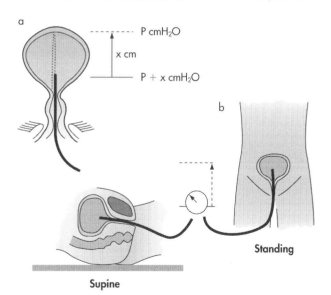

Figure 6 Effect of catheter position in bladder on recorded pressure. (**A**) Effect of intravesical catheter position of microtip pressure transducer. (**B**) Effect of relative position of external pressure transducer.

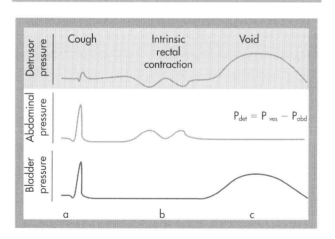

Figure 7 Subtraction cystometry with detrusor pressure calculated from difference between vesical and rectal pressure measurement. (**A**) Cough appears in both P_{ves} and P_{abd} and therefore no P_{det}. (**B**) Intrinsic bowel contraction appears in P_{abd} only; therefore, P_{det} shows inverse trace. (**C**) Bladder contraction activity appears in P_{ves} alone and therefore in P_{det}.

cystometry is performed with the patients lying either supine or semirecumbent and then raised to sitting or standing position for voiding cystometry (see later in this section).

Urethral Pressure Profilometry

This technique is used to determine the intraluminal pressure along the length of the urethra, during the storage phase. This investigation has lost favor among some clinicians, probably as a result of its relative complexity and inaccuracy if not performed correctly. However, knowledge of urethral resistance can be useful in identifying urethral incompetence (as in anatomical obstruction by stricture, benign prostatic hyperplasia (BPH), or active dyssynergic sphincters). There are two principal techniques for measuring UPP: fluid perfusion profilometry (5) and solid-state microtip pressure transducers.

The perfusion technique is based on the pressure required to perfuse fluid through a catheter at a constant rate; this is best achieved with a syringe driver rather than a peristaltic pump. A catheter with side holes is introduced into the urethra and zeroed in the standard way, and the catheter is attached via a three-way tap to a pressure transducer and an infusion pump. The pressure recorded is defined as the resistance the urethral wall produces to the perfusing fluid. The catheter is then withdrawn slowly along the length of the urethra, thus giving a pressure profile. A profile can also be obtained by withdrawing a solid-state pressure tip transducer at a constant rate (Fig. 8).

There are a number of factors that must be taken into account when performing UPP to ensure accuracy. As described earlier, pressure has no direction, and therefore measuring in a particular orientation along the urethral wall may introduce errors because of position of side holes or transducer sensors. In addition, bladder volume, patient position and artefacts caused by movement or abdominal straining can also introduce errors.

Urethral pressure profiles can be measured in steady-state or static conditions, or, alternatively, under conditions of stress such as coughing or straining.

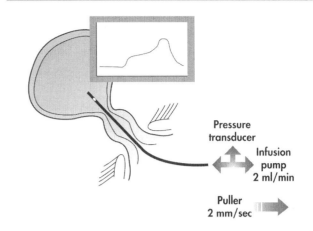

Figure 8 Brown-Wickham perfusion technique for measurement of urethral pressure profile.

Flowmetry

Of all urodynamic tests, this is the least invasive and easiest to perform with modern flow rate recorders and should certainly be the first line of investigation for suspected voiding problems. As described in the previous section, the flow rate of urine from the bladder is dependent on both the driving force of the pressure generated in the bladder and the resistance of the urethra. A simple flow rate measurement cannot accurately distinguish the relative importance of these two factors; therefore, accurate diagnosis is often not possible without measuring both bladder pressure and flow rate simultaneously. Even then, the effect of urethral resistance may be an important additional factor.

There are a number of techniques available for measuring urine flow, based on the different principles described in Table 2.

Modern electronic devices can output a number of parameters based on the voiding characteristics. However, a single flow rate on a single occasion is unlikely to be of much diagnostic value, and a number of factors should be taken into account when performing meaningful flowmetry. The bladder volume at

Table 2 Methods of Measuring Urine Flow

Type of flowmeter	Principle	Comments
Weight transducer	Weight of urine voided measured and differentiated with respect to time to calculate flow rate.	
Rotating disc	A servomotor rotates the disc at a constant rate, but rate of urine flow tends to slow the disc, requiring greater power to keep at a constant speed. Power consumption of servomotor is proportional to flow rate and can be integrated for voided volume.	"Cruising" (moving urine stream over disc and sides of collecting container) can cause artifact.
Capacitance	A capacitor comprised of a metal strip is placed vertically in the collecting vessel. As volume of urine increases, the level of urine on the strip changes and capacitance decreases. The signal is proportional to voided volume and can be differentiated for flow rate.	Urinating on to capacitance strip may cause artifact.

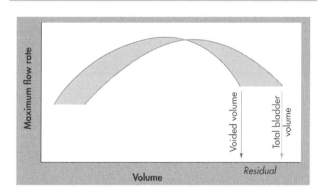

Figure 9 The relationship between maximum flow rate out of the bladder and bladder volume, demonstrating the reduction in flow rate at bladder volumes significantly larger or smaller than the functional volume.

which the flow rate was measured is extremely important, especially with respect to the force-length curve of the detrusor muscle. An over- or understretched bladder will not be capable of generating the maximal force to expel urine and thus may give a lower than optimal flow rate (Fig. 9). The urethral resistance may also change with bladder volumes and also give rise to different flow rates.

It is important to estimate the total bladder volume not only from the voided volume but also taking into account any residual volume in the bladder. This can be calculated by ultrasound or by catheter. In unfamiliar surroundings, a patient may feel uncomfortable, be inhibited or strain during voiding, and this may lead to an unnatural flow pattern and incomplete voiding. Technical artefacts can occur if the stream of flow is not aimed directly into the flow meter, and "cruising" or moving the stream across the flow meter can lead to abnormal traces. Flowmetry can also now be carried out with portable devices at home. This can lead to more accurate results, as the patient is more comfortable and multiple measurements can be recorded.

The ideal situation in which to carry out flowmetry is in conjunction with cystometry, so that voiding pressure and flow rate can be measured simultaneously, although the delay in urine flow exiting the bladder and reaching the flow meter must be taken into account. Pressure-flow studies can, for example, help to identify whether a low flow rate is due to a urethral obstruction or a hypocontractile bladder; this information could not be inferred from a flow rate alone.

INTERPRETATION: ART OR SCIENCE?

Interpretation of urodynamic investigations is very much dependent on both a proper understanding of the physiological factors controlling and affecting the lower urinary tract and the technical aspects of urodynamic technique. This is particularly important if the interpreters did not undertake the investigations themselves, Table 3 summarizes some important factors which may influence urodynamic findings.

The diagnostic potential of urodynamic studies relies on a number of measures, which should be quantified and standardized to minimize subjective interpretation. The ICS Standardization Committee has been pivotal in introducing procedures and guidelines for the standardization of terminology of lower urinary tract function, dysfunction and rehabilitation, including derived parameters and indices of function (6). However, it should be appreciated that rather little of this standardization has been based on comparative control data from healthy volunteers. Therefore, interpretation of urodynamic data on patients, in the hope of providing definitive diagnosis, can still remain unclear.

Filling Cystometry

From the filling cystometrogram, we can determine information about bladder compliance, the incidence of "unstable" detrusor activity, and the sensations perceived by subjects as the bladder volume increases to capacity.

As described in the previous section, bladder compliance is defined as the ratio of volume change

Table 3 Potential Factors That May Lead to Inaccuracies in Urodynamic Findings

Problem	Artefact and possible effects
Transducer zeroing and position	Incorrect pressure with respect to reference and poor subtraction of P_{ves} and P_{abd}.
Poor subtraction	Incorrect P_{det} recording, best checked by continuous coughing, which should show equal pressure changes on P_{ves} and P_{abd}.
Patient position	May not reproduce patients' symptoms and give false pressure.
Filling medium, temperature, viscosity, pH	May cause irritation, increasing sensations and possibly provoking overactivity.
Filling rate	Filling too fast may provoke unstable contractions and underestimate compliance.
Catheter size	A large catheter may cause irritation and partial obstruction.
Air bubbles in water-filled lines	This will cause a damped pressure recording and incorrect pressure values.
Misplaced catheter	Will not represent true P_{ves} or P_{det}; that is, catheter being expelled during voiding or coughing.
Overfilling of bladder	May reduce ability to void, especially in patients with reduced sensation or outflow obstruction.
Presence of infection	May increase urgency symptoms.
Concomitant medication	May affect symptoms.

to pressure change—$\Delta V/\Delta P$. For a normal healthy bladder, the maximum capacity should be reached with only a small change in bladder pressure, to give a high value for compliance (about 40 mL/cmH$_2$O). As the bladder becomes stiffer, particularly toward maximum capacity, the pressure per unit volume can increase, and the compliance becomes smaller in a nonlinear fashion. It is important to recognize the effect that the rate that bladder filling can have on compliance, and in some cases it may be necessary to stop the fill and wait until the bladder pressure has returned to its stress-relaxed state before calculating a value for compliance. This might be particularly important in the pathologically small bladder where fibrosis, a reduction in elasticity and other factors might be expected to reduce compliance severely. Indeed, in the neurogenic bladder of spinal cord injury, the rate of filling cystometry is usually kept low at 10 to 20 mL/min.

During filling, the normal bladder should remain stable up to full bladder capacity, showing little or no activity. Unlike the slow rises in detrusor pressure associated with lowered bladder compliance, detrusor overactivity is characterized by phasic events which rise relatively and then fall again within a few tens of seconds. Bladder activity can also be provoked by rapid filling (e.g., 10 mL/sec) or ice water, and these may be more useful provocative tests than the standard filling cystometrogram in some patients, such as those with a neurological cause for their overactive detrusor, as in spinal cord injury. Although it is not common practice in routine urodynamic laboratories, quantifying detrusor overactivity is important if a proper assessment of interventions is to be made. Various approaches have been adopted, including measuring the peak pressure, calculating the area under the unstable contraction and recording the frequency of events. For many urodynamic tests, overactivity presents itself as a single "end-fill" event, which occurs when the bladder reaches its maximum cystometric volume (Fig. 10).

The sensations recorded by subjects during a filling cystometrogram usually receive much less attention than the occurrence of abnormal pressure changes. The standard technique for monitoring bladder sensations is the use of markers for the first sensation (FS), first desire to void (FDV), and strong desire to void (SDV) (7), which is sometimes described as strong urge and occasionally associated with severe discomfort and pain, though it is not always associated with changes in detrusor pressure. However, these markers may be very subjective, variable and susceptible to prompting by the investigator. Bladder sensations may also be confused because of interference from catheterization, nonphysiological fill rates and embarrassment.

With the development of a new technique for investigating bladder sensations during cystometry, it may now become possible to determine the relevance of urodynamics and symptomatology more objectively particularly when determining the effects of interventions such as drugs or neuromodulation (8). This will be especially useful in conditions such as urgency, frequency and urge incontinence where overactivity cannot always be reliably demonstrated even at full capacity.

The maximum capacity of the bladder is described as the volume at which patients feel they can no longer delay micturition. This measure can be very different in the same individual in everyday life and probably depends on many factors. Of course, functional bladder capacity, rather than maximum capacity, may be more accurately reflected in frequency-volume diaries. However, in the relatively controlled environment of the urodynamics laboratory, repeated cystometries can give a reasonable indication of a person's maximum capacity. Of course this is more difficult to determine in patients with poor or absent sensation such as those with a neurological cause for their bladder problems. In these patients, it is possible to get a reasonable estimate of maximum capacity by filling until detrusor overactivity occurs. Interestingly, patients who present with intractably small bladder capacities are sometimes found to have relatively normal capacities when tested under general anesthesia.

Urethral Pressure Profiles

A number of parameters can be derived from the static urethral pressure profile, including maximum urethral pressure (MUP), maximum urethral closure pressure (MUCP), and functional profile length (FPL) (Fig. 11). Although the FPL may not be diagnostically useful in itself, it can be used to calculate a further index by multiplying it with MUP. This index has been used to diagnose stress incontinence.

The stress UPP can be used to determine the decrease in transfer of abdominal pressures to the urethra during maneuvers such as the Valsalva and cough to determine degree of stress incontinence.

However, it has been shown that the position of the patient during these studies can dramatically alter

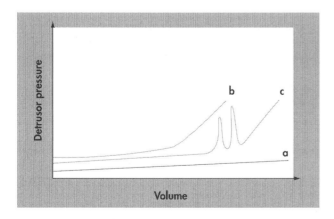

Figure 10 Typical filling cystometrogram traces illustrating **(A)** normal bladder, **(B)** bladder with loss of compliance at end fill and **(C)** instability and end-fill loss of compliance.

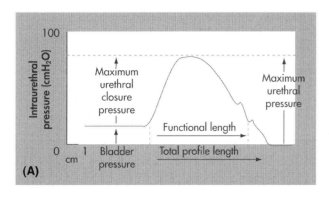

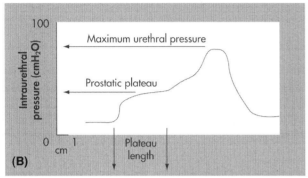

Figure 11 Typical urethral pressure profiles in (**A**) female and (**B**) male subjects.

the results. Diagnostic interpretations of urethral function can also be made from the characteristic shape of the UPP. However, it should be noted that there are a number of differences caused by both age and sex that may lead to inaccuracies in these interpretations. For example, the MUP often decreases with age, and, in women, it often decreases, especially after the menopause. The MUP is often lower in patients with stress incontinence, though the findings are not always consistent with symptoms reported by the patient, and there is a significant overlap in the values found in incontinent and continent subjects.

Flowmetry and Voiding Cystometry

The most useful voiding study involves the simultaneous measurement of voiding pressure and flow rate. This allows the derivation of a number of factors that may be useful in the diagnosis of lower urinary tract dysfunction, particularly obstructive disorders. However, if flowmetry alone is undertaken, there are a number of factors that are measured, including maximum flow rate, average flow rate, flow time, voiding time, voided volume and time to maximum flow. Several nomograms have been developed for determining the degree of obstruction from flow rate alone. These include the Liverpool nomogram, which was constructed after analyzing flow rates and bladder volumes collected from many hundreds of

patients (9). The shape of the normal flow curve is near Gaussian and deviations from this shape may suggest pathology; for example, a low flat curve may be indicative of a stricture, while an intermittent flow with low flow rate may indicate obstruction. It is also important during uroflowmetry to determine the residual volume; this can be calculated most accurately by catheterizing the patient, or by ultrasonography.

Pressure-flow studies are carried out to determine whether the low flow rate recorded during flowmetry is attributable to a high urethral resistance or a low bladder pressure. The interrelationship between these variables means that accurate diagnosis of dysfunction requires simultaneous measurement of flow rate and detrusor pressure. The most common variables measured are the maximum flow rate (Q_{max}) and the detrusor pressure at this flow rate ($P_{det}Q_{max}$). As for simple flowmetry, a number of nomograms have been derived for these variables to identify patients with obstructive disorders (Fig. 12) (10,11).

It is important to note that nearly all of these nomograms have a large equivocal region, which makes a definitive diagnosis impossible.

If a low flow rate is also associated with a low detrusor pressure, it is may be necessary to determine the contractility of the detrusor muscle. Detrusor contractility is an important parameter that is relatively complicated to measure and understand. An isometric detrusor contraction can be produced by asking a patient to stop voiding as soon as the maximum flow rate is reached. As the detrusor muscle continues to contract against a closed outlet, the contraction is assumed to be isometric, the resulting pressure is defined as $P_{det.iso}$. A single stop test is often used, and a single value for $P_{det.iso}$ is derived from this. However, the definition of contractility includes a dependence on the muscle length. The serial stop

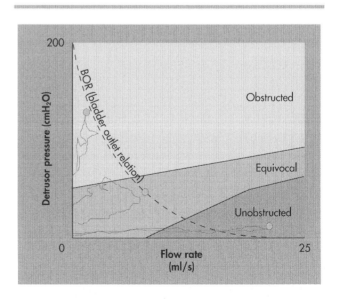

Figure 12 Nomogram for determining bladder outlet obstruction.

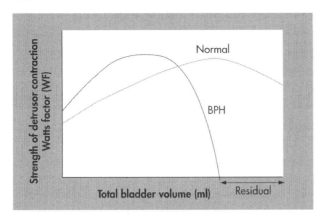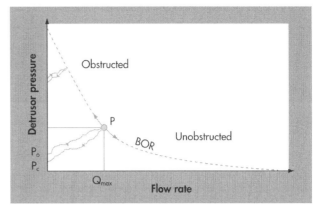

Figure 13 Graphs illustrating derived bladder parameters Watts factor (WF) and bladder output relationship (BOR).

test has therefore been suggested as a more accurate method for determining a true contractility curve (12,13).

In this way, the detrusor force at each given volume can be determined for each stop test. It should be noted that patients with severe stress incontinence may not be able to stop urine flow sufficiently, and there is the theoretical possibility that repeated cessation may cause an inhibition of detrusor contraction.

The Watts factor (WF) developed by Griffiths (14) is an alternative method for deriving a continuous calculation of detrusor contractility. The WF is defined as the power per unit area of bladder and is numerically equal to isometric detrusor pressure throughout voiding (Fig. 13).

ADVANCED TECHNIQUES AND NEW DEVELOPMENTS

In some centers, more specialized techniques to assist diagnosis have been introduced into the practice of urodynamics. Of these, the videocystometrogram (VCMG), in which X-ray imaging of the urinary tract with a contrast medium is combined with urodynamic measurements, is the most common (Fig. 14). Although it can yield valuable information about bladder morphology, urethral dysfunction (e.g., in assessing dyssynergic sphincters or bladder neck obstruction) and ureteral reflux (important to identify and eliminate for the preservation of renal function), which cannot be obtained with urodynamics alone, it has the danger of overexposure to X-rays and is relatively expensive, thus precluding frequent use. However, some patient groups, for example, those with a neurogenic bladder will particularly benefit from the additional information video urodynamics can yield.

Another technique gaining much favor is ambulatory urodynamics, where bladder pressure, rectal pressure and leakage can be monitored continuously over a long period on a portable data-logger to assess the effects of "normal" activities on lower urinary

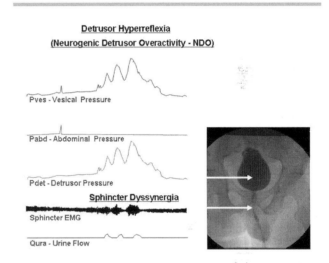

Figure 14 Videourodynamics from a case of spinal cord injury.

tract function. Considerable technical back up is required for this type of study, and much time and care are needed in data analysis, especially for the identification and elimination of artefacts. Although expensive, it is said to be a valuable aid in diagnosing conditions such as idiopathic instability where standard urodynamics has been unsuccessful.

Newer methods are now being investigated which may overcome some of the problems associated with conventional voiding cystometry for investigating obstructive disorders such as benign prostatic hypertrophy. As we have seen, bladder pressure is conventionally measured by catheterization with the attendant risk of traumatizing the urethra and introducing infection into the bladder (estimated to occur in about 1–5% of urodynamic investigations), so by eliminating the need for catheters in the bladder, this morbidity could be reduced. One such technique to do this is noninvasive urodynamics first demonstrated in an objective test of the effects of atropine on the

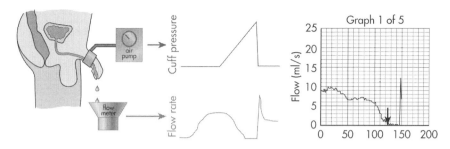

Figure 15 The principles of "noninvasive" urodynamics using the Mediplus CT3000. Isometric bladder pressure is indirectly measured by monitoring the pressure of an inflatable cuff, applying compression to the urethra, at the point where urine flow ceases.

bladder in man where an inflating cuff around the penis was used to indirectly measure isometric bladder pressure at the point when urine flow stopped (15), similar to reverse sphygmomanometry. This early technique has more recently been developed into a practical clinical test (Fig. 15) (16), which is now commercially available (CT3000—Mediplus Ltd., U.K.). Another technique along similar lines uses a condom and external catheter, the urine flow is interrupted by an external valve and isovolumetric bladder pressure measured (17). Such noninvasive bladder pressure measuring techniques could provide a more cost-beneficial diagnostic method for selecting patients for surgery as well as lowering morbidity through infection.

Ultrasonography has been used more widely in a number of clinics. The most common use is as a measure of residual urine although reliability can be very variable. Measurements of bladder wall thickness and bladder weight have also been reported as a diagnostic tool for determining bladder outlet obstruction (18).

Future developments include the use of functional magnetic resonance imaging (fMRI) to produce high-quality anatomical characterization of the function of the bladder, urethra and pelvic floor. However, the use of MRI combined with urodynamics is still in an experimental phase (19), but it has the potential for giving three-dimensional views of the bladder and urethra during filling and voiding. More recently, positron emission tomography (PET) studies have been used to determine which areas of the brain are responsible for sensations of bladder filling (20). It is likely that this technique will remain a research tool for the foreseeable future but the results will help to increase our knowledge and understanding of the control of the micturition cycle at a cerebral level.

SYMPTOMS AND URODYNAMICS

Although we may now have a good scientific understanding of the basis of urodynamics, the question still remains: "What exactly is the relationship between urinary symptomatology and urodynamics?" There have been many studies and papers written about this topic but without a firm conclusion as to whether they do correlate in any urological problem.

In a recent study of women questioned about their complaints of urinary incontinence, it was found that not only were the subjective answers by patients not helpful in differentiating the etiology of incontinence but also that almost no questions were helpful in predicting which patients would have normal video urodynamics (21). Interestingly, questions about nocturia, frequency, urgency and urge incontinence, among others, were not statistically significant for any group. If there is so little correlation between symptoms and urodynamics, what is the purpose of urodynamics? If it is the symptoms that drive patients to seek help in the first place, what additional information is urodynamics providing? Are the rather nonphysiological techniques used in urodynamics part of the problem?

Perhaps for some urological problems, such as urge incontinence, the difficulty in urodynamics has to do with measuring the sensations during bladder filling and urge itself rather than looking just for instability as a cause for their symptoms. Diaries show that these patients void frequently, suggesting that they may be having strong sensations of urge (or perhaps more correctly "urgency"?) and the desire to void at relatively low bladder volumes.

During urodynamics, patients are asked through dialogue to report on any sensations; for example, the standard measures are "FS of filling," "FDV," and, finally, "SDV." Prompting the patient for answers probably helps to undermine the value of these measures of sensation, and this may be very important if we are trying to get an accurate picture of the bladder volume at the time. Perhaps we should pay more attention to the sensations experienced by patients during urodynamics and get accurate measures of bladder volumes for each level of reported sensation (Fig. 16) (8).

So, in urge (urgency?) incontinence at least, there may be a more positive correlation between symptoms and the semi-objectively measured sensations during urodynamics, which would be important information when we are assessing the impact of interventions such as neuromodulation (22).

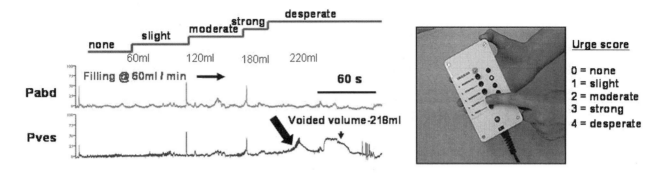

Figure 16 The "urge keypad" is shown on the right. Operating independently of investigator prompting, subjects press buttons indicating five levels on the scale, 0 (none), (*i*) (slight; FSF), (*ii*) (moderate; first desire to void), (*iii*) (strong; strong desire to void), and (*iv*) (desperate), as their subjective sensations change during bladder filling. Only one button can be pressed at a time. An electrical output from the keypad for each level of sensation can be recorded alongside the other cystometrogram traces shown on the left.

CONCLUSION: URODYNAMICS—ART OR SCIENCE?

This chapter has outlined the scientific basis of urodynamics and how simple physical principles can be applied to explain the functions of the bladder during filling and voiding cystometry. The techniques for measuring and recording pressure changes and flow accurately are described together with how we can relate these measurements to some functions of the lower urinary tract. For the urologist, it is important to know when and in what ways the lower urinary is dysfunctional, so comparisons with "normal function" are crucial. There are some tabulated examples of normal versus patient data in the form of nomograms or charts, such as flow versus voided volume (23) or detrusor pressure (24). From these charts, clinicians can relate their findings on urodynamics to the variation of the "normal population" and draw conclusions about departure of their patients from normality. Even more sophisticated graphs have evolved which describe the contractility and urethral resistance (25) calculated as derivations from pressure, volume and flow measured during urodynamics. Applying these graphs "blindly" and without full appreciation of urodynamic techniques, their errors and their artefacts is very likely to lead to false information about a patient's true lower urinary tract function.

Finally, if we are to relate some types of urinary symptoms with urodynamics, we must include more objective ways of recording the sensations of filling and urge in our studies (7). Reading urodynamic records in an intelligent way is both an art form and a science requiring considerable experience to reach a high standard of interpretation.

FURTHER READING

Abrams P. Urodynamics. 3rd ed. London: Springer, 2006.
Chapple CR, MacDiarmid SA, Patel A. Urodynamics Made Easy. 3rd ed. London: Churchill Livingstone Elsevier, 2009.

Griffiths D. The Mechanics and Hydrodynamics of the Lower Urinary Tract. Medical Physics Handbooks 4. Bristol: Adam Hilger Limited, 1980.
Mundy AR, Stephenson TP, Wein AJ, eds. Urodynamics: Principles, Practice and Application. 2nd ed. New York: Churchill Livingstone, 1994.
Sand PK, Ostergard DR. Urodynamics and the Evaluation of Female Incontinence. London: Springer-Verlag, 1997.

REFERENCES

1. Schafer W. Urethral resistance. Urodynamic concepts of physiological and pathological bladder outlet function during voiding. Neurourol Urodyn 1985; 4:161–201.
2. van Mastrigt R, Coolsaet BL, van Duyl WA. Passive properties of the urinary bladder in the collection phase. Med Biol Eng Comput 1978; 16:471–482.
3. Zinner NR, Sterling AM, Ritter RC. Role of inner urethral softness in urinary continence. Urology 1980; 16:115–117.
4. Hill AV. The heat of shortening and the dynamic constants of muscle. Proc R Soc Lond B Biol Sci 1938; 126:136–195.
5. Brown M, Wickham JE. The urethral pressure profile. Br J Urol 1969; 41:211–217.
6. Abrams P, Cardozo L, Fall M, et al. The standardisation of terminology in lower urinary tract function: report from the standardisation sub-committee of the International Continence Society. Urology 2003; 61:37–49.
7. Wyndaele JJ. The normal pattern of perception of bladder filling during cystometry studied in 38 young healthy volunteers. J Urol 1998; 160:479–481.
8. Oliver SE, Fowler CJ, Mundy AR, et al. Measuring the sensations of urge and bladder filling during cystometry in urge incontinence and the effects of neuromodulation. Neurourol Urodyn 2003; 22:7–16.
9. Haylen BT, Parys BT, Anyaegbunam WI, et al. Urine flow rates in male and female urodynamic patients compared with the Liverpool nomograms. Br J Urol 1990; 65:483–487.
10. Griffiths D, Hofner K, van Mastrigt R, et al. Standardisation of terminology of lower urinary tract function: pressure-flow studies of voiding, urethral resistance, and urethral obstruction. International Continence Society Sub-Committee on Standardisation of Terminology of Pressure-Flow Studies. Neurourol Urodyn 1997; 16:1.
11. Schafer W. Analysis of bladder outlet function with the linearized passive urethral resistance relation, linPURR

and a disease specific approach for grading obstruction: from complex to simple. World J Urol 1995; 13:47.

12. Susset JG, Brissot RB, Regnier RB. The stop-flow technique: a way to measure detrusor strength. J Urol 1982; 127: 489–494.

13. Craggs MD, Knight SL, McFarlane JA. Detrusor force measured by serial stop-tests in healthy volunteers. Neurourology Urodyn 1998; 17:1–2.

14. Griffiths DJ. Mechanics of micturition. In: Yalla SV, McGuire EJ, Elbadawi E, et al., eds. Neurology and Urodynamics: Principles and Practice. New York: Macmillan, 1988.

15. Brindley GS, Craggs MD. The effect of atropine on the urinary bladder of the baboon and of man. J Physiol 1975; 256:55.

16. Griffiths CJ, Rix D, MacDonald AM, et al. Noninvasive measurement of bladder pressure by controlled inflation of a penile cuff. J Urol 2002; 167:1344–1347.

17. Rikken B, Pell JJ, van Mastrigt R. Repeat noninvasive bladder pressure measurements with an external catheter. J Urol 1999;162(2):474–479.

18. Oelke M, Höfner K, Jonas U, et al. Diagnostic accuracy of noninvasive tests to evaluate bladder outlet obstruction in men: detrusor wall thickness, uroflowmetry, postvoid residual urine, and prostate volume. Eur Urol 2007; 52(3): 827–834.

19. Simmons A, Williams SC, Craggs M, et al. Dynamic multiplanar EPI of the urinary bladder during voiding with simultaneous detrusor pressure measurement. Magn Reson Imaging 1997; 15:295–300.

20. Athwal BS, Berkley KJ, Hussain I, et al. Brain responses to changes in bladder volume and urge to void in healthy men. Brain 2001; 124(pt 2):369–377.

21. Amundsen C, Lau M, English SF, et al. Do urinary symptoms correlate with urodynamic findings? J Urol 1999; 161:1871–1874.

22. Craggs MD. Objective measurement of bladder sensation: use of a new patient-activated device and respons to neuromodulation. BJU Int 2005; 96(suppl 1):29–36.

23. Haylen BT, Ashby D, Sutherst JR, et al. Maximum and average urine flow rates in normal male and female populations – the Liverpool nonograms. Br J Urol 1989; 64(1):30–38.

24. Abrams PH, Griffiths DJ. The assessment of prostatic obstruction from urodynamic measurements and from residual urine. Br J Urol 1979; 51:129–134.

25. Schaefer W. Basic principles and clinical application of advance analysis of bladder voiding function. Urol Clin N Am 1990; 17:553–566.

17

Scientific Basis of Male Hypogonadism

Thang S. Han and Pierre-Marc G. Bouloux

*Department of Endocrinology, Royal Free and University College Hospital Medical School,
Royal Free Hospital, London, U.K.*

BACKGROUND

Definition of Male Hypogonadism

Male hypogonadism is a multisystem clinical syndrome that results from subphysiological circulating levels of testosterone because of disruption of one or more levels of the hypothalamic-pituitary-testicular (HPT) axis (1). Defective androgen receptor (AR) or specific converting enzymes at target organs also results in hypogonadism.

An Overview of Key Factors Controlling Hypothalamic-Pituitary-Testicular Axis

The HPT axis is a closed loop system interlinking the central hypothalamic-pituitary components to the testis by means of various hormones. It is considered to be the core of the reproductive endocrine system, regulating not only classic sexual function but also a host of vital bodily functions. The axis is activated by constant changes of ambience signaled by neuronal and hormonal activities (Fig. 1). Centrally, hypothalamic production of gonadotrophin-releasing hormone (GnRH) is regulated by cortical neurotransmitters, including γ-aminobutyric acid (GABA), catecholamines, and endorphins. Pulsatile GnRH secretion stimulates pituitary synthesis and secretion of gonadotrophins, luteinizing hormone (LH), and follicle-stimulating hormone (FSH). In turn, gonadotrophins act on the testis to initiate biosynthesis of testosterone and spermatogenesis. Testicular hormones produced in the Sertoli and Leydig cells, in turn, exert a negative feedback control on the central components to complete the closed loop of HPT axis.

Testicular hormones exert their effects soon after conception, stimulating the formation of both external and internal male sex organs while inhibiting the differentiation of the internal female Müllerian structures (Fig. 2). During puberty they induce secondary sexual characteristics and, in adulthood, are responsible for sexual function as well as maintaining long-term health of vital organs and general well-being. Defects of the HPT axis lead to variable clinical features of hypogonadism, depending on the timing of disease onset. Correct diagnosis of the defect is important for appropriate treatment: optimal development in the young and ensuring of long-term health in adults.

ANATOMY AND PHYSIOLOGY OF THE TESTIS

Anatomy of the Testis

The testes function as both an endocrine and exocrine organ, and lie within the scrotum, encapsulated by tunica albuginea. Each testis is divided into approximately 300 lobules by thin connective tissue septa. Each lobule contains two to three very convoluted seminiferous tubules, in which gametes are produced by spermatogenesis. In the intertubular regions lie the steroid-producing Leydig cells. Tubuli recti are the terminal ends of the seminiferous lobules, which extend into the mediastinum of the testis, anastomosing to form the rete testis (Fig. 2). From the rete testis, a series of 6 to 12 fine efferent ducts join to form the duct of the epididymis. The distal pole of the epididymis gives rise to the vas deferens, which ends as the ampulla of the vas at the posterior aspect of the bladder, where it joins the seminal vesicular duct, forming the ejaculatory duct that passes through the prostate to enter the prostatic urethra. Together the seminal vesicles and prostate contribute approximately 90% to 95% of the volume of the ejaculate. In health, each testis can produce between 10 and 200 million gametes a day.

Spermatogenesis

Spermatogenesis involves a complex series of cell divisions, transforming spermatogonia to mature spermatozoa (Fig. 3). Until spermiation, the gametes are nursed by Sertoli cells, which regulate the internal environment of the seminiferous tubule under the influence of FSH and testosterone. This environment is created by the formation of inter-Sertoli cell junctions where processes of Sertoli cell cytoplasm from adjacent cells merge. The junctions are predominantly located at the basolateral regions of the cell to create occluding-type junctions, the anatomical basis of the blood-testis barrier. As a result, intercellular transport between the Sertoli cell and spermatogonia is possible, but this barrier is impermeable to macromolecules.

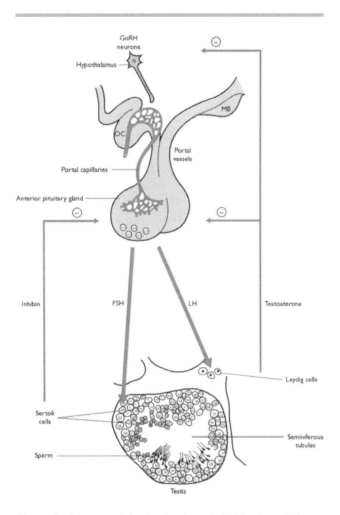

Figure 1 Diagram of the feedback control of the hypothalamo-pituitary-testicular axis. *Source*: Adapted from Ref. 2 with permission.

During the fetal stage of sexual differentiation, the Sertoli cells produce the polypeptide anti-Müllerian hormone (AMH) that inhibits the formation of internal female genitalia (uterus and Fallopian tubes) from the Müllerian duct. Sertoli cells also produce the hormones inhibin and activin, which exert feedback action on FSH secretion.

ENDOCRINE REGULATION OF MALE REPRODUCTIVE SYSTEM

Regulation and Action of Gonadotrophin-Releasing Hormone

Embryologically, GnRH neurons are born in the nasal pit. Under the influence of adhesion molecules they migrate alongside the vomeronasal nerve into their final destination in the septopreoptic area of the anterior hypothalamus. Their axons innervate the median eminence and secrete pulsatile GnRH into the pituitary portal system. GnRH is initially produced as a 92 amino acid (AA) pre-pro-GnRH (Fig. 4), which is encoded by the *GnRH* gene mapped to 8p21-p11.2. Posttranslational cleavage by prohormone

convertase-1 of the leading 23 AAs ("pre" portion) and the supporting gonadotrophin-associated peptide (GAP) 56 AAs ("pro" portion) results in the decapeptide GnRH.

GnRH neurons discharge at an intrinsic frequency of 90 to 120 minutes, releasing GnRH in a pulsatile manner. The amplitude and frequency of discharge are modulated by cortical neurotransmitters (Fig. 4). The α-adrenergic impulses have a stimulatory action and β-adrenergic, dopamine, and endorphins impulses have an inhibitory action on GnRH secretion. Testosterone and progesterone, probably via β-endorphins, attenuate pulse frequency.

It is well recognized that stress can have an adverse effect on reproductive function. Many factors are involved in this process, including corticotrophin-releasing hormone (CRH), which inhibits GnRH through direct neuronal contact between the paraventricular nucleus and preoptic region. Elevated prolactin levels, in response to stress, further suppress GnRH pulsatility. Observations in a wide variety of species indicate that intermediary cytokines such as interleukin 1 (IL-1) or tumor necrosis factor-α (TNF-α) may also have an inhibitory effect (3,4).

Leptin, a hormone produced by adipocytes whose gene was cloned by Friedman's group, is another hormone that influences GnRH secretion probably indirectly via neuropeptide Y by intervening with the feedback mechanism (5). It acts on the hypothalamus via specific leptin receptors to signal the nutritional status (adipose tissue reserve). Leptin may be involved in the initiation of puberty. In anorexia nervosa, low leptin levels are associated with reduced GnRH levels, an effect that can be reversed by leptin administration (6).

The G protein–coupled receptor 54 (GPR54, also known as KISS1R) and its natural ligand kisspeptin, are encoded by *KISS1R* and *KiSS1* genes (7). The kisspetin/GPR54 system is expressed in the arcuate and anteroventral periventricular nuclei of the forebrain and implicated in the neuroendocrine regulation of reproduction. GPR54$^{-/-}$ mice and compound heterozygote missense mutations of the GPR54 in humans have hypogonadotrophic hypogonadism (8,9). A study of healthy male volunteers has shown that kisspeptin administration increases levels of gonadotrophins and testosterone (10). Hypothalamic levels of *KiSS1* and *GPR54* mRNA increase dramatically at puberty, suggesting that kisspeptin signaling could mediate the neuroendocrine events that trigger its onset. A study of primary culture of human fetal GnRH-secreting neuroblasts (FNC-B4) has shown that kisspeptin-induced GnRH secretion and kisspeptin per se are decreased by oestradiol and stimulated by androgens. Furthermore, leptin was also shown to increase KiSS1/GPR54 expression in FNC-B4 (11). Together, these observations indicate that interactions between metabolic and sexual hormones may trigger the KiSS1/GPR54 signaling to GnRH neurons to regulate reproductive activity.

GnRH has specific receptors (G protein–bound receptors with seven transmembrane loops) on pituitary gonadotrophs. Binding of GnRH to these specific

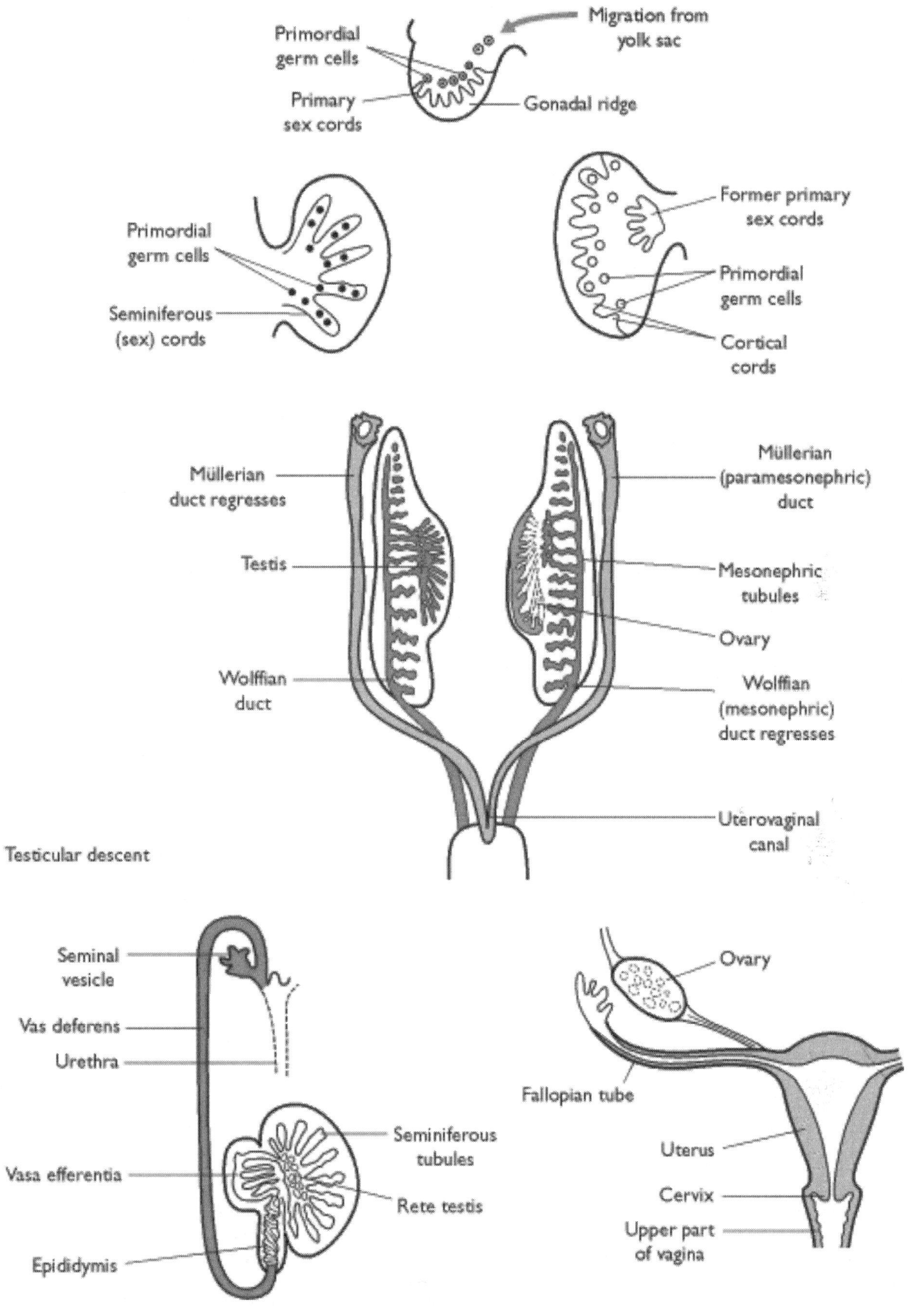

Figure 2 Schematic overview of the differentiation of the internal male and female (for comparison) reproductive tracts from the Wolffian and Müllerian ducts. *Source*: Adapted from Ref. 2 with permission.

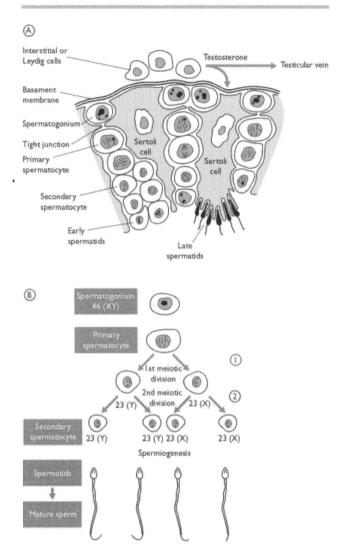

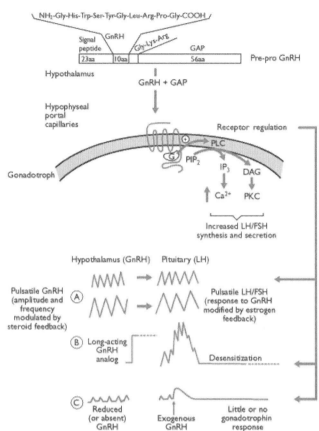

Figure 3 Diagram of the structural organization of the human seminiferous tubule and the stages of spermatogenesis. (**A**) Spermatogonia push their way through the tight junctions between adjacent Sertoli cells and become primary spermatocytes. (**B**) In the first meiotic division (1) each of the 46 chromosomes doubles up and then forms a pair with another doubled-up chromosome during which time there is exchange of genetic material (crossing over). The cell divides and each daughter cell contains one of the pairs of chromosomes. In the second meiotic division (2) each double chromosome simply separates producing genetically identical secondary spermatocytes. *Source*: Adapted from Ref. 2 with permission.

Figure 4 Synthesis of GnRH and its actions on pituitary gonadotrophs. GnRH is synthesized as a large prohormone and released with gonadotrophin-associated peptide. It acts on the gonadotroph via a G protein–linked receptor that activates phospholipase C, which stimulates the inositol signaling pathway. (**A**) GnRH is secreted in a pulsatile manner with one pulse occurring approximately each hour. (**B**) Administration of long-acting agonist analogues induces an initial stimulation of LH (and follicle-stimulating hormone) but over a few days causes complete desensitization of the pituitary gonadotroph. (**C**) Loss of endogenous GnRH secretion induces loss of GnRH receptors and the LH response to a bolus injection of GnRH is very low. *Abbreviations*: PIP_2, phosphatidylinositol 4,5-bisphosphate; IP_3, inositol 1,4,5-trisphosphate; DAG, diacylglycerol; PKC, protein kinase C; GnRH, gonadotrophin-releasing hormone; LH, luteinizing hormone. *Source*: Adapted from Ref. 2 with permission.

receptors initiates gene expression of α- and β-chains of FSH and LH and promotes their secretion by inducing inositol-1,4,5,-triphosphate (IP_3) and diacylglycerol (DAG), resulting in mobilizing of intracellular calcium and protein kinase C (PKC), respectively.

Pulsatile exposure of gonadotrophs to GnRH is essential for gonadotrophin secretion: Continuous exposure to GnRH attenuates gonadotrophin secretion because of GnRH receptor downregulation. This is exploited in the treatment of steroid-dependent conditions such as endometriosis, prostate carcinoma,

and precocious puberty where long-acting potent GnRH analogues are used. In contrast, correct pulsatile administration of GnRH induces LH and FSH release and thus normalizes reproductive function, forming the basis of one form of treatment for secondary hypogonadal conditions such as Kallmann's syndrome (KS).

Regulation and Action of Luteinizing Hormone

Like thyroid-stimulating hormone (TSH) and human chorionic gonadotrophin (hCG), LH and FSH are large glycoproteins. They have a common noncovalent binding of two peptide chains (α and β) to form a heterodimer. The α-chain is identical in all four glycoprotein hormones, the β-chain only mediating the biological effect. The α-chain is encoded by a gene on 6q12.21, FSH-β on 11p13 and LH-β and hCG-β on 19q13.32. The genes of LH and FSH receptors both locate to chromosome 2.

LH binds to specific GPRs on the surface of Leydig cells, activating adenyl cyclase and generating the intracellular second messenger cyclic adenosine monophosphate (cAMP), which, acting via PKA, leads to steroid biosynthesis. LH influences the conversion of cholesterol to pregnenolone, the most critical step of testosterone biosynthesis, via two mechanisms: cAMP-mediated stimulation of the synthesis and activity of cytochrome P450scc (side chain cleavage) enzyme, and a PKC-mediated increase in the production of cholesterol by activation of hydrolase.

Regulation and Action of Follicle-Stimulating Hormone

FSH binds to specific receptors on Sertoli cells to promote spermatogenesis. Sertoli cells stimulate the activity of aromatase, an enzyme catalyzing the conversion of testosterone to oestradiol. The hormones inhibin B and activin are formed in Sertoli cells in an FSH-dependent manner. Inhibin B is a heterodimeric glycoprotein hormone comprising α and β subunits; the latter has two variants (β_A and β_B). Homodimers of the β-chains are called activin A (β_A-β_A) and activin B (β_B-β_B). On one hand, inhibin B exerts a specific negative feedback inhibition on pituitary FSH secretion. Loss of inhibin B in conditions such as Sertoli-cell-only syndrome, or following radiotherapy or chemotherapy, augments FSH levels while LH remains unchanged. On the other hand, both activins A and B stimulate FSH secretion. A structurally unrelated protein termed follistatin has the capacity to suppress FSH, probably through the binding and neutralizing the actions of activin. Testosterone and oestradiol inhibit FSH either directly or through GnRH suppression.

Testosterone and Androgen Effect

Testosterone Biosynthesis

Central to the male reproductive system is testosterone, secreted by Leydig cells of the testis at about 5 to 7 mg a day. The regulation of testosterone biosynthesis and metabolism involves a complex system interlinking the HPT axis and target organs. Testosterone synthesis per se requires multienzymatic action and its bioavailability is modulated by circulating binding proteins such as sex hormone–binding globulin (SHBG) and albumin and the sensitivity of the target organs.

Leydig cells have a large endoplasmic reticulum and high density of mitochondria. The precursor of testosterone synthesis is cholesterol, synthesized mainly by the Leydig cells with a very small amount taken up from the circulation and stored as esters in Leydig cell fat vacuoles. The 29 carbon atom cholesterol is hydrolyzed to the 19 carbon atom testosterone, through five enzymatic stages (Fig. 5). Defects in any of these steps result in primary hypogonadism.

The most significant rate-limiting step is the conversion from cholesterol to pregnenolone, which takes place on the inner mitochondrial membrane, where cytochrome P450scc catalyzes in three consecutive stages: first hydroxylation on atom C20, then C22 and thereafter, cleavage between C20 and C22 to produce pregnenolone and isocaproic acid. Cytochrome P450scc (also known as 20,22-desmolase), encoded by a gene on chromosome 15, is the crucial enzyme in all steroid-producing tissues, such as the adrenal gland and ovary. Pregnenolone is the parent substance of all biologically active steroid hormones. It diffuses across the mitochondria into the endoplasmic reticulum where further processing occurs. There are two pathways (Δ^4 or Δ^5) depending on whether the double bond is located in ring A or B. The Δ^5 synthesis pathway is preferred in human. Accordingly, hydroxylation frequently occurs first in position C17 by the action of P450c17 (17α-hydroxylase), to 17α-hydroxypregnenolone. The weak androgens dehydroepiandrosterone (DHEA) and androstenediol are produced by the enzymes 17,20-desmolase and 17β-hydroxysteroid dehydrogenase consecutively. A further important step is the conversion of the less biologically active Δ^5 steroids 17α-pregnenolone, DHEA and androstenediol, to the corresponding more effective Δ^4 steroids 17α-progesterone, androstenedione and testosterone. This step is catalyzed by the enzyme 3β-hydroxysteroid dehydrogenase, and comprises oxidation of the 3β-hydroxyl group to a ketone group, with subsequent transfer of the double bond from C5-C6 on ring B to C4-C5 on ring A (Δ^5-Δ^4 isomerization). The majority of testosterone produced this way is immediately released into the circulation via the spermatic vein, with small amounts via lymphatic system.

Testosterone and its metabolite oestradiol exert negative feedback action on LH secretion, by both inhibiting GnRH production and action through diminution of GnRH pulse frequency, but not pulse amplitude. Downregulation of GnRH receptors also occurs. Oestradiol has an inhibitory effect predominantly on the pituitary where it decreases LH pulse amplitude without changing pulse frequency.

Transport of Testosterone in the Circulation

The bioavailability of testosterone is modulated by its binding to circulating SHBG (10^{-9} M affinity binding) and albumin (10^{-6} M affinity binding) and the sensitivity of the target organs. Testosterone, a lipophilic molecule, diffuses freely across Leydig cell membranes into the circulation where 60% is bound with high affinity to SHBG and 38% is loosely bound to albumin, leaving only 2% free testosterone available for biological activity.

Most of the SHBG is produced by liver, with small amounts derived from prostate and mammary glands. SHBG is a large glycoprotein (92.5 kD)

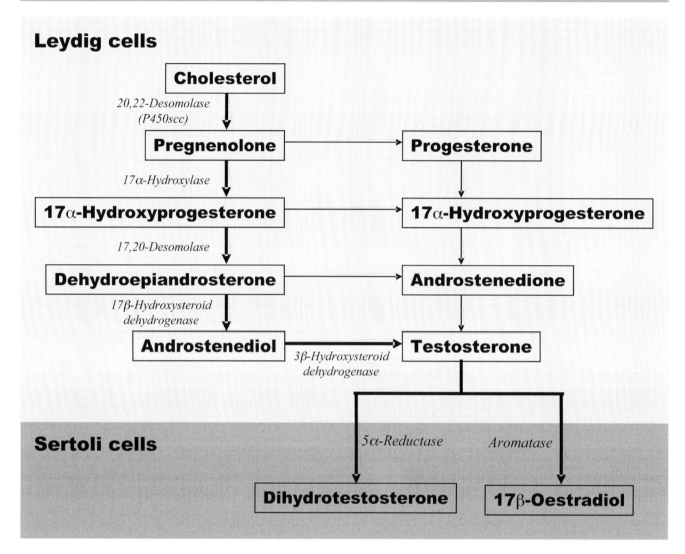

Figure 5 The major human testicular steroidogenic pathway.

encoded by a gene located on 17p13.1. It circulates in the serum as homodimer, and carries two binding sites for sex steroids with high affinity for testosterone and dihydrotestosterone (DHT), and relatively lower affinity for oestradiol. Circulating SHBG concentrations determine free testosterone levels: As a corollary, reproductive function is greatly influenced by various conditions that affect SHBG levels (Table 1).

Table 1 Factors Altering Concentrations of Serum SHBG

Elevation of SHBG	Suppression of SHBG
Estrogen use	Androgen therapy
Androgen deficiency	Obesity
Growth hormone deficiency	Acromegaly
Hyperthyroidism	Hypothyroidism
Hepatitis	Nephrotic syndrome
Liver cirrhosis	Corticosteroids
Phenytoin	Hyperinsulinism
	Gestagens

Abbreviation: SHBG, sex hormone–binding globulin.

Metabolism of Testosterone

Testosterone can also act as a prohormone for DHT and oestradiol (Fig. 5), and diffuses into target cells where conversion to 5α-DHT or 17β-oestradiol occurs, depending on the presence of metabolizing enzymes. There are two high homology isoenzymes of 5α-reductase responsible for testosterone conversion to DHT. Type I 5α-reductase is encoded by a gene on chromosome 5, expressed mainly in skin and liver. A gene on chromosome 2 encodes type II 5α-reductase, which is expressed predominantly in prostate, adrenal gland, seminal vesicle, genital skin, hair follicles, and cerebral cortex. About 80% of circulating DHT is produced peripherally and 20% directly secreted by the testes.

Testosterone and DHT bind to the identical AR, but DHT is more potent, having a 10-fold greater affinity for the receptor and slower dissociation. About 30 μg of oestradiol a day is generated by extratesticular aromatization of testosterone and androstenedione in adipose tissue, osteocytes, and

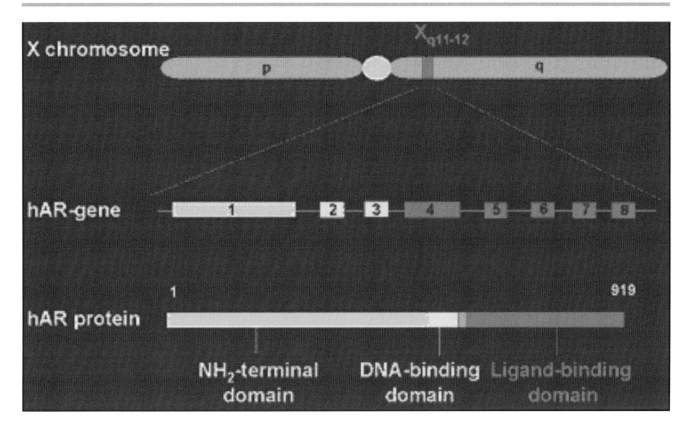

Figure 6 The human androgen receptor gene. Reprinted with permission from WWW.ENDOTEXT.ORG, the free on-line Endocrinology textbook, in Androgen Physiology: Receptor and Metabolic Disorders by AO Brinkmann, L J De Groot, Editor, Version November 2009, published by MDTEXT.COM, South Dartmouth, MA, USA.

prostate. An additional 10 µg of oestradiol is secreted directly by Leydig cells. In physiological concentrations, testosterone and its metabolites complement one another during normal sexual development and virilization at puberty.

Testosterone and DHT are catabolized in the liver first by oxidation, reduction, or hydroxylation, and second by conjugation with glucuronic acid or sulfation at positions C3 or C17. Elimination takes place via urine as the corresponding 17-ketosteroid and sulfate (e.g., androsterone, etiocholanolone, epiandrosterone, and epitestosterone). Despite being bound to transport proteins in the circulation, elimination of testosterone from the serum by liver is very efficient as reflected by a short half-life (10 minutes) of free testosterone in the blood.

Structure and Function of the Androgen Receptor

The AR belongs to the steroid and thyroid hormone receptor family and encoded by eight exons of a gene located proximal to the centromere on the long arm of the X chromosome (Xq11–12) (Fig. 6). It encodes a 919 AA polypeptide with a conceptual molecular weight of 98.5 kD. AR is a DNA-binding protein and its activity is ligand dependent and transcription regulating.

AR has three domains with different functions. The amino-terminal (*N*-terminal) segment (exon A) of the receptor contains a polymorphic polyglutamine (CAG) tract with variable repeat sequences (normally 8–35 repeats) lying inside a split *N*-terminal transactivation domain (Fig. 7). The number of CAG repeats affects the transcription intensity of the receptor. Longer CAG repeats are associated with weaker activation of the AR-mediated transcription (12). Coactivators and androgens tend to bind more

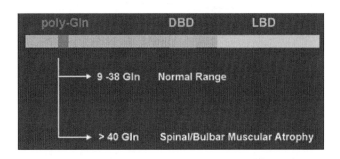

Figure 7 Variation of the sequences of CAG repeats in the gene encoding androgen receptor. Reprinted with permission from WWW.ENDOTEXT.ORG, the free on-line Endocrinology textbook, in Androgen Physiology: Receptor and Metabolic Disorders by AO Brinkmann, L J De Groot, Editor, Version November 2009, published by MDTEXT.COM, South Dartmouth, MA, USA.

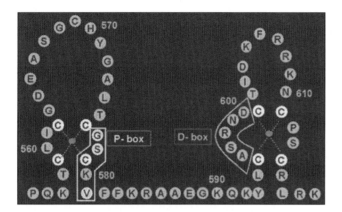

Figure 8 DNA-binding domain of androgen receptor. Reprinted with permission from WWW.ENDOTEXT.ORG, the free on-line Endocrinology textbook, in Androgen Physiology: Receptor and Metabolic Disorders by AO Brinkmann, L J De Groot, Editor, Version November 2009, published by MDTEXT.COM, South Dartmouth, MA, USA.

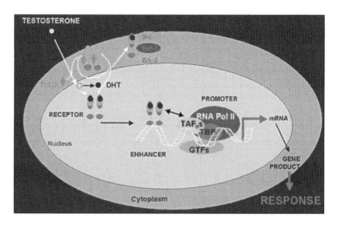

Figure 9 Molecular mechanism of testosterone action on target cell. Reprinted with permission from WWW.ENDOTEXT.ORG, the free on-line Endocrinology textbook, in Androgen Physiology: Receptor and Metabolic Disorders by AO Brinkmann, L J De Groot, Editor, Version November 2009, published by MDTEXT.COM, South Dartmouth, MA, USA.

strongly to an AR with short CAG sequences, resulting in stronger androgen effects. Short CAG repeat sequences (less than 22) are associated with increased risk of prostate carcinoma (13), whereas sequences greater than 38 have been shown to relate to androgen resistance and Kennedy's syndrome, an X-linked degenerative spinal/bulbar muscular atrophy (14) associated with gynecomastia, testicular atrophy, impotence, and remarkably high incidence of diabetes (15).

The centrally located hydrophilic DNA-binding domains (DBDs), exons B and C, carry two zinc fingers, which bind to specific sections of DNA in or next to androgen-sensitive genes and thus influence transcription (Fig. 8). The DBDs of the steroid hormone receptors are largely similar (40–90%), gene specificity being conferred by the ligand-binding site.

The carboxy-terminal (C-terminal) end (exons (D-H) carries the hydrophobic androgen-binding domain responsible for testosterone and DHT binding. This domain has 40% to 50% similarity with the AA sequence of the corresponding domains of the progesterone, mineralocorticoid, and corticosteroid receptors. However, there is only a slight similarity with the ligand-binding domain of the estrogen receptor.

The unliganded AR is stabilized by its association with a heat shock protein (HSP 90) acting as a molecular chaperone. Binding of testosterone or DHT to AR induces a conformational change, causing AR to dissociate from HSP 90, thereby becoming activated. The ligand-bound AR dimerizes, which increases its DNA-binding activity. The dimerized AR tandems target specific DNA sections of androgen response elements (AREs) in the promoter region of the androgen-sensitive genes, thereby initiating gene transcription. The first zinc finger is responsible for specificity of DNA binding. The second zinc finger stabilizes AR binding. Binding of AR to DNA influences transcription of androgen-sensitive genes, which lie downstream (3′) of the AREs. The

transcriptional activity of the AR involves recruitment of coactivators that link AR to components of the transcription machinery such as RNA-polymerase II (RNA-Pol II), TATA box-binding protein (TBP), TBP-associating factors, and general transcription factors. This communication triggers mRNA and protein synthesis, which consequently results in an androgen response (Fig. 9).

Biological Effects of Testosterone

Testosterone is essential for development of the male phenotype and optimal male function. In addition to its role in reproductive function, testosterone activates many other tissues, including bone, bone marrow, kidney, liver, breast, skin, skeletal muscle, and brain. The actions of testosterone depend on the stage of development. During sexual differentiation, testosterone induces development and growth of the Wolffian duct structures (epididymis, vas deferens, and seminal vesicle) (Fig. 10). During puberty, testosterone induces virilization, leading to development of secondary sexual characteristics. In the adult male, testosterone maintains the male phenotype, sexual function and exerts anabolic effects. It has an indirect effect on the prostate and external genitalia, following conversion to DHT (Fig. 10). If no testosterone is produced, these organs regress, with failed seminal vesicle and prostate development, leading to aspermia.

In the embryo, growth of the external genitalia is dependent on the concentration of DHT generated in situ from testosterone. A lack of DHT due to reduced testosterone production or 5α-reductase enzymatic conversion to DHT leads to an intersexual state, with associated absent phallic development. During puberty, increase in androgens causes penile growth. After puberty, negligible androgen-induced penile growth occurs because of downregulation of ARs (16). Conversely, androgen deficiency in adult does not result in reduction of penile size.

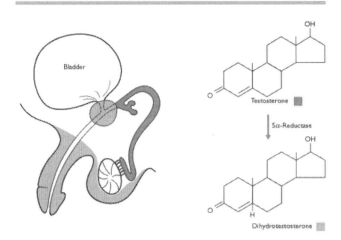

Figure 10 Upon entering the target cells, testosterone (T) binds directly to the AR and the complex T-AR binds to specific DNA sequences and regulates gene transcription, resulting in initiation and regulation of spermatogenesis and in differentiation and development of the Wolffian duct. Testosterone is also metabolized to DHT by 5α-reductase type II, which binds directly to the AR and the complex DHT-AR interacts to specific DNA sequences and regulates gene transcription, resulting in differentiation and development of the prostate and external genitalia. *Abbreviation*: AR, androgen receptor; DHT, dihydrotestosterone. *Source*: Adapted from Ref. 2 with permission.

Testosterone and Cardiovascular System

Androgens may play an important role in the increased risk of cardiovascular disease in men. Testosterone is an important determinant of cardiovascular health, having positive effects on several features of the metabolic syndrome, inducing a reduction in waist circumference, lipids, and inflammatory markers (17). Although testosterone overreplacement in hypogonadal men reduces high-density lipoprotein (HDL) and elevates low-density lipoprotein (LDL) cholesterol, this effect may be counteracted by reduction in plasminogen activator inhibitor favoring increased fibrinolysis.

Testosterone and Central Nervous System

ARs are found in the hypothalamus, pituitary, cerebellar tonsil, and septum of the central nervous system (18). In the hypothalamus and pituitary, androgens exert a negative feedback effect on GnRH and gonadotrophin secretion. In addition, aromatase and 5α-reductase are expressed in all regions of the brain at varying density. Androgens exert a number of effects on higher function, including drive, libido, and possible effects on visuospatial recognition. Conversely, testosterone deficiency is associated with depression and lack of motivation.

DEVELOMENT OF MALE HYPOGONADISM

Clinical Presentation of Male Hypogonadism

Fetal Stage

Androgen deficiency during sexual differentiation (9th–14th week of gestation) leads to a disorder of sexual development with insufficient masculinization of male external genitalia, ranging from a completely female phenotype to external male genitalia with distal hypospadias. During fetal development, androgen deficiency also results in malpositioning of the testes and microphallus.

Before Puberty

Testosterone deficiency occurring during this period leads to inadequate virilization, resulting in the syndrome of eunuchoidism with typical long limbs and increased arm span due to late epiphyseal fusion of the appendicular skeleton. The rate of long bone growth is faster than that of the spine, resulting in a high ratio of lower body to upper body length. Maldevelopment of other androgen-dependent organs such the larynx (high-pitched voice) occurs and there is reduced facial and pubic hair growth and testes remain small.

Adulthood

Although voice, body proportions, and size of the penis are unaffected by androgen deficiency at this stage, body and facial hair growth dwindles, requiring infrequent shaving. Symptoms include decreased sexual potency, loss of libido, and infertility. Testicular size may be reduced. Long-term health complications include osteoporosis because of a lack of stimulation of osteoblasts by androgens and estrogen, and anemia as a result of decreased stimulation of erythropoiesis by testosterone. Quality of life is also impaired because of loss of strength from muscle atrophy and reduced vitality. Subfertility occurs because of loss of testosterone action on spermatogenesis.

Etiology of Male Hypogonadism

Hypogonadism can be primary (testicular in origin: hypergonadotrophic hypogonadism) or secondary, (hypothalamic or pituitary in origin: hypogonadotrophic hypogonadism). This classification has therapeutic implications, because fertility may be restored with appropriate hormonal stimulation in patients with secondary hypogonadism, though not in primary. Fertility options for men with primary testicular failure may include the use of donor sperm, adoption, or intracytoplasmic sperm injection (ICSI). Either type of hypogonadism may be caused by congenital or acquired conditions (Table 2). Other causes of male hypogonadism result from defects of AR or in the enzymes that metabolize testosterone within the target organ.

Congenital Causes of Hypogonadotrophic Hypogonadism

Idiopathic hypogonadotrophic hypogonadism and Kallmann's syndrome. Both idiopathic hypogonadotrophic hypogonadism (IHH) and KS are caused by insufficient secretion of hypothalamic GnRH, leading to a loss of stimulation of the pituitary production of gonadotrophins. As a consequence, androgen production and spermatogenesis by the testes are impaired.

Table 2 Etiology of Male Hypogonadism

I. Hypogonadotrophic hypogonadism

Congenital
 Idiopathic hypogonadotrophic hypogonadism
 Kallmann's syndrome
 Fertile eunuch syndrome
 Genetic defects of gonadotrophin subunits
 Prader-Willi's syndrome
 Laurence-Moon-Bardet-Biedl's syndrome
 Defective genes of pituitary differentiation (*PIT-1* and *PROP-1*)
 Mutations and deletions genes of gonadotrophin-releasing hormone–producing neurons (*DAX-1* gene)

Acquired
 Tumor: Pituitary adenomas, residual cell tumors (craniopharyngiomas, epidermoid tumors, Rathke's pouch tumors), gamete tumors
  (germinomas, teratomas, dysgerminomas), metastases
 Infiltrative: Sarcoidosis, hemochromatosis, histiocytosis-X, tuberculosis
 Infection: Tuberculosis, HIV/AIDS, fungal, syphilis
 Trauma: Contusion, skull fracture, pituitary stalk transection
 Vascular: Ischemia, Sheehan's syndrome
 Stress: Excessive exercise, mental stress, severe dieting (anorexia nervosa, anorexia bulimia), malnourishment
 Illness: Diabetes, nephrotic syndrome, obesity, primary hypothyroidism, critical illness, sickle cell disease, thalassemia
 Medical use and abuse: Radiation, anabolic steroids, glucocorticoids, narcotics, alcoholism, hypophysectomy
 Aging

II. Hypergonadotrophic hypogonadism

Congenital
 Klinefelter's syndrome (47, XXY)
 47,XYY syndrome
 Testicular dysgenesis
 Noonan's syndrome
 Defective androgen synthesis (enzyme deficiency):
  20α-Hydroxylase
  17,20-Demolase
  3β-Hydoxysteroid dehydrogenase
  17-Hydroxylase
  17-Ketosteroid reductase (also known as17β-hydroxysteroid dehydrogenase)

Acquired
 Infection: Mumps orchitis, HIV/AIDS, tuberculosis
 Medical use and abuse: Opiates, chemotherapy, radiation, glucocorticoids, alcoholism, castration (gender reassignment)
 Neoplastic: Testicular cancer
 Trauma: Injury, orchidoplexy, crypto-orchidism, vanishing testes syndrome, seminiferous tubule failure
 Illness: Cirrhosis, chronic renal failure, myotonic dystrophy, hyperthyroidism, autoimmune disease, Sertoli cell syndrome, diabetes,
  metabolic syndrome, cystic fibrosis, sickle cell disease, thalassemia major
 Others: Idiopathic

III. Defects in target organs

 5α-Reductase (pseudovaginal perineoscrotal hypospadias)
 Aromatase deficiency
 Complete androgen insensitivity syndrome
 Partial androgen insensitivity syndrome:
  Rosewater's syndrome, Reifenstein's syndrome, Gilbert-Dreyfus' syndrome, Lub's syndrome

KS is a congenital disorder inherited as a sporadic condition or as an X-linked recessive trait occurring in about 1 in 10,000 male births. The gene *KALIG-1* located in the regions of Xp22.3 for classic KS (19) and associated anosmia has been cloned (20).

The *KALIG-1* gene encodes anosmin 1, a cell adhesion protein involved in the coordinated migration of GnRH-producing neurons and olfactory neurons. Born in the nasal pit, GnRH neurons migrate to the hypothalamus during early fetal development under the influence of anosmin 1. This process is impaired in KS because of inactivating mutations of the *KALIG-1* gene (21). The concurrent underdeveloped olfactory tract can be identified by magnetic resonance imaging (MRI) scanning (22). Manifestations of X-linked KS include bimanual synkinesis and unilateral renal agenesis. Other defects such as cerebellar dysfunction, cleft palate, and congenital deafness may also be present in autosomal dominant forms of KS because of mutations of FGFR1. Recent studies have revealed other candidate genes for KS including NELF, FGF8, PKR2, and PK2 (23). Failure of gonadotrophin-induced testosterone production results in testicular maldescent. Partial pubertal development may be present in patients with partial defects, making early diagnosis difficult.

GnRH-producing neurons also appear to be affected by mutations and deletions of the *DAX-1* gene (dosage-sensitive sex reversal, adrenal hypoplasia congenita critical region on the X chromosome gene 1). *DAX-1* is located on Xp21 and expressed in the hypothalamus, pituitary, adrenal gland, gonads, and gonadal structures during fetal development. It encodes a 470 AA orphan receptor related to the steroid receptor family. It regulates expression of hormones involved in sexual differentiation. Mutations in the *C*-terminal end of *DAX-1* lead to hypogonadotrophic hypogonadism as well as adrenal hypoplasia congenita (24).

Fertile eunuch syndrome. This syndrome is a variant of IHH, also known as Pasqualini's syndrome. Patients have reduced GnRH secretion, though just enough to stimulate pituitary FSH and a minute amount of LH secretion. The small amount of LH is sufficient to raise intratesticular testosterone levels but not extratesticular testosterone; thus, these patients are fertile, as spermatogenesis is intact, but they acquire eunuchoid body segments.

Prader-Willi's syndrome. Prader-Willi's syndrome (PWS) results from a genetic imprinting defect caused by a seven-exon gene deletion or inactivation of the paternally inherited chromosome 15 (15q11–13), whereby the maternally inherited copy is silent. PWS may also be caused by uniparental disomy from inheritance of two copies of the inactive maternal gene. The incidence is 1 in 15,000 to 20,000 live births. The syndrome is characterized by hypotonia at birth, hypogonadism, short stature, facial dysmorphism, learning difficulties, hyperphagia, and obesity (25). Hypogonadism in such patients is due to a disturbance in GnRH secretion, resulting in undescended testes and microphallus at birth, as well as failure of onset of puberty. Hyperphagia leads to childhood obesity, and up to 10% go on to develop diabetes (26).

Laurence-Moon-Bardet-Biedl's syndrome. Laurence-Moon-Bardet-Biedl's syndrome (LMBBS) is rare autosomal recessive heterogeneous genetic disorder (prevalence <1:100,000). At least 12 of the genes (BBS) responsible for LMBBS have been identified. LMBBS is characterized by learning difficulties, retinitis pigmentosa, polydactyly, obesity, diabetes, renal abnormalities, and hypogonadism secondary to hypothalamic dysfunction. There has been longstanding uncertainty as to whether the Laurence-Moon's syndrome and the Bardet-Biedl's syndrome are two separate conditions. Klein and Ammann suggested that the patients of Laurence and Moon represented a distinct disorder with paraplegia and without polydactyly and obesity (27), but a 22-year prospective cohort study of 46 patients from 26 Newfoundland families conducted by Moore et al. found no correlation between clinical/dysmorphic features and genotype (28).

Defective genes of pituitary differentiation. The pituitary transcription factor-1 (PIT-1) and prophet of PIT-1 (PROP1) play an important role in the ontogenesis, differentiation, and function of somatotrophic, lactotrophic, thyrotrophic and gonadotrophic cells. Mutations in these factors result in pituitary hormone deficiencies (gonadotrophins, growth hormone, prolactin, and TSH) and delayed puberty and hypogonadism (29). Other factors that regulate pituitary differentiation include LHX3, a homeodomain transcription factor, and HESX-1 gene expressed in embryonic brain and pituitary. Mutations of HESX-1, a transcription factor and homeobox gene, cause septo-optic dysplasia (30), a syndrome characterized by panhypopituitarism, optic nerve atrophy, and midline defects of the cerebrum (corpus callosum agenesis). Another genetic cause of pituitary failure is due to inactivating mutations of LH β-chain, which results in LH deficiency and thus androgen deficiency and infertility.

Acquired Causes of Hypogonadotrophic Hypogonadism

Pituitary disorders. Benign adenoma of the anterior lobe of the pituitary is the most common cause of pituitary insufficiency. Prolactinoma is the most frequent, followed by nonfunctioning adenomas. Growth hormone and ACTH-secreting tumors are less common hormone-secreting adenomas causing acromegaly and Cushing's disease, respectively. Gonadotrophin and thyrotrophin-secreting tumors are even rarer causes. Pituitary disease may also occur with granulomatous and infiltrative disorders, cranial trauma with or without pituitary stalk transection, irradiation, and hypophysitis.

Serious illness, acquired immune deficiency syndrome, and stress. Transient hypogonadotrophic hypogonadism may occur in patients with serious disorders or malnutrition. Testosterone levels in patients with (acquired immune deficiency syndrome) AIDS may be suppressed and associated with low gonadotrophin levels (suggestive of hypothalamic-pituitary involvement) or elevated gonadotrophin levels (suggestive of primary testicular disease).

Aging. The concept of a male andropause is debatable (31). There is evidence to suggest that some aging males with reduced production of testosterone acquire clinical features of hypogonadism, increased risk of myocardial infarction, and osteoporosis. Levels of SHBG need to be taken into account as they usually increase with advancing age, probably related to higher serum oestradiol levels from increased adiposity and from a fall in IGF-1. Often the FSH and LH levels are mildly increased, suggesting that a primary testicular disorder may also be present. The circadian variation in serum testosterone levels may be lost with aging. Management of such individuals may be guided by recommendations prepared together by several groups of endocrinologists and urologists (32).

Congenital Causes of Hypergonadotrophic Hypogonadism

Klinefelter's syndrome. This condition is most commonly caused by an extra X chromosome as the result of nondysjunction during the first meiotic division of the maternal gamete, and occurs in 1 in 400 live births (33), the incidence increasing with older maternal age. Up to 90% of men with Klinefelter's syndrome have the classic 47,XXY karyotype, but mosaicism is occasionally present (34). Less than 5% are due to nondysjunction during zygotic mitosis. Others variants may be due to an additional Y chromosome such as 48,XXXY or 48,XXYY.

Patients with Klinefelter's syndrome present with small (<5 mL) firm testes, gynecomastia, eunuchoid habitus, and raised gonadotrophin levels. Despite low testosterone production, high levels of SHBG may result in "normal range" testosterone levels in about 40% of patients. Azoospermia is common, but those with mosaicism may have some spermatogenesis and be potentially fertile. Histologically, there is hyaline degeneration of the germinal epithelium with few intact gametes (35) and immature Leydig cells (36). Virilization, libido, and sexual potency may develop initially, but wane by the age of 25 to 35 years as Leydig cells begin to fail. High gonadotrophin levels hyperstimulate testicular aromatase activity leading to elevated oestradiol levels, causing gynecomastia in 50% of patients. Enlarged breasts are unsightly and patients are predisposed to a 3% to 5% risk of breast cancer. Patients are usually eunuchoid and have an increased risk of osteoporosis, learning disabilities as manifested by dyslexia, and attention deficit disorder. There is increased incidence of autoimmune disorders, such as systemic lupus erythematosus, rheumatoid arthritis, and Sjögren's syndrome. The underlying cause may be due to lower autoimmune-protecting testosterone and higher autoimmune-promoting estrogen levels in Klinefelter's patients. These autoimmune disorders may become attenuated following initiation of testosterone therapy (37).

47,XYY syndrome. An extra Y chromosome from paternal meiosis results in 47,XYY syndrome, occurring in about 0.1% of newborn males. There are few clinical signs other than a relatively tall stature. Testicular function is mildly impaired with normal Leydig cell function, and thus the levels of testosterone and LH are within reference range. Although, most patients are fertile, a proportion may be azoospermic because of germinal epithelium maturation arrest. Serum FSH levels are usually increased, and cognitive abilities may be reduced in some men. It was originally thought that patients with 47,XYY syndrome have aggressive behavior (38), but there has been no consistent evidence to support this notion.

Testicular dysgenesis. Testicular (gonadal) dysgenesis is a heterogeneous disorder with both Y-linked and non-Y-linked forms. The underlying sex chromosome abnormality includes XO, mixed XO/XY karyotype, or pure XY karyotype with streak gonads (39).

Swyer's syndrome is a condition of pure testicular dysgenesis in association with an XY karyotype (40). Eighty percent of patients with sporadic or familial 46, XY gonadal dysgenesis do not have a mutation or deletion of the SRY gene, indicating that other autosomal or X-linked genes have a role in sex determination. In about 10% of these patients, defects are present in the gene on the Y chromosome responsible for differentiation of the testes (SRY) (40,41). Gonadal dysgenesis has also been shown to be caused by duplication (41) or deletion mutation (42) of *DAX-1* on Xp21.2. Steroidogenic factor 1 (SF1/AdBP4/FTZF1, *NR5A1*) is a nuclear receptor transcription factor involved in the regulation of adrenal and gonadal development, steroidogenesis, and reproduction (43). A recent study identified heterozygous missense mutations in *NR5A1* in 4 out of 30 individuals with XY gonadal dysgenesis. These mutations (V15M, M78I, G91S, L437Q) were shown to impair transcriptional activation through abnormal DNA binding (V15M, M78I, G91S), altered subnuclear localization (V15M, M78I), or disruption of the putative ligand-binding pocket (L437Q) (44). Such patients usually have ambiguous genitalia, requiring surgical repair to the assigned gender (45). Streak gonads are associated with an increased risk of gonadoblastoma, and gonadectomy is usually performed at an early age with immediate estrogen replacement therapy as these patients are often raised as females (46).

Enzyme defects of testosterone biosynthesis. Biosynthesis of testosterone from cholesterol is catalyzed in the Leydig cells by five different enzymes (Fig. 5). Defects in any of these enzymes lead to failure of testosterone biosynthesis (Table 3). Defect of an enzyme characteristically leads to reduction of testosterone with an excessive production of its substrate. The Wolffian duct fails to differentiate into the male sexual organs and feminization of the external genitalia occurs. The phenotype of the individual depends on the residual activity of the defective enzyme. If a complete enzyme block occurs, female genitalia are formed with a blind vaginal pouch, absent uterus, Fallopian tubes, and ovaries because of the expression of anti-Müllerian hormone. The condition is found occasionally when patients undergo investigations for hernias but turn out to be abdominal or inguinal testes. The enzyme defect is normally discovered during investigations for primary amenorrhea. As testicular and adrenal steroid biosynthesis shares many enzymes in common, defects may lead to symptoms of hypogonadism and adrenocortical insufficiency simultaneously.

Table 3 Enzyme Defects Affecting Androgen Biosynthesis

Enzymatic defect	Cortisol	Androstenedione	Testosterone	Pregnenolone	Progesterone	17α-Hydroxy-progesterone
20α-Hydroxylase	↓	↓	↓	↓	↓	↓
17,20-Demolase	↓	↓	↓	↓	↓	↓
3β-Hydoxysteroid dehydrogenase	↔	↓	↓	↔ or ↑	↔ or ↑	↔ or ↑
17-Hydroxylase	↓	↓	↓	↑	↑	↓
17β-Hydroxysteroid dehydrogenase[a]	↔	↑	↓	↔	↔	↔
5α-Reductase	↔	↔	↔	↔	↔	↔

[a]Also known as 17-ketosteroid reductase.

Acquired Causes of Hypergonadotrophic Hypogonadism

Myotonic dystrophy. Myotonic dystrophy is an autosomal dominant disorder, characterized by hypogonadism, muscle weakness, and frontal balding. Repeat sequences of CTG in an untranslated region of the DMPK gene have been identified in many of these patients, but the disorder seems to be genetically and phenotypically heterogeneous. Testicular failure usually occurs after age 40 years; thus, they often have children who may inherit the disease. Testosterone levels may be variably decreased in the presence of azoospermia and high gonadotrophin levels.

Cryptorchidism. Cryptorchidism may occur unilaterally or bilaterally in about 3% to 4% at birth. Since most testes descend with age, the one-year incidence is reduced to less than 1%. Because normal testicular descent requires normal pituitary function and DHT levels, the incidence of cryptorchidism is increased in patients with KS. It is vital to distinguish cryptorchidism from retractile testes so that the treatment with hCG or orchidoplexy is applied correctly. The aim is to bring down the undescended testes into the scrotum before one to two years of age to improve fertility potential. In prepubertal boys, a four-week trial of hCG may be used to determine whether testicular descent can occur before considering surgical intervention.

Vanishing testes syndrome (congenital anorchism or prepubertal functional castrate). The initial presentation of vanishing testes syndrome is sexual immaturity in a male patient with impalpable testes. The condition may arise from fetal testicular torsion after sufficient testosterone exposure to complete reproductive tract development. The levels of testosterone are low with elevated gonadotrophins. If the LH levels are only minimally increased, hCG stimulation testing of the gonad may help diagnosis. An absent testosterone response to hCG stimulation suggests the vanishing testes syndrome. A response to hCG stimulation may indicate the presence of intraabdominal testes and requires further assessment by MRI scanning.

Other acquired causes of hypergonadotrophic hypogonadism. These include trauma, mumps orchitis, radiation and chemotherapy, and Sertoli-cell-only syndrome. Recent evidence has suggested that in utero exposure to maternal toxic substances such as cigarette smoking and alcohol may have long-lasting adverse effects on the reproductive system, including reduced testicular size and sperm production in adult males (47) and cryptorchidism in newborn boys (48). The underlying mechanism is not clear, but toxins and hypoxia may be important factors interfering with androgen activity and/or their modulators. In rats, androgen action blockade by flutamide results in cryptorchidism and hypospadias, but only within a critical programming window for reproductive tract masculinization, equating to 8 to 14 weeks of gestation in humans (49).

Hypogonadism Secondary to Target Organ Defects

Target organ defects are disorders in which testicular hormones testosterone and/or its metabolites (DHT and oestradiol), and AMH do not function, despite intact testicular function. The disorders may be due to defects of the corresponding receptor or the enzymes (5α-reductase or aromatase).

Androgen insensitivity syndrome (AIS) is caused by sporadic or familial loss of function mutations of the AR and affects 1 in 20,000 to 90,000 births. More than 600 mutations have been documented in the AR gene, located on Xp11 to 12, 200 in exons B-H carrying steroid and DBDs. Although there are only 23 mutations in exon A, a complete loss of receptor function occurs compared with slight receptor dysfunction in mutations of other exons. The N-terminal section (exon A) of the AR is very variable, containing a polymorphic polyglutamine (CAG) repeat sequences comprising 8 to 35 repeats (Fig. 7). Excess number of CAG repeats (>38) results in androgen resistance because coactivators and androgens bind less strongly to AR with long CAG sequences. The severity of androgen resistance is reflected by the variety of clinical phenotype of affected individuals. Testosterone levels may be within or slightly above the male testosterone reference range with modestly elevated gonadotrophin levels.

Complete androgen insensitivity syndrome. Complete AIS is the most severe form of AR resistance. These patients have a 46(XY) karyotype and are phenotypically female, with normal pubertal development including unambiguous female external genitalia, but lack Müllerian duct structures and androgen-dependent body hair. They typically present with inguinal hernia during infancy or with primary amenorrhea in adolescence. The testes may reside in the abdomen, groin, or labia majora, and secrete androgen and AMH. Testosterone has no effects on target organs; thus, the Wolffian structures fail to differentiate, leading to the absence of epididymis, seminal vesicle, duct, and prostate. Testicular AMH inhibits the differentiation of Müllerian structures resulting in the absence of the uterus, Fallopian tubes and ovaries, and a short blind pouch vagina. Osteopenia or osteoporosis occurs in about a quarter of individuals with complete AIS (46) and estrogen replacement has been shown to improve bone mineral density (BMD).

Reifenstein's syndrome. Partial AR defect in this disorder results in a male phenotype at birth with variable pseudohermaphroditism. The testes are often not descended completely and small in size with resultant atrophy of the germinal epithelium and azoospermia. The lack of feedback inhibition of the pituitary by testosterone results in elevated LH levels, and as a consequence, hyperstimulation of Leydig cells occurs. FSH may be normal or slightly increased. The external genitalia are insufficiently masculinized, ranging from incomplete labioscrotal fusion with formation of a pseudovagina, through perineoscrotal hypospadia, to slight penile hypospadia. Sometimes, the only signs are revealed at puberty, with gynecomastia and azoospermia. The Wolffian duct structures may be normal or hypoplastic. Virilization may be delayed with normal pubic and axillary hair distribution, but body hair is sparse and the voice may not break. Gynecomastia in these patients, unlike those with Klinefelter's syndrome, is not predisposed to increased risk of breast cancer.

5α-Reductase deficiency. This is an autosomal recessive condition caused by various types of mutations including substitution and deletion of the 5α-reductase type 2 (*SRD5A2*) gene, leading to 5α-reductase deficiency in the background of a XY genotype (50). The degrees of masculinization defects correlate weakly with genotype defects. External female genitalia are present at birth and these individuals are often raised as girls until puberty, when the underlying condition is revealed by developing male secondary characteristics. The diagnosis is based on clinical manifestations and an increased testosterone to DHT ratio, both after puberty and in response to hCG before puberty. Sexual reassignment is a major issue, and patients would benefit from clinical psychological assessment before proceeding to corrective surgery.

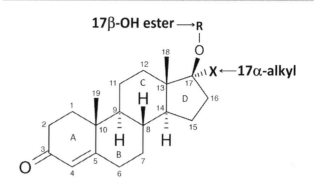

Figure 11   Testosterone and its derivatives.

TESTOSTERONE THERAPY

Goals of Testosterone Therapy

Ideally, long-term testosterone replacement therapy (TRT) should be safe, potent with a high tissue-specific selectivity, convenient and inexpensive with long-acting properties. Maximal efficacy within adequate safety limits should be taken into consideration and cost-effectiveness compared with other drugs. The aim of treating testosterone deficiency is to restore and maintain stable, physiological concentrations of serum testosterone for prolonged periods using convenient formulations that facilitate compliance, and avoid wide fluctuations of androgen levels. Ultimately, the outcome of treatment is to improve mortality, but it appears that attaining morbidity benefits is more realistic, aiming to improve quality of life, symptoms of hypogonadism, prevention of long-term health sequelae, development of secondary sex characteristics, and restoration of fertility in cases of hypogonadotrophic hypogonadism. The adverse effects of testosterone therapy should be considered (Table 4). Because of the stimulatory effects on androgen-dependent tumor growth, treatment with testosterone, pulsatile GnRH, and gonadotrophin are contraindicated in those with prostate cancer, male breast cancer, or untreated prolactinoma. Relative contraindications are applied to those with sleep apnea and polycythemia because of the risk of hyperviscosity. Because testosterone treatment tends to reduce sperm counts and testicular size, it is not recommended for men who are seeking fertility.

Testosterone Therapy in Adult Males with Hypogonadism

For reasons of safety and ease of monitoring, testosterone rather than synthetic androgens is used. It has a short circulating half-life or transit time and low oral bioavailability due to rapid hepatic oxidation and glucuronidation to biologically inactivate metabolites. This has led to the development of parenteral depot formulations (injectable, implantable, and transdermal), products bypassing the hepatic portal system (sublingual, buccal, gut lymphatic absorption) and orally active synthetic androgens (51). Testosterone is the prototype androgen with a 19-carbon, four-ring steroid structure and two oxygens (3-keto, 17β-hydroxy) including a Δ^4 nonaromatic A ring (Fig. 11).

Testosterone therapy aims to attain a physiological range of serum testosterone (9–42 nmol/L), DHT and oestradiol levels, to gain optimal virilization and normal sexual function. Testosterone therapy can be used in the male patient with hypogonadism who is not seeking fertility or is not able to achieve fertility and late teenage males with delayed puberty. The approved preparations of testosterone for clinical use include long-acting and short-acting intramuscular preparations, scrotal and transdermal patches, transdermal gel, and orally administered agents (Table 5). Orally administered testosterone such as testosterone undecanoate is available, but it undergoes hepatic metabolism rapidly (52), thus requiring frequent dosing. As a result, the levels of testosterone are often erratic. For patients with hypogonadotrophic hypogonadism requiring fertility, hCG with or without

Table 4   Common Adverse Effects of Testosterone Replacement Therapy and Recommended Monitoring Tests During the Course of Therapy

System/organ	Adverse effect	Monitoring during therapy
Prostate	Benign prostate hypertrophy	Digital rectal examination, prostate specific antigen
Hematological	Polycythemia, hyperviscosity	Hemoglobin, hematocrit
Lipids	Dyslipidemia	Fasting lipid profile
Spermatogenesis	Reduced sperm counts	Sperm counts
Respiratory	Sleep apnea	Clinical symptoms, sleep study

Table 5 Currently Available Testosterone Preparations

Route	Generic name	Trade name	Dosage	Adverse effects
Transdermal	Testosterone patch	Androderm	2 × 5 mg/day	Contact dermatitis
	TTS scrotal	Testoderm	1 membrane/day	Supraphysiological dihydrotestosterone levels
	Testosterone gel	Testogel, Androtop gel	25–50 mg/day	
	Testosterone gel	Testim	50 mg/day	Potential partner transfer
Parenteral	Testosterone enanthate	Testosterone Depot	1 ampoule (250 mg) every 2–3 wk	Fluctuating symptoms
	Testosterone undecanoate	Nebido	1 ampoule (1 g) every 12 wk	Deep and slow intragluteal injection
Implants	Testosterone	Testosterone implants	6 implants (1.2 g) every 6 mo	Specialist minor surgical implantation
Oral	Testosterone undecanoate	Andriol Testocaps	2–4 capsules (40 mg) daily	Variable testosterone levels
Buccal	Testosterone	Striant	1 tablet (30 mg) twice daily	Gum/buccal irritation

human menopausal gonadotrophin (hMG) or pulsatile GnRH therapy with or without assisted reproduction are considered (53).

Transdermal Testosterone

Pharmacogenetics and metabolism. About 10% to 15% of the transdermal testosterone is absorbed and the remaining 85% to 90% is lost, some of which may be because of metabolism by 5-α reduction, while factors such as variation in the clearance rate of testosterone, which could be a function of skin blood flow, skin temperature, or perspiration may also contribute. Short-term application (7–14 days) of 5 to 10 g of 1% transdermal testosterone gel (5 g gel contains 50 mg testosterone as active ingredient) results in peak serum testosterone levels between 18 and 24 hours (54), with a steady state achieved after application of the testosterone gel after 7 to 14 days. Studies have shown that DHT and oestradiol levels increased steadily after the first application (55). Long-term evaluation over one, three, and six months of treatment showed steady serum testosterone, DHT, and oestradiol levels similar to that of short-term pharmacokinetics, with only small and variable peaks of serum testosterone after each daily application. Suspension of testosterone application leads to a gradual fall in serum testosterone levels between 48 and 96 hours, indicating the presence of a testosterone reservoir that is a unique feature of this form of delivery (54). With continued application of testosterone gel, accumulation rates showed no further increases, providing further reassurance on the safety of this delivery system (55).

Serum DHT concentrations increase threefold after application of 50 mg of testosterone in 5 g gel and nearly fivefold with 100 mg of testosterone in 10 g gel, a higher increase than that observed with patches (56). This could be the consequence of both a higher delivery of bioavailable testosterone and a higher conversion of testosterone to DHT in the skin where high 5-α reductase activity is expressed as well as the larger area of skin surface exposed to the testosterone gel compared with testosterone patch. DHT levels are nonetheless much lower than that observed with scrotal patches.

Clinical efficacy. The average recommended dose of transdermal testosterone is 50 mg (in 5 g of gel)/day, but about a fifth of patients may not achieve stable serum testosterone concentration in the young adult reference range (300–100 ng/dL or 10.4–34.7 mmol/L). It is uncertain whether lower responders are less compliant or are biologically different in that they might have low absorption and/or high clearance of testosterone. In such patients, a trial of injectable testosterone may be desirable (57).

A dose of 1% testosterone gel has been shown to have positive benefits on sexual function, mood, muscle strength, body composition, and BMD in men with various forms of hypogonadism over a considerable time (54,58). Increases of about 1% to 2% in BMD after six months of treatment appeared to relate to the testosterone level achieved (58). In patients with treatment-resistant depression, 1% testosterone gel added to existing antidepressant regimens resulted in reduced symptoms of depression (59). After about three years of treatment, levels of total LDL and HDL cholesterol and triglycerides remained unchanged (54). For this reason, testosterone gel is considered an appropriate therapy for patients with hypogonadism as well as age-related male hypogonadism (60).

Scrotal testosterone patches are available in 40 and 60 cm² sizes, delivering 4 and 6 mg of testosterone daily, respectively. Scrotal skin absorbs testosterone better than does nonscrotal skin, but may be reduced if the scrotum is small or has abnormal skin surface. Because genital skin contains high concentrations of 5α-reductase, DHT levels are often persistently elevated (61). The HDL to total cholesterol ratio does not change by this route of testosterone therapy. The long-term potential effects of increased levels of DHT are currently unknown but may cause benign prostate hypertrophy (BPH). The cost of using the scrotal patch is expensive but is convenient to use.

Parenteral Testosterone Preparations

Enanthate and cypionate testosterone. The absorption of these esters is prolonged by suspension in oil. After intramuscular injection, peak levels occur in about 72 hours and a slow decline occurs during the following one to two weeks. A steady state of plasma testosterone between injections can be achieved by doses between 50 and 100 mg of testosterone administered intramuscularly at 7 to 10 days intervals. Higher doses of 100 to 150 mg of testosterone every two weeks can also be used, but the use of 300 mg injections every three weeks is associated with wider fluctuations of testosterone levels, wider swings between peak and nadir, resulting in fluctuating symptoms.

Lower doses of testosterone are used in adult male patients with prepubertal onset of hypogonadism who are going through puberty for the first time during therapy. The starting testosterone dose of 50 mg every three to four weeks with a gradual increment during subsequent months until full replacement is achieved within 12 months. It may take three to four years to attain full virilization. Men with BPH who have hypogonadism and prostatic symptoms may be given 50 to 100 mg of testosterone every two weeks as an initial regimen with careful monitoring of urinary symptoms and prostate examinations.

Undecanoate preparations. Nebido® is a testosterone undecanoate preparation suspended in castor oil for intramuscular injection. This testosterone ester had been used in oral capsules since the 1970s, but had obviously already been applied as intramuscular injections in China for several years, with a long half-life (62). The vehicle was changed from Chinese teaseed oil to castor oil in Europe (61,63,64). When compared with testosterone enanthate, serum testosterone levels remain in the normal range for long periods of time (64). Some patients have now been followed for up to eight years, with good substitution and no serious side effects (65). Treatment necessitates 1000 mg injections every 10 to 14 weeks, following a loading dose at 6 weeks (32,66). Adjustments of injection intervals may be scheduled according to serum testosterone levels determined from serum samples taken just before the next injection. In addition to its use in hypogonadism, testosterone undecanoate has become a valuable asset in male contraception trials and, as such, has outlived testosterone enanthate and buciclate. Testosterone undecanoate has the potential to be combined with norethisterone enanthate (NETE) into one contraceptive regimen, and in combination with subcutaneous etonorgestrel implants, it is currently being tested in Europe by Schering and Organon in multicenter trials for male contraception (67). Since this preparation in teaseed oil has a shorter half-life than its European variant in castor oil, it needs to be injected more frequently than Nebido. However, a trial involving 308 couples in China, using monthly injections of 500 mg testosterone undecanoate, resulted in 97% of men showing azoospermia with complete contraceptive protection.

Gonadal Stimulation in Hypogonadotrophic Hypogonadism

Because gonadotrophin or GnRH therapy is effective only in hypogonadotrophic hypogonadism, this diagnosis must be established before consideration of therapy. Although these agents may also be used to induce puberty in boys and to treat androgen deficiency in hypogonadotrophic hypogonadism, the major use of these preparations is in the initiation and maintenance of spermatogenesis in hypogonadotrophic men who desire fertility.

Gonadotrophin Therapy in Testosterone Deficiency

Because of its ability to bind to LH receptors on Leydig cell, hCG can stimulate the production of testosterone. Peripubertal boys with hypogonadotrophic hypogonadism and delayed puberty can be treated with hCG instead of testosterone to induce pubertal development. The initial regimen of hCG is usually 1000 to 2000 IU administered intramuscularly once to twice a week. The clinical response is monitored, and testosterone levels are measured about every two to three months for optimal dose adjustments. High doses of hCG may reduce testicular stimulation by downregulating the end organ. The advantages of hCG over testosterone include its long half-life and the stimulation of testicular growth, and maintenance of greater stability of testosterone levels, resulting in fewer fluctuations in hypogonadal symptoms. In addition, hCG treatment is necessary for stimulating enough intratesticular testosterone to allow the initiation of spermatogenesis. The disadvantages of hCG include the need for more frequent injections and greater cost.

Gonadotrophin Therapy for Induction of Spermatogenesis

Male patients with onset of hypogonadotrophic hypogonadism before completion of pubertal development may have testes generally smaller than 5 mL. These patients usually require therapy with both hCG and hMG (or FSH) to induce spermatogenesis. Men with partial gonadotrophin deficiency or who have previously (peripubertally) been stimulated with hCG may initiate and maintain production of sperm with hCG therapy alone. Men with postpubertal acquired hypogonadotrophic hypogonadism and who have previously had normal production of sperm can also generally initiate and maintain spermatogenesis with hCG treatment alone. Fertility may be possible at much lower sperm counts (less than 1 million/mL) than what would otherwise be considered fertile. Therapeutic dose of hCG starts at 1000 to 2000 IU intramuscularly twice a week with monthly monitoring of testosterone levels for appropriate dose adjustments, which may take two to three months to achieve. When normal levels of testosterone are attained, monthly assessment of testicular growth and sperm counts is carried out during a 12-month period. Because of the high cost of hMG (or FSH) preparations, hCG usually is the initial therapy of choice for at least 6 to 12 months. In general, the response to hCG therapy is greater in those with large initial testicular volume. In completely hypogonadotrophic men, combining purified FSH and testosterone without LH or hCG does not stimulate spermatogenesis. If spermatogenesis has not been initiated by the end of 6 to 12 months of therapy with hCG or LH, administration of an FSH-containing preparation is initiated in a dosage of 225 IU intramuscularly three times a week along with the hCG injections. If pregnancy occurs, the patient's regimen can be switched to hCG only to allow continued spermatogenesis for subsequent potential pregnancies. If no further pregnancies are desired, testosterone therapy can be used, or long-term hCG therapy can be continued with appropriate contraceptive measures. Rarely, antibodies against hCG may arise, rendering therapy ineffective; in such situations, human LH may be used as alternative.

Gonadotrophin-Releasing Hormone Therapy

In patients with hypothalamic hypogonadism (intact pituitary gland), synthetic GnRH can be given in a pulsatile fashion subcutaneously through a pump every two hours. Response to GnRH therapy reflected by two weekly LH, FSH, and testosterone levels. GnRH therapy can be used to initiate pubertal development, maintain virilization and sexual function, and initiate and maintain spermatogenesis. In most patients, these effects may take from 3 to 15 months to achieve sperm production. Fertility can be achieved with very low sperm counts (<1 million/mL). GnRH may be more effective than gonadotrophin stimulation in increasing testicular size and initiating spermatogenesis in many patients with hypogonadotrophic hypogonadism.

Assisted Reproductive Technology

ICSI directly into the egg by a single sperm or immature form retrieved from the testis is sufficient to fertilize an egg. In vitro fertilization with ICSI may be a viable option in many men with hypogonadism who cannot otherwise be induced to produce enough sperm as well as in the presence of a female factor that may further make pregnancy by the couple impossible. The procedure is expensive and the low-cost intrauterine insemination may be more suitable when the patient has mild to moderate oligospermia.

Pituitary Tumors

Patients with acquired hypogonadotrophic hypogonadism may require assessment for a possible pituitary tumor with appropriate pituitary imaging studies, such as MRI, and assessment of full pituitary function to provide the correct diagnosis and therapy. If a prolactinoma is present, medical therapy with bromocriptine, pergolide, or cabergoline would be the first approach to reduce prolactin levels sufficiently to allow gonadal function to resume or allow stimulation with gonadotrophins. Even when prolactin levels cannot be normalized, hCG therapy alone or combined with hMG (or FSH) therapy may stimulate spermatogenesis. Surgical therapy may be considered for significant pituitary tumors that are not prolactin-secreting microadenomas, and only those with prolactin-secreting microadenomas who cannot tolerate medical treatment because of adverse effects.

FUTURE RESEARCH AND DEVELOPMENT

Testosterone Therapy in Combination with Phosphodieterase Type 5 Inhibitors

The use of testosterone to treat human erectile dysfunction (ED) has proved controversial because of conflicting findings. For example, it has been found that erectile function remains intact in some severely hypogonadal men who have reduced libido; on the other hand, testosterone therapy in hypogonadal men with ED leads to improvement of erectile function (68). Testosterone probably has a complex interaction with the penile system through its influences on the metabolism of mediators such as nitric oxide (NO) and cyclic guanosine monophosphate (cGMP), as well as its action on phosphodieterase type 5 (PDE5). The normal erectile function involves the synthesis of the neurotransmitter NO and the subsequent accumulation of cGMP (69). The NO formation, which leads to erection, is regulated by the activity of NO synthase (NOS) isoenzymes, whereas cGMP degradation, which promotes smooth muscle tone and terminates erection, is specifically controlled by PDE5. The regulation of the activity of these two counteracting enzymes allows the penis to be contracted for the majority of the time. Androgens play a pivotal role in these mechanisms by regulating both NOS and PDE5 activity (70). In castrated mice testosterone replacement induces de novo DNA synthesis in the smooth muscle cells and blood vessels, with a pancellular proliferative effect in the penis and endothelial NOS expression (71). Testosterone also induces second messenger signal transduction cascades, including increases in cytosolic calcium and activation of PKA, PKC, and mitogen-activated protein kinase (MAPK), leading to smooth muscle relaxation, neuromuscular and junctional signal transmission, and neuronal plasticity (72).

PDE5 inhibitors such as sildenafil enhance vasodilatation by blocking the inactivation of cGMP, resulting in increased smooth muscle relaxation and better erections in the presence of sexual stimulation. It has been shown that the efficacy of sildenafil is improved by the presence of testosterone (69,71). The idea of combining therapy of testosterone with PDE5 inhibitors is based on several reasons. First, there is a large proportion (up to 50%) of hypogonadal men with ED who do not respond to monotherapy of PDE5 inhibitor (73), and second, the presence of a consensus sequence for the AR in the 5'-flanking region of the PDE5 promoter suggests that testosterone could regulate PDE5 expression (72). In a clinical setting, it has been demonstrated that TRT improves ED in partial androgen-deficient aging men (74), renal transplant or dialyzed patients (75), and in patients with type 2 diabetes (76) who fail monotherapy of sildenafil.

Pharmacogenetics

Original research on X-linked spinal and bulbar muscular atrophy (Kennedy's disease) suggested a mutation at the *N*-terminus of the AR gene exon 1, involving

Table 6 Diseases Related to Abnormally Short or Long Polymorphic Polyglutamine (CAG) Sequences of the *N*-Terminal Section (Exon A) of the Androgen Receptor

Consequences of short CAG sequences	Reference
Prostate hypertrophy	Zitzmann et al. (80)
Prostate cancer	Bratt et al. (81)
Coronary artery disease	Alevizaki et al. (82)
Breast cancer	Suter et al. (83)
Increased erythropoiesis	Zitzmann (84)
Consequences of long CAG sequences	
Androgen insensitivity	Crabbe et al. (85)
Osteoporosis	Zitzmann et al. (86)

amplification of CAG (polyglutamine) repeats as the underlying cause (77), probably because of the neurotoxicity of the polyglutamine-expanded gene products (78). Subsequent studies have identified a number of candidate genes for this CAG triplet polymorphism of the AR (79). It appears that a normal length of CAG repeats is between 8 and 35. Abnormally shorter sequences or longer sequences than this range are associated with increased risk of diseases that are androgen dependent (Table 6) (80–86). This relationship has been explained by the fact that the length of the CAG repeats of the AR determines the transactivation activity of the receptor (87), such that shorter CAG repeats are associated with stronger and longer CAG repeats with weaker activation of the transcription triggered by the AR. The underlying mechanism may lie in the unfolded state of the sequence when it exceeds a critical length (87,88).

The potential for pharmacogenetic tailoring of TRT dose to an individual's genetic background of androgen sensitivity and potential adverse effects may be based on CAG triplets and metabolic characteristics of each patient to enhance effectiveness and avoid unwanted effects (12,84). Testosterone treatment of hypogonadal men with shorter CAG repeat lengths exhibits a more pronounced increase in prostate volume and hematocrit than men with longer CAG repeat lengths. Furthermore, patients with long CAG repeats have been shown to respond better to endocrine therapy (81). On the basis of this evidence, it would be plausible to select a shorter-acting formulation to treat hypogondal men with a shorter CAG repeat length, as they give more flexibility for monitoring and dose adjustments. The dose of testosterone in a particular formulation may also have an impact. For example, higher dose of testosterone may benefit men with a longer CAG repeat length (more resistant to testosterone) but contraindicated in those with a shorter CAG repeat length (increased risk of prostate cancer and polycythemia).

Synthetic Androgens and Elective Androgen Receptor Modulators

In the past 40 years, more than a thousand testosterone derivatives have been synthesized to enhance intrinsic androgenic potency, prolong duration of action, and/or improve oral bioavailability of synthetic androgens. Major structural modifications of testosterone include 17β-esterification, 19-nor methyl, 17-α alkyl, 1-methyl, 7-α methyl, and D-homo-androgens (Fig. 11); most of these are unavailable for clinical use because of hepatotoxicity (89), especially 17α-alkyl and 7α-methyl derivatives. Only a few synthetic androgens are currently being investigated in clinical trials, including 7α-methyl-19-nortestosterone (MENT), which is not hepatotoxic (90). MENT is a nandrolone derivative with high tissue-specific selectivity as it is preferably metabolized by aromatization rather than 5α-reduction. MENT is more potent than testosterone; it is therefore being considered as transdermal formulation or for long-term use in subdermal implants as well as for male contraception. Evidence from preclinical trials has demonstrated that it has less effects on the prostate than testosterone but has little effects on BMD in hypogonadal males (91).

Current research on steroids with tissue specificity is being extended to the search for selective androgen receptor modulators. The compounds are structurally modified so that the nonsteroidal molecules avoid intrinsic aromatization or 5α-reduction (92) and may produce agonistic effects in desired target tissues, with minimal unwanted adverse effects. Such compounds have a potential for treating certain groups of patients such as hypogonadal men with osteoporosis, BPH, or hyperviscosity.

REFERENCES

1. American Association of Clinical Endocrinologists. American Association of Clinical Endocrinologists Medical Guidelines for clinical practice for the evaluation and treatment of hypogonadism in adult male patients—2002 update. Endocr Pract 2002; 8:440–456.
2. Nussey SS, Whitehead SA. Endocrinology: an integrated approach. Oxford: BIOS: Taylor & Francis, 2001.
3. Kalra PS, Sahu A, Kalra SP. Interleukin-1 inhibits the ovarian steroidinduced luteinizing hormone surge and release of hypothalamic luteinizing hormone-releasing hormone in rats. Endocrinology 1990; 126:2145–2152.
4. Yoo MJ, Nishihara M, Takahashi M. Tumor necrosis factor-α mediates endotoxin induced suppression of gonadotropin-releasing hormone pulse generator activity in the rat. Endocr J 1997; 44:141–148.
5. Zhang Y, Proenca R, Maffei M, et al. Positional cloning of the mouse obese gene and its human homologue. Nature 1994; 372:425–432.
6. Baranowska B, Baranowska-Bik A, Bik W, et al. The role of leptin and orexins in the dysfunction of hypothalamo-pituitary-gonadal regulation and in the mechanism of hyperactivity in patients with anorexia nervosa. Neuro Endocrinol Lett 2008; 29:37–40.
7. Kotani M, Detheux M, Vandenbogaerde A, et al. The metastasis suppressor gene KiSS-1 encodes kisspeptins, the natural ligands of the orphan G protein-coupled receptor GPR54. J Biol Chem 2001; 276:34631–34636.
8. de Roux N, Genin E, Carel JC, et al. Hypogonadotrophic hypogonadism due to loss of function of the KiSS1-derived peptide receptor GPR54. Proc Natl Acad Sci U S A 2003; 100:10972–10976.
9. Seminara SB, Messager S, Chatzidaki EE, et al. The GPR54 gene as a regulator of puberty. N Engl J Med 2003; 349:1614–1627.

10. Dhillo WS, Chaudhri OB, Thompson EL, et al. Kisspeptin-54 stimulates gonadotropin release most potently during the preovulatory phase of the menstrual cycle in women. J Clin Endocrinol Metab 2007; 92(10):3958–3966.

11. Morelli A, Marini M, Mancina R, et al. Sex steroids and leptin regulate the "first kiss" (KiSS 1/G-protein-coupled receptor 54 system) in human gonadotropin-releasing-hormone-secreting neuroblasts. J Sex Med 2008; 5: 1097–1113.

12. Zitzmann M, Nieschlag E. Androgen receptor gene CAG repeat length and body mass index modulate the safety of long-term intramuscular testosterone undecanoate therapy in hypogonadal men. J Clin Endocrinol Metab 2007; 92:3844–3853.

13. Ferro P, Catalano MG, Dell'Eva R, et al. The androgen receptor CAG repeat: a modifier of carcinogenesis? Mol Cell Endocrinol 2002; 193:109–120.

14. Dejager S, Bry-Gauillard H, Bruckert E, et al. A comprehensive endocrine description of Kennedy's disease revealing androgen insensitivity linked to CAG repeat length. J Clin Endocrinol Metab 2002; 87:3893–3901.

15. Berkhoff M, Sturzenegger M, Spiegel R, et al. X-chromosomal bulbospinal muscular atrophy (Kennedy syndrome). Schweiz Med Wochenschr 1998; 128:817–823.

16. Baskin LS, Sutherland RS, DiSandro MJ, et al. The effect of testosterone on androgen receptors and human penile growth. J Urol 1997; 158:1113–1118.

17. Saad F, Gooren L, Haider A, et al. A dose-response study of testosterone on sexual dysfunction and features of the metabolic syndrome using testosterone gel and parenteral testosterone undecanoate. J Androl 2008; 29:102–105.

18. Sarkey S, Azcoitia I, Garcia-Segura LM, et al. Classical androgen receptors in non-classical sites in the brain. Horm Behav 2008; 53:753–764.

19. Hardelin JP, Levilliers J, Young J, et al. Xp22.3 deletions in isolated familial KS. J Clin Endocrinol Metab 1993; 76: 827–831.

20. Franco B, Guioli S, Pragliola A, et al. A gene deleted in KS shares homology with neural cell adhesion and axonal path-finding molecules. Nature 1991; 353:529–536.

21. Layman LC. Genetics of human hypogonadotrophic hypogonadism. Am J Med Genet 1999; 89:240–248.

22. Klingmüller D, Dewes W, Krahe T, et al. Magnetic resonance imaging of the brain in patients with anosmia and hypothalamic hypogonadism (Kleinfelter syndrome). J Clin Endocrinol Metab 1987; 65:581–584.

23. Cadman SM, Kim SH, Hu Y, et al. Molecular pathogenesis of Kallmann's syndrome. Horm Res 2007; 67:231–242.

24. Calvari V, Alpigiani MG, Poggi E, et al. X-linked adrenal hypoplasia congenita and hypogonadotrophic hypogonadism: report on new mutation of the DAX-1 gene in two siblings. J Endocrinol Invest 2006; 29:41–47.

25. Gunay-Aygun M, Cassidy SB, Nicholls RD. Prader–Willi and other syndromes associated with obesity and mental retardation. Behav Genet 1997; 27:307–324.

26. Nagai T, Mori M. Prader–Willi syndrome, diabetes mellitus and hypogonadism. Biomed Pharmacother 1999; 53:452–454.

27. Klein D, Ammann F. The syndrome of Laurence–Moon–Bardet–Biedl and allied diseases in Switzerland. Clinical, genetic and epidemiological studies. J Neurol Sci 1969; 9:479–513.

28. Moore SJ, Green JS, Fan Y, et al. Clinical and genetic epidemiology of Bardet–Biedl syndrome in Newfoundland: a 22-year prospective, population-based, cohort study. Am J Med Genet A 2005; 132:352–360.

29. Pfäffle RW, Blankenstein O, Wüller S, et al. Combined pituitary hormone deficiency: role of Pit-1 and Prop-1. Acta Paediatr Suppl 1999; 88:33–41.

30. Dattani MT, Martinez-Barbera JP, Thomas PQ, et al. Mutations in the homeobox gene HESX1/Hesx1 associated with septo-optic dysplasia in human and mouse. Nat Genet 1998; 19:125–133.

31. Morales A. Andropause (or symptomatic late-onset hypogonadism): facts, fiction and controversies. Aging Male 2004; 7:297–303.

32. Nieschlag E. Testosterone treatment comes of age: new options for hypogonadal men. Clin Endocrinol 2006; 65:275–281.

33. Hamerton JL, Canning N, Ray M, et al. A cytogenetic survey of 14,069 newborn infants. I. Incidence of chromosome abnormalities. Clin Genet 1975; 8:223–243.

34. Huckins C, Bullock LP, Long JL. Morphological profiles of cryptorchid XXY mouse testes. Anat Rec 1981; 199: 507–518.

35. Paulsen CA, Gordon DL, Carpenter RW, et al. Klinefelter's syndrome and its variants: a hormonal and chromosomal study. Recent Prog Horm Res 1968; 24:321–363.

36. Nistal M, Paniagua R, Abaurrea MA, et al. 47,XXY Klinefelter's syndrome with low FSH and LH levels and absence of Leydig cells. Andrologia 1980; 12:426–433.

37. Bizzarro A, Valentini G, Di Martino G, et al. Influence of testosterone therapy on clinical and immunological features of autoimmune diseases associated with Klinefelter's syndrome. J Clin Endocrinol Metab 1987; 64:32–36.

38. Santen RJ, DeKretser DM, Paulsen CA, et al. Gonadotrophins and testosterone in the XYY syndrome. Lancet 1970; 2(7668):371.

39. Sarafoglou K, Ostrer H. Clinical review 111. Familial sex reversal: a review. J Clin Endocrinol Metab 2000; 85:483–493.

40. Hawkins JR, Taylor A, Goodfellow PN, et al. Evidence for increased prevalence of SRY mutations in XY females with complete rather than partial gonadal dysgenesis. Am J Hum Genet 1992; 51:979–984.

41. Barbaro M, Oscarson M, Schoumans J, et al. Isolated 46,XY gonadal dysgenesis in two sisters caused by a Xp21.2 interstitial duplication containing the DAX1 gene. J Clin Endocrinol Metab 2007; 92:3305–3313.

42. Smyk M, Berg JS, Pursley A, et al. Male-to-female sex reversal associated with an approximately 250 kb deletion upstream of NR0B1 (DAX1). Hum Genet 2007; 122:63–70.

43. Lin L, Gu WX, Ozisik G, et al. Analysis of DAX1 (NR0B1) and steroidogenic factor-1 (NR5A1) in children and adults with primary adrenal failure: ten years' experience. J Clin Endocrinol Metab 2006; 91:3048–3054.

44. Lin L, Philibert P, Ferraz-de-Souza B, et al. Heterozygous missense mutations in steroidogenic factor 1 (SF1/Ad4BP, NR5A1) are associated with 46,XY disorders of sex development with normal adrenal function. J Clin Endocrinol Metab 2007; 92:991–999.

45. Minto CL, Liao KL, Conway GS, et al. Sexual function in women with complete androgen insensitivity syndrome. Fertil Steril 2003; 80:157–164.

46. Han TS, Goswami D, Trikudanathan S, et al. Comparison of bone mineral density and body proportions between women with complete androgen insensitivity syndrome and women with gonadal dysgenesis. Eur J Endocrinol 2008; 159:179–185.

47. Jensen TK, Jørgensen N, Punab M, et al. Association of in utero exposure to maternal smoking with reduced semen quality and testis size in adulthood: a cross-sectional study of 1,770 young men from the general population in five European countries. Am J Epidemiol 2004; 159:49–58.

48. Damgaard IN, Jensen TK, Petersen JH, et al. Cryptorchidism and maternal alcohol consumption during pregnancy. Environ Health Perspect 2007; 115:272–277.

49. Welsh M, Saunders PT, Fisken M, et al. Identification in rats of a programming window for reproductive tract

masculinization, disruption of which leads to hypospadias and cryptorchidism. J Clin Invest 2008; 118:1479–1490.

50. Hackel C, Oliveira LE, Ferraz LF, et al. New mutations, hotspots, and founder effects in Brazilian patients with steroid 5alpha-reductase deficiency type 2. J Mol Med 2005; 83:569–576.

51. Korbonits M, Slawik M, Cullen D, et al. A comparison of a novel testosterone bioadhesive buccal system, striant, with a testosterone adhesive patch in hypogonadal males. J Clin Endocrinol Metab 2004; 89:2039–2043.

52. Frey H, Aakvaag A, Saanum D, et al. Bioavailability of testosterone in males. Eur J Clin Pharmacol 1979; 16:345–349.

53. Pitteloud N, Hayes FJ, Dwyer A, et al. Predictors of outcome of long-term GnRH therapy in men with idiopathic hypogonadotrophic hypogonadism. J Clin Endocrinol Metab 2002; 87:4128–4136.

54. Swerdloff RS, Wang C, Cunningham G, et al. Long-term pharmacokinetics of transdermal testosterone gel in hypogonadal men. J Clin Endocrinol Metab 2000; 85:4500–4510.

55. Mazer N, Bell D, Wu J, et al. Comparison of the steady-state pharmacokinetics, metabolism, and variability of a transdermal testosterone patch versus a transdermal testosterone gel in hypogonadal men. J Sex Med 2005; 2:213–226.

56. Dean JD, Carnegie C, Rodzvilla J, et al. Long-term effects of Testim® 1% testosterone gel in hypogonadal men. Rev Urol 2004; 6(suppl 6):S22–S29.

57. Jockenhövel F. Testosterone supplementation: what and how to give. Aging Male 2003; 6:200–206.

58. Wang C, Cunningham G, Dobs A, et al. Long-term testosterone gel (AndroGel) treatment maintains beneficial effects on sexual function and mood, lean and fat mass, and bone mineral density in hypogonadal men. J Clin Endocrinol Metab 2004; 89:2085–2098.

59. Pope HG, Jr, Cohane GH, Kanayama G, et al. Testosterone gel supplementation for men with refractory depression: a randomized, placebo-controlled trial. Am J Psychiatry 2003; 160:105–111.

60. Han TS, Bouloux PMG. Transdermal testosterone gel treatment of hypogonadal men. Aging Health 2008; 4:517–528.

61. Behre HM, Abshagen K, Oettel M, et al. Intramuscular injection of testosterone undecanoate for the treatment of male hypogonadism: phase I studies. Eur J Endocrinol 1999; 140:414–419.

62. Wang L, Shi DC, Lu SY, et al. The therapeutic effect of domestically produced testosterone undecanoate in Klinefelter syndrome. N Drugs Mark 1991; 8:28–32.

63. Nieschlag E, Büchter D, von Eckardstein S, et al. Repeated intramuscular injections of testosterone undecanoate for substitution therapy in hypogonadal men. Clin Endocrinol 1999; 51:757–763.

64. Schubert M, Minnemann T, Hübler D, et al. Intramuscular testosterone undecanoate: pharmacokinetic aspects of a novel testosterone formulation during long-term treatment of men with hypogonadism. J Clin Endocrinol Metab 2004; 89:5429–5434.

65. Zitzmann M, Saad F, Nieschlag E. Longterm experience of more than 8 years with a novel formulation of testosterone undecanoate (Nebido) in substitution therapy of hypogonadal men. Endocr Abstr 2006; 11:178.

66. Morales A, Nieschlag E, Schubert M, et al. Clinical experience with the new long-acting injectable testosterone undecanoate. Report on the educational symposium on the occasion of the 5th World Congress on the Aging Male, 9–12 February 2006, Salzburg, Austria. Aging Male 2006; 9:221–227.

67. Aaltonen P, Amory JK, Anderson RA, et al. 10th Summit Meeting consensus: recommendations for regulatory approval for hormonal male contraception. J Androl 2007; 28:362–363.

68. Aversa A, Isidori AM, Spera G, et al. Androgens improve cavernous vasodilation and response to sildenafil in patients with erectile dysfunction. Clin Endocrinol 2003; 58:632–638.

69. Morelli A, Vignozzi L, Filippi S, et al. Erectile dysfunction: molecular biology, pathophysiology and pharmacological treatment. Minerva Urol Nefrol 2005; 57:85–90.

70. Aversa A, Isidori AM, De Martino MU, et al. Androgens and penile erection, evidence for a direct relationship between free testosterone and cavernous vasodilation in men with erectile dysfunction. Clin Endocrinol 2000; 5:517–522.

71. Burnett AL. The role of nitric oxide in erectile dysfunction: implications for medical therapy. J Clin Hypertens (Greenwich) 2006; 8(suppl 4):53–62.

72. Heinlein CA, Chang C. The roles of androgen receptors and androgen-binding proteins in nongenomic androgen actions. Mol Endocrinol 2002; 16:2181–2187.

73. Hwang TI, Chen HE, Tsai TF, et al. Combined use of androgen and sildenafil for hypogonadal patients unresponsive to sildenafil alone. Int J Impot Res 2006; 18: 400–404.

74. Shamloul R, Ghanem H, Fahmy I, et al. Testosterone therapy can enhance erectile function response to sildenafil in patients with PADAM: a pilot study. J Sex Med 2005; 2:559–564.

75. Chatterjee R, Wood S, McGarrigle HH, et al. A novel therapy with testosterone and sildenafil for erectile dysfunction in patients on renal dialysis or after renal transplantation. J Fam Plann Reprod Health Care 2004; 30:88–90.

76. Kalinchenko SY, Kozlov GI, Gontcharov NP, et al. Oral testosterone undecanoate reverses erectile dysfunction associated with diabetes mellitus in patients failing on sildenafil citrate therapy alone. Aging Male 2003; 6:94–99.

77. La Spada AR, Wilson EM, Lubahn DB, et al. Androgen receptor gene mutations in X-linked spinal and bulbar muscular atrophy. Nature 1991; 352:77–79.

78. Thomas PS, Jr, Fraley GS, Damian V, et al. Loss of endogenous androgen receptor protein accelerates motor neuron degeneration and accentuates androgen insensitivity in a mouse model of X-linked spinal and bulbar muscular atrophy. Hum Mol Genet 2006; 15:2225–2238.

79. Butland SL, Devon RS, Huang Y, et al. CAG-encoded polyglutamine length polymorphism in the human genome. BMC Genomics 2007; 8:126.

80. Zitzmann M, Depenbusch M, Gromoll J, et al. Prostate volume and growth in testosterone-substituted hypogonadal men are dependent on the CAG repeat polymorphism of the androgen receptor gene: a longitudinal pharmacogenetic study. J Clin Endocrinol Metab 2003; 88:2049–2054.

81. Bratt O, Borg A, Kristoffersson U, et al. CAG repeat length in the androgen receptor gene is related to age at diagnosis of prostate cancer and response to endocrine therapy, but not to prostate cancer risk. Br J Cancer 1999; 81:672–676.

82. Alevizaki M, Cimponeriu AT, Garofallaki M, et al. The androgen receptor gene CAG polymorphism is associated with the severity of coronary artery disease in men. Clin Endocrinol 2003; 59:749–755.

83. Suter NM, Malone KE, Daling JR, et al. Androgen receptor (CAG)n and (GGC)n polymorphisms and breast cancer risk in a population-based case–control study of young women. Cancer Epidemiol Biomarkers Prev 2003; 12:127–135.

84. Zitzmann M. Mechanisms of Disease: pharmacogenetics of testosterone therapy in hypogonadal men. Nat Clin Pract Urol 2007; 4:161–166.

85. Crabbe P, Bogaert V, De Bacquer D, et al. Part of the interindividual variation in serum testosterone levels in healthy men reflects differences in androgen sensitivity and feedback set point: contribution of the androgen

receptor polyglutamine tract polymorphism. J Clin Endocrinol Metab 2007; 92:3604–3610.

86. Zitzmann M, Brune M, Kornmann B, et al. The CAG repeat polymorphism in the androgen receptor gene affects bone density and bone metabolism in healthy males. Clin Endocrinol 2001; 55:649–657.

87. Walcott JL, Merry DE. Trinucleotide repeat disease. The androgen receptor in spinal and bulbar muscular atrophy. Vitam Horm 2002; 65:127–147.

88. Chen YW. Local protein unfolding and pathogenesis of polyglutamine-expansion diseases. Proteins 2003; 51: 68–73.

89. Kopera H. The history of anabolic steroids and a review of clinical experience with anabolic steroids. Acta Endocrinol Suppl (Copenh) 1985; 271:11–18.

90. Edelstein D, Dobs A, Basaria S. Emerging drugs for hypogonadism. Expert Opin Emerg Drugs 2006; 11:685–707.

91. Qoubaitary A, Swerdloff RS, Wang C. Advances in male hormone substitution therapy. Expert Opin Pharmacother 2005; 6:1493–1506.

92. Bhasin S, Calof OM, Storer TW, et al. Drug insight: testosterone and selective androgen receptor modulators as anabolic therapies for chronic illness and aging. Nat Clin Pract Endocrinol Metab 2006; 2:146–159.

18

Male Sexual Function

Giulio Garaffa, Suks Minhas, and David J. Ralph
Department of Urology, University College London Hospitals, London, U.K.

INTRODUCTION

This chapter describes the development of the male reproductive system and the role of the male hormone, Testosterone. The physiological mechanisms of erection, causes and treatment of erectile dysfunction (ED) and male fertility are also reviewed.

THE DEVELOPMENT OF THE MALE REPRODUCTIVE SYSTEM

The establishment of the male reproductive system involves the formation of the testis and the maintenance and differentiation of the Wolffian duct. Both events are crucial for normal sexual function.

The presence of the Y chromosome, and in particular of the sex determining region of the Y chromosome (SRY) gene, activates a cascade of molecular and cellular events leading to the differentiation of cells of the primitive genital ridge into Leydig and Sertoli cells and the organization of the testis structure (Figs. 1 and 2).

Furthermore, increasing evidence indicates that SRY induces Sertoli cells differentiation via another transcription factor, the SRY box containing gene 9 (SOX9). On the other hand, Leydig cells start to differentiate after Sertoli cells appear. This suggests that their differentiation is regulated indirectly by paracrine factors secreted by Sertoli cells.

Sertoli cells ensure the production of Mullerian inhibitory factor (MIF), which is responsible for the regression of the Mullerian duct, the precursor of the female reproductive tract.

The Leydig cells produce testosterone and insulin-like factor 3 (ILF3). Androgens are important for differentiation of the Wolffian duct, also known as mesonephric duct, to form the body and tail of the epididymis, the vas deferens and the seminal vesicles. Moreover, androgens and ILF3 are required for testicular descent (1,2).

Besides male sexual differentiation and the development of testicular tissue, the descent of the testes from an intra-abdominal into a scrotal position is an essential prerequisite for spermatogenesis to occur. Cryptorchdism (Greek: hidden testis) is regarded the most frequent pediatric complication and affects 3% of the male newborns. While this decreases to 1% in boys aged one year, the prevalence rate of this condition is 30% in premature boys. Conditions like low birth weight, small size for gestational age, maternal exposure to estrogens during the first trimester of pregnancy is associated with a higher frequency of undescended testicle.

Genetic factors also play an important role in this condition, as demonstrated in inherited X chromosome–linked anomalies associated with cryptorchisdism (Table 1) (3). If left untreated, cryptorchisdism may lead to disturbed spermatogenesis, impaired fertility, and a higher incidence of testicular cancer (up to 33-fold for bilateral cryptorchisdism), which is likely a consequence of exposure of the testis to the increased intra-abdominal temperatures (4).

Testicular descent can be subdivided in two separate phases, an intra-abdominal and inguino-scrotal phase. The first phase is initiated at about 10 to 14 weeks of gestation and lasts to about week 20 to 23. This phase is mediated by ILF3 factor, that is, structurally closely related to relaxin and that stimulates gubernaculum mesenchymal cells. However, androgens don not play any role during the phase of intra-abdominal descent (5). The second phase of descent is usually completed by week 35 in the human and is mediated by the action of androgens on the gubernaculum and the cranial suspensory ligament of the testis. Above all, the androgen-mediated regression of the cranial suspensory ligament is a condition sine qua non for a complete testicular descent. The androgens also affect the second phase of the testicular descent by inducing the masculinization of the sensory nucleus of the genitofemoral nerve. Furthermore, the sensory branch of this nerve, when adequately stimulated by androgens, acts via the calcitonin gene related transmitter inducing the migration of the gubernaculums testis and transection of this nerve causes ipsilateral cryptorchisdism (6).

The male external genitalia originate from the genital tubercle that develops following the formation of the urethral plate and urethral tube (see chapter). The genital tubercle consists of the lateral plate mesoderm, surface ectoderm, and endoderm urethral

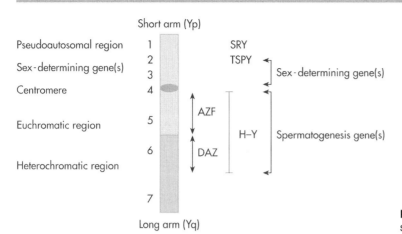

Figure 1 The Y chromosome is critical for normal male sexual determination.

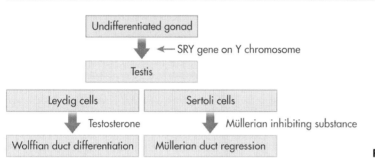

Figure 2 Male genital development in the fetus.

Table 1 Syndromes Associated with Cryptorchisdism

Chromosomal location	Name of the syndrome
Xq 11-q 12	Testicular feminization
Xq 12-q 21.31	FG syndrome
Xq 25-q 27	Dandy Walker syndrome
Xp 21.1	Aarskorg Scott syndrome
Xq 28	Torcicollis, renal dysplasia, cryptorchisdism
Xp 22.31	X-linked Kallmann syndrome
Xp 11.3-q 11.2	Arthrogryphosis multiplex congenital
Xq 28	Frontometaphyseal dysplasia
Xp 22.32	Ichthyosis
Xq 26.1	Lowe oculocerebrorenal syndrome
Xp 21.1-p 11.22	X-linked dysmorphism
Xq 27-q 28	Lenz dysplasia
Xp 11.4-p 21.2	
1p 22-p 21	Zellweger syndrome
3p 22-p 26	Fanconi anemia
	Denys-Drash syndrome
11p 13	WAGR syndrome (Wilms tumor, aniridia, genitourinary anomalies, mental retardation)
15q 11-q13	Prader-Willy
16p 13	Rubinstein-Taybi syndrome

epithelium derived from the urogenital sinus. The first phase of the genital tubercle growth is androgen independent and relies on the activity of a growth factor known as sonic hedgehog (Shh). Shh orchestrates, directly or indirectly, the activity of numerous genes that play a role in the outgrowth and differentiation of the genital tubercle (7).

After Shh has promoted the formation of a sexually dimorphic genital tubercle, starting from the seventh to eighth gestational week, exposure to androgens masculinizes the genitalia. The enzyme 5α-reductase converts testosterone in dihydrotestosterone (DHT), the most potent androgen to cause virilization of the developing external genitalia in

Table 2 Causes of Male Pseudohermaphroditism

Defect in the formation of the testis
Hypoplastic testicular Leydig cells
Insufficient secretion of LH
Insufficiency of the LH receptor
P450 deficiency
3β-Hydroxysteroid-dehydrogenase type II deficiency
17α-Hydroxylase/17,20-lyase deficiency
17β-Hydroxysteroid-dehydrogenase type III deficiency
5α-Reductase deficiency
Functional androgen receptor deficiency

the human fetus. DHT induces rapid elongation of the genital tubercle to form a phallus, the closure of the opposing urethral folds to form the penile urethra and the formation of the scrotum by fusion of the genital swelling.

Disruption of androgen signaling can result in feminization of the genitalia, which may include hypospadias, which affects one in every 125 male births and accounts for the most common genital malformation (8). More severe disturbances in androgen biosynthesis result in the clinical condition of pseudohermaphroditism, which is characterized by a genotypic sex masked by a phenotypic appearance closely resembling the other sex. Causes of male pseudohermaphroditism are reported in Table 2 (9).

THE HYPOTHALAMIC-PITUITARY-TESTICULAR AXIS

The hypothalamus interacts with the pituitary gland via a portal vascular system and by neural pathways of particular relevance are the preoptic area and the medial basal region of the hypothalamus that contain neurons that secrete gonadotropin-releasing hormone (GnRH) in a pulsatile fashion, the so-called GnRH pulse generator. Several hormones, neurotrasmitters and cytokines modulate GnRH secretion.

GnRH, whose precursor gene has been identified and mapped on the chromosome 8p, is a decapeptide released into the pituitary-portal system every 90 to 140 minutes.

The pulsatile secretion of GnRH in turn stimulates pulsatile secretion of luteinizing hormone (LH) and follicle-stimulating hormone (FSH) by the gonadotrophs of the anterior pituitary. The pulsatile release of GnRH is essential for the stimulation of LH and FSH release; in fact a continuous of GnRH or GnRH agonists inhibits gonadotropin release.

GnRH binds to cell surface receptors on the pituitary and enhances the secretion of both LH and FSH by a calcium dependent mechanism that is independent of cyclic AMP (cAMP).

LH and FSH are composed of two glycoproteins chains and have a molecular weight of about 30,000 d. The α subunit of the two hormones is identical and the distinct immunological and functional characteristics of the two hormones are conveyed by the unique β subunits.

LH interacts with cell membrane receptors on Leydig cells to stimulate adenyl cyclase and enhance

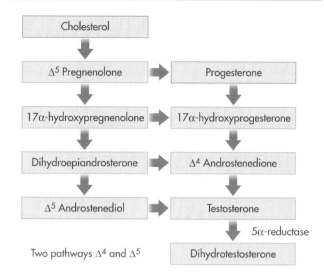

Figure 3 The metabolic pathway for androgen production.

the formation and release of cAMP. This second messenger binds to the regulatory subunit of a protein kinase and activates the production of testosterone from cholesterol. The conversion of cholesterol to pregnenolone by the activity of the cytochrome p450 is the rate-limiting step in the synthesis of testosterone (Fig. 3). However, in the vast majority of cases, the rate of conversion is determined by the rate of delivery of cholesterol to the enzyme in the inner mitochondrial membrane by the steroidogenic acute regulatory protein (StAR), a process that may be the main site of action of LH (10). Additional factors that may influence Leydig cell function include insulin-like growth factor I, transforming growth factor α and β, epidermal growth factor and fibroblast growth factor.

Despite of a pulsatile release of FSH, LH and testosterone, FSH and testosterone pulses are not apparent in normal men because of the slower secretion of newly synthesized rather than stored hormone, and the longer circulating half lives.

FSH interacts with receptors on the basal aspect of the Sertoli cell membrane and activates the production of cAMP that as a second messenger activates protein kinase activity. The end result is an increased secretion of several Sertoli cell proteins, including androgen-binding protein (ABP) and the aromatase enzyme (CYP 19) that converts testosterone in estradiol. The mechanism by which FSH regulates spermatogenesis is still poorly understood.

LH secretion is regulated primarily by negative feedback independently by testosterone and estradiol. estradiol instead appears to be the primary steroid regulator of FSH secretion.

Testosterone exerts his action of negative feedback directly at the level of the hypothalamic pulse generator and of the pituitary. These effects may be mediated by the local conversion of testosterone in estradiol. Estrogens instead exert their negative feedback by decreasing GnRH pulse frequency at the level of the hypothalamus and by reducing the amplitude of LH pulses via decreased pituitary responsiveness to GnRH (11).

The feedback regulation of the secretion of FSH instead involves both steroid hormones and the gonadal peptide inhibin. The latter, is a peptide produced by the germ cells starting from puberty and consists of two subunits (α and β). Since the β subunit can exist in two different forms, there are two forms of inhibin, inhibin A and inhibin B. Inhibin B is the active form and exerts its activity by inhibiting the release of FSH form the pituitary; the level of inhibin B correlates with the presence of germ cells in early spermatogenesis in the adult men and with the presence of Sertoli cells before puberty (12).

The hypothalamic-pituitary-gonadal axis is also influenced by physical stress, such as illness and fasting. In case of stress, the increased levels of corticotropins and cytokines exert an inhibitory effect on the axis, with consequent reduction of the testosterone levels. In particular, on fasting, the inhibition of the axis is consequence to the reduced plasmatic levels of leptins that are required for a normal pulse generator activity (13).

THE EFFECTS OF TESTOSTERONE

Testosterone is the most important circulating androgen in men and is bound to sex hormone–binding globulin (SHBG) and albumin. Usually around 2% of testosterone is free, 60% is bound to SHBG and 38% to albumin. Albumin binds with low affinity to all steroids whereas SHBG has a high affinity for testosterone. Because of the low affinity for steroids, all the testosterone bound to albumin is available for tissue uptake, and therefore, the bioavailable testosterone in plasma approximates the sum of free and albumin bound hormone (14).

Testosterone can be converted to 5α-DHT, which promotes male sexual differentiation and virilization, or can be aromatized to estrogens by aromatase enzymes.

Conversion of testosterone in DHT occurs mainly in the target tissues and accounts for 6% to 8% of testosterone metabolism; the process is carried out by the group of 5α-reductase isoenzymes. Isoenzyme 1 is present in the liver and in the skin with the exception of the genital area. The isoenzyme 2 instead is expressed in the urogenital tract and skin and liver and is defective in subjects with 5α-reductase deficiency.

About 85% of the conversion of testosterone to estradiol is carried out in the peripheral tissue and the remaining in the testis. The process is catalyzed by aromatase enzyme (CYP 19) that is primarily expressed in adipose tissue. Furthermore, the conversion of testosterone to estradiol increases with increasing adipose tissue and advancing age.

In addition to regulating the hypothalamic-pituitary system via negative feedback, Androgens initiate and maintain spermatogenesis, promote the formation of the male phenotype during embryogenesis and are responsible for sexual maturation at puberty and its maintenance thereafter.

Moreover testosterone exerts an important function on protein synthesis and bone maturation.

Both testosterone and DHT bind to the same high affinity androgen receptor (AR) that is located in the target cells nucleus and that is coded by a gene located in the long arm of the X chromosome. The binding activates the AR that interacts and with a variety of cofactors and stimulates the transcription of genes under androgen control (15). Almost all effects of androgens are exerted through the same high affinity androgen receptor.

DHT creates a more amplified androgen signal, when compared with testosterone; this is probably due to a higher affinity of DHT for the AR (16).

However, even if the vast majority of the effects of the androgens are mediated by direct interaction with the AR, androgens may also indirectly influence the expression of a variety of genes. These effects may involve modulation the expression and activity of secondary transcription factors, the production of growth factors, or changes in the expression of other hormones (17).

THE PHYSIOLOGICAL MECHANISMS OF ERECTILE FUNCTION AND THE PATOPHYSIOLOGY OF ERECTILE DYSFUNCTION

Penile erection is a complex neurovascular process involving relaxation of the smooth muscle inside the corpora cavernosa, increased arterial inflow into the penis, and restricted venous outflow from the organ. The corporeal bodies of the penis are surrounded by both a superficial and deep layer of fascia that is continuous with the fascia of the perineum. The deeper layer is known as Buck's fascia and is encircled by a soft connective layer, the Dartos fascia and by the skin (Figs. 4–6).

The arterial blood supply to the penis is derived from the internal pudendal arteries, branch of the hypogastric arteries. The pudendal arteries trifurcate into the spongiosal artery, cavernosal artery, and dorsal artery, which supply the spongiosum, corpora cavernosa, and glans, respectively. The cavernosal arteries course through each corpus cavernosum longitudinally and form helicine arteries, which are responsible for the flow in the vascular spaces of the corpora cavernosa, causing engorgement leading to erection. The dorsal arteries of the penis travel under Buck's fascia giving circumflex branches to the corpora cavernosa and spongiosa. The venous drainage of the penis can be divided in superficial and deep system. The superficial system drains all the tissue superficial to the Buck's fascia into the saphenous vein. The deep venous system instead drains into the pudendal plexus. The deep dorsal vein that runs on the dorsal aspect of the penis drains the blood from the corpora cavernosa, the spongiosum, and the glans. In particular, the venous drainage from the corpora cavernosa occurs through the subtunical veins that are compressed and occluded by the expansion of the sinusoidal spaces during erection. The compression of the subtunical veins is condition sine qua non for an adequate erection and is called "veno-occlusive mechanism" (Fig. 7).

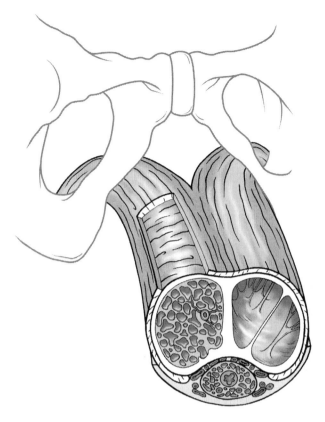

Figure 4 The structure of the penis.

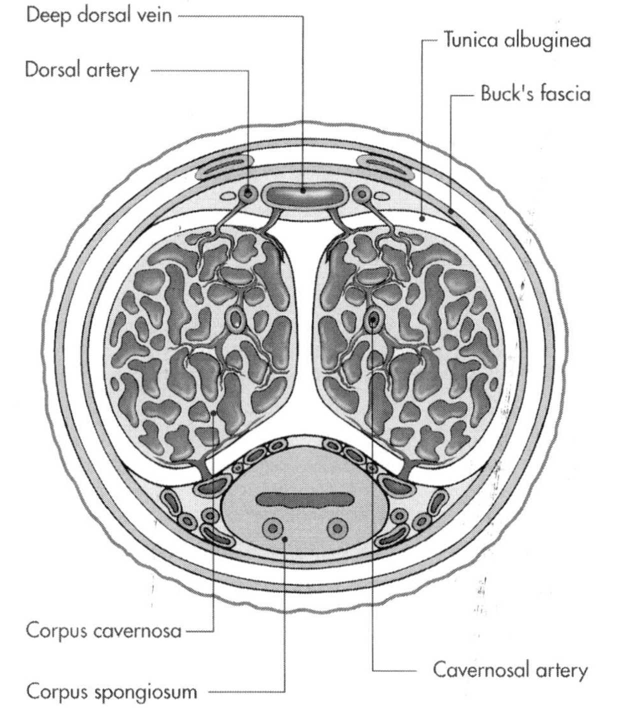

Figure 5 Cross-sectional anatomy of the human penis.

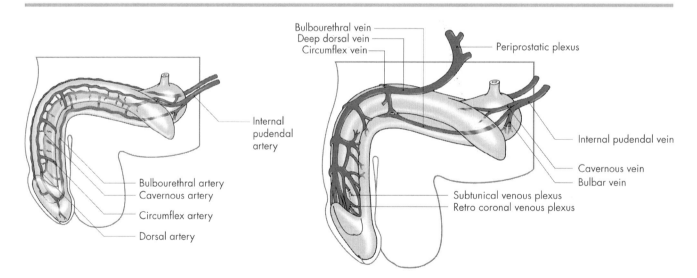

Figure 6 Arterial supply and venous drainage of the human penis.

The Phases of Erection

During erection, the relaxation of the smooth muscle of the arterioles supplying the sinusoidal spaces results in an increase in blood flow into the corpora cavernosa. Penile detumescence is also an active process that requires the contraction of the cavernosal smooth muscle under the influx of sympathetic stimulation. All these changes in the smooth muscle tone translate into modifications in the flow in the cavernosal arteries that can be recorded with an eco color ultrasound (ECDUS). Ultrasonography is the ideal investigation to study systolic and diastolic velocities and spectral waveform changes before and during

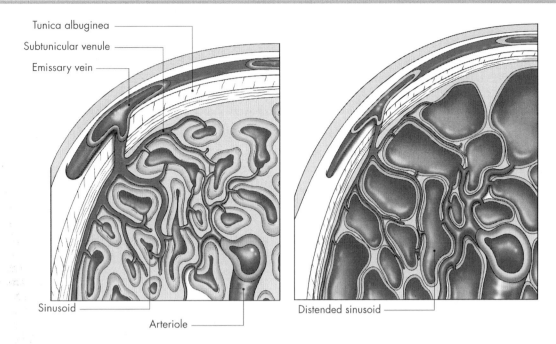

Figure 7 Veno-occlusive mechanism. During sexual stimulation, the smooth muscle surrounding the sinusoidal spaces relaxes leading to engorgement of the spaces with blood. This leads to compression of subtunical venules and emissary veins, causing penile erection.

erection because of its ability to visualize small vessels with low flow.

The variation in systolic and diastolic velocities and the consequent modification of spectral waveform allow the subdivision of erection in the following phases (Fig. 8).

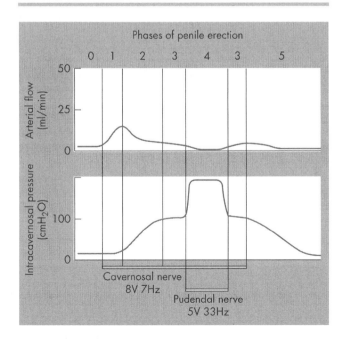

Figure 8 The hemodynamic phases of penile erection.

Phase 1

This phase is characterized by a progressive relaxation of the arterial smooth muscle with a resulting rapid inflow of blood into the corpora cavernosa. The inflow is continuous for the duration of the cardiac cycle and leads initially to an isometric filling (phase 1A) and then to a progressive increase of intracorporeal pressure from 11 mmHg, the normal value during the flaccid state, to around 25 mmHg (phase 1B).

The arterial blood flow is characterized by a peak systolic velocity that progressively increases up to 35 cm/sec and by a positive end diastolic velocity.

During this phase there is only a slight elongation and fullness of the penis.

Phase 2

As the inflow of blood continues, it becomes associated with increasing cavernous pressure, which grows from 25 mmHg to approximately 40 mmHg. The onset of this phase is heralded by a progressive decrease in the end diastolic velocity because of the increased intracorporeal pressure. Ultimately, the end diastolic velocity becomes 0 when the intracavernosal pressure equals the diastolic pressure. There is also a decrease in the peak systolic velocity.

Phase 3

This phase is identified when end diastolic flow reaches 0. The continued inflow of blood and the progressive distension of the sinusoidal spaces compress the subtunical venous plexuses against the noncompliant tunical albuginea. This phenomenon, which is also known as the veno-occlusive mechanism, impedes the outflow of blood through the emissary veins and leads to a further increase of intracavernosal pressures. This leads to a progressive reduction in the duration of systolic inflow and peak systolic velocity during this phase that translates into narrower, sharper-peaked and lower waveforms at the ECDUS.

Phase 4

This phase is characterized by reversed diastolic flow that initially develops at the end of diastole as the intracavernosal pressure becomes higher than diastolic pressure. As intracorporeal pressure increases, the reverse flow becomes evident throughout diastole. During this phase the systolic waveform becomes narrower and sharply peaked, and its duration continues to reduce.

Phase 5

This phase is characterized by the progressive loss of both systolic and diastolic flow signals. The loss becomes complete when the intracavernosal pressure reaches the systolic pressure. The first half of this phase is defined by the loss of both forward systolic and reverse diastolic flow components. Loss of reversal flow is initially noted during end diastole, while velocity and duration of the systolic component decrease continuously.

The second half of the phase is the end stage of the flow cycle and is characterized by the loss of both systolic and diastolic flow and by a further increase of the intracavernosal pressure de to a contraction of the ischiocavernosus muscles. During this half of the phase, the corpora cavernosa become functionally dead spaces with hardly any inflow or outflow (18–20).

The Phases of Detumescence

Detumescence is initiated by the relaxation of the ischiocavernosus muscles and is consequence of the active contraction of the cavernosal smooth muscle under sympathetic nervous stimulation.

Detumescence can be subdivided into three phases; the first is characterized by a transient increase of intracavernosal pressure, because of the contraction of the smooth muscle against a closed venous system. The second phase instead is characterized by a progressive slow decrease of pressure leading to the slow reopening of the venous channels with resumption of the basal level of arterial inflow. The last phase is characterized by a fast reduction of intracavernosal pressure because of a fully restored venous outflow capacity (21).

The Neurophysiology of Penile Erection

The penis receives a complex autonomic and somatic innervation. The autonomic innervation, which can be subdivided in sympathetic and parasympathetic, derives from the neurons in the spinal cord and peripheral ganglia (Fig. 9). Autonomic nerves form

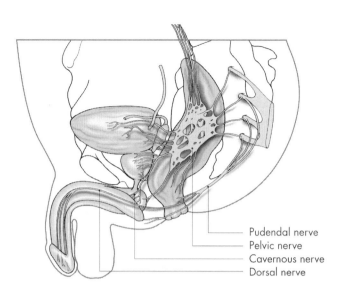

— Pudendal nerve
— Pelvic nerve
— Cavernous nerve
— Dorsal nerve

Figure 9 The autonomic and somatic innervation of the penis.

the cavernous nerves, which enter the corpora cavernosa and the corpus spongiosum to initiate the neurovascular events that lead to erection and detumescence. Somatic innervation, instead, consists of sensory fibers that carry sensory stimuli from the genitalia and of motor fibers that induce the contraction of bulbocavernosus and ischiocavernosus muscles.

The sympathetic pathway arises from the eleventh thoracic to the second lumbar spinal segment (T11-L2) and its fibers are carried through the white rami to reach the sympathetic chain ganglia. Some of these fibers then travel via the lumbar splanchnic nerves to the superior and inferior hypogastric plexuses. Some fibers originated from the superior hypogastric plexus form the hypogastric nerve and reach the pelvic plexus.

In the vast majority of cases, the T10-T12 segments are the origin of the sympathetic fibers, and the chain ganglia cells projecting to the penis are located in the sacral and caudal ganglia.

The parasympathetic pathway originates from neurons located in the intermediolateral cell columns of the second, third, and forth sacral spinal cord segments. The preganglionic fibers form the pelvic nerves that reach the pelvic plexus, where they join the sympathetic nerves derived from the superior hypogastric plexus. From the pelvic plexus originate the cavernous nerves that innervate the corpora cavernosa and spongiosa. These nerves are located in close proximity to the prostatic capsule and are easily damaged in case of radical excision of rectum, bladder and prostate.

A parasympathetic input along the cavernous nerves induces relaxation of the cavernosal smooth muscle and ultimately an erection. On the other hand, the stimulation of the hypogastric nerve or of the sympathetic trunk induces contraction of the cavernosal smooth muscle and leads to penile detumescence.

Table 3 Central Neurotransmitters Involved in Penile Erection

Neurotransmitter pathways	Effect on erection
Dopamine	Excitatory
Serotonin	Mainly inhibitory
Noradrenaline	Excitatory
GABA	Inhibitory
Oxytocin	Inhibitory
Nitric oxide	Excitatory

The cerebral impulses originate presumably from the medial preoptic area (MPOA) that is under the control of hypothalamic nuclei. In particular, central dopaminergic neurons with projections to the MPOA and paraventricular nucleus have been identified in hypothalamic nuclei. Dopaminergic hypothalamic neurons also project to the lumbar spine and may be involved with the erectile process. The key role played by dopamine in the central nervous system has been confirmed in the animal model by the induction of the erections following intrathecal administration of this neuromediator. Central noradrenergic neurons, largely represented in the MPOA, seem to play also a key role in the regulation of erections, but in contrast to peripheral neural pathways, appear to facilitate penile erection. Serotoninergic neurons are also well represented in the MPOA and in the paraventricular areas of the hypothalamus where they play a key role in the inhibition of sexual drive. Central neurotrasmitters involved in penile erection are reported in Table 3.

Cerebral impulses travel in sympathetic, parasympathetic and somatic pathways to regulate the erectile process.

The somatosensory pathway originates from the sensory receptors located in the penile skin, corpora, glans and urethra. The fibers originated from the receptors form the dorsal nerves of the penis that then becomes part of the pudendal nerve. The stimulation of these receptors triggers the release of messages of pain, temperature, and touch that via the pudendal nerve, the spinal cord and spinothalamic tract reaching the thalamus and the sensory cortex. Onuf's nucleus that is located in the second to fourth sacral spinal segment is the center of somatomotor penile innervation. From this nucleus derive the nerve fibers that travel in the sacral nerve and then in the pudendal nerve to reach the ischiocavernosus and bulbospongiosus muscles. The contraction of the ischiocavernosus muscle is responsible of the onset of the phase 5 of the erection while the rhythmic contraction of the bulbocavernosus muscle is part of the mechanisms of ejaculation.

The above described nervous structures are responsible for the three types of erection: psychogenic, reflexogenic and nocturnal. Psychogenic erection is the consequence of audiovisual stimuli and of the fantasy and is consequence of the direct activation of the cerebral nuclei that modulate the spinal cord centers to activate the erectile process.

Reflexogenic erection is on the other hand as a consequence of tactile stimuli to the genitals that reach the spinal erection centers via the dorsal and pudendal nerve where they activate the autonomic nuclei. The activation of the autonomic nuclei subsequently induces the release of NO and acetylcholine from the terminations of the cavernosal nerves and the consequent relaxation of the cavernosal smooth muscle.

Nocturnal erection instead occurs during the rapid eye movement (REM) phase of the sleep and its mechanisms are still obscure (22).

Neurotransmitters Involved in Penile Erection and Detumescence

Detumescence and flaccidity are mainly mediated by the release of norephinephrine by the adrenergic nerve endings in the corporeal tissue. The vasoconstrictive effect of noradrenaline is mediated by its interaction with adrenergic receptors that are well represented in the cavernosal artery wall as well as in the cavernous trabeculae (23,24). In particular, among the adrenergic receptor subtypes, the α-adrenoreceptors seem to be the main responsible of the smooth muscle contraction, since they are represented ten fold more than their β-receptor counterpart in the corpora cavernosa.

Despite noradrenaline playing the key role in the control of smooth muscle contraction, many other agents are known to induce detumescence.

Among those, endothelin, tromboxane A2, prostaglandin F2 and leukotrienes are potent vasoconstrictors produced by the endothelial lining of the vessels that may play a role inducing smooth muscle contraction in the corpora cavernosa (25,26).

Vasoconstriction is partially mediated by the activation of a GTPase, RhoA, and its downstream effector, Rho kinase. The final result is a calcium dependent activation of myosin light chain and actin/myosin assembly.

Penile erection is a complex neurovascular process involving relaxation of the corpus cavernosal smooth muscle (Fig. 10). The nerves, endothelium of sinusoids and blood vessels, and smooth muscle cells in the penis produce transmitters and modulators that control the erect versus the flaccid state of the penis. Acetylcholine and NO are of critical importance to the physiological induction and maintenance of erections. The key role played by acetylcholine is confirmed by the fact that cholinergic nerve endings are well represented within the cavernosal smooth muscle and surrounding penile arteries. Acetylcholine induces relaxation of the smooth muscle directly via a stimulation of nicotinic receptors that, when activated induce an intracellular cascade of second messengers. However, acetylcholine acts in an indirect way by stimulating the endothelium to release NO.

NO also plays a key role in the induction of the relaxation of corporeal smooth muscle. In particular, this molecule can be derived from different pathways. There is a constitutive endothelial synthesis of NO via the enzyme endothelial NO synthase (eNOS) and a neuronal synthesis of the mediator via the neuronal NO synthase (nNOS) located in the nerve endings of the nonadrenergic/noncholinergic (NANC) system. NO production can

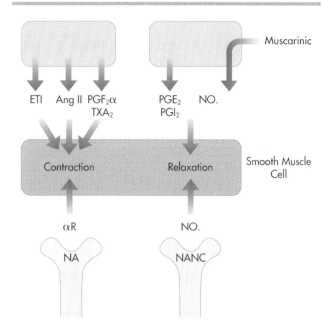

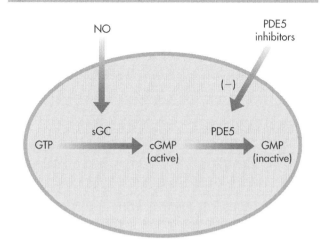

Figure 12 The cellular action of NO incorporal smooth muscle (sGC-soluble guanylate cyclase).

Figure 10 Diagram depicting the functional anatomy of the corpus cavernosum and the main vasoactive factors involved in penile erection.

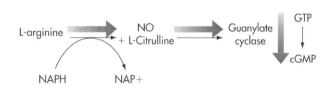

Figure 11 Biosynthesis of prostanoids.

be also induced by various stimuli that activate another form of NOS, the inducible NOS (iNOS) (Fig. 11).

eNOS and nNOS are two isoforms of the same enzyme and are tightly regulated and produce physiologically relevant levels of NO in the endothelial cells and autonomic nerve endings of the penis. There is increased evidence that both isoforms of the enzyme

play an important rule in the mechanisms of erection as documented by the complex and delicate regulation of eNOS and nNOS that involves multiple molecular mechanisms that act in concert to both positively and negatively affect the function of these enzymes (27).

eNOS is an important mediator of both physiological and pathological responses of the penis. In case of normal endothelial function, NO has vasodilatatory and counterbalances RhoA/Rho kinase mediated vasoconstriction.

NO causes relaxation of the corporeal smooth muscle via the production of cGMP, its active intracellular second messenger (Fig. 12). The activity of cGMP is terminated by its conversion in GMP, which is catalyzed by enzymes called phosphodiesterases (PDE). A large variety of PDE isoenzymes have been identified within human tissues, however the type 5 isoenzyme appears to be the most important in the human penis (Table 4).

Other mediators that may play a role in smooth muscle relaxation are the vasoactive intestinal peptide (VIP), calcitonine gene related peptide (CGRP), histidine, methionine, and some prostaglandins. In particular, VIP immunoreactive fibers have been identified within the corpus cavernosus trabeculae and surrounding penile arteries and the administration of VIP

Table 4 Pharmacology and Localization of Phosphodiesterases

Isoenzyme	Substrate	Tissue
PDE 1	cAMP/cGMP	Brain, heart, vascular smooth muscle
PDE 2	cAMP/cGM	Brain, heart, vascular smooth muscle, skeletal muscle, adrenal cortex
PDE 3	cAMP/cGMP	Smooth muscle, platelet, liver
PDE 4	cAMP	Brain, heart, vascular smooth muscle, skeletal muscle, adrenal cortex, lung, testis
PDE 5	cGMP	Vascular smooth muscle, platelet
PDE 6	cGMP	Retina
PDE 7	cAMP	Skeletal muscle, heart
PDE 8	cAMP	Testis, ovary, intestinal tract
PDE 9	cAMP	Spleen, intestinal tract
PDE 10	cAMP/cGMP	Brain, testis, thyroid
PDE 11	cAMP/cGMP	Vascular smooth muscle, brain, hearth

antagonists has been proven to prevent smooth muscle relaxation (28).

Pathophysiology of Organic Erectile Dysfunction

Erections are neurovascular phenomena modulated by hormonal stimuli, local biochemical interactions and biochemical mechanisms; as a consequence, all conditions that affect the hemodynamic of erectile response may be responsible of the onset of ED that is defined as the inability to achieve and maintain a penile erection adequate for satisfactory sexual intercourse.

Since erection is a neurovascular event, ED can be consequence of disease of the brain, spinal cord, cavernous and pudendal nerves and receptors in the terminal arterioles and cavernosal smooth muscles. In particular, lesions affecting the brain, such as strokes, Alzheimer's or Parkinson's diseases, tumor, or trauma cause ED through a derangement of the hypothalamic centers or overinhibition of the spinal center. Dysfunction at the spinal cord level may affect either the afferent or efferent nerve pathways. The peripheral neuropathy seen in alcoholism, vitamin deficiency, diabetes as well as nerve lesions typical of trauma and pelvic surgery may disrupt the neural pathway. With the exception of when the nerves are transacted from radical surgery and injury, most neurological dysfunctions are partial.

ED can be also consequence of disease of terminal aorta, hypogastric, pudendal and penile arteries. Although trauma or a congenital anomaly may cause arterial insufficiency, in the majority of cases arteriogenic impotence is a consequence of a generalized atherosclerotic process. Associated risk factors include hypercholesterolemia, obesity, smoking, diabetes, radiation, hypertension, and perineal trauma. In case of arteriogenic impotence, the initial symptoms are characterized by a progressive delay in the onset of erection and early detumescence. With progressive reduction of luminal diameter, partial to complete ED ensues.

ED can also be consequence of the lack of the veno-occlusive mechanism due to the presence of abnormal venous channels, tunical abnormalities or functional impairment of the erectile tissue.

Endocrine factors play a role in approximately 3% of all organic ED cases. In particular, hypogonadism, hypothyroidism, hyperthyroidism, pituitary tumors, and hyperprolactinemia are well known causes of ED (29).

ED might also be consequence of impairment of erectile tissue due to Peyronie's disease, traumas, fibrosis, diabetes, tumor infiltration and scleroderma.

Finally many medications may induce ED, in particular some classes of antihypertensive drugs and antiandrogens (Table 5). Hypnotics and major tranquillizers may exert their effects by elevating plasma prolactin as well as depressing the libido. Centrally acting antihypertensives instead, are thought to exert their effect on erectile function by their central actions on α-receptors (Fig. 13).

Table 5 Drug That May Be Responsible for Erectile Dysfunction

Psychotropic drugs
Benzodiazepines, butyrophenones
Antidepressants
Tryciclics, monoamine oxidase inhibitors
Anthypertensives
β-blockers, spironolactone
Endocrine drugs
Cyprotherone acetate, LHRH analogues, estrogens
Anticholinergic drugs
Atropine
Others
Cimetadine, digoxin, alcohol, some recreational drugs

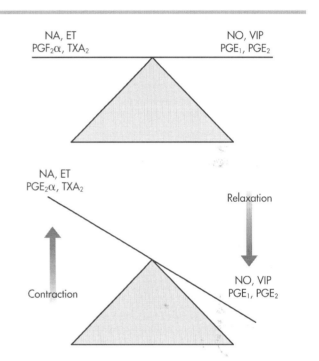

Figure 13 Pathophysiological mechanism of erectile dysfunction. Under physiological conditions, corporeal smooth muscle is maintained by relaxatory factors acting in opposition to contractile factors. In disease states, the balance is tipped to favor contractile factors. This may be secondary to increased formation/uninhibited activity of these factors or secondary to reduced production/activity of relaxatory factors.

Pharmacological Treatment of Erectile Dysfunction

The pharmacological treatment of ED has been revolutionized in recent years, particularly with the introduction of PDE inhibitors. The pharmacotherapy for ED is based on the principles of stimulating central or peripheral proerectile pathways or inhibiting antierectile mechanisms. In particular, drugs enhancing peripheral nitrergic-mediated pathways have been developed, and PDE inhibitors, such as Viagra, deserve a special mention. The medications currently available for treating ED are reported in Table 6.

Table 6 Currently Available Pharmacological Treatments for Male Erectile Dysfunction

Oral treatments	Mechanism of action
Sildenafil citrate (Viagra™)	PDE 5 inhibitor
Tadalafil (Cialis™)	PDE 5 inhibitor
Vardenafil hydrochloride	PDE 5 inhibitor
Apomorphine sublingual (Uprima™)	Dopamine agonist
Yohimbine	α-Adrenoceptor antagonist
Phentolamine (Vasomax™)	α-Adrenoceptor antagonist
Prazosin and Doxazosin	α-Adrenoceptor antagonist
L-arginine	NO precursor
Intracavernosal agents	Mechanism of action
PGE1 (Alprostadil)	Increase in intracellular cAMP
Papaverine	Nonselective PDE inhibitor
Vasoactive intestinal polypeptide	Increase in intracellular cAMP
Linsidomine chlorhydrate	NO donor
Phentolamine	α-Adrenoceptor antagonist
Topical agents used for the treatment of MED	**Mechanism of action**
Transdermal nitroglycerin	NO donor
Intraurethral PGE1 (MUSE)	Increase in intracellular cAMP
Topical PGE1	Increase in intracellular cAMP

Table 7 Pharmacokinetic Profiles of Available PDE 5 Inhibitors

Drug	C_{max} (ng/mL)	T_{max} (hr)	$T_{1/2}$ (hr)
Sildenafil	560	0.8	3.7
Vardenafil	209	0.7	3.9
Tadalafil	378	2.0	17.5

Phosphodiesterase 5 Inhibitors

Drugs such as Sildenafil and the novel PDE 5 inhibitors Vardenafil and Tadalafil are referred to as competitive inhibitors of PDE 5, as such, they have a similar chemical structure to cGMP. As mentioned before, PDE inhibitors inhibit the breakdown of cGMP to 5-GMP, leading to an increase in corporeal smooth muscle relaxation.

Pharmacological Concepts of Potency and Selectivity of a Drug

An ideal drug for the treatment of a medical condition should be potent and have a high selectivity toward its target tissue. In pharmacological terminology, drug potency is defined as the concentration of a drug required to inhibit an enzyme or receptor in vitro. Potency under these conditions is expressed as the IC_{50} of the drug; that is, the concentration of the drug in vitro required to inhibit 50% of a measured response, such as enzyme activity. Thus, in the case of PDE 5 inhibitors, the lower the IC_{50} value, the more potent the drug is in vitro. This is purely a pharmacological concept meaning that less of the drug is required to produce a desired effect in vitro. In other words, the lower IC_{50} value of a PDE inhibitor, the more potent, theoretically, the drug is. However, a low IC_{50} does not always indicate that a drug is more potent and thus has greater efficacy. The efficacy of a drug is a measure of its clinical or in vivo effects and therefore does depend simply on the potency of the drug in vitro, but also on its pharmacokinetic profile, that is, its absorption, distribution, and metabolism within the body (Table 7).

The selectivity of a drug is its relative activity between different receptor types or isoenzymes. For competitive antagonists such as the PDE inhibitors, selectivity can be expressed by the ratio of IC_{50} values for each PDE isoenzyme. Selectivity is the main factor determining the side-effect profile of a drug (Table 8).

PDE inhibitors used for MED should have a high selectivity for PDE 5, thereby minimizing their side effects on other PDEs present in the body. The side effects of PDE 5 inhibitors are related to their effects on other PDEs around the body. This accounts for the commonly observed adverse events ascribed to these drugs, including headache, facial flushing and dyspepsia.

Table 8 Properties of the PDE 5 Inhibitors

	Sildenafil	Tadalafil	Vardenafil
Time to onset	60 min	45 min	25–40
Duration of action	4–8 hr	24–36 hr	Not known
IC50 PDE 5 (nM)	3.5	0.9	0.7
Selectivity ratio			
PDE 1	80	10 000	257
PDE 2	1000	10 000	10 000
PDE 3	1000	10 000	10 000
PDE 4	10 000	10 000	10 000
PDE 5	1	1	1
PDE 6	10	780	16

Table 9 Medical Treatment for Peyronie's Disease

Medication	Mechanism of action
Vitamine E	Antioxidant and anti-inflammatory effect
Colchicine	Inhibition of deposition of collagene, anti-inflammatory
POTABA	Inhibition of deposition of fibrosis
Carnitine	Promotes cell regeneration
L-arginine	Induces the production of NOS, inhibition of deposition of fibrosis
Tamoxifen	Antiestrogen inhibits the release of TGF1
Pentoxyphilline	Reduces the deposition of collagen
Verapamil	Increases collagenase activity
Corticosteroids	Anti-inflammatory, reduces the deposition of collagen
Interferons	Decrease proliferation of fibroblasts

Peyronie's Disease

Peyronie's disease (PD) is a condition that manifests as a fibrous scar of the tunica albuginea that may determine penile deformity, penile curvature, hinging, narrowing and painful erections. This condition is also frequently associated with ED; it is still unclear whether ED predisposes to PD or is a consequence of the contracture of the tunica albuginea.

Although the exact mechanisms responsible of the onset of this disease are still unclear, it is widely accepted that PD is a disorder of wound healing that derives from an imbalance between profibrotic and antifibrotic agents. Among the profibrotic factors, transforming growth factor 1 (TGF1), normally released by neutrophils and macrophages during the acute and proliferative phases of wound healing, is overexpressed in PD plaques where it induces deposition of collagen. However, other profibrotic enzymes may also play a role in the pathogenesis of PD promoting the deposition of collagen or inhibiting the breakdown of collagen mediated by the matrix metalloproteinases (MMP).

Since the exact mechanisms of PD is not known, there is still no effective medical treatment for this condition and the only management is surgical The type of surgical procedure varies according to the degree of deformity, the quality of the erection and the penile length. Surgery may involve plication of the tunica albuginea, plaque incision/excision associated with grafting of the consequent defect, a combination of the previous techniques, or the insertion of a penile prosthesis.

The medical treatments available for PD are outlined in Table 9 (30).

FERTILITY

Development of the Testicle and Spermatogenesis

Male fertility depends on the successful integration of a series of physiological events, starting from sperm production and ending with the successful fertilization of the oocyte. This multi step process is reported in Table 10.

Table 10 Sequence of Events Leading to the Fertilization of the Oocyte

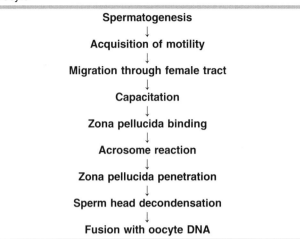

Spermatogenesis
↓
Acquisition of motility
↓
Migration through female tract
↓
Capacitation
↓
Zona pellucida binding
↓
Acrosome reaction
↓
Zona pellucida penetration
↓
Sperm head decondensation
↓
Fusion with oocyte DNA

An adequate development of the testicles is a condition sine qua non for the process of sperm production.

During childhood, the testes are small and contain the seminiferous tubules, that at this stage appear as solid, cord-like structures containing spermatocytes and Sertoli cells. The seminiferous tubules progressively then acquire a lumen as the spermatocytes start to differentiate under the influence of testosterone and FSH. In particular, FSH acts through the Sertoli cells to stimulate the germ cells to manufacture sperm. The Sertoli cells, when spermatogenesis proceeds, are responsible of the secretion of inhibin B that constitutes the negative feedback mechanism for the production of FSH.

Spermatogenesis is a complex process that starts after puberty and involves two cell divisions, meiosis I and II, that starting from a diploid cell, the spermatogonium, leads to the formation of a haploid cell, known as the gamete.

In particular, each spermatogonium undergoes cell division to produce type A spermatogonia, which, in turn produce intermediate and then type B spermatogonia. Subsequently, each spermatogonia undergoes meiosis I to become primary spermatocytes. Each spermatogonia gives rise to 16 primary spermatocytes. Each primary spermatocyte enters meiosis II to give rise to four spermatids and finally four spermatozoa. Thus, each of the 3 million spermatogonia that begin the process every day gives rise to 64 spermatozoa. The spermatogenic cycle in the testis lasts approximately 16 days, however, the complete process, from the commencement of spermatogenesis to emission, lasts around 72 days.

Sertoli cells play a key role in the process of spermatogenesis since they provide support and nourishment for the germ cells. They are irregular columnar cells that extend from the basal lamina to the lumen to provide structural organization to the tubule.

Important functions of Sertoli cells are the synthesis of ABP, which helps to maintain the high androgen levels inside the seminiferous tubules, and the creation of the blood testis barrier, that subdivides the seminiferous tubules into a basal compartment containing spermatogonia, and a luminal compartment that contains spermatocytes and spermatids.

Hormonal Control of Spermatogenesis

FSH and testosterone are the main hormones that control spermatogenesis; FSH receptors are well represented on Sertoli cells and spermatogonia while the AR are located on Sertoli cells, Leydig cells and myoid peritubular cells. FSH stimulates Sertoli cells to produce ABP and inhibin B. In particular, ABP maintains testosterone levels approximately 100 times higher than in the systemic circulation, conditions required for meiosis II (31).

There is also in vitro evidence that local autocrine and paracrine factors such as neuropeptides, vasoactive peptides, growth factors, and immune derived cytokines play regulatory functions in the seminiferous tubules (Fig. 14) (32,33).

Spermatozoa

Transformation of the human spermatid into a mature sperm involves reorganization of the nucleus and cytoplasm and the development of a flagellum. Mature spermatozoa have an oval head, which contains a nucleus The anterior halve is surrounded by the acrosomal cap, a midpiece, which is characterized by the presence of mitochondria, and a tail or flagellum.

The acrosome contains lytic enzymes that are essential for the penetration in the zona pellucida, while the tail provides the progressive movement that allows the sperm to reach the ampullar portion of the tube.

The head is characterized by the presence of condensed nuclear chromatin, which represents the haploid chromosome complement. The nucleus relocates to occupy an eccentric position at the head of the spermatid that is covered by an acrosomal cap. The flagellum has a complex structure that consists of nine outer microtubules, disposed in a circular fashion, and two inner microtubules. This proteic core is surrounded by mitochondria, which provide the energy necessary for movement, in the middle section, and only by a cell membrane in the tail. Sperm motility is consequence of the sliding action of the microtubules in the axial structure of the tail thanks to the action of the protein nexin that forms bridges between the tubules via its dynein arms.

Male Infertility

Male infertility can be considered a syndrome since it may result from a variety of congenital or acquired conditions.

The ejaculate can be abnormal because of a primary testicular dysfunction, to an impaired stimulation of otherwise normal testis or to an abnormal development of the sperm or to a defect of migration. Impairment of the seminal parameters might also be consequence of inflammation or infection of the reproductive tract due to the detrimental effects of mediators of the inflammatory response and of the free radicals on the semen. Moreover, men who produce normal sperm may be infertile because o ejaculatory or ED.

According to their etiopathogenesis, the disorders of spermatogenesis can be subdivided in the following categories:

Idiopathic

The cause of infertility remains unexplained in up to 50% of infertile men. It is likely that the impairment of the seminal parameters are consequence of an alteration in the process of maturation due to the presence of high levels of reactive oxygen species (ROS) that

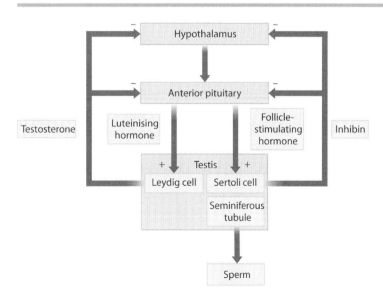

Figure 14 Hormonal regulation of testicular function.

leads to oxidative damage to the acrosome and impairment in the motility (34).

Primary Testicular Failure

This condition, also known as hypergonadotropic hypogonadism, is characterized by small size testicles, impaired spermatogenesis and elevated levels of FSH. The condition may be associated with androgen deficiency.

Genetic Abnormalities

The incidence of genetic abnormalities, that is, less than 0.1% in the normal population, is 2.2% in men attending fertility clinics and raises to 15.4% in those men that are azoospermic. The most common abnormality is Klinenfelther's syndrome that consist in a disomy of the X chromosome (XXY) and that accounts for almost 50% of all abnormalities. Also some microdeletions of the Y chromosome are associated with defective spermatogenesis. In particular, the lack of the AZF gene is associated with total lack of spermatogenesis.

Testicular Maldescent

This condition, also known as cryptorchisdism, might be consequence of an intrinsic testicular defect or be due to multiple environmental factors. Usually these testicles have a normal number of Leydig cells and therefore testosterone secretion is normal. The germinal epithelium instead tends to be partially or completely atrophied.

Sertoli-Cell-Only Syndrome

This condition is characterized by the complete absence of any spermatogenic epithelium. The only cells present in the seminiferous tubules are the Sertoli cells. The condition not necessarily involves the entire testicle, since tubules with normal spermatogenesis and with Sertoli only syndrome may coexist in the same gonad.

Acquired Testicular Failure

Acquired testicular failure can be consequence of a variety of condition. Testicular torsion, epididymoorchitis, radiation therapy and chemotherapy are among the most common causes.

Secondary Testicular Failure

This condition, also known as hypogonadotrophic hypogonadism, is consequence of a deficiency of hypothalamic releasing or pituitary hormones. The latter can be a complete deficiency of pituitary hormones, a combined loss of both FSH and LH, or an isolated loss of LH or FSH. The condition may be secondary to a direct damage of the pituitary gland by a trauma, a vascular event or an expansive process, or consequence of a hyper production of prolactin. Recognition of hypogonadotrophic hypogonadism is of particular importance since it is the only cause of azoospermia amenable to hormonal treatment.

Obstructive Azoospermia

This condition should be suspected in patients with bilateral normal sized testis, normal FSH, LH and testosterone. The obstruction can be anywhere in between the testis and the ejaculatory ducts. In particular, obstruction of the epididymis might be congenital (Young's syndrome) or consequence of recurrent episodes of epididymitis. Obstruction of the vas can be postinfective or iatrogenic. Accidental division of the vas can has been reported during inguinal hernia repair. The congenital absence of the vas can be indicative of Wolffian duct abnormality; in this case the condition is unilateral and can be associated with malformation of the genitalia, in particular hypospadias, and with ipsilateral malformations of the upper urinary tract such as absence of the renal aplasia. Instead, bilateral absence of the vas deferens is a common finding in patients carrier of the cystic fibrosis gene.

The congenital obstruction of the ejaculatory ducts may be due to Mullerian ducts cysts or Wolffian ducts abnormalities. Malignancy and lithiasis account for the most common acquired causes.

Sperm Maturation

When they pass from rete testis to the caput of the epididymis, spermatozoa are still functionally immature and immotile; their maturation occurs when they pass through the epididymis. The epididymis secretes a variety of substances and actively reabsorbs testicular fluid under the direct control of adrenergic and androgenic stimuli. In particular, the secretion of glycerophosphorylcholine, inositol, and carnitine create a favorable environment where spermatozoa can complete their maturation, which involves acquisition of motility and of fertilizing capacity. From a morphological point of view, the cytoplasmatic droplets decrease in size and migrate distally along the midpiece, the acrosomal membrane swells and the epididymal glycoproteins are incorporated in the plasma membrane. An increase in the S-S bonds in the flagellum and in the intracytoplasmatic concentration of ATP is also noted (Fig. 15).

The normal site where mature sperms are stored is the tail of the epididymis; spermatozoa are not usually found in the seminal vesicles except in case of ejaculatory duct obstruction.

Ejaculation

The process of ejaculation is probably triggered by the hypothalamus and consists of two consecutive phases, emission and ejaculation proper. Emission consists of the propulsion of the semen in the bulbar urethra and is a consequence of the sequential contraction of the epididymis, vas, seminal vescicles, prostate, and bladder neck under the influence of thoracic sympathetic outlets (T10-L2) through the hypogastric nerve.

Ejaculation proper instead consists in the expulsion of the semen from the bulbar urethra to the outside. This process, which is an involuntary spinal

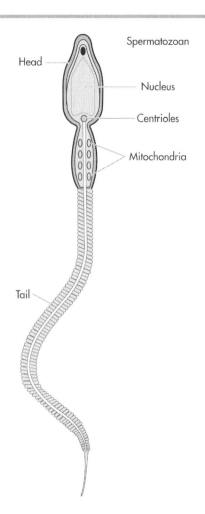

Figure 15 A mature human spermatozoon.

Table 11 Advanced Semen Analysis Tests

A. Optional tests
   Computer-aided semen analysis
   Culture studies
   Chemical studies
   Chromatin studies
B. Sperm function tests
   Sperm-mucus interaction
   Sperm capacitation
   Zona binding and acrosome reaction
   Sperm-ovum interaction

evaluate the sperm concentration, motility, viability, morphology and agglutination and search for the presence of antibodies anti sperm and nonsperm cells.

Although the semen analysis represents the cornerstone of the evaluation of the infertile male, it is generally inadequate to establish a definitive diagnosis or predict a prognosis. Furthermore, even if conducted according to World Health Organization (WHO) criteria, the basic parameters measured in this analysis, such as the sperm concentration, motility and morphology are highly dependent on subjective factors. Therefore a number of advanced sperm tests have been developed in an attempt to overcome the limitations and the drawback of the standard semen analysis (Table 11). These advanced sperm tests depend on the evaluation of sperm functions by precise and objective techniques and their interactions inside the female genital tract till the stage of fertilization. Unfortunately, there is still no single sperm function test that can evaluate all sperm functions.

Currently, all the advanced sperm tests are still considered optional or research test by the WHO.

somatic reflex, is a consequence of the rhythmic contraction of the pelvic floor and perineal muscles ischiocavernosum and bulbocavernosum and is mediated by motor fibers of the pudendal nerve (S2–S4).

The bulk of the ejaculate consists of secretions of the seminal vesicles (65%) and prostate. The testicles contribution accounts for less than 1% of the entire ejaculate. The secretions of the seminal vesicles are rich in fructose, coagulates and bicarbonates that are responsible for the typical alkaline pH. On the other hand, the prostatic secretions contain proteolytic enzymes that liquefy the coagulated proteins of the ejaculated semen, and are rich in zinc, citric acid and acid phosphatase that confer the characteristic acid pH. An obstruction of the seminal vesicles or bilateral vasal aplasia can be easily recognized by the presence of acid pH and by the absence of fructose in the ejaculate.

Semen Analysis

The standard semen analysis involves a chemical and microscopic examination. The chemical examination evaluates color, odor, volume, liquefaction, viscosity and pH. While the microscopic examination aims to

REFERENCES

1. Barsoum I, Hung-Chang YH. The road to maleness: from testis to Wolffian duct. Trends Endocrinol Metab 2006; 17(6): 223–228.
2. Foresta C, Bettella A, Vinanzi C, et al. Insulin like factor 3: a novel circulating hormone of testicular origin in humans. J Clin Endocrinol Metab 2004; 89:5952–5928.
3. Saifi GM, Chandra HS. An apparent excess of sex- and reproduction-related genes on the human X chromosome. Proc Biol Sci 1999; 266(1415):203–209.
4. Benson RC, Beard CM, Kelalis PP, et al. Malignant potential of the cryptorchid testis. Proc Mayo Clin 1991; 66:372–378.
5. Adham IM, Steding G, Thamm T, et al. The overexpression of INSL3 in female mice causes descent of the ovaries. Mol Endocrinol 2002; 16:244–252.
6. Hrabovsky Z, Farmer PJ, Hutson JM. Undescended testis is accompanied by calcitonin gene related peptide accumulation within the sensory nucleus of the genitofemoral nerve in trans-scrotal rats. J Urol 2001; 165:1015–1018.
7. Haraguchi R, Mo R, Hui C, et al. Unique functions of Sonic hedgehog signalling during external genitalia development. Development 2001; 128:4241–4250.
8. Boehmer ALM, Nijman RJM, Lammers BAS, et al. Etiological studies of severe o familiar hypospadias. J Urol 2001:1246–1254.
9. Klonisch T, Fowler PA, Hombach-Klonsch S. Molecular and genetic regulation of testis descent and external genitalia development. Dev Biol 2004; 270:1–18.

10. Stocco DM, Clark BJ. The role of the steroidogenic acute regulatory protein in steroidogenesis. Steroids 1997; 62(1): 29–36.

11. Hayes FJ, Decruz S, Seminara SB, et al. Differential regulation of gonadotropin secretion by testosterone in the human male: absence of a negative feed back effect of testosterone on follicle-stimulating hormone secretion. J Clin Endocrinol Metab 2001; 86(1):53–58.

12. Andersson AM, Skakkebaek NE. Serum inhibin B levels during male childhood and puberty. Mol Cell Endocrinol 2001; 180(1–2):103–107.

13. Chan Jl, Heist K, DePaoli AM, et al. The role of falling leptin in the neuroendocrine and metabolic adaptation to short-term starvation in healthy men. J Clin Invest 2003; 111(9):1409–1421.

14. Pardridge WM, Landaw EM. Testosterone transport in brain: primary role of plasma protein-bound hormone. Am J Physiol 1985; 249(5):E534–E542.

15. Lee DK, Chang C. Molecular communication between androgen receptor and general transcription machinery. J Steroid Biochem Mol Biol 2003; 84(1):41–49.

16. Griffin JE, Mc Paul MJ, Russell DW, et al. The androgen resistance syndromes: steroid 5-α-reductase 2 deficiency, testicular feminization, and related disorders. In: Scriver CR, Beaudet AL, Sly WS, et al., eds. The Metabolic and Molecular Bases of Inherited Disease. 8th ed. New York: McGraw-Hill, 2001:4117.

17. Heemers HV, Verhoeven G, Swinnen JV. Androgen activation of the sterol regulatory element binding protein pathway: current insights. Mol Endocrinol 2006; 20:2265.

18. Schwartz AN, Wang KY, Mack LA, et al. Evaluation of normal erectile function with color flow Doppler sonography. AJR Am J Roentgenol 1989; 153:1155–1160.

19. Chiou RK, Pomeroy BD, Chen WS, et al. Hemodynamic patterns of pharmacologically induced erection: evaluation by color Doppler sonography. J Urol 1998; 59:109–112.

20. Chung WS, Park YY, Kwon SW. The impact of aging on penile hemodynamics in normal responders to pharmacological injection: a Doppler sonographic study. J Urol 1997; 157:2129–2131.

21. Bosh RJ, Bernard F, Aboseif SR, et al. Penile detumescence: characterization of the three phases. J Urol 1991; 146:867–871.

22. El Sakka AI, Lue TF. Physiology of penile erection. Sci World J 2004; 4(S1):128–134.

23. Hedlund H, Andersson K. Comparison of responders to drug acting on adrenoreceptors and muscarinic receptors in human isolated corpus cavernosum and cavernous artery. J Auton Pharmacol 1985; 5:81.

24. Diederch W, Stief CG, Lue TF, et al. Norepinephrine involvement in penile detumescence. J Urol 1990; 143(6): 1264–1266.

25. Hedlund H, Andersson K, Fovaeus M, et al. Characterization of contraction-mediating prostanoid receptors in human penile erectile tissues. J Urol 1989; 141(1):182–186.

26. Azadzoi KM, Kim N, Brown ML, et al. Endothelium derived nitric oxide and cycloxygenase products modulate corpus cavernosum smooth muscle tone. J Urol 1992; 147(1): 220–225.

27. Musicki B, Burnett AL. eNOS function and dysfunction in the penis. Exp Biol Med 2006; 231:154–165.

28. Ottesen B, Wagner G, Virag R, et al. Penile erection: possible role of for vasoactive intestinal polypeptide as a neurotransmitter. Br Med J 1984; 288(6410):9–11.

29. Burnett Al. Erectile dysfunction. J Urol 2006; 175(S1): S25–S31.

30. Taylor FL, Levine L. Non-surgical therapy of Peyronie's Disease. Asian J Androl 2008; 10(1):79–87.

31. De Gendt K, Swinnen JV, Saunders PT. A Sertoli cell-sensitive knockout of the androgen receptor causes spermatogenic arrest in meiosis. Proc Natl Acad Sci U S A 2004; 101:1327.

32. Gnessi L, Fabbri A, Spera G. Gonadal peptides as mediators of development and functional control of the testis: an integrated system with hormones and local environment. Endocr Rev 1997; 18(4):541–609.

33. Schlatt S, einhardt A, Nieshlag E. Paracrine regulation of cellular interactions in the testis: factors in search of a function. Eur J Endocrinol 1997; 137(2):107–117.

34. Iamarrone E, Balet R, Lower AM, et al. Male infertility. Best Pract Res Clin Obstet Gynaecol 2003; 17(2):211–229.

19

The Prostate and Benign Prostatic Hyperplasia

Mark Feneley and Anthony R. Mundy
Institute of Urology, University College Hospital, London, U.K.

Mark Emberton
*Department of Urology, Division of Surgical and Interventional Sciences,
University College London, London, U.K.*

THE PROSTATE

An average urologist spends about 30% of his or her time dealing with problems related to the prostate. Surprisingly, for a structure that attracts so much of our attention, we know very little about why the prostate is there and what it does. It is one of four accessory sex glands or pairs of glands; the other three are the seminal vesicles, Cowper's glands, and the glands of Littre. If we know little about the prostate, we know even less about the others. The seminal vesicles, which are secretory glands and not storage organs for semen as their name implies, contribute substantially to the volume of seminal fluid and produce one or two substances that we know about, notably fructose and glyceryl phosphocholine. However, the other two structures are something of a mystery. The embryological development of these organs reflects notable gender-specific differences and contrasts substantial species-specific differences in the structural and functional development of the mammalian male genital tract.

We do know that the prostate is intimately related anatomically to the bladder neck and plays an integral part in ensuring antegrade ejaculation. We know it contains a substantial amount of smooth muscle as well as glandular tissue and that this smooth muscle is under α-adrenergic control and is thought somehow to be involved in the process of seminal emission prior to ejaculation. We know that the prostate contributes various substances to the ejaculate, some of which are present in unusually high concentrations, notably zinc, citrate, and polyamines. Prostatic-specific antigen is an enzyme involved in the liquifaction of the seminal coagulum, and has acquired great medical importance as a serum marker for prostate cancer, as well as being a prognostic indicator in benign prostatic hyperplasia (BPH). We know that the development and function of the prostate are under hormonal control; in other words, it is a secondary sex organ.

We do not know, however, what part if any the prostate plays in continence in normal individuals. The mechanism of emission and ejaculation is uncertain (in humans), and we do not know why the prostatic secretion contains so much zinc, citrate and polyamines, or what the roles are of these and the various other substances that the prostate secretes. We also do not understand why prostatic diseases of benign hyperplasia and cancer occur naturally only in the human and dog, or why these pathologies do not develop in other male secondary sexual organs.

The Structure of the Prostate

The prostate has been described as having a lobar structure, first, because of the endoscopic appearance of "lobes" in patients with BPH and in the pathological specimen after retropubic prostatectomy, and second, on embryological grounds in which the prostate is seen to develop from five distinct ductal systems (1). More recently, the morphology of the prostate has been described on the basis of the predisposition of parts of its structure to various pathological processes, and to McNeal we owe our current understanding of the structure of the prostate (Fig. 1) (2–5).

McNeal noted that the nodules of BPH began in the periurethral glandular area within the collar of the preprostatic sphincter in the supramontanal part of the prostate. Subsequently, he noted that these microscopic nodules were principally concentrated just below the distal margin of the preprostatic sphincter, and he named that area the transition zone. The transition zone only accounted for about 2% of the glandular tissue of the normal prostate but accounted for much more as the hyperplastic nodules coalesced, became macroscopic, and tended to displace the normal prostate away from the urethra.

McNeal noted that about 25% of prostatic cancer originated within the transition zone, whereas 75% of cancers and almost all instances of prostatitis arose in the so-called peripheral zone. The peripheral zone forms a posteriorly and inferiorly orientated cup that encloses the central zone, through the center of which are transmitted the ejaculatory ducts. McNeal

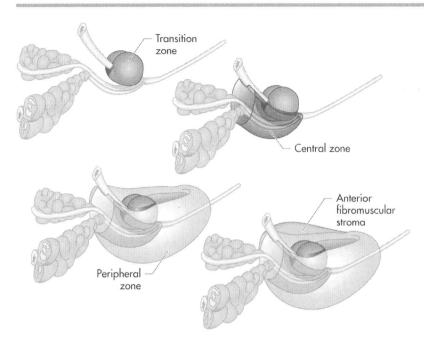

Figure 1 Zones of the prostate.

noted the comparative absence of disease in the central zone by comparison with the other glandular areas of the prostate and likened it to the seminal vesicles, which are also comparatively free of disease. He speculated further that both these structures might arise embryologically from the Wolffian ducts and noted some histological similarities between the central zone and the seminal vesicles to support this contention (5).

Completing the anterior aspect of the substance of the prostate where the peripheral zone peters out on either side is the anterior fibromuscular stroma of the prostate. Most of the glandular tissue of the prostate is in the peripheral zone, which accounts for 75% of the total, the remaining 25% of the glandular tissue of the prostate being in the central zone. It is not known whether the three zones of glandular tissue—transition, central, and peripheral—have different secretory functions.

Embryological Development of the Prostate

As mentioned above, the seminal vesicles (and possibly the central zone of the prostate) arise from the Wolffian ducts along with the vasa and their ampullae and the epididymes. Their embryological development is under the control of testosterone. Otherwise, the rest of the prostate and other secondary sexual organs develop by ductal outbudding from the urethra into surrounding urogenital sinus mesenchyme. The embryological and pubertal development of the prostate is in contrast principally under the control of dihydrotestosterone. These distinctions in tissue androgen sensitivity are evident from abnormalities of prostatic and secondary sexual organ development that occur with congenital 5-α reductase deficiency and androgen insensitivity syndromes. Differences of

embryological origin and hormonal control may also account for the observation that, whereas the prostate is commonly involved in disease, the structures of Wolffian duct origin rarely are.

Endocrinology of the Prostate

The normal prostate develops and functions in response to dihydrotestosterone produced within prostate cells from circulating testosterone (Fig. 2). Circulating testosterone is derived principally from testicular Leydig cell secretion; the testis produces 6 to 7 mg a day under the influence of luteinizing hormone, which in turn is produced by the pituitary in response to the pulsatile release of luteinizing hormone–releasing hormone from the hypothalamus. The adrenal glands secrete essential steroid hormones including testosterone and also androgens of lesser activity that alone or by peripheral interconversion may be metabolically important in target tissues. Without sufficient testicular testosterone synthesis, however, the adult prostate undergoes partial involution.

Testosterone is insoluble in water and is carried in the circulation bound principally to sex hormone–binding globulin, also somewhat loosely to albumen, leaving a small but physiologically important fraction of free circulating testosterone. Free testosterone is a lipid-soluble molecule derived from cholesterol that transfers across lipid cell membranes with ease. Testosterone stimulates androgen signaling principally through binding the androgen receptor, though it may also have cell surface interactions with intracellular signaling pathways. It also serves as a precursor for other steroid hormones through irreversible metabolic conversion within target tissues, principally to either dihydrotestosterone (by 5-α reductase) or estradiol (by aromatase).

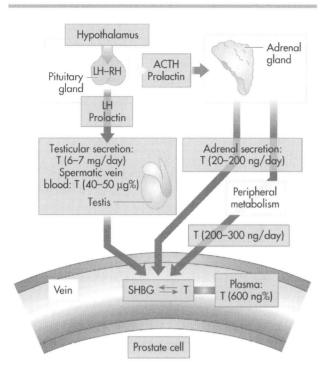

Figure 2 Endocrinological influences on the prostate. Pulsatile release of LH-RH from the hypothalamus causes the release of luteinizing hormone (LH) from the anterior pituitary, which circulates to the Leydig cells of the testis, which produce testosterone (T). Testosterone circulates from the testis bound to sex hormone–binding globulin (SHBG) and is available to the prostate. Circulating testosterone has a negative feedback inhibition of the hypothalamic release of LH-RH. Adrenal secretion and peripheral steroid metabolism are other sources of circulating androgens. *Abbreviation:* LH-RH, luteinizing hormone–releasing hormone.

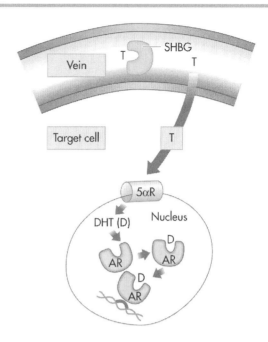

Figure 3 Testosterone (T) dissociates from its protein binding and translocates across the cell membrane. Intracellularly, it is converted to dihydrotestosterone (DHT) and binds to the androgen receptor (AR), from where it translocates to the nucleus.

In the prostate, intracellular 5-α reductase irreversibly converts testosterone to dihydrotestosterone. Dihydrotestosterone binds the androgen receptor with higher affinity and stimulates greater receptor activation than its precursor testosterone. Prostatic dihydrotestosterone is predominantly synthesized in situ, whereas circulating dihydrotestosterone is derived principally from 5-α reductase type 1 activity in the skin and liver. By an alternative pathway, testosterone may be converted irreversibly to estradiol through aromatization, a much less active pathway in the prostate but may be relevant in the development of BPH and prostatic inflammation.

There are two 5-α reductase isozymes, type 1 and type 2. In the prostate, the type 2 isozyme is predominantly expressed and therefore the more important. Finasteride and dutasteride are both 5-α reductase inhibitors used for treatment of BPH. Finasteride specifically inhibits 5-α reductase type 2, whereas dutasteride inhibits both isozymes (6). It is a deficiency of the type 2 isozyme that is responsible for the intersex state first noted by Imperato-McInley in the Dominican Republic in which apparently normal girls change to boys at puberty (7).

In cells that express androgen receptor, intracellular androgen binds the androgen receptor, which then translocates to the nucleus and forms a complex that binds DNA to initiate transcription. Binding of the androgen receptor with androgen involves various coactivators, copressors, dimerization, and conformational changes of the receptor that determines its molecular activity as a transcription factor. Through binding of the receptor DNA-binding domain to specific target DNA, androgen-sensitive gene transcription is initiated (Fig. 3).

Within the prostate, there are intracellular differences in 5-α reductase and androgen receptor expression according to cell type and epithelial differentiation reflecting dynamic cellular interactions that are involved in tissue regulation and function. Both epithelial cells and stromal cells contain 5-α reductase enzymes (8). The type 2 isozyme provides the majority of this enzymatic activity, and is present predominantly in stromal cells, which are therefore the principal source of prostatic androgen, dihydrotestosterone. Small amounts of the type 1 isozyme are expressed by glandular epithelial cells. Similarly, both epithelial and stromal cells contain androgen receptors. Within glandular structures, androgen receptor is expressed at relatively low levels in the basal epithelial cell layer (representing the stem cell and proliferating compartments), contrasting much greater expression in the luminal secretory cells. This reflects the dependence of glandular differentiation and epithelial secretion on androgen signaling. Prostatic androgen receptor is more consistently present in the stromal cells where

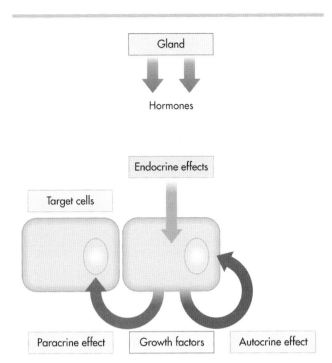

Figure 4 The effect of androgens in the stroma is to cause the release of growth factors that have an autocrine effect on themselves and a paracrine effect on epithelial cells.

they stimulate transcription of various growth factors that drive both the epithelial cells and the stromal cells themselves to grow and develop (9,10). It is this interaction between the stroma and the epithelium that is thought to account not only for development and for normal function but also, when the interaction is deranged, for the process leading to BPH.

Thus, several processes are active within the prostate. The endocrine effect of testosterone leads to the intracrine effect of dihydrotestosterone, which generates the autocrine and paracrine effects of growth factors on both the stroma and the epithelium of the prostate (Fig. 4). These growth factors, responsible for the autocrine and paracrine effects, act principally during the G1 phase of the cell cycle and have various effects, mainly stimulatory but in some instances inhibitory, leading generally to the entry of the cell into the S phase and ultimately then to mitosis.

The normal adult prostate should not be thought of as being an entirely static structure. There is a turnover of cells throughout life and this turnover is heterogeneous (11). Those glandular cells further out in the periphery of the gland away from the urethra show little in the way of secretion and most in the way of mitotic activity within the prostate, resembling basal or stem cells. At an intermediate level along the prostatic duct, the epithelial cells show less mitosis but almost all of the secretory activity of the prostate. These two types of acinar cells are tall and columnar and show no evidence of cell death. More centrally, close to the urethra, the epithelial cells are lower,

flatter, and without any secretory activity, and programmed cell death (apoptosis) is readily visible. In relation to these different epithelial cell types, there are differences in the underlying extracellular matrix that probably reflect the driving force for epithelial differentiation (12). In addition, there are the neuro-endocrine cells described below.

Growth Factors in the Prostate

It has been known for many years that prostatic cells could only proliferate in vitro in the presence of serum. The factors that were present in serum were not present in plasma and so it seemed that whatever was necessary to stimulate cell growth in vitro was derived from the process of blood coagulation and most probably liberated from platelets. Thus, one of the first "growth factors" to be identified was called platelet-derived growth factor. Various other factors were subsequently identified as being growth factors for various different cell types in vitro and have derived their names from the circumstances under which they were isolated. These substances may have effects other than being growth factors, and most have many different roles in stimulating cellular growth both in vitro and in vivo (chapter 1).

Other factors that are known to be important in the normal growth and development in the prostate have been (a) derived from the mouse submaxillary gland [epidermal growth factor (EGF)]; (b) shown to have a very characteristic and strong tendency to bind to heparin (fibroblast growth factor, one of the so-called heparin-binding growth factors); or (c) biochemically related to proinsulin [insulin-like growth factor (IGF)]. Hence, the origin of names that are somewhat confusing to the uninitiated.

Typically, growth factors are grouped into families of factors having similar effects and there is an EGF family, a fibroblast growth factor family, a transforming growth factor β (TGF-β) family (TGF-α—somewhat confusingly—is a member of the EGF family), and the IGF family. There are other growth factor families as well, but these are the ones that are thought to be important in the normal prostate.

Of these various growth factors, the most important stimulatory ones are EGF and TGF-α, both of which are derived from the EGF family, and basic fibroblast growth factor (bFGF) of the fibroblast growth factor family. Of these, bFGF and EGF are thought to account for 80% and TGF-α for 20% of the stimulatory growth factor effect in health (13). The other important growth factor is TGF-β, whose effects are complex but generally inhibitory (14).

Other growth factors such as IGF are thought to be principally "permissive" in the same sense that androgens are permissive. IGF and testosterone have to be present in vivo and in vitro, but adding more and more of either does not produce a corresponding parallel proliferation of the prostate in vitro, whereas adding EGF, TGF, or bFGF does. The effects of some of these factors are only or principally apparent at different stages of development. EGF and bFGF are predominant in the adult (developed) prostate. On the other hand, TGF and another member of the fibroblast growth factor family, acidic fibroblast growth factor, are principally evident in fetal life (15).

Most of the growth factors alluded to above act to increase gene expression, although the TGF-β family is notable for generally producing inhibition. Most growth factors act through single-pass transmembrane receptors with tyrosine kinase activity that, through a transduction pathway, induce mitogen-activated protein kinases, which produce the increase in gene expression.

The Role of the Prostate in Continence

One could be forgiven for thinking that the prostate has a major role in continence by virtue of its situation around the bladder neck, but of course the female of the species manages perfectly well without it.

In individuals of either sex there is a change in the orientation of the smooth muscle bundles of the detrusor as they approach the region of the bladder neck, with a tendency to become more oblique in disposition, smaller and more finely interspersed in a more dense connective tissue framework (Fig. 5) (16). In males, but not in females, there is a quite definitely circular/oblique orientation of smooth muscle bundles around the area just below the bladder neck and within the substance of the prostate, with a dense adrenergic innervation that can be demonstrated by immunofluorescence (Fig. 6) (17). Elsewhere in the bladder in both sexes and in the female urethra, α-adrenergic innervation is only seen in relation to blood vessels, although α-adrenergic receptors may be more widely distributed. This ring of smooth muscle around the supramontanal prostatic urethra, between the bladder neck and the site of drainage of the prostatic ducts and ejaculatory ducts into the urethra, is called the preprostatic sphincter. It is present to ensure antegrade ejaculation (see below).

Elsewhere within the prostate, particularly within the prostatic capsule but distributed throughout the stroma, there are smooth muscle cells that

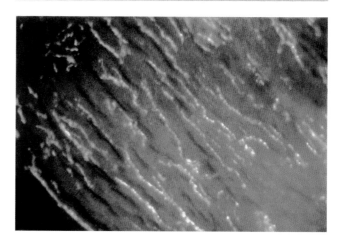

Figure 6 Immunofluorescence photomicrograph to show the presence of noradrenergic nerves interspersed between the smooth muscle bundles at the bladder neck.

amount to about 50% of the total mass of the stroma of the prostate (18). These cells also have (mainly) an α-adrenergic innervation (19).

Classical pharmacological studies were able to distinguish between α- and β-adrenergic activities and, later, between α-1 receptors (postjunctional α-adrenoceptors that mediate the effector response) and α-2 receptors (prejunctional α-adrenoceptors that regulate neurotransmitter release). Further, pharmacological α-1 subtypes are now distinguished by the selective effects of antagonists. The International Union of Pharmacology classification of α-receptors clarified the nomenclature used to describe native as distinct from cloned receptors (20). The majority of the adrenergic receptors are of the α-adrenergic type, 98% of which are located within the stroma, of which 90% are of the α-1 subtype. Only 10% of α receptors and neurons are of the α-2 subtype. Of the α-1, the α-1A type accounts for 60%, and it is these that characterize the cells that have been targeted pharmacologically by drugs such as indoramin, terazosin, doxazosin, alfuzosin, and tamsulosin in an attempt to reverse some of the features of bladder outflow obstruction due to BPH (21).

This adrenergic innervation is not the only form of innervation to the prostate or even the only innervation of prostatic smooth muscle cells. There is a cholinergic innervation thought to control epithelial secretion (22), and there are a number of different nonadrenergic, noncholinergic nerve or receptor types as well. The latter include serotonin (5-hydroxytryptamine), dopamine β hydroxylase, vasoactive intestinal polypeptide, neuropeptide Y, leu-encephalin, met-encephalin, calcitonin gene–related peptide, and substance P (23). What these are all doing is by no means clear.

Some of the nonadrenergic, noncholinergic substances listed above are present in so-called "neuroendocrine cells" (24). The principal neuroendocrine

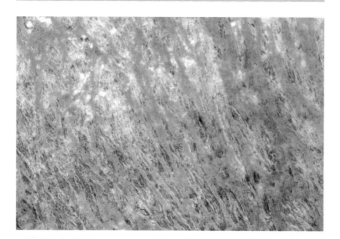

Figure 5 The orientation of smooth muscle bundles at the bladder neck to form the preprostatic sphincter.

cell types are cells that secrete serotonin and thyroid-stimulating hormone. Other cells contain calcitonin or the calcitonin gene–related peptide and somatostatin. It is not clear what these do, but they are thought to be involved in the regulation of secretion or cell growth. The function of the other neurons or receptors is completely unknown; they may not actually have any function. As has been pointed out elsewhere in this volume, the presence of neurons does not necessarily imply the presence of receptors for those neurons and vice versa, and even if both are present, that does not necessarily mean that there is a neural pathway, and if there is, it does not necessarily follow that that pathway has a physiological significance even if it has a pathological significance.

Thus, there is no evidence that the prostate plays any active role in continence, although in disease it may interfere with normal continence. There is no evidence that the male bladder neck in the strict sense is any different from the female bladder neck except that it simply has a preprostatic sphincter superimposed on the common bladder neck pattern. All the evidence is that the prostatic smooth muscle and its innervation and the other nerve supply to the prostate are involved in glandular secretion and the process of emission.

EMISSION AND EJACULATION

Ejaculation in human beings remains a mystery, in part as it is so difficult to study because of the problems of sexual sensibilities. In animals this is less of a problem; indeed, because of the financial implications of breeding in animal husbandry, ejaculation in some species has been studied in considerable detail.

We have known for some time from so-called split ejaculate studies in humans that spermatozoa and prostatic fluid are ejaculated first, followed by seminal vesicle fluid later (25). We also know that ejaculation is antegrade in the presence of a competent bladder neck despite the competence of the urethral sphincter mechanism, which therefore must be overcome actively or reflexly to enable ejaculation to occur. It is also common male experience that voiding is difficult with an erection and for a while after ejaculation.

The latter has been shown to be because of tightening of the "bladder neck"—more accurately, of the preprostatic sphincter—on erection, which becomes more marked in the period leading up to ejaculation. This has been shown both in urethral pressure profile studies, which show enhancement of the pressure zone produced by the bladder neck (Fig. 7), and in transrectal ultrasound studies, which demonstrate the preprostatic sphincter quite clearly and which show it to become more marked in the pre-ejaculatory period (26).

The next step, also shown on transrectal ultrasound (26) (and radiographically in some animal species), is the transportation of spermatozoa from the ampullae of the vasa into the prostatic urethra. This process of filling of the inframontanal prostatic urethra, below the occluding preprostatic sphincter, is known as emission, as distinct from the process by which the seminal fluid is transported to the outside world, which is ejaculation. The mechanism for this is not clear. Once it occurs, ejaculation is imminent. Next is a contraction of the prostatic smooth muscle including the preprostatic sphincter, which is presumably under α-1A adrenergic control.

Synchronously but not in any coordinated fashion, there is a sequence of five or six contractions of the bulbospongiosus muscle. The first generally occurs before any of the seminal fluid has entered the bulbar urethra, and the last occurs after pulsatile ejaculation ceases. Neither is the mechanism for this clear, nor is the means by which the urethral sphincter mechanism is overcome. It used to be thought that it was overcome passively by the sheer pressure that prostatic emission generates. But the recent transrectal ultrasound studies referred to above suggest that this is probably not the case. Urethral sphincter studies to look for a relaxation mechanism have not been useful in providing an alternative explanation. In any case, a postulated urethral sphincter relaxation mechanism would tend to flounder on the observation that after transurethral resection, men are not incontinent during sexual activity when the bladder neck mechanism has been ablated.

Once emission and ejaculation have begun, there is further contraction of the prostate and of the seminal vesicles until the process is complete. There is therefore an important role for the prostate in the process of emission leading to ejaculation, irrespective of the content of prostatic secretion added.

The Physiological Function of Prostatic Secretion

In an average ejaculate, 2 mL is contributed by the secretion of the seminal vesicles, 0.5 mL is contributed by the secretion of the prostate, and Cowper's glands and the glands of Littre contribute 0.1 mL (27). The contribution of the sperm cells themselves is insignificant. Although the function of these various secretions is not clear, epididymal sperm can fertilize an ovum but not as well as ejaculated sperm, so presumably their function is to maximize the potential for fertilization. This may be by having a protective effect during the onward journey of the sperm until its contact with the ovum, or an effect to enhance motility and sperm survival more directly, or a role to increase the fertilizing effect of the sperm when it reaches the ovum. There are various pieces of evidence to support a role in each of these three areas, but details are distinctly lacking.

These various secretions also have a protective role in the lower urinary tract itself. The sheer presence of the fluid provides lubrication both of the urethra itself and, through the pre-ejaculatory fluid, for penetration, although penetration has often occurred long before most human males produce pre-ejaculatory fluid. Nonetheless, this may at least be the role of the glands of Littre. It would be nice to think they were there for some purpose!

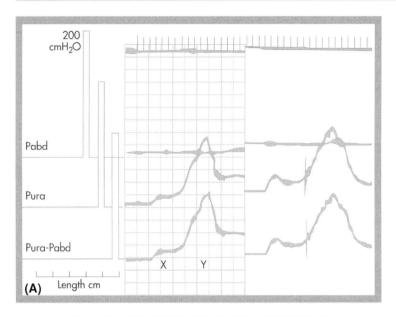

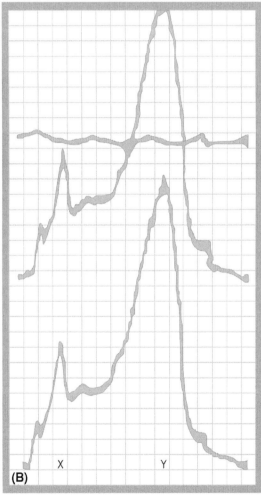

Figure 7 (**A**) A urethral pressure profile of the bladder neck (where x is the site of the bladder neck and y is the site of the urethral sphincter mechanism). (**B**) A urethral pressure profile during erection to show the enhanced pressure zone at the bladder neck.

A protective effect on the lower urinary tract by the biological effects of some of the components of seminal fluid may be more important, indeed much more important than just the mechanical washing of the urethra. In fact, it has been argued that the principal function of the prostate and the other sexual secondary sex organs is to protect the integrity of the spermatozoa. Zinc has a strong antimicrobial action;

spermine less so. Immunoglobulins of various types could have a similar biological role. All this is, however, unproven.

One substance known to enhance the fertilizing capacity of ejaculated sperm cells after ejaculation is fertilization-promoting peptide, which is structurally similar to thyrotrophin-releasing hormone (28). Neither is its mode of action nor whether there are other compounds with a similar action is known. EGF has a high concentration in seminal fluid, second only to colostrum in fact, and it may be that this reflects a role in fertilization.

Numerous compounds are produced by the prostate, most of which have no obvious function. Acid phosphatase splits glycerylphosphocholine produced by the seminal vesicles to produce glycerylphosphate ultimately, and it may be that glycerylphosphate is important in sperm protection. It may be more than just coincidental that in a laboratory setting glycerin is used for this sort of purpose. Polyamines are the strongest known cationic substances in nature and they may have an important role in transcription and translation (29). Alternatively, these two observations may be no more than just coincidence. Prostate-specific antigen is a serine protease that has a role in sperm liquefaction (30). Sperm coagulation and liquefaction have an important role in small mammals such as rats and mice, but their role in humans is unclear.

More interesting perhaps, because of their high concentration within the prostate, are zinc and citrate. Citrate is present in 240 to 1300 times the concentration found elsewhere (31), and zinc is present in about 30 times the concentration elsewhere; (32) it seems likely that there is a reason for this and for the uniquely high concentrations of polyamines. There appears to be a close correlation between all three, and it has long been suspected that citrate is there as a ligand for zinc (33). It is thought that the zinc is there to help maintain the quaternary structure of sperm chromatin (34) in addition to the biological protective effect mentioned above. It now seems likely that the complex of zinc and citrate and polyamines forms a structure that has electrochemical neutrality and therefore buffers the citrate (35), although this does seem an extremely energy-inefficient way of achieving this effect. An alternative, or additional, explanation is that the complex is there not just to protect the zinc (so to speak) but to hold the citrate there (36). The optimum pH for the activity of acid phosphatase is much lower than the natural pH of seminal fluid, and if acid phosphatase does indeed have an important biological role, this may be facilitated by the availability of large amounts of citrate. This, however, is pure speculation at present.

One of the problems is that most of these substances have only been investigated from the point of view of their concentrations in disease to serve as a marker for a disease state rather than to investigate their physiological role. Until the thrust of research is redirected, the function of these various components of prostatic and seminal vesicular secretion will continue to remain obscure.

BENIGN PROSTATIC HYPERPLASIA

Having discussed some of the aspects of our current understanding of the prostate in health, we now turn to a consideration of the disorders of the prostate seen in BPH.

The general impression generated in many reviews is that BPH is a generalized and diffuse disease of the prostate that occurs as a result of some sort of hormonal derangement that leads to hyperplasia of the prostate, producing enlargement of the gland as a whole, which in turn leads to compression of the prostatic urethra and a progressive occlusion of the bladder outflow and the clinical syndrome of "prostatism." None of this is true.

BPH is very unusual in that it only occurs in human beings and dogs. The same is true of carcinoma of the prostate. Despite this and the fact that both diseases are common, most authorities suggest that there is no direct link between the two diseases (37). Recently, however, there has been a suggestion that the two are related: that a series of genetic "hits" gives rise to BPH, and further hits to prostate cancer (38). In this hypothesis, BPH would represent an early stage in the development of prostate cancer; however, benign hyperplasia itself is not a premalignant pathological abnormality.

BPH seems to be a disease (also like carcinoma of the prostate) that any human adult male can expect to get if he lives long enough with functioning testes and if his prostate was normal to start off with. It is clearly important, therefore, to distinguish between the clinical conditions associated with the histological disease of BPH and other clinical conditions affecting the lower urinary tract in aging males.

The recent interest in symptom scores and in the effects of aging on the bladder in individuals of either sex seems to make it clear that there are symptoms arising from the lower urinary tract, and particularly from the bladder, that are related to aging, which need to be distinguished from those symptoms related to histological BPH in males. Furthermore, many of the features of the BPH clinical symptom complex are difficult to explain in relation to histological BPH alone. Acute retention can be explained when it is secondary to urinary tract infection, severe constipation, or sympathetic stimulation in hypothermia and psychological stress, but otherwise its nature is somewhat elusive, although it may be due to prostatic infarction or some other prostatic "vascular accident" (39). The "urge" symptom complex related to secondary detrusor instability is more easy to explain (40), but bladder decompensation is more difficult given our present knowledge of clinical BPH and the experimental effects of obstruction on bladder function (41), unless this is related more to the coincidentally aging bladder than to BPH per se. It is, in fact, difficult to explain how BPH causes obstruction at all. Squeezing on a hosepipe is a very inefficient way of stopping the water emerging from the end, and a very marked restriction of the caliber of the hosepipe has to be produced before there is any overt change in flow. Obstruction by urethral constriction is easily understood in relation to urethral stricture disease, but it is much more difficult to argue for a similar effect in the prostatic urethra in BPH when a large resectoscope can be passed through and into the bladder with ease. It may, therefore, be that it is distortion of the prostatic urethra that is more important in producing outflow obstruction than compression or constriction, as it is distortion of a hosepipe by kinking that is more likely to stop flow.

Etiology

It has already been mentioned that the only proven risk factors for developing BPH are aging and the presence of functioning testes (42), assuming that the prostate was normal to start off with—in other words, if 5-α reductase is present to convert testosterone to dihydrotestosterone, and functioning androgen receptors are available for binding the dihydrotestosterone.

Various factors have been investigated such as dietary factors, alcohol, and cirrhosis of the liver (43), all of which may indirectly support the hypothesis of an endocrine imbalance in parallel with age-related declining circulating androgen levels or a relative decrease with respect to estrogen, but without substantive evidence at tissue level. Inherited factors may also predispose to the development of the disease in families and at a younger than usual age (44). More recently, BPH has been shown to be associated broadly with erectile and ejaculatory dysfunction, with the possibility of common underlying mechanisms involving molecular signaling (particularly upregulation of the RhoA/Rho-kinase pathway). Its

association with aging, endocrinological changes, and vascular disease may also account for observed associations with hypertension, metabolic syndrome, and type II diabetes (45,46). The presence of nitric oxide in prostate and bladder, and their deficiency in outflow obstruction, as well as the responsiveness of both voiding symptoms and erectile dysfunction to α-receptor blockade (perhaps reflecting hyperadrenergic status), suggests certain commonalities in etiology and therapeutic opportunity at least in some cases (47,48).

Pathogenesis

It has been pointed out that androgens (in other words, functioning testes) are permissive for prostatic growth and development in health, and the same is true for the prostate in vitro. Androgens (and IGF and other "factors") have to be present for prostate cells to grow, but once the critical "permissive" concentration has been reached, there is no extra growth produced by adding more.

Also discussed above was the concept of a stromal-epithelial interaction in which testosterone production by the epithelial cells leads to the elaboration of growth factors by the stromal cell that act in both an autocrine and paracrine fashion to produce further growth and differentiation in both the stroma and the epithelium. This stromal-epithelial interaction was most clearly demonstrated by Cunha (Fig. 8), who implanted embryonic urogenital sinus mesenchyme and adult bladder epithelial cells from a normal

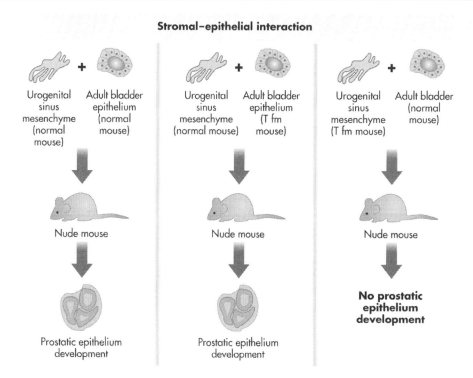

Stromal–epithelial interaction

Figure 8 Cunha's experiments showing the importance of stroma (in this case urogenital sinus mesenchyme) in epithelial differentiation. *Abbreviation:* T fm, testicular feminization.

mouse under the renal capsule of a nude mouse and showed that the urogenital sinus mesenchyme induced prostatic epithelial differentiation of the bladder epithelium (10). Cunha also showed that normal prostatic differentiation could be induced from the bladder epithelium taken from a mouse with androgen receptor deficiency as long as the urogenital sinus mesenchyme was taken from a normal mouse. Prostatic epithelial differentiation did not occur when the urogenital sinus mesenchyme was taken from a mouse with androgen receptor deficiency, whatever the androgen receptor status of the bladder epithelium. In this way, Cunha demonstrated the importance of the androgen receptor in the prostatic stroma (derived from urogenital sinus mesenchyme) as well as the importance of the stromal-epithelial interaction in producing epithelial and glandular development.

In BPH, the stromal:epithelial ratio increases (18). Normally, it is something in the region of 2:1, but in BPH it increases to 3:1 or 4:1. As mentioned above, there is a substantial smooth muscle component to the stroma in health and in BPH, but the majority of the stroma is made up of connective tissue such that about 50% of BPH is connective tissue, 25% is smooth muscle, and 25% is epithelium (19).

The first discernible sign of BPH is the presence of microscopic nodules of fibromuscular hyperplasia with a variable epithelial cell component. These nodules are found initially in the transition zone just below the smooth muscle collar of the preprostatic sphincter (Fig. 9) (49). The transition zone is found on either side of the urethra, and nodules in this area are a mixture of glandular and epithelial hyperplasia. The nodules of BPH also form, with lesser frequency, in the periurethral glandular tissue within the smooth muscle collar of the preprostatic sphincter. Here, these nodules develop principally posteriorly and have no epithelial or glandular component, consisting entirely of connective tissue (50,51). Within these nodules, most unusual changes can be seen, notably fibroblasts transforming themselves into smooth muscle cells. It was this observation that led McNeal to suggest that the nodules of BPH, wherever they occurred, were the

result of an "embryonic reawakening" as a consequence of localized changes in the normal stromal-epithelial interaction (49,52).

The so-called lateral lobes of BPH are derived from micronodule formation and coalescence and further growth within the transition zone, whereas the so-called middle lobe is derived from nodule formation and development within the periurethral glandular sleeve posteriorly. The remainder of the prostate—as has been well recognized for many years—is compressed outward to form a false capsule posteriorly (53).

In other words, BPH is not a diffuse and generalized disease of the prostate but is a highly localized disease of the smallest area of the prostate (the transition zone and the periurethral gland area) (54). Whereas the description embryonic reawakening may not be entirely accurate, the disease does seem to be related to an abnormal stromal-epithelial interaction confined to this small area of the prostate, in which both increased cell growth and reduced cell death—that is to say, programmed cell death (apoptosis)—are equally important components (55). It was mentioned above that along the prostatic duct, from the urethra out to the periphery, the most distal glands were dividing while the most proximal ones (nearest the urethra) were undergoing apoptosis. The epithelial cells of the more distal or peripheral glands, which have been noted to be more mitotically active, seem to be related to underlying smooth muscle cells that are vimentin positive, whereas those that are proximal or central, which tend to show apoptosis, are related to smooth muscles that are actin positive (12,56). Perhaps vimentin-positive smooth muscle cells tend to be more stimulatory, whereas those that are actin positive produce inhibitory growth factors or growth factors that tend to promote apoptosis. Alterations in growth factor expression have, indeed, been identified in BPH, although it is not yet possible to say with confidence that these growth factors are the cause of this histological condition, and that their effects are confined to the transition zone and not present elsewhere within the prostate (57).

In the normal prostate, the main stimulatory growth factors are EGF and TGF-α, the former being principally active in adults and the latter in growth and differentiation of the prostate. Neither of these appears to play any part in BPH, although the EGF expression appears to be reduced (58). Another growth factor family with an important role in the normal prostate is the fibroblast growth factor family. Like TGF-α, acidic fibroblast growth factor is predominantly active in growth and differentiation (15). It is bFGF that is the main stimulatory growth factor of this group in adults. All members of the fibroblast growth factor family have a variety of actions on a variety of different cell types, including producing angiogenesis and remodeling the extracellular matrix by producing modulating proteases and inducing the synthesis of fibronectin (14,59). Members of the fibroblast growth factor family are abundant in the extracellular matrix, where they bind heparin avidly. Basic fibroblast growth factor is interesting because it is not secreted;

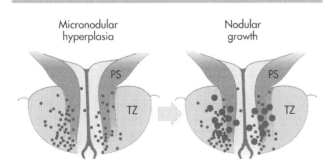

Figure 9 The siting of early nodules in benign prostatic hyperplasia: just below and within the collar of the preprostatic sphincter (PS) in the general area of the transitional zone (TZ).

it is only released from cells by injury or cell death, although it may, of course, have intracrine activity (60). However, there is another member of this family, called keratinocyte growth factor (KGF) (61). This is a truly paracrine substance that is secreted only by stromal cells but for which there are receptors only on epithelial cells. It may be that some of the stimulatory activity previously ascribed to bFGF is, in fact, more related to KGF. Both bFGF and KGF appear to have a role in BPH as both show increased expression (62).

The TGF-β family is the family of growth factors that are generally inhibitory for epithelial cells. It is more true to say that they may be inhibitory or stimulatory depending on the cell type, the state of differentiation, and the circumstances (14,63), but in general they are inhibitory for epithelial cells and stimulatory for stromal cells. They also increase angio-genesis and extracellular matrix formation (64,65). This family is interesting, first because these growth factors have receptors that are serine/threonine kin-ases rather than tyrosine kinases, which are usual with growth factor receptors (65), and second, because they can inhibit the transition from the G1 phase to the S phase of the cell cycle and thereby override the action of mitogens, including the growth factors alluded to above (14,66).

There are five isoforms of TGF-α, but only three have been found in mammals (α-1– α-3) and only α-1 and α-2 have been investigated in BPH. TGF-α-1 is negatively regulated by androgen: a fall in androgen leads to increased expression of the growth factor, and vice versa (65). It also seems that bFGF and KGF expression is regulated by TGF-β (14). As a result, fibroblast growth factor expression is regulated by androgen indirectly by the androgen effect on TGF-α expression.

The fibroblast growth factors—bFGF and KGF—are stimulatory growth factors and TGFs α-1 and α-2 are inhibitory. Stromal cells produce both fibroblast growth factors and TGF-α-1 (14,57). Epithelial cells produce TGF-α-2 (67). bFGF acts on both epithelial cells and stromal cells but principally on stromal cells because that is where it is released. KGF, on the other hand, can only act on epithelial cells because only epithelial cells have receptors for it. The TGFs α-1 and α-2 act on both epithelial and stromal cells (Fig. 10).

Thus, KGF stimulates and TGF-β inhibits epithe-lial cells, and bFGF stimulates and TGF-β inhibits stromal cells; in the normal prostate, a steady state exists in which each pair is in balance. It is believed (68) that in BPH, the fibroblast growth factors tend to override the TGF-α and there is therefore a prolifera-tion of epithelial and stromal cells and, in addition, because of the effect on extracellular matrix compo-nents, an increased activity there as well.

If one assumes that this hypothesis is true, there is still a need to identify the cause of the changes outlined above. It has been suggested that declining androgen levels could account for the increasing expression of TGF-α (69), but that would not explain the localized nature of the disease process. An alter-native explanation is that repeated microtrauma or inflammation produced by repeated (lifelong) voiding

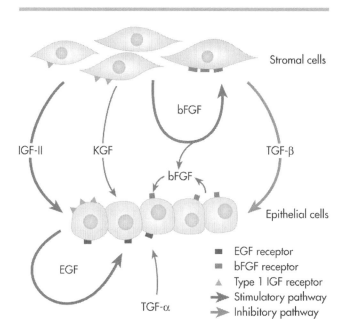

Figure 10 The interaction of growth factors in benign prostatic hyperplasia. *Abbreviations:* bFGF, basic fibroblast growth factor; IGF-II, insulin-like growth factor II; KGF, keratinocyte growth factor; TGF-β, transforming growth factor β; TGF-α, transforming growth factor α; EGF, epidermal growth factor.

and ejaculation, acting, as they do, on the point of angulation of the prostatic urethra, which is where the transition zone is situated, leads to cell damage at that site, which in turn leads to the release of bFGF, which starts the whole process off (70).

Whether or not the details given above and the hypothesis outlined in the last few paragraphs prove ultimately to be true, it is quite clear that BPH is not a diffuse generalized disease of glandular epithelium due to androgen imbalance within the glandular epi-thelium or due to systemic changes in the androgen: estrogen ratio. It is a focal, stromal-induced disease affecting the transition and periurethral zones, pro-ducing micronodule formation by a stromal-epithelial interaction that appears to be mediated by growth factors. Androgen appears to act through TGF-α expression to regulate the expression of other growth factors. The micronodules enlarge and coalesce, per-haps with an altered balance between cell growth and programmed cell death, which is also mediated by growth factor activity. This, in turn, produces an effect on the prostatic urethra, possibly by distortion, to produce bladder outflow obstruction. This, however, is only one of the symptom complexes found in aging patients who have histological BPH, and in some, nonobstructive BPH may well produce symptoms by means that are not entirely clear. Others, possibly as a result of a vascular accident within the prostate or otherwise because of sympathetic stimulation or super-added obstruction by external compression in consti-pation or by epithelial edema in urinary infection, develop acute retention. Others develop detrusor instability as a consequence of the secondary changes induced by obstruction in the detrusor cells, although many patients with BPH will have detrusor instability coincidentally as a result of this. Still others, possibly as a result of the coincidence of BPH in conjunction with the impaired detrusor contractility that is commonly seen with the aging bladder, develop detrusor decompensation and the symptom complex that leads ultimately to chronic retention and overflow incontinence. In some of these patients, the obstructive element causes high intravesical pressures, leading to structural and functional abnormalities of the upper urinary tract and thus to renal impairment and renal failure.

It should again be stated that some of the changes outlined in the last paragraph are hypothetical and unproven, but are nonetheless more likely to be accurate than the rather simplistic ideas hitherto promulgated on the basis of "prostatic enlargement," "urethral compression," and "obstruction" leading to "prostatism."

A more pragmatic approach considers the clinical impact of lower urinary tract symptoms (whether directly or indirectly related to BPH, or due to other disease or aging processes) in relation to the natural history of BPH or its treatment. The clinical diagnosis of BPH is made by demonstrating prostatic enlargement in the presence of typical symptoms, and exclusion of other significant urinary tract disease (71). Its diagnosis represents opportunity for various management options with various efficacy, risks, and side effects. Symptom scores that are valid for BPH tend therefore to be used for initial assessment of symptoms but may in fact reflect changes due to various underlying pathophysiologies. Flow rate and residual volume assessment should be carried out according to practice guidelines (72). Serum creatinine measurement is generally recommended in view of associated chronic renal disease (73), and PSA is measured principally for prostate cancer risk assessment.

Therapeutic objectives including symptom reduction and improved quality of life are consistently achieved in the majority of men with uncomplicated BPH by pharmacological treatment, particularly α blockade, 5-α reductase inhibition, or their combination (74,75). The Medical Therapy of Prostatic Symptoms (MTOPS) study was a landmark in demonstrating the utility of combined α-blockade and 5-α reductase inhibition, particularly for men with higher symptom score (mean IPSS 17), larger prostate volume (mean 32 cc), and higher PSA level (>1.5 ng/mL) (74). The success of these treatments lies in their achieving overall benefit, and providing acceptable balance between therapeutic convenience and its side effects (whether or not presenting symptoms were specifically obstructive or even directly due to BPH). Recent interest has arisen in alternative pharmacological interventions including muscarinic blockade (76), botulinum toxin (77), and other lower urinary tract receptor (78).

In recommending treatment, it is important to understand the natural history of the untreated disease. The Olmsted County Study of Urinary Symptoms and Health Status Among Men was an important longitudinal, community, cohort study demonstrating progressive prostatic growth, decline in flow rate, and increasing prostate-related symptoms with age (79). The development of prostatic enlargement and its relationship with baseline PSA level, with higher PSA levels predicting enlargement, was shown in the Baltimore Longitudinal Study of Aging (80). Prior historical studies of the natural history of untreated BPH had emphasized that clinical deterioration in symptomatic men was by no means inevitable, that the clinical course of BPH may be episodic, and that spontaneous improvement may occur in a significant proportion of those not proceeding to surgery (81). The trend for improvement may also be seen with symptomatic improvement after lifestyle modification, or with symptomatic improvement within the placebo arm of randomized trials, or more simply with statistical regression toward the mean when observing a highly selected population. These considerations, taken together with an association between sexual dysfunction and BPH (82), indicate that some aspects of lower urinary tract function relate to modifiable risk factors, for which lifestyle, diet and physical exercise may be important. Their modifications may also have a wider impact on men's health, aging, cardiovascular disease, and autonomic nervous system activity (83,84).

In recent years, increasing interest has focused on the progressive course of benign hyperplasia and its risk factors. In the Olmsted County Study and the Health Professionals Followup Study, the risk of retention was 6.8/1000 and 4.5/1000, respectively (85,86). While recognizing the importance of observational community studies, present understanding has been substantially influenced by placebo arms of pharmacotherapy trials where outcomes of interest include symptom deterioration, incontinence, acute urinary retention, development of urinary tract infection or renal insufficiency, and need for surgical treatment. Taking these as indicators of clinical progression, symptom deterioration is by far the most frequent, representing around 80% of events (87). Progression overall, however, is relatively uncommon, as defined by all indicators. In the MTOPS study, the risk of clinical progression in the placebo arm was 4.5 per 100 man-years, representing a total risk of 17% at 4 years, including symptom deterioration in 14%, retention in 2%, and surgery in 5% (88). Clinical progression in men with BPH is predicted by baseline prostate volume, and serum PSA, impacting risk of symptom deterioration, flow rate decline, urinary retention, and need for surgery (87,89). In contrast to treatment with the 5-α reductase inhibitor finasteride that reduces all these measures of progression, alfuzosin reduces all except urinary retention (90).

Particular concern has focused on the risk of developing acute urinary retention. Pharmaceutical trials have emphasized that retention develops more frequently when the clinical diagnosis of BPH is associated with certain baseline characteristics that include large prostate volume, elevated PSA not due to prostate cancer, prostatic inflammation, lower maximum flow rate, higher postvoid residual volume, previous acute retention, older age, and symptom deterioration (86,88,91–93). Review of reported pharmacotherapy trials indicates spontaneous acute urinary retention rates in placebo arms of between 0.9% and 5.2%, though comparison or extrapolation of such figures are of little validity owing to variability in trial duration, individual enrollment, and follow-up (94). Furthermore, the significance of acute retention may vary as clinical outcomes and potential to restore spontaneous voiding may relate to prostate size (95) and whether retention is precipitated or spontaneous—spontaneous retention reportedly having a greater need for surgery (96). Finally, the likelihood of successful voiding trial after a first episode of retention may be further modified by treatment, particularly with α-blockers (97).

Treatment with a 5-α reductase inhibitor alone may reduce the risk of retention or surgery by at least 55% (98), or more in high-risk individuals (89). The clinical impact of 5-α reductase inhibition and combination therapy relates to prostate volume at baseline. Medications with adrenergic or anticholinergic activity may increase the risk of acute urinary retention (86). The association of inflammation with aging, lower urinary tract symptoms, progression of benign hyperplasia and its relationship to the development of malignant prostatic disease is attracting interest (91,99), and may indicate a role for estrogen, estrogen receptors α and β, and selective estrogen receptor modulators in the prostate (100,101).

A hypothesis proposing that clinical progression is specifically attributable to progression of benign hyperplasia would be supported where treatment that specifically targets the prostate pathology also reduces the risk of adverse clinical outcomes; in contrast, failure to prevent clinical progression might indicate the impact of other pathophysiology. Indeed, symptom deterioration on treatment with alfuzosin has been shown to be associated with higher baseline post-void residuals and their progressive worsening, as well as a greater risk of BPH-related endpoints (102). The failure of BPH therapy to prevent clinical progression indicates the need for more precise understanding of lower urinary tract pathophysiology as well as optimal treatment for risk reduction and prevention of retention (103,104).

Thus, there is an uncertain relation between histological BPH, lower urinary tract symptoms, response to treatments for BPH, and pathophysiological events underlying clinical progression. Advances have principally been in symptom management rather than overall or long-term strategic therapy for BPH. Further research may identify markers for more efficacious strategies (105).

Urodynamic Aspects

It has already been suggested that BPH may be asymptomatic or symptomatic, and that symptoms may arise purely and simply from the condition itself by virtue of its effects on the prostate alone or from its secondary obstructive effect on the prostatic urethra. Mention has been made of the secondary effects that obstruction can have on the previously normal bladder, leading to detrusor instability, and on the aging bladder, hastening the process begun by aging and leading through progressive degrees of detrusor decompensation to chronic retention with overflow; and that in the latter category high intravesical pressures can lead to obstructive changes in the upper tracts, leading ultimately to renal failure. Also mentioned have been those factors that can act in BPH to cause acute retention.

Symptom severity, which is increasingly being defined by symptom scores (106–108), can be used as selection criteria for surgery. When symptom scores are high, 90% of men will experience substantial improvement in symptoms after surgery, even in the absence of proven urodynamic obstruction (109,110). In addition, the symptoms of BPH in obstructed patients seem to be relieved by thermotherapy and other recent "alternative treatments" for this condition without any effect on flow (111).

Urinary symptoms may equally be the result of detrusor instability that has developed as a consequence of obstruction, in which case the patient may have both obstructive and irritative symptoms, and they might equally be relieved by transurethral resection of the prostate if relief of the obstruction causes the detrusor to return to normal function.

Unfortunately, those same urinary symptoms may occur as a result of "idiopathic" detrusor instability that the patient has developed for some entirely different reason, and the fact that he might coincidentally have histological BPH is irrelevant. Such a patient will not benefit from transurethral resection of the prostate because the instability will persist.

Similarly, a patient with a poorly contractile bladder may have it in association with, or even, perhaps, as a consequence of, outflow obstruction due to BPH and might therefore benefit from transurethral resection of the prostate. But, equally, the poorly contractile bladder may be an age-related phenomenon and coincidental BPH may not be causing any symptoms, in which case transurethral resection of the prostate would not be helpful (112,113).

Clearly, therefore, BPH is not always obstructive but may nonetheless cause symptoms, generally of an irritative nature, and, equally, those symptoms may occur for other reasons than BPH, generally arising in the bladder smooth muscle as an age-related or other phenomenon, causing detrusor instability or impaired detrusor contractility or a combination of the two.

Somehow, these different phenomena have to be dissected out to determine the cause of a patient's symptoms and to decide how best to treat him, and urodynamic studies of various different types are the means by which this is done in clinical practice.

Historically, only bladder outflow obstruction was considered of any significance. Indeed, 50 years ago, treatment was only considered in the presence of urinary retention or when there was evidence of impaired function of the upper urinary tract and kidneys. More recently, detrusor instability has been recognized as an entity, but even so, detrusor instability and bladder decompensation leading to chronic retention and overflow incontinence were both thought of only as consequences of obstruction rather than conditions that might arise per se. Irritative symptoms in the absence of obstructive instability were largely ignored. It is only the recent interest in symptom scores, in alternative treatments for BPH that reduce symptoms without any effect on urodynamic variables, and in the effect of aging on the bladder that has led to a reconsideration of this historical attitude. Nonetheless, the attitude that only obstruction mattered has established the primacy of the pressure-flow relationship in the objective assessment of BPH in clinical practice.

Urinary obstruction can be regarded as being present when intravesical pressure has to be raised to maintain the urinary flow rate. When an elevated intravesical pressure can no longer maintain the urinary flow rate, the flow rate begins to decline. Thus, in the first stage of obstruction, voiding detrusor pressure is raised above the upper limit of normal (which is about 50 cm H_2O), but the peak urinary flow rate is still greater than 15 mL/sec, which is the lower limit of normal. In the second stage of obstruction, the peak urinary flow rate drops below 15 mL/sec.

This relationship between pressure and flow was likened by Griffiths (114) to the Hill equation, which was a well-established and widely accepted means of describing the relationship between the force of contraction and the speed of shortening of skeletal muscle. Griffiths, by relating detrusor pressure to flow rate in what he called the "bladder output relation," showed that the two relationships were very similar. He also introduced the concept of the "urethral resistance relationship" by relating flow rate to detrusor pressure throughout the period of a voiding detrusor contraction (115). In this way, he was able to distinguish graphically (Fig. 11) between an obstructed system, in which pressure was high and flow was low, and an unobstructed system, in which pressure was low and flow was high. In practice, rather than plot the continuous relationship graphically, Abrams and Griffiths (116) devised a nomogram on which could be plotted the single point of detrusor pressure at maximum urinary flow rate (Fig. 12). Several other physicists, notably Schafer, have devised more sophisticated techniques for the analysis of pressure-flow data, but they are all based on the same principles (117,118).

The two main reasons why physicists are continuing to analyze this pressure-flow relationship are, first, to be able to express it in a single term rather than as a relationship between two variables, particularly if this could be determined noninvasively, and, second, to minimize the equivocal zone.

The desire to find a noninvasive way of extrapolating the pressure-flow relationship is obviously commendable but has so far been unsuccessful. Nonetheless, in the interests of patient comfort and as it is a quick, simple, cheap, and easy test to use, the problem has been circumvented in routine clinical practice by measuring flow rate alone and by inferring the pressure-flow relationship from this measurement (116). In this way, most unobstructed patients with normal flow

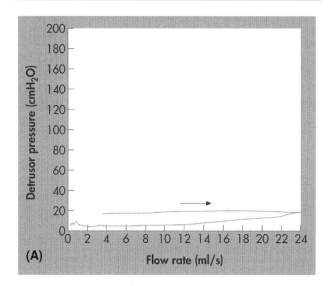

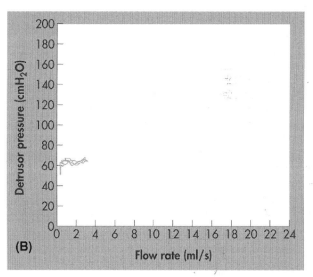

Figure 11 (**A**) A dynamic pressure-flow plot during voiding to illustrate normal emptying with low pressure and high flow. (**B**) A dynamic pressure-flow plot of so-called compressive bladder outflow obstruction due to benign prostatic hyperplasia—with high pressure and low flow.

rates can be saved from ineffective and inappropriate obstruction-relieving surgery. Unfortunately, a low flow rate is not exclusively due to high pressure–low flow outflow obstruction; a low flow rate may also be due to a poorly contracting detrusor.

Poor detrusor contractility also accounts for most of the equivocal results on pressure-flow analysis. Poor detrusor contractility characteristically shows normal or low detrusor pressure and low flow, and this is very common, with an incidence that increases with age. Indeed, as a general rule, all men over the age of 80 have a maximum flow rate of less than 10 mL/sec (119).

Thus, we appear to have three independent variables determining the clinical picture—symptoms, BPH, and bladder outflow obstruction—each of

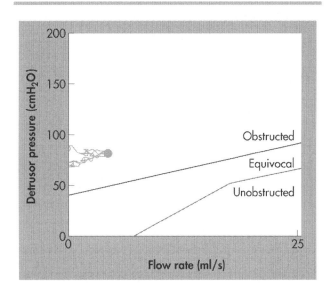

Figure 12 An obstructive pressure-flow plot, similar to Figure 12 in Chapter 16, superimposed on the Abrams-Griffiths nomogram. Normally, only the detrusor pressure at maximum flow (dot) would be marked on the plot—this figure illustrates the principle.

which, as has been said, may be confounded by two age-related abnormalities of detrusor contractility—impaired detrusor contractility and detrusor instability. Irritative symptoms in men with or without BPH correlate strongly with the presence of detrusor instability on urodynamic evaluation (120), and this presumably accounts, at least in part, for the observation that symptom scores are the same in an unselected population of elderly women (in whom detrusor instability is equally common) as they are in an unselected population of elderly men (121). By contrast, objectively demonstrable obstruction correlates poorly with symptoms (122), presumably because obstructive symptoms are less ''bothersome,'' although those with bothersome obstructive symptoms who have objectively demonstrable obstruction, rather than low pressure–low flow bladders because of impaired detrusor contractility, do best after transurethral resection of the prostate (123).

Detrusor instability is clearly an important factor in the patient with BPH, whether it is a secondary consequence of obstruction or coincidental. Nocturia and daytime urgency and frequency are the commonest reasons why elderly men seek medical attention (124), and although there are other causes of these symptoms, detrusor instability is the commonest reason for all these symptoms being present together.

It is generally thought that most instances of detrusor instability in patients with BPH are secondary to obstruction, and that 70% or so will improve symptomatically after transurethral resection of the prostate because the obstruction has been relieved, allowing the detrusor to recover and the pathophysiological changes to reverse. Various experimental studies support this view (125), although they have failed to show complete recovery after relief of obstruction, only a tendency to improve. The alternative view is that detrusor instability in these patients is an entirely age-related phenomenon in both sexes that coincidentally develops at the same time as BPH in men, and that the reason why so many men improve after transurethral resection of the prostate is related to denervation (or de-afferentation, to be more accurate) produced by this surgical procedure (126,127).

Impaired detrusor contractility is more problematic. Like detrusor instability, this is common in the elderly of both sexes and is a regular cause of dissatisfaction in male patients who have undergone transurethral resection of the prostate because they were thought to be obstructed (128). Unlike detrusor instability, which regularly seems to resolve after this operation, impaired detrusor contractility rarely, if ever, improves. This is the first reason for suggesting that impaired detrusor contractility is an independent age-related condition rather than secondary to obstruction, as has always been assumed. The second reason is that experimental models of obstruction cause a thick-walled, trabeculated, high-pressure, unstable bladder, and not chronic retention (129). Thus, the view that impaired contractility—causing residual urine initially, progressing eventually to chronic retention with overflow incontinence—arises as a result of decompensation of the detrusor in the face of continuing obstruction after an initial phase of compensation seems flawed. It may be that if obstruction is superimposed on impaired detrusor contractility, the consequences are correspondingly more severe, and it may be that these patients are prone to high-pressure retention and renal impairment as a result. Either way, impaired detrusor contractility is common in elderly men and women, and may be complicated by superadded detrusor instability in some (130), suggesting that in many, if not all, males with BPH, impaired contractility is an independent variable unrelated to obstruction in its cause.

And so the diagnostic quandary persists. Obstruction is still the only problem that can reliably and predictably be treated, and urodynamic studies that measure both detrusor pressure and urinary flow during voiding are still the only way to diagnose obstruction reliably. With a clinical problem that is so common, this poses logistic problems and, as obstruction is only one part of the picture, the problems are compounded. Nonetheless, a normal flow rate will virtually exclude obstruction, and such patients might be treated by any of the various non-surgical treatments currently available and discussed in detail elsewhere. Otherwise, these patients might benefit from simple reassurance and discussion. Those with a reduced flow rate and a little or no residual urine can confidently be diagnosed as obstructed and treated accordingly. Those with a substantial residual urine volume (250 mL or more on repeated assessment) may have an obstructive component to their symptoms but are more likely to have impaired detrusor contractility, and the likelihood of this increases as the residual urine volume and the patient's age increase, and the likelihood that transurethral resection of the prostate will help these patients symptomatically or objectively decreases accordingly. There are various caveats to these generalizations, but at least they form a basis for considering the problems in clinical practice.

REFERENCES

1. Lowsley O. The development of the human prostate gland with reference to the development of other structures at the neck of the urinary bladder. Am J Anat 1912; 13:299–346.
2. McNeal JE. The zonal anatomy of the prostate. Prostate 1981; 2:35–49.
3. McNeal JE. The prostate gland: morphology and pathology. Monogr Urol 1983; 4:3–6.
4. McNeal JE. The prostate gland: morphology and pathobiology. Monogr Urol 1988; 9:3–4.
5. McNeal JE. Normal histology of the prostate. Am J Surg Pathol 1988; 12:619–633.
6. Marberger M. Drug insight: 5-alpha-reductase inhibitors for the treatment of benign prostatic hyperplasia. Nat Clin Pract Urol 2006; 3(9):495–503.
7. Wilson J, Griffin J, Russell D. Steroid five alpha reductase (II) deficiency. Endocr Rev 1993; 14:577–593.
8. Schweikert H, Totzauer P, Rohr H, et al. Correlated biochemical and stereological studies on testosterone metabolism in the stromal and epithelial compartment of human benign prostatic hyperplasia. J Urol 1985; 134:403–407.
9. Camps JL, Chang SM, Hsu TC, et al. Fibroblast-mediated acceleration of human epithelial tumour growth in vivo. Proc Natl Acad Sci U S A 1990; 87:75–79.
10. Cunha GR, Battle E, Young P, et al. Role of epithelial–mesenchymal interactions in the differentiation and spatial organisation of visceral smooth muscle. Epithelial Cell Biol 1992; 1:76–83.
11. Bruchovski N, Lesser B, Van Doorn E, et al. Hormonal effects on cell proliferation in rat prostate. Vitam Horm 1975; 33:61–102.
12. Lee C, Sensibar JA, Dudek SM, et al. Prostatic ductal system in rats: regional variation in morphological and functional activities. Biol Reprod 1990; 43:1079–1086.
13. Begun FP, Story MT, Hopp KA, et al. Regional concentration of basic fibroblast growth factor in normal and benign hyperplastic human prostates. J Urol 1995; 153:839–843.
14. Story MT, Hopp KA, Meier DA, et al. Influence of transforming growth factor beta 1 and other growth factors on basic fibroblast growth factor level and proliferation of cultured human prostate-derived fibroblasts. Prostate 1993; 22:183–197.
15. Taylor TB, Ramsdell JS. Transforming growth factor alpha and its receptor are expressed on the epithelium of the rat prostate gland. Endocrinology 1993; 113:1306–1308.
16. Gosling JA, Dixon DS. The structure and innervation of smooth muscle in the wall of the bladder neck and proximal urethra. Br J Urol 1975; 47:549–552.
17. Hedlund H, Anderson K, Larsson B. Alpha adrenoceptors and muscarinic receptors in the isolated human prostate. J Urol 1985; 134:1291–1293.
18. Bartsch G, Muller H, Oberholzer M, et al. Light microscopic and stereological analysis of the normal human prostate and of benign prostatic hyperplasia. J Urol 1979; 122:487–491.
19. Shapiro E, Hartanto V, Lepor H. The response to alpha blockade in benign prostatic hyperplasia is related to the percent area density of prostate smooth muscle. Prostate 1992; 21:297–307.
20. Bylund DB, Eikenberg DC, Hieble JP, et al. International Union of Pharmacology nomenclature of adrenoceptors. Pharmacol Rev 1994; 46:121–136.
21. Forray C, Bard JA, Wetzel JM, et al. The alpha-1 adrenergic receptor that mediates smooth muscle contraction in the human prostate has the pharmacological properties of the cloned human alpha-1c subtype. Mol Pharmacol 1994; 45:703–709.
22. Lieberman C, Nogimori T, Wu CF, et al. TRH pharmacokinetics and nerve stimulation evoked prostatic fluid secretion during TRH infusion in the dog. Acta Endocrinol (Copenh) 1989; 120:134–142.
23. Gu J, Polak JM, Probert L, et al. Peptidergic innervation of the human male genital tract. J Urol 1983; 130:386–391.
24. Crowe R, Chapple C, Burnstock G. The human prostate gland: a histochemical and immunohisto chemical study of neuropeptides, serotonin, dopamine beta hydroxylase and acetylcholinesterase in autonomic nerves and ganglia. Br J Urol 1991; 68:53–61.
25. Brindley G. Pathophysiology of erection and ejaculation. In: Hendry W, Whitfield H, eds. A Textbook of Genitourinary Surgery. London: Churchill Livingstone, 1988:1083–1094.
26. Gil-Vernet J, Alvarez-Vijande R, Gil-Vernet J, Jr. Ejaculation in men: a dynamic endorectal ultrasonographical study. Br J Urol 1994; 73:442–448.
27. Tauber PF, Zaneveld LJD, Propping D, et al. Components of human split ejaculate. J Reprod Fertil 1975; 43:249–267.
28. Kennedy AM, Morrell JM, Siviter RJ, et al. Fertilisation promoting peptide in reproductive tissues and semen of the male marmoset. Mol Reprod Dev 1997; 47:113–119.
29. Williams-Ashman HG, Cannellakis ZN. Polyamines in mammalian biology and medicine. Perspect Biol Med 1979; 22:421–453.
30. Lilja H. Structure and function of prostatic and seminal vesicle-secreted proteins involved in the gelatin and liquefaction of human semen. Scand J Clin Lab Invest Suppl 1988; 48:13–17.
31. Coffey DS. Physiology of male reproduction: the biochemical and physiology of the prostate and seminal vesicles. In: Harrison JH, Gittes RF, Perlmutter AD, et al., eds. Campbell's Urology, Vol. 1. 4th ed. Philadelphia: WB Saunders, 1978:61–94.
32. Fair WR, Wehner N. The prostatic antibacterial factor: identity and significance. In: Marberger H, ed. Prostatic Disease, Vol. 6. New York: Alan R Liss, 1976:383.
33. Grayhack JT, Kropp KA. Changes with aging in prostatic fluid: citric acid and phosphatase and lactic dehydrogenase concentration in man. J Urol 1965; 56:6–11.
34. Kvist U. Reversible inhibition of nuclear chromatin decondensation (NCD) ability of human spermatozoa induced by prostatic fluid. Acta Physiol Scand 1980; 109:73–78.
35. Kvist U. Importance of spermatozoal zinc as temporary inhibitor of sperm nuclear chromatin decondensation ability in man. Acta Physiol Scand 1980; 109:79–84.
36. Kvist U, Kjellberg J, Bjorndahl L, et al. Seminal fluid from men with agenesis of the Wolffian ducts: zinc binding properties and effects on sperm chromatin stability. Int J Androl 1990; 13:245–252.
37. Greenwald P, Kirmes V, Polan A, et al. Cancer of the prostate among men with BPH. J Natl Cancer Inst 1974; 355:53–56.
38. Carter H, Plantadosi S, Isaacs J. Clinical evidence for and implications of the multistep development of prostate cancer. J Urol 1990; 143:742–746.
39. Spiro L, Labay G, Orkin L. Prostatic infarction: role in acute urinary retention. Urology 1974; 3:345–347.
40. Cuchi A. The development of detrusor instability in prostatic obstruction in relation to sequential changes in voiding dynamics. J Urol 1994; 51:1342–1344.

41. Levin RM, Longhurst PA, Monson FC, et al. Effect of bladder outlet obstruction on the morphology, physiology and pharmacology of the bladder. Prostate Suppl 1990; 3:9–26.

42. Glynn R, Campion E, Bouchard G, et al. The development of benign prostatic hyperplasia among volunteers in the normative aging study. Am J Epidemiol 1985; 121:78–90.

43. Adlercreutz H. Western diet and Western diseases: some hormonal and biochemical mechanisms and associations. Scand J Clin Invest Suppl 1990; 50:3–23.

44. Sanda M, Beatty T, Stautzman R. Genetic susceptibility of benign prostatic hyperplasia. J Urol 1994; 151:115–119.

45. Rosen RC, Giuliano F, Carson CC. Sexual dysfunction and lower urinary tract symptoms (LUTS) associated with benign prostatic hyperplasia (BPH). Eur Urol 2005; 47(6): 824–837.

46. McVary K. Lower urinary tract symptoms and sexual dysfunction: epidemiology and pathophysiology. BJU Int 2006; 97(suppl 2):23–28.

47. Yassin A, Saad F, Hoesl CE, et al. Alpha-adrenoceptors are a common denominator in the pathophysiology of erectile function and BPH/LUTS—implications for clinical practice. Andrologia 2006; 38(1):1–12.

48. Giuliano F. Lower urinary tract symptoms and sexual dysfunction: a common approach. BJU Int 2008; 101 (suppl 3):22–26.

49. McNeal JE. Origin and evolution of benign prostatic enlargement. Investig Urol 1978; 15:340–345.

50. Eble JN, Tejada E. Prostatic stromal hyperplasia with bizarre nuclei. Arch Pathol Lab Med 1991; 115:87–89.

51. Leong SS, Vogt PF, Yu GM. Atypical stroma with muscle hyperplasia of the prostate. Urology 1988; 31:163–167.

52. McNeal JE. The pathobiology of nodular hyperplasia. In: Bostwick DG, ed. Pathology of the Prostate. New York: Churchill Livingstone, 1990:31–36.

53. Franks LM. Benign nodular hyperplasia of the prostate: a review. Ann R Coll Surg Engl 1954; 14:92–106.

54. Partin AW, Oesterling JE, Epstein JI, et al. Influence of age and endocrine factors on the volume of benign prostatic hyperplasia. J Urol 1991; 145:405–409.

55. Isaacs JT. Antagonistic effect of androgen on prostatic cell death. Prostate 1984; 5:545–547.

56. Sensibar JA, Griswold MD, Sylvester SR, et al. Prostatic ductal system in rats: regional variation in localisation of an androgen-repressed gene product, sulphated glycoprotein-2. Endocrinology 1991; 128:2091–2102.

57. Steiner MS. Review of peptide growth factors in benign prostatic hyperplasia and urological malignancy. J Urol 1995; 153:1085–1096.

58. Gregory H, Willshire IR, Kavanagh JP, et al. Urogastrone–epidermal growth factor concentrations in prostatic fluid of normal individuals and patients with benign prostatic hypertrophy. Clin Sci 1986; 70:359–363.

59. Folkman J, Klagsbrun M, Sasse J, et al. Heparin-binding angiogenic protein—basic fibroblast growth factor—is stored within the basement membrane. Am J Pathol 1988; 130:393–400.

60. Ku PT, D'amore P. Regulation of fibroblast growth factor (bFGF) gene and protein expression following its release from sublethally injured endothelial cells. J Cell Biochem 1995; 58:328–343.

61. Yan G, Fukaborvi Y, Nikolaropoulos S, et al. Heparin-binding keratinocyte growth factor is a candidate for stromal to epithelial andromedin. Mol Endocrinol 1992; 6:2123–2128.

62. Yan G, Fukabori Y, McBride G, et al. Exon switching and activation of stromal and embryonic fibroblast growth factor (FGF)–FGF-receptor genes in prostate epithelial cells accompany stromal independence and malignancy. Mol Cell Biol 1993; 13:4513–4522.

63. Sporn MB, Roberts AB. TFT-beta: problems and prospects. Cell Regul 1990; 1:875–882.

64. Brogli E, Wu T, Namiki A, et al. Indirect angiogenic cytokines upregulate VEGF and bFGF gene expression in vascular smooth muscle cells, whereas hypoxia upregulates VEGF expression only. Circulation 1994; 90: 649–652.

65. Roberts AB, Sporn MB. Physiological actions and clinical applications of transforming growth factor-beta (TGF-β). Growth Factors 1993; 8:1–9.

66. Timme TL, Truong LD, Merz VW, et al. Mesenchymal epithelial interactions and transforming growth factor beta expression during mouse prostate morphogenesis. Endocrinology 1994; 134:1039–1045.

67. Millan FA, Denhez F, Kondaiah P, et al. Embryonic gene expression patterns of TGF beta-1, beta-2 and beta-3 suggest different development functions in vivo. Development 1991; 111:131–143.

68. Sporn MB, Roberts AB. Interactions of retinoids and transforming growth factor beta in regulation of cell differentiation and proliferation. Mol Endocrinol 1991; 5:3–7.

69. Katz AE, Benson MC, Wise GJ, et al. Gene activity during the early phase of androgen-stimulated rat prostatic regrowth. Cancer Res 1989; 49:5889–5894.

70. Cho KS, Kim J, Choi YD, et al. The overlooked cause of benign prostatic hyperplasia: prostatic urethral angulation. Med Hypotheses 2008; 70(3):532–535.

71. Madersbacher S, Alivizatos G, Nordling J, et al. EAU 2004 guidelines on assessment, therapy and follow-up of men with lower urinary tract symptoms suggestive of benign prostatic obstruction (BPH guidelines). Eur Urol 2004; 46(5): 547–554.

72. Gravas S, Tzortzis V, Melekos MD. Translation of benign prostatic hyperplasia guidelines into clinical practice. Curr Opin Urol 2008; 18(1):56–60.

73. Rule AD, Lieber MM, Jacobsen SJ. Is benign prostatic hyperplasia a risk factor for chronic renal failure? J Urol 2005; 173(3):691–696.

74. McConnell JD, Roehrborn CG, Bautista OM, et al. The long-term effect of doxazosin, finasteride, and combination therapy on the clinical progression of benign prostatic hyperplasia. N Engl J Med 2003; 349(25):2387–2398.

75. McVary KT. A review of combination therapy in patients with benign prostatic hyperplasia. Clin Ther 2007; 29(3): 387–398.

76. Kaplan SA, Roehrborn CG, Rovner ES, et al. Tolterodine and tamsulosin for treatment of men with lower urinary tract symptoms and overactive bladder: a randomized controlled trial. JAMA 2006; 296(19):2319–2328.

77. Antunes AA, Srougi M, Coelho RF, et al. Botulinum toxin for the treatment of lower urinary tract symptoms due to benign prostatic hyperplasia. Nat Clin Pract Urol 2007; 4(3): 155–160.

78. Andersson KE. LUTS treatment: future treatment options. Neurourol Urodyn 2007; 26(6 suppl):934–947.

79. Roberts RO, Jacobsen SJ, Jacobson DJ, et al. Longitudinal changes in peak urinary flow rates in a community-based cohort. J Urol 2000; 163(1):107–113.

80. Wright EJ, Fang J, Metter EJ, et al. Prostate specific antigen predicts the long-term risk of prostate enlargement: results from the Baltimore Longitudinal Study of Aging. J Urol 2002; 167(6):2484–2487.

81. Ball AJ, Feneley RCL, Abrams PH. The natural history of untreated "prostatism." Br J Urol 1981; 53:613–616.

82. Gur S, Kadowitz PJ, Hellstrom WJ. Guide to drug therapy for lower urinary tract symptoms in patients with benign

prostatic obstruction: implications for sexual dysfunction. Drugs 2008; 68(2):209–229.

83. Parsons JK, Kashefi C. Physical activity, benign prostatic hyperplasia, and lower urinary tract symptoms. Eur Urol 2008; 53(6):1228–1235.

84. McVary KT, Rademaker A, Lloyd GL, et al. Autonomic nervous system overactivity in men with lower urinary tract symptoms secondary to benign prostatic hyperplasia. J Urol 2005; 174(4 pt 1):1327–1433.

85. Jacobsen SJ, Jacobson DJ, Girman CJ, et al. Natural history of prostatism: risk factors for acute urinary retention. J Urol 1997; 158(2):481–487.

86. Meigs JB, Barry MJ, Giovannucci E, et al. Incidence rates and risk factors for acute urinary retention: the health professionals followup study. J Urol 1999; 162(2):376–382.

87. Roehrborn CG. Alfuzosin 10 mg once daily prevents overall clinical progression of benign prostatic hyperplasia but not acute urinary retention: results of a 2-year placebo-controlled study. BJU Int 2006; 97(4):734–741.

88. Crawford ED, Wilson SS, McConnell JD, et al. Baseline factors as predictors of clinical progression of benign prostatic hyperplasia in men treated with placebo. J Urol 2006; 175(4):1422–1426.

89. Roehrborn CG, McConnell JD, Lieber M, et al. Serum prostate-specific antigen concentration is a powerful predictor of acute urinary retention and need for surgery in men with clinical benign prostatic hyperplasia. PLESS Study Group. Urology 1999; 53(3):473–480.

90. Kaplan SA, McConnell JD, Roehrborn CG, et al. Combination therapy with doxazosin and finasteride for benign prostatic hyperplasia in patients with lower urinary tract symptoms and a baseline total prostate volume of 25 ml or greater. J Urol 2006; 175(1):217–220.

91. Nickel JC, Roehrborn CG, O'Leary MP, et al. The relationship between prostate inflammation and lower urinary tract symptoms: examination of baseline data from the REDUCE trial. Eur Urol 2008; 54(6):1379–1384.

92. Emberton M, Elhilali M, Matzkin H, et al. Symptom deterioration during treatment and history of AUR are the strongest predictors for AUR and BPH-related surgery in men with LUTS treated with alfuzosin 10 mg once daily. Urology 2005; 66(2):316–322.

93. Kefi A, Koseoglu H, Celebi I, et al. Relation between acute urinary retention, chronic prostatic inflammation and accompanying elevated prostate-specific antigen. Scand J Urol Nephrol 2006; 40(2):155–160.

94. Roehrborn CG. Reporting of acute urinary retention in BPH treatment trials: importance of patient follow-up after discontinuation and case definitions. Urology 2002; 59(6):811–815.

95. McNeill AS, Rizvi S, Byrne DJ. Prostate size influences the outcome after presenting with acute urinary retention. BJU Int 2004; 94(4):559–562.

96. Roehrborn CG, Bruskewitz R, Nickel GC, et al. Urinary retention in patients with BPH treated with finasteride or placebo over 4 years. Characterization of patients and ultimate outcomes. The PLESS Study Group. Eur Urol 2000; 37(5):528–536.

97. McNeill SA, Hargreave TB, Roehrborn CG. Alfuzosin 10 mg once daily in the management of acute urinary retention: results of a double-blind placebo-controlled study. Urology 2005; 65(1):83–89.

98. McConnell JD, Bruskewitz R, Walsh P, et al. The effect of finasteride on the risk of acute urinary retention and the need for surgical treatment among men with benign prostatic hyperplasia. Finasteride Long-Term Efficacy and Safety Study Group. N Engl J Med 1998; 338(9):557–563.

99. Mishra VC, Allen DJ, Nicolaou C, et al. Does intraprostatic inflammation have a role in the pathogenesis and progression of benign prostatic hyperplasia? BJU Int 2007; 100(2):327–331.

100. Prins GS, Korach KS. The role of estrogens and estrogen receptors in normal prostate growth and disease. Steroids 2008; 73(3):233–244.

101. Sciarra A, Mariotti G, Salciccia S, Gomez AA, Monti S, Toscano V, et al. Prostate growth and inflammation. J Steroid Biochem Mol Biol 2008; 108(3–5):254–260.

102. Roehrborn CG. BPH progression: concept and key learning from MTOPS, ALTESS, COMBAT, and ALF-ONE. BJU Int 2008; 101(suppl 3):17–21.

103. Khastgir J, Khan A, Speakman M. Acute urinary retention: medical management and the identification of risk factors for prevention. Nat Clin Pract Urol 2007; 4(8): 422–431.

104. Parsons JK. Modifiable risk factors for benign prostatic hyperplasia and lower urinary tract symptoms: new approaches to old problems. J Urol 2007; 178(2):395–401.

105. Mullins C, Lucia MS, Hayward SW, et al. A comprehensive approach toward novel serum biomarkers for benign prostatic hyperplasia: the MPSA Consortium. J Urol 2008; 179(4):1243–1256.

106. Boyarski S, Jones G, Paulson DF, et al. A new look at bladder neck obstruction by the Food and Drug Administration regulators: guidelines for the investigation of benign prostatic hypertrophy. Trans Am Assoc Genitourin Surg 1977; 68:29–32.

107. Madsen PO, Iversen P. A point system for selecting operative candidates. In: Hinman F Jr., ed. Benign Prostatic Hypertrophy. New York: Springer-Verlag, 1983: 763–765.

108. Barry MJ, Fowler FJ, O'Leary MP, et al. The American Urological Association symptom index for benign prostatic hyperplasia. J Urol 1992; 148:1549–1557.

109. McConnell JD, Barry MJ, Bruskewitz RC, et al. Benign prostatic hyperplasia: diagnosis and treatment. In: Clinical Practice Guidelines, No. 8. Rockville: U.S. Department of Health and Human Services1994:99–103.

110. Emberton M, Neal DE, Black N, et al. The effect of prostatectomy on symptom severity and quality of life. Br J Urol 1996; 77:233–247.

111. Tubaro A, Ogden C, de la Rosette J, et al. The prediction of clinical outcome from thermotherapy by pressure flow study. Results of a European multicentre study. World J Urol 1994; 12:352–356.

112. Neal DE, Styles RA, Powell PH, et al. Relationships between detrusor function and residual urine in men undergoing prostatectomy. Br J Urol 1987; 60:560–566.

113. George NJR, Feneley RCL, Roberts JBM. Identification of the poor risk patient with prostatism and detrusor failure. Br J Urol 1986; 58:290–295.

114. Griffiths DJ. Urodynamics: the Mechanics and Hydrodynamics of the Lower Urinary Tract. Medical Physics Handbook 4. Bristol: Adam Hilger, 1980.

115. Griffiths DJ. Urethral resistance to flow: the urethral resistance relation. Urol Int 1975; 30:28.

116. Abrams PH, Griffiths DJ. The assessment of prostatic obstruction from urodynamic measurements and from residual urine. Br J Urol 1979; 51:129–134.

117. Van Mastrigt R, Rollema HJ. Urethral resistance and urinary bladder contractility before and after transurethral resection as determined by the computer program CLIM. Neurourol Urodyn 1988; 7:226–230.

118. Schafer W. Principles and clinical application of advanced urodynamic analysis of voiding function. Urol Clin North Am 1990; 17:553–566.

119. Jorgensen JB, Jensen KME, Morgensen P. Age-related variation in urinary flow variables and flow cure patterns in elderly males. Br J Urol 1992; 69:265–271.

120. Olssen CA, Goluboft ET, Chang DT, et al. Urodynamics and the etiology of post-prostatectomy incontinence. J Urol 1994; 151:2063–2065.

121. Lepor H, Machi G. Comparison of AUA symptom index in unselected males and females between fifty-five and seventy-nine years of age. Urology 1993; 42:36–40.

122. Barry MJ, Cockett ATK, Holtgrewe HL, et al. Relationship of symptoms of prostatism to commonly used physiological and anatomical measures of the severity of benign prostatic hyperplasia. J Urol 1993; 150:351–356.

123. Abrams P. In support of pressure flow studies for evaluating men with lower urinary tract symptoms. Urology 1994; 44:153–155.

124. Roberts RO, Rhodes T, Panser LA. Natural history of prostatism: worry and embarrassment of firm urinary symptoms and health care-seeking behaviour. Urology 1994; 43:621–628.

125. Malkowiez SB, Wein AJ, Elbadawi A, et al. Acute biochemical and functional alterations in the partially obstructed rabbit urinary bladder. J Urol 1986; 136:1324–1329.

126. Susset JG. The effect of aging and prostatic obstruction on detrusor morphology and function. In: Hinman C Jr., ed. Benign Prostatic Hypertrophy. New York: Springer-Verlag, 1985:653–665.

127. Luutzeyer W, Hannapel J, Schafer W. Sequential events in prostatic obstruction. In: Hinman C Jr., ed. Benign Prostatic Hypertrophy. New York: Springer-Verlag, 1985: 693–700.

128. Schafer W, Rubben H, Noppeney R, et al. Obstructed and unobstructed prostatic obstruction. A plea for urodynamic objectivation of bladder outflow obstruction in benign prostatic hyperplasia. World J Urol 1989; 6:198–203.

129. Dixon JS, Gilpin CJ, Gilpin SA, et al. Sequential morphologic changes in the pig detrusor in response to chronic partial urethral obstruction. Br J Urol 1989; 64:385–390.

130. Coolsaet BRLA, Blok C. Detrusor properties related to prostatism. Neurourol Urodyn 1986; 5:435–441.

20

Genetic and Biological Alterations in Cancer

Vincent J. Gnanapragasam

Uro-oncology Group, Department of Oncology, Hutchinson MRC Research Centre,
University of Cambridge, Cambridge, U.K.

INTRODUCTION

The hallmark of the cancer cell is its ability to escape from the normal regulatory mechanisms that control cellular biology. Thousands of research studies have been published on the changes that occur in the cancer cell that might facilitate this process. While some changes are generic to many tumor types, others are specific. Changes are known to occur at all levels of the cell and can influence events from the DNA code right up to its posttranslational modification into a functional protein. The serial accumulation of genetic and biological changes is thought to drive the transition from normal to dysplastic and eventually malignant cells. Collectively genes that increase the potential for tumorigenesis at any level of cell function are termed oncogenes while those whose loss facilitates cancer are termed tumor suppressor genes. In this chapter, only the principles of genetic and biological changes will be discussed with salient examples in urological cancers (Fig. 1). A full list of all the known alterations would take many books to cover.

GENETIC CHANGES IN CANCER

The basis of all function in the cell is the data contained in the genome. It is clear that the coding sequences, which are transcribed into mRNA represent only a part of the known human genome. The non-coding DNA is now thought to contain putative regulatory elements whose function in controlling gene expression is not fully understood. Indeed, in recent studies important predisposition loci for prostate cancer have been identified in so called gene poor regions and their function in the cell is unclear (1). Within the genome the genetic alterations that can occur and predispose to cancer can include rearrangements and polymorphisms, which alter the normal coding reading sequence.

Chromosomal Rearrangements

Chromosomal rearrangements include translocations, deletions, duplications and inversions. Each of this can be caused by breakage of DNA in the genome followed by rejoining of the broken ends to produce a new chromosomal structure. There are two types of rearrangements. In balanced rearrangements the chromosomal gene order is changed but there is no duplication or removal of any of the DNA. Examples of this include inversion and reciprocal translocations. In imbalanced rearrangements there is a change in the total number of genes in the affected chromosome such as a loss of one copy or the addition of a copy. Examples of these are deletions and duplications. In bladder cancer the most well known is the loss of chromosome 9 (either the p or q arm) (2). In clear cell renal caner the loss of 3p by deletion or translocation can be found in over two thirds of tumors (3). In papillary renal cancers trisomies of chromosome 7,12,16,17 and 20 have all been shown to occur albeit at low frequencies. In testicular germ cell tumors the only consistent abnormality is iso-chromosome 12p where an extra short arm is present. In prostate cancer the most common genetic event to date are gene fusions involving the 5' untranslated region of the androgen dependent TMPRSS2 gene and the ETS family of transcription factors. These changes are though to occur in over 50% of clinical prostate cancers (4).

DNA Polymorphisms

Polymorphisms are sequence variations in the DNA code such as nucleotide substitutions, deletions, insertions and duplications. These alterations may or may not result in changes in protein phenotype and function. Polymorphisms in genes that code for enzymes, for example, have been associated with cancer risk and progression. In bladder cancer polymorphisms in the N-acetyltransferase 1 and 2 enzymes result in amino acid changes that reduce their efficiency in de-activating potential bladder carcinogens (5). Similar polymorphic changes in DNA repair genes can change the cell's ability to repair damaged DNA. The accumulation of damaged DNA can then lead to genetic instability and carcinogenesis. Examples of this include polymorphisms in the XP (xeroderma pigmentosa) and XRCC (X-ray repair cross-complementary) genes that have been detected in bladder and prostate cancer (6).

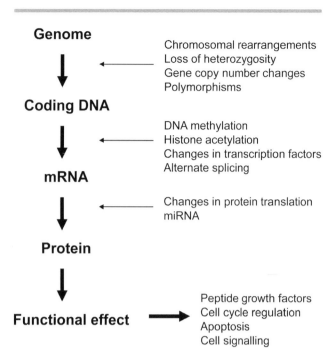

Figure 1 Summary chart of genetic and biological alterations that can occur in cancer cells.

Loss of Heterozygosity

LOH describes the loss of the normal two heterogeneous allele configurations at a gene locus. This can occur through chromosomal rearrangements or polymorphisms. LOH can be detected by using microsatellite analysis (with known simple sequence repeats) or by looking for single nucleotide polymorphisms (SNP). This latter technique can now be done using very large SNP arrays that can screen for thousands of polymorphisms simultaneously. A good example of LOH in a urological cancer is the Wilms tumor. The WT 1 gene is located on chromosome 11p13. Loss of 1 allele at 11p13 has been found in over 40% of tumors suggesting that inactivation of this gene is a critical step in Wilm's tumor development (7). In bladder cancer LOH at 3p, 8p, 13q and 17p have been identified in carcinoma in situ as well as muscle invasive tumors but not in superficial disease highlighting the differences in these tumor types (8).

Gene Copy Number Changes

Increases or loss of expression of a particular molecule can be due to changes at any level. At the most basic is an alteration in the number of gene copies available for transcription. Gene copy number changes are well described in many malignancies. The c-myc gene for instance which encodes a nuclear transcription factor is known to be amplified by an increase in copy number in many tumors including pancreatic, breast and brain cancer. In bladder cancer the ERBB2 receptor gene is known to be amplified at 17q in 10% to 14%

of high-grade cancers (8). Amplification of the androgen receptor (AR) gene is thought to occur in castration resistant prostate cancer and may be an important mechanism by which prostate cancer cells respond to very low levels of androgens (9).

EPIGENETIC CHANGES IN DNA

DNA Methylation

Methylation results in gene silencing by the process of adding a methyl group on a cytosine in the context of a Cytosine-Guanine rich DNA sequence (called CpG islands). CpG islands are frequently found in the promoter region of genes and are usually unmethylated to allow efficient gene transcription. Methylation at CpG islands therefore results in transcriptional silencing by preventing the binding of transcription factors. Methylation also enhances chromatin folding and condensation thus making the gene promoter inaccessible to the transcription machinery. Both abnormal hypermethylation and hypo-methylation can occur in cancer cells. Many tumor suppressor genes have been shown to be silenced by the mechanism of DNA methylation. Numerous studies have been performed to investigate methylated targets in urological cancers. In renal cell cancers a number of genes have been shown to be inactivated by methylation including VHL and RASS1FA. These events occur in between 20% and 30% of cancers (10). In bladder cancer hypermethylation at 5 gene loci including RASS1FA and E Cadherin have been associated with an increased risk of tumor progression (11). Analysis of cell free serum DNA in men with bladder cancer has also suggested that hypermethylation of the APC gene was associated with a poorer clinical outcome following radical cystectomy (12). Gene methylations have also been identified in prostate cancer. One of the most frequent is hypermethylation of the GSTPI gene, which is involved in detoxification by conjugation with glutathione. GSTP1 methylation has been reported in biopsies of over 70% of prostate cancers and also in the serum and urine of patients. These results have prompted its potential use as a tumor marker for prostate cancer detection (13).

Histone Acetylation

Efficient RNA transcription is dependent on the ability of the transcriptional machinery to gain access to the tightly packed DNA. In the normal state DNA is supercoiled around histone proteins which allow the long DNA strand to be compacted. The combination of DNA and histones together comprise the chromatin. Histones proteins are subject to posttranslational modification, which can affect how efficiently the DNA coiled around them is transcribed. Histones consist of a globular domain and a charged NH2 terminal tail and it is this section that is the prime site for protein modification. An important modification is the process of acetylation, which is mediated by histone acetyl transferases (HAT), while deacetylation is mediated by histone deacetylases (HDAC). Acetylation of histone proteins at lysine residues removes positive charges, and reduces the affinity between histones and DNA. This then allows easier access of the transcriptional machinery to gene promoter regions. Histone acetylation therefore enhances transcription while deacetylation represses it. Upregulation of HDAC proteins has been demonstrated in disease progression to androgen insensitive prostate cancer and is associated with a shorter time to biochemical relapse following radical surgery (14,15). Preclinical studies have shown good efficacy of HDAC inhibitors in blocking cell proliferation and inducing growth arrest as well as apoptosis in in vitro and in vivo models of prostate cancer (16,17). These promising results have prompted phase I and II trials into the use of HDAC inhibitors in clinical cancers.

TRANSCRIPTION FACTORS IN CANCER

The transcriptional machinery binds to the promoter of genes and initiates the process of gene transcription. This process is facilitated by transcription factors, which have cognate binding sites at the gene promoter. A complex of more than 20 individual transcription factors can make up the transcriptional engine together with RNA polymerase II. Upregulation of transcription factors is a principal hallmark of cancer biology and a major class of oncogenes. Activation of transcription factors is also the final end point of many signal transduction and stress response pathways. There are numerous families of transcription factors and considerable functional redundancy between them. Specific factors however have been strongly associated with individual urological cancers. Hypoxia inducible factors (HIF) are transcription factors that function to promote cell survival in hypoxic conditions by increasing expression of genes involved in glycolysis as well as new vessel formation. HIF factors are themselves regulated by the VHL protein, which targets them for protein degradation. Mutations of VHL in renal cancer are common events occurring in up to 70% of cases (18,19). This results in increased stability of HIF transcription factors and enhanced expression of its target genes.

Nuclear factor κ B (NF-κB) is a family of at least 6 transcription factors which have an important role in regulating cell proliferation and inhibiting apoptosis. They are activated by a range of mechanisms including interleukin, growth factors and in stress response. In the inactivate state they are maintained at the cell membrane by inhibitors [inhibitors of κ B (IκBs)]. In bladder cancer the level of NF-κB expression is significantly associated with histological grade and tumor stage (20). In renal cell cancers use of a NF-κB inhibitor has shown promising results in blocking tumor growth by inducing cell apoptosis (21). In prostate cancer cell lines androgen-independent prostate tumor cells demonstrate constitutive activation of NF-κB while IκB expression levels were low. In contrast, androgen-sensitive prostate cell lines

expressed low levels of NF-κB (22). Early phase clinical studies with an NF-κB inhibitor (bortezomib) in combination with docetaxel in men with prostate cancer have shown early promise in reducing PSA levels (23).

The ETS family is one of the biggest groups of transcription factors and is involved in many key cellular processes including differentiation, proliferation, migration and angiogenesis. Gene fusions of members of the ETS family have been reported in many tumor types with the best know being the fusion of the FLI-1 transcription factor to the EWS gene in Ewing's sarcoma (24). In 2005 Tomlins et al. published a seminal paper describing the fusion of the androgen regulated TMPRSS2 gene with the ERG and ETV-1 ETS members in a large number of prostate cancers (4). Since then numerous variants of gene fusions between TMPPRSS2 and ETS family members have been reported (25,26). These fusions have been found in between 40% to 60% of primary clinical prostate cancers. This finding provides a strong link between the androgen receptor and a transcription factor in the initiation and progression of prostate cancer. The TMPRS22: ETS fusion has also been proposed as a putative prognostic marker of a poorer outcome following radical prostatectomy and a urine-based assay has shown promise as a potential cancer detection tool (27,28).

ALTERNATIVE SPLICING IN CANCER CELLS

The first step in transcription is the production of pre-mRNA which contains both intron and exon sequences. Splicing occurs when introns are removed and exons are joined to produce the final mRNA for protein translation. Alternative (as opposed to constitutive) splicing allows pre-mRNA to be processed into different final mRNA sequences and hence proteins which may have different functional effects. The process of splicing is performed in the nucleus by the spliceosome (a large multi-protein complex) and is regulated by enhancers and silencers, which identify the exon-intron boundary. It has become recently evident that the process of splicing can be significantly altered in the cancer cell. This may be the result of a mutation in the enhancers and repressors of splicing or due to changes in the splicing machinery itself (29). In bladder cancer, for example, different FGFR3 transcript has been observed in benign as opposed to cancer cells as a result of alternate splicing at the pre-mRNA stage (30). Alternative splicing of fibroblast growth factors (FGF) receptors has also been reported in prostate cancer cells and clinical tissue (31). High throughput techniques have now been introduced to look for global splicing changes in cancer ad other diseases. Li et al. have recently determined mRNA isoform specific signatures for prostate cancers using a large custom made splicing array (32). The significance of splicing changes and their exploitation for therapy is still at an early stage but is an area of active interest among cancer biologists.

CHANGES IN PROTEIN TRANSLATION IN CANCER

Translation is the process by which the information encoded in the mRNA is used to produce the protein. Alterations in the expression or function of the translational machinery can lead to marked changes in protein synthesis, which ultimately is the functional product of the gene. This process occurs at the ribosome where the translation initiation complex binds to mRNA and reads the tri-nucleotide sequence. The initiator complex consists of transfer RNA (tRNA), 40 and 60S ribosomal units and translation factors, which assemble the complex at the 5′ end of the mRNA sequence. Key translation factors in this complex include the eIF family, which has five members with each having a distinct role in translation. eIF4e in particular has a crucial role in translational regulation. Expression of eIF4e is regulated through many different signal transduction pathways including ERK and p38. eIF4e is also regulated by binding proteins such as 4E-BP1, which inactivate its function. Phosphorylation of binding proteins reduces their interaction with eIF4e and results in increased protein translation. One important mechanism is through the mammalian target of rapamycin (mTOR) protein kinase. Rapamycin which inhibits mTOR is used in transplant immuno-suppression to block T cell activation. It has been recently advocated as a promising new anticancer therapy (33). eIF4E itself has been shown to be overexpressed in many cancers including prostate cancer (34). Another mechanism of regulation is by the phosphorylation of the ribosomal 40S protein by S6 kinase (S6K). Phosphorylation of S6K is regulated by among others, the PI3K and mTOR pathways. Translation factors are therefore common targets of signal transduction pathways, which are themselves dysregulated in cancer (see below). Finally protein translation in cancer can also be altered by inherent mutations in the transcribed RNA. This can result in a mutated protein or abnormal protein production. A classic example of this is the BRCA1 protein. In malignant cells the transcript has a longer 5′ untranslated region compared with BRCA 1 in normal mammary tissue. The modified transcript is less efficient during translation and results in a reduction in BRCA1 protein expression.

MicroRNA

miRNA are small single stranded RNA molecules of about 21 to 23 nucleotides. These do not code for proteins and are members of the large family of noncoding RNA which have regulatory functions in the cell. miRNA are a relatively new discovery in gene regulation but are a fast growing family of molecules. They function as regulators of translation by annealing to mRNA and inhibiting the translational machinery. This is achieved through miRNA incorporation into a RNA induced silencing complex (35). This complex then localizes to mRNA with a complimentary strand and cleaves it. This effectively blocks protein translation either with or without associated degradation of the mRNA. To date over 500 hundred miRNAs have been discovered and this number is likely to grow with increasing understanding of their importance and function. miRNAs have been implicated in the regulation of many cellular processes and their role in cancer is unsurprisingly is the subject of intense research. Urological cancers have all been shown to harbour abnormal expression of miRNAs (36,37). Gottardo et al. have shown that 4 miRNAs (mir-28, miR-185, miR-27, and let-7f2) are significantly increased in renal cell carcinoma. In bladder cancer a panel of 10 miRNAs were shown to be increased in comparison with normal controls. In prostate cancer a microarray approach detected 51 miRNAs that were altered between benign and malignant tissue with 37 downregulated (resulting in increased target mRNA translation) and 14 upregulated (reduced target mRNA translation) (38). The authors further proposed that patterns of miRNA expression could distinguish between androgen dependent and independent prostate cancers. The field of cancer relevant miRNA (called OncomiRs) is growing rapidly and is very likely to lead to new therapeutic targets in the near future.

PEPTIDE GROWTH FACTORS IN CANCER

Peptide growth factors play an important role in carcinogenesis and are currently the best exploited in terms of new drug development. Ligands bind to their cognate receptors at the cell membrane and initiate a cascade of downstream signalling that is in general promitogenic and antiapoptotic. The key growth factors implicated in cancer include fibroblast growth factors (FGF), epidermal growth factor (EGF), insulin-like growth factor (IGF), vascular endothelial growth factor (VEGF), platelet derived growth factor (PDGF), and transforming growth factor (TGF). In cancer cells, alterations at every level of growth factor regulation have been found. In prostate cancer both growth factor ligands and receptors have been shown to be upregulated in carcinogenesis and tumor progression (39–41). In the FGF axis for instance, ligands including FGF1, 2, 8, and 17 have been shown to be increased in high-grade and high-stage disease (42–44). FGF10 has been recently implicated as an important stromal-epithelial initiator of prostate tumor development (45). FGF receptor (FGFR)1 is known to be overexpressed as an early event in clinical prostate cancer, and induced expression is causative in the development and progression of tumor in a mouse model (46,47). FGFR4 in contrast is preferentially overexpressed in more advanced tumors.

In bladder cancer the EGF system has emerged as an important target for therapy. EGF receptor (also known as Her 1) is over-expressed in a large number of tumors and expression is associated with tumor grade and stage (48). Another member of the EGF receptor family is the Her 2 receptor, which has no known ligand (termed an orphan receptor) but functions by binding as a homodimer to other EGF receptors. Her 2 has been found to be overexpressed in breast cancer and targeting this receptor (by the Her 2 antibody, Herceptin) has emerged as a promising new therapy. Crucially it is primarily effective in tumors that are known to be Her 2 positive. Her 2 is also known to be over-expressed in bladder cancer but to date the benefits of Herceptin in this tumor have not been encouraging (49,50). Activating mutations of FGFR3 have emerged as a common feature in many bladder cancers. The principal mutation occurs in the extracellular domain, which allows ligand independent dimerization and constitutive activation of the receptor. Intriguingly these mutations are most commonly found in low-grade superficial tumors and are much less apparent in muscle invasive disease. The prognostic significance of FGFR mutations as well as its therapeutic value is currently the subject of much research (51).

In renal cancer VEGF has emerged as the most important growth factor axis in the terms of novel therapy. Up-regulation of VEGF is a key feature in many renal cell cancers. Bevacizumab, an antibody against the VEGF-A isoform has shown clinical efficacy in advanced renal cancer and prolongs time to disease progression in combination with interferon (52). The multiple growth factors that are active in cancers have made it difficult to gain therapeutic benefit from blocking just one axis. This has led to the concept of using inhibitors against multiple targets. An example of this is the multi tyrosine kinase inhibitor sorafenib. This drug is an inhibitor of Raf kinase, PDGF, VEGF receptors 2 and 3 and the c Kit receptor. Initial studies have shown that sorafenib can prolong progression-free survival in patients with advanced clear-cell renal-cell carcinoma in whom previous therapy has failed (53). Sorafenib is currently being evaluated in a multinational randomized trial coordinated by the Medical Research Council in the U.K.

SIGNAL TRANSDUCTION CHANGES IN CANCER

The effect of extracellular stimuli in promoting cell growth and differentiation is mediated through intracellular signalling pathways. These include among others the mitogenic activated protein kinases (MAPK), phosphoinositol 3 kinase (PI3K), and phospholipase C (PLC) pathways. The PI3K pathway is involved in promoting cell survival and anti-apoptosis. One of the key genes lost in prostate cancer, Phosphatase and tensin homologue deleted on chromosome 10 (PTEN) is an inhibitor of PI3K signalling. PTEN loss has been shown to directly contribute to an aggressive and invasive tumor phenotype through enhanced PI3 signalling (54). A principal target of PI3K is Akt, which is turn is known to activate the serine threonine kinase mTOR, which as previously discussed is an important regulator of protein translation. The MAPK family consist of 3 members; extracellular related kinase (ERK), p38 and Jun N-terminal kinase (JNK) also known as stress-activated protein kinase (SAPK). The ERK pathway in particular has an important role in tumor biology and is the principle mediator of the mitogenic effect of many growth factors. In cancer cells this pathway can be switched on inappropriately by a constitutively active upstream component or by continuous or enhanced exposure to the stimulus. A good example of the former is the effect of the Ras oncogenes. Ras is a small GTPase protein that is membrane bound and an upstream component of the ERK cascade. In the normal state it is activated by guanine exchange factors, which are targets of mitogenic stimuli (e.g., phosphorylated growth factor receptors). Mutations in Ras can result in a constitutively active protein in the absence of a stimulus and this induces sustained activation of ERK. Ras mutations have been detected in between 10% to 20% of prostate cancers and 13% of bladder cancers (55,56). Signalling pathways are however more commonly hyper-activated through increased activity of exogenous stimuli, for example, increased growth factor ligands and receptors as previously discussed. EGF mediated ERK activation for instance is responsible for reducing the cytotoxic effect of radiation and increasing clonogenic survival and repopulation following irradiation (57). Inhibition of this pathway has been shown to radiosensitize tumor cells and enhance cell kill. Recently, a separate layer of endogenous regulators of ERK pathway has been reported. These act as negative feedback inhibitors of ERK activity and serve a homeostatic function in normal cells to control the intensity and duration of signalling. Members of this group include Sprouty, similar expression to FGF (Sef) and Spred. Recent work has shown that these inhibitors are downregulated in urological cancers and can result in unattenuated enhanced signalling (58,59).

CELL CYCLE REGULATION CHANGES IN CANCER

The normal cell cycle consists of mitosis (nuclear and cytoplasmic division), G1 (First growth phase), S (DNA synthesis and chromosome replication) and G2 (second growth phase). When the cell is quiescent it is said to enter the G0 phase (out of the cell cycle). This process is controlled by cyclins in complex with cyclin-dependent kinases (CDK) as well as other proteins, which regulates the progression through the cell cycle. The retinoblastoma protein (Rb) functions as an inhibitor of cell cycling by blocking progression into the S phase. Its normal function is to prevent replication of damaged DNA. Loss of Rb therefore results in increased progression through the cell cycle. In bladder cancer Rb deletions or mutations have been detected in up to 30% of muscle invasive tumors (8). In prostate cancer loss of Rb has been suggested as an independent predictor of disease specific survival (54). Other studies have suggested that levels of Cyclin D1 (which phosphorylates and reduces Rb activity) are also expressed at higher levels in prostate cancer (60). p53 is a well-characterized tumor suppressor and has many known functions including DNA repair, initiating apoptosis after DNA damage and cell cycle progression. Its function in regulating the cell cycle is achieved through transcriptional regulation of p21 (also known as CDK inhibitor 1A). p21 inhibits cell cycling by forming a complex with CDK 2 and preventing progression into the S phase of the cycle. Mutations in the p53 gene results in increased expression of a non-functional protein. As a result of this there is reduced p21 expression and increased progression through the cell cycle. In bladder cancer high levels of p53 have been positively correlated with a poorer disease specific outcome for muscle invasive disease (8). p21 loss has also been reported as a frequent finding in aggressive bladder cancers (61). Tumors with a coordinated dysregulation of different cell cycle regulators (such as combined loss of p53 and Rb) seem to exhibit even poorer survival outcomes (62,63).

APOPTOSIS IN CANCER CELLS

There are two basic apoptotic pathways in the cell. In the mitochondrial (or intrinsic) pathway cellular damage stimulates migration of the proapoptotic proteins Bad and Bax to the mitochondrial surface where it binds and inhibits antiapoptotic Bcl 2. This allows the release of cytochrome C, which is the first step in the assembly of the apoptosome complex. This complex then activates caspase 9, which in turn triggers the activation of other caspase and ultimately leads to destruction of cellular proteins as well as DNA degradation. The second mechanism is through the activation of death receptors (extrinsic pathway). These include the Fas, tumor necrosis factor (TNF) and tumor necrosis factor–related apoptosis inducing ligand (TRAIL) receptors. Following binding of their respective ligands these receptors mediate the assembly of a death-inducting signal complex (DISC), which activates caspase 8 and in turn triggers the caspase cascade resulting in cell death. Bcl 2 has been shown to be reduced in androgen dependent prostate cancer but is over-expressed in androgen-independent disease (64). These and similar findings in other cancers has led the development of targeted therapy against Bcl 2. Oblimersen is a Bcl 2 antisense oligonucleotide and a potent inhibitor of its expression. Studies in preclinical models have shown that cotreatment of prostate cancer cells can enhance the cytotoxic effects of chemotherapy (65). Phase II studies have also shown promising results in combining oblimersen with docetaxel for men with hormone refractory disease in prolonging survival (66). Bcl 2 has also been tested as a target in renal cell cancers. Downregulation in in vitro cultured renal cancer cell has been shown to enhance sensitivity to Fas receptor-mediated apoptosis (67). A recent phase I/II trial of oblimersen as an adjunct to interferon therapy in renal cell cancer however has failed to show any significant clinical benefit (68). In the extrinsic pathway loss of FAS expression has been demonstrated in bladder and renal tumors (69,70). Decoy receptors are also known to exist for the Fas and TRAIL axis. These are produced by tumor tissue and block ligands from binding to the membrane bound receptors. High levels of Fas decoy receptors have been reported in the serum of patients with renal and prostate cancers (71,72). Osteoprotegerin can act as a decoy for TRAIL and has been implicated in bladder and prostate cancer. In bladder cancer low levels of Osteoprotegerin have been linked to a favorable outcome in muscle invasive bladder cancer while in prostate cancer high levels have been associated with disease progression (73,74). There are as yet no clinical trials exploiting the death receptors in cancers. Of note, TRAIL is already an exploited target as BCG immunotherapy is thought to act in part by activating these receptors and inducing immune mediated cell death (75).

CONCLUSION

Alteration can occur at every level in the cell processes in cancer biology and it has only been possible here to highlight important changes in urological cancers. Common themes occur in different malignancies but some alterations may be more relevant depending on the tumor type. The goal for the next generation of cancer drugs will be to define the key alterations that are relevant for a specific tumor type and target these using novel therapies. This is already occurring with novel VEGF targeted therapy in renal cancers and early clinical studies of HDAC inhibitors in prostate cancers. It is highly likely however that a combination of drugs directed at different targets will be most likely to have the optimal therapeutic effect. Moreover drug combinations may well be tailored for a specific patient on the basis of the unique set of genetic and biological alterations identified in their particular tumor.

REFERENCES

1. Eeles RA, Kote-Jarai Z, Giles GG, et al. Multiple newly identified loci associated with prostate cancer susceptibility. Nat Genet 2008; 40(3):316–321.
2. Fadl-Elmula I. Chromosomal changes in uroepithelial carcinomas. Cell Chromosome 2005; 4:1.
3. Kardas I, Mrózek K, Babinska M, et al. Cytogenetic and molecular findings in 75 clear cell renal cell carcinomas. Oncol Rep 2005; 13(5):949–956.
4. Tomlins SA, Mehra R, Rhodes DR, et al. Whole transcriptome amplification for gene expression profiling and development of molecular archives. Neoplasia 2006; 8(2):153–162.
5. Hung RJ, Boffetta P, Brennan P, et al. GST, NAT, SULT1A1, CYP1B1 genetic polymorphisms, interactions with environmental exposures and bladder cancer risk in a high-risk population. Int J Cancer 2004; 110:598–604.
6. Franekova M, Halasova E, Bukovska E, et al. Gene polymorphisms in bladder cancer. Urol Oncol 2008; 26(1):1–8.
7. Huff V. Wilms tumor genetics. Am J Med Genet 1998; 79(4):260–267.
8. Knowles MA. What we could do now: molecular pathology of bladder cancer. Mol Pathol 2001; 54:215–221.
9. Gnanapragasam VJ, Robson CN, Leung HY, et al. Androgen receptor signalling in the prostate. BJU Int 2000; 86(9):1001–1013.
10. Morris MR, Hesson LB, Wagner KJ, et al. Multigene methylation analysis of Wilms' tumor and adult renal cell carcinoma. Oncogene 2003; 22(43):6794–6801.

11. Yates DR, Rehman I, Abbod MF, et al. Promoter hypermethylation identifies progression risk in bladder cancer. Clin Cancer Res 2007; 13(7):2046–2053.

12. Ellinger J, El Kassem N, Heukamp LC, et al. Hypermethylation of cell-free serum DNA indicates worse outcome in patients with bladder cancer. J Urol 2008; 79(1):346–352.

13. Harden SV, Guo Z, Epstein JI, et al. Quantitative GSTP1 methylation clearly distinguishes benign prostatic tissue and limited prostate adenocarcinoma. J Urol 2003; 169:1138–1142.

14. Weichert W, Röske A, Gekeler V, et al. Histone deacetylases 1, 2 and 3 are highly expressed in prostate cancer and HDAC2 expression is associated with shorter PSA relapse time after radical prostatectomy. Br J Cancer 2008; 98(3):604–610.

15. Halkidou K, Gaughan L, Cook S, et al. Upregulation and nuclear recruitment of HDAC1 in hormone refractory prostate cancer. Prostate 2004; 59(2):177–189.

16. Qian DZ, Wei YF, Wang X, et al. Antitumor activity of the histone deacetylase inhibitor MS-275 in prostate cancer models. Prostate 2007; 67(11):1182–1193.

17. Arts J, Angibaud P, Mariën A, et al. R306465 is a novel potent inhibitor of class I histone deacetylases with broad-spectrum antitumoral activity against solid and haematological malignancies. Br J Cancer 2007; 97(10):1344–1353.

18. Wiesener MS, Münchenhagen PM, Berger I, et al. Constitutive activation of hypoxia-inducible genes related to overexpression of hypoxia-inducible factor-1alpha in clear cell renal carcinomas. Cancer Res 2001; 61(13):5215–5222.

19. Kaelin WG Jr. The von Hippel-Lindau tumor suppressor protein and clear cell renal carcinoma. Clin Cancer Res 2007; 13(2 pt 2):680s–684s.

20. Levidou G, Saetta AA, Korkolopoulou P, et al. Clinical significance of nuclear factor (NF)-kappaB levels in urothelial carcinoma of the urinary bladder. Virchows Arch 2008; 452(3):295–304.

21. Sourbier C, Danilin S, Lindner V, et al. Targeting the nuclear factor-kappaB rescue pathway has promising future in human renal cell carcinoma therapy. Cancer Res 2007; 67(24):11668–11676.

22. Palayoor ST, Youmell MY, Calderwood SK, et al. Constitutive activation of IkappaB kinase alpha and NF-kappaB in prostate cancer cells is inhibited by ibuprofen. Oncogene 1999; 18(51):7389–7394.

23. Price N, Dreicer R. Phase I/II trial of bortezomib plus docetaxel in patients with advanced androgen-independent prostate cancer. Clin Prostate Cancer 2004; 3(3):141–143.

24. Sorensen PH, Lessnick SL, Lopez-Terrada D, et al. A second Ewing's sarcoma translocation, t(21;22), fuses the EWS gene to another ETS-family transcription factor, ERG. Nat Genet 1994; 6(2):146–151.

25. Tomlins SA, Laxman B, Dhanasekaran SM, et al. Distinct classes of chromosomal rearrangements create oncogenic ETS gene fusions in prostate cancer. Nature 2007; 448(7153):595–599.

26. Helgeson BE, Tomlins SA, Shah N, et al. Characterization of TMPRSS2:ETV5 and SLC45A3:ETV5 gene fusions in prostate cancer. Cancer Res 2008; 68(1):73–80.

27. Attard G, Clark J, Ambroisine L, et al. Transatlantic Prostate Group. Duplication of the fusion of TMPRSS2 to ERG sequences identifies fatal human prostate cancer. Oncogene 2008; 27(3):253–263.

28. Nam RK, Sugar L, Yang W, et al. Expression of the TMPRSS2:ERG fusion gene predicts cancer recurrence after surgery for localised prostate cancer. Br J Cancer 2007; 97(12):1690–1695.

29. Faustino NA, Cooper TA. Pre-mRNA splicing and human disease. Genes Dev 2003; 17:419–437.

30. Li HR, Wang-Rodriguez J, Nair TM, et al. Two-dimensional transcriptome profiling: identification of messenger RNA isoform signatures in prostate cancer from archived paraffin-embedded cancer specimens. Cancer Res 2006; 66(8):4079–4088.

31. Tomlinson DC, L'Hôte CG, Kennedy W, et al. Alternative splicing of fibroblast growth factor receptor 3 produces a secreted isoform that inhibits fibroblast growth factor-induced proliferation and is repressed in urothelial carcinoma cell lines. Cancer Res 2005; 65(22):10441–10449.

32. Kwabi-Addo B, Ropiquet F, Giri D, et al. Alternative splicing of fibroblast growth factor receptors in human prostate cancer. Prostate 2001; 46(2):163–172.

33. Tolcher AW. Novel therapeutic molecular targets for prostate cancer: the mTOR signaling pathway and epidermal growth factor receptor. J Urol 2004; 171(2 pt 2):S41–S43.

34. De Benedetti A, Graff JR. eIF-4E expression and its role in malignancies and metastases. Oncogene 2004; 23(18):3189–3199.

35. Cho WC. OncomiRs: the discovery and progress of microRNAs in cancers. Mol Cancer 2007; 6:60.

36. Gottardo F, Liu CG, Ferracin M, et al. Micro-RNA profiling in kidney and bladder cancers. Urol Oncol 2007; 25(5):387–392.

37. Ozen M, Creighton CJ, Ozdemir M, et al. Widespread deregulation of microRNA expression in human prostate cancer. Oncogene 2008; 27(12):1788–1793.

38. Porkka KP, Pfeiffer MJ, Waltering KK, et al. MicroRNA expression profiling in prostate cancer. Cancer Res 2007; 67(13):6130–6135.

39. Mimeault M, Pommery N, Hénichart JP. New advances on prostate carcinogenesis and therapies: involvement of EGF-EGFR transduction system. Growth Factors 2003; 21(1):1–14.

40. Fürstenberger G, Senn HJ. Insulin-like growth factors and cancer. Lancet Oncol. 2002; 3(5):298–302.

41. Kwabi-Addo B, Ozen M, Ittmann M. The role of fibroblast growth factors and their receptors in prostate cancer. Endocr Relat Cancer 2004; 11(4):709–724.

42. Dorkin TJ, Robinson MC, Marsh C, et al. aFGF immunoreactivity in prostate cancer and its co-localization with bFGF and FGF8. J Pathol 1999; 189(4):564–569.

43. Gnanapragasam VJ, Robinson MC, Marsh C, et al. FGF8 isoform b expression in human prostate cancer. Br J Cancer 2003; 88(9):1432–1438.

44. Heer R, Douglas D, Mathers ME, et al. Fibroblast growth factor 17 is over-expressed in human prostate cancer. J Pathol 2004; 204(5):578–586.

45. Memarzadeh S, Xin L, Mulholland DJ, et al. Enhanced paracrine FGF10 expression promotes formation of multifocal prostate adenocarcinoma and an increase in epithelial androgen receptor. Cancer Cell. 2007; 12(6):572–585.

46. Sahadevan K, Darby S, Leung HY, et al. Selective overexpression of fibroblast growth factor receptors 1 and 4 in clinical prostate cancer. J Pathol 2007; 213(1):82–90.

47. Acevedo VD, Gangula RD, Freeman KW, et al. Inducible FGFR-1 activation leads to irreversible prostate adenocarcinoma and an epithelial-to-mesenchymal transition. Cancer Cell 2007; 12(6):559–571.

48. Sriplakich S, Jahnson S, Karlsson MG. Epidermal growth factor receptor expression: predictive value for the outcome after cystectomy for bladder cancer? BJU Int 1999; 83(4):498–503.

49. Latif Z, Watters AD, Dunn I, et al. HER2/neu gene amplification and protein overexpression in G3 pT2 transitional cell carcinoma of the bladder: a role for anti-HER2 therapy? Eur J Cancer 2004; 40(1):56–63.

50. Hussain MH, MacVicar GR, Petrylak DP, et al. Trastuzumab, paclitaxel, carboplatin, and gemcitabine in advanced human

epidermal growth factor receptor-2/neu-positive urothelial carcinoma: results of a multicenter phase II National Cancer Institute trial. J Clin Oncol 2007; 25(16):2218–2224.

51. Black PC, Agarwal PK, Dinney CP. Targeted therapies in bladder cancer–an update. Urol Oncol 2007; 25(5):433–438.

52. Escudier B, Pluzanska A, Koralewski P, et al. AVOREN Trial investigators. Bevacizumab plus interferon alfa-2a for treatment of metastatic renal cell carcinoma: a randomised, double-blind phase III trial. Lancet 2007; 370(9605): 2103–2111.

53. Escudier B, Eisen T, Stadler WM, et al. TARGET Study Group. Sorafenib in advanced clear-cell renal-cell carcinoma. N Engl J Med 2007; 356(2):125–134.

54. van der Poel HG. Molecular markers in the diagnosis of prostate cancer. Crit Rev Oncol Hematol 2007; 61(2): 104–139.

55. Anwar K, Nakakuki K, Shiraishi T, et al. Presence of ras oncogene mutations and human papillomavirus DNA in human prostate carcinomas. Cancer Res 1992; 52: 5991–5996.

56. Jebar AH, Hurst CD, Tomlinson DC, et al. FGFR3 and Ras gene mutations are mutually exclusive genetic events in urothelial cell carcinoma. Oncogene 2005; 24(33): 5218–5225.

57. Dent P, Yacoub A, Fisher PB, et al. MAPK pathways in radiation responses. Oncogene 2003; 22(37):5885–5896.

58. McKie AB, Douglas DA, Olijslagers S, et al. Epigenetic inactivation of the human sprouty2 (hSPRY2) homologue in prostate cancer. Oncogene 2005; 24(13):2166–2174.

59. Darby S, Sahadevan K, Khan MM, et al. Loss of Sef (similar expression to FGF) expression is associated with high grade and metastatic prostate cancer. Oncogene 2006; 25(29):4122–4127.

60. Han EK, Lim JT, Arber N, et al. Cyclin D1 expression in human prostate carcinoma cell lines and primary tumors. Prostate 1998; 35(2):95–101.

61. Stein JP, Ginsberg DA, Grossfeld GD, et al. Effect of p21WAF1/CIP1 expression on tumor progression in bladder cancer. J Natl Cancer Inst 1998; 90:1072–1079.

62. Grossman HB, Liebert M, Antelo M, et al. p53 and RB expression predict progression in T1 bladder cancer. Clin Cancer Res 1998; 4:829–834.

63. Cordon-Cardo C, Zhang ZF, Dalbagni G, et al. Cooperative effects of p53 and pRB alterations in primary superficial bladder tumors. Cancer Res 1997; 57:1217–1221.

64. McDonnell TJ, Troncoso P, Brisbay SM, et al. Expression of the protooncogene bcl-2 in the prostate and its association with emergence of androgen-independent prostate cancer. Cancer Res 1992; 52(24):6940–6944.

65. Leonetti C, Biroccio A, D'Angelo C, et al. Therapeutic integration of c-myc and bcl-2 antisense molecules with docetaxel in a preclinical model of hormone-refractory prostate cancer. Prostate 2007; 67(13):1475–1485.

66. Tolcher AW, Chi K, Kuhn J, et al. A phase II, pharmaco-kinetic, and biological correlative study of oblimersen sodium and docetaxel in patients with hormone-refractory prostate cancer. Clin Cancer Res 2005; 11(10):3854–3861.

67. Kelly JD, Dai J, Eschwege P, et al. Downregulation of Bcl-2 sensitises interferon-resistant renal cancer cells to Fas. Br J Cancer 2004; 91(1):164–170.

68. Margolin K, Synold TW, Lara P, et al. Oblimersen and alpha-interferon in metastatic renal cancer: a phase II study of the California Cancer Consortium. J Cancer Res Clin Oncol 2007; 133(10):705–711.

69. Sejima T, Isoyama T, Miyagawa I. Alteration of apoptotic regulatory molecules expression during carcinogenesis and tumor progression of renal cell carcinoma. Int J Urol 2003; 10:476–479.

70. Maas S, Warskulat U, Steinhoff C, et al. Decreased Fas expression in advanced-stage bladder cancer is not related to p53 status. Urology 2004; 63:392–396.

71. Furuya Y, Nagakawa O, Fuse H. Prognostic significance of serum soluble Fas level and its change during regression and progression of advanced prostate cancer. Endocr J 2003; 50:629–633.

72. Kimura M, Tomita Y, Imai T, et al. Significance of serum-soluble CD95 (Fas/APO-1) on prognosis in renal cell cancer patients. Br J Cancer 1999; 80:1648–1651.

73. Mizutani Y, Matsubara H, Yamamoto K, et al. Prognostic significance of serum osteoprotegerin levels in patients with bladder carcinoma. Cancer 2004; 101:1794–1802.

74. Eaton CL, Wells JM, Holen I, et al. Serum osteoprotegerin (OPG) levels are associated with disease progression and response to androgen ablation in patients with prostate cancer. Prostate 2004; 59:304–310.

75. Ludwig AT, Moore JM, Luo Y, et al. Tumor necrosis factor-related apoptosis inducing ligand a novel mechanism for Bacillus Calmette-Guerin-induced antitumor activity. Cancer Res 2004; 64:3386–3394.

21

General Biology of Cancer and Metastasis

David E. Neal

Department of Oncology, University of Cambridge, Addenbrooke's Hospital, Cambridge, U.K.

CANCER

An understanding of cancer is important to the urologist, not only because it is common, but also because its study provides insight into normal and abnormal cellular function. One in five adults dies of cancer (Tables 1 and 2), and about 30% to 50% of common, solid epithelial tumors are advanced and incurable when first detected clinically. So far as urological tumors are concerned, prostate, bladder, and kidney cancers are common, and while testis cancer is rare, it is important because, even when advanced, it is frequently curable and because it occurs in young men with an otherwise full life expectancy.

It is thought that individual cancers arise from a single cell following a set of genetically determined events. The evidence for this monoclonal origin lies in findings, first, that all cells in a tumor often contain specific point mutations in genes, which would be unlikely to arise by chance in several cells, and, second, that in women, in whom one X chromosome is inactivated in a mosaic and apparently random fashion throughout the body, one particular X chromosome is inactivated throughout the tumor.

CHEMICAL CARCINOGENESIS

Many different chemicals have been shown to be carcinogenic (Table 3). The best known historical example is that of scrotal cancer, in which Percival Pott demonstrated through epidemiological observations that boys who had been employed as chimney sweeps were likely to develop this disease as adults. He hypothesized that chemicals in soot caused the problem. Tobacco use (mainly cigarette smoking) was later shown to be clearly associated with cancers of the mouth, larynx, trachea, lung, kidney, and bladder.

Evidence of a chemical cause for bladder cancer was found by Rehn in 1894, when he recorded a series of such tumors occurring in workers in aniline dye factories. Hueper was subsequently able to show that 2-naphthylamine was carcinogenic in dogs, and further investigation demonstrated that a variety of chemicals may be carcinogenic.

Common factors in most human cancers include damage to several genes (rather than one) resulting from point mutations, insertions, or deletions in certain genes known as oncogenes or tumor suppressor genes. Even recently, chemical causes of urothelial cancers have been shown to be important. Balkan nephropathy exists in certain defined parts of the Balkans. A herb found in these places, and also used widely in Chinese medicine, contains aristocholic acid and this chemical is nephrotoxic and carcinogenic.

Occupations that have been reported to have a significantly excess risk of bladder cancer are shown in Table 4.

Historically, chemicals have been classified into those that produced mutations in DNA on first application (initiators), but that themselves were usually insufficient to cause cancer unless there was further exposure to the initiator or unless initiator application was followed by a promoter. Promoters are compounds that do not cause cancer, however, often they are applied, but they will cause the development of cancer when there has been previous application of an initiator. Promoters include chemicals such as phorbol esters, which stimulate protein kinase C (PKC). PKC phosphorylates several proteins on serine and threonine residues and activates MAP kinase, which is also activated by the ras pathway (see Chapter 22 for "Ras").

Most carcinogens are genotoxic and cause damage to DNA. It is thought that there is also a class of nongenotoxic carcinogens that, in mice, cause peroxisome proliferation, and that may activate agents that interfere with the cell cycle or apoptosis. It is uncertain whether this mechanism is active in man.

GENETIC POLYMORPHISMS

Many genotoxic carcinogens are inactive and require to be converted into active agents by acetylation or hydroxylation (Fig. 1). Mammalian cells have developed a complex system for detoxifying external biologically active chemicals known as xenobiotics. These enzymes, which also detoxify drugs and carcinogens, include the following:

- Hydroxylation by means of the cytochrome P450 system (CYP), which is found on the microsomal fraction of cells (particularly in the liver)

Table 1   Common Causes of Human Cancer

- Ionizing radiation (hematopoietic cells, bone)
- Sunlight (malignant melanoma, squamous cell carcinoma of the skin)
- Familial genetic causes (certain types of breast, colon, kidney, and prostate cancer)
- Familial cancer predispositions due to altered activity in detoxifying or activating enzymes such as *N*-acetyltransferase 2 and glutathione transferase M (bladder, lung, and colon cancer)
- Chemicals from occupations and smoking (bladder, larynx, and lung cancer)
- Chronic inflammation (squamous cell carcinoma arising in a chronic ulcer, schistosomal bladder cancer, tumors in ulcerative colitis, and adenocarcinoma arising in Barrett esophagus)
- Viral infection: DNA viruses: penile and cervical cancer (papovavirus), liver cancer (Hep B and C), Epstein-Barr virus (Burkitt's lymphoma, nasopharyngeal cancer); RNA viruses: human T-cell leukemia (HTLV-1), Kaposi's sarcoma (HIV-1)

Table 2   Cancer Incidence and Death in the United States

Type of cancer	New cases per year	Percentage	Deaths per year	Percentage
Total	1,170,000	100	528,300	100
Mouth and pharynx	29,800	3	7,700	1
Colon and rectum	152,000	13	57,000	11
Stomach	24,000	2	13,600	3
Pancreas	27,700	2	25,000	5
Lung	170,000	15	149,000	28
Breast	183,000	16	46,300	9
Malignant melanoma	32,000	3	6,800	1
Prostate	185,000	14	35,000	7
Ovary	22,000	2	13,300	3
Cervix	13,500	1	4,400	1
Uterus	31,000	3	5,700	1
Bladder	52,300	4	9,900	2
Kidney	21,200		8,300	
Hematopoietic	93,000	8	50,000	9
CNS	18,250	2	12,350	2
Testis	5,100		210	
Sarcomas	8,000	1	4,150	1

Table 3   Compounds Associated with Bladder Cancer

2-Naphthylamine	Chlornaphazine	4,49-Methylene bis (2-choloranliline)
4-Aminobiphenyl	4-Chloro-O-toluidine	Methylene dianiline
Benzidine	o-toluidine	Benzidine-derived azo dyes

Table 4   Occupations Associated with Bladder Cancer

Textile workers	Leather workers	Lorry drivers
Dye workers	Shoe manufacturers and cleaners	Drill press operators
Tyre rubber and cable workers	Painters	Chemical workers
Petrol workers	Hairdressers	Rodent exterminators and sewage workers

- Glutathione transferases, which couple glutathione to water-insoluble chemicals and which are classified into families (α, υ, μ, π)
- *N*-acetyltransferase pathway (NAT-1 and NAT-2)

Some individuals are more at risk than others after exposure to a carcinogen because of genetic polymorphisms. This arises because each individual carries two alleles for each gene, but within a population there may be many alleles. Some combinations will lead to an individual's having enzymes that may be more or less active than those found in other individuals. Polymorphic genes of interest in bladder cancer include *N*-acetyltransferase types 1 and 2 (NAT-1, NAT-2), glutathione transferase M1 and p (GSTM1 and GSTp),

and several cytochrome P450s (CYP2D6: debrisoquine hydroxylase; and CYP1A1). Individuals who have high levels of NAT-2 or GSTM1 may be less likely to develop cancer after exposure to smoking because they can detoxify the mutagen, whereas those with high levels of CYP2D6 may be more likely to develop cancer because they convert inactive to active forms of the mutagen. Similarly, some individuals may be generally resistant to carcinoma formation because they have polymorphisms that produce protective compounds. It should be noted that some enzymes will have a dual effect; for instance, NAT-2 in the liver will detoxify some carcinogens, but may activate others. This explains the paradox that fast acetylators are less likely to develop bladder cancer, but may be more likely to develop colon

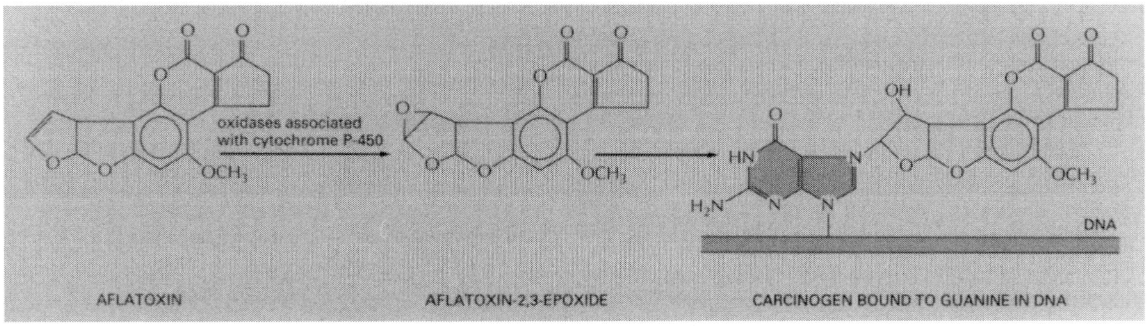

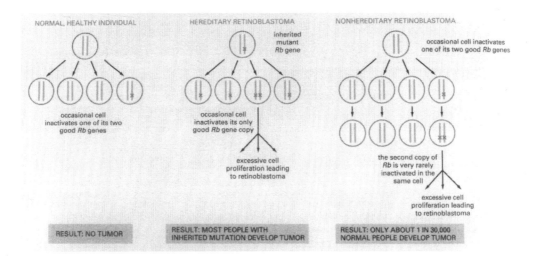

Figure 1 showing structures labeled AFLATOXIN, with arrow "oxidases associated with cytochrome P-450" to AFLATOXIN-2,3-EPOXIDE, then to CARCINOGEN BOUND TO GUANINE IN DNA.

Figure 1 Metabolic activation of a carcinogen. Many chemical carcinogens have to be activated by a metabolic transformation before they will cause mutations by reacting with DNA. The compound illustrated here is aflatoxin B1, a toxin made from a mold (*Aspergillus flavus-oryzae*) that grows on grain and peanuts stored under humid tropical conditions. It is thought to be a contributory cause of liver cancer in the tropics and is associated with specific mutations of the p53 gene.

cancer. NAT-1 is found in high levels in the bladder urothelium, and nontoxic metabolites produced by NAT-2 in the liver and excreted in the urine can be taken into the urothelial cells and converted by NAT-1 into active carcinogens that produce genotoxic damage in the bladder cell.

Cancer Is a Multistep Process

Human cancer requires several mutations to occur before a tumor develops clinically. One reason for supporting this view is that cancer incidence increases markedly with age, and this would be unlikely if tumors simply arose from a single gene mutation. Instead, tumorigenesis would be more likely to occur randomly throughout life. Recent molecular biological studies have supported the view that cancer arises only when there has been an accumulation of several genetic events.

Cancer Genes

Several tumors have a strong genetic component, including retinoblastoma (Rb gene), Wilms' tumor (WT gene), familial forms of prostate cancer (unknown gene, possibly on chromosome 1), breast cancer (BRCA1 and BRCA2 genes and mutations in p53 in Li-Fraumeni families), familial adenomatosis polyposis (APC gene), hereditary nonpolyposis colon cancer (HNPCC) (MSH1 gene), and von Hippel–Lindau disease (VHL gene). These tumors have proven to be instructive because in most cases they appeared to be inherited clinically in a dominant fashion. Nevertheless, biochemically, these genes act in a recessive fashion because, although the disease is caused by an inherited mutation in one allele of a tumor suppressor gene, cancer develops only when the other normal allele becomes deleted or mutated by chance (Fig. 2). Why tumors in such patients appear only in certain

Figure 2 The genetic mechanisms underlying retinoblastoma. In the hereditary form, all cells in the body lack one of the normal two functional copies of a tumor suppressor gene, and tumors occur where the remaining copy is lost or inactivated by a somatic mutation. In the nonhereditary form, all cells initially contain two functional copies of the gene, and the tumor arises because both copies are lost or inactivated through the coincidence of two somatic mutations in one cell.

tissues is uncertain when tumor suppressor genes are inactivated in most cells. Methylation in the prompter of such genes can also, through epigenetic mechanisms, functionally inactivate such genes. The impact of oncogenes and tumor suppressor genes is dealt with in other chapters in this book.

Other tumors can arise in patients whose DNA repair machinery is deficient (xeroderma pigmentosa, ataxia telangiectasia, and HNPCC).

DNA Repair Genes

Mismatch Repair

Patients with HNPCC have tumors in which there are a large number of microsatellites in the genome of the tumor. Microsatellites are short (two to four nucleotides; e.g., CACA on one strand and GTGT on the other), noncoding, tandem repeats of DNA, which are found throughout the genome and which show pronounced polymorphism. Abnormalities in microsatellites have been found in Huntington's chorea, the fragile X syndrome, and spinobulbar atrophy, in which, over several generations, there is a progressive expansion of the nucleotide repeats in the genes of interest. This leads to disease, but it is found that with each succeeding generation there is an increased severity of the disease because the microsatellites become longer. This phenomenon is called *genetic anticipation*. In HNPCC, microsatellite instability is thought to be the result of failure to correct replication errors that occur during cell division. This failure is caused by hereditary defects in the enzymes responsible for the repair of these replication mismatch errors. These enzymes include MSH2, MLH1, GTBP, and PMS1.

Nucleotide Excision Repair

Abnormal nucleotide insertions can occur during DNA replication and are excised by mechanisms that are deficient in xeroderma pigmentosa.

CELLULAR CHARACTERISTICS OF CANCER

Not all features of cancer cells are caused directly by abnormal genes; some abnormalities are due to failure to regulate genetically normal genes (Table 5). These epigenetic events include upregulation of enzymes that can dissolve the basement membrane (such as cathepsins and plasminogen activators) and may predispose the cell to metastasize; changes in expression of cell surface molecules (such as HLA antigens) that may allow the cancer cell to escape detection by the body's immunosurveillance; loss of molecules responsible for intercellular adherence, leading the cell to be more likely to metastasize (such as E-cadherin); upregulation of growth factors or their receptors, allowing the cell to become self-reliant (such as epidermal growth factor and its receptor, EGFr); and upregulation of molecules that detoxify anticancer drugs (such as the multitumor-suppressor gene—MDR-1).

Table 5 Characteristics of the Transformed Cell

Plasma membrane abnormalities
  Increased transmembrane transport (as for glucose and calcium)
  Excessive endocytosis and blebbing
  Increased mobility
Adhesion molecules
  Decreased adhesion
  Failure of organization of actin into stress fibers
  Reduced fibronectin expression
  Increased expression of enzymes such as cathepsin, plasminogen activators, and metalloproteinases
Growth
  Growth to high density (lack of density-dependent inhibition)
  Decreased requirement for added growth factors
  Anchorage-independent growth
  Immortal
  Can cause animal tumors

ANGIOGENESIS

Angiogenesis is the process of new blood-vessel formation, which is found in a number of diseases, including cancer, diabetic retinopathy, and inflammatory arthritides. The initiation of angiogenesis in tumors is dependent on the coordinated expression of several factors (Table 6). Angiogenesis requires dilatation of vessels, breakdown of perivascular stroma, migration and proliferation of endothelial cells, and canalization of endothelial buds. Potent inhibitors of angiogenesis include angiostatin (which, paradoxically, is secreted by some primary tumors) and thrombospondin (which is involved in the binding of macrophages to apoptotic cells, and which is also upregulated by normal p53). A potent stimulus of angiogenesis is hypoxia, which upregulates the expression of vascular endothelial growth factor (VEGF). This occurs through the upregulation of the intermediate hypoxia-inducible factors (HIF) (Fig. 3).

VEGF is a specific mitogen for endothelial cells. It exists in four forms (121-, 165-, 189-, and 206-aa peptides) and is secreted by a number of cell types. VEGFr, which is a tyrosine kinase, is found on endothelial cells in two forms (Flt-1 and Flk-1).

RENAL CELL CANCER

A good example of how modern molecular biology has helped to unravel the causes and different phenotypes of cancer is kidney cancer. Renal cancer is not

Table 6 Peptides Associated with Angiogenesis

Vascular endothelial growth factor (VEGF)
FGFs
PDGF
Tumor necrosis factor α
Angiogenin
EGF
TGF-α and TGF-β
Platelet-derived endothelial cell growth factor or thymidine phosphorylase

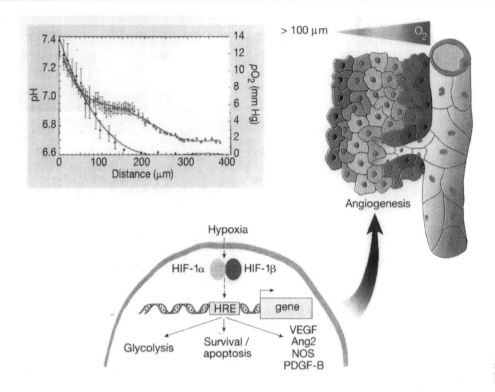

Figure 3 Factors controlling angiogenesis. Hypoxia induces transcription of hypoxia-inducible factors (HIF) that act on HIF-responsive elements in the promoter region of genes such as VEGF.

a single disease; it is comprised of several different types of cancer, each with a different histology, a different clinical course, and different genetic changes. For these different tumor types, hereditary, familial, and sporadic forms exist. Most of our current knowledge was originally derived from studies on familial forms of the disease, but subsequent studies of sporadic cancers found similar changes. Recent developments in genetics and molecular biology have led to an increasing knowledge of the origin and biology of renal cell carcinoma (RCC).

Chromosome 3 Changes: the von Hippel–Lindau Tumor Suppressor

Clear cell RCCs are characterized by nonhomologous chromatid exchange, leading to loss of genetic material from the short (p) arm of chromosome 3 and gains of material from the long (q) arm of chromosome 5. Loss of heterozygosity studies in sporadic RCCs identified three common regions of allelic loss: 3p12–14, 3p21–22, and 3p25–26.

Loss of 3p and gain of 5q implicate genes within these regions as being involved in clear cell RCC tumorigenesis. Tumor suppressor genes are likely to be found in areas of chromosomal loss (3p) and oncogenes found in areas of chromosomal gain (5q). The only gene definitively shown to be involved in the development of such tumors is the VHL, located at

3p25, a documented tumor suppressor. Renal cell cancers found in VHL follow Knudson's theory of the two hit model of carcinogenesis. The VHL gene is inactivated in patients with VHL and in almost 100% of sporadic clear cell RCC.

The inactivation of VHL is accomplished by mutation, deletion, or methylation. Mutations of the VHL gene seen in sporadic RCC differ from those seen in RCC associated with VHL disease. In sporadic RCC, 45% of the mutations are clustered in the second exon, although abnormalities are seen in all three exons. Large deletions are not observed, and 48% of the mutations are microdeletions or insertions, resulting in frame shifts of the protein-coding sequence.

VHL encodes two different protein isoforms. Both isoforms are capable of suppressing RCC growth in vivo and will be referred as pVHL. pVHL functions as a component of an ubiquitin ligase complex (VBC complex) and its best understood function relates to its ability to target specific proteins for destruction. pVHL forms stable complexes that contain other proteins called elongin B, elongin C, Cul2, and Rbx1. These complexes are capable of directing the covalent attachment of polyubiquitin tails to specific proteins, which serves as a signal for such proteins to be degraded by the proteasome. Several pVHL targets have been identified, including the members of the HIF-α family (HIF-1α, HIF-2α, and HIF-3α). HIF-1α and HIF-2α, when bound to a HIF-β member (such as

Table 7 Main Protein Targets of the VHL Protein

Target protein	Function
Hypoxia-inducible factors (HIF-1 and HIF-2)	Protein transcription
Vascular endothelial growth factor (VEGF)	Angiogenesis
Glucose transporter protein (Glut-1)	Glucose transport
Platelet-derived growth factor (PDGF-β)	Angiogenesis, mitogenesis
Transforming growth factor (TGF-α, TGF-β)	Epithelial proliferation, mitogenesis
Intracellular fibronectin	Epithelial proliferation
Erythropoietin	Erythropoiesis
Carbonic anhydrase 9 and 12	Extracellular pH control
Chemokine receptor (CXCR4)	Metastasis

HIF-1β, also called ARNT), form a sequence-specific, DNA-binding transcription factor called HIF. Ordinarily, the HIF-α members are highly unstable except under low-oxygen conditions. In the presence of oxygen, these proteins become hydroxylated on conserved prolyl residues in a reaction catalyzed by members of the EGLN family. pVHL recognizes the hydroxylated HIF-α species and orchestrates their destruction through ubiquitination (Table 7).

Since the 1990s, evidence has continued to accumulate demonstrating that hypoxia is a common consequence of the rapid growth of many solid tumors, including tumors such as kidney cancer. Studies of renal cell biology also provide evidence that hypoxia is an important regulator of a network of gene expression with the ability to both stimulate and inhibit individual genes and to effect their expression on both posttranscriptional and posttranslational levels. When there is normoxia, the VHL complex targets HIF and degrades it. In cells that lack pVHL, or when oxygen is limiting, the complex cannot degrade HIF; HIF-1α and HIF-2α are upregulated through the phosphatidylinositol 4,5-bisphosphate-AKT-mammalian target of rapamycin pathway (P13K-AKT-mTOR) and Ras/Raf/MEK/mitogen-activated protein kinase (MAPK) pathway and they then form the transcription factor HIF. HIF is free to accumulate intracellularly and activates the transcription of a cadre of genes that encode proteins essential to cancer cell functions under hypoxic conditions.

Included among these genes are genes that control glucose uptake and metabolism [such as the Glut1 (glucose transporter protein) and various glycolytic enzymes], extracellular pH (such as carbonic anhydrase IX), angiogenesis (such as VEGF), erythropoiesis (such as erythropoietin), and mitogenesis [such as transforming growth factor-α (TGF-α) and platelet-derived growth factor-β (PDGF-β)]. Signaling occurs through various cell surface receptors, including EGFR, HER2, VEGFR, and type I insulin-like growth factor receptor. These considerations explain the frequent overproduction of HIF, as well as its downstream targets, in RCC. pVHL binds to other cellular proteins, some of which may also be polyubiquitinated or in some other way modulated by pVHL. These proteins include the atypical protein kinase C family members, Sp1, heteronuclear ribonucleoprotein hnRNP A2, specific RNA Pol II subunits (Rpb1 and hsRBP7), Jade-1, Vdu1/2, fibronectin, proteins associated with microtubules, nuclear factor kappa B, and metalloproteinases (MMPs).

Although our knowledge of the functions of pVHL is still incomplete, studies conducted thus far highlight its role as an inhibitor of HIF, and dysregulation of HIF is likely to contribute to the development of RCC.

METASTASIS

This is the process by which cells from the primary tumor enter the circulation and seed elsewhere in the body to produce secondary tumors. It is the usual cause of death in cancer. It is a series of linked processes, but it is thought that only some subclones of cells are capable of spreading. Most cells entering the circulation do not survive. There are intriguing features; some tumors have preferential sites for metastasis—the prostate or bone, for example. Experimental data have shown that subclones of cells, produced from the same tumor, may have very different capacities for metastasis (Fig. 4). The following steps are thought to be important in metastasis:

- Angiogenesis
- Invasion and degradation
- Altered adhesion
- Migration and circulation
- Tumor cell attachment
- Invasion and degradation
- Migration
- Colonization of the secondary site

Degradation of Extracellular Matrix Barriers

Metastasis requires cancer cells to penetrate extracellular matrix barriers. This involves the proteolytic degradation of extracellular matrix components. MMPs are a family of zinc-dependent endopeptidases (gelatinases) known to degrade extracellular matrix components. Their activity is inhibited by tissue inhibitors of MMPs (TIMPs). High levels of TIMP-2 immunoreactivity, detected both in tumor cells and in stroma, have been reported to be associated with cancer-specific death. This is somewhat surprising, given that TIMPs inhibit the degradation of the extracellular matrix. However, recent studies have shown that, under certain circumstances, TIMP-2 can also activate MMP-2. Other enzymes include the plasminogen activators. These enzymes may be expressed by host stromal around a tumor merely as an indicator of tissue remodeling (Fig. 5). Hence, they have not shown consistent usefulness as prognostic markers.

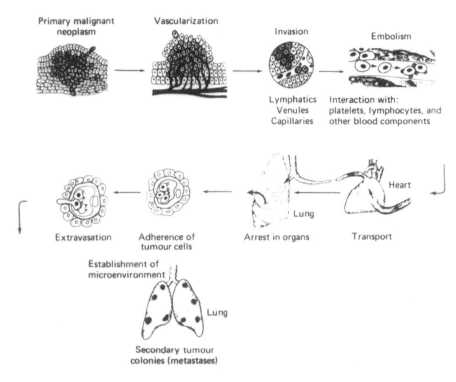

Figure 4 Factors involved in metastasis.

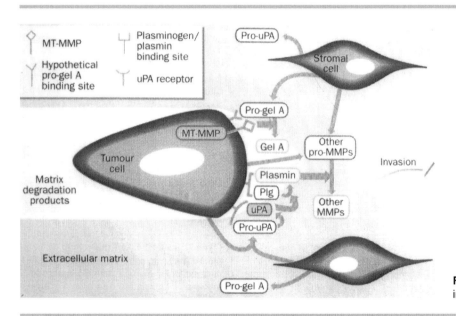

Figure 5 Secretion of proteases (and their inhibitors) by tumor and stroma.

Altered Cell Adhesion

Decreased intercellular adhesiveness favors detachment of tumor cells, and this may play a role in regression to metastatic disease. At least four families of cell adhesion molecules are thought to be involved in cell-cell adhesion (cadherins, selectins, immunoglobulins, and integrins). The most widely studied have been E-cadherin, a cell surface glycoprotein restricted

to epithelial tissue, which is involved in calcium-dependent homotypic cell-cell adhesion, and the vascular cell adhesion molecules, E-selectin, vascular cell adhesion molecule-1 (VCAM-1), and intercellular adhesion molecule-1 (ICAM-1). The regulation of the expression of E-cadherin on tumor cells is unclear. Posttranslational modification of the protein product may affect function. It is known that three molecules (a, b, and c catenins) form bridges between the cytoplasmic tail of E-cadherin and the cytoskeleton, a bridging that may be necessary for E-cadherin to function normally.

Migration and Circulation

Tumor cells have increased motility that allows them to insinuate between the components of the extracellular matrix. They then reach the basement membranes of capillaries or lymph vessels, which they lyse to enter the circulation. This process is likely to be controlled in part by the secretion of cytokines, chemokines, and growth factors by tumor or stromal cells.

Attachment and Colonization

Most tumor cells do not survive. From experimental studies, we know that less than 1% survive and less than 0.1% will grow and proliferate. We know that growth in animal models is far more complex than that produced by the same cells in tissue culture. Attachment of tumor cells is controlled by various factors. Shear forces at the bifurcation of vessels increase the risk that tumor cells will become attached. Certain tumors may induce the formation of distant fibrin clots that makes it more likely that tumor cells will stick. Tumor cells that possess the capacity to invade and migrate are more likely to spread in secondary sites. Capillaries, lymph vessels, and veins are more susceptible than arteries to invasion by tumor cells, as they lack protease inhibitors.

The site of metastasis can be typical. For instance, bone stroma is likely to be the site of secondary spread from prostate cancer. This occurs because of the secretion of particular growth factors that encourage the survival of prostate cells. Other sites, such as the spleen, are very unlikely to be invaded by tumor cells. The immunological factors in tumor control are discussed elsewhere in the book.

ACKNOWLEDGMENT

Artwork reproduced from Alberts B, Johnson A, Lewis J, et al., eds. Molecular Biology of the Cell. 4th ed. New York: Garland Science, 2002.

22

Tumor Suppressor Genes and Oncogenes

David E. Neal

Department of Oncology, University of Cambridge, Addenbrooke's Hospital, Cambridge, U.K.

ONCOGENES

What have sometimes been referred to as "recessive oncogenes" are now more commonly called tumor suppressor genes. Many DNA viruses produce proteins that directly perturb the function of tumor suppressor genes (e.g., large T antigen of SV40 binds p53 and Rb; E6 and E7 of the papilloma virus bind p53 and Rb; the E1A protein of adenovirus binds Rb).

The term "oncogene" was originally used to describe those genes carried by viruses (most of them being retroviruses), which were found to be the cause of transmissible forms of cancer in animals. These retroviral oncogenes (v-oncs) were closely related to normal host cellular genes called proto-oncogenes. Cellular oncogenes found in cancer (c-oncs) were shown to be normal proto-oncogenes that had become "activated" by a variety of mechanisms, including point mutations, deletion, insertional mutagenesis, translocation, and overexpression—often associated with gene amplification. The initial techniques involved in identifying these genes (transfection of tumor DNA into NIH 3T3 fibroblasts) tended to select dominantly acting transforming genes, which are now generally known as "oncogenes."

As the number of known oncogenes increased and their functions became known, they were classified into families defined by their normal cellular counterparts. These include growth factors and their receptors, nuclear regulators of gene transcription and DNA replication, and signal transduction proteins, which couple cell surface receptors and the nucleus. More than 60 oncogenes have now been identified. The types of oncogenes and some of their functions are shown in Figure 1. Their transfection into cells causes transformation (Table 1).

A cellular proto-oncogene can be converted to an oncogene in the following ways:

- Insertion of a section of DNA into the promoter region of the gene (insertional mutagenesis, e.g., Wnt-1)
- Deletion [conversion of epidermal growth factor receptor (EGFr) to v-erbB-2]
- Translocation or chromosomal rearrangement (Philadelphia chromosome) (Fig. 2)
- Point mutation (H-ras)
- Gene amplification (EGFr in brain tumors)

G Proteins and Ras

Proteins that bind and hydrolyze guanidine triphosphate (GTP) are found commonly in the cell and play a crucial role in cell signaling. When GTP (which is found in large excess in the cell compared with GDP) is bound to such G proteins, the protein becomes activated and initiates a cascade of events. However, GTP-binding proteins also rapidly hydrolyze GTP to GDP, thereby rendering themselves inactive. Other proteins can control the activity of GTP binding to such proteins, including one called GTPase-activating protein (GAP), which binds to G proteins, inducing them to convert GTP to GDP and become inactive. Another protein called guanine nucleotide–releasing protein (GNRP) binds to G proteins, inducing them to release GDP and bind GTP (which is present in large amounts in the normal cell), converting it into an active form. G proteins are classified into the following:

- Monomeric G proteins (such as ras, rac, and rho)
- Heterotrimeric G proteins (often directly coupling cell surface receptors to intracellular receptors, such as adrenoreceptors or muscarinic acetylcholine receptors to adenyl cyclase and phospholipase C, respectively)

Ras Family

The human *ras* gene family consists of three closely related genes: H-ras, K-ras, and N-ras, which encode 21-kDa signal transduction G proteins involved in the transmission of signals from cell surface receptors. Ras proteins belong to the monomeric family of G proteins as distinct from the trimeric family that couple cell surface receptors (such as adrenergic receptors) to intracellular events. Other monomeric G proteins include the rho and rac family, which, like ras proteins, are involved in the relay of signals from the cell membrane. Activation of ras by mutation occurs as a result of a single amino acid change as a consequence of single nucleotide mutations. Activated H-ras has been found in bladder carcinomas, Ki-ras in lung and colon carcinomas, and N-ras in hematological malignancies. H-ras is a monomeric G protein. In its mutated (H-ras) form, it contains a single-point mutation, leading to the conversion of a glycine to a valine

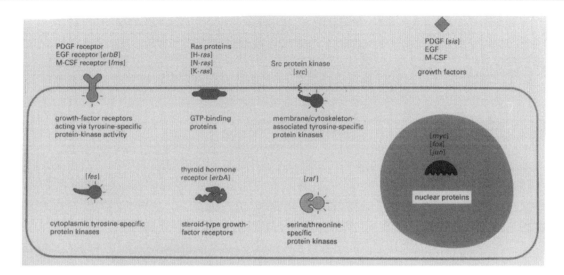

Figure 1 The activities and cellular locations of the products of the main classes of known proto-oncogenes. Some representative proto-oncogenes in each class are indicated in brackets.

Table 1 Some Oncogenes

Oncogene	Proto-oncogene	Source of virus	Virus-induced tumor
Abl	Tyrosine kinase	Mouse	Leukemia
erbB	Tyrosine kinase (EGFr, c-erbB2, etc.)	Chicken	Erythroleukemia
Fes	Tyrosine kinase	Cat	Sarcoma
Fms	Tyrosine kinase (M-CSM factor)	Cat	Sarcoma
Fos	AP-1 protein	Mouse	Osteosarcoma
Jun	AP-1 protein	Chicken	Fibrosarcoma
raf (MAP kinase kinase kinase)	Serine kinase activated by ras	Chicken	Sarcoma
Myc	Transcription factor	Chicken	Sarcoma
H-ras	GTP (G)-binding protein	Rat	Sarcoma
K-ras	G protein	Rat	Sarcoma
Rel	NFκB transcription factor	Turkey	Reticuloendotheliosis
Sis	PDGF	Monkey	Sarcoma
Src	Tyrosine kinase	Chicken	Sarcoma

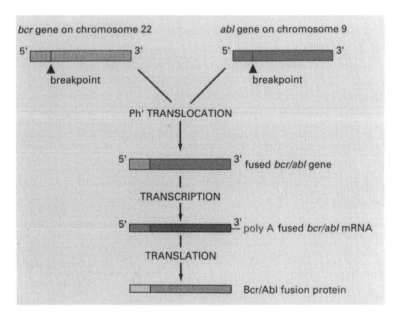

Figure 2 The translocation between chromosomes 9 and 22 responsible for chronic myelogenous leukemia. The smaller of the two resulting abnormal chromosomes is called the Philadelphia chromosome, after the city where the abnormality was first recorded.

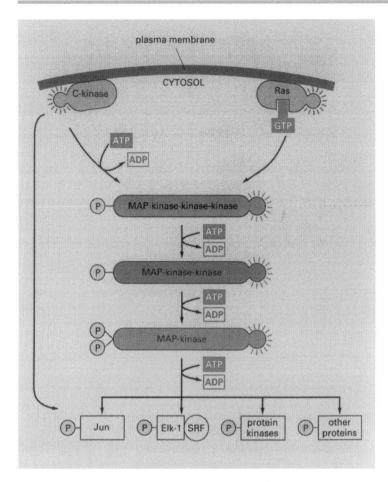

Figure 3 The serine/threonine phosphorylation cascade activated by ras and C kinase. In the pathway activated by receptor tyrosine kinases via ras, the MAP kinase kinase kinase is often a serine/threonine kinase called Raf, which is thought to be activated by the binding of activated ras. In the pathway activated by G protein–linked receptors via C kinase, the MAP kinase kinase kinase can either be Raf or a different serine/threonine kinase. A similar serine/threonine phosphorylation cascade involving structurally and functionally related proteins operates in yeasts and in all animals that have been studied, where it integrates and amplifies signals from different extracellular stimuli. Receptor tyrosine kinases may also activate a more direct signaling pathway to the nucleus by directly phosphorylating, and thereby activating, gene regulatory proteins that contain SH2 domains.

residue at codon 12. Mutated H-ras is constitutively active whether GTP is bound or not.

Ras helps to link activated tyrosine kinase receptors to downstream events by acting as a molecular switch. It is in the "off" position when bound to GDP and in the "on" position when bound to GTP. Some tyrosine kinase receptors phosphorylate themselves on tyrosine residues, which then bind to other proteins that have SH2 domains that dock to phosphorylated tyrosine residues. These proteins with SH2 domains then link to other proteins (such as Sos) that activate ras. Activated ras initiates a serine/threonine phosphorylation cascade, which eventually activates a kinase called mitogen-activated protein kinase (MAP kinase). Eventually, such activation stimulates the action of a number of transcription factors, including jun and elk-1 (Fig. 3). Figure 3 shows another important point: namely, that protein kinase C can also activate MAP kinase.

Heterotrimeric G Proteins

A large number of membrane-bound receptors function by activating downstream trimeric G proteins, which initiate a phosphorylation cascade stimulating certain enzymes. The trimeric G proteins consist of three parts (α, β, and γ) that disassemble when activated. The a-subunit bound to GTP activates nearby enzymes such as adenyl cyclase, which synthesizes cyclic AMP (Fig. 4), or phospholipase C, which forms inositol triphosphate (IP_3), and diacylglycerol from inositol biphosphate found in the cell membrane (Fig. 5). IP_3 causes calcium release from various intracellular stores and diacylglycerol activates protein kinase C, which is a serine/threonine kinase (Fig. 6) that, as pointed out above, can also stimulate MAP kinase.

Examples of receptors linked by G proteins to phospholipase C include the muscarinic receptor. Activation of the muscarinic receptor causes an increase in transmembrane calcium flux and also release of IP_3, which further releases calcium from the endoplasmic reticulum. Receptors linked by G proteins to adenyl cyclase include the β-adrenergic receptor (stimulation of cyclic AMP) and the α2-receptor (inhibition of cyclic AMP). The α1-receptor stimulates phospholipase C as well as inhibits adenyl cyclase. Thus, although a wide variety of receptors are coupled to different G proteins, the exact consequences of receptor activation depend on the specific G protein, which couples the receptor to downstream intracellular signaling mechanisms.

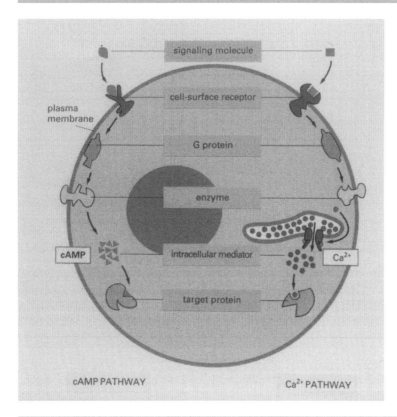

Figure 4 Two major pathways by which G protein–linked cell surface receptors generate small intracellular mediators. In both cases, the binding of an extracellular ligand alters the conformation of the cytoplasmic domain of the receptor, causing it to bind to a G protein that activates (or inactivates) a plasma membrane enzyme. In the cAMP pathway, the enzyme directly produces cAMP. In the Ca^{2+} pathway, the enzyme produces a soluble mediator (inositol trisphosphate) that releases Ca^{2+} from the endoplasmic reticulum. Like other small intracellular mediators, both cAMP and Ca^{2+} relay the signal by acting as allosteric effectors: they bind to specific proteins in the cell, altering their conformation and thereby their activity. *Abbreviation*: cAMP, cyclic AMP.

Tyrosine Kinase Growth Factor Receptors

Many cell surface receptors for growth factors contain a tyrosine kinase domain as part of the protein, which is similar to the src family of oncogene tyrosine kinase (including Src, Yes, Fgr, Lck, Lyn, Hck, and Blk) and contain SH2 domains facing the internal portion of the cell. Other growth factor receptors are closely associated with separate tyrosine kinase proteins that are not an intrinsic part of the receptor protein itself. Most of the transforming growth factor receptors [EGFr, insulin-like growth factor I receptor (IGF-Ir), nerve growth factor receptor (NGFr), platelet-derived growth factor receptor (PDGFr), fibroblast growth factor receptor (FGFR), and vascular endothelial growth factor receptor (VEGFr)] contain an intrinsic tyrosine kinase domain, with an exception for transforming growth factor-β (TGF-β), which contains a serine/threonine kinase. When activated by ligand binding, tyrosine kinase receptors autophosphorylate at several phosphorylation sites and can then act as docking sites for a small set of intracellular proteins that recognize tyrosine-associated phosphate sites via their SH2 domains (such as SOS and GrB2). Activation of the EGFr produces dimerization of the receptor, autophosphorylation of tyrosine residues, and phosphorylation of target proteins. EGFr activation is linked to the ras signal transduction pathway via two proteins (Sos and Grb2), which, when EGFr is activated, link via Raf (MAP kinase kinase kinase) to the downstream signals of the ras pathway such as MAP kinase.

In many growth factor receptors, ligand binding induces dimerization, a conformational change takes place, and the tyrosine kinase domain is activated. Some mutated growth factor receptors are constitutively active, whereas other receptors can become activated in the absence of ligand if the receptor protein is found at very high levels. Such receptors can also form heterodimers [such as c-erbB-2 with c-erbB-3 or with c-erbB-1 (EGFr)]. It should be noted that herceptin has recently been introduced as cancer treatment in advanced breast cancer; it is a "humanized" antibody against c-erbB2. It is proof of the principle that novel treatments against some of these targets can be clinically useful.

Epidermal Growth Factor and the EGF Receptor

EGF is a 53–amino acid peptide with mitogenic activity whose action is mediated by binding to a membrane-bound receptor. EGF was originally isolated from murine submaxillary gland extracts, and its distribution is widespread, with high levels of milk, prostatic fluid, and urine. The detection of high levels of EGF in urine prompted studies of EGFr levels in bladder cancer.

EGFr is a 175-kDa transmembrane protein with an extracellular EGF-binding domain, a small hydrophobic region that spans the plasma membrane, and an intracellular domain, which has tyrosine kinase activity as well as target tyrosine residues for autophosphorylation. EGFr (*c-erbB-1* gene) has considerable sequence homology with the gp65^{erbB} protein

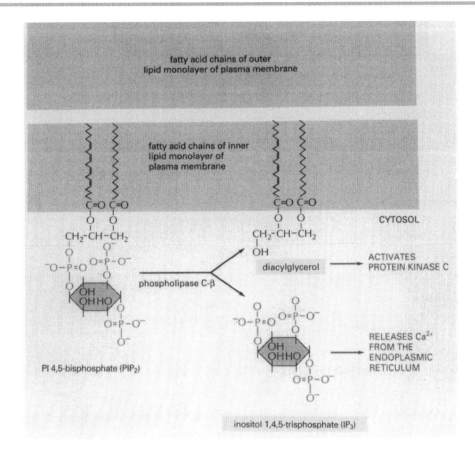

Figure 5 The hydrolysis of PIP$_2$. Two intracellular mediators are produced when PIP$_2$ is hydrolyzed: inositol triphosphate (IP$_3$), which diffuses through the cytosol and releases Ca^{2+} from the ER, and diacylglycerol, which remains in the membrane and helps activate the enzyme protein kinase C. There are at least three classes of phospholipase C—β, γ, and δ—and it is the β class that is activated by G protein–linked receptors. We shall see later that the γ class is activated by a second class of receptors, called *receptor tyrosine kinases*, that activate the inositol phospholipid signaling pathway without an intermediary G protein.

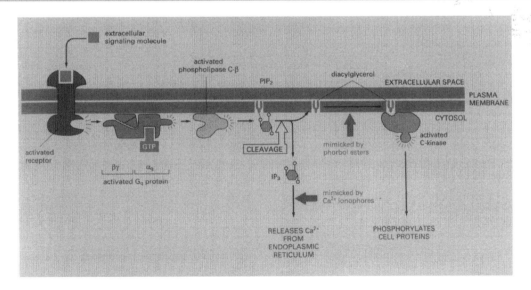

Figure 6 The two branches of the inositol phospholipid pathway. The activated receptor binds to a specific trimeric G protein (G$_q$), causing the α subunit to dissociate and activate phospholipase C-β, which cleaves PIP$_2$ to generate IP$_3$ and diacylglycerol. The diacylglycerol (together with bound Ca^{2+} and phosphatidylserine—not shown) activates C kinase. Both phospholipase C-β and C kinase are water-soluble enzymes that translocate from the cytosol to the inner face of the plasma membrane in the process of being activated. The effects of IP$_3$ can be mimicked experimentally in intact cells by treatment with Ca^{2+} ionophores, while the effects of diacylglycerol can be mimicked by treatment with phorbol esters, which bind to C kinase and activate it.

from the avian erythroblastosis virus. EGFr is also the target for the peptide growth factor TGF-α, which is synthesized by a wide range of common epithelial tumors, including transitional cell carcinomas (TCC) of the urinary bladder, renal, and prostate.

EGFr is distributed throughout the body and is present on normal fibroblasts, corneal cells, kidney cells, basal prostate epithelium, and basal urothelium. Increased expression of EGFr protein is transforming in some cell lines, and some human solid tumors, including TCC, have increased levels of EGFr protein. This appears to be achieved by a variety of mechanisms, including gene amplification, upregulation of mRNA, and increased translation or posttranslational modification of the protein.

C-erbB-2

The proto-oncogene c-erbB-2 (also known as neu or HER-2) encodes a transmembrane glycoprotein, which is related to the EGFr. Several groups have reported a candidate ligand for the c-erbB-2 receptor, and elucidation of its structure (neu differentiation factor or heregulin-α) reveals it to be an additional member of the EGF family. Two further members of the erbB receptor family are HER3/p160[erbB-3] and HER4/p180[erbB-4]. Recent evidence suggests, however, that heregulin is the physiological ligand for c-erbB-3 and that for c-erbB-2 is as yet unidentified.

Fibroblast Growth Factors

The FGFs are a family of peptides related by sequence similarity that have been implicated in the regulation of cell proliferation, angiogenesis, embryonal development, differentiation, and motility. The family includes FGF (aFGF; FGF-1), basic FGF (bFGF; FGF-2), int-2 (FGF-3), hst (FGF-4), FGF-5, hst2 (FGF-6), keratinocyte growth factor (KGF; FGF-7), androgen-inducible growth factor (AIGF; FGF-8), and FGF-9. They bind with varying degrees of specificity to a family of tyrosine kinase receptors (FGFRs). bFGF has been shown to transform mouse fibroblasts in vitro, int-2 (FGF-3) is the human homologue of one of the common integration sites of mouse mammary tumor virus, and hst (FGF-4) is the most frequently detected human transforming gene after ras in the NIH 3T3 assay. These two genes were reported to be amplified in 3/43 (7%) of bladder tumors and 41/238 (17%) of breast carcinomas.

Basic FGF has been identified in both benign and malignant human prostate. Immunohistochemistry has identified FGF-2 predominantly in not only prostatic stroma but also epithelial cells. FGF-1 is also present in the prostate but at a lower level than FGF-2. In addition, in a prostate stromal cell culture model, there is evidence for the interaction of FGF-2 and TGF-β1, resulting in positive and negative proliferative effects, respectively. Besides potential autocrine loop activation, FGFs may also contribute to the pathophysiology of the prostate via paracrine activity. FGF-7, or KGF, is synthesized and secreted by stromal cells, being thought to act on FGF receptor–bearing epithelial cells, resulting in cellular proliferation. It is also interesting to note that, in a transgenic mouse system, overexpression of FGF-3 or int-2, alterations to the prostate of the male progeny, were dramatic and involved only hyperplasia, without evidence of malignant transformation.

The FGFrs share structural similarities in both the extracellular domains that bind FGFs and the intracellular domains that activate the signal transduction pathway. The four FGFRs, FGFR-1 to FGFR-4, display different binding affinities for the different FGFs. FGF-1 binds to all four receptors, while FGF-2 is more restricted and binds only to the first three FGFRs. Receptor-receptor interactions are known to occur and may have a role in the development of both benign hyperplasia and carcinoma of the prostate. To date, the expression of FGFs and their receptors is not fully understood, but there does appear to be a major difference between benign and malignant prostate in the activity of the FGF system. Splice variants occur in the FGFRs. It is likely that subtle changes occur in the FGF system during malignant progression. This has been demonstrated elegantly in a mouse prostate cancer model. During progression from the benign to the malignant phenotype, the prostate epithelial cells display a switch of expression of FGFR splice variants, conferring a switch of high-affinity binding from FGF-7 to FGF-2. FGF-2 was also concomitantly upregulated along with FGF-3 and FGF-5. Further evidence supporting a role for FGFs in the development of malignancy is that transformation of BHK-21 (baby hamster kidney) cells with plasmids carrying the bFGF coding sequence results in cells that exhibit the transformed phenotype. The prostatic cancer cell lines DU145 and PC-3 produce active FGF-2 and express large amounts of FGFR-2. However, only the DU145 cell line, and not the PC-3 cell line, has been shown to respond to exogenous FGF-2.

The interaction between the androgen receptor and growth factor systems is important. It is known that certain growth factors, including FGF-7/KGF, IGFs, and EGF, may activate androgen-dependent gene expression in the absence of androgen, and this may represent a mechanism for the development of hormone insensitivity in prostate tumors.

Insulin-Like Growth Factors

IGF-I is a 70-amino acid polypeptide with functional homology to insulin. The mitogenic effect of IGF-I is due to its ability to facilitate the transfer of cells from the G1 phase to the S phase in the cell cycle. IGF-I and the closely related IGF-II are present in biological fluids and tissue extracts, and are usually bound to an IGF-binding protein (IGF-BP). There are two types of receptors for the IGFs. The type 1 receptor is a tyrosine kinase and binds both IGF-I and IGF-II. The type 2 receptor is structurally distinct and binds primarily IGF-II. The majority of the mitogenic effects of the IGFs appear to be mediated via the type 1 IGF receptor.

The growth of normal prostatic epithelial cells in culture is dependent on the presence of IGF-I and II. The response is most marked with IGF-I. The type 1 IGF receptor has been identified in normal, benign, and malignant prostatic tissues. It is preferentially expressed in the basal cells. Production of IGF-II has been demonstrated by prostatic fibroblasts, but IGF-I has not been identified as being produced by either prostatic fibroblasts or epithelial cells. However, IGF-I mRNA has been identified in stromal cells from benign prostatic hyperplasia (BPH) specimens. The mechanism of IGF-II-mediated stimulation of prostatic epithelial cells in BPH appears to be similar to that in normal prostate, although the expression of IGF-II mRNA is 10-fold higher in fibroblasts from BPH tissues. This led to the hypothesis that such cells may be ''reverting to a fetal-like state,'' where IGF-II expression is normally high, causing stimulation of proliferation and the development of BPH.

Transforming Growth Factor β

TGF-β_1 is the predominant species in the TGF-β superfamily, which includes several modulators of growth, differentiation, and morphogenesis (including bone morphogenetic proteins). TGF-β_1 is classically regarded as a stimulator for mesenchyme cells and an inhibitor for epithelial cells. Five isoforms of TGF-β have so far been identified, of which only the first three occur in mammals. TGF-β_1 is a homodimer of two 112-amino acid subunits linked by disulfide bonds. Cellular receptors for TGF-β_1 have been identified in the rat ventral prostate where they are negatively regulated by androgens and involved in the mechanism of castration-induced prostatic cell death. Receptors for TGF-β_1 have been identified in the human prostate cancer cell lines DU145 and PC-3. TGF-β_1 has been shown to have an inhibitory effect on human prostatic fibroblasts and epithelial cells in culture. It has been suggested that TGF-β_1 causes inhibition of proliferation by preventing phosphorylation of the protein product of the retinoblastoma gene (pRB) by upregulation of p15, which is a cyclin-dependent kinase inhibitor, and by stabilization of the p27 protein. The TGF-β receptor is a serine protease and links to downstream signals, including SMAD2.

TUMOR SUPPRESSOR GENES

Evidence for the existence of tumor suppressor genes has come from several sources, although the significance of the observations was not appreciated at the time. Experiments dating back to the 1960s, involving the fusion of normal and transformed cells, had shown that normal genes can suppress transformation and malignancy in cell lines.

The second line of evidence came from an analysis of the inheritance of rare hereditary childhood cancers. On the basis of retinoblastoma, Knudson proposed a two-hit inactivation process in which both copies of a critical gene had to be inactivated for the disease to be manifest. That these hereditary cancers are often associated with predisposition to a wide range of sporadic tumors of other tissues led to the further suggestion that somatic mutation or loss of these same genes was probably involved in the genesis of a wide range of cancers, including bladder cancer. This also provided a possible explanation for the observation of the nonrandom chromosome deletions seen in sporadic tumors. This concept in turn led to the identification of the p53 gene as a tumor suppressor gene.

Cytogenetic studies have shown that frequent nonrandom chromosome alterations occur in cancer. For instance, in bladder cancer, these involve chromosomes 1p, 3p, 9p, 10q, 11, 13q, 17p, and 18q. Loss of one copy of chromosome 9p was found as an early event in low-stage, low-grade tumors, unlike other chromosome losses, which appeared to be more prevalent in advanced tumors. The high frequency of chromosome 9p losses in bladder cancer is not seen in other tumor types, suggesting the possible location of a tumor suppressor gene specific to bladder cancer.

The p53 Tumor Suppressor Gene

The human p53 gene, located on the short arm of chromosome 17, encodes a nuclear phosphoprotein, which binds to specific DNA sequences in the human genome and appears to play a key role in the control of DNA replication and hence cellular proliferation. Nonrandom chromosome 17 losses involving the p53 locus are commonly found in human tumors, including bladder cancer, and the loss of one copy of the p53 gene has been found to be frequently accompanied by mutation of the remaining allele. Transfection studies have shown that the wild-type protein is able to suppress cell proliferation and transformation. It thus acts in such circumstances as a tumor suppressor gene, which can contribute to tumor formation by deletions or loss of function mutations. Germline mutations of the p53 gene have been found in certain inherited predispositions to cancer (Li-Fraumeni syndrome, in which there is clustering of soft tissue and bone sarcomas at any age; and cancers under the age of 45 in breast, brain, adrenal cortex, and lung) and somatic cell mutations have frequently been detected in a wide range of common sporadic tumors, including breast, colon, brain, and lung tumors, as well as bladder cancer. These mutations are predominantly of the point missense type and occur at many different locations within four highly conserved regions of the gene (codons 117–142, 171–181, 234–258, and 270–286) located in exons 4 to 9 of the p53 gene.

The p53 protein has three parts: a central DNA-binding domain in which mutations are usually of the missense type, a transcription domain (*N*-terminus) and a regulatory domain (*C*-terminus) in which mutations result in nonsense or stop codons. The protein murine double minute-2 (mdm-2) binds near the *N*-terminus of the protein. One of the genes activated by p53 is the p21 protein (WAF1), which inhibits the activity of cyclin-dependent kinases and which also binds to PCNA. Other genes include gadd45 and the protein bax (which promotes apoptosis).

The p53 protein has a short half-life, measured in the order of minutes, and is normally present at low levels not detectable by immunohistochemistry. One of the remarkable features of the p53 gene is that a broad spectrum of mutations can lead to an altered conformation and inactivation of the protein product with an increased cellular half-life, resulting in accumulation in the cell to levels that are readily detectable by immunohistochemical staining. Although this initially led to suggestions that positive detection of p53 by immunohistochemistry was synonymous with the detection of mutations, this is now realized not to be the case. Moreover, some mutations do not result in accumulation of the altered protein product, and these have to be screened for by alternative complementary methods such as single-strand conformation polymorphism assays to obtain a more complete picture. However, even combined, these techniques are, at best, a way of trawling for mutations rather than a way of systematically screening for all possible mutations. The definitive method of establishing the presence of a mutation in a sample is by DNA-sequencing procedures.

Inactivation of Normal p53 in Tumors

Some proteins have been shown to bind to p53 and inactivate it. For instance, in sarcomas, it has been shown that p53 mutations are rare, but there is increased expression of a protein called mdm-2, which, like the large T antigen of the SV40 virus, binds to p53, inactivates it, and stabilizes it. This confirms the frequent involvement of the p53 pathway in many human tumors.

p53 and G1 Arrest

Irradiation of cells has been shown to result in marked upregulation of the wild-type p53 protein. It may be that the primary event is DNA repair following radiotherapy, which then activates p53. However, upregulation of p53 switches on downstream genes such as p21, which is a potent inhibitor of cell division, and places them into G1 arrest, allowing completion of DNA repair if this is possible.

p53 and Apoptosis

Some authors believe that increased levels of p53 can, if DNA damage is too severe to repair during G1 arrest, force the cell into apoptosis. There is no doubt that with severe DNA damage there is an initial attempt at DNA repair followed by upregulation of p53, stimulation of p21, and cell cycle arrest. With more severe DNA damage or with less severe damage in certain types of cells (such as thymocytes), this process may be followed by apoptosis, but, currently, it is controversial as to whether p53 is directly responsible for apoptosis in such circumstances. Certainly, p53 can upregulate bax (a promoter of apoptosis), but it is also certain that in some cells apoptosis can occur without recourse to the p53-bax pathway.

mdm-2 Oncogene

The *mdm-2* gene is located on chromosome 12q13–14 and encodes a 90-kDa nuclear protein. The mdm-2 protein may act as an oncoprotein when overexpressed, by binding to the "guardian of the genome," wild-type p53 protein, and abrogating its functions.

Retinoblastoma Gene

The *Rb1* gene encodes a 105- to 115-kDa nuclear phosphoprotein, which binds to DNA and appears to be involved in growth regulation in a wide variety of cell types. There are related p107 and p130 proteins, whose function in man has not been elucidated but which may have overlapping actions. The Rb1 gene product binds to the transforming proteins of several DNA tumor viruses, including adenovirus E1A, SV40 large T antigen, and human papilloma virus E7 proteins. Abnormalities in the Rb gene were first reported in patients with inherited retinoblastoma who had one abnormal copy of the gene in all retinal cells; it is thought that subsequent "spontaneous" alterations in the remaining copy of the Rb gene causes tumor formation.

The Rb protein is central to the function of the cell cycle; it is inactive when phosphorylated or when bound to inactivating proteins. It is the target of cyclin-dependent kinases and cyclin D. When it is activated, it stimulates the E2F family of transcription factors (myc and jun are among them): it is a negative regulator of the cell cycle. Disruption of this pathway is central to many tumors. The cyclin-dependent kinase inhibitor p16 is particularly linked to Rb, so when p16 is upregulated, the activity of cdk2 is inhibited. The Rb protein is not phosphorylated, so it binds to DNA and inhibits transcription, and the E2F family of transcription factors is switched off.

A wider role for the Rb1 gene was suggested by the observation that those who inherit the mutant allele have a higher incidence of not only a wide range of nonocular second tumors, particularly osteosarcomas, but also lung melanoma and bladder cancer.

Initial studies with the Rb1 cDNA probe, based mainly on tumor cell lines, reported frequent structural abnormalities of the gene and absence of Rb1 mRNA. Subsequent extensions of these studies with polyclonal antisera indicated that absence or abnormal forms of the Rb protein are almost universal in small-cell lung cancer cell lines and present in one-third of bladder carcinoma cell lines, while being infrequent in colonic, breast, and melanoma cell lines. Studies on primary bladder tumors have shown that loss of heterozygosity for Rb1-linked markers is associated with the development of invasive lesions. The overall frequency of Rb1 allelic loss in bladder cancer was 3/63 (5%) for superficial (pTa/pT1) and 30/58 (53%) for invasive (T2–T4) tumors. Major rearrangements of the remaining Rb1 gene were detected in only a small proportion of these cases, suggesting that generally more subtle small deletions or point mutations are involved that have yet to be characterized. Altered Rb protein expression is associated with a poor outcome in several tumor types, including bladder.

von Hippel–Lindau Disease

This is inherited as a dominant abnormality and consists of retinal cysts, cerebellar hemangioblastomas, pancreatic cysts, pheochromocytomas, renal cysts, and renal cancer. The VHL gene is situated on chromosome 3p and also affects many sporadic renal cancers. It encodes a small protein (213 aa) with three exons, and in the human gene there are eight penta-peptide repeats in exon 1. Most mutations in VHL are found at the carboxy terminus of exon 1 and at the beginning of exon 3. Similar mutations are found in sporadic tumors, but, in addition, mutations are found in exon 2, a rare event in VHL. The VHL protein binds to the elongation factors elongin B and C, which help in the synthesis of mRNA; it is thought that the VHL/ elongin B and C complex moves from the nucleus into the cytoplasm as a response to cell/cell contacts. VHL also upregulates the peptide VEGF (see next section), a feature that may be responsible for angiogenesis in renal cancer

Genes Associated with Chemoresistance

Chemotherapy with epirubicin or mitomycin C is increasingly used for recurrent superficial papillary tumors. In muscle-invasive disease, adjuvant and neo-adjuvant chemotherapy regimens are currently being tested in clinical trials. Molecular mechanisms that mediate cellular drug resistance may play a role in the differential responsiveness of individual bladder tumous to chemotherapy. Transcript levels of the multidrug resistance (*mdr1*) gene have been found to vary 34-fold in high-grade muscle-invasive bladder tumors. In addition, renal cell carcinomas have very high levels of this gene, perhaps explaining why it is chemoresistant.

ACKNOWLEDGMENT

Artwork reproduced from Alberts B, Johnson A, Lewis J, et al., eds. Molecular Biology of the Cell. 4th ed. New York: Garland Science, 2002.

23

The Molecular Genetics and Pathology of Renal Cell Carcinoma

Maxine G. B. Tran

Department of Urology, Addenbrooke's Hospital, Cambridge, U.K.

Tim O'Brien

Department of Urology, Guy's and St Thomas' Hospital, London, U.K.

Patrick H. Maxwell

Division of Medicine, University College Hospital, London, U.K.

INTRODUCTION

Renal cell carcinoma (RCC) is the commonest malignancy of the kidney and represents 2% to 3% of all adult cancers. Each year in the United Kingdom, more than 6600 patients are diagnosed with kidney cancer, and over half will die of the disease. The highest prevalence is in the 6th decade of life, with a male: female ratio of approximately 2:1.

Although RCC is a relatively rare malignancy, the incidence is steadily increasing at a rate of approximately 2% per year worldwide, in part but not entirely due to increased use of imaging modalities leading to recognition of tumors that were previously undiagnosed (1,2). Incidentally discovered renal masses now account for 48% to 66% of RCC diagnoses (3). In the United States the incidence rates in black Americans have increased rapidly surpassing the incidence rate of white Americans. Large epidemiological studies have established cigarette smoking, western style diet, obesity and hypertension as main risk factors in both sexes for the development of RCC; while recreational exercise is associated with decreased risk (1,4). Diuretic use is associated with an increased risk in females, and alcohol consumption is inversely associated with risk in men (5,6). A positive family history of RCC is associated with a two- to threefold increase in risk, while the inherited forms of RCC account for 2% of all cases.

THE PATHOLOGICAL AND GENETIC CLASSIFICATION OF ADULT RENAL EPITHELIAL NEOPLASMS

A workshop held in Heidelberg in 1996 culminated in the widely accepted Heidelberg classification of adult renal epithelial neoplasms (7) (Table 1). The Union Internationale Contre le Cancer (UICC) and the American Joint Committee on Cancer (AJCC) held a workshop in Minnesota the following year and proposed a very similar classification system (8). More recently, the World Health Organisation (WHO) in 2004 introduced a new classification of adult renal epithelial neoplasms that is more comprehensive and includes new diagnostic categories (9) (Table 2).

These new classification systems reflect our increased understanding of the molecular pathology of renal neoplasms, the close correlation between specific genetic abnormalities and histological subgroups, and differ from the older systems, which were essentially based on architectural and cytological subtypes (10). Importantly, they allow the majority of cases to be classified by routine H&E light microscopy, with more specialized molecular genetic studies reserved for a minority of atypical cases; in addition the classification systems have prognostic utility (11,12).

Having once been considered a single disease entity, it is now clear that there are a number of different types of kidney cancer, each with a different histological pattern, clinical behavior, prognosis, and each caused by abnormalities of different genes (11,13).

The major clinical and histopathological features of the main adult renal epithelial neoplasms will be reviewed in this chapter. We will then consider our current understanding of the molecular and genetic basis of renal neoplasm development, how these relate to the current classification of renal epithelial neoplasms, and finally how this improved insight has led to the development of new management strategies in renal cancer.

Table 1 The Heidelberg Classification of Adult Renal Epithelial Neoplasms

Benign tumors	Malignant tumors
Papillary renal adenoma	Conventional renal cell carcinoma
Metanephric adenoma	Papillary renal cell carcinoma
Oncocytoma	Chromophobe renal cell carcinoma
	Collecting duct carcinoma (including renal medullary carcinoma)
	Renal cell carcinoma, unclassified

Source: From Ref. 7.

Table 2 WHO Classification of Kidney Tumors

Familial renal cancer

Renal Cell tumors
  Malignant
    Clear cell renal cell carcinoma
    Multilocular clear cell renal cell carcinoma
    Papillary renal cell carcinoma
    Chromophobe renal cell carcinoma
    Carcinoma of the collecting ducts of Bellini
    Renal medullary carcinoma
    Xp11 translocation carcinomas
    Carcinoma associated with neuroblastoma
    Mucinous tubular and spindle cell carcinoma
    Renal cell carcinoma unclassified
  Benign
    Papillary adenoma
    Oncocytoma
Metanephric tumors
  Metanephric adenoma
  Metanephric adenofibroma
  Metanephric stromal tumors
Mixed mesenchymal and epithelial tumors
  Cystic nephroma
  Mixed epithelial and stromal tumor
  Synovial sarcoma
Nephroblastic tumors
  Nephrogenic rests
  Nephroblastoma
  Cystic partially differentiated nephroblastoma
Neuroendocrine tumors
  Carcinoid
  Neuroendocrine carcinoma
  Primitive neuroectodermal tumor
  Neuroblastoma
  Phaeochromocytoma
Other tumors
  Mesenchymal tumors
  Hematopoietic and lymphoid tumors
  Germ cell tumors
  Metastatic tumors

Source: From Ref. 9.

THE CLINICAL AND HISTOPATHOLOGICAL FEATURES OF ADULT RENAL EPITHELIAL NEOPLASMS

Benign Renal Tumors

Papillary Renal Adenoma: the Macroscopic and Microscopic Appearances of Papillary Renal Adenoma and Its Association with Papillary Adenocarcinoma

Papillary adenomas are very common lesions, affecting 40% of the general population and are usually an incidental finding at autopsy or in nephrectomies. They are almost always multiple in number, averaging eight lesions per kidney in specimens removed for papillary renal cell carcinoma (PRCC) (14). Papillary adenomas are histologically, immunohistochemically and cytogenetically very similar to low-grade PRCCs; being differentiated principally by size so that an adenoma must be less than 5 mm in maximum diameter. Lesions greater than 5 mm are considered as having malignant potential. Histologically, papillary adenomas are characterized by a tubulopapillary architecture formed by cuboidal cells with scant basophilic cytoplasm. There should not be any evidence of nuclear pleomorphism, significant mitotic activity or vasculolymphatic invasion (15). Because of the similarities between papillary adenomas and PRCCs, it has been proposed that they may represent a continuum of a malignant process (16), although it is unclear what percentage of renal adenomas will progress to carcinomas.

Metanephric Adenoma: Epidemiology, Macroscopic and Microscopic Appearances

Metanephric adenomas are rare tumors of the kidney that have an invariably benign clinical course. They are twice as common in females compared with males, with a mean age at presentation of 41 years (15). They are usually an incidental finding, although they can present with the classical triad of hematuria, loin pain and palpable mass. An unusual paraneoplastic feature of this tumor is polycythaemia, due to erythropoietin and other cytokines produced by the metanephric tumor cells (17). The erythrocytosis resolves following tumor resection.

Histologically, metanephric adenomas are composed of predominantly small tubules lined by cuboidal epithelial cells, and glomeruloid bodies reminiscent of embryonic metanephric tissue are also seen. In the past they have been confused with and misclassified as Wilm's tumor, nephroblastomatosis, or variants of tubular carcinoma or PRCC.

Oncocytoma: Epidemiology, Macroscopic and Microscopic Appearances

Renal oncocytomas was first reported by Zippel in 1942 (18), and account for approximately 2% to 7% of renal neoplasms. There is a male to female ratio of 2.5:1, with a mean age of 65 years at presentation. Renal oncocytomas are usually asymptomatic and are diagnosed incidentally during investigations for other medical problems. Historically they are said to have a characteristic radiological appearance of a cartwheel peripheral vascular arrangement with a central star on angiography, although a recent small series has reported that this could also be a feature of chromophobe RCC and is thus unreliable (19).

Oncocytomas, by and large, are discrete unilateral benign masses, although bilateral and multifocal tumors have been reported (20). Metachronous tumor development has been described to occur in 5% of patients, and they coexist with RCC in 10% (20). On gross pathological examination, oncocytomas appear solid, spherical, are well circumscribed, un-encapsulated, homogenous, tan-brown in color and range in size averaging about 7 cm. A central, stellate, fibrous scar can be found in approximately a third of cases (21), and hemorrhage can occasionally be seen, though cystic change and necrosis is rare (Fig. 1A).

Oncocytomas are thought to arise from the intercalated cells of the collecting duct (22). Histologically, the classic oncocyte consists of polygonal or round cells with abundant eosinophilic cytoplasm, arranged in nests or trabeculae separated by hypocellular, hyalinized stroma (Fig. 1B). By definition, areas of papillary or clear cell differentiation are not allowed. The nuclei appear smooth and round with evenly dispersed chromatin. There is a minimal degree of nuclear atypia and mitotic activity. Ultrastructurally the tumor cells are packed with mitochondria accounting for the eosinophilic appearance of the cells seen on light microscopy.

Occasionally oncocytomas may show atypical features including nuclear polymorphism, prominent nucleoli, and adjacent renal parenchymal and perinephric fat involvement. Oncocytomas are benign tumors and prognosis following resection is excellent (21,23). Malignant variants of oncocytomas have been reported in the literature, however many of these case reports predate the recognition and distinction of chromophobe carcinoma, and it is likely that the majority of the previously so-called malignant oncocytomas would be reclassified as eosinophilic variants of chromophobe or conventional renal cell carcinoma (CRCC).

Malignant Tumors (Renal Cell Carcinoma)

Conventional RCC (CRCC): Epidemiology, Macroscopic and Microscopic Appearances

CRCC is the most common form of renal cancer, accounting for approximately 75% of cases (7). CRCC is also known as "clear cell renal cell carcinoma" (CCRCC) and "hypernephroma." There is a male to female ratio of 2:1. The great majority of CRCC are diagnosed "incidentally" by imaging for nonurological symptoms. The classic presentation with the triad of hematuria, flank pain and loin mass is now rare. Notwithstanding this, one third of patients have metastases on presentation and are considered incurable by surgery alone. Most CRCC are solitary cortical neoplasms although multicentricity (4%) and bilaterality (0.5–3%) may occur (9). The peak incidence of CRCC is ten years earlier than prostate or bladder cancer, occurring most commonly in the sixth decade.

Architecturally, CRCCs commonly have both solid and cystic regions and are typically uniformly golden yellow in color, but larger tumors may have a variegated appearance with a mixture of viable, necrotic and hemorrhagic areas (Fig. 1C).

Historically, CRCC is thought to arise from the proximal tubule, although this is now disputed with recent evidence pointing to a distal tubular origin (24,25). The great majority of CRCC are comprised predominantly of neoplastic cells with abundant clear cytoplasm, a low nuclear/cytoplasm ratio, and nuclei with prominent nucleoli (Fig. 1D). The clear cytoplasm is due to the presence of intracytoplasmic lipid and glycogen. The cells are usually organized in sheets and trabeculae separated by a rich vascular fibrous stroma, or are arranged in a pseudoglandular or cystic pattern. Multilocular cystic renal cell carcinoma (MCRCC) is a subtype of CRCC, where the tumor is composed almost entirely of cysts. The cysts are of variable size and are lined by a single layer of clear cells (9), they are separated by fibrous septa which may also contain nests of clear cells. MCRCC has an excellent prognosis (26) and is recognized as a separate entity in the current WHO classification (27) (Table 2).

Sarcomatoid change occurs in approximately 5% of CRCC cases (28). On immunohistochemistry, CRCC cells stain positive for vimentin, CD10, Glutathione S-transferase α (GST-α) and Cytokeratin 8 and 18, which can be helpful in the differential diagnosis between different subgroups of RCC (29,30).

Papillary Adenocarcinoma: Epidemiology, Macroscopic and Microscopic Appearances

PRCC is the second commonest form of renal cancer, comprising 10% to 15% of cases in most surgical series, and has been known as "chromophil carcinoma" and "tubulopapillary carcinoma" in the past. PRCC is commoner in males with a male to female ratio of 1.5:1. Presentation can occur over a wide age range, though most cases present in the sixth decade. The most important clinical feature of PRCC is that they are often multifocal and bilateral, and frequently are accompanied by multiple renal adenomata in the ipsilateral or contralateral kidney (31). Patients with end-stage kidney disease (ESKD) have an increased risk of developing RCC, and the incidence of PRCC is significantly higher (1.4% compared with 0.04% and 57% compared with 10%, respectively) compared with the general population (32). Radiologically, PRCCs are often hypovascular and so contrast enhancement on CT imaging may be minimal (<10 Hounsfield units) (33,34). Tumor calcification also occurs more frequently in PRCC than in other subtypes.

Macroscopically, PRCCs are usually small (<4cm) and are typically well circumscribed and organ confined (Fig. 1E). Larger tumors tend to have areas of necrosis and hemorrhage rather than being a solid tumor mass.

Histologically, these tumors are characterized by the presence of lipid-laden macrophages ("foamy macrophages") and small calcific concretions (psammomma bodies) in the papillary cores. By definition, over 70% of the tumor must exhibit papillary or tubulopapillary architecture (35) (Fig. 1F).

Two distinct subtypes with prognostic implications have been described; type 1 PRCC consists of basophilic cells with scant cytoplasm covering thin papillae and type 2 PRCC consists of eosinophilic cells with abundant granular cytoplasm, larger nuclei and

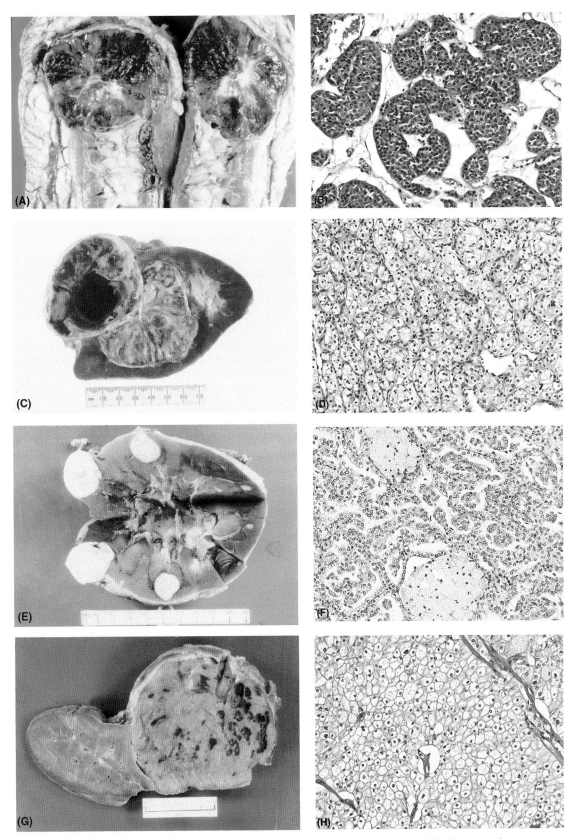

Figure 1 Macroscopic and histological appearances of adult renal epithelial neoplasms. (**A**) Macroscopic appearance of renal oncocytoma, showing tan-brown cut surface and prominent central fibrous scar. (**B**) Typical histological appearance of oncocytoma, with nests of eosinophilic cells in hyalinized stroma. (**C**) Macroscopic appearance of CRCC with prominent cystic degeneration and hemorrhage. (**D**) Histology of conventional RCC with clear cell morphology. (**E**) Macroscopic image of nephrectomy specimen bearing multiple PRCCs. (**F**) Histological appearance of type 1 PRCC with tubulopapillary architecture. Collections of foamy macrophages were a prominent feature in this case. (**G**) Macroscopic appearance of chromophobe RCC with a beige cut surface. (**H**) Chromophobe RCC characterized by large polygonal cells with prominent cell borders.

pseudostratification. Type 1 tumors are twice as common and are associated with a better prognosis than type 2 PRCC (36). CK7 immunoreactivity has been reported in the vast majority of PRCC and can be a useful diagnostic tool. Overall, considering stage for stage and grade for grade, PRCC has a better five-year survival than CRCC (37).

Chromophobe RCC: Epidemiology, Macroscopic and Microscopic Appearances

Chromophobe RCC is the third most common carcinoma of the kidney and accounts for approximately 5% in most surgical series. They are slow growing tumors, are usually organ confined at presentation and have a better prognosis than CRCC. There is a slight male predominance, with a mean age of presentation in the sixth decade although there is a wide age range of 31 to 75 years (38). Chromophobe RCCs average 8 cm in size, with a range from 1.3 to 20 cm. Grossly, the cut surface is solid, and less variegated than CRCC, and is usually beige/light brown or gray in color (Fig. 1G). Histologically, the cells have variable amounts of pale or eosinophilic cytoplasm staining blue with Hale's colloidal iron stain. Two variants of chromophobe RCC are recognized: classical and eosinophilic. The classical type is composed of large polygonal tumor cells with an abundant fine granular cytoplasm that tends to condense near the cell membrane, arranged in a compact solid architecture. This classical form of chromophobe RCC can mimic CRCC phenotypically. The eosinophilic variant is composed of small tumor cells with abundant eosinophilic granular cytoplasm and shares a similar phenotype with renal oncocytoma. Diagnostic distinction between the two can be made with Hale's colloidal iron stain or cytokeratin (7) immunohistochemistry. The relationship between chromophobe RCC and oncocytoma is still being investigated with oncocytomas postulated to be the benign counterpart. Both are thought to arise from the intercalated cells of the collecting duct and both have mitochondrial abnormalities.

Ultrastructurally, the cytoplasm of the cells contain numerous microvesicles 150 to 300 nm in diameter, that are oval or round in shape and often have the complex appearance of a vesicle within a vesicle.

Genetically, chromophobe RCCs display characteristic monosomy of multiple chromosomes (1,2,6,10, 13,17,21).

Collecting Duct Carcinoma: Epidemiology, Macroscopic and Microscopic Appearances

Collecting duct carcinoma (CDC) is a rare tumor and accounts for less than 1% of renal malignancies in surgical series. There is a slight male predominance and average age at presentation is 55 years. These tumors arise from the collecting ducts, especially the papillary ducts (Bellini ducts) hence they are also called Bellini duct carcinomas. They are centrally located in the kidney, averaging 5 cm though range in size from 2.5 to 12 cm, and the cut surface appears solid with a gray-white color. Patients may present with hematuria, flank pain and mass. Urine cytology

may be positive (39) and imaging studies may suggest urothelial malignancy.

Histologically, the tumor is composed of infiltrating glands lined by pleomorphic cells which lie in a desmoplastic stroma (40). These tumor cells show positive immunoreactivity to epithelial membrane antigen, vimentin, Leu-1, high–molecular weight cytokeratins (CK8 and CK19) and mucin (40–42).

Renal medullary carcinoma is an aggressive variant of CDC that is predominantly seen in young males with sickle cell trait. These are very poorly differentiated tumors and have a poor prognosis (27).

Sarcomatoid Change in Renal Cell Carcinoma

Sarcomatous change can occur in all histological subtypes of renal carcinoma, and is now recognized as dedifferentiation of carcinoma cells and not a distinct histological entity. The incidence of finding a sarcomatoid component is approximately 5% to 8% in CRCC, 3% in PRCC and 9% in chromophobe RCC. The significance of finding sarcomatoid change in RCC is that after adjusting for stage, tumor size and presence of necrosis, sarcomatous differentiation portends a worse prognosis (43,44). It is not clear whether the primary histological subtype affects the poor clinical outcome.

THE MOLECULAR GENETICS OF RENAL EPITHELIAL NEOPLASIA DEVELOPMENT

Inherited Cancer Predisposition Syndromes Identify Genes Involved in RCC Development

Recent years have seen a significant increase in our understanding of the molecular genetics of renal epithelial neoplasia development. While 98% of RCCs are sporadic in nature, 2% of cases arise in individuals with an inherited predisposition and it is studies on these individuals and rare families at high risk of developing kidney cancer that has provided significant insights into the molecular mechanisms of RCC tumorigenesis which are also relevant to sporadic kidney cancer. Strikingly, mutations in completely different genes are now implicated in different histological types of kidney cancer (13). These provide good illustrations of different genetic mechanisms contributing to cancer development, including loss of function of tumor suppressor genes (e.g., *VHL* in CRCC), and also activation of proto-oncogenes (e.g., *c-Met* in type 1 papillary renal cell carcinoma).

Von Hippel–Lindau Disease and Familial CRCC

Von Hippel-Lindau (VHL) disease is an autosomal dominant inherited multicancer syndrome that affects approximately 1 in 36,000 of live births. Affected individuals have a very high lifetime risk (c.70%) of developing renal cancer, which is always CRCC, and is commonly multifocal, bilateral and of early onset compared with sporadic cases. Other aspects of the syndrome include hypervascular tumors of the CNS and retina, pheochromocytomas, endolymphatic sac tumors, pancreatic cysts, pancreatic islet cell tumors and epididymal cystadenomas.

The first description of this syndrome was probably by Treacher Collins in 1894, who detailed his observations of bilateral retinal angiomas in two siblings (45). Ten years later, von Hippel, a German ophthalmologist noted retinal angiomas in two of his patients (46). Later still, in 1927, the Swedish pathologist Arvid Lindau described the association of retinal lesions with increased risk of developing haemangioblastomas of the brain and spinal cord (47) and the eponym "von Hippel–Lindau disease" was finally coined by Charles Davison in 1936 (48).

The protean manifestations of VHL mean that patients can present in a variety of ways. Common symptoms include: loss of vision, neurological deficits, paroxysmal raised blood pressure and local pain. Individuals with a positive family history of VHL can be diagnosed as affected on the basis of a single typical VHL tumor such as a retinal or cerebellar hemangioma, CRCC or pheochromocytoma (49). The presence of endolymphatic sac tumors and multiple pancreatic cysts which are uncommon in the general population are also highly suggestive of VHL disease in the context of a positive family history. In contrast, renal and epididymal cysts occur very frequently in the general population are therefore not reliable indicators of *VHL* status.

In the absence of a positive family history, clinical diagnosis of VHL disease can be made with the detection of two or more haemangioblastomas, or a single hemangioblastoma in association with a visceral manifestation (49). Diagnosis of VHL can be confirmed by molecular genetic analysis of the *VHL* gene which is informative in virtually all VHL families (50). Family members of confirmed VHL patients are offered genetic counseling and testing, and are enrolled into clinical monitoring programs if found to be carriers of a germline mutation in *VHL*.

Clinically, VHL families can be broadly grouped on the basis of the absence (type 1) or presence (type 2) of a risk of developing pheochromocytoma. Type 2 VHL families are further subdivided into type 2A (low risk of developing CRCC), type 2B (high risk of developing CRCC), and type 2C (risk of developing pheochromocytoma alone). Recently a third subtype of VHL disease has been recognized, type 3 VHL disease, also known as Chuvash polycythaemia, as it was originally described as being a condition endemic in the Chuvash region of Central Russia. Type 3 disease differs from the other variants of VHL disease by the autosomal recessive rather than dominant mode of inheritance, and is characteristically not associated with CRCC, or other manifestations of classical VHL disease (Table 3) (51).

Identification of the VHL Tumor Suppressor Gene

Linkage analysis of VHL kindreds mapped the *VHL* locus to the short arm of chromosome 3 in 1988, and the *VHL* gene was cloned in 1993 ($3p^{25-26}$) after a concerted international effort (52). Improved molecular technology means that a germline *VHL* mutation or

deletion can be demonstrated in virtually all individuals with a clinical diagnosis of VHL disease (50). Approximately 20% to 37% of patients have large or partial germline deletions, 30% to 38% have missense mutations, and 23% to 27% have nonsense or frameshift mutations (49,50). Intriguingly, clear genotype-phenotype correlations have emerged indicating that different *VHL* mutations predispose to particular types of tumor development. Type 1 VHL disease families tend to have deletions and truncations, and these patients have a low risk of developing pheochromocytoma (53,54). Families affected by type 2 VHL disease, with a high risk of pheochromocytoma, have missense mutations in the *VHL* gene (54), while type 3 VHL families (autosomal recessive erythrocytosis) usually have a specific 598C>T mutation (51). It is rare for specific groups of mutations to be so well correlated with phenotypic manifestations and distinguishes *VHL* from many other tumor suppressor gene syndromes, where a mutation causes loss of tumor suppressor function with a single phenotypic result, for example, retinoblastoma.

The great majority of affected individuals have inherited an inactivated *VHL* allele, with de novo mutations accounting for only about 20% of cases (55). Somatic inactivation of the remaining wild-type *VHL* allele is necessary to initiate the tumorigenic process in VHL disease. Thus at a cellular level, VHL disease is recessive requiring a second hit mutation, which more often than not is a deletion (56), for phenotypic manifestations to occur.

*The VHL Tumor Suppressor Gene
in Sporadic CRCC Tumorigenesis*

Soon after the *VHL* gene was isolated from studying VHL families (52), it was shown that the *VHL* gene is mutated in 50% to 60% of sporadically occurring CRCC (57) and silenced by hypermethylation in a further 19% of cases (58). Human renal cancer cell lines isolated from sporadic CRCC usually have defects in VHL function, and reexpression of a wild-type *VHL* gene is effective at suppressing their growth as tumors in nude mice (59). Thus, *VHL* is a classical two-hit gatekeeper tumor suppressor gene (TSG), conforming to Knudson's two-hit criteria, and is conclusively implicated in the majority of sporadic and hereditary CRCCs (Table 4).

The Function of the VHL Tumor Suppressor Gene Product

The VHL gene contains three exons, the mRNA is ubiquitously expressed and encodes two proteins with relative molecular masses of approximately 30kDa ($pVHL_{30}$) and 19kDa ($pVHL_{19}$). The smaller polypeptide arises as a result of an alternate translation initiation site at Met 54 of $pVHL_{30}$ (60,61).

The VHL proteins can be found in both the nucleus and the cytoplasm, where they have been variously reported to be associated with the endoplasmic reticulum, microtubules and mitochondria (62–64). A larger proportion of $pVHL_{19}$ is found in the nucleus compared with $pVHL_{30}$, although the relevance of

Table 3 Familial RCC: Syndrome, Gene Implicated, Renal Tumor Subtype, and Clinical Features

Syndrome	Gene	Gene location	Renal tumor subtype	Other clinical features
Von Hippel–Lindau	VHL	3p25	CRCC	Retinal hemangiomas, CNS haemangioblastomas, pheochromocytoma
Chromosomal 3 translocations	FHIT	3p14	CRCC	
	RASSF1A	3p21	CRCC	
Familial CRCC	unknown	unknown	CRCC	
Hereditary papillary RCC (HPRC1)	c-MET	7q31.1-4	PRCC (type 1)	
Hereditary Leimyomatosis RCC (HPRC2)	FH	1q42-43	PRCC (type 2)	Uterine leimyosarcoma, cutaneous leiomyomata
Birt-Hogg-Dubé	BDH	17p11.2	chromophobe RCC oncocytoma	Multiple lipoma Pulmonary cysts
Hyperparathyroidism-jaw tumor	unknown	1q21-31	PRCC	Parathyroid adenoma/carcinoma Ossifying jaw tumors
Tuberous sclerosis	TSC1	9q34	CRCC	Angiomyolipoma
	TSC2	16p13	CRCC	seizures, mental retardation

Table 4 Common Chromosomal Abnormalities Detected in Sporadic RCC

RCC subtype	DNA losses	DNA gains	Chromosomal rearrangements
Conventional (rearrangements)	3, 14	-	3p (translocations), 5q
Papillary	Y	3q, 7,12,16,17,20	t(X;1) translocation
Chromophobe	1,2,6,10,13,17,21,Y	-	-
Oncocytoma	1	-	11q13 region (translocation)

subcellular localization and/or trafficking of VHL is not yet clear. Both forms of pVHL are biologically active and behave similarly in most biochemical assays.

The complex genotype-phenotype associations observed in VHL disease (see above) indicate that the VHL gene product has multiple and tissue-specific functions (65). It is clear that the tumor suppressor role of VHL is that of a gatekeeper. It satisfies genetic criteria since inactivation of VHL is a rate-limiting step in CRCC development, and it also satisfies functional criteria as reintroduction of a wild-type VHL allele suppresses the ability of VHL-defective cells to form tumor xenografts in nude mice (59).

The best-established function of VHL is its central role in cellular oxygen sensing (66). The VHL gene product has been shown to be the recognition component of a multiprotein complex composed of elongins B/C, cul-2 and Rbx (67–70). In normoxic conditions, this functions as an E3 ubiquitin ligase that binds and targets the prolyl-hydroxylated hypoxia-inducible factor (HIF) α subunits for polyubiquitination. The polyubiquitin-tagged HIF α subunits are subsequently captured by the 26S proteosome for degradation.

The transcription factor HIF is a master regulator of the cells adaptive response to reduced oxygen availability and has a key role in the regulation of genes involved in glycolytic pathways and angiogenesis (71). A HIF complex consists of a heterodimer of an oxygen regulated α subunit and a constitutively expressed stable β subunit (72). Inactivation of pVHL results in elevated intracellular levels of HIFα, allowing dimerization with the β subunit and formation of an active HIF complex that can then drive the transcription of target genes including VEGFA and EPO (73–75). This results in broadly adaptive changes in gene expression that normally occur in response to hypoxia, including promoting glucose uptake and angiogenesis (66). There is an abundance of evidence indicating that the HIF transcriptional pathway is involved in mediating at least some significant aspects of renal cancer tumorigenesis (24,76–80). Consequences of HIF activation include constitutively high levels of glycolytic enzyme expression and angiogenic growth factor signaling thus providing a plausible explanation for the highly vascular nature of VHL associated tumors.

There are two main isoforms of HIF, HIF1α and HIF2α. Interestingly, the role of HIF2α seems to be unusually prominent relative to HIF1α in VHL-defective renal cancer (78,80,81). Potential insight into HIF's role in CRCC development also comes from genotype-phenotype studies. To date, all CRCC associated VHL mutations disrupt the ability of pVHL to regulate HIF (53). However, some mutations which deregulate HIF carry a low risk of CRCC (type 2A or type 3 VHL disease), suggesting that HIF dysregulation may be necessary but not sufficient to drive CRCC development.

Other putative VHL pathways have been shown to be involved in the tumor suppressor action of VHL in the kidney. For example, pVHL has been shown to have a direct role in fibronectin matrix assembly (82), and interacts with the oncogenic β-catenin signaling pathway (83). Biochemical studies have suggested that

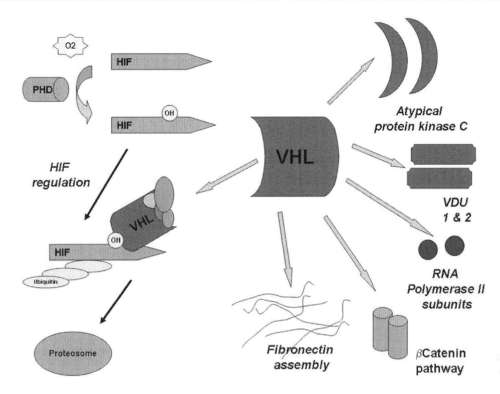

Figure 2 Schematic diagram showing the role of VHL in HIF regulation and other putative interactions such as with Atypical protein kinase C, VDU 1 and 2, RNA polymerase II subunits, fibronectin assembly, and the β-catenin signaling pathway.

pVHL has other protein substrates such as atypical protein kinase C, de-ubiquinating enzymes (VDU-1 and VDU-2) and RNA polymerase II subunits (84–86). The function of the VHL protein is summarized in Figure 2.

Chromosome 3 translocations, VHL-competent CRCC and non-VHL-familial CRCC. An inherited predisposition to CRCC has been associated with balanced translocations involving the short arm of chromosome 3, although this is rare. Several reports have identified a variety of chromosomal breakpoints such as t(3;8)(p14, q24) (87), t(3;8)(p13,q24.1) (88), t(3;6)(p13;q25) (89), t(2;3)(q35;q21) (90) and t(3;12)(q35;q21) (89). Analysis of tumors from patients with chromosome 3 translocations has demonstrated loss of the derivative chromosome by random nondisjunction, and somatic mutation of the *VHL* gene in the remaining chromosome, rendering these tumors *VHL null* (90,91).

A common feature of CRCC, regardless of *VHL* status, is chromosome 3p allele loss (92). Loss of heterozygosity analysis in sporadic CRCC samples has implicated several candidate TSG sites: 3p21.3 (lung cancer tumor suppressor gene region 1—*LCTSGR1*), 3p12 (*LCTSGR2*) and 3p14 (fragile histidine triad gene-*FHIT*) (92,93). These studies are consistent with experiments showing suppression of renal tumor cell growth mediated by transfer of fragments of chromosome 3p regions not containing the *VHL* gene (94). RAS association domain family 1A (*RASSF1A*) gene which resides at 3p21.3 has been shown to be frequently hypermethylated or epigenetically silenced in both *VHL*-defective and *VHL*-competent CRCC (95–97). Interestingly, hypermethylation of *RASSF1A* has also been reported in 40% of PRCC, in the absence of deletions of Chromosome 3p (96). Taken together, these findings indicate that additional non-*VHL* TSGs residing on chromosome 3p have crucial roles in renal cancer development in both *VHL*-defective and *VHL*-competent CRCC.

Families with high risk of CRCC but without any other manifestation of VHL disease and that do not harbor *VHL* germline mutations, are very rare and they are termed non-VHL familial CRCC (FCRC). They have a dominantly inherited susceptibility to CRCC but the molecular mechanisms underlying this are still unclear and they do not have evidence of mutations in *VHL, MET, CUL2* or chromosome 3 translocations (98).

The MET proto-oncogene and familial type 1 papillary RCC (HPRC1). In a similar way to CRCC, studies of families with hereditary forms of PRCC have provided insights into the underlying genetic pathways (13,99). Hereditary papillary renal carcinoma (HPRC) is a rare dominantly hereditary form of type 1 PRCC of reduced penetrance, affecting approximately 1 per 10 million of the population. It is characterized by the development of multiple type 1 PRCC, affecting both kidneys. Genetic linkage studies on HPRC kindreds led to the identification of the proto-oncogene *c-MET* on chromosome 7 as the gene responsible for HPRC (100). HPRC associated tumors are also characterized by trisomy 7 caused by nonrandom duplication of the chromosome bearing the mutated *MET* gene (101). Activating missense mutations have been found in the tyrosine kinase domain of *c-MET* in both the germline of affected individuals with HPRC, and in 13% of patients with sporadic type 1 PRCC (102).

c-MET acts as a cell-surface receptor for the hepatocyte growth factor/scatter factor (HGF/SF), and normally is involved in diverse biological events such as cell growth, migration and morphogenesis. Upon stimulation by HGF/SF, the c-MET receptor kinase undergoes autophosphorlyation on multiple tyrosine residues and recruits a number of signal transducers and adapter proteins to its cytoplasmic domain and multiple docking sites (such as growth factor receptor-bound protein 2 (Grb2), Gab1, phosphatidylinositol 3-kinase (PI3K), phospholipase C-γ, Shc and Src) (103). This results in the activation of several downstream signaling pathways resulting in pleotropic effects. For example, the direct binding of Grb2 to c-MET activates the Ras/mitogen-activated pathway regulating cell-cycle progression (103) and Gab1 is involved in initiating morphogenesis, cell motility and apoptosis (104).

The Fumurate Hydratase Gene and Hereditary Leiomyomatosis Renal Cell Carcinoma/Familial Type 2 Papillary RCC (HPRC2)

Hereditary leiomyomatosis renal cell carcinoma (HLRCC) is an autosomal dominant hereditary form of type 2 PRCC accompanied by uterine fibroids and cutaneous leiomyomatosis lesions. HLRCC patients in contrast to VHL and HPRC1 patients may have solitary tumors, although bilaterality and multifocality has recently been reported (105). The renal tumors in HLRCC are significantly more aggressive than other hereditary forms of kidney cancer, with even small tumors being associated with nodal and metastatic disease.

HLRCC is caused by mutations in the gene that codes for the Krebs' cycle enzyme, fumarate hydratase (*FH*) (106). The *FH* gene has been mapped to chromosome 1q42.3-q43 and mutations are thought to be inactivating and include both deletions and missense mutations (107). *FH* satisfies some important criteria of a tumor suppressor gene, as germline mutations are found in HLRCC kindreds and loss of the second allele has been detected in kidney tumor tissue from patients with HLRCC (108).

The molecular mechanism underlying HLRCC tumorigenesis and the role of *FH* mutations in sporadic kidney cancer is not yet defined, although FH has recently been shown to increase the stability of the transcription factor HIF suggesting a VHL and hypoxia independent mechanism for HIF accumulation in HLRCC renal tumors (109).

Birt-Hogg-Dubé gene and familial chromophobe RCC/renal oncocytoma. Birt-Hogg-Dubé (BHD) syndrome is an autosomal dominant hereditary cancer syndrome, in which affected individuals have susceptibility to develop hamartomatous tumors of the hair follicle (fibrofolliculloma), pulmonary cysts, and bilateral, multifocal renal tumors (110–112). The renal tumors that can occur in BHD are varied, they may

be chromophobe RCC (33%), mixed chromophobe/oncocytic (50%), oncocytoma (7%) or conventional RCC (5%). Genetic linkage studies in BHD kindreds led to the localization and identification of the *BHD* gene on chromosome 17p11.2 in 2002 (113). *BHD* mutations can be variable and include frameshift or nonsense mutations, although insertion or deletion of a cytosine in exon 11 has been detected in over half of BHD families (114). Most mutations are predicted to truncate the BHD protein, folliculin, which is highly conserved across species. Somatic *BHD* mutations or loss of heterozygosity at the BHD locus has been detected in 70% of RCCs from BHD patients supporting its probable tumor suppressor function (115). Further studies on the genotype-phenotype correlations and characterization of *BHD* mutations are required to better understand the molecular mechanisms of BHD tumorigenesis.

Familial PRCC and hyperparathyroidism-jaw tumor syndrome/familial papillary thyroid cancer. Familial hyperparathyroidism-jaw tumor syndrome is an autosomal dominant inherited disease characterized by primary hyperparathyroidism due to either parathyroid adenoma or carcinoma, and ossifying fibroma of the jaw, and the gene has been mapped to chromosome 1q21-q31 (116). Affected individuals commonly have renal cysts, but renal cortical adenoma and type 1 PRCC has also been described in a large kindred (117).

Malchoff et al. (118) described PRCC arising in two family members with familial papillary thyroid cancer, and linkage analysis in this family mapped the gene to chromosome 1q21. Therefore, evidence from these two syndromes suggests the presence of an as yet unidentified PRCC susceptibility locus in the 1q.21 region.

Tuberous sclerosis. Tuberous sclerosis (TSC) is an autosomal dominant inherited syndrome characterized by seizures, mental retardation, and multiple hamartomas. Renal manifestations of TSC occur in over half of affected individuals and include angiomyolipoma (AML) in 85%, renal cysts in 45%, and renal cell carcinoma in 4% (119). AMLs are yellow and gray in color, and composed microscopically of adipocytes, sheets of smooth muscle and blood vessels. Two genes implicated in TSC have been identified, *TSC1* and *TSC2*, and these have been mapped to chromosomes 9q34 (120) and 16p13.3, respectively (121). *TSC1* encodes a protein called hamartin, which is involved in cell adhesion through the ezrin-radixin-moesin (ERNM) family of actin binding proteins (122), and *TSC2* encodes tuberin, a GTPase activating protein for Rap1, a member of the Ras-related superfamily (123). Both AML and renal cysts are more common and numerous in patients with *TSC2* mutations compared with *TSC1* (119).

Genetic Insights and Molecular Targeting Enable the Development of New Therapeutic Strategies in RCC

RCC has an excellent prognosis if detected in the early organ-confined stages, with surgical excision usually being curative therapy in stages I-III. However, approximately a third of patients present with metastatic disease, which has a dismal prognosis with a median survival of 6 to 10 months and 10% to 20% survival at two years (124). RCC is notorious for being largely chemotherapy and radiotherapy resistant. Many systemic agents have been trialled, including capecitabine, thalidomide, fluorouracil and medroxyprogesterone acetate, and have yielded disappointing results (125,126). This is thought to be due to high levels of expression of the multidrug resistant gene (MDR) product P-glycoprotein by renal tumor cells. Radiotherapy is ineffective as suggested by in vitro studies which have shown renal cancer cells to be the least radiosensitive of 76 human cell types (127), so its use is mainly limited to palliative treatment.

Until very recently, IFN-α and/or IL-2 have been the only widely established effective treatment in advanced renal cancer, with high-dose IL-2 being shown to have an overall response rate of 15% to 20% (128,129).

Improved understanding of the genetic basis and the activating mechanisms underlying renal cancer has contributed to the development of much needed new approaches in the management of advanced RCC. There has been an abundance of research since the elucidation of the role of the VHL-HIF pathway in renal tumorigenesis. Activation of the transcription factor HIF mediates the transcription of target genes normally involved in the cellular response to hypoxic stress, including *VEGFA, EGFR, TGF-α* and *EPO*. HIF has also been shown to be upregulated by other growth factor and cell signaling pathways, including the PI3K/AKT/mTOR and Ras/Raf/MAPK pathways. Various treatment strategies targeting both upstream and downstream of these signaling pathways have yielded exciting results. Bevacizumab is a neutralizing antibody to VEGFA, and was the first of the new line of molecular therapies that has been shown to be effective in advanced RCC, significantly prolonging the time to progression (4.8 months compared with 2.5 months placebo) (130). Sunitinib is an inhibitor of multiple tyrosine kinases including VEGFR and PDGF. It has the added advantage of being orally administered, and has shown encouraging results in a recent large phase III trial, with a mean progression-free survival of 11 months compared with 5 months in the IFN treated patients (131). Sorafenib is another multitarget kinase inhibitor, having VEGFR, PDGF and Raf signaling inhibitory effects; and has also shown positive results in a large randomized phase III trial, with significant progression-free survival benefit of 24 weeks in treated patients compared with 12 weeks in the placebo group (132). Other promising new treatments include Temsirolimus and the orally active Everolimus, which are inhibitors of the mTOR pathway which is upstream of HIF (133).

SUMMARY

Advances in molecular techniques have allowed the elucidation of specific genetic events involved in the development of RCC. Our increased understanding of the genetic basis of kidney cancer has enabled the diagnostic classification of renal tumors into specific subtypes on the basis of clinical, histopathological, and genetic criteria. It is now clear that each RCC subtype represents a distinct entity characterized by specific genetic alterations leading to dysregulation of critical molecular pathways underlying their tumorigenesis.

Further progress in dissecting the genetic basis of renal tumorigenesis will no doubt identify other putative RCC genes, and clarifying their functional roles will increase our understanding further. So far, our studies of familial renal tumors have provided significant insight into the molecular pathways involved in both inherited and sporadic RCC. This has already resulted in the development of exciting therapeutic strategies in the form of small molecular inhibitors in the management of advanced RCC, and will undoubtedly continue to direct future novel therapies which will ultimately improve our diagnosis and management of familial and nonfamilial RCC.

REFERENCES

1. Murai M, Oya M. Renal cell carcinoma: etiology, incidence and epidemiology. Curr Opin Urol 2004; 14(4):229–233.
2. Chow WH, Devesa SS, Warren JL, et al. Rising incidence of renal cell cancer in the United States. JAMA 1999; 281(17):1628–1631.
3. Volpe A, Jewett MA. The natural history of small renal masses. Nat Clin Pract Urol 2005; 2(8):384–390.
4. Bergstrom A, Pisani P, Tenet V, et al. Overweight as an avoidable cause of cancer in Europe. Int J Cancer 2001; 91(3):421–430.
5. McLaughlin JK, Lipworth L, Tarone RE. Epidemiologic aspects of renal cell carcinoma. Semin Oncol 2006; 33(5):527–533.
6. Setiawan VW, Stram DO, Nomura AM, et al. Risk factors for renal cell cancer: the multiethnic cohort. Am J Epidemiol 2007; 166(8):932–940.
7. Kovacs G, Akhtar M, Beckwith BJ, et al. The Heidelberg classification of renal cell tumours. J Pathol 1997; 183(2):131–133.
8. Storkel S, Eble JN, Adlakha K, et al. Classification of renal cell carcinoma: Workgroup No. 1. Union Internationale Contre le Cancer (UICC) and the American Joint Committee on Cancer (AJCC). Cancer 1997; 80(5):987–989.
9. Eble JN, Sauter G, Epstein JI, et al. Pathology and Genetics. Tumors of the Urinary System and Male Genital Organs. Lyon: IARC Press 2004.
10. Thoenes W, Storkel S, Rumpelt HJ, et al. Cytomorphological typing of renal cell carcinoma—a new approach. Eur Urol 1990; 18 (suppl 2):6–9.
11. Moch H, Gasser T, Amin MB, et al. Prognostic utility of the recently recommended histologic classification and revised TNM staging system of renal cell carcinoma: a Swiss experience with 588 tumors. Cancer 2000; 89(3):604–614.
12. Amin MB, Amin MB, Tamboli P, et al. Prognostic impact of histologic subtyping of adult renal epithelial neoplasms: an experience of 405 cases. Am J Surg Pathol 2002; 26(3):281–291.
13. Linehan WM, Walther MM, Zbar B. The genetic basis of cancer of the kidney. J Urol 2003; 170(6 pt 1):2163–2172.
14. Xipell JM. The incidence of benign renal nodules (a clinicopathologic study). J Urol 1971; 106(4):503–506.

15. Grignon DJ, Eble JN. Papillary and metanephric adenomas of the kidney. Semin Diagn Pathol 1998; 15(1):41–53.

16. Wang KL, Weinrach DM, Luan C, et al. Renal papillary adenoma–a putative precursor of papillary renal cell carcinoma. Hum Pathol 2007; 38(2):239–246.

17. Yoshioka K, Miyakawa A, Ohno Y, et al. Production of erythropoietin and multiple cytokines by metanephric adenoma results in erythrocytosis. Pathol Int 2007; 57(8): 529–536.

18. Zippel L. Zur Kenntnis der Oncocytem. Virch Arch 1942; 308:360.

19. Kondo T, Nakazawa H, Sakai F, et al. Spoke-wheel-like enhancement as an important imaging finding of chromophobe cell renal carcinoma: a retrospective analysis on computed tomography and magnetic resonance imaging studies. Int J Urol 2004; 11(10):817–824.

20. Dechet CB, Bostwick DG, Blute ML, et al. Renal oncocytoma: multifocality, bilateralism, metachronous tumor development and coexistent renal cell carcinoma. J Urol 1999; 162(1):40–42.

21. Perez-Ordonez B, Hamed G, Campbell S, et al. Renal oncocytoma: a clinicopathologic study of 70 cases. Am Jo Surg Pathol 1997; 21(8):871–883.

22. Storkel S, Pannen B, Thoenes W, et al. Intercalated cells as a probable source for the development of renal oncocytoma. Virchows Arch B Cell Pathol Incl Mol Pathol 1988; 56(3):185–189.

23. Amin MB, Crotty TB, Tickoo SK, et al. Renal oncocytoma: a reappraisal of morphologic features with clinicopathologic findings in 80 cases. Am J Surg Pathol 1997; 21(1):1–12.

24. Mandriota SJ, Turner KJ, Davies DR, et al. HIF activation identifies early lesions in VHL kidneys: evidence for site-specific tumor suppressor function in the nephron. Cancer Cell 2002; 1(5):459–468.

25. Esteban MA, Tran MG, Harten SK, et al. Regulation of E-cadherin expression by VHL and hypoxia-inducible factor. Cancer Res 2006; 66(7):3567–3575.

26. Webster WS, Thompson RH, Cheville JC, et al. Surgical resection provides excellent outcomes for patients with cystic clear cell renal cell carcinoma. Urology 2007; 70(5): 900–904; discussion 4.

27. Lopez-Beltran A, Scarpelli M, Montironi R, et al. 2004 WHO classification of the renal tumors of the adults. Eur Urol 2006; 49(5):798–805.

28. Renshaw AA. Subclassification of renal cell neoplasms: an update for the practising pathologist. Histopathology 2002; 41(4):283–300.

29. Avery AK, Beckstead J, Renshaw AA, et al. Use of antibodies to RCC and CD10 in the differential diagnosis of renal neoplasms. Am J Surg Pathol 2000; 24(2):203–210.

30. Liu L, Qian J, Singh H, et al. Immunohistochemical analysis of chromophobe renal cell carcinoma, renal oncocytoma, and clear cell carcinoma: an optimal and practical panel for differential diagnosis. Arch Pathol Lab Med 2007; 131(8):1290–1297.

31. Renshaw AA, Corless CL. Papillary renal cell carcinoma. Histology and immunohistochemistry. Am J Surg Pathol 1995; 19(7):842–849.

32. Farivar-Mohseni H, Perlmutter AE, Wilson S, et al. Renal cell carcinoma and end stage renal disease. The Journal of urology 2006; 175(6):2018–2020; discussion 21.

33. Blei CL, Hartman DS, Friedman AC, et al. Papillary renal cell carcinoma: ultrasonic/pathologic correlation. J Clin Ultrasound 1982; 10(9):429–434.

34. Press GA, McClennan BL, Melson GL, et al. Papillary renal cell carcinoma: CT and sonographic evaluation. AJR Am J Roentgenol 1984; 143(5):1005–1009.

35. Bostwick DG, Murphy GP. Diagnosis and prognosis of renal cell carcinoma: highlights from an international consensus workshop. Semin Urol Oncol 1998; 16(1):46–52.

36. Pignot G, Elie C, Conquy S, et al. Survival analysis of 130 patients with papillary renal cell carcinoma: prognostic utility of type 1 and type 2 subclassification. Urology 2007; 69(2):230–235.

37. Amin MB, Corless CL, Renshaw AA, et al. Papillary (chromophil) renal cell carcinoma: histomorphologic characteristics and evaluation of conventional pathologic prognostic parameters in 62 cases. Am J Surg Pathol 1997; 21(6):621–635.

38. Crotty TB, Farrow GM, Lieber MM. Chromophobe cell renal carcinoma: clinicopathological features of 50 cases. J Urol 1995; 154(3):964–967.

39. Nguyen GK, Schumann GB. Cytopathology of renal collecting duct carcinoma in urine sediment. Diagn Cytopathol 1997; 16(5):446–449.

40. Kennedy SM, Merino MJ, Linehan WM, et al. Collecting duct carcinoma of the kidney. Hum Pathol 1990; 21(4):449–456.

41. Srigley JR, Eble JN. Collecting duct carcinoma of kidney. Semin Diagn Pathol 1998; 15(1):54–67.

42. Kim MK, Kim S. Immunohistochemical profile of common epithelial neoplasms arising in the kidney. Appl Immunohistochem Mol Morphol 2002; 10(4):332–338.

43. Cheville JC, Lohse CM, Zincke H, et al. Sarcomatoid renal cell carcinoma: an examination of underlying histologic subtype and an analysis of associations with patient outcome. Am J Surg Pathol 2004; 28(4):435–441.

44. de Peralta-Venturina M, Moch H, Amin M, et al. Sarcomatoid differentiation in renal cell carcinoma: a study of 101 cases. Am J Surg Pathol 2001; 25(3):275–284.

45. Collins E. Intra-ocular growths (two cases, brother and sister, with peculiar vascular new growth, probably retinal, affecting both eyes). Trans Ophthalmol Soc UK 1894; 14:141–149.

46. Hippel Ev. Ueber eine sehr seltene Erkrankung der Nethaut. Graefe Arch Ophthalmol 1904; 59:83–106.

47. lindau A. Zur frage der angiomatosis retinai und ihrer hirncomplikation. Acta Ophthalmol 1927; 4:193–226.

48. Davison C BS, Cyke CG. Retinal and central nervous haemangioblastomatosis with visceral changes (von Hippel-Lindau's disease). Bull Neurol Inst New York 1936; 5:72–93.

49. Maher ER, Kaelin WG Jr. von Hippel-Lindau disease. Medicine (Baltimore) 1997; 76(6):381–391.

50. Stolle C, Glenn G, Zbar B, et al. Improved detection of germline mutations in the von Hippel-Lindau disease tumor suppressor gene. Hum Mutat 1998; 12(6):417–423.

51. Ang SO, Chen H, Gordeuk VR, et al. Endemic polycythemia in Russia: mutation in the VHL gene. Blood Cells Mol Dis 2002; 28(1):57–62.

52. Latif F, Tory K, Gnarra J, et al. Identification of the von Hippel-Lindau disease tumor suppressor gene. Science 1993; 260(5112):1317–1320.

53. Clifford SC, Cockman ME, Smallwood AC, et al. Contrasting effects on HIF-1alpha regulation by disease-causing pVHL mutations correlate with patterns of tumourigenesis in von Hippel-Lindau disease. Hum Mol Genet 2001; 10(10):1029–1038.

54. Chen F, Kishida T, Duh FM, et al. Suppression of growth of renal carcinoma cells by the von Hippel-Lindau tumor suppressor gene. Cancer Res 1995; 55(21):4804–4807.

55. Sgambati MT, Stolle C, Choyke PL, et al. Mosaicism in von Hippel-Lindau disease: lessons from kindreds with germline mutations identified in offspring with mosaic parents. Am J Hum Genet 2000; 66(1):84–91.

56. Glasker S, Sohn TS, Okamoto H, et al. Second hit deletion size in von Hippel-Lindau disease. Ann Neurol 2006; 59(1): 105–110.

57. Gnarra JR, Tory K, Weng Y, et al. Mutations of the VHL tumour suppressor gene in renal carcinoma. Nat Genet 1994; 7(1):85–90.

58. Herman JG, Latif F, Weng Y, et al. Silencing of the VHL tumor-suppressor gene by DNA methylation in renal carcinoma. Proc Natl Acad Sci U S A 1994; 91(21):9700–9704.

59. Iliopoulos O, Kibel A, Gray S, et al. Tumour suppression by the human von Hippel-Lindau gene product. Nat Med 1995; 1(8):822–826.

60. Iliopoulos O, Ohh M, Kaelin WG Jr. pVHL19 is a biologically active product of the von Hippel-Lindau gene arising from internal translation initiation. Proc Natl Acad Sci U S A 1998; 95(20):11661–11666.

61. Schoenfeld A, Davidowitz EJ, Burk RD. A second major native von Hippel-Lindau gene product, initiated from an internal translation start site, functions as a tumor suppressor. Proc Natl Acad Sci U S A 1998; 95(15): 8817–8822.

62. Shiao YH, Resau JH, Nagashima K, et al. The von Hippel-Lindau tumor suppressor targets to mitochondria. Cancer Res 2000; 60(11):2816–2819.

63. Schoenfeld AR, Davidowitz EJ, Burk RD. Endoplasmic reticulum/cytosolic localization of von Hippel-Lindau gene products is mediated by a 64-amino acid region. Int J Cancer 2001; 91(4):457–467.

64. Hergovich A, Lisztwan J, Barry R, et al. Regulation of microtubule stability by the von Hippel-Lindau tumour suppressor protein pVHL. Nat Cell Biol 2003; 5(1):64–70.

65. Clifford SC, Maher ER. Von Hippel-Lindau disease: clinical and molecular perspectives. Adv Cancer Res 2001; 82:85–105.

66. Maxwell PH, Wiesener MS, Chang GW, et al. The tumour suppressor protein VHL targets hypoxia-inducible factors for oxygen-dependent proteolysis. Nature 1999; 399(6733): 271–275.

67. Iwai K, Yamanaka K, Kamura T, et al. Identification of the von Hippel-lindau tumor-suppressor protein as part of an active E3 ubiquitin ligase complex. Proc Natl Acad Sci U S A 1999; 96(22):12436–12441.

68. Kamura T, Koepp DM, Conrad MN, et al. Rbx1, a component of the VHL tumor suppressor complex and SCF ubiquitin ligase. Science 1999; 284(5414):657–661.

69. Lisztwan J, Imbert G, Wirbelauer C, et al. The von Hippel-Lindau tumor suppressor protein is a component of an E3 ubiquitin-protein ligase activity. Genes Dev 1999; 13(14): 1822–1833.

70. Cockman ME, Masson N, Mole DR, et al. Hypoxia inducible factor-alpha binding and ubiquitylation by the von Hippel-Lindau tumor suppressor protein. J Biol Chem 2000; 275(33):25733–25741.

71. Maxwell PH. Hypoxia-inducible factor as a physiological regulator. Exp Physiol 2005; 90(6):791–797.

72. Wang GL, Jiang BH, Rue EA, et al. Hypoxia-inducible factor 1 is a basic-helix-loop-helix-PAS heterodimer regulated by cellular O2 tension. Proc Natl Acad Sci U S A 1995; 92(12):5510–5514.

73. Forsythe JA, Jiang BH, Iyer NV, et al. Activation of vascular endothelial growth factor gene transcription by hypoxia-inducible factor 1. Mol Cell Biol 1996; 16(9): 4604–4613.

74. Beck I, Ramirez S, Weinmann R, et al. Enhancer element at the 3′-flanking region controls transcriptional response to hypoxia in the human erythropoietin gene. J Biol Chem 1991; 266(24):15563–15566.

75. Semenza GL, Nejfelt MK, Chi SM, et al. Hypoxia-inducible nuclear factors bind to an enhancer element

located 3′ to the human erythropoietin gene. Proc Natl Acad Sci U S A 1991; 88(13):5680–5684.

76. Krieg M, Haas R, Brauch H, et al. Up-regulation of hypoxia-inducible factors HIF-1alpha and HIF-2alpha under normoxic conditions in renal carcinoma cells by von Hippel-Lindau tumor suppressor gene loss of function. Oncogene 2000; 19(48):5435–5443.

77. Kondo K, Klco J, Nakamura E, et al. Inhibition of HIF is necessary for tumor suppression by the von Hippel-Lindau protein. Cancer Cell 2002; 1(3):237–246.

78. Turner KJ, Moore JW, Jones A, et al. Expression of hypoxia-inducible factors in human renal cancer: relationship to angiogenesis and to the von Hippel-Lindau gene mutation. Cancer Res 2002; 62(10):2957–2961.

79. Zimmer M, Doucette D, Siddiqui N, et al. Inhibition of hypoxia-inducible factor is sufficient for growth suppression of VHL-/- tumors. Genetic and clinical aspects of familial renal neoplasms. The molecular basis of von Hippel-Lindau disease. Mol Cancer Res 2004; 2(2):89–95.

80. Raval RR, Lau KW, Tran MG, et al. Contrasting properties of hypoxia-inducible factor 1 (HIF-1) and HIF-2 in von Hippel-Lindau-associated renal cell carcinoma. Mol Cell Biol 2005; 25(13):5675–5686.

81. Kondo K, Kim WY, Lechpammer M, et al. Inhibition of HIF2alpha is sufficient to suppress pVHL-defective tumor growth. PLoS Biol 2003; 1(3):E83.

82. Ohh M, Yauch RL, Lonergan KM, et al. The von Hippel-Lindau tumor suppressor protein is required for proper assembly of an extracellular fibronectin matrix. Mol Cell 1998; 1(7):959–968.

83. Peruzzi B, Athauda G, Bottaro DP. The von Hippel-Lindau tumor suppressor gene product represses oncogenic beta-catenin signaling in renal carcinoma cells. Proc Natl Acad Sci U S A 2006; 103(39):14531–14536.

84. Okuda H, Saitoh K, Hirai S, et al. The von Hippel-Lindau tumor suppressor protein mediates ubiquitination of activated atypical protein kinase C. J Biol Chem 2001; 276(47): 43611–43617.

85. Kuznetsova AV, Meller J, Schnell PO, et al. von Hippel-Lindau protein binds hyperphosphorylated large subunit of RNA polymerase II through a proline hydroxylation motif and targets it for ubiquitination. Proc Natl Acad Sci U S A 2003; 100(5):2706–2711.

86. Li Z, Wang D, Na X, et al. Identification of a deubiquitinating enzyme subfamily as substrates of the von Hippel-Lindau tumor suppressor. Biochem Biophys Res Commun 2002; 294(3):700–709.

87. Cohen AJ, Li FP, Berg S, et al. Hereditary renal-cell carcinoma associated with a chromosomal translocation. N Engl J Med 1979; 301(11):592–595.

88. Melendez B, Rodriguez-Perales S, Martinez-Delgado B, et al. Molecular study of a new family with hereditary renal cell carcinoma and a translocation t(3;8)(p13;q24.1). Hum Genet 2003; 112(2):178–185.

89. Kovacs G, Hoene E. Loss of der(3) in renal carcinoma cells of a patient with constitutional t(3;12). Hum Genet 1988; 78(2):148–150.

90. Bodmer D, Eleveld MJ, Ligtenberg MJ, et al. An alternative route for multistep tumorigenesis in a novel case of hereditary renal cell cancer and a t(2;3)(q35;q21) chromosome translocation. Am J Hum Genet 1998; 62(6): 1475–1483.

91. Schmidt L, Li F, Brown RS, et al. Mechanism of tumorigenesis of renal carcinomas associated with the constitutional chromosome 3;8 translocation. Cancer J Sci Am 1995; 1(3):191–195.

92. Clifford SC, Prowse AH, Affara NA, et al. Inactivation of the von Hippel-Lindau (VHL) tumour suppressor gene

and allelic losses at chromosome arm 3p in primary renal cell carcinoma: evidence for a VHL-independent pathway in clear cell renal tumourigenesis. Genes Chromosomes Cancer 1998; 22(3):200–209.

93. Martinez A, Fullwood P, Kondo K, et al. Role of chromosome 3p12-p21 tumour suppressor genes in clear cell renal cell carcinoma: analysis of VHL dependent and VHL independent pathways of tumorigenesis. Mol Pathol 2000; 53(3):137–144.

94. Sanchez Y, el-Naggar A, Pathak S, et al. A tumor suppressor locus within 3p14-p12 mediates rapid cell death of renal cell carcinoma in vivo. Proc Natl Acad Sci U S A 1994; 91(8):3383–3387.

95. Dreijerink K, Braga E, Kuzmin I, et al. The candidate tumor suppressor gene, RASSF1A, from human chromosome 3p21.3 is involved in kidney tumorigenesis. Proc Natl Acad Sci U S A 2001; 98(13):7504–7509.

96. Morrissey C, Martinez A, Zatyka M, et al. Epigenetic inactivation of the RASSF1A 3p21.3 tumor suppressor gene in both clear cell and papillary renal cell carcinoma. Cancer Res 2001; 61(19):7277–7281.

97. Yoon JH, Dammann R, Pfeifer GP. Hypermethylation of the CpG island of the RASSF1A gene in ovarian and renal cell carcinomas. Int J Cancer 2001; 94(2):212–217.

98. Woodward ER, Clifford SC, Astuti D, et al. Familial clear cell renal cell carcinoma (FCRC): clinical features and mutation analysis of the VHL, MET, and CUL2 candidate genes. J Med Genet 2000; 37(5):348–353.

99. Zbar B, Tory K, Merino M, et al. Hereditary papillary renal cell carcinoma. J Urol 1994; 151(3):561–566.

100. Schmidt L, Duh FM, Chen F, et al. Germline and somatic mutations in the tyrosine kinase domain of the MET proto-oncogene in papillary renal carcinomas. Nat Genet 1997; 16(1):68–73.

101. Zhuang Z, Park WS, Pack S, et al. Trisomy 7-harbouring non-random duplication of the mutant MET allele in hereditary papillary renal carcinomas. Nat Genet 1998; 20(1):66–69.

102. Schmidt L, Junker K, Nakaigawa N, et al. Novel mutations of the MET proto-oncogene in papillary renal carcinomas. Oncogene 1999; 18(14):2343–2350.

103. Zhang YW, Vande Woude GF. HGF/SF-met signaling in the control of branching morphogenesis and invasion. J Cell Biochem 2003; 88(2):408–417.

104. Rosario M, Birchmeier W. How to make tubes: signaling by the Met receptor tyrosine kinase. Trends Cell Biol 2003; 13(6):328–335.

105. Grubb RL 3rd, Franks ME, Toro J, et al. Hereditary leiomyomatosis and renal cell cancer: a syndrome associated with an aggressive form of inherited renal cancer. J Urol 2007; 177(6):2074–2079; discussion 9–80.

106. Delahunt B, Eble JN. Papillary renal cell carcinoma: a clinicopathologic and immunohistochemical study of 105 tumors. Mod Pathol 1997; 10(6):537–544.

107. Tomlinson IP, Alam NA, Rowan AJ, et al. Germline mutations in FH predispose to dominantly inherited uterine fibroids, skin leiomyomata and papillary renal cell cancer. Nat Genet 2002; 30(4):406–410.

108. Toro JR, Nickerson ML, Wei MH, et al. Mutations in the fumarate hydratase gene cause hereditary leiomyomatosis and renal cell cancer in families in North America. Am J Hum Genet 2003; 73(1):95–106.

109. Isaacs JS, Jung YJ, Mole DR, et al. HIF overexpression correlates with biallelic loss of fumarate hydratase in renal cancer: novel role of fumarate in regulation of HIF stability. Cancer Cell 2005; 8(2):143–153.

110. Birt AR, Hogg GR, Dube WJ. Hereditary multiple fibrofolliculomas with trichodiscomas and acrochordons. Arch Dermatol 1977; 113(12):1674–1677.

111. Toro JR, Glenn G, Duray P, et al. Birt-Hogg-Dube syndrome: a novel marker of kidney neoplasia. Arch Dermatol 1999; 135(10):1195–1202.

112. Zbar B, Alvord WG, Glenn G, et al. Risk of renal and colonic neoplasms and spontaneous pneumothorax in the Birt-Hogg-Dube syndrome. Cancer Epidemiol Biomarkers Prev 2002; 11(4):393–400.

113. Nickerson ML, Warren MB, Toro JR, et al. Mutations in a novel gene lead to kidney tumors, lung wall defects, and benign tumors of the hair follicle in patients with the Birt-Hogg-Dube syndrome. Cancer Cell 2002; 2(2):157–164.

114. Schmidt LS, Nickerson ML, Warren MB, et al. Germline BHD-mutation spectrum and phenotype analysis of a large cohort of families with Birt-Hogg-Dube syndrome. Am J Hum Genet 2005; 76(6):1023–1033.

115. Vocke CD, Yang Y, Pavlovich CP, et al. High frequency of somatic frameshift BHD gene mutations in Birt-Hogg-Dube-associated renal tumors. J Natl Cancer Inst 2005; 97(12):931–935.

116. Szabo J, Heath B, Hill VM, et al. Hereditary hyperparathyroidism-jaw tumor syndrome: the endocrine tumor gene HRPT2 maps to chromosome 1q21-q31. Am J Hum Genet 1995; 56(4):944–950.

117. Haven CJ, Wong FK, van Dam EW, et al. A genotypic and histopathological study of a large Dutch kindred with hyperparathyroidism-jaw tumor syndrome. J Clin Endocrinol Metab 2000; 85(4):1449–1454.

118. Malchoff CD, Sarfarazi M, Tendler B, et al. Papillary thyroid carcinoma associated with papillary renal neoplasia: genetic linkage analysis of a distinct heritable tumor syndrome. J Clin Endocrinol Metabol 2000; 85(5):1758–1764.

119. Rakowski SK, Winterkorn EB, Paul E, et al. Renal manifestations of tuberous sclerosis complex: incidence, prognosis, and predictive factors. Kidney Int 2006; 70(10):1777–1782.

120. Fryer AE, Chalmers A, Connor JM, et al. Evidence that the gene for tuberous sclerosis is on chromosome 9. Lancet 1987; 1(8534):659–661.

121. Kandt RS, Haines JL, Smith M, et al. Linkage of an important gene locus for tuberous sclerosis to a chromosome 16 marker for polycystic kidney disease. Nat Genet 1992; 2(1):37–41.

122. Lamb RF, Roy C, Diefenbach TJ, et al. The TSC1 tumour suppressor hamartin regulates cell adhesion through ERM proteins and the GTPase Rho. Nat Cell Biol 2000; 2(5):281–287.

123. Identification and characterization of the tuberous sclerosis gene on chromosome 16. Cell 1993; 75(7):1305–1315.

124. Campbell SC, Flanigan RC, Clark JI. Nephrectomy in metastatic renal cell carcinoma. Curr Treat Options Oncol 2003; 4(5):363–372.

125. Yagoda A, Petrylak D, Thompson S. Cytotoxic chemotherapy for advanced renal cell carcinoma. Urol Clin North Am 1993; 20(2):303–321.

126. Motzer RJ, Russo P. Systemic therapy for renal cell carcinoma. J Urol 2000; 163(2):408–417.

127. Deschavanne PJ, Fertil B. A review of human cell radiosensitivity in vitro. Int J Radiat Oncol, Biol, Phys 1996; 34(1):251–266.

128. Fyfe G, Fisher RI, Rosenberg SA, et al. Results of treatment of 255 patients with metastatic renal cell carcinoma who received high-dose recombinant interleukin-2 therapy. J Clin Oncol 1995; 13(3):688–696.

129. Yang JC, Sherry RM, Steinberg SM, et al. Randomized study of high-dose and low-dose interleukin-2 in patients with metastatic renal cancer. J Clin Oncol 2003; 21(16): 3127–3132.

130. Yang JC, Haworth L, Sherry RM, et al. A randomized trial of bevacizumab, an anti-vascular endothelial growth factor antibody, for metastatic renal cancer. N Engl J Med 2003; 349(5):427–434.

131. Motzer RJ, Hutson TE, Tomczak P, et al. Sunitinib versus interferon alfa in metastatic renal-cell carcinoma. N Engl J Med 2007; 356(2):115–1124.

132. Escudier B, Eisen T, Stadler WM, et al. Sorafenib in advanced clear-cell renal-cell carcinoma. N Engl J Med 2007; 356(2):125–134.

133. Atkins MB, Hidalgo M, Stadler WM, et al. Randomized phase II study of multiple dose levels of CCI-779, a novel mammalian target of rapamycin kinase inhibitor, in patients with advanced refractory renal cell carcinoma. J Clin Oncol 2004; 22(5):909–918.

24

Transitional Cell Carcinoma of the Bladder

T. R. Leyshon Griffiths
*Urology Group, Department of Cancer Studies and Molecular Medicine,
University of Leicester, Leicester, U.K.*

Nick Mayer
University Hospitals of Leicester, Leicester, U.K.

INTRODUCTION

Each year in the United Kingdom, approximately 10,100 people are diagnosed with bladder cancer and 4700 people die from the disease. The male to female ratio is 5:2. Although it is ranked the fourth most common cancer in men and the eleventh most common cancer in women (1), bladder cancer is an enormous burden on the health economy because of its prevalence and duration. In the United Kingdom it has been estimated that the cost of treatment for bladder cancer to the National Health Service is approximately £200 million per annum, making it the most expensive cancer to treat (2).

The age-specific bladder cancer incidence rates in Great Britain show a consistent decrease since the early 1990s for all age groups under age 85. While some of this can be attributed to coding changes, reduction in smoking and reduced exposure to occupational carcinogens may also have played a role, especially as mortality rates have also decreased (3). In the developed world, transitional cell carcinoma (TCC), rather than squamous or adenocarcinoma, is responsible for 90% of bladder cancers. About 25% of newly diagnosed cancers are muscle invasive (T2–T4); the remainder are non–muscle invasive (70%) and classified as noninvasive (pTa), lamina propria–invasive (pT1), or in situ (Tis [CIS, carcinoma in situ]—5%).

ETIOLOGY

Smoking

Smoking cigarettes is the principal preventable risk factor for bladder cancer in both men and women. In Europe, it is estimated that up to half the bladder cancer cases in men and a third in women are caused by cigarette smoking (4,5). A causal relationship has been established between an exposure to tobacco and cancer studies in which chance, bias, and confounding factors can be controlled with reasonable confidence (6). Current smokers have around three times the risk of never-smokers of developing bladder cancer, while ex-smokers have double the risk of never-smokers (7). Risk positively associates with both increasing dose and duration of smoking (4,5). Passive smoking may also increase risk. In a recent European study, exposure to environmental tobacco during childhood (but not adulthood) increased the risk of bladder cancer (8).

Smoking cessation reduces risk by 40% within 1 to 4 years and reaches 60% after 25 years (4,5). The alleged carcinogenic constituents of tobacco smoke include arylamines (particularly 4-aminobiphenyl), polycyclic aromatic hydrocarbons (PAHs), N-nitroso compounds, heterocyclic amines, and various epoxides. Studies show that risk varies by type of tobacco, with a higher risk for black "air-cured" than blond "flue-cured" tobacco. Smoking also leads to higher mortality from bladder cancer during long-term follow-up (9).

Occupation

Occupational exposure to chemicals in Europe accounts for up to 10% of male bladder cancers. Most carcinogens have a latent period of 15 to 20 years between exposure and the development of tumors. The proportion may be higher in countries with less-regulated industrial processes. Bladder cancer has an important place in the history of occupational disease. In 1895, Rehn reported cases of bladder cancer in a German aniline dye factory. In 1938, Hueper produced the first experimental evidence showing that the aromatic amine, β-naphthylamine, could induce bladder cancer in dogs (10). Following this and other reports, a full epidemiological survey conducted by Case showed that exposure to α-naphthylamine, β-naphthylamine, or benzidine, rather than to aniline itself, was the main factor associated with the development of bladder cancer (11). Aromatic amines were widely used in the manufacture of dyes and pigments for textiles, paints, plastics, paper and hair dyes, in drugs, pesticides and as anticipated in the rubber industry. In 1952, production of β-naphthylamine ceased in the United Kingdom, and in 1953 bladder cancer became a prescribed industrial disease (12).

It is calculated that approximately 4% of bladder cancer cases in European men are because of exposure to PAHs, by-products of the catabolic process (13).

Hair Dyes

Occupational studies of hairdressers have produced conflicting results. However, a recent study in Sweden suggested that modern hair dyes are not carcinogenic (14). Within the European Union, the Scientific Committee on Cosmetic Products and Non-food products (ISCCNFP) aims to set up a "high-risk" permanent and semipermanent register of hair dye formulations.

Drugs

In the 1950s and 1960s, analgesic abuse was rife in Australia and New Zealand. Both upper tract and bladder TCC were linked to the aniline derivative, phenacetin. Cyclophosphamide has also been shown to induce bladder cancer; the increased risk of TCC has been calculated as ninefold (15). In comparison to other carcinogenic agents, the latency period is relatively short. Acrolein, a metabolite of cyclophosphamide, is responsible for this increase, which is independent of the occurrence of hemorrhagic cystitis.

Pelvic Irradiation

Patients who are treated with pelvic radiotherapy for cervical carcinoma have a two- to fourfold increased risk of developing bladder cancer (16). In patients treated for prostate cancer, the incidence of bladder cancer was significantly higher in patients treated with external beam radiotherapy than those treated with radical prostatectomy (17).

Food and Drink

Several dietary factors have been related to bladder cancer, but the results of different studies have been controversial. A meta-analysis of 38 articles supported the hypothesis that vegetable and fruit intake reduced the risk of bladder cancer (18).

Genetic Polymorphisms

Drug- and carcinogen-metabolizing enzymes are important in the processing of lipophilic chemicals to products that are more water soluble and can be excreted. These enzymes systems are partly controlled by genetic polymorphism. In the liver, chemicals are oxidized by the cytochrome P450 superfamily and detoxified by *N*-acetylation, predominantly by *N*-acetyltransferases (NAT). Aromatic amines are usually detoxified by NAT2. Certain allelic combinations result in the slow acetylation phenotype. Studies have suggested that people who carry the "slow" variant are at increased risk of bladder cancer (relative risk 1.4), and this may be especially true in smokers (19). Approximately 50% of Caucasians and 25% of Asians are slow acetylators. Glutathione *S*-transferase (GST)

is the product of the *GSTM1* gene and is involved in the detoxification of PAHs. Approximately 50% of Caucasians and Asians have a homozygous deletion of *GSTM1* gene, which is associated with a relative risk of 1.4 (20).

PATHOLOGY

The urinary collecting system, which extends from the renal calyces to the urethra, is lined by a specialized epithelium with unique morphological and ultrastructural features known as transitional epithelium or urothelium.

Tumors of the bladder are roughly 50 times more common than those of the upper tracts, the vast majority (>90%) are TCCs that are usually "pure" but can show a range of divergent differentiation including squamous (20%), glandular (6%), and rarer forms such as trophoblastic. Pure squamous carcinoma and adenocarcinoma (urachal and nonurachal) also occur but are rare. Primary bladder adenocarcinoma has to be distinguished from direct or metastatic spread from a variety of other sites, including the colorectum, prostate, ovary, breast, and stomach. This distinction usually requires clinical and radiological correlation.

Tumor Grade

For more than three decades the preferred grading system in the United Kingdom for invasive and non-invasive TCC has been the World Health Organization (WHO) 1973 classification (21), which has been repeatedly validated and shown to be of clinical relevance for treatment and prognosis. WHO 1973 divides TCC into three grades on the basis of cytological and architectural disorder: grade 1 being well differentiated, grade 2 moderately differentiated, and grade 3 poorly differentiated. However, the classification has been criticized for imprecise definitions, resulting in poor reproducibility between pathologists and for having the majority of tumors in the middle grade (grade 2), which as a group therefore shows considerable variability in clinical behavior. In 1998, the WHO/International Society of Urological Pathology (ISUP) consensus classification was published by a group of expert uropathologists (22), notably without input from urologists, which was intended to replace the original WHO 1973 classification. The 1998 classification has subsequently been adopted in the most recent WHO 2004 classification (23). The main differences are two grades of carcinoma (high grade and low grade) in the WHO 2004 classification and the introduction of the term papillary urothelial neoplasm of low malignant potential, to replace the best differentiated grade 1 tumors, avoiding the term carcinoma for tumors with low risk of either recurrence or progression (Fig. 1). However, there has been considerable resistance in the United Kingdom to adopting the WHO 2004 classification, which was not prospectively validated prior to its introduction and has subsequently not demonstrated either improved reproducibility or clinical relevance over WHO 1973 (25). A

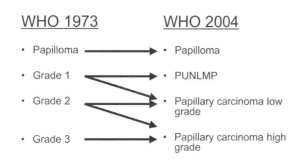

WHO 1973   WHO 2004

- Papilloma ⟶ • Papilloma
- Grade 1 ⟶ • PUNLMP
- Grade 2 ⟶ • Papillary carcinoma low grade
- Grade 3 ⟶ • Papillary carcinoma high grade

Figure 1 World Health Organization (WHO) 1973 versus 2004 classifications. *Source*: Adapted from Ref. 24.

Table 1 TNM Classification of Urinary Bladder Cancer (2002)

T (Primary tumor)
  TX Primary tumor cannot be assessed
  T0 No evidence of primary tumor
    Ta Noninvasive papillary carcinoma
    Tis Carcinoma in situ ("flat tumor")
  T1 Tumor invades subepithelial connective tissue
  T2 Tumor invades muscle
    T2a Tumor invades superficial muscle (inner half)
    T2b Tumor invades deep muscle (outer half)
  T3 Tumor invades perivesical tissue:
    T3a Microscopically
    T3b Macroscopically (extravesical mass)
  T4 Tumor invades any of the following: prostate, uterus, vagina, pelvic wall, abdominal wall
    T4a Tumor invades prostate, uterus, or vagina
    T4b Tumor invades pelvic wall or abdominal wall

N (Lymph nodes)
  NX Regional lymph nodes cannot be assessed
  N0 No regional lymph node metastasis
  N1 Metastasis in a single lymph node 2 cm or less in greatest dimension
  N2 Metastasis in a single lymph node more than 2 cm but not more than 5 cm in greatest dimension, or multiple lymph nodes, none more than 5 cm in greatest dimension
  N3 Metastasis in a lymph node more than 5 cm in greatest dimension

M (Distant metastasis)
  MX Distant metastasis cannot be assessed
  M0 No distant metastasis
  M1 Distant metastasis

Source: From Ref. 28.

particular uncertainty is whether all patients in the high-grade group will benefit from intravesical BCG therapy or be exposed to unnecessary side effects. Current reporting guidelines therefore recommend providing the urologist with both classifications (26,27).

Tumor Stage

Bladder tumors are often separated into non–muscle invasive (CIS, pTa, pT1) or muscle invasive (T2, T3, T4) to aid clinical management. Clinical stage is based on a combination of histopathological assessment, bimanual clinical examination, and imaging studies. The International Union Against Cancer (UICC) 2002 is the most recent pathological TNM staging system (Table 1) (28). For transurethral (TUR) resection specimens, showing lamina propria invasion (pT1), the pathologists should provide some indication of the extent and/or depth of invasion, as this correlates with outcome and may influence whether to perform a reresection. It is important for the pathologists to comment on whether detrusor muscle is present in pT1 tumors. Those lacking detrusor and/or those who are high-grade normally require reresection because of the significant risk of understaging. It is useful for the urologists to send the deep or base biopsies in a separate specimen pot, to aid the histological identification of detrusor muscle in TUR specimens. In patients being considered for cystectomy with orthotopic urinary reconstruction, TUR biopsies from the prostatic urethra are also usually submitted to exclude CIS. It is of interest that of those apparently organ-confined (clinical stage T2) tumors, 40% to 50% are more advanced on pathological examination of the radical cystectomy specimen.

Histological Variants

Several histological variants of TCC are now well described that are relevant to prognosis and treatment. The micropapillary variant of TCC was first described in 1994 (29) and histologically resembles ovarian serous carcinoma. It is rare, accounting for about 1% of TCC with a strong male predominance. It can involve either the surface or invasive components of the tumor (Figs. 2 and 3). The micropapillary phenotype is often associated with advanced clinical stage at presentation, including a propensity for lymph node metastasis (30). There is evidence that for non–muscle invasive micropapillary disease, BCG therapy is often ineffective (31) and therefore radical treatment should be offered early.

The nested variant of TCC also shows a marked male predominance. It is unusual in having very bland cytomorphology, particularly in the superficial tumor (Fig. 4). However, it is usually clinically aggressive and often muscle invasive at presentation (32).

The sarcomatoid variant of TCC is a biphasic tumor displaying malignant epithelial and mesenchymal morphologies. The latter can include divergent differentiation into tissues not normally found in the bladder such as bone, cartilage, and skeletal muscle, so-called heterologous differentiation. There is sometimes a history of previous external beam radiotherapy or cyclophosphamide treatment. These tumors are often advanced at presentation and are associated with poor survival (33).

Small cell carcinoma (SCC) of the bladder is morphologically identical to its pulmonary counterpart and usually neuroendocrine differentiation is demonstrable with immunohistochemistry (Fig. 5). In roughly half of cases there is coexistent TCC

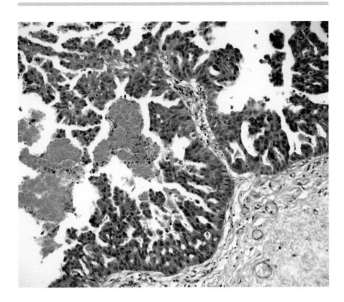

Figure 2 Noninvasive micropapillary TCC showing the characteristic filiform arrangement of micropapillae, without fibrovascular cores. Note the high-grade cytomorphology that is typical of this variant; there is also focal necrosis. *Abbreviation*: TCC, transitional cell carcinoma.

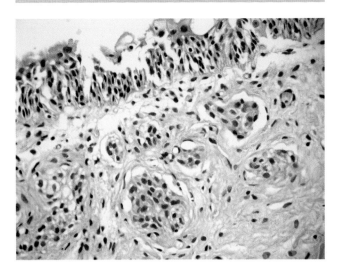

Figure 4 Nested variant of TCC. In small biopsies, because of the bland cytological features, the invasive nests of malignant cells in the lamina propria can be confused histologically with hyperplastic Von Brunn's nests or other benign transitional cell proliferations. The overlying flat urothelium here is normal; note that the cells in the invasive nests are very similar in size. There is usually more obvious cellular atypia in the more deeply invasive tumor, but this is not always represented in superficial resections. *Abbreviation*: TCC, transitional cell carcinoma.

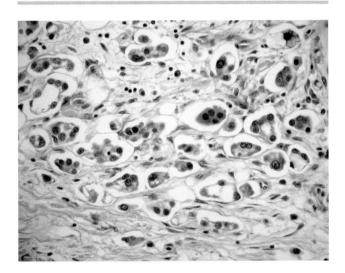

Figure 3 Invasive micropapillary TCC comprising small compact aggregates of cells infiltrating the lamina propria and demonstrating prominent lacunae (retraction spaces around the invasive nests), which should not be confused with lymphovascular space invasion. *Abbreviation*: TCC, transitional cell carcinoma.

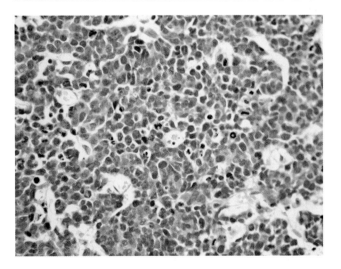

Figure 5 Small cell carcinoma. The cells have negligible cytoplasm, and as a consequence the nuclei are closely packed and show prominent "nuclear moulding." There is a high mitotic and apoptotic rate, and although it is not demonstrated here, necrosis is usually prominent. The tumors are typically positive with the neuroendocrine immunohistochemical markers synaptophysin and chromogranin-A and also with CD56 and TTF-1.

and/or CIS and this has been cited as evidence for a transitional cell origin (34), although others have proposed alternative origins from stem cells or bladder neuroendocrine cells. Metastatic disease is usually present (~70% cases) at diagnosis, and the disease is generally managed as a systemic disease

with similar cisplatin-based chemotherapy regime as for pulmonary SCC. There is no apparent survival difference for control of local disease between radiotherapy and radical cystectomy (35,36).

Premalignant Conditions

Keratinizing squamous metaplasia (KSM) is rare and sometimes referred to clinically as leukoplakia. It is usually associated with some form of chronic inflammatory process, for example, infections (usually *Escherichia coli*, *Streptococcus faecalis*, or *Proteus*), indwelling catheters, stones, or parasitic eggs. In contrast to its nonkeratinizing counterpart, KSM is a risk factor for the development of invasive malignancy, which is usually squamous cell carcinoma. The more extensive the changes found at cystoscopy, the greater the risk of malignant transformation (37). Small areas of KSM can be managed by TUR resection and cystoscopic follow-up; extensive disease, particularly in younger patients, merits radical cystectomy.

Urothelial dysplasia (low-grade intraurothelial neoplasia) is defined morphologically as "cytological and architectural changes felt to be preneoplastic but which fall short of carcinoma in situ" (23). Urothelial dysplasia is most commonly diagnosed in mucosa adjacent to invasive and high-grade TCC. Although it has been argued that dysplasia represents a risk factor for recurrence and progression (38), it is not clear whether dysplasia develops before or concomitantly with clinically manifest TCC. Furthermore, in many clinical studies that have shown risk of progression, dysplasia has not been separated from CIS.

CLINICAL FEATURES

Natural History

The natural history of bladder cancer can be classified as follows:

- No further recurrence
- Local recurrence, which can occur on a single occasion or on multiple occasions; it can involve single or multiple tumor recurrences, but recurrent tumors are usually of the same stage and grade as the primary tumor
- Local progression—an increase in local stage with time, the appearance of distant metastases, and subsequent death

Predicting Recurrence/Progression in Non–Muscle Invasive (pTa, pT1) Tumors

Of newly diagnosed non–muscle invasive tumors, approximately 30% are multifocal at presentation. The classic way to categorize patients with pTa/pT1 tumors is to divide them into risk groups on the basis of prognostic factors derived from univariate analyses and in some studies multivariate analyses (39–44). In each of these studies, multifocality is consistently a predictor of recurrence. Prior recurrence rate (43,44) and positive three-month check cystoscopy (39,40) are also key predictors. Histological grade is consistently a predictor of progression to muscle invasive disease (41–44). The poor prognosis of pT1G3 TCC is well described, with 50% progression rate if associated with concomitant CIS (41,45).

A British study proposed a cystoscopic follow-up plan based on the risk of recurrence determined from two objective parameters: solitary or multifocal at presentation and tumor-free/recurrence at first three-month check cystoscopy (46) (Table 2). Sixty percent of non–muscle invasive tumors are low-risk, 30% intermediate-risk, and 10% high-risk for recurrence. In a meta-analysis of seven randomized trials with one immediate postoperative instillation of chemotherapy, ideally within 6 hours but if not within 24 hours of TUR bladder tumor, the risk of recurrence was decreased by 39%. The benefit was confirmed in both solitary and multifocal tumors (47). However, of those with multifocal tumors, 65% still had a recurrence at a median follow-up of 3.4 years despite immediate-dose chemotherapy. For these patients, European Association of Urology (EAU) Guidelines recommend additional adjuvant intravesical instillations. The duration and frequency of additional instillations remain controversial. In a multivariate study, patients were divided into three groups at low-, intermediate-, and high-risk of recurrence and progression (42). However, this did not differentiate the risk of recurrence and progression. Some patients may have a high risk of recurrence but not progression, whereas others may have a high risk of recurrence and progression.

To separately predict the short-term and long-term risks of recurrence and progression in individual patients, the European Organisation for Research and Treatment of Cancer (EORTC) developed a scoring system (Table 3) and risk tables (Table 4) (48). The

Table 2 Prognostic Groups, Their Relationship to Risk of Recurrence and Recommended Management Plans for pTa and pT1 (G1 and G2) (WHO, 1973) Tumors

Prognostic groups	Cystoscopic findings	Management plan
Group 1	Solitary tumor at presentation, no tumor recurrence at 3 mo (20% risk of recurrence at 1 yr)	Followed up safely by annual flexible cystoscopy
Group 2	Solitary tumor at presentation, tumor recurrence at 3 mo; multiple tumors at presentation, no tumor recurrence at 3 mo (40% risk of recurrence at 1 yr)	Followed up 3-monthly by flexible cystoscopy for the first year; then annually if no recurrence
Group 3	Multiple tumors at presentation, tumor recurrences at 3 mo (90% risk of recurrence at 1–2 yrs)	3-monthly rigid cystoscopic assessment under general anesthesia for 2 yr; then annually if no recurrence

Source: From Refs. 39, 46.

Table 3 Weighting Used to Calculate Recurrence and Progression Scores

Factor	Recurrence	Progression
Number of tumors		
Single	0	0
2–7	3	3
≥8	6	3
Tumor diameter		
<3 cm	0	0
≥3 cm	3	3
Prior recurrence rate		
Primary	0	0
≤1 recurrence/year	2	2
>1 recurrence /year	4	2
Category		
Ta	0	0
T1	1	4
Concomitant CIS		
No	0	0
Yes	1	6
Grade (1973 WHO)		
G1	0	0
G2	1	0
G3	2	5
Total score	0–17	0–23

Abbreviation: CIS, carcinoma in situ.
Source: From Ref. 48.

basis for these tables was the EORTC database, which provided individual data for 2591 patients diagnosed with pTa/pT1 tumors who were randomized in seven EORTC trials. Patients with primary CIS were excluded.

Primary CIS

Patients presenting with bladder pain, dysuria, and positive urine cytology are likely to harbor primary CIS. If primary CIS is diffuse, 50% of these patients die of metastatic TCC within a year or two if aggressive intravesical therapies are not instituted (49). Currently, these patients are usually offered maintenance intravesical BCG.

Muscle Invasive Disease

Over 50% of patients with muscle invasive disease have occult metastatic disease at presentation; its presence is strongly related to initial tumor stage, being most frequent in T4 disease. Among patients with muscle invasive bladder cancer thought to have negative nodes on preoperative computerized tomography, around one-fifth are found to have metastatic nodal disease when managed by radical cystectomy and bilateral lymphadenectomy alone. The presence of concomitant CIS and/or upper tract dilatation is associated with less good outcomes following radiotherapy, and consequently these patients are usually offered radical cystectomy. Neoadjuvant chemotherapy has become standard in many centers prior to radical cystectomy or radiotherapy following the publication of two meta-analyses, one showing a 5% overall survival benefit (50), the other showing a 6.5% survival benefit (51).

MOLECULAR PATHOGENESIS OF BLADDER TCC

Molecular biology is paramount to our understanding of bladder cancer pathogenesis. Although great insights have been made into our ability to predict recurrence and progression using established prognostic markers, they are not sufficiently sensitive or specific to predict individual prognosis. Understanding the molecular profile of individual patients could usher us into an era of improving prediction of the natural history of the disease and providing a more personalized and tailored treatment. It should also facilitate the development of novel targeted treatments. Multiple genetic and epigenetic alterations have been described in bladder cancer, including those that affect signal transduction, the cell cycle, invasion, angiogenesis, and apoptosis.

Model for Bladder TCC Progression

Current evidence suggests that genetic alterations on chromosome 9 are an early event in bladder tumor formation. Chromosome 9 loss of heterozygosity

Table 4 Probability of Recurrence and Progression According to Total Score

Recurrence score	Probability of recurrence at 1 yr		Probability of recurrence at 5 yr		Recurrence risk group
	%	(95% CI)	%	(95% CI)	
0	15	(10–19)	31	(24–37)	Low
1–4	24	(21–26)	46	(42–49)	Intermediate
5–9	38	(35–41)	62	(58–65)	Intermediate
10–17	61	(55–67)	78	(73–84)	High

Progression score	Probability of progression at 1 yr		Probability of progression at 5 yr		Progression risk group
	%	(95% CI)	%	(95% CI)	
0	0.2	(0–0.7)	0.8	(0–1.7)	Low
2–6	1	(0.4–1.6)	6	(5–8)	Intermediate
7–13	5	(4–7)	17	(14–20)	High
14–23	17	(10–24)	45	(35–55)	High

Source: From Ref. 48.

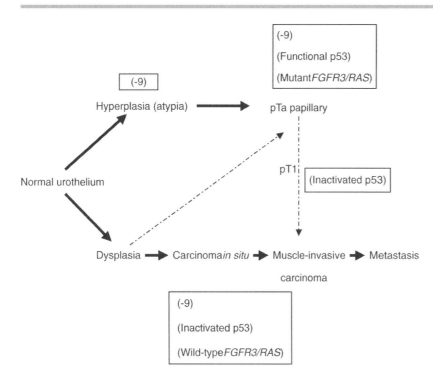

Figure 6   A simplified genetic model for bladder tumor development. Minus signs indicate copy number losses or loss of heterozygosity.

(LOH) is found in more than 50% of all bladder tumors, regardless of stage and grade. It has also been identified in hyperplastic urothelium. Low-grade pTa tumors usually have alterations in the RAS-MAP kinase signal transduction pathway, the most frequent being fibroblast growth factor receptor 3 (*FGFR3*) mutations on chromosome 4p (52). Most genetic events to date have been identified in high-grade and muscle invasive tumors. Many of these events are also found in CIS, confirming the likely progression to muscle invasive TCC via CIS. Muscle invasive tumors and CIS frequently have alterations in the p53 and retinoblastoma (pRb) pathways that control the cell cycle. Although almost certainly too simplistic, this model does provide a useful basis for further genetic studies (Fig. 6). There are clearly some gaps in our knowledge. For example, no significant molecular differences have yet been found among CIS, muscle invasive TCC, and the metastases that develop from them. Moreover, we are unsure whether pT1 tumors represent a distinct group or are merely caught in their journey to muscle invasion.

Molecular Basis of Metachronous and Synchronous Bladder TCC

Two theories have arisen from the observation that patients with bladder cancer often present with metachronous tumors that develop at different times and sites within the bladder: the field change (oligoclonal) and monoclonal theories (53). The field change theory attributes multifocality to individual transformation of urothelial cells at a number of sites where there is dysplasia or CIS. In contrast, at least in some cases,

molecular biological studies support a common clonal origin for concomitant urothelial tumors. This was first demonstrated in methylation studies of the X chromosome (54). For each of four female patients with multiple bladder tumors, it was found that all the tumors from a given individual had inactivation of the same X chromosome. Lateral intraepithelial spread and dispersal of transformed cells are possible mechanisms underlying the monoclonal theory. Current evidence suggests that oligoclonal tumors might be more common in precursor lesions and early tumor stages. The frequent monoclonality found in patients with advanced tumors could be because of outgrowth of one tumor clone with specific genetic alterations (53).

SPECIFIC GENETIC ALTERATIONS IDENTIFIED IN TCC

The key genetic alterations identified in bladder TCC are in the following subsections.

Oncogenes

Several known oncogenes are altered in TCC. They contribute to the malignant phenotype in a dominant manner. This is achieved either by overexpression of the gene product, or, less commonly, by expression of the mutant protein product with altered function.

FGFR3, RAS, and PI3 Kinase

The *FGFR3* gene found on chromosome 4 (4p16) encodes a glycoprotein that belongs to a family of

Table 5 Frequency of *FGFR3* Mutations in Bladder Tumors

Tumor	*FGFR3* mutation frequency (%)
Papilloma	~75
Ta	>60
T1	20–25
CIS	0
Muscle invasive	~16

Abbreviation: CIS, carcinoma in situ.
Source: From Ref. 52.

structurally related tyrosine kinase receptors. Activating point mutations of *FGFR3* have been identified in approximately 40% of bladder tumors overall (Table 5). The only other malignancy in which significant involvement of *FGFR3* has been reported is multiple myeloma. A large study of more than 700 tumors recently found that *FGFR3* mutation was associated with a high recurrence rate in TaG1 tumors (55). Mutant *FGFR3* is predicted to activate the RAS-MAP kinase pathway. *FGFR3* and *RAS* gene mutations are mutually exclusive in bladder cancer, as expected if each has the same signaling consequences. *RAS* mutations are found in 13% of bladder TCC and 85% of low-grade pTa tumors were found to have a *RAS* or a *FGFR3* mutation (56).

RAS can also activate the PI3 kinase pathway. Mutations of the α-catalytic subunit of PI3 kinase have recently been identified. Interestingly, 26% of *FGFR3* mutant tumors were also PI3 kinase mutant compared with 7% of *FGFR3* wild-type tumors. The functional relationship between these events is not yet known (57).

EGFR, ErbB2 (HER2)

Overexpression of genes that encode receptor tyrosine kinases such as EGFR (epidermal growth factor receptor) and the ErbB2 receptor have been reported in TCC of the bladder. In a prospective study, the overexpression of EGFR correlated not only with higher tumor stage and grade but also with patient survival (58). Mechanisms underlying EGFR overexpression in bladder cancer are not clear, although gene amplification is not the principal mechanism.

The *ErbB2* gene encodes a 185-kDa cell surface glycoprotein with extensive homology to EGFR (59). Overexpression of the gene in the absence of gene amplification has been described (59). Although associations between gene amplification, protein overexpression, and death from bladder cancer have been reported, the prognostic significance of ErbB2 overexpression has not been fully explored.

**Tumor Suppressor Genes
and Cell Cycle Regulators**

In the mammalian cell cycle, functional inactivation of these genes either by mutation, deletion, or DNA hypermethylation contributes to the development of cancer. The key tumor suppressor genes altered in bladder cancer are *TP53* and *RB1*. The p53 pathway

markers are p53, p21, MDM2, and p14. The pRb pathway markers are pRb, E2F1, cyclins, cyclin kinases, p27, and p16.

TP53

The *TP53* gene has been mapped to chromosome 17q13. *TP53* gene mutations are associated with high-grade and high-stage TCC. Around 50% of muscle invasive TCCs harbor *TP53* gene mutations (60). Overall, p53 protein accumulation is associated with *TP53* gene mutation. Mutant p53 has an increased half-life and can be detected with ease, whereas normal physiological concentrations of the wild-type protein are undetectable. Most studies have therefore used immunohistochemical detection of p53 protein as a surrogate for *TP53* gene mutation. However, microdissection studies of p53-immunopositive and immunonegative regions have demonstrated that p53 accumulation is not a reliable method of screening for *TP53* gene mutations in TCC (61). Clearly p53 accumulation can arise by alternate methods of p53 inactivation or by upregulation of functional wild-type p53. One such mediator of p53 inactivation in TCC is the MDM2 protein.

Despite studies correlating p53 immunohistochemistry with progression, meta-analysis of 117 studies concluded that there is insufficient evidence to infer that p53 by itself is a good prognostic marker for bladder cancer, previously because of small study cohorts and heterogeneity in laboratory and statistical methods (62). Finally, a recent prospective trial found no clinical utility for p53 expression in predicting survival in high-risk patients with pT1 tumors although this may have been affected by the low event rate related to treatment efficacy (63).

RB1

The *RB1* gene located at chromosome 13q14 was the first tumor-suppressor gene isolated. Structural alterations to the *RB1* gene by mutation or deletion are associated with muscle invasive TCC and have been reported in up to half of these tumors. Studies have shown that alterations in p53 and pRb pathways act in cooperative or synergistic ways to promote bladder cancer progression (64).

Tumor Invasion and Metastasis

As an initial step, cancer cells must detach from their original site before they can invade the surrounding tissue and metastasize to distant organs. The main families of adhesion molecules are the cadherins, integrins, members of the immunoglobulin superfamily, and selectins. This diverse system of transmembrane glycoproteins mediates cell–extracellular matrix adhesion and intercellular matrix adhesion.

Cadherins are the main mediators of cell-cell adhesion in epithelial tissues, being major components of both the adherens junction and desmosomes. Adhesion is achieved by homodimeric interactions between the extracellular domains of classical cadherins (E-cadherin, P-cadherin, and N-cadherin) on neighboring cells. Catenins (α-, β-, and γ-catenin and p120) anchor the cadherins to the cell cytoskeleton. In bladder TCC, reduced E-cadherin and β-catenin expression is associated with high grade and stage. Although E-cadherin has been shown to be an independent prognostic factor on multivariate analysis (65), many other studies have disputed its independent prognostic value for progression. Mutations, hypermethylation, and transcriptional repression of the *E-cadherin* gene may play a role in reduced expression.

The ability of tumor cells to degrade tissue extracellular matrix and basement membrane components is a prerequisite for invasion and metastasis. Such functions can be performed by a family of zinc-dependent proteolytic enzymes called matrix metalloproteinases (MMPs). A balance is maintained by tissue inhibitors of metalloproteinases. In bladder cancer, MMP-2 and MMP-9 expression is associated with higher tumor stage and grade. MMP-2 expression is associated with decreased survival (66).

Angiogenesis

Angiogenesis, the growth of new blood vessels from existing vessels, is essential to meet the metabolic requirements for tumor growth. Angiogenesis is controlled by the balance of pro- and antiangiogenic signals. Promoters of angiogenesis in bladder cancer include vascular endothelial growth factor receptor (VEGFR), thymidine phosphorylase, acidic and basic fibroblast growth factors (FGF1 and 2), and cyclooxygenase (COX)-2. An inhibitor of angiogenesis is thrombospondin. Both promoters and inhibitors have been shown to have an impact on clinical outcomes such as recurrence, progression, and survival (67). Increased microvessel density, a histological surrogate for angiogenesis, is a significant independent prognostic indicator of recurrence and poor survival (68).

COX is a key enzyme in the synthesis of prostaglandins from arachidonic acid. The inducible form of COX, COX-2, produces prostaglandins E1 and E2, which are considered to be angiogenic stimulators. COX-2 is rarely detected in normal urothelium. Although elevated COX-2 expression correlates with high-grade and muscle invasive TCC (69), COX-2 appears to have limited prognostic potential (70).

Apoptosis

Apoptosis is a unique form of cell death in which the cell activates a self-destruct mechanism, causing its death. Suppression of apoptosis can facilitate accumulation of gene mutations. Genes responsible for the regulation of apoptosis interact in a cascade that can be divided into initiation, regulation, and degradation phases. Initiators include p53 and cytokines such as tumor necrosis factor-α and fas ligand. The key regulators are the Bcl-2 family of proteins and survivin. The degradation stage of apoptosis is primarily mediated by a family of 10 or more proteolytic enzymes called caspases. They are expressed as precursors that are activated when cleaved. Caspases target proteins that

are integral to the cell structure and repair processes. Activated caspase-3 can inhibit the cyclin-dependent kinase activity of p27 by cleaving it into two fragments.

A recent study evaluated p53, Bcl-2, caspase-3, and survivin in patients treated with radical cystectomy. Multivariate analysis showed that changed expression of all four markers has an independent prognostic value for recurrence and survival (71).

URINARY BIOMARKERS OF TCC

Urine Cytology

Urine cytology was first described by Papanicolaou and Marshall in 1945. The median specificity is >95% when obvious cancer cells are identified. However, the median sensitivity of cytology is only 35% (72). The main limitation is that low-grade tumors often shed cytologically normal–appearing cells. Urine cytology is more sensitive in patients with high-grade tumors and CIS.

New Urinary Biomarkers

Novel urinary biomarkers have been developed to aid diagnosis of bladder cancer and to reduce the check cystoscopic burden (72). However, none to date has had sufficient sensitivity to replace cystoscopy at diagnosis. Moreover, no single marker has been shown to aid the decision making with regard to the frequency of surveillance cystoscopies. Current FDA-approved tests are nuclear matrix protein-22 (NMP-22), UroVysion™/fluorescence in situ hybridization (FISH), ImmunoCyt™, BTA stat, BTA TRAK, and fibrin-fibrinogen degradation products. Other key biomarkers under investigation include microsatellite analysis, telomerase, hyaluronic acid and hyaluronidase, BLCA-4, cytokeratins, and survivin.

At present the three most commonly used novel biomarkers are NMP-22 (sensitivity 49–65%; specificity 40–87%), UroVysion (sensitivity 69–87%; specificity 89–96%), and ImmunoCyt (sensitivity 38–100%; specificity 73–84%). NMP-22 is an important regulator of mitosis. In tumor cells, the nuclear mitotic apparatus is elevated and NMP-22 is released from cells in detectable levels; it is a point-of-care test. The UroVysion test utilizes FISH technology with probes for chromosome 3, 7, 17 and a locus for 9p21. In the ImmunoCyt assay, three fluorescently marked antibodies label two mucin-like proteins and a high molecular weight form of carcinoembryonic antigen.

The development of urinary markers for the detection of bladder cancer is a dynamic field, but the perfect marker with high sensitivity, specificity, and point-of-care results is still to be found. An important issue will be the financial cost-benefit ratio.

TRIALS ASSESSING INHIBITORS OF MOLECULAR TARGETS AND COX-2

Trials are ongoing or planned for tyrosine kinase inhibitors, targeting EGFR and ErbB2 (such as lapatinib), VEGFR (such as sorafenib and sunitinib), and farnesyl transferase (such as SCH66336). Monoclonal antibody studies include those using cetuximab that targets EGFR, trastuzumab that targets the ErbB2 receptor, and bevacizumab that targets VEGFR (73). Most targeted treatments are predominantly cytostatic, resulting in stable disease in some cases for variable periods if given alone. There is therefore great interest in combining targeted treatments with combination chemotherapy regimens or radiotherapy. In vitro studies suggest that precise scheduling of targeted agents and chemotherapy is important and is likely to influence outcome (74).

The BOXIT trial sponsored by the National Cancer Research Institute (NCRI) has commenced in the United Kingdom. The primary objective of this phase 3 trial is to determine if the addition of the oral COX-2 inhibitor celecoxib to standard therapy is more effective in terms of disease recurrence at three years compared with standard therapy alone for the treatment of non–muscle invasive TCC of the bladder in intermediate or high-risk groups.

NEW TECHNOLOGIES IN THE DIAGNOSIS OF BLADDER CANCER

Photodynamic Diagnosis

The use of white light cystoscopy alone at the time of TUR bladder tumor may miss lesions that are present but not visible. Fluorescence cystoscopy is performed using blue-violet light after intravesical instillation of photosensitizer, usually 5-aminolevulinic acid (5-ALA) or hexaminolevulinate (HAL). 5-ALA fluorescence cystoscopy has been shown to detect more CIS and papillary tumors (75). In a randomized trial, 5-ALA fluorescence cystoscopy at the time of diagnostic TUR bladder tumor was associated with reduced residual disease (76). Of those who underwent fluorescence cystoscopy at initial TUR bladder tumor, 4.5% had residual disease compared with 25% who underwent white light cystoscopy. In the same trial, fluorescence cystoscopy at diagnostic TUR bladder tumor reduced the recurrence rate. Eight years after initial TUR bladder tumor, 29% of those who underwent 5-ALA fluorescence cystoscopy developed a recurrence compared with 55% in the white light cystoscopy arm. HAL fluorescence cystoscopy has also been shown to improve the detection of CIS and papillary tumors.

Although very promising, its value remains to be proven with regard to reducing progression rates and improving survival. Moreover, although 5-ALA fluorescence cystoscopy reduced recurrence rates by 64%, patients did not routinely receive a single dose of intravesical chemotherapy within 24 hours of initial TUR bladder tumor in this trial (76). The question therefore remains whether photodynamic diagnosis gives added value if immediate-dose intravesical chemotherapy is administered. The additional costs of the equipment need to be considered in any health economic model.

Principles

Fluorescence occurs when a molecule absorbs one color of light, and emits another color; this is termed Stokes shift. The molecule absorbs the photon; an electron is elevated to an excited state and then returns to its resting state. The photon is then emitted with less energy and so has a longer wavelength. Porphyrins absorb violet-blue light and emit red light.

5-ALA is an initial substrate of heme biosynthesis. Exogenous application of 5-ALA induces an accumulation of fluorescent porphyrins, predominantly protoporphyrin IX (PPIX) in epithelial tissue. Using a blue-violet light with a wavelength of 400 nm, PPIX appears as fluorescent red while normal urothelium appears blue. This is because PPIX accumulates up to 10 times more in neoplastic cells than in normal tissue. The mechanism of accumulation of fluorescent PPIX in urothelial cancer is unclear. Several theories, including a difference in the metabolic rate of neoplastic tissue, hyperproliferation, and inflammation-induced increased permeability to ALA, have been proposed. These are supported by the observations that increased PPIX can be detected in urothelial hyperplasia, inflammation, and granulation tissue. 5-ALA absorption is limited because of its positive electric charge. The esterification of 5-ALA as HAL makes ALA more lipophilic, which enables it to cross the cell membrane more easily. A consequence of this is more rapid cellular uptake and higher fluorescence than ALA. HAL therefore needs to be administered only one hour before cystoscopy compared with two hours before for 5-ALA. The procedure requires special telescopes with a filter to reduce autofluorescence, and a specific light source.

THE FUTURE

Technologies such as high-throughput transcript profiling, microarrays, and proteomics are facilitating the comprehensive identification of molecular pathways and targets that are active in bladder cancer. This will also enable the development of novel targeted treatments. Future management of bladder cancer will employ molecular profiling that will be able to provide accurate predictions of prognosis and chemotherapeutic response in individual patients.

REFERENCES

1. CancerStats. Available at: http://info.cancerresearchuk.org/cancerstats/.
2. Whelan P. Bladder cancer—contemporary dilemmas in its management. Eur Urol 2008; 53(1):24–26.
3. Pelucchi C, Bosetti C, Negri E, et al. Mechanisms of disease: the epidemiology of bladder cancer. Nat Clin Pract Urol 2006; 3:327–340.
4. Brennan P, Bogillot O, Cordier S, et al. Cigarette smoking and bladder cancer in men: a pooled analysis of 11 case-controlled studies. Int J Cancer 2000; 86:289–294.
5. Brennan P, Bogillot O, Greiser E, et al. The contribution of cigarette smoking to bladder cancer in women (pooled European data). Cancer Causes Control 2001; 12:411–417.
6. IARC Working Group on the Evaluation of Carcinogenic Risks to Humans. Tobacco smoke and involuntary smoking. IACR Monogr Eval Carcinog Risks Hum 2004; 83:1438.

7. NICE Guidance on Cancer Services. Improving Outcome in Urological Cancers. National Institute for Clinical Excellence, 2002.

8. Bjerregaard BK, Raaschou-Nielsen O, Sørensen M, et al. Tobacco smoke and bladder cancer—in the European Prospective Investigation into Cancer and Nutrition. Int J Cancer 2006; 119:2412–2416.

9. Aveyard P, Adab P, Cheng KK, et al. Does smoking status influence the prognosis of bladder cancer? A systematic review. BJU Int 2002; 90:228–239.

10. Hueper WC, Wiley FH, Wolfe HD. Experimental production of bladder tumours in dogs by administration of beta-naphthylamine. J Ind Hyg Toxicol 1938; 20:46–84.

11. Case RAM, Hosker ME. Tumour of the urinary tract as an occupational disease in the rubber industry in England and Wales. Br J Prev Soc Med 1954; 8:39–50.

12. BAUS Subcommittee on Industrial Bladder Cancer. Occupational bladder cancer: a guide for physicians. Br J Urol 1988; 61:183–191.

13. Kogevinas M, 't Mannetje A, Cordier S, et al. Occupation and bladder cancer among men in Western Europe. Cancer Causes Control 2003; 14:907–914.

14. Czene K, Tiikkaja S, Hemminki K, et al. Cancer risks in hairdressers: assessment of carcinogenicity of hair dyes and gels. Int J Cancer 2003; 105:108–112.

15. Fairchild WV, Spence CR, Solomon HD, et al. The incidence of bladder cancer after cyclophosphamide therapy. J Urol 1979; 122:163–164.

16. Duncan RE, Bennett DW, Evans AT, et al. Radiation-induced bladder tumours. J Urol 1977; 118:43–45.

17. Boorjian S, Cowan JE, Konety BR, et al. Cancer of the prostate Strategic Urologic Endeavor Investigators. Bladder cancer incidence and risk factors in men with prostate cancer: results from Cancer of the Prostate Strategic Urologic Research Endeavor. J Urol 2007; 177:883–887.

18. Steinmaus CM, Nunez S, Smith AH. Diet and bladder cancer: a meta-analysis of six dietary variables. Am J Epidemiol 2000; 151:693–702.

19. Garcia-Closas M, Malats N, Silverman D, et al. NAT2 slow acetylation, GSTM1 null genotype, and risk of bladder cancer: results from the Spanish Bladder Cancer Group and meta-analyses. Lancet 2005; 366:649–659.

20. Engel LS, Taioli E, Pfeiffer R, et al. Pooled analysis and met-analysis of glutathione S-transferase M1 and bladder cancer: a HuGe review. Am J Epidemiol 2002; 156:95–109.

21. Mostofi F. International histologic classification of tumours. A report by the Executive Committee of the International Council of Societies of Pathology. Cancer 1973; 33:1480–1484.

22. Epstein JI, Amin MB, Reuter VR, et al. The World Health Organisation/International Society of Urological Pathology consensus classification of urothelial (transitional cell) neoplasms of the urinary bladder. Bladder Consensus Conference Committee. Am J Surg Pathol 1998; 22:1435–1448.

23. Eble JN, Sauter G, Epstein JI, et al. World Health Organisation Classification of Tumours. Pathology and Genetics of Tumours of the Urinary System and Male Genital Organs. Lyon, France: IACR Press, 2004:89–158.

24. Epstein JI, Amin MB, Reuter VE. Bladder Biopsy Interpretation. Philadelphia: Lippincott, Williams and Wilkins, 2004:40.

25. Harnden P. A critical appraisal of the classification of urothelial tumours: time for a review of the evidence and a radical change? BJU Int 2007; 99:723–725.

26. Lopez-Beltran A, Montironi R. Non-invasive urothelial neoplasms: according to the most recent WHO classification. Eur Urol 2004; 46:170–176.

27. Standards and datasets for reporting cancers. Dataset for tumours of the urinary collecting system (renal pelvis, ureter, bladder, and urethra). Royal College of Pathologists, January 2007. Available at: http://www.rcpath.org/resources/pdf/G044TumoursurinaryCollectingSystemFINAL.pdf.

28. Sobin DH, Witteking CH, eds. TNM Classification of Malignant Tumours. 6th ed. New York: Wiley-Liss, 2002.

29. Amin AB, Ro JY, el-Sharkawy T, et al. Micropapillary variant of transitional cell carcinoma of the urinary bladder. Histologic pattern resembling ovarian papillary serous carcinoma. Am J Surg Pathol 1994; 18:1224–1232.

30. Kamat AM, Dinney CP, Gee JR, et al. Micropapillary bladder cancer: a review of the University of Texas M.D. Anderson Cancer Center experience with 100 consecutive patients. Cancer 2007; 110:62–67.

31. Kamat AM, Gee JR, Dinney CP, et al. The case for early cystectomy in the treatment of nonmuscle invasive micropapillary bladder carcinoma. J Urol 2006; 175:881–885.

32. Drew PA, Furman J, Civantos F, et al. The nested variant of transitional cell carcinoma: an aggressive neoplasm with innocuous histology. Mod Pathol 1996; 9:989–994.

33. Wright JL, Black PC, Brown GA, et al. Differences in survival among patients with sarcomatoid carcinoma, carcinosarcoma and urothelial carcinoma of the bladder. J Urol 2007; 178:2302–2306.

34. Wang X, MacLennan GT, Lope-Beltran A, et al. Small cell carcinoma of the urinary bladder—histogenesis, genetics diagnosis, biomarkers, treatment and prognosis. Appl Immunohistochem Mol Morphol 2007; 15:8–18.

35. Sved P, Gomez P, Manoharan, et al. Small cell carcinoma of the bladder. BJU Int 2004; 94:12–17.

36. Abol-Enein H, Kava BR, Carmack AJ. Nonurothelial cancer of the bladder. Urology 2007; 69:93–104.

37. Khan MS, Thornhill JA, Gaffney E, et al. Keratinising squamous metaplasia of the bladder: natural history and rationalisation of management based on review of 54 years experience. Eur Urol 2002; 42:469–474.

38. Cheng L, Cheville JC, Neumann RM, et al. Natural history of urothelial dysplasia of the bladder. Am J Surg Pathol 1999; 23:443–447.

39. Parmar MK, Freedman LS, Hargreave TB, et al. Prognostic factors for recurrence and follow-up policies in the treatment of superficial bladder cancer: report from the British Medical Research Council Subgroup on Superficial Bladder Cancer (Urological Cancer Working Party). J Urol 1989; 142:284–288.

40. Fitzpatrick JM, West AB, Butler MR, et al. Superficial bladder tumours (stage pTa, grades 1 and 2): the importance of recurrence pattern following initial resection. J Urol 1986; 135:920–922.

41. Heney NM, Ahmed S, Flanagan MJ, et al. Superficial bladder cancer: progression and recurrence. J Urol 1983; 130:1083–1086.

42. Millan-Rodriguez F, Chechile-Toniolo G, Salvador-Bayarri J, et al. Primary superficial bladder cancer risk groups according to progression, mortality and recurrence. J Urol 2000; 164:680–684.

43. Kurth KH, Denis L, Bouffioux C, et al. Factors affecting recurrence and progression in superficial bladder tumours. Eur J Cancer 1995; 31A:1840–1846.

44. Lutzeyer W, Rubben H, Dahm H. Prognostic parameters in superficial bladder cancer: an analysis of 315 cases. J Urol 1982; 127:250–252.

45. Jakse G, Loidl W, Seeber G, et al. Stage T1 grade G3 transitional cell carcinoma of the bladder: an unfavourable tumour? J Urol 1987; 137:39–43.

46. Hall RR, Parmar MK, Richards AB, et al. Proposal for changes in cystoscopic follow-up of patients with bladder

cancer and adjuvant intravesical chemotherapy. BMJ 1994; 308:257–260.

47. Sylvester RJ, Oosterlinck W, van der Meijden AP. A single immediate postoperative instillation of chemotherapy decreases the risk of recurrence in patients with stage Ta T1 bladder cancer: a meta-analysis of published results of randomised clinical trials. J Urol 2004; 171:2186–2190.

48. Sylvester RJ, Oosterlinck W, van der Meijden AP, et al. Predicting recurrence and progression in individual patients with stage TaT1 bladder cancer using EORTC risk tables: a combined analysis of 2596 patients from seven EORTC trials. Eur Urol 2006; 49:466–477.

49. Utz DC, Farrow GM. The management of carcinoma in situ of the urinary bladder: the case for surgical management. Urol Clin North Am 1980; 7:533–541.

50. Advanced Bladder Cancer (ABC) Meta-analysis Collaboration. Neoadjuvant chemotherapy in invasive bladder cancer: update of a systematic review and meta-analysis of individual patient data advanced bladder cancer (ABC) meta-analysis collaboration. Eur Urol 2005; 48:202–205.

51. Winquist E, Kirchner TS, Segal R, et al. Genitourinary Cancer Disease Site Group, Cancer Care Ontario program in Evidence-based Care practice Guidelines Initiative. Neoadjuvant chemotherapy for transitional cell carcinoma of the bladder: a systemic review and meta-analysis. J Urol 2004; 171:561–569.

52. Knowles MA. Novel therapeutic targets in bladder cancer: mutation and expression of FGF receptors. Future Oncol 2008; 4:71–83.

53. Hafner C, Knuechel R, Stoehr R, et al. Clonality of multifocal urothelial carcinomas: 10 years of molecular genetic studies. Int J Cancer 2002; 101:1–6.

54. Sidransky D, Von Eschenbach A, Oyasu R, et al. Clonal origin bladder cancer. N Engl J Med 1992; 326:737–740.

55. Hernandez S, Lopez-Knowles E, Lloreta J, et al. Prospective study of FGFR3 mutations as a prognostic factor in non-muscle invasive urothelial bladder carcinomas. J Clin Oncol 2006; 24:3664–3671.

56. Jebar AH, Hurst CD, Tomlinson DC, et al. FGFR3 and Ras gene mutations are mutually exclusive genetic events in urothelial cell carcinoma. Oncogene 2005; 24:5218–5225.

57. Lopez-Knowles E, Hernandez S, Malats N, et al. PIK3CA mutations are an early genetic alteration associated with FGFR3 mutations in superficial papillary bladder tumours. Cancer Res 2006; 66:7401–7404.

58. Mellon K, Wright C, Kelly P, et al. Long-term outcome related to epidermal growth factor receptor status in bladder cancer. J Urol 1995; 153:919–925.

59. Sauter G, Moch D, Moore P, et al. Heterogeneity of erbB-2 gene amplification in bladder cancer. Cancer Res 1993; 53:2199–2203.

60. Spruck CHR, Ohneseit PF, Gonzalez-Zulueta M, et al. Two molecular pathways to transitional cell carcinoma of the bladder. Cancer Res 1994; 54:784–788.

61. Abdel-Fattah R, Challen C, Griffiths TRL, et al. Alterations of TP53 in microdissected transitional cell carcinoma of the human bladder: high frequency of TP53 accumulation in the absence of detected mutations is associated with poor prognosis. Br J Cancer 1998; 77:2230–2238.

62. Malats N, Bustos A, Nascimento CM, et al. P53 as a prognostic marker for bladder cancer: a meta-analysis and review. Lancet Oncol 2005; 6:678–686.

63. Dalbagni G, Parekh DJ, Ben-Porat L, et al. Prospective evaluation of p53 as a prognostic marker in T1 transitional cell carcinoma of the bladder. BJU Int 2007; 99:281–285.

64. Chatterjee SJ, Datar R, Youssefzadeh D, et al. Combined effects of p53, p21, and pRb expression in the progression of bladder transitional cell carcinoma. J Clin Oncol 2004; 22:1007–1013.

65. Byrne RR, Shariat SF, Brown R, et al. E-cadherin immunostaining of bladder transitional cell carcinoma, carcinoma in situ and lymph node metastases with long-term follow-up. J Urol 2001; 165:1473–1479.

66. Papathoma AS, Petraki C, Grigorakis A, et al. Prognostic significance of matrix metalloproteinases 2 and 9 in bladder cancer. Anticancer Res 2000; 20:2009–2013.

67. Charlesworth PJ, Harris AL. Mechanisms of disease: angiogenesis in urologic malignancies. Nat Clin Pract Urol 2006; 3:157–169.

68. Bochner BH, Cote RJ, Weidner N, et al. Angiogenesis in bladder cancer: relationship between microvessel density and tumour prognosis. J Natl Cancer Inst 1995; 87:1603–1612.

69. Yoshimura R, Sano H, Mitsuhashi M, et al. Expression of cyclooxygenase-2 in patients with bladder carcinoma. J Urol 2001; 165:1468–1472.

70. Shariat SF, Matsumoto K, Kim J, et al. Correlation of cyclooxygenase-2 expression with molecular markers, pathological features and clinical outcome of transitional cell carcinoma of the bladder. J Urol 2003; 170:985–989.

71. Karam JA, Lotan Y, Karakiewicz PI, et al. Use of combined apoptosis biomarkers for prediction of bladder cancer recurrence and mortality after radical cystectomy. Lancet Oncol 2007; 8:128–136.

72. Vrooman OP, Witjes JA. Urinary markers in bladder cancer. Eur Urol 2008; 53:909–916.

73. Sonpavde G, Ross R, Powles T, et al. Novel agents for muscle-invasive and advanced urothelial cancer. BJU Int 2008; 101:937–943.

74. McHugh LA, Kriajevska M, Mellon JK, et al. Combined treatment of bladder cancer cell lines with lapatinib and varying chemotherapy regimens—evidence of schedule-dependent synergy. Urology 2007; 69:390–394.

75. Hungerhuber E, Stepp H, Kriegmair M, et al. Seven years' experience with 5-aminolevulinic acid in detection of transitional cell carcinoma of the bladder. Urology 2007; 69:260–264.

76. Denzinger S, Burger M, Walter B, et al. Clinically relevant reduction in risk of recurrence of superficial bladder cancer using 5-aminolevulinic acid-induced fluorescence diagnosis: 8-year results of prospective randomized study. Urology 2007; 69:675–679.

25

Prostate Cancer

Freddie C. Hamdy
Nuffield Department of Surgery, University of Oxford, Oxford, U.K.

Craig N. Robson
Northern Institute for Cancer Research, The Medical School, University of Newcastle, Newcastle, U.K.

> As the eyes grow dim, the trunk bends, the cartilages ossify, and the arteries change in their coats, so the prostate is supposed to grow large and hard...
> *James Miller, 1864*

INTRODUCTION

Prostate cancer is the most common malignancy in Western countries. In the United States, 186,320 cases were diagnosed in 2008 and there were 28,660 deaths from the disease (1). In England and Wales, there were 13,481 cases registered in 1990, rising to 34,302 new cases in 2005 with 10,000 prostate cancer deaths (2). Public awareness about the disease is clearly on the increase, partly because of media interest and growing general interest in men's health issues. While incidence has been increasing gradually, this has not corresponded to a paralleled increase in death rates, but there is a striking reduction, both in the United States and England and Wales, which appears to be of slightly higher magnitude in the United States compared to the United Kingdom (3). This observation is difficult to interpret, and although screening using prostate-specific antigen (PSA) testing in asymptomatic men has been shown recently to reduce prostate cancer–specific mortality (4), it alone cannot explain this reduction because of the very low opportunistic PSA-testing patterns in the United Kingdom (5). The reasons are undoubtedly multifactorial, such as screening, the earlier detection and aggressive treatment of nonmetastatic locally advanced disease, and improved diet as well as general environmental issues.

Evidence of carcinoma has been found in postmortem studies in approximately 30% of men aged 50 years, and 70% of men over the age of 80 years (6), but only a small proportion of these tumors progress to become clinically significant. With well-conducted screening programs, it is now possible to detect small volume tumors amenable to cure. However, clinicians are still unable to predict which tumor is likely to progress and which will remain quiescent.

ETIOLOGY

Prostate cancer results from a complex and yet unclear interaction between aging, genetic factors, hormones, growth factors, and the environment, including an increasing body of evidence incriminating dietary fat (7).

Prostate cancer can be sporadic: familial with clustering of disease within families and exposure to common risk factors; or hereditary, with typical characteristics of early age onset and an autosomal dominant inheritance pattern. The latter is likely to be triggered by a single gene passed along families, yet to be discovered and possibly located in chromosome 1 (8). It has been estimated that men who have three first-degree relatives have a 10.9-fold increase in risk of developing the disease (9). An increased risk of prostate cancer has also been associated with familial breast cancer (7). It is generally accepted that prostate cancer is not divided into latent and clinically significant tumor, but that its very long natural history, coupled with cumulative genetic and biological changes, eventually leads to progressive disease. It is the length of this natural history that allows more men to die *with* the disease than *from* it.

PATHOLOGY

Adenocarcinoma arising from the prostatic epithelium accounts for about 95% of prostatic malignancies and is usually composed of small glandular acini that infiltrate in an irregular haphazard manner. The critical feature in prostatic adenocarcinoma is absence of the basal cell layer (Fig. 1), which may be detected immunohistochemically by using monoclonal antibodies against high–molecular weight cytokeratin.

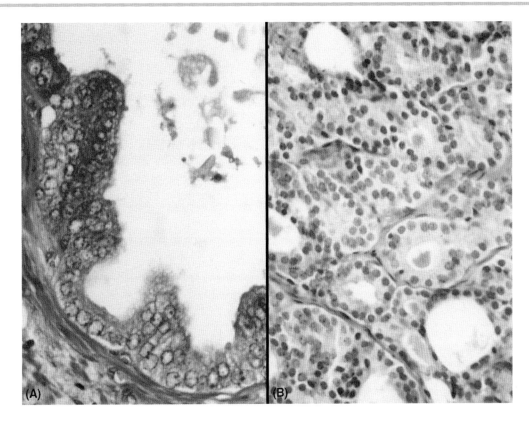

Figure 1 (**A**) A photomicrograph of the prostate demonstrating high-grade prostatic intraepithelial neoplasia with dysplastic changes, nuclear enlargement, hyper chromatism, prominent nuclei, cellular crowding, overlapping nuclei, and epithelial hyperplasia *H&E staining; magnification approximately 400×). (**B**) A photomicrograph of the prostate demonstrating adenocarcinoma with small glandular acini infiltrating in an irregular haphazard manner. The acini are composed of a single layer of cells showing nuclear enlargement with prominent nucleoli. The critical diagnostic feature in prostatic adenocarcinoma is absence of the basal layer (H&E staining; magnification approximately 400×).

Perineural and microvascular invasion may be seen, the latter correlating with histological grade.

Prostatic adenocarcinoma originates in the peripheral zone in approximately 75% of cases, with the rest originating in the transition zone (10). The tumors arising from these separate zones have different pathological features and clinical behavior. Transition zone tumors arise in or near foci of benign prostatic hyperplasia (BPH) and are usually smaller and better differentiated (Gleason pattern 1 and 2). Peripheral zone cancers are often less well differentiated (Gleason pattern 2, 3, or 4), larger in volume then transition zone tumors, and are frequently associated with greater stromal fibrosis, extracapsular extension, seminal vesicle invasion, and lymph node metastases.

Histological Grading

There are numerous grading systems, but the accepted standard is that developed by Gleason (11). The system is based on the degree of architectural differentiation, and individual cell cytology does not play a role. The system identifies five patterns that are often seen in prostatic adenocarcinoma, and to accommodate this, a primary and secondary pattern are assigned and the Gleason score is given as their sum, ranging from 2 to 10, with the dominant pattern recorded first, for example, 3 + 4 = 7 (Fig. 2). Gleason score correlates strongly with crude survival, tumor-free survival, and cause-specific survival, and is a significant predictor of time to recurrence following radical prostatectomy (12).

Grading errors are common in needle biopsy specimens of the prostate, with underestimation of the grade in 40% of cases, and overestimation in 25% when compared with the whole specimen following prostatectomy. This occurs more readily in biopsies containing small foci and low-grade cancers, reflecting sampling error and tumor heterogeneity. Nevertheless, useful predictive information can be provided by Gleason grading needle biopsies (13). More recently, tertiary Gleason grades were introduced, and defined as Gleason grade pattern 4 or greater for Gleason score 6 and Gleason grade pattern 5 for Gleason score 7 or 8. They are not at present consistently reported by pathologists, and although advocated as an important set of information in the evaluation of a patient's disease, to date consensus has not been reached regarding its interpretation and impact on management (14).

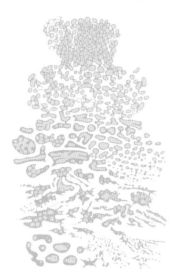

Grade	Margins	Gland pattern	Gland size	Gland distribution
1	Well defined	Single, separate, round	Medium	Closely packed
2	Less defined	Same as one but more variable	Medium	Spaced up to one gland apart
3	Poorly defined	Single, separate, irregular rounded masses of cribriform epithelium	Small, medium or large	Spaced more than one gland apart, rarely packed
4	Ragged infiltrating	Fused glandular masses	Small	Fused ragged masses
5	Ragged infiltrating. Poorly defined	Almost absent, few tiny glands or signet ring cells	Small	Ragged anaplastic masses of epithelium

Figure 2 The Gleason system of grading adenocarcinoma of the prostate.

Table 1 TNM Classification of Prostate Cancer

Tumor	Tx	Primary tumor cannot be assessed
	T0	No evidence of primary tumor
	T1	Tumor clinically unapparent, not palpable nor visible by imaging
	T1a	Incidental finding following TURP in up to 5% of tissue
	T1b	Incidental finding following TURP in more than 5% of tissue
	T1c	Tumor identified by needle biopsy (e.g., because of elevated PSA)
	T2	Tumor confined to the prostate, palpable or visible by imaging
	T2a	Tumor involves one lobe
	T2b	Tumor involves both lobes
	T3	Locally advanced tumor
	T3a	Extracapsular extension
	T3b	Invasion of the seminal vesicle
		Invasion into the prostatic apex or into (but not beyond) the prostatic capsule is not classified as T3, but as T2
	T4	Tumor is fixed or invades adjacent structures other than seminal vesicles; i.e., bladder neck, external sphincter, rectum, levator muscles, and/or pelvic wall
Nodes	Nx	Regional lymph nodes cannot be assessed
	N0	No regional lymph node metastases
	N1	Regional lymph node metastases
Metastasis	Mx	Presence of distant metastases cannot be assessed
	M0	No distant metastases
	M1	Distant metastases present
	M1a	Nonregional lymph nodes
	M1b	Skeletal metastases
	M1c	Other sites

Tumor Staging

The TNM system is the most common classification used worldwide (Table 1). Clinical staging is limited by a number of factors including understaging with digital rectal examination (DRE) and TURP specimens, limited accuracy of imaging, and the wide pathological variation of tumors identified on needle biopsy (stage T1c). The inaccuracy of clinical staging is especially important when comparing nonsurgical treatment methods (observation or radiotherapy) with pathologically staged disease following radical prostatectomy.

Prostate cancer commonly spreads to the pelvic lymph nodes, bones, especially the axial skeleton, and lung. Unlike most other malignancies, skeletal metastases from prostate cancer are osteoblastic in over 80% of cases, and despite the increase in bone formation they lead to disturbance in the normal skeletal architecture and subsequent pathological fractures if left untreated.

Putative Premalignant Lesions of the Prostate

Prostatic Intraepithelial Neoplasia and Atypical Small Acinar Proliferation

Prostatic intraepithelial neoplasia (PIN) is believed to be the preinvasive end of a morphological continuum of cellular proliferation affecting prostatic ducts, ductules, and acini. It tends to be multifocal and occurs in the peripheral zone, as does prostate cancer. PIN is divided into two groups: low and high grade. The continuum from normal prostatic epithelium through low- and high-grade PIN to invasive cancer is characterized by increased epithelial dysplasia within the luminal secretory cell layer. The dysplastic changes with increasing grade of PIN include nuclear enlargement, hyperchromatism, prominent nucleoli, cellular crowding with overlapping nuclei, and epithelial hyperplasia (Fig. 1). The basal cell layer remains intact though there may be some disruption in high-grade PIN. There is strong clinical, histological, and molecular evidence linking high-grade PIN with prostate cancer. High-grade PIN is seen in up to 16% of needle biopsies in men over 50 years of age. In malignant prostates, PIN is more frequent and of higher grade than in glands without cancer. The incidence of PIN increases with age, with low-grade PIN occurring in men in their third and fourth decade and high-grade PIN occurring in their fifth decade. Its association with cancer when repeat biopsies are performed is in the range of 0% to 24% (15). Atypical small acinar proliferation, on the other hand, does not appear to be a specific entity but a diagnostic category, including a number of atypical lesions that are suspicious for but not diagnostic of prostate cancer. The incidence of ASAP on prostate biopsy has been reported to be between 2.5% and 9.0% with a firm diagnosis of cancer in 30% to 60% of those cases (16).

Prostate-Specific Antigen

PSA is a serine protease and organ-specific glycoprotein (molecular weight 34,000) that originates in the cytoplasm of ductal cells of the prostate. It belongs to the family of glandular kallikreins of which 15 are known to date and are clustered in a locus on chromosome 19q133-4 (17). PSA is responsible for liquefaction of seminal coagulation. The measurement of serum PSA concentrations is now well established as a useful investigation in the diagnosis and follow-up of patients with prostate cancer (18). The greatest limitation of PSA is that it is *tissue* and not *tumor* specific in the prostate. However, PSA concentrations are the best overall predictor of bone scan findings and can be used as a screening test for prostate cancer (19,20). PSA circulates in blood mainly bound to protease inhibitors, including α-1-antichymotrypsin (ACT) and α-2-macroglobulin (AMG); only a small fraction of the total PSA exists in a free state. While AMG encapsulates all epitopes of the PSA protein, ACT leaves some exposed; therefore, immunoassay techniques have been developed to assess free PSA and PSA bound to ACT but not to AMG (21). It has been demonstrated that the free/total (f/t) PSA ratio in patients with BPH is significantly higher than in prostate cancer, but its role is not established in diagnosing the disease. Several studies report various optimal cutoff levels, largely because of the different nature of assays used (22). A study using the Hybritech assay

(Hybritech Inc., California, U.S.) demonstrated a sensitivity of 90% in diagnosing prostate cancer in the total PSA range of 2.6 to 4.0 ng/mL, while sparing approximately 18% of patients from having prostatic biopsies (23). The use of f/t PSA ratios in routine clinical practice remains to be determined. If measured before the age of 50 years, PSA levels appear to be a strong predictor of the incidence of prostate cancer later in life (24). PSA kinetics is determined as changes of PSA over time, represented either as PSA velocity, or PSA doubling time. PSA kinetics appears to be associated with diagnosis and disease recurrence/progression after treatment, although its interpretation remains unclear in monitoring patients who receive active monitoring and attempts are made to adjust changes observed to rising concentration for noncancerous changes such as age and BPH (25). For many years, the "normal" PSA threshold below which men were not recommended prostate biopsy varied between 3 and 4 ng/mL in an age group starting at approximately 50 years. However, results from the Prostate Cancer Prevention Trial (PCPT) in men receiving the 5-α reductase inhibitor finasteride versus placebo for prostate cancer chemoprevention showed through end-of-study biopsies that 15% of men had PSA levels less than 4 ng/mL (26). There is therefore no PSA threshold below which a man can be told that he does not have prostate cancer histologically. Furthermore, it has been demonstrated that using lower PSA threshold such as 1.5 ng/mL and a lower cutoff age of 45 years, the positive predictive value of PSA was 21.3%, with half the detected patients exhibiting clinically significant disease (27).

Circulating Tumor Cells

Clinically localized prostate cancers are frequently understaged in over 50% of cases, with resulting positive surgical margins, extracapsular extension, and potential treatment failure. This has stimulated researchers to detect circulating micrometastases prior to the establishment of overt secondaries, to avoid unnecessary radical treatment. Metastasis does not rely on the random survival of cells released from the primary tumor, but from the selective growth of specialized subpopulations of highly metastatic cells endowed with properties that will allow them to successfully complete each step of the metastatic cascade (28,29). Over the years, technologies such as flow cytometry and the reverse transcription polymerase chain reaction (RT-PCR) have given researchers the opportunity of detecting circulating tumor cells (CTCs) with high levels of sensitivity. In that sense, prostate cancer has a significant advantage over other malignancies, because of the specificity of PSA as a reliable marker, although additional identifying markers are being used, including cytokeratins. However, it has to be emphasized again that PSA is not tumor specific—a major drawback of all techniques attempting to detect CTCs. A PSA-positive cell in the peripheral blood, therefore, does not necessarily mean a prostate tumor cell, but a cell expressing PSA, which is likely to be of prostatic origin, in particular if the cell is found to express the gene constitutively, that is, mRNA for PSA. On the basis of these principles, analytical flow cytometry and RT-PCR have been used in an attempt to detect and isolate CTCs from patients with prostate cancer. Studies have shown that although quantification of circulating PSA-positive cells by FC was a better predictor of skeletal metastases than isotope bone scanning, the majority of these cells were not of prostatic origin, raising important questions regarding the role of nonprostatic circulating PSA-positive cells in patients with prostate cancer (30,31). RT-PCR methods, on the other hand, are considerably more sensitive in detecting circulating PSA-positive cells, relying on the identification of mRNA for PSA, an unequivocal proof that the cells are of prostatic origin. A number of studies demonstrated the ability of RT-PCR to detect circulating prostate cells in patients with apparently localized disease, undergoing radical prostatectomy, and some found a strong correlation between a positive PCR reaction, capsular tumor penetration, and positive surgical margins, suggesting the potential of this technique to be used for "molecular staging" of prostate cancer (32). Other workers used nested RT-PCR to compare the sensitivity of PSA with a different marker, prostate-specific membrane antigen (PSMA), in the detection of circulating prostatic cells (33). The authors of all these studies assume that circulating PSA-positive cells are endowed with metastatic propensity, despite the fact that the results only demonstrate the presence of cells of prostatic origin. Furthermore, the specificity of PSA mRNA in identifying cells of prostatic origin has been questioned (34). More recently, novel sensitive methods of capturing these cells were developed, using immunomagnetic bead technology, such as CellSearch and CellTracks systems (Veridex, Raritan, New Jersey, U.S.) (35), and enumerating CTCs has been advocated as a useful prognostic marker in castration-resistant patients (36). As technology advances further, it will be possible to determine the phenotype, genotype, and biological significance of CTCs in the future.

SCREENING FOR EARLY PROSTATE CANCER

Primum non nocere

Hippocrates

There has been an apparent consensus, on the basis of the evidence, that there is no justification to introduce population screening for prostate cancer. However, this consensus has been put to question by recently published results from the European Randomised Study of Screening for Prostate Cancer (4). In this large study with a median follow-up of 9 years, 72,952 men aged 55 to 69 years were randomized to screening and there were 89,435 age-matched controls. At follow-up to date, there was a relative risk reduction of 0.80 for dying of prostate cancer, and in absolute terms, 1410 men needed to be screened, and, of these, 48 men needed to receive treatment to prevent one man from dying of prostate cancer. So despite the fact that screening has now been shown to reduce prostate cancer mortality, it appears to be at a significant cost of overdetection and overtreatment.

Until such time that methods of active monitoring/surveillance are refined to prevent low-risk patients from being overtreated, and reliable biomarkers are identified to stratify patients into appropriate risk categories, it will be difficult for any health provider to advocate PSA-testing as a mass screening public health policy (37). The classic triad of detection tests consists of serum PSA measurement, DRE and transrectal ultrasound (TRUS) of the prostate and biopsy, which detect up to 6% of a screened population as having prostate cancer. However, methods of screening are changing rapidly, and when the results of these studies are available, it may well be that urologists will be detecting a different category of disease altogether compared with current screening modalities.

CLINICAL PRESENTATION

We found the patient complaining of excruciating pains in various parts of the body, which could be compared to nothing except the pains under which persons afflicted with carcinoma occasionally labour. He could void no urine without the assistance of a catheter. The prostate gland, examined by the rectum was found to be much enlarged and of a stony hardness. I continued to visit him in consultation for nearly a year, at the end of which time he suddenly lost the use of the muscles of his lower limbs and died a fortnight afterwards.

Sir Benjamin Brodie, 1842

Early prostate cancer is asymptomatic. The above description by Benjamin Brodie, over 150 years ago, illustrates all the relevant symptoms in advanced prostate cancer. Patients with symptomatic disease can present in a variety of ways, including bladder outflow obstruction, irritative bladder symptoms secondary to trigonal involvement, and hematuria. Metastatic disease may present with skeletal pain, spinal cord compression secondary to collapsed vertebrae, and pathological fractures; or with general systemic manifestations, including weight loss, weakness, and anorexia. With locally advanced disease, prostate cancer may manifest itself as renal failure secondary to bilateral ureteric orifices involvement.

TREATMENT

The more resources we have, and the more complex they are, the greater are the demands on our clinical skill. These resources are calls upon our judgment, and not substitutes for it.

Sir Francis Walsh

For the sake of simplicity, prostate cancer can be classified into early organ-confined and advanced disease when treatment is discussed.

Organ-Confined Prostate Cancer

Over the past decade, it has become evident that many cancers diagnosed through PSA testing in asymptomatic men are of low risk, with little potential to progress and become lethal disease. Patients with newly diagnosed clinically localized prostate cancer can thus be categorized into low-, intermediate-, and high-risk disease, following several analyses of data by a number of researchers (38). However, most data concern disease that has been already treated rather than patients receiving observation only. Historical cohort studies have been undertaken in the United States and Europe, confirming the observation that competing morbidity is an important factor in many men with early prostate cancer, linked to their age, serum PSA at diagnosis, and Gleason grading (39).

Conventional "curative" treatments of localized disease includes surgery in the form of radical prostatectomy through the open retropubic and perineal routes, laparoscopic and more recently robot-assisted laparoscopic intraperitoneal or extraperitoneal approaches; radiotherapy with its variations, including external beam conformal approaches, intensity modulated techniques, mostly in combination with neoadjuvant androgen suppression for a period of three to six months; and radioactive seed implantation otherwise known as brachytherapy. These treatments carry relatively low morbidity in experienced hands and a high cure rate. Active monitoring also known as active surveillance remains a reasonable option in many men with low-risk disease. Radical interventions are not recommended for men who are likely to have a life expectancy of less than 10 years because of competing morbidities and the likelihood that treatment will not benefit the patient. Studies indicate that selected groups of men may benefit from radical intervention, particularly those who are youngest and fittest, and have high-grade tumors.

High-level evidence concerning the effectiveness of treatments is limited at present to one randomized controlled trial of watchful waiting versus radical prostatectomy performed in Scandinavia, which showed successively a reduction in mortality from prostate cancer in favor of radical prostatectomy at 6-, 8-, and 10-year median follow-up, with a decrease in disease progression and development of metastases (40–42). However, the study was performed before the PSA era, and most tumors treated were of higher volume and stage than contemporary series. Addressing the same issues, PIVOT (The Prostate Cancer Intervention Versus Observation Trial) in the United States has closed to recruitment, comparing watchful waiting to surgery, as well as the ProtecT study in the United Kingdom, comparing active monitoring, surgery, and external beam radiotherapy (43,44). Results are awaited. In observational studies, survival following treatment for localized prostate cancer is good for all modes of treatment: 85% to 90% for radical prostatectomy, 65% to 90% for radiotherapy, and 70% to 90% for conservative management. This major issue of treatment efficacy in early prostate cancer is likely to be resolved once the results from both the PIVOT and ProtecT studies are reported in due course.

Advanced Prostate Cancer

Locally Advanced Disease

For many years, external beam irradiation has been widely accepted in treating locally advanced prostate cancer, and its combination with androgen suppression for three years has been shown to improve survival (45). A study by the Medical Research Council has closed to recruitment recently, comparing androgen suppression alone and in combination with radiotherapy. The results are awaited. To determine the benefits of immediate versus deferred treatment in asymptomatic men with nonmetastatic advanced prostate cancer, a further study by the Medical Research Council suggested that there is a small but significant advantage in treating these patients early, albeit to delay or prevent the advent of serious morbidity and complications from progressive disease. (46). Downstaging of extracapsular disease has also been attempted in a number of studies, whereby androgen ablation is performed for three to six months prior to radical prostatectomy. Although the incidence of positive margins decreases in clinically T2 tumors, there is no apparent change in T3 disease, and disease-free survival is not affected (47,48). In general, radical prostatectomy is not recommended for non–organ confined disease, but there appears to be an increasing tendency to offer surgery to patient with high-risk disease and/or clinically operable extracapsular tumors, although the evidence of benefits to such patients from surgical intervention remains to be demonstrated through well-conducted clinical trials.

Metastatic Disease

In 1940, Charles Huggins discovered the beneficial effects of androgen deprivation in patients with metastatic prostate cancer (49). Since then, hormonal manipulation has remained the mainstay of treatment in advanced stages of the disease. It is still expected that about 80% of all patients with advanced prostate cancer will respond to androgen blockade. Patients will show both subjective and objective responses, manifested by considerable and rapid symptomatic improvement, particularly in metastatic skeletal pain, together with local and distant regression of the disease. This is complemented by normalization of serum tumor markers. Relapse, however, is common at a mean interval of two years following initiation of treatment. The disease is then hormone resistant and prognosis becomes extremely poor. Methods of hormonal manipulation include bilateral orchidectomy and estrogen preparations, which are rarely prescribed nowadays, in view of the serious cardiovascular side effects encountered with the recognized 3 mg daily dose, to achieve castrate levels. The use of the smaller dose of 1 mg daily remains controversial, as castrate levels are not reached in 30% of patients. Alternative therapy includes the use of analogues of the hypothalamic luteinizing hormone-releasing hormone (LHRH). These occupy the receptors of LHRH in the pituitary, initially stimulating the release of luteinizing hormone and then blocking the subsequent stimulation of the receptors by the endogenous pulsatile secretion of luteinizing hormone. More recently, a new class of drugs, the GnRH antagonists, has been shown to immediately block the GnRH receptor and thus produce rapid AD without the ensuing testosterone surge, removing the need for administering antiandrogens to prevent testosterone flare. To date, results from randomized controlled trials comparing analogues with antagonists of LHRH report equivalent results in achieving castrate testosterone levels (50). In the late 1980s, total androgen blockade has been advocated to prevent the effect of the nontesticular circulating testosterone formation by the adrenals. After initial enthusiasm, further studies failed to show any survival advantage in patients treated with maximum androgen blockade (51,52), although a recent study from Japan reports that overall survival in such patients is indeed improved with maximum blockade compared with monotherapy using LHRH analogues (53). But this was achieved in a relatively small series of patients, and the debate continues.

In men with castration-resistant prostate cancer, taxanes have been shown to improve survival and quality of life in two randomized controlled trials undertaken simultaneously in North America (54,55). Docetaxel has now been adopted in men with these advanced stages of prostate cancer and low comorbidity as a palliative treatment option. More recently, a novel agent, abiraterone acetate, which is a potent, selective, and orally available inhibitor of CYP17 and the key enzyme in androgen and estrogen biosynthesis, has been shown to be of significant benefit in men with castration-resistant prostate cancer (56), and is being investigated further.

Awareness about the effects of androgen ablation on the skeleton has increased considerably over recent years, in particular loss of bone mineral density, which appears to occur mostly in the first 12 months of treatment, and could lead to osteopenia and osteoporosis, which may compound the effect of metastatic disease (57). Bone protection agents are therefore being tested to prevent these complications, such as bisphosphonates and RANK-ligand inhibitors that both act on reducing osteoclast activity. A recent study of a RANK-L inhibitor showed that it reduces the incidence of skeletal events in such patients (58). In men with skeletal metastases and castration-resistant disease, potent bisphosphonates such as zoledronic acid were shown to reduce and delay the incidence of skeletal-related events if given irrespective of the patient's symptoms with a sustained effect over time (59,60).

Novel Therapies in Prostate Cancer

The development of new therapeutic approaches in prostate cancer will rely on continuing progress made in three specific areas: (*i*) imaging of the prostate and identification of cancerous lesions; (*ii*) the delivery of different forms of energy to achieve safe and targeted tissue ablation; and (*iii*) understanding the biology of prostate cancer from its early genetic alterations to the molecular changes responsible for tumor progression.

On the basis of modern TRUS technology, two distinct modes of energy delivery systems for tissue ablation have been revived in recent years: cryotherapy and high-intensity focused ultrasound (HIFU).

Cryotherapy

The in situ destruction of tumors by the application of low temperatures was first developed in the 1970s to treat localized prostate cancer with reasonable success. Cryoablation had a number of advantages over other forms of treatment, but suffered from many limitations. Equipment was cumbersome, probes were placed mostly transurethrally under digital rectal guidance, temperature control was poor, and damage to adjacent tissue was common. The ability of real-time TRUS to guide cryoprobe placement and accurately monitor the freezing process, in addition to the development of urethral warming devices, encouraged clinicians to attempt again the destruction of prostate cancer by freezing. A number of studies on humans followed the animal work, and results are slowly emerging (61,62).

High-Intensity Focused Ultrasound

The technique consists of delivering ultrasonic energy with resultant heat and tissue destruction to a discrete point without damaging intervening tissue. Much higher temperatures are generated at the focal point using HIFU (approximately 98°C) than diffuse ultrasound hyperthermia (approximately 42°C), leading to complete tumor necrosis. After evaluating the technique initially in animal models and in vitro using cell lines, its use was reported in the treatment of BPH without significant side effects as a minimally invasive therapeutic option in symptomatic patients. The relative safety of HIFU coupled with its documented ability to cause targeted tissue necrosis prompted researchers to extrapolate its application to the treatment of prostate cancer, as an alternative to surgery and radiotherapy (63).

Photodynamic Therapy

Gene Therapy

Since the discovery of DNA and its structure by James Watson and Francis Crick in 1953, our knowledge of the molecular basis and human genetics in health and disease has made giant steps forward, bringing closer the "double helix" to the bedside of patients where every other conventional treatment may be failing. Advances in molecular biology, particularly in recombinant DNA technology, have paved the way to unlimited possibilities in predicting, controlling, and preventing disease at its molecular origin.

The prostate is a prime target in the development of successful gene therapy for the following reasons: (*i*) prostate cancer is slow growing; (*ii*) tumor burden can be significantly reduced by surgery; and (*iii*) the prostate expresses unique antigens, including PSA and PSMA.

The most significant limitation of gene therapy is the difficulty in gene delivery to the relevant cells.

Gene transfer can be achieved in vitro or in vivo. In vitro methods can be chemical through calcium-phosphate transfection, physical through electroporation or microinjection, by fusion with liposomes, through receptor-mediated endocytosis, or using recombinant viruses. In vivo methods include direct injection of DNA either naked, contained in liposomes, conjugated to a carrier (e.g., antibodies to a specific cell surface protein), or by particle bombardment (64).

Gene-directed enzyme prodrug therapy (GDEPT) is based on the potential use of prodrugs that are essentially inert, but can be converted in vivo to highly toxic, active species with the aim of specifically destroying tumor cells. Activation can be the result of metabolism by an enzyme that is either unique to the target organ, or present at much higher concentrations compared to other tissues. Tumor destruction involves two essential steps: (*i*) specific targeting of malignant cells with the gene encoding enzyme, which can also be under the control of a specific promoter (e.g., PSA or PSMA in the prostate), and (*ii*) administration of the prodrug, which will be activated into its toxic derivative by the appropriate enzyme *within* the target tissue concerned, with little or no systemic consequences (65,66).

Tumor vaccines represent a different potential treatment modality. There are three basic approaches to construct cancer vaccines: (*i*) whole tumor cells or nonpurified cellular extracts preparations, in an attempt to include relevant tumor antigens that can stimulate protective immune responses; (*ii*) partially purified preparations, enriched in the cellular fraction most likely to contain relevant tumor antigens; and (*iii*) preparations from highly purified tumor antigens. The development of these "vaccines" depends on expression of a family of genes reported to encode antigens recognized by autologous cytotoxic T lymphocytes. Such genes have now been identified in melanoma cells (*MAGE-1*, *MAGE-3*, *BAGE*, *GAGE*) as well as in head and neck tumors, non–small cell lung cancers, and bladder carcinomas. Work from Chen et al. (67) demonstrated the presence of two genes (*PAGE* and *GAGE-7*) expressed in the LNCaP cell line that may be specific to prostate cancer and serve as a potential target for tumor immunization.

Every technique mentioned above has specific advantages and disadvantages, the details of which are beyond the scope of this chapter. Experimental studies of gene therapy in prostate cancer are emerging in the literature at an increasing frequency.

ANDROGEN REGULATION

Androgens are important male sex hormones that, in addition to being essential for the growth and differentiation of all male sex accessory organs, are strongly associated with the development and progression of prostate cancer. Androgen action in prostate cancer is mediated through the androgen receptor (AR), a ligand-dependent transcription factor that is a member of the steroid/thyroid hormone receptor gene superfamily. The mitogenic effects of androgens on prostatic growth appear to be mediated through the action of soluble peptide growth factors, acting in either an autocrine or paracrine manner. Various model systems for prostate cancer have shown fibroblast growth factor 7 (FGF-7) and transforming growth factor-β1 (TGF-β1) to be paracrine mediators of androgen action and FGF-2 to be an androgen-mediated autocrine growth factor.

Androgen depletion prolongs the disease-free interval for prostate cancer patients, indicating that the cancer cells are androgen sensitive for growth. However, this treatment is only palliative because androgen-insensitive clones of cancer cells expand and progress. This observation has been made in almost every case of prostate cancer. These androgen-insensitive (or castrate-resistant) cells acquire the ability to proliferate in the absence of androgen through genetic mutations. Mutations may result in changes in the function/expression of AR protein or growth factors and their receptors.

Androgen Receptor

The AR can be structurally divided into three domains: a transcriptional activation domain, a DNA-binding domain, and a ligand-binding domain (68) (Fig. 3). Cellular signaling occurs following androgen binding to the AR and translocation of the receptor to the nucleus. This activated complex associates with androgen responsive elements contained in the DNA sequence of a number of target genes to affect their transcriptional activity. The possible presence in vivo of alternate AR isoforms, the extent of AR phosphorylation, the

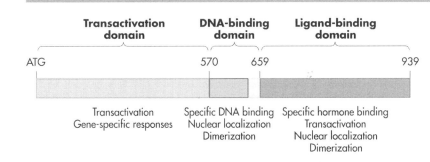

Figure 3 Functional organization of the androgen receptor.

association with other proteins, and the presence of polymorphic glutamine and glycine regions may provide additional levels of control for AR action.

Radioligand-binding studies and immunohistochemistry have been used to detect AR protein expression. Both primary and metastatic prostate cancer show elevated AR by ligand-binding assays when compared to nonmalignant prostate tissue (69). Immunohistochemistry supports elevated AR in prostate cancer with strong nuclear staining, mostly of a heterogeneous nature in hormone-relapsed and in primary and metastatic hormone-refractory prostate cancer (70).

A number of studies have suggested that a high frequency of amino acid substitutions occur in the AR protein (25–50%) for advanced prostate cancer and in hormone-relapsed tumors from primary and metastatic sites. Functional analysis of these mutations has revealed alterations in ligand binding and transcriptional activation. Additionally, AR gene amplification has been identified in 30% of recurrent prostate tumors (71). Examination of the corresponding primary tumor prior to initiation of hormone therapy showed no evidence of amplification, suggesting that amplification occurred during androgen deprivation, conferring a growth advantage on the prostate cancer cells. Variation in the length of a polyglutamine stretch in the N-terminal domain of the AR protein, causing an alteration in AR function, has been suggested as a contributory factor toward an increased lifetime risk for the development of prostate cancer.

RECURRENT GENE REARRANGEMENTS IN PROSTATE CANCER

In late 2006, Arul Chinnaiyan's research group identified the first recurrent gene fusions in the majority of prostate cancers (72). The major fusion identified comprised a fusion of the 5′ promoter region of the TMPRSS2 gene (a prostate-specific, androgen-responsive gene) to an Ets family (oncogenic transcription factor) gene. The resulting fusions result in the overexpression of an oncogenic Ets family transcription factor. These findings have been confirmed by several research groups, and additional, less common gene rearrangements have further been identified (73). These recurrent fusions appear to correlate with prostate cancer development and progression. Circulating prostate cancer cells from serum have been identified using FISH to detect these fusion genes, opening up many opportunities to exploit these gene rearrangements as powerful biomarkers to study prostate cancer response to therapy.

MOLECULAR PROFILING IN PROSTATE CANCER

Extensive investigations have been conducted to profile the genes that are aberrantly expressed in prostate cancer to help elucidate those oncogenes and tumor suppressor genes that contribute toward development and progression of the disease. The complexity and heterogeneous nature of prostate tumors have further complicated data analysis. However, mRNA molecular profiling of the full human genome using microdissected tumor material has identified small groups of genes, so-called gene signatures, that correlate with the Gleason grading system, providing several potential targets for therapeutic intervention. Increased expression of the AR is consistently associated with progression to hormone refractory prostate cancer, highlighting the important, central role of the AR in the hormone refractory phenotype (74,75).

Micro-RNAs are a group of small, noncoding, single-stranded RNAs of approximately 22 nucleotides that repress protein production by targeting specific mRNAs. Recent research has highlighted the widespread altered expression of these micro-RNAs in cancer. Several hundreds of different micro-RNAs have been identified; each micro-RNA can repress the expression of multiple proteins. In common with many cancers, many micro-RNAs have been demonstrated to be overexpressed in prostate cancer (76,77). Two micro-RNAs, miR-15a and miR-16-1, are shown to act as tumor suppressor genes in prostate cancer by controlling proliferation, invasion, and cell survival (78). Interestingly, a number of micro-RNAs have been shown to be androgen regulated, again highlighting the important role of the AR signaling pathway in prostate cancer (79).

APOPTOSIS-REGULATING GENES IN PROSTATE CANCER

Apoptosis

Hormone ablation in prostate cancer achieves its effect by activation of apoptosis (programmed cell death) (80,81), which is a distinct mode of cell death that occurs in both normal physiological conditions and the diseased state, and is frequently dysregulated in disease, including cancer (82). Apoptosis is an active process mediated by a family of cysteine proteases (caspases) and is characterized by distinct morphological changes in individual cells, with compaction and margination of nuclear chromatin, cytoplasmic condensation, and convolution of nuclear and cell outlines (83). Later changes involve nuclear fragmentation and budding of the cell with the development of membrane-bound apoptotic bodies, which are removed by phagocytosis. In contrast to necrosis, which is a passive process, there is no associated inflammation.

A number of genes are involved in the control of apoptosis including the proto-oncogene Bcl-2 on chromosome 18q21 (84,85) and the tumor suppressor gene p53 on chromosome 17p13 (86).

Bcl-2

The Bcl-2 gene was initially identified in B cell lymphomas (87), and the gene product was shown to act by inhibiting cell death without directly affecting cell proliferation. The Bcl-2 protein family has at least 20 members, comprising two functionally antagonistic groups controlling the balance between cell death and survival. Bax and Bak are proapoptotic Bcl-2 family members that induce mitochondrial outer membrane permeabilization, promoting release of caspase-activating proteins and other cell death mediators. The antiapoptotic proteins, including Bcl-2, oppose this action and preserve the integrity of the outer membrane (88,89).

In the prostate Bcl-2 is normally expressed in basal epithelial cells, seminal vesicles, and ejaculatory ducts. In primary prostate cancer Bcl-2 is expressed in around 25% of cases (90). Bcl-2 overexpression is associated with increasing tumor stage and the development of hormone refractory disease (91,92). In high-grade prostatic intraepithelial neoplasia (HGPIN) the reported expression of Bcl-2 has shown a wide variation from 0% to 100%. The largest study reported Bcl-2 expression in 4/24 (17%) cases of HGPIN (90,93,94).

p53

Inactivation of the tumor suppressor gene p53 is the most common mutation identified in human cancers (95). Functional (wild-type) p53 protein has DNA-binding properties and forms a key part of the mechanism by which mammalian cells undergo growth arrest or apoptosis in response to DNA damage. Mutation of p53 may result in loss of its normal function. Mutations in the p53 gene are most frequently detected in the highly conserved exons 5, 6, 7, and 8. In most cases one allele is completely deleted with a missense mutation in the remaining allele. Mutant p53 protein has a prolonged half-life compared to the wild-type p53 protein, and its nuclear accumulation is detectable by immunohistochemistry.

In benign prostatic epithelium p53 positivity is absent. In primary prostate cancer p53 nuclear positivity is present in around 20% of cases (96,97). p53 protein accumulation appears to be a late event, being associated with advanced stage, high Gleason tumor grade, hormonal resistance, poor survival, DNA aneuploidy, and high cell proliferation rate (98–101). A good correlation is observed between p53 immunoreactivity in prostate cancer and direct evidence of gene mutation using the polymerase chain reaction, single-strand conformational polymorphism and direct sequencing (102). p53 positivity is infrequent in HGPIN, the largest study showing strong nuclear staining to be 14% (103).

Wild-type p53 may participate with Bcl-2 and Bax in a common pathway, regulating cell death by decreasing the expression of Bcl-2 while simultaneously increasing the expression of Bax, resulting in apoptosis (104). The combination of Bcl-2 overexpression and nuclear accumulation of p53 protein in human prostate cancer has been shown to correlate with the development of hormone refractory disease (96), and are independent prognostic markers for postradical prostatectomy recurrence (92,105).

ANGIOGENESIS

Microvessel Density

The ability of a tumor to grow and metastasize depends on the induction of a tumor vasculature, referred to as the "angiogenic switch." The quantification of new microvessels within a tumor is commonly performed using antibodies against factor VIII to identify endothelial cells. Increasing microvessel density correlates with increasing Gleason score, presence of metastases, and is an independent predictor of progression after radical prostatectomy for Gleason score 5 to 7 tumor (106,107).

Vascular Endothelial Growth Factor

Angiogenesis is controlled by a group of substances termed angiogenic factors. Vascular endothelial growth factor (VEGF) is a potent inducer of endothelial cell growth and is expressed in a variety of tumors. VEGF expression is increased in prostate cancer compared to benign prostatic epithelium (108). Targeting the tumor vasculature with angiogenic inhibitors presents an attractive therapy to limit growth of the primary cancer and prevent cancer recurrence or metastases (109).

GROWTH FACTORS

Growth factors may act as positive or negative effectors of various cellular processes, including proliferation, differentiation, and cell death. Interaction occurs with specific membrane receptors, which results in the transmission of signals through an intracellular protein cascade and the activation or the repression of a number of target genes. Several growth factors have been associated with prostatic growth, including TGF-α and TGF-β, FGFs, insulin-like growth factors (IGFs), epidermal growth factor (EGF), nerve growth factor, and various cytokines.

Growth factors act primarily over short distances in either an autocrine or paracrine manner. In addition, growth factors may act through an endocrine pathway affecting target cells at distant sites. Many growth factors possess a mitogenic activity that is mediated through a membrane-bound receptor. Interaction occurs with an extracellular ligand-binding domain leading to a change in receptor conformation, resulting in the activation of an intracellular tyrosine kinase domain. Tyrosine phosphorylation of specific intracellular proteins is responsible for the mitogenic signal. In many cases the protein components of the intracellular cascade remain to be elucidated (110). Aberrant signaling may result from mutation in growth factors or their downstream effector proteins, leading to either loss of growth factor function, that is, switching off the signaling pathway, or uncontrolled expression or activation, that is, permanently switched on signaling pathway. Such changes are commonly associated with the malignant state and the aggressive phenotypes of cancer cells. Given the important role of growth factor receptor signaling in cell proliferation and their frequent alterations in cancer, the receptors provide attractive targets for therapeutic intervention using small molecule inhibitors and antibodies (111).

Transforming Growth Factor-β1

TGF-β1 belongs to a superfamily of structurally related regulatory polypeptides that includes activins/inhibins and bone morphogenetic proteins (BMPs). TGF-β1 is a pleiotropic growth factor that acts through type I and II receptor kinases to regulate multiple cellular mechanisms including proliferation, angiogenesis, immune response, and cell differentiation. Generally, TGF-β1 functions as a mitogen for various mesenchymal cells and a potent growth inhibitor of lymphoid, endothelial, and epithelial cells. TGFβ-1 and -2 have been implicated in the development of prostatic disease (112). TGF-β1 has been detected using immunohistochemistry in both human prostatic stromal and epithelial cells, and TGF-β2 mRNA has been identified in normal and malignant human prostate. Addition of TGF-β1 to cultured prostatic epithelial and stromal cells inhibits proliferation (113).

Bone Morphogenetic Proteins

The term BMP refers to an activity derived from bone that induces ectopic bone formation in vivo (114). The BMPs belong to the TGF-β superfamily that have the capability of inducing ectopic and de novo bone formation in vivo, as well as having roles in chondrogenesis, differentiation, and development. To date, few efforts were made to link BMP activity with the development and progression of cancer. This is not surprising because the majority of bony secondaries result in osteolytic lesions, with increased bone resorption and osteoclastic activity, unlike prostatic secondaries that are mostly osteoblastic. A number of studies have shown an association between BMP expression and skeletal metastases in prostate cancer. BMP-6, in particular, is expressed in the majority of primary prostate cancers with established skeletal secondaries, and rarely in localized disease. Overexpression of BMP-6 is associated with a more invasive phenotype (115). Primary and secondary prostate cancer expresses BMP-6, which is found infrequently in skeletal metastases from other human malignancies. BMP-6 may have a role in the initiation of skeletal secondaries, and the osteoblastic reaction commonly seen in these deposits (116).

Fibroblast Growth Factors

The FGF family of polypeptide growth factors has diverse physiologic and pathologic functions including development, wound healing, angiogenesis, and tumorigenesis (117). The human FGFs comprise at least 23 highly conserved genes and the receptor family comprises four members, FGFR-1 to -4. Multiple ligands and receptors allow interaction between a single receptor and several ligands, and between different receptor monomers through heterodimerization following activation by FGF (118) to modulate a range of biologic effects including mitogenesis, motility, invasion, and differentiation. Multiple FGFs are expressed at elevated levels in prostate cancer, including FGF-1, -2, -6, and -8 (119) acting as both paracrine and autocrine growth factors.

Basic FGF (FGF-2) is secreted by prostatic fibroblasts in response to androgen and acts in an autocrine fashion to stimulate fibroblast cell growth (120). Stromal-derived keratinocyte growth factor (KGF/ FGF-7) is upregulated in hormone-resistant prostate cancer and has a role as a potential paracrine growth factor on epithelial cells (121). KGF has a potent mitogenic action on epithelial cells and is proposed to act as an androgen-regulated mediator of epithelial cell growth (122). A similar paracrine action applies to FGF-8 (androgen-induced growth factor), which is secreted in response to androgens and can stimulate growth of epithelial and fibroblast cells. FGFR-1 to -3 can undergo alternative splicing to generate two alternative exons (IIIb and IIIc) that generate receptor isoforms with variant binding specificity. Differential expression of the four FGFRs and a switch in the expression of alternate spliced variants of FGFR2 are documented (123). Given the importance of FGF signaling in mediating epithelial-stromal interactions during prostate carcinogenesis (124) and the aberrant expression of many components of the FGF-FGFR system in prostate cancer, this highlights the great potential for therapeutic intervention in this pathway (125).

Insulin-Like Growth Factors

IGF-1 and -2 are potent mitogens that mediate normal and neoplastic cell growth. The IGFs bind to specific receptors, designated type I and II IGF receptors (IGFR). Type I IGFR is a transmembrane heterotetramer tyrosine kinase that primarily mediates the mitogenic actions of IGFs. IGFs are two of the most abundant growth factors in bone (126), the preferential site for metastatic prostate cancer. Type I IGFR is expressed by prostate cancer cells that could facilitate the development of bone metastases, and several population studies suggest that elevated serum IGF-1 levels increase the risk of prostate cancer (127).

IGFs also have high affinity for a family of at least six IGF-binding proteins (IGFBPs) that act to regulate their bioavailability (128). The levels of circulating IGFBPs are regulated by endocrine factors and by specific proteases that cleave IGFBPs to small inactive peptides. IGFBPs are believed to modulate proliferative and mitogenic effects of IGFs as well as modulating cell growth independently of IGF. Although all IGFBPs have high affinity for IGFs, IGFBP-3 is the major transporter of IGFs in serum. A number of studies have suggested that IGFBPs may be involved in growth modulation of prostate malignancy. One study showed that IGFBP-2 was an androgen-dependent predictor for prostate cancer survival (129).

Epidermal Growth Factor

Binding of EGF to the extracellular domain of its receptor, EGFR, results in activation of the receptor's cytoplasmic tyrosine kinase, phosphorylation of substrate proteins, and stimulation of cell proliferation. Members of the EGF family play a role in modulation of prostatic growth. Withdrawal of androgen from the rodent prostate leads to reduced expression of EGF, which is a potent mitogen for epithelial cells (130). Thus, the continued presence of androgens within the prostate helps maintain epithelial cell proliferation mediated through the expression of EGF. Increased EGF receptor signaling has been demonstrated in prostate cancer and progression (131), and more recently missense mutations of the EGF receptor tyrosine kinase domain have been identified that have oncogenic properties (132).

CELL ADHESION

Cell adhesion is of fundamental importance in establishing and maintaining tissue form and function. Several adhesion molecules, including cadherins, integrins, selectins, and members of the immunoglobulin superfamily, are involved in the mechanisms by which a cell maintains contact with other cells and interacts with the extracellular matrix (133,134). Fibronectin, collagen, laminin, and vitronectin are major components of this complex extracellular matrix that interact with their cognate receptors, most of which are integrins. Integrins function as heterodimeric membrane glycoproteins, the combination of α and β subunits determining the ligand specificity. Differential expression of members of the large integrin family allows the cell to modulate its interaction with other cells and the extracellular matrix. Integrins are important components of cellular signal transduction, mediating cell-matrix interactions, while cadherins principally mediate intercellular interactions.

Cadherins are a large family of calcium-dependent morphoregulatory proteins. The best studied proteins within this family are E- and N-cadherin. Membrane-associated cadherins require members of the catenin family of proteins to mediate their interaction with the cytoskeleton. Catenins probably act by oligomerizing proteins to which they bind and/or to attach them to the actin cytoskeleton.

E-cadherin

The E-cadherin gene plays a critical role in embryogenesis and organogenesis, and membrane-bound E-cadherin protein mediates epithelial cell-cell recognition and adhesion (135). E-cadherin complexes are important in maintaining the normal differentiated phenotype of epithelial cells. Downregulation of E-cadherin is observed in many cancers, and for prostate cancer dysregulation of E-cadherin is associated with an invasive phenotype (136). The intracellular domain of E-cadherin is anchored to the actin cytoskeleton via three cytoplasmic proteins, α-, β- and γ-catenin, and the integrity of the cadherin-catenin complex is regulated by phosphorylation. Protein kinase D1 (PKD1) phosphorylates E-cadherin and stabilizes cadherin-catenin complexes (137). Downregulation of PKD1 is observed in prostate cancer (138), and its effects on E-cadherin likely contribute toward metastatic progression.

Aberrant E-cadherin staining is a powerful predictor of poor outcome, both in terms of disease progression and patient survival (136).

CD44

The CD44 gene is an integral transmembrane glycoprotein involved in specific cell-cell and cell-extracellular matrix interactions (139). The gene is encoded by 20 exons, at least 10 of which are differentially expressed because of alternative splicing of mRNA (140). CD44 is expressed on the plasma membrane of prostatic glandular cells. It is involved in cell adhesion because it acts as a receptor for the extracellular matrix components hyaluronic acid and osteopontin. CD44 is believed to play a major role in tumor metastases; alternative splice variants of the receptor differ in their capacity to enhance or decrease metastatic potential. In human prostate cancer CD44 downregulation is correlated with high tumor grade, aneuploidy, and distant metastases (141).

PROLIFERATION

The hallmark of malignancy is uncontrolled growth. It is therefore logical to assume that measuring proliferative capacity within a tumor may indicate its invasive potential and ability to progress. Several methods are available to assess proliferation, including determination of S-phase fraction by flow cytometry, labeling of replicating DNA with bromodeoxyuridine (BrdU), and application of immunohistochemistry using antibodies against proliferation-related antigens (Ki67 and MIB-1) (142,143). Their use in clinical practice, however, remains to be determined.

TUMOR PLOIDY AND NUCLEAR MORPHOMETRY

Nuclear DNA content, otherwise known as ploidy, can be studied by flow cytometry and image or static cytometry. Tumors can be broadly classified as diploid, tetraploid, or aneuploid, with accompanying variations in view of the well-documented heterogeneity of prostatic adenocarcinoma. Several reports have correlated DNA ploidy with prognosis in prostate cancer. The results are conflicting, and only half the studies published confirm ploidy to be an independent prognostic marker (144). A more modern and sensitive method of assessing ploidy has been developed, using fluorescent (FISH) and nonfluorescent DNA in situ hybridization of interphase cells. These techniques visualize individual chromosomes by specific binding of a labeled probe to a particular DNA sequence, mostly localized at the centromere region. There is good correlation with flow cytometry, but FISH appears to be more sensitive (145). FISH analysis is beginning to impact on clinical practice, for example, in assessing the HER2 gene copy number in breast cancer stratification of patients.

GENETIC FACTORS

Genetic alterations are important contributory events in neoplasia. A variety of genes have been identified that are associated with predisposition or progression for most of the common epithelial neoplasms. Most known oncogenes and suppressor genes have been screened for their importance in primary prostate cancer, but no common mutations have been identified. p53 mutations are rare in early prostate cancer but have been observed in almost 50% of advanced, metastatic disease (100). Mutations in the retinoblastoma (Rb) gene and deletion or methylation of p16^{INK4a} (CDKN2), two genes intimately linked to cell cycle progression, have been described in a few prostate tumors and cell lines.

Allelic loss, defined by the absence of one of the two copies of an autosomal locus present in somatic cells, commonly occurs in prostate cancer. Loss of heterozygosity and comparative genomic hybridization analyses have revealed frequent loss of genetic material from chromosome regions 7q, 8p, 10pq, 13q, 16q, 17p, and 18q in primary and metastatic prostate cancer. Specific gene loci have also been identified as metastatic suppressors in prostate cancer. Introduction of the genes for KAI1 (chromosome 11p11.2), E-cadherin (chromosome 16q22), or CD44 (chromosome 11p13) into prostate cancer cells have been shown to suppress metastatic ability.

Hereditary prostate cancer has been reported to account for some 9% of all prostate cancer and more than 40% of early onset disease (146). A number of studies revealed a familial clustering for prostate cancer, supporting a genetic predisposition to the disease. A risk factor of between 2 and 3 has been indicated in first-degree relatives of affected men. This is further increased when they are diagnosed at an earlier age (147).

More recent work using genome-wide association analysis of thousands of men investigating the frequency of small nucleotide polymorphisms have identified multiple genetic loci (located on chromosomes 2, 3, 6, 7, 10, 11, 17, 19, and X) that are associated with susceptibility to developing prostate cancer (148–150).

MATRIX METALLOPROTEINASES AND THEIR INHIBITORS

Tumor invasion and metastasis represent key events in the natural history of cancer. To complete the different steps involved in the metastatic cascade of events, a malignant cell has to overcome a number of natural barriers, including extracellular matrix and basement membranes. This can be partly achieved through excess production of proteolytic enzymes either by the tumor cells themselves, or through stimulation of surrounding stromal cells to secrete such enzymes (151). The matrix metalloproteinases (MMPs) are a large family (23 in humans) of extracellular zinc enzymes that mediate a number of tissue-remodeling processes, and have been strongly associated with cancer invasion and metastasis because of their capacity to degrade the extracellular matrix. A number of malignancies including prostate cancer have been shown to differentially express MMPs that correlated strongly with aggressive disease (152–154). MMPs are tightly regulated by their inhibitors called tissue inhibitors of metalloproteinases that bind in a 1:1 stoichiometry to inactivate the MMPs. Past clinical evaluation of small molecule inhibitors of the MMPs has been unrewarding, partly a consequence of treating patients with advanced, metastatic disease. However, several novel inhibitors of MMPs have been synthesized and they may still provide a useful therapeutic approach for prostate tumors that have not metastasized (155).

IN VITRO AND IN VIVO MODELS OF PROSTATE CANCER

To investigate the biology of prostate cancer, a number of models have been developed over the years. The three most widely used cell lines are LNCaP, an AR-positive epithelial prostate cancer cell line originating from a metastatic lymph node; PC-3, an AR-negative epithelial prostate cancer line originating from metastatic bone secondaries; and DU-145, an AR-negative epithelial prostate cancer line originating from metastatic brain secondaries (156–158). A wide range of murine in vivo experimental models are used to study tumor initiation, growth, and metastatic progression in prostate cancer. These models frequently employ gene "knockout," "knock-in" or conditional regulation of individual gene expression (oncogenes, growth factors, cell cycle regulators), or combinations of genes (159,160). These models are extremely useful in studying a variety of factors thought to affect the development and progression of prostate cancer (161). The recent ability to alter the expression of a specific gene in a single tissue cell type in a temporal fashion will greatly facilitate our studies to accurately model sporadic tumor formation for this disease in a whole animal (162).

REFERENCES

1. Jemal A, Siegel R, Ward E, et al. Cancer statistics 2008. CA Cancer J Clin 2008; 58:71–96.
2. Cancer Research UK statistics. Available at: http://info. cancerresearchuk.org/cancerstats/types/prostate/.
3. Collin SM, Martin RM, Metcalfe C, et al. Prostate-cancer mortality in the US and UK in 1975–2004: an ecological study. Lancet Oncol 2008; 9:445–452.
4. Schröder FH, Hugosson J, Roobol MJ, et al. ERSPC Investigators. Screening and prostate-cancer mortality in a randomized European study. N Engl J Med 2009; 360 (13):1320–1328.
5. Melia J, Moss S, Johns L. Rates of prostate-specific antigen testing in general practice in England and Wales in asymptomatic and symptomatic patients: a cross-sectional study. BJU Int 2004; 94:51–56.

6. Muir CS, Nectoux J, Statzsewski J. The epidemiology of prostatic cancer. Acta Oncol 1991; 30:133–140.

7. Pienta KJ, Esper PS. Risk factors for prostate cancer. Ann Intern Med 1993; 118:793–803.

8. Smith JR, Freije D, Carpten JD, et al. Major susceptibility locus for prostate cancer on chromosome 1 suggested by a genome-wide search. Science 1996; 274:1371–1374.

9. Bova GS, Beaty TH, Steinberg GD, et al. Hereditary prostate cancer: epidemiologic and clinical features. J Urol 1993; 150:797–802.

10. McNeal JE, Redwine EA, Frieha FS, et al. Zonal distribution of prostatic adenocarcinoma: correlation with histologic pattern and direction of spread. Am J Surg Pathol 1988; 12:897–906.

11. Gleason DF. Histologic grading of prostate cancer: a perspective. Hum Pathol 1992; 23: 273–279.

12. Humphrey PA, Frazier HA, Vollmer RT, et al. Stratification of pathologic features in radical prostatectomy specimens that are predictive of elevated initial postoperative serum prostate-specific antigen levels. Cancer 1993; 71:1821–1827.

13. Bostwick DG. Gleason grading of prostatic needle biopsies: correlation with grade in 316 matched prostatectomies. Am J Surg Pathol 1994; 18:796–803.

14. Trock BJ, Guo CC, Gonzalgo ML, et al. Tertiary Gleason patterns and biochemical recurrence after prostatectomy: proposal for a modified Gleason scoring system. J Urol 2009; 182(4):1364–1370.

15. Epstein JI. Precursor lesions to prostatic adenocarcinoma. Virchows Arch 2009; 454(1):1–16.

16. Girasole CR, Cookson MS, Putzi MJ, et al. Significance of atypical and suspicious small acinar proliferations, and high grade prostatic intraepithelial neoplasia on prostate biopsy: implications for cancer detection and biopsy strategy. J Urol 2006; 175(3 pt 1):929–933; discussion 933.

17. Lundwall A, Clauss A, Olsson AY. Evolution of kallikrein-related peptidases in mammals and identification of a genetic locus encoding potential regulatory inhibitors. Biol Chem 2006; 387:243–249.

18. Lilja H, Ulmert D, Vickers AJ. Prostate-specific antigen and prostate cancer: prediction, detection and monitoring. Nat Rev Cancer 2008; 8(4):268–278.

19. Chybowski FM, Larson Keller JJ, Beerstralh EH, et al. Predicting radionuclide bone scan findings in patients with newly diagnosed, untreated prostate cancer: prostate specific antigen is superior to all other clinical parameters. J Urol 1991; 145:313–318.

20. Catalona WJ, Ritchie JP, Ahmann FB, et al. Comparison of digital rectal examination and serum prostate specific antigen in the early detection of prostate cancer: results of a multicentre clinical trial of 6,630 men. J Urol 1994; 151:1283–1290.

21. Christensson A, Bjork T, Nilsson O, et al. Serum prostate specific antigen complexed to alpha-1-antichymotrypsin as an indicator of prostate cancer. J Urol 1993; 150:100–105.

22. Leung H, Lai L, Day J, et al. Serum free PSA in the diagnosis of prostate cancer. Br J Urol 1997; 80:256–259.

23. Catalona WJ, Smith DS, Ornstein DK. Prostate cancer detection in men with serum PSA concentrations of 2.6 to 4.0 ng/mL and benign prostate examination: enhancement of specificity with free PSA measurements. JAMA 1997; 227:1452–1455.

24. Lilja H, Ulmert D, Bjork T, et al. Long-term prediction of prostate cancer up to 25 years before diagnosis of prostate cancer using prostate kallikreins measured at age 44 to 50 years. J Clin Oncol 2007; 25:431–436.

25. Tilling K, Garmo H, Metcalfe C, et al. Development of a new method for monitoring prostate-specific antigen changes in men with localised prostate cancer: a comparison of observational cohorts. Eur Urol 2009; 57:446–452.

26. Thompson IM, Pauler DK, Goodman PJ, et al. Prevalence of prostate cancer among men with a prostate-specific antigen level < or = 4.0 ng per milliliter. N Engl J Med 2004; 350(22):2239–2246.

27. Lane JA, Howson J, Donovan J, et al. Prostate cancer detection in an unselected young population: experience of the ProtecT study. BMJ 2007; 335:1139–1143.

28. Fidler IJ. Metastasis: quantitative analysis of distribution and fate of tumour emboli labelled with ^{125}I-5-iodo-2'-deoxyuridine. J Natl Cancer Inst 1970; 45:773–782.

29. Fidler IJ, Hart IR. Biological diversity in metastatic neoplasms: origins and implications. Science 1982; 217:998–1003.

30. Hamdy FC, Lawry J, Anderson JB, et al. Circulating prostate-specific antigen-positive cells correlate with metastatic prostate cancer. Br J Urol 1992; 69:392–396.

31. Fadlon EJ, Rees RC, Lawry J, et al. Detection of circulating PSA-positive cells in patients with prostate cancer by flow cytometry and reverse transcription polymerase chain reaction. Br J Cancer 1996; 74:400–405.

32. Katz AE, Olsson CA, Raffo AJ, et al. Molecular staging of prostate cancer with the use of an enhanced reverse transcriptase-PCR assay. Urology 1994; 43:765–774.

33. Israeli RS, Miller WH, Su SL, et al. Sensitive nested reverse transcription polymerase chain reaction detection of circulating prostatic tumor cells: comparison of prostate-specific membrane antigen and prostate-specific antigen-based assays. Cancer Res 1994; 54:6306–6310.

34. Smith MR, Biggar S, Hussain M. Prostate specific antigen messenger RNA is expressed in non-prostate cells: implications for the detection of micrometastases. Cancer Res 1995; 55:2640–2644.

35. Tibbe AG, de Grooth BG, Greve J, et al. Optical tracking and detection of immunomagnetically selected and aligned cells. Nat Biotechnol 1999; 17:1210–1213.

36. Scher HI, Jia X, de Bono JS, et al. Circulating tumour cells as prognostic markers in progressive, castration-resistant prostate cancer: a reanalysis of IMMC38 trial data. Lancet Oncol 2009; 10(3):233–239.

37. Neal DE, Donovan JL, Martin RM, et al. Screening for prostate cancer remains controversial. Lancet 2009; 374 (9700):1482–1483.

38. D'Amico AV, Whittington R, Malkowicz SB, et al. Biochemical outcome after radical prostatectomy, external beam radiation therapy, or interstitial radiation therapy for clinically localized prostate cancer. JAMA 1998; 280:9.

39. Albertsen PC, Hanley JA, Fine J. 20-year outcomes following conservative management of clinically localized prostate cancer. JAMA 2005; 293(17):2095–2101.

40. Holmberg L, Bill-Axelson A, Helgesen F, et al. Scandinavian Prostatic Cancer Group Study Number 4. A randomized trial comparing radical prostatectomy with watchful waiting in early prostate cancer. N Engl J Med 2002; 347 (11):781–789.

41. Bill-Axelson A, Holmberg L, Filén F, et al. Scandinavian Prostate Cancer Group Study Number 4. Radical prostatectomy versus watchful waiting in localized prostate cancer: the Scandinavian Prostate Cancer Group-4 randomized trial. J Natl Cancer Inst 2008; 100(16):1144–1154.

42. Bill-Axelson A, Holmberg L, Ruutu M, et al. Scandinavian Prostate Cancer Group Study No. 4. Radical prostatectomy versus watchful waiting in early prostate cancer. N Engl J Med 2005; 352(19):1977–1984.

43. Wilt TJ, Brawer MK, Barry MJ, et al. The Prostate cancer Intervention Versus Observation Trial: VA/NCI/AHRQ Cooperative Studies Program #407 (PIVOT): design and baseline results of a randomized controlled trial

comparing radical prostatectomy to watchful waiting for men with clinically localized prostate cancer. Contemp Clin Trials 2009; 30(1):81–87.

44. Donovan J, Mills N, Smith M, et al. Improving the design and conduct of randomised trials by embedding them in qualitative research: the ProtecT study. Br Med J 2002; 325 (7367):766–770.

45. Bolla M, de Reijke TM, Van Tienhoven G, et al. EORTC Radiation Oncology Group and Genito-Urinary Tract Cancer Group. Duration of androgen suppression in the treatment of prostate cancer. N Engl J Med 2009; 360(24): 2572–2574.

46. Adib RS, Anderson JB, Ashken MH, et al. Immediate versus deferred treatment for advanced prostatic cancer: initial results of the Medical Research Council trial. Br J Urol 1997; 79:235–246.

47. Abbas F, Scardino PT. Why neoadjuvant androgen deprivation prior to radical prostatectomy is unnecessary. Urol Clin North Am 1996; 23(4):587–604.

48. Witjes WP, Schulman CC, Debruyne FM. Preliminary results of a prospective randomized study comparing radical prostatectomy versus radical prostatectomy associated with neoadjuvant hormonal combination therapy in T2-T3 N0 M0 prostatic carcinoma. The European study group on neoadjuvant treatment of prostate cancer. Urology 1997; 49:(3A suppl):65–69.

49. Huggins C, Hodges CV. Studies on prostate cancer. The effect of castration, of oestrogen and of androgen injection on serum phosphatase in metastatic carcinoma of the prostate. Cancer Res 1941; 1:293–297.

50. Klotz L, Boccon-Gibod L, Shore ND, et al. The efficacy and safety of degarelix: a 12-month, comparative, randomized, open-label, parallel-group phase III study in patients with prostate cancer. BJU Int 2008; 102:1531–1538.

51. Maximum androgen blockade in advanced prostate cancer: an overview of 22 randomised trials with 3283 deaths in 5710 patients. Prostate Cancer Trialists' Collaborative Group. Lancet 1995; 346:265–269.

52. Caubet JF, Tosteson TD, Dong EW, et al. Maximum androgen blockade in advanced prostate cancer: a meta-analysis of published randomized controlled trials using nonsteroidal antiandrogens. Urology 1997; 49:71–78.

53. Akaza H, Hinotsu S, Usami M, et al. Study Group for the Combined Androgen Blockade Therapy of Prostate Cancer. Combined androgen blockade with bicalutamide for advanced prostate cancer: long-term follow-up of a phase 3, double-blind, randomized study for survival. Cancer 2009; 115(15):3437–3445.

54. Petrylak DP, Tangen CM, Hussain MH, et al. Docetaxel and estramustine compared with mitoxantrone and prednisone for advanced refractory prostate cancer. N Engl J Med 2004; 351(15):1513–1520.

55. Tannock IF, de Wit R, Berry WR, et al. TAX 327 Investigators. Docetaxel plus prednisone or mitoxantrone plus prednisone for advanced prostate cancer. N Engl J Med 2004; 351(15):1502–1512.

56. Attard G, Reid AH, A'Hern R, et al. Selective inhibition of CYP17 with abiraterone acetate is highly active in the treatment of castration-resistant prostate cancer. J Clin Oncol 2009; 27(23):3742–3748.

57. Shahinian VB, Kuo YF, Freeman JL, et al. Risk of fracture after androgen deprivation for prostate cancer. N Engl J Med 2005; 352(2):154–164.

58. Smith MR, Egerdie B, Hernández Toriz N, et al. Denosumab HALT Prostate Cancer Study Group. Denosumab in men receiving androgen-deprivation therapy for prostate cancer. N Engl J Med 2009; 361(8):745–755.

59. Saad F, Gleason DM, Murray R, et al. Zoledronic Acid Prostate Cancer Study Group. A randomized, placebo-controlled trial of zoledronic acid in patients with hormone-refractory metastatic prostate carcinoma. J Natl Cancer Inst 2002; 94(19):1458–1468.

60. Saad F, Gleason DM, Murray R, et al. Zoledronic Acid Prostate Cancer Study Group. Long-term efficacy of zoledronic acid for the prevention of skeletal complications in patients with metastatic hormone-refractory prostate cancer. J Natl Cancer Inst 2004; 96(11):879–882.

61. Pisters LL, Leibovici D, Blute M, et al. Locally recurrent prostate cancer after initial radiation therapy: a comparison of salvage radical prostatectomy versus cryotherapy. J Urol 2009; 182(2):517–525.

62. Finley DS, Osann K, Skarecky D, et al. Hypothermic nerve-sparing radical prostatectomy: rationale, feasibility, and effect on early continence. Urology 2009; 73(4):691–696.

63. Ahmed HU, Zacharakis E, Dudderidge T, et al. High-intensity-focused ultrasound in the treatment of primary prostate cancer: the first UK series. Br J Cancer 2009; 101 (1):19–26.

64. Culver KW. Gene Therapy. A Handbook for Physicians. New York: Liebert MA, 1994.

65. Connors TA. The choice of prodrugs for gene directed enzyme prodrug therapy of cancer. Gene Ther 1995; 2:702–709.

66. Both GW. Recent progress in gene-directed enzyme prodrug therapy: an emerging cancer treatment. Curr Opin Mol Ther 2009; 11(4):421–432.

67. Chen ME, Sikes RA, Troncoso P, et al. PAGE and GAGE-7 are novel genes expressed in the LNCaP prostatic carcinogenesis model that share homology with melanoma associated antigens. J Urol 1996; 155:642A.

68. O'Malley B. The steroid receptor superfamily: more excitement predicted for the future. Mol Endocrinol 1990; 4:363–369.

69. Brolin J, Skoog L, Elman P. Immunohistochemistry and biochemistry in detection of androgen, progesterone, and estrogen receptors in benign and malignant human prostatic tissue. Prostate 1992; 20:281–295.

70. Masai M, Sumiya H, Akimoto S, et al. Immunohistochemical study of androgen receptor in benign hyperplastic and cancerous human prostates. Prostate 1990; 17:293–300.

71. Visakapori T, Hyytinen E, Koivisto P, et al. In vivo amplification of the androgen receptor gene and progression of human prostate cancer. Nat Genet 1995; 9:401–406.

72. Tomlins SA, Mehra R, Rhodes DR, et al. TMPRSS2:ETV4 gene fusions define a third molecular subtype of prostate cancer. Cancer Res 2006; 66(7):3396–3400.

73. Kumar-Sinha C, Tomlins SA, Chinnaiyan AM. Recurrent gene fusions in prostate cancer. Nat Rev Cancer 2008; 8(7): 497–511.

74. True L, Coleman I, Hawley S, et al. A molecular correlate to the Gleason grading system for prostate adenocarcinoma. Proc Natl Acad Sci U S A 2006; 103(29):10991–10996.

75. Tamura K, Furihata M, Tsunoda T, et al. Molecular features of hormone-refractory prostate cancer cells by genome-wide gene expression profiles. Cancer Res 2007; 67(11):5117–5125.

76. Ozen M, Creighton CJ, Ozdemir M, et al. Widespread deregulation of microRNA expression in human prostate cancer. Oncogene 2008; 27(12):1788–1793.

77. Porkka KP, Pfeiffer MJ, Waltering KK, et al. MicroRNA expression profiling in prostate cancer. Cancer Res 2007; 67(13):6130–6135.

78. Bonci D, Coppola V, Musumeci M, et al. The miR-15a-miR-16-1 cluster controls prostate cancer by targeting multiple oncogenic activities. Nat Med 2008; 14(11): 1271–1277.

79. Ambs S, Prueitt RL, Yi M, et al. Genomic profiling of microRNA and messenger RNA reveals deregulated

microRNA expression in prostate cancer. Cancer Res 2008; 68(15):6162–6170.

80. Kyprianou N, English HF, Isaacs JT. Programmed cell death during regression of PC-82 human prostate cancer following androgen ablation. Cancer Res 1990; 50: 3748–3753.

81. Colombel M, Symmans F, Gil S, et al. Detection of the apoptosis-suppressing oncoprotein bc1-2 in hormone-refractory human prostate cancers. Am J Pathol 1993; 143:390–400.

82. Kerr JFR, Winterford CM, Harmon BV. Apoptosis. Its significance in cancer and cancer therapy. Cancer 1994; 27:2013–2026.

83. Riedl SJ, Shi Y. Molecular mechanisms of caspase regulation during apoptosis. Nat Rev Mol Cell Biol 2004; 5 (11):897–907.

84. Hockenbery D, Nunez G, Milliman C, et al. Bcl-2 is an inner mitochondrial membrane protein that blocks programmed cell death. Nature 1990; 348:334–336.

85. Lu QL, Abel P, Foster CS, et al. bcl-2: role in epithelial differentiation and oncogenesis. Hum Pathol 1996; 27:102–110.

86. Lane DP. p53, guardian of the genome. Nature 1992; 358:15–16.

87. Vaux DL, Cory S, Adams JM. Bcl-2 gene promotes haemopoietic cell survival and cooperates with c-myc to immortalize pre-B cells. Nature 1988; 335(6189):440–442.

88. Kroemer G. The proto-oncogene Bcl-2 and its role in regulating apoptosis. Nat Med 1997; 3:614–620.

89. Yip KW, Reed JC. Bcl-2 family proteins and cancer. Oncogene 2008; 27(50):6398–6406.

90. Bauer JJ, Sesterhenn IA, Mostofi FK, et al. Elevated levels of apoptosis regulator proteins p53 and bcl-2 are independent prognostic biomarkers in surgically treated clinically localised prostate cancer. J Urol 1996; 156:1511–1516.

91. McDonnell TJ, Troncoso P, Brisbay SM, et al. Expression of the proto-oncogene bcl-2 in the prostate and its association with emergence of androgen-independent prostate cancer. Cancer Res 1992; 52:6940–6944.

92. Apakama I, Robinson MC, Walter NM, et al. bcl-2 overexpression combined with p53 protein accumulation correlates with hormone-refractory prostate cancer. Br J Cancer 1996; 74:1258–1262.

93. Krajewski M, Krajewski S, Epstein JI, et al. Immunohistochemical analysis of bcl-2, bax, bcl-X and mcl-1 expression in prostate cancers. Am J Pathol 1996; 148:1567–1576.

94. Stattin P, Damber JE, Karlberg L, et al. Bcl-2 immunoreactivity in prostate tumourigenesis in relation to prostatic intraepithelial neoplasia, grade, hormonal status, metastatic growth and survival. Urol Res 1996; 24:257–264.

95. Vogelstein B, Kinzler KW. p53 function and dysfunction. Cell 1992; 70:523–526.

96. Mellon K, Thompson S, Charlton RG, et al. p53, c-erbB-2 and the epidermal growth factor receptor in the benign and malignant prostate. J Urol 1992; 147:496–499.

97. Thomas DJ, Robinson M, King P, et al. p53 expression and clinical outcome in prostate cancer. Br J Urol 1993; 72:778–781.

98. Visakorpi T, Kallioniemi OP, Heikkinen A, et al. Small subgroup of aggressive, highly proliferative prostatic carcinomas defined by p53 accumulation. J Natl Cancer Inst 1992; 84:883–887.

99. Kallakury BV, Figge J, Ross JS, et al. Association of p53 immunoreactivity with high Gleason tumor grade in prostatic adenocarcinoma. Hum Pathol 1994; 25:92–97.

100. Heidenberg HB, Sesterhenn JP, Gaddipati JP, et al. Alteration of the tumour suppressor gene p53 in a high fraction of hormone refractory prostate cancer. J Urol 1995; 154:414–421.

101. Porkka KP, Visakorpi T. Molecular mechanisms of prostate cancer. Eur Urol 2004; 45(6):683–691.

102. Navone NM, Troncoso P, Pisters LL, et al. p53 protein accumulation and gene mutation in the progression of human prostate carcinoma. J Natl Cancer Inst 1993; 85:1657–1669.

103. Humphrey PA, Swanson PE. Immunoreactive p53 protein in high-grade prostatic intraepithelial neoplasia. Pathol Res Pract 1995; 191:881–887.

104. Miyashita T, Reed JC. Tumor suppressor p53 is a direct transcriptional activator of the human bax gene. Cell 1995; 80:293–299.

105. Moul JW, Bettencourt MC, Sesterhenn IA, et al. Protein expression of p53, bcl-2 and KI-67 (MIB-1) as prognostic biomarkers in patients with surgically treated, clinically localized prostate cancer. Surgery 1996; 120:159–166.

106. Weidner N, Carroll PR, Flax J, et al. Tumour angiogenesis correlates with metastasis in invasive prostate carcinoma. Am J Pathol 1993; 143:401–409.

107. Silberman MA, Partin AW, Veltri RW, et al. Tumour angiogenesis correlates with progression after radical prostatectomy but not with pathologic stage in Gleason sum 5 to 7 adenocarcinoma of the prostate. Cancer 1997; 79:772–779.

108. Ferrer FA, Miller LJ, Andrawis RI, et al. Vascular endothelial growth factor (VEGF) expression in human prostate cancer: in situ and in vitro expression of VEGF by human prostate cancer cells. J Urol 1997; 157:2329–2333.

109. Faivre S, Demetri G, Sargent W, et al. Molecular basis for sunitinib efficacy and future clinical development. Nat Rev Drug Discov 2007; 6(9):734–745.

110. Yarden Y, Sliwkowski MX. Untangling the ErbB signalling network. Nat Rev Mol Cell Biol 2001; 2(2):127–137.

111. Sachdev D, Yee D. Disrupting insulin-like growth factor signaling as a potential cancer therapy. Mol Cancer Ther 2007; 6(1):1–12.

112. Shariat SF, Shalev M, Menesses-Diaz A, et al. Preoperative plasma levels of transforming growth factor beta(1) (TGFbeta(1)) strongly predict progression in patients undergoing radical prostatectomy. J Clin Oncol 2001; 19:2856–2864.

113. Byrne RL, Leung H, Neal DE. Peptide growth factors in the prostate as mediators of stromal epithelial interaction. Br J Urol 1996; 77(5):627–633.

114. Urist MR. Bone formation by autoinduction. Science 1965; 150:893–899.

115. Darby S, Cross SS, Brown NJ, et al. BMP-6 over-expression in prostate cancer is associated with increased Id-1 protein and a more invasive phenotype. J Pathol 2008; 214(3):394–404.

116. Hamdy FC, Autzen P, Wilson Horne CH, et al. Immunolocalization and mRNA expression of bone morphogenetic protein-6 in human benign and malignant prostate tissue. Cancer Res 1997; 57:4427–4431.

117. Basilico C, Moscatelli D. The FGF family of growth factors and oncogenes. Adv Cancer Res 1992; 59:115–165.

118. Leung HY, Hughes CM, Kloppel G, et al. Expression and functional activity of fibroblast growth factors and their receptors inhuman pancreatic cancer. Int J Oncol 1994; 4:1219–1223.

119. Kwabi-Addo B, Ozen M, Ittmann M. The role of fibroblast growth factors and their receptors in prostate cancer. Endocr Relat Cancer 2004; 11(4):709–724.

120. Story MT. Regulation of prostate growth by fibroblast growth factors. World J Urol 1995; 13:297–305.

121. Leung HY, Mehta P, Gray LB, et al. Keratinocyte growth factor expression in hormone insensitive prostate cancer. Oncogene 1997; 15:1115–1120.

122. Tanaka A, Miyamoto K, Matsuo H, et al. Human androgen-induced growth factor in prostate and breast cancer

cells: its molecular cloning and growth properties. FEBS Letters 1995; 363:226–230.

123. Sahadevan K, Darby S, Leung HY, et al. Selective over-expression of fibroblast growth factor receptors 1 and 4 in clinical prostate cancer. J Pathol 2007; 213(1):82–90.

124. Abate-Shen C, Shen MM. FGF signaling in prostate tumorigenesis—new insights into epithelial–stromal interactions. Cancer Cell 2007; 12(6):495–497.

125. Gowardhan B, Douglas DA, Mathers ME, et al. Evaluation of the fibroblast growth factor system as a potential target for therapy in human prostate cancer. Br J Cancer 2005; 92 (2):320–327.

126. Yoneda T, Sasaki A, Mundy GR Osteolytic bone metastasis in breast cancer. Breast Cancer Res Treat 1994; 32: 73–84.

127. Oliver SE, Gunnell D, Donovan J, et al. Screen-detected prostate cancer and the insulin-like growth factor axis: results of a population-based case-control study. Int J Cancer 2004; 108(6):887–892.

128. Gennigens C, Menetrier-Caux C, Droz JP. Insulin-like growth factor (IGF) family and prostate cancer. Crit Rev Oncol Hematol 2006; 58(2):124–145.

129. Inman BA, Harel F, Audet JF, et al. Insulin-like growth factor binding protein 2: an androgen-dependent predictor of prostate cancer survival. Eur Urol 2005; 47(5): 695–702.

130. Denmeade SR, Lin XS, Isaacs JT. Role of programmed (apoptotic) cell death during the progression and therapy for prostate cancer. Prostate 1996; 28:251–265.

131. Ratan HL, Gescher A, Steward WP, et al. ErbB receptors: possible therapeutic targets in prostate cancer? BJU Int 2003; 92(9):890–895.

132. Cai CQ, Peng Y, Buckley MT, et al. Epidermal growth factor receptor activation in prostate cancer by three novel missense mutations. Oncogene 2008; 27(22):3201–3210.

133. Cavallaro U, Christofori G. Cell adhesion and signalling by cadherins and Ig-CAMs in cancer. Nat Rev Cancer 2004; 4(2):118–132.

134. Guo W, Giancotti FG. Integrin signalling during tumour progression. Nat Rev Mol Cell Biol 2004; 5(10):816–826.

135. Takeichi M. Cadherin cell adhesion receptors as a morphogenetic regulator. Science 1991; 251:1451–1455.

136. Umbas R, Isaacs WB, Bringuier PB, et al. Decreased E-cadherin expression is associated with poor prognosis in patients with prostate cancer. Cancer Res 1994; 54:3929–3933.

137. Jaggi M, Rao PS, Smith DJ, et al. E-cadherin phosphorylation by protein kinase D1/protein kinase C{mu} is associated with altered cellular aggregation and motility in prostate cancer. Cancer Res 2005; 65(2):483–492.

138. Jaggi M, Rao PS, Smith DJ, et al. Protein kinase C mu is down-regulated in androgen-independent prostate cancer. Biochem Biophys Res Commun 2003; 307(2):254–260.

139. Gunthert U, Stauder R, Mayer B, et al. Are CD44 variant isoforms involved in human tumour progression? Cancer Surv 1995; 24:19–42.

140. Ponta H, Sherman L, Herrlich PA. CD44: from adhesion molecules to signalling regulators. Nat Rev Mol Cell Biol 2003; 4(1):33–45.

141. De Marzo AM, Bradshaw C, Sauvageot J, et al. CD44 and CD44v6 downregulation in clinical prostatic carcinoma: relation to Gleason grade and cytoarchitecture. Prostate 1998; 34(3):162–168.

142. Cattoretti G, Becker MHG, Key G, et al. Monoclonal antibodies against recombinant parts of Ki-67 antigen detect proliferating cells in microwave-processed formalin-fixed paraffin sections. J Pathol 1992; 168:357–363.

143. Noordzij MA, van der Kwast TH, van Steenbrugge GJ, et al. Determination of Li-67 in formalin-fixed, paraffin-embedded prostatic cancer tissues. Prostate 1995; 27:154–159.

144. Adolfsson J. Prognostic value of deoxyribonucleic acid content in prostate cancer: a review of current results. Int J Cancer 1994; 58:211–216.

145. Persons DL, Takai K, Gibney DJ, et al. Comparison of fluorescence in situ hybridisation with flow cytometry and static image analysis in ploidy analysis of paraffin-embedded prostate adenocarcinoma. Hum Pathol 1994; 25:678–683.

146. Carter BS, Beaty TH, Steinberg GD, et al. Mendelian inheritance of familial prostate cancer. Proc Natl Acad Sci U S A 1992; 89:3367–3371.

147. Edwards SM, Eeles RA. Unravelling the genetics of prostate cancer. Am J Med Genet C Semin Med Genet 2004; 129C(1):65–73.

148. Eeles RA, Kote-Jarai Z, Giles GG, et al. Multiple newly identified loci associated with prostate cancer susceptibility. Nat Genet 2008; 40(3):316–321.

149. Gudmundsson J, Sulem P, Rafnar T, et al. Common sequence variants on 2p15 and Xp11.22 confer susceptibility to prostate cancer. Nat Genet 2008; 40(3):281–283.

150. Thomas G, Jacobs KB, Yeager M, et al. Multiple loci identified in a genome-wide association study of prostate cancer. Nat Genet 2008; 40(3):310–315.

151. Liotta LA. Tumor invasion and metastases—role of the extracellular matrix: Rhoads Memorial Award lecture. Cancer Res 1986; 46(1):1–7.

152. Hamdy FC, Fadlon EJ, Cottam DW, et al. Matrix metalloproteinase-9 expression in human prostatic adenocarcinoma and benign prostatic hyperplasia. Br J Cancer 1994; 69:177–182.

153. Wood M, Fudge K, Mohler JL, et al. In situ hybridization studies of metalloproteinases 2 and 9, and TIMP-1 and TIMP-2 expression in human prostate cancer. Clin Exp Metastasis 1997; 15:246–258.

154. Still K, Robson C, Neal DE, et al. The ratio of tissue matrix metalloproteinase-2 (MMP-2) to tissue inhibitor of matrix metalloproteinase (TIMP-2) is increased in high-grade prostate cancer. J Urol 1997; 157:25A.

155. Overall CM, Kleifeld O. Towards third generation matrix metalloproteinase inhibitors for cancer therapy. Br J Cancer 2006; 94(7):941–946.

156. Kaighn ME. Establishment and characterization of a human prostatic carcinoma cell line (PC-3). Invest Urol 1979; 17:16–23.

157. Stone KR, Mickey DD, Wunderli H, et al. Isolation of a human prostate carcinoma cell line (DU-145). Int J Cancer 1978; 21:274–281.

158. Horoszewicz JS, Leong SS, Kawinski E, et al. LNCaP model of tumor prostatic carcinoma. Cancer Res 1983; 43:1809–1818.

159. Ahmad I, Sansom OJ, Leung HY. Advances in mouse models of prostate cancer. Expert Rev Mol Med 2008; 10:e16.

160. Majumder PK, Grisanzio C, O'Connell F, et al. A prostatic intr neoplasia-dependent p27 Kip1 checkpoint induces senescence and inhibits cell proliferation and cancer progression. Cancer Cell 2008; 14(2):146–155.

161. Abate-Shen C, Shen MM. Mouse models of prostate carcinogenesis. Trends Genet 2002; 18(5):S1–S5.

162. Jonkers J, Berns A. Conditional mouse models of sporadic cancer. Nat Rev Cancer 2002; 2(4):251–265.

26

Testis Cancer

Danish Mazhar
Department of Medical Oncology, Addenbrooke's Hospital, Cambridge, U.K.

Michael Williams
Department of Clinical Oncology, Addenbrooke's Hospital, Cambridge, U.K.

INTRODUCTION

Testis cancer is a malignancy whose management has been transformed over the last 40 years. This chapter provides the scientific background to these clinical developments. Germ cell malignancies of the testis are categorized into seminoma and nonseminoma germ cell tumor (NSGCT). In addition there are rarer stromal cell tumors and lymphoma, which are not discussed further.

Testis cancers occur predominantly between the ages of 20 and 40 and are the commonest malignancy in men of that age group. However, exquisite sensitivity to cytotoxic chemotherapy means that this malignancy has a limited impact in terms of mortality. In the United Kingdom, there were 2005 cases diagnosed in the year 2000 but only 74 deaths recorded in 2002 (1). The five year–age standardized relative survival was 95% in 1996 to 1999 and has shown a progressive improvement since 1986 (1).

NSGCT has long been recognized as an anomalous malignancy because it manifests spontaneous remission and because disseminated metastatic disease has been found to be curable both with wide-field radiotherapy and with single-agent chemotherapy. There have been a number of reports of spontaneous remission (2). These were based on the diagnostic standards of the day (3) and histological proof of metastatic disease has rarely been obtained. It has been argued that the level of proof required should be the same as that required to initiate treatment (4).

Before the development of effective chemotherapy, radiotherapy was used to treat para-aortic nodal metastases (5,6); local control and cure rates depended on the bulk of disease treated (7). More surprisingly, selected patients with three or fewer lung metastases were successfully treated with whole lung radiotherapy and a boost to the tumor nodules. For these highly selected patients, this policy resulted in a 40% cure rate (5,8).

Nevertheless, for the majority of patients metastatic disease was a death sentence, even though it had become clear in the 1960s that the disease was chemosensitive. The first major breakthrough occurred when Samuels described combination therapy with vinblastine and bleomycin. This treatment was extremely toxic by the standards of the time with a substantial mortality but a complete remission rate of 35% (9). The next major advance was the addition of cisplatin to develop PVB chemotherapy (platinum, vinblastine, bleomycin), first described by Einhorn (10). The BEP regimen (bleomycin, etoposide, platinum) was described by Peckham (11) and was subsequently shown in a clinical trial to be less toxic and at least as efficacious as PVB, and possibly more so in adverse subgroups (12).

Patients with stage I disease and no demonstrable metastases have a high risk of relapse. In Europe they were managed with adjuvant radiotherapy (5,6,13) but in North America retroperitoneal lymph node dissection (RPLND) was the favored approach (14). The development of effective chemotherapy led to the investigation of surveillance with chemotherapy held in reserve (15). This study transformed the management of stage I patients in Europe and they are now usually offered surveillance. There have been a number of studies to define the risk of relapse in such patients (16,17) and adjuvant chemotherapy has been offered to such patients resulting in very low relapse rates (18), but exposure to significant short-term toxicity and to the long-term hazards of chemotherapy (19,20). In North America RPLND continues to be the standard therapy for clinical stage I nonseminoma, although it is accepted that the options to be discussed with the patient should include surveillance or nerve sparing RPLND (14). The short-term morbidity of RPLND has improved with modern techniques (21), and, of those found histologically to have lymph node involvement (stage II), 50% to 75% are cured by surgery alone (14).

Seminoma of the testis occurs in older men with a peak age of incidence of about 30 years. It has a lower metastatic potential than NSGCT. The predominant site of metastasis is the para-aortic region and adjuvant radiotherapy is an effective treatment, which has been refined in a series of trials (22,23). In many centers, this treatment has now been replaced by a

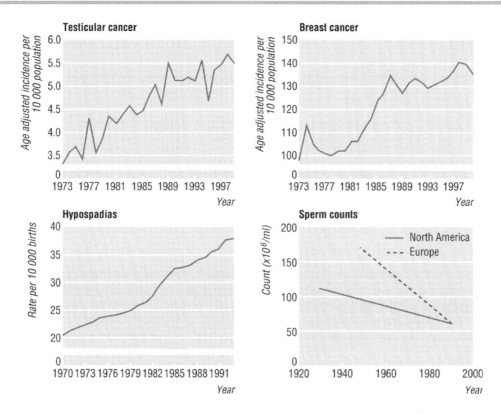

Figure 1 Trends in reproductive health in the United States. *Source*: From Ref. 34.

single dose of carboplatin (24). This does not have the well-established carcinogenic risks of wide-field radiotherapy which carries a 1.4 fold relative risk of second cancer approximating to an increase in incidence of 2% per decade of follow-up (25,26). However, although carboplatin has been in use in the management of seminoma for 15 years, there are limited data on long-term late effects (27). This has led some authors to continue to recommend radiotherapy despite its known long-term carcinogenic hazards (28). In addition, continued follow-up is required as late relapse can occur and has been reported up to four years later (29).

EPIDEMIOLOGY/RISK FACTORS

Epidemiology

The incidence of testis cancer in the United Kingdom is 6/100,000 population (1). In the United Kingdom, it has shown a gradual increase over the last 20 years and more dramatic changes have been seen in some other countries particularly Denmark and Sweden (30,31). The incidence varies between different countries and races. Black populations show a low prevalence (1/100,000) both in Africa and the United States indicating the predominance of genetic rather than environmental factors (32). Complex changes occurring in the years before the Second World War (1935–1945) have been reported in some Nordic countries but not in

other Eastern European countries. It has been speculated that this may imply etiological factors affecting the early years of life or even growth in utero (33).

Environmental Factors

Figure 1 shows changes in the incidence of breast and testicular cancer in the United States over the past 30 years. This has led to speculation that these changes are related to increasing levels of exogenous oestrogens or exposure to other synthetic man-made chemicals in environment (34).

Social Class

The effect of social class is complex: some studies have shown an association with higher social class (35), but the relationship has diminished in the West. Studies in Finland have shown a reduction from a five-fold risk for social class one in the early 1970s (compared with social classes four and five) down to a two-fold risk more recently (36). It has been hypothesized that there may be a dietary basis for this (37) or else that it may relate to the earlier age of puberty (38,39). There are also links to congenital abnormalities, infertility and low amounts of exercise (39).

Family History

A large number of studies have suggested a link to family history. A British study found that having a brother with the condition is associated with a relative risk of eight and having a father with the condition with a relative risk of four (40). This issue is discussed in detail later in this article.

Testicular Maldescent

There is a well-established association between testicular maldescent and testis cancer. The testis cancer risk applies to both testes and not only the one that was affected by maldescent. Although only 1% to 2% of cryptorchid boys go on to develop testis cancer, the relative risk is increased about fivefold. In a U.K. study the relative risk was 7.5 and did not decrease with younger age at orchidopexy. In addition, testicular biopsy was identified as a strong risk factor for the subsequent development of a tumor (41). A more recent Swedish study has shown that those who underwent orchidopexy before 13 years of age had a relative risk of 2.2 but for those operated on later the relative risk was 5.4 (42). It is now recommended that the procedure is performed on patients before the age of two years, or even as young as six months old (43–46).

Testicular Atrophy

Testicular atrophy is associated with maldescent, infertility and testis cancer. In patients who have already had one testicular cancer, the overall risk of second malignancy in the contralateral testis is 2% to 3% (47,48). However, in patients who have a remaining testis of 12 mL or less, onset of the first malignancy below the age of 31 and a history of maldescent, the risk has been shown in one study to be 34% and contralateral testicular biopsy has therefore been advocated to detect carcinoma in situ (49). Testicular microlithiasis has been shown to be associated with carcinoma in situ in subfertile men and this may provide an additional tool for the early diagnosis of this disease (50).

TUMOR MARKERS

A high proportion of patients with testicular tumors show abnormal proteins in the plasma. This does not necessarily indicate that they have metastatic disease because production may be solely from the primary tumor in the testis. These proteins are useful in the clinical management of the disease and 80% of patients with NSGCT will show abnormal levels of either AFP or hCG (13).

α-Fetoprotein

Raised levels of AFP are found in 60% of NSGCT patients (13). Physiologically, large amounts of AFP are produced by yolk sac and by the liver during gestation, but production ceases after birth. Adult levels are usually designated as 1 to 10 kU/L.

It is important to be aware that there is a subgroup of patients who have congenital elevation of AFP up to a level of about 25 (51–53). This has no significance but may cause diagnostic confusion.

In addition, liver injury can cause elevation of AFP. This can be caused by the chemotherapy used to treat the patient or by other toxins, for example, alcohol (53). Such effects can lead to inappropriate recommendations for further treatment whereas a period of observation will allow the level to fall to normal (53).

Other causes of elevated AFP levels are hepatocellular carcinoma and some gastro-intestinal tumors. In addition, AFP may be raised in patients with liver metastases from any primary tumor. With these caveats in mind, a raised AFP level can be diagnostic in a patient with metastatic malignancy from an unknown primary.

Human Chorionic Gonadotropin

hCG comprises an α and a β subunits. The α subunit is identical to that of lutenizing normal, follicular stimulation hormone and thyroid stimulating hormone. This can have importance in interpreting elevated levels in some patients depending on the assay used. The β subunit is specific to hCG and can be secreted either bound to the α subunit or as free β. This small molecule has a high clearance rate. This is important in a complete understanding of a patient's tumor markers as discordant responses between different hCG assays have been reported (54). hCG is elevated in 55% of NSCGT patients and in 20% of seminoma. Levels of greater than 500 IU/L in patients with seminoma warrant careful clinical consideration as this may indicate the presence of nonseminomatous elements (55).

Congenital elevation of hCG has not been reported but it can be produced by some tumors of non–germ cell origin, particularly bladder and pancreatic cancers and colon carcinoma. It may rarely be produced in inflammatory bowel disease.

Lactate Dehydrogenase

Elevated LDH is a nonspecific marker of cell turnover and is of prognostic significance in the staging of lymphoma (56). It is not specific for testis cancer but it has a strong association with prognosis and is a key element of the staging system devised by the International Germ Cell Cancer Collaborative Group (IGCCCG) (57) (Table 1). It is of limited value in follow-up because of limited sensitivity, specificity and a low positive predictive value for detecting relapse of testicular germ cell tumors (GCTs); false-positive increases are common (58). It does not add to the early detection of relapse in surveillance of stage 1 patients (59).

Placental Alkaline Phosphatase

PLAP staining can be useful histologically in confirming the germ cell origin of a tumor. Elevated levels of serum PLAP are seen in about half of patients with metastatic seminoma but it is not a reliable test and elevations are also seen in smokers (60). This serum marker is therefore little used clinically.

Table 1 IGCCCG Prognostic Scoring System for NSGCT Including Marker Levels

Good prognosis
Nonseminoma

- Testis/retroperitoneal primary
- No nonpulmonary visceral metastases
- Good markers—all of:

    α-Fetoprotein less than 1000 ng/mL
    Human chorionic gonadotropin less than 5000 IU/mL
        (1000 ng/mL)
    Lactate dehydrogenase less than 1.5 × the upper limit of
        normal

Seminoma

- Any primary site
- No nonpulmonary visceral metastases
- Normal AFP, any hCG, any LDH

Intermediate prognosis
Nonseminoma

- Testis/retroperitoneal primary
- No nonpulmonary visceral metastases
- Intermediate markers—any of:

    AFP 1,000 to 10,000 ng/mL
    hCG 5,000 IU/L to 50,000 IU/L
    LDH 1.5-10 × upper normal level

Seminoma

- Any primary site
- Nonpulmonary visceral metastases
- Normal AFP, any hCG, any LDH

Poor prognosis
Nonseminoma:

- Mediastinal primary
- Nonpulmonary visceral metastases
- For markers—any of:

    AFP more than 10,000 ng/mL
    hCG more than 50,000 IU/mL (10,000 ng/mL)
    LDH more than 10 × the upper limit of normal

Seminoma

- No patients are classified as poor prognosis

Prognostic Significance

Staging by anatomical site of involvement is still used clinically but its prognostic significance has become much less with the development of effective chemotherapy. IGCCCG performed a multivariate analysis on 5862 patients and used the level of AFP, hCG and LDH as key elements in categorizing patients into good, intermediate and poor risk cases (57). This has been extremely important in providing a reliable framework for clinical trials (Table 1), separating patients with five-year progression free survival of 91% (good), 79% (intermediate) and 48% (poor) (57).

Rate of Tumor Growth

It has been shown in a small study of 58 patients, in whom sequential pretreatment measurements were available, that marker production doubling time is a surrogate for tumor growth rate and carries a poor prognosis in patients with nonseminoma treated with BEP chemotherapy (61). The practical difficulties of this technique mean that it has not been taken forward.

Response to Therapy

In patients who are ultimately shown to have stage I disease with no distant metastases then after orchidectomy AFP should fall with a half-life of five to seven days (13) and hCG with a half-life of 24 to 36 hours (13). A prolonged half-life suggests the possibility of metastatic disease but it is now widely accepted that relapse should only be diagnosed when there is sustained and progressive elevation of tumor marker levels (4).

Occasional patients present with surges of marker levels following pulses of chemotherapy (62).

It is an attractive hypothesis to assume that the rate of fall of tumor markers may have prognostic significance and this has been shown in one study (63). However, other studies have found that marker half-life does not predict patients at high risk of progression after front-line therapy and that it is a poor guide to long-term prognosis (64).

Persistently elevated tumor markers after the completion of induction chemotherapy may indicate residual active disease, but the alternative causes indicated above need to be considered. In addition, it is now widely accepted that a sustained and progressive rise in tumor markers should be documented before second-line chemotherapy is offered. Patients with residual cystic masses may have elevated tumor markers, which return to normal after RPLND (65).

By contrast, patients with normal markers can have enlarging masses of growing teratoma. These should be managed surgically (66).

MOLECULAR BIOLOGY OF TESTICULAR GERM CELL TUMORS

GCTs are a heterogeneous group of neoplasms that arise mainly in the gonads and more rarely from extragonadal sites along the midline including the retroperitoneum, sacrum, mediastinum and pineal gland. This pattern of distribution is thought to reflect the route of migratory primordial germ cells to the genital ridge.

It is possible to define three diverse groups of testicular germ cell tumors (TGCTs). The first group includes teratomas and yolk sac tumors of neonates and infants. The second group includes seminomas and nonseminomatous GCTs in postpubertal patients, by far the commonest form of TGCT, and occurring usually between the ages 15 and 40 years. The final group is spermatocytic seminoma, which usually occurs in an older group.

Carcinoma in situ or intratubular germ cell neoplasia (ITGCN) is commonly found in testes containing a GCT, and is regarded as a premalignant lesion. In patients with ITGCN, the cumulative probability for development of a testicular GCT is 70% after seven years (67). Five percent of patients with testicular tumors harbor ITGCN within the contralateral testis, detectable by open biopsy in 99% of cases. For patients with testicular volume <12 mL and an age at diagnosis <30 years, the risk of ITGCT in the contralateral testis is >34% (49,68,69). Contralateral testicular biopsy should be discussed with patients at high risk of ITGCT. If it is to be performed, it should be carried out preferably at the time of orchidectomy. Biopsies to identify ITGCT must be preserved in Strieve's or Bouin's solution (70).

There is debate as to the initiating genetic events that lead to ITGCN and subsequent invasive GCT. One theory postulates the most likely target cell for transformation is the zygotene-pachytene spermatocyte where there appears to be a ''recombination checkpoint.'' At this stage, there is replicated DNA and upregulated p53, the latter to allow prolongation of the phase and recombination. If unresolved, DNA strand breaks occur and the elevated wild-type p53 can trigger apoptosis. Aberrant chromatid exchange events associated with crossing-over may lead to increased chromosome 12p copy number. Possibly through the oncogenic affect of cyclin D2, this aberrant genomically unstable cell is now able to escape the apoptotic effects of p53 and may reenter the cell cycle, now as a neoplastic cell (71).

The second and more widely accepted hypothesis, based on immunohistochemical data linking gonocytes to ITGCN, developmental abnormalities associated with GCT and epidemiological data, suggests that primordial germ cells may undergo abnormal cell division (polyploidization) because of mostly environmental factors in utero and give rise to ITGCN (40,72,73).

The three distinct categories of GCT described above, have separate genetic characteristics. Most is known about the adult seminomas and nonseminomas. The DNA content of ITGCN and seminoma is hypertriploid and that of nonseminoma is hypotriploid. The characteristic genetic abnormality of these tumors is excess genetic material of the short arm of chromosome 12, usually in the form of an isochromosome i12p (74,75). Approximately 80% of cases have i12p and the remainder have excess 12p genetic material in derivative chromosomes (76). The consistent gain of 12p genetic material is supported by gene array and comparative genomic hybridization data (77,78). The presence of i12p in ITGCN is a matter of controversy with most investigators suggesting it is not present (79,80), supporting the hypothesis that polyploidization is an initiating event followed by i12p formation in the invasive phenotype.

The consistent gain of genetic material from chromosome 12 seen in these tumors suggests that it has a crucial role in their development. Some investigators have identified an amplified region at 12p11.2-12.1. Several genes of interest are located in this region including SOX5, JAW1 and K-RAS (79). However, data suggests that this minimally deleted region applies preferentially to seminomas, suggesting that the search for putative relevant genes should not be restricted to this region. For example, Houldsworth et al. have implicated cyclin D2, which is

mapped to region 12p13, as the most likely gene to be involved (81).

A few studies have suggested the presence of relevant tumor suppressor genes but the data have not been consistent. Extensive molecular analyses have identified genomic and/or functional (expression) loss of several known tumor suppressor genes such as RB1, WT1 and p16, although no firm data are available to date linking these genes with tumor development and/or progression (79,80). Mutation of p53 is a rare event in GCT, though some have suggested this event in some chemotherapy-resistant tumors (82).

GCTs in infants and adults are genetically distinct (80,83–87). While virtually all-adult cases are aneuploid, pediatric cases are mostly diploid, particularly, teratomas, although yolk sac tumors may be nondiploid. Amplification of i12p and 12p are rare in childhood GCTs. On the other hand, such tumors are characterized by deletions of 1p, particularly region p36, loss of 6q, and structural abnormalities of chromosome 2 and 3p. Published reports suggest a significant heterogeneity in the structural chromosomal constitution of infantile teratomas. Spermatocytic seminoma may be either diploid or aneuploid, and have losses of chromosome 9 rather than i12p (80).

Given the observation that amongst the two strongest associations with testis cancer are having a brother (relative risk 8) and having a father (relative risk 4) (40,88–90) with the condition, investigators have sought to find a heritable susceptibility gene. A genetic component of TGCT is supported by demonstration of a higher risk to monozygotic twins of TGCT patients than to dizygotic twins (91) and by the observation that the frequency of bilateral disease is higher among cases with a family history than those without (88,89).

A segregation analysis using Scandinavian TGCT patients has suggested that the best model for a TGCT susceptibility locus is a major gene with a recessive mode of inheritance, an estimated gene frequency of 3.8% and a lifetime risk of developing TGCT of 43% among homozygous men (92). A recessive model was also suggested by Nicholson and Harland (93) who performed an analysis based on age at onset of TGCT and the frequency of bilateral disease. However, in both studies genetic heterogeneity and other models of inheritance could not be excluded.

In 1994, the International Testicular Cancer Linkage Consortium was established to collect a sufficiently large set of multiple case families for linkage analysis. This group includes essentially all groups in the world working in the field of TGCT susceptibility. A genomewide linkage study for TGCT susceptibility loci on 237 pedigrees with two or more cases of the disease was recently completed, which found no statistically significant regions of linkage (94). Moreover, a previous report of linkage to a region of Xq27 was not replicated (95). The results demonstrate that TGCT susceptibility cannot be caused by a single major gene. A U.K. collaborative genetics of testicular cancer study is now underway which aims at collecting samples from 3000 patients with TGCT and their parents, and performing genomewide single nucleotide polymorphism analysis.

INTRATUBULAR GERM CELL NEOPLASIA

ITGCN as a preinvasive malignancy was first suggested by Skakkebaek in 1972 (96). It is present in up to 4% of cryptorchid patients, in up to 5% of contralateral gonads in patients with unilateral GCT and in up to 1% of patients biopsied for oligospermic infertility. Its association with TGCT arising in prepubertal patients is still a source of controversy (97,98).

Microscopically, ITGCN is composed of atypical germ cells situated at the periphery of seminiferous tubules. It is rarely demonstrated immunocytochemically in tubules showing spermatogenesis, presumably reflecting pagetoid spread (i.e., along the basement membrane). The abnormal germ cells comprising ITGCN have ballooned clear cytoplasm (containing fat and glycogen) and a large hyperchromatic nucleus, which may show mitotic figures. These appearances are identical in ITGCN adjacent to seminoma and nonseminomatous GCT.

The age at which the morphological features of ITGCN can be recognized is another area of contention. Observation that ITGCN in adults displays markers and some ultrastructural features seen in fetal germ cells has been interpreted as evidence that ITGCN originates in the fetus. However, markers seen in the fetus may be displayed in adult tumors in the absence of intervening lesions. Also, in contrast to the high incidence of ITGCN seen in adult GCTs, it is a rare observation in childhood tumors (98,99), and was not identified in the orchidectomy specimens from pubertal GCT patients (97,100). In a review of biopsies from mal-descended testes, ITGCN was identified only in the testis of a 16-year-old and not from biopsies taken from children aged 9, 10, and 14 years in whom GCT subsequently developed (101).

Placental alkaline phosphatase (PLAP) and CD117 (c-kit) are used in diagnostic histopathology. Positive staining is seen in a paranuclear and cytoplasmic membrane distribution. Other antibodies, which immunoreact with ITGCN but are rarely used in practice, include M2A and 43-F (102,103). Oct 3/4 is also expressed in ITGCN (104).

Microlithiasis (microcalcification) was identified in one study in 39% of specimens showing ITGCN compared with an incidence 2% of 429 nonmalignant testicular disorders (105). In a sonographic series of 528 symptomatic patients, 48 (9%) had microlithiasis of which 13 (27%) had testicular cancer (106). Of the remaining 480 patients without microlithiasis, 38 (8%) had cancer. Thus, of those with cancer, about 25% have microlithiasis, and of those with microlithiasis, a similar proportion will have cancer.

However, the situation in healthy men is different. A prospective study of testicular sonography on 1504 healthy men aged 18 to 35 years revealed microlithiasis in 84 (5.6%). For black Americans the prevalence was 14%, and this higher proportion in a low risk population would seem to deny a close association between microlithiasis and TGCT (107).

About one-third of patients with extragonadal germ cell cancer harbor ITGCN within one or both testicles which otherwise appear normal. The cumulative risk of developing a metachronous testicular cancer 10 years after diagnosis and treatment of extragonadal GCTs is only 10%, and higher among patients with nonseminomatous histology or retroperitoneal location than among patients with pure seminomatous histology (1.4%) or primary mediastinal location (6.2%) (48). However, since all patients with extragonadal germ cell cancer will receive platinum-based chemotherapy which will eliminate a substantial percentage of ITGCN, a routinely performed bilateral testicular biopsy is not recommended. Nevertheless, if a biopsy is planned in patients with a higher risk for ITGCT following an extragonadal GCT, this should be preferably performed prior to chemotherapy. If performed thereafter, testicular biopsy should not be considered earlier than six months after the completion of chemotherapy (108–113).

HISTOLOGICAL EXAMINATION OF GERM CELL CANCER

TGCTs are a heterogeneous group of neoplasms with diverse histopathology and variable clinical course and prognosis. This diversity is reflected in various systems offered to classify these tumors. Currently the most comprehensive and widely accepted system of classification is the one proposed by the World Health Organization (114), which is summarized in Table 2. TGCTs are broadly divided into seminoma and nonseminoma for treatment planning because seminomatous types of testicular cancer are more sensitive to radiation therapy.

Table 2   World Health Organization Histological Classification of Germ Cell Testis Tumors (2004)

Intratubular germ cell neoplasia, unclassified

Tumors of 1 histological type (pure forms)

- Seminoma
- Seminoma with syncytiotrophoblastic cells
- Spermatocytic seminoma
- Spermatocytic seminoma with sarcoma
- Embryonal carcinoma
- Yolk sac tumor
- Trophoblastic tumors
- Choriocarcinoma
- Trophoblastic neoplasms other than choriocarcinoma
- Monophasic choriocarcinoma
- Placental site trophoblastic tumor
- Teratoma
- Dermoid cyst
- Monodermal teratoma
- Teratoma with somatic type malignancies

Tumors of more than 1 histological type (mixed forms)

- Mixed embryonal carcinoma and teratoma
- Mixed teratoma and seminoma
- Choriocarcinoma and teratoma/embryonal carcinoma
- Others

It is recommended to completely laminate the testicular specimen in transverse sections. Additional sections have to be taken from the spermatic cord. For a full histological examination of the tumor, it is necessary to obtain one block per centimeter of tumor, not less than a total of three blocks, as well as blocks from the peritumoral region and of remote testicular tissue. Further samples have to be taken from the resection margin and from the spermatic cord with 1 cm distance to the testicle. Immunohistology can include cytokeratin for the detection of non-seminomatous elements, PLAP for the identification of ITGCN, CD31/factor VIII for the identification of vessel endothelium as well as AFP and β-HCG. ITGCN may be identified using H&E preparations, PLAP staining or by semithin-section technique.

Histopathological reporting should address the following issues: localization and size of the tumor, multiplicity, tumor extension (rete testis, tunica albuginea, tunica vaginalis, epididymis, spermatic cord, scrotum), pT category according to the UICC classification (115), histological type (WHO-ICD-O), the presence or absence of ITGCN, as well as the presence or absence of invasion of blood or lymphatic vessels.

After chemotherapy for metastatic nonseminomatous GCT, if tumor markers are within normal limits but residual masses remain, resection is performed as a diagnostic and therapeutic procedure. Postoperative disease course depends on a number of factors including number and site of metastases (116), completeness of resection as assessed intraoperatively (117–119). The content of the mass, and the presence of viable GCT (undifferentiated teratoma/embryonal carcinoma, yolk sac tumor and trophoblastic tumor) is prognostic (118–120).

In nine series each reporting residual masses from over 50 patients, malignant GCT components were found in 6% to 28% (mean 17%), fibrosis and necrosis only in 22% to 65% (mean 45%), and differentiated teratoma (plus or minus necrosis/fibrosis) in 22% to 57% (mean 36%) (119). The two-year progression free survival rate for patients whose masses included malignant GCT elements was 12.5% compared with 88% in patients where these components were absent (119). Nonoperative predictors have been sought with a view to leaving appropriate masses in situ. It has been demonstrated that shrinkage of the mass during chemotherapy to a size of ≤ 1.5 cm, high serum LDH, and normal serum AFP and HCG levels before chemotherapy, and absence of differentiated teratoma from the primary are indicative of necrotic tissue only in the residual mass (121,122). The development of non-GCT malignancies (such as sarcoma, adenocarcinoma and squamous carcinoma) within the resected specimen is associated with a poor prognosis (123).

STAGING PROCEDURES AND PROGNOSTIC INFORMATION

To define the clinical stage of a patient with a gonadal GCT the TNM classification of the UICC should be used (115). In addition, most patients with metastatic disease are classified according to the classification of IGCCCG (57), which is also incorporated into the TNM classification. The individual treatment strategy is based on both the TNM classification and the IGCCCG prognostic factor–based classification which includes histology, location of primary tumor, location of metastases and level of AFP, β-HCG and LDH as prognostic markers to categorize patients into "good," "intermediate," and "poor" prognosis groups (Table 1). For patients presenting with primary extragonadal GCTs, a different prognostic outcome model has been developed (124) but is not in routine use. For clinical stage 1 seminoma, although no prognostic classification system has been prospectively validated so far, there is evidence that the size of the primary tumor (<4 cm vs. ≥4 cm) and the infiltration of the rete testis are independent prognostic indicators for occult metastases (125). Patient age (<34 vs. ≥34 yr) and the presence of vascular invasion (VI) are of equivocal prognostic relevance (125–128). For clinical stage 1 nonseminoma, infiltration of the primary tumor by venous blood vessels or lymphatic infiltration (vascular invasion, VI) are the most important prognostic indicators for occult metastases (129–134). Without adjuvant treatment 48% of patients with VI will develop metastases while only 14% to 22% of those without will relapse (135). The proliferation rate, as well as the percentage of embryonal carcinoma in relation to the total tumor volume, are further prognostic indicators (133,135,136). However, these markers do not contribute independent prognostic information in addition to the factor of vascular invasion.

Computerized tomography (CT), with oral and intravenous contrast, of the chest, abdomen and pelvis is required for initial staging. For the evaluation of the lung and mediastinum, chest CT is more sensitive than plain X-ray films (137–139). Ultrasonography of the retroperitoneum is less sensitive than CT (140). Magnetic resonance imaging (MRI) of the abdomen and pelvis, does not provide additional information and should be restricted to patients to whom intravenous contrast media cannot be (141,142). The role of PET is controversial (143), and such scans are not recommended outside clinical trials as part of routine initial staging. Bone scans should be obtained in patients with elevated levels of alkaline phosphatase or if bone metastases are clinically suspected. Imaging of the brain by CT or MRI is required in patients with clinical signs potentially indicating brain metastases, or in patients with extensive lung and/or retroperitoneal disease.

BASIS FOR CHEMOSENSITIVITY AND CHEMORESISTANCE OF GERM CELL TUMORS

Germ cell cancer has become the model for a curable solid malignancy. Around 95% of newly diagnosed GCT patients are cured, and in patients with advanced disease requiring initial cisplatin-based chemotherapy, close to 80% are cured. The molecular basis for this exquisite sensitivity to cytotoxic treatment probably resides in inherent biological features involved in cell growth, cell death, differentiation pathways, and cellular response to DNA damage.

Normal tissues react to DNA damage by increasing the amount of p53 in cells. This induces the transcription of other proteins, notably Waf-1 and Mdm-2. Waf-1 is a potent inhibitor of cyclin-dependent kinases (144,145) and can cause cell cycle arrest in G1. G1 arrested cells have the opportunity to recover from genotoxic damage. Alternatively, particularly when myc, myb, or E2F are overexpressed, an elevated p53 expression may lead to apoptosis (146,147).

Normal germ cells contain high levels of wild-type p53. GCT are similar and do not have mutations in the p53 gene (148–150). When GCT lines are exposed to etoposide, p53 protein is increased, but Waf-1 only modestly so, and apoptosis ensues (151). This is different to many other cancers, where either the p53 protein remains at low level, possibly because of the presence of a p53 mutation, or p53 induction takes place and the associated Waf-1 induction causes G1 arrest. The sensitivity of GCT to cytotoxic agents is therefore associated with the apoptotic response to genotoxic damage. This, in turn, is in part attributed to the high levels of wild-type p53, the absence of p53 mutations and only a modest level of Waf-1 induction.

GCT cell lines have relatively high levels of apoptosis-promoting proteins Bax and low levels of the suppressors of apoptosis, Bcl-2 (151). The Bax:Bcl ratio may be of importance in determining whether the response to cell damage is apoptosis or repair. The role of p53 in affecting this ratio in GCT is uncertain.

The basis for cisplatin sensitivity observed in germ cell cancers has been the subject of investigation. Exposure of cells to cisplatin causes crucial intrastrand cross-links, and this is followed by nuclear excision repair (NER). Testis cancer cells have been shown to be deficient in this process. NER is complex and includes the recognition of DNA damage by high mobility group (HMG) proteins. There is a testis-specific HMG protein. When this has been transfected into HeLa cells, the amount of apoptosis following cisplatin exposure was increased in some cases (152). Of the other proteins involved in the NER, the xeroderma pigmentosum group A (XPA) protein and the ERCC1-XPF endonuclease complex are present in low levels in testis cancer cells. When these proteins were added to testis tumor cell extracts, full NER capacity was restored (153), suggesting a pivotal role for these proteins.

Sensitive testis cancer cells do not have higher levels of p53 than resistant ones, though, since it is likely that resistant cell lines had been derived from tumors heavily exposed to chemotherapeutic agents in vivo, other resistance mechanisms may be operative. Studies have implicated failure to activate caspase-9 (154) or failure to induce expression of FAS and recruitment of FADD and caspase-8 to FAS (155) as a possible means by which GCTs subvert the inherent capacity of these cells to rapidly activate cell death pathways. High-level gene amplification, a genetic feature often associated in other tumor types with a poorer prognosis, has been implicated (156).

Amplification of genetic material at multiple sites other than 12p was observed in 5 of 17 GCTs not cured by cisplatin-based therapy, but not in 17 cured GCTs. Expression studies aimed at identifying markers of resistance not restricted to regions identified by molecular genetic studies provide an exciting opportunity to utilize a group of expression identifiers together with clinical parameters for risk stratification of patients.

REFERENCES

1. Toms JR, ed. CancerStats Monograph 2004. London: Cancer Research UK, 2004.
2. Huddart R, Moore NR, Williams MV, et al. Difficulties in the diagnosis of metastatic testicular teratoma. Br J Radiol 1990; 63:569–572.
3. Franklin CIV. Spontaneous remission of metastases from testicular tumours. A report of six cases from one centre. Clin Radiol 1977; 28:499–502.
4. Benstead K, Williams MV, Dixon A. Spontaneous regression of metastatic teratoma teratoma (letter). Clin Oncol 1991; 3:357.
5. Van der Werf-Messing B. Radiotherapeutic treatment of testicular tumours. Int J Radiat Oncol Biol Phys 1976; 1:235–248.
6. Peckham MJ. An appraisal of the role of radiation therapy in the management of nonseminomatous germ cell tumors of the testis in the era of effective chemotherapy. Cancer Treat Rep 1979; 63:1653–1658.
7. Tyrell CJ, Peckham MJ. The response of lymph node metastases of testicular teratoma to radiation therapy. Brit J Urol 1976; 48:363–370.
8. Van der Werf-Messing B. The treatment of pulmonary metastases of malignant teratoma of the testis. Clin Radiol 1973; 24:121–123.
9. Samuels ML, Lanzotti VJ, Holoye PY, et al. Combination chemotherapy in germinal cell tumours. Cancer Treat Rev 1976; 3:185–204.
10. Einhorn LH, Donohue J. Diamminedichloroplatinum, Vinblastine and Bleomycin combination chemotherapy in disseminated testicular cancer. Ann Intern Med 1977; 87:293–298.
11. Peckham MJ, Barrett A, Liew KH, et al. The treatment of metastatic germ-cell testicular tumours with Bleomycin, Etoposide and Cis-platin (BEP). Br J Cancer 1983; 47:613–619.
12. Williams SD, Birch R, Einhorn LH, et al. Treatment of disseminated germ-cell tumors with Cisplatin, Bleomycin and either Vinblastine or Etoposide. N Engl J Med 1987; 316:1435–1440.
13. Peckham MJ, ed. The Management of Testicular Tumours. London: Edward Arnold, 1981.
14. Foster RS, Donohue JP. Retroperitoneal lymph node dissection for the management of clinical stage I non-seminoma. J Urol 2000; 163:1788–1792.
15. Peckham MJ, Barrett A, Husband JE, et al. Orchidectomy alone in testicular stage I non-seminatous germ cell tumours. Lancet 1982; 2:678–680.
16. Freedman LS, Parkinson MC, Jones WG, et al. Histopathology in the prediction of relapse of patients with stage I testicular teratoma treated by orchidectomy alone. Lancet 1987; 2(8554):294–298.
17. Alexandre J, Fizazi K, Mahé C, et al. Stage I non-seminomatous germ-cell tumours of the testis: identification of a subgroup of patients with a very low risk of relapse. Eur J Cancer. 2001; 37:576–582.

18. Cullen MH, Stenning SP, Parkinson MC, et al. Short-course adjuvant chemotherapy in high-risk stage I nonseminomatous germ cell tumors of the testis: a Medical Research Council report. J Clin Oncol 1996; 14:1106–13.

19. Huddart RA, Norman A, Shahidi M, et al. Cardiovascular disease as a long-term complication of treatment for testicular cancer. J Clin Oncol 2003; 21(8):1513–1523.

20. van den Belt-Dusebout AW, de Wit R, Gietema JA, et al. Treatment-specific risks of second malignancies and cardiovascular disease in 5-year survivors of testicular cancer. J Clin Oncol 2007; 25:4370–4378.

21. Beck SDW, Peterson MD, Bihrle R, et al. Short-term morbidity of primary retroperitoneal lymph node dissection in a contemporary group of patients. J Urol 2007; 178:504–506.

22. Fossa SD, Horwich A, Russell JM, et al. Optimal planning target volume for stage I testicular seminoma: a Medical Research Council randomised trial. J Clin Oncol 1999; 17:1146–1154.

23. Jones WG, Fossa SD, Mead GM, et al. Randomised trial of 30 versus 20 Gy in the adjuvant treatment of stage I testicular seminoma: a report on Medical Research Council Trial TE18, European Organisation for the Research and Treatment of Cancer Trial 30942 (ISRCTN 18525328). J Clin Oncol 2005; 23:1200–1208.

24. Oliver RTD, Mason MD, Mead GM, et al. Radiotherapy versus single-dose Carboplatin in adjuvant treatment of stage I seminoma: a randomised trial. Lancet 2005; 366:293–330.

25. Travis LB, Curtis RE, Storm H, et al. Risk of second malignant neoplasm among long-term survivors of testicular cancer. J Natl Cancer Inst 1997; 89:1429–1439.

26. Zagars GK, Ballo MT, Lee AK, et al. Mortality after cure of testicular seminoma. J Clin Oncol 2004; 22:640–647.

27. Powles T, Robinson D, Shamash J, et al. The long-term risks of adjuvant carboplatin treatment for stage I seminoma of the testis. Ann Oncol 2008; 19:443–447.

28. Loehrer PJ, Bosl GJ. Carboplatin for stage I seminoma and the sword of Damocles. C Clin Oncol 2005; 23:8566–8569.

29. Raj S, Williams MV, Dixon AK, et al. Late relapse of stage 1 seminoma following single-agent carboplatin. Oncology 2008; 73(5–6):419–421.

30. Moller H. Clues to the aetiology of testicular germ cell tumours from descriptive epidemiology. Eur Urol 1993; 23:8–15.

31. Bergstrom R, Adami HO, Mohner M, et al. Increase in testicular cancer incidence in 9 European countries: a birth cohort phenomenon. J Natl Cancer Inst 1996; 88:727–733.

32. Ekbom A, Akre O. Increasing incidence of testis cancer: a birth cohort effect. In: Rajpert De Meyts E, Grigor KM, Skakkebaek NE, eds. Neoplastic transformation of testicular germ cells. APMIS 1998; 106:225–229.

33. Freeman A, Harland SJ. Testis cancer. In: Mundy AR, Fitzpatrick JM, Neal DE, et al. eds. Scientific Basis of Urology. 2nd ed., London: Taylor and Francis, 2004.

34. Sharpe RM, Irvine DS. How strong is the evidence of a link between environmental chemicals and adverse effects on human reproductive health? BMJ 2004; 328:447–451.

35. Ross RK, McCurtis JW, Henderson BE, et al. Descriptive epidemiology of testicular and prostatic cancer in Los Angeles. Br J Cancer 1979; 39:284–292.

36. Pukkala E, Wiederpass E. Socio-economic differences in incidence rates of cancers of the male genital organs in Finland, 1971–1995. Int J Cancer 2002; 102:643–648.

37. Prattala R, Berg MA, Puska P. Diminishing or increasing contrasts? Social class variation in Finnish food consumption patterns, 1979–1990. Eur J Clin Nutr 1992; 46:279–287.

38. Tanner JM. Trend towards earlier menarche in London, Oslo, Copenhagen, The Netherlands and Hungary. Nature 1973; 243:96–97.

39. Forman D, Pike MC, Davey G, et al. Aetiology of testicular cancer: association with congenital abnormalities, age at puberty, infertility and exercise. BMJ 1994; 308:1393–1399.

40. Forman D, Gallagher R, Moller H, et al. Aetiology and epidemiology of testicular cancer: report of consensus group. Prog Clin Biol Res 1990; 357:245–253.

41. Swerdlow AJ, Higgins CD, Pike MC. Risk of testicular cancer in cohort of boys with cryptorchidism. BMJ 1997; 314:1507–1511.

42. Pettersson MD, Lorenzo R, Nordenskjold A, et al. Age at surgery for undescended testis and risk of testicular cancer. N Engl J Med 2007; 356:1835–1841.

43. Timing of elective surgery on the genitalia of male children with particular reference to the risks, benefits and psychological effects of surgery and anaesthesia. Paediatrics 1996; 97:590–594.

44. Hutson JM, Hasthorpe S. Abnormalities of testicular descent. Cell Tissue Res 2005; 322:155–158.

45. Hutson JM, Hasthorpe S. Testicular descent and cryptorchidism: the state of the art in 2004. J Paediatr Surg 2005; 40:297–302.

46. McCabe JE, Kenny SE. Orchidopexy for undescended testis in England: is it evidence based? J Paediatr Surg 2008; 43:353–357.

47. Sokal M, Peckham MJ, Hendry WF. Bilateral germ cell tumours of the testis. Br J Urol 1980; 52:158–162.

48. Hartmann JT, Fossa SD, Nichols CR, et al. Incidence of metachronous testicular cancer in patients with extragonadal germ cell tumors. J Natl Cancer Inst 2001; 93: 1733–1738.

49. Harland SJ, Cook PA, Fossa SD, et al. Intratubular germ cell neoplasia of the contralateral testis in testicular cancer: defining a high risk group. J Urol 1998; 160:1353–1357.

50. de Gouveia Brazao CA, Pierik FH, Oosterhuis JW, et al. Bilateral testicular microlithiasis predicts the presence of the precurs testicular germ cell tumours in subfertile men. J Urol 2004; 171:158–160.

51. Schefer H, Mattman S, Joss RA. Hereditary persistence of alpha-fetoprotein. Case report and review of the literature. Ann Oncol 1998; 9:667–672.

52. Greenburgh F, Alpert E, Rose E. Hereditary persistence of alpha fetoprotein. Gastroenterology 1990; 1998:1083–1085.

53. Pandha HS, Wasan HS, Harrington K, et al. The failure of normalisation of alpha fetoprotein concentration after successful treatment of teratoma. BMJ 1995; 311:434–435.

54. Summers J, Wraggatt P, Pratt J, et al. Experience of discordant beta-hCG results by different assays in the management of non-seminomatous germ cell tumours of the testis. Clin Oncol 1999; 11:388–392.

55. Bjurlin MA, August CZ, Weldon-Linne M, et al. Histologically pure stage I seminoma with an elevated beta-hCG of 4497 IU/I. Urology 2007; 70:1007.e13–1007.e15.

56. A predictive model for aggressive Non-Hodgkin's Lymphoma. The International Non-Hodgkin's Lymphoma Prognostic Factors Project. N Engl J Med 1993; 329: 987–994.

57. International Germ Cell Cancer Collaborative Group. International germ cell consensus classification: a prognostic factor-based staging system for metastatic germ cell cancers. J Clin Oncol 1997; 15:594–603.

58. Venkitaraman R, Johnson B, Huddart RA, et al. The utility of lactate dehydrogenase in the follow-up of testicular germ cell tumours. BJU Int 2007; 100:30–32.

59. Ackers C, Rustin GJ. Lactate dehydrogenase is not a useful marker for relapse in patients on surveillance for stage I germ cell tumours. Br J Cancer 2006; 94:1231–1232.

60. Stinghen ST, Moura JF, Zancanella P, et al. Specific immunoassays for placental alkaline phosphatase as a tumor marker. J Biomed Biotechnol 2006; 2006(5):56087.

61. Price P, Hogan SJ, Bliss JM, et al. The growth rate of metastatic non-seminomatous germ cell testicular tumours measured by marker production doubling time – II. Prognostic significance in patients treated by chemotherapy. Eur J Cancer 1990; 26:453–457.

62. Al-Karim HA, Bryce C, Mulhall P, et al. Repeated AFP surge: an unusual and potentially misleading tumour marker phenomenon. Clin Oncol 2002; 14:294–295.

63. Toner GC, Geller NL, Tan C, et al. Serum tumor marker half-life during chemotherapy allows early prediction of complete response and survival in non-seminomatous germ cell tumours. Cancer Res 1990; 50:5904–5910.

64. Stephens MJ, Norman AR, Dearnaley DP, et al. Prognostic significance of early serum tumour marker half-life and life in metastatic testicular teratoma. J Clin Oncol 1995; 13:87–92.

65. Beck SDW, Patel MI, Sheinfeld J. Tumour markers levels in post-chemotherapy cystic masses: clinical implications for patients with germ cell tumours. J Urol 2004; 171:168–171.

66. Logothetis CJ, Samuels ML, Trindade A, et al. The growing teratoma syndrome. Cancer 1982; 50:1629–1635.

67. Skakkebaek NE, Berthelsen JG, Müller J. Carcinoma in situ of the undescended testis. Urol Clin North Am 1982; 9:377–385.

68. von der Maase H, Rorth M, Walbom-Jorgensen S, et al. Carcinoma in situ of contralateral testis in patients with testicular germ cell cancer: study of 27 cases in 500 patients. Br Med J (Clin Res Ed) 1986; 293:1398–1401.

69. Dieckmann KP, Loy V. Prevalence of contralateral testicular intraepithelial neoplasia in patients with testicular germ cell neoplasms. J Clin Oncol 1996; 14:3126–3132.

70. Giwercman A, Andrews PW, Jorgensen P, et al. Immunohistochemical expression of embryonal marker TRA-1-60 in carcinoma in situ and germ cell tumors of the testis. Cancer 1993; 72:1308–1314.

71. Chaganti RS, Houldsworth J. Genetics and biology of adult human male germ cell tumours. Can Res 2000; 60:1475–1482.

72. Grigor KM, Skakkebaek NE. Pathogenesis and cell biology of germ cell neoplasia: general discussion. Eur Urol 1993; 23:46–53.

73. Looijenga LH, de Munnik H, Oosterhuis JW. A molecular model for the development of germ cell cancer. Int J Cancer 1999; 83:809–814.

74. Bosl GJ, Ilson DH, Rodriguez E, et al. Clinical relevance of the i(12p) marker chromosome in germ cell tumors. J Natl Cancer Inst 1994; 86:349–355.

75. Rodriguez E, Mathew S, Mukherjee AB, et al. Analysis of chromosome 12 aneuploidy in interphase cells from human male germ cell tumors by fluorescence in situ hybridization. Genes Chromosomes Cancer 1992; 5:21–29.

76. Rodriguez E, Houldsworth J, Reuter VE, et al. Molecular cytogenetic analysis of i(12p)-negative human male germ cell tumors. Genes Chromosomes Cancer 1993; 8:230–236.

77. Rodriguez S, Jafer O, Goker H, et al. Expression profile of genes from 12p in testicular germ cell tumors of adolescents and adults associated with i(12p) and amplification at 12p11.2–p12.1. Oncogene 2003; 22:1880–1891.

78. Kraggerud SM, Skotheim RI, Szymanska J, et al. Genome profiles of familial/bilateral and sporadic testicular germ cell tumors. Genes Chromosomes Cancer 2002; 34: 168–174.

79. Skotheim RI, Lothe RA. The testicular germ cell tumour genome. APMIS 2003; 111:136–150; discussion 50–51.

80. Oosterhuis JW, Looijenga LH. Current views on the pathogenesis of testicular germ cell tumours and perspectives for future research: highlights of the 5th Copenhagen Workshop on Carcinoma in situ and Cancer of the Testis. APMIS 2003; 111:280–289.

81. Houldsworth J, Reuter V, Bosl GJ, et al. Aberrant expression of cyclin D2 is an early event in human male germ cell tumorigenesis. Cell Growth Differ 1997; 8:293–299.

82. Houldsworth J, Xiao H, Murty VV, et al. Human male germ cell tumor resistance to cisplatin is linked to TP53 gene mutation. Oncogene 1998; 16:2345–2349.

83. Schneider DT, Schuster AE, Fritsch MK, et al. Multipoint imprinting analysis indicates a common precursor cell for gonadal and nongonadal pediatric germ cell tumors. Cancer Res 2001; 61:7268–7276.

84. Bussey KJ, Lawce HJ, Himoe E, et al. Chromosomes 1 and 12 abnormalities in pediatric germ cell tumors by interphase fluorescence in situ hybridization. Cancer Genet Cytogenet 2001; 125:112–118.

85. Silver SA, Wiley JM, Perlman EJ. DNA ploidy analysis of pediatric germ cell tumors. Mod Pathol 1994; 7:951–956.

86. Jenderny J, Koster E, Borchers O, et al. Interphase cytogenetics on paraffin sections of paediatric extragonadal yolk sac tumours. Virchows Arch 1996; 428:53–57.

87. Stock C, Strehl S, Fink FM, et al. Isochromosome 12p and maternal loss of 1p36 in a pediatric testicular germ cell tumor. Cancer Genet Cytogenet 1996; 91:95–100.

88. Forman D, Oliver RT, Brett AR, et al. Familial testicular cancer: a report of the UK family register, estimation of risk, and an HLA class 1 sib-pair analysis. Br J Cancer 1992; 65:255–262.

89. Heimdal K, Olsson H, Tretli S, et al. Familial testicular cancer in Norway and southern Sweden. Br J Cancer 1996; 73:964–969.

90. Hemminki K, Li X. Familial risk in testicular cancer as a clue to a heritable and environmental aetiology. Br J Cancer 2004; 90:1765–1770.

91. Swerdlow AJ, De Stavola BL, Swanwick MA, et al. Risks of breast and testicular cancers in young adult twins in England and Wales: evidence on prenatal and genetic aetiology. Lancet 1997; 350:1723–1728.

92. Heimdal K, Olsson H, Tretli S, et al. A segregation analysis of testicular cancer based on Norwegian and Swedish families. Br J Cancer 1997; 75:1084–1087.

93. Nicholson PW, Harland SJ. Inheritance and testicular cancer. Br J Cancer 1995; 71:421–426.

94. Crockford GP, Linger R, Hockley S, et al. Genome-wide linkage screen for testicular germ cell tumour susceptibility loci. Hum Mol Genet 2006; 15:443–451.

95. Rapley EA, Crockford GP, Teare D, et al. Localization to Xq27 of a susceptibility gene for testicular germ cell tumours. Nat Genet 2000; 24:197–200.

96. Skakkebaek NE. Possible carcinoma in situ of the testis. Lancet 1972; 2:516.

97. Manivel JC, Simonton S, Wold LE, et al. Absence of intratubular germ cell neoplasia in testicular yolk sac tumors in children. A histochemical and immunohistochemical study. Arch Pathol Lab Med 1988; 112:641–645.

98. Hu LM, Phillipson J, Barsky SH. Intratubular germ cell neoplasia in infantile yolk sac tumor. Verification by tandem repeat sequence in situ hybridization. Diagn Mol Pathol 1992; 1:118–128.

99. Stamp IM, Barlebo H, Rix M, et al. Intratubular germ cell neoplasia in an infantile testis with immature teratoma. Histopathology 1993; 22:69–72.

100. Soosay GN, Bobrow L, Happerfield L, et al. Morphology and immunohistochemistry of carcinoma in situ adjacent to testicular germ cell tumours in adults and children: implications for histogenesis. Histopathology 1991; 19:537–544.

101. Ramani P, Yeung CK, Habeebu SSM. Testicular intratubular germ cell neoplasia in children and adolescents with intersex. Am J Surg Pathol 1993; 17:1124–1133.

102. Giwercman A, Lindenberg S, Kimber SJ, et al. Monoclonal antibody 43-9F as a sensitive immunohistochemical

marker of carcinoma in situ of human testis. Cancer 1990; 65:1135–1142.

103. Marks A, Sutherland DR, Bailey D, et al. Characterization and distribution of an oncofetal antigen (M2A antigen) expressed on testicular germ cell tumours. Br J Cancer 1999; 80:569–578.

104. Looijenga LH, Stoop H, de Leeuw HP, et al. POU5F1 (OCT3/4) identifies cells with pluripotent potential in human germ cell tumors. Cancer Res 2003; 63:2244–2250.

105. Kang JL, Rajpert-De Meyts W, Giwercmann A, et al. The association of testicular carcinoma in situ with intratubular microcalcifications. J Urol Pathol 1994; 2:235–242.

106. Bach AM, Hann LE, Hadar O, et al. Testicular microlithiasis: what is its association with testicular cancer? Radiology 2001; 220:70–75.

107. Peterson AC, Baumann JM, Light DE, et al. The prevalence of testicular microlithiasis in an asymptomatic population of men 18 to 35 years old. J Urol 2001; 166:2061–2064.

108. Bassetto MA, Pasini F, Franceschi T, et al. Extragonadal germ cell tumour: a clinical study. Anticancer Res 1995; 15:2751–2754.

109. Casella R, Rochlitz C, Sauter G, et al. "Burned out" testicular tumour: a rare form of germ cell neoplasias. Schweiz Med Wochenschr 1999; 129:235–240.

110. de Takats PG, Jones SR, Penn R, et al. a-Foetoprotein heterogeneity: what is its value in managing patients with germ cell tumours? Clin Oncol (R Coll Radiol) 1996; 8:323–326.

111. Dueland S, Stenwig AE, Heilo A, et al. Treatment and outcome of patients with extragonadal germ cell tumours: the Norwegian Radium Hospital's experience 1979–1994. Br J Cancer 1998; 77:329–335.

112. Hartmann M, Pottek T, Bussar-Maatz R, et al. Elevated human chorionic gonadotropin concentrations in the testicular vein and in peripheral venous blood in seminoma patients. An analysis of various parameters. Eur Urol 1997; 31:408–413.

113. van de Gaer P, Verstraete H, De Wever I, et al. Primary retroperitoneal extragonadal germ cell tumour. J Belge Radiol 1998; 81:221–222.

114. Eble JN, Sauter G, Epstein JI, et al. World Health Organization Classification of Tumours: Pathology and Genetics of Tumours of the Urinary System and Male Genital Organs. Lyon, France: IARC Press, 2004:218–249.

115. Sobin LH, Wittekind CH, eds. UICC: TNM Classification of Malignant Tumours. 6th ed. New York: Wiley-Liss, 2002.

116. Steyerberg EW, Keiser HJ, Zwartendijk J, et al. Prognosis after resection of residual masses following chemotherapy for metastatic non-seminomatous testicular cancer: a multivariate analysis. Br J Cancer 1993; 68:195–200.

117. Hendry WF, A'Hern RP, Hetherington JW, et al. Paraaortic lympadenectomy after chemotherapy for metastatic non-seminomatous germ cell tumours: prognostic value and therapeutic benefits. Br J Urol 1993; 71:208–213.

118. Gerl A, Clemm C, Schmeller N, et al. Outcome analysis after post-chemotherapy surgery in patients with non-seminomatous germ cell tumours. Ann Oncol 1995; 6: 483–488.

119. Stenning SP, Parkinson MC, Fisher C, et al. Postchemotherapy residual masses in germ cell tumour patients: content, clinical features, and prognosis. Medical Research Council Testicular Tumour Working Party, Cancer 1998; 83:1409–1419.

120. Hendry WF. Decision-making in abdominal surgery following chemotherapy for testicular cancer. Eur J Cancer 1995; 31A:649–650.

121. Toner GC, Panicek DM, Heelan RJ, et al. Adjunctive surgery after chemotherapy for non-seminomatous testicular cancer: recommendations for patient selection. J Clin Oncol 1990; 8:1683–1694.

122. Steyerberg EW, Keizer HJ, Stoter G, et al. Predictors of residual mass histology following chemotherapy for metastatic non-seminomatous testicular cancer: a quantitative overview of 996 resections. Eur J Cancer 1994; 30A:1231–1239.

123. Little JS, Foster RS, Ulbright TM, et al. Unusual neoplasms detected in testis cancer patients undergoing post-chemotherapy retroperitoneal lymphadenectomy. J Urol 1994; 152:1144–1149.

124. Hartmann JT, Nichols CR, Droz JP, et al. Prognostic variables for response and outcome in patients with extragonadal germ-cell tumors. Ann Oncol 2002; 13: 1017–1028.

125. Warde P, Specht L, Horwich A, et al. Prognostic factors for relapse in stage I seminoma managed by surveillance. J Clin Oncol 2002; 20:4448–4452.

126. Warde P, Gospodarowicz MK, Banerjee D, et al. Prognostic factors for relapse in stage I testicular seminoma treated with surveillance. J Urol 1997; 157:1705–1710.

127. Weissbach L, Bussar-Maatz R, Löhrs U, et al. Prognostic factors in seminomas with special respect to HCG: results of a prospective multicenter study. Eur Urol 1999; 36:601–608.

128. Horwich A, Alsanjari N, A'Hearn R, et al. Surveillance following orchiectomy for stage I testicular seminoma. Br J Cancer 1992; 65:775–778.

129. Albers P, Siener R, Kliesch S, et al. Risk factors for relapse in clinical stage I non-seminomatous testicular germ cell tumors: results of the German Testicular Cancer Study Group trial. J Clin Oncol 2003; 21:1505–1512.

130. Bohlen D, Borner M, Sonntag RW, et al. Long term results following adjuvant chemotherapy in patients with clinical stage I testicular non-seminomatous malignant germ cell tumors with high risk factors. J Urol 1999; 161:1148–1152.

131. Klepp O, Dahl O, Flodgren P, et al. Risk-adapted treatment of clinical stage I non-seminoma testis cancer. Eur J Cancer 1997; 33:1038–1044.

132. Kratzik Ch, Höltl W, Albrecht W, et al. Risk adapted management for NSGCT stage 1: long-term results of a multicenter study. J Urol 1996; 157:547A.

133. Ondrus D, Matoska J, Belan V, et al. Prognostic factors in clinical stage I non-seminomatous germ cell testicular tumors: rationale for different risk-adapted treatment. Eur Urol 1998; 33:562–566.

134. Pont J, Holtl W, Kosak D, et al. Risk-adapted treatment choice in stage I non-seminomatous testicular germ cell cancer by regarding vascular invasion in the primary tumor: a prospective trial. J Clin Oncol 1990; 8:16–19.

135. Read G, Stenning SP, Cullen MH, et al. Medical Research Council prospective study of surveillance for stage I testicular teratoma. Medical Research Council Testicular Tumors Working Party. J Clin Oncol 1992; 10:1762–1768.

136. Albers P, Ulbright TM, Albers J, et al. Tumor proliferative activity is predictive of pathological stage in clinical stage A non-seminomatous testicular germ cell tumors. J Urol 1996; 155:579–586.

137. White PM, Howard GC, Best JJ, et al. The role of computed tomographic examination of the pelvis in the management of testicular germ cell tumours. Clin Radiol 1997; 52:124–129.

138. White PM, Adamson DJA, Howard GCW, et al. Imaging of the thorax in the management of germ cell testicular tumours. Clin Radiol 1999; 54:207–211.

139. Meyer CA, Conces DJ. Imaging of intrathoracic metastases of non-seminomatous germ cell tumors. Chest Surg Clin N Am 2002; 12:717–738.

140. Krug B, Heidenreich A, Dietlein M, et al. Lymphknotenstaging maligner testikularer Keimzelltumoren. Fortschr Rontgenstr 1999; 171:87–94.

141. Bellin M, Roy C, Kinkel K, et al. Lymph node metastases: safety and effectiveness of MR imaging with ultrasmall superparamagnetic iron oxide particles: initial clinical experience. Radiology 1998; 207:799–808.

142. Hogeboom WR, Hoekstra HJ, Mooyart EL, et al. Magnetic resonance imaging of retroperitoneal lymph node metastases of non-seminomatous germ cell tumors of the testis. Eur J Surg Oncol 1993; 19:429–437.

143. Lassen U, Daugaard G, Eigtved A, et al. Wholebody positron emission tomography (PET) with FDG in patients with stage I non-seminomatous germ cell tumours (NSGCT). Eur J Nucl Med Imaging 2003; 30: 396–402.

144. El-Deiry WS, Harper JW, O'Connor PM, et al. WAF1/CIPI is induced in p53-mediated G1 arrest and apoptosis. Cancer Res 1994; 54:1169–1174.

145. Canman CE, Gilmer TM, Coutts SB, et al. Growth factor modulation of p53-mediated growth arrest versus apoptosis. Genes Dev 1995; 9:600–611.

146. Wagner AJ, Kokontis JM, Hay N. myc-mediated apoptosis requires wild-type p53 in a manner independent of cell cycle arrest and the ability of p53 to induce p21 waf1/cip1. Genes Dev 1994; 8:2817–2830.

147. Lin D, Fiscella M, O'Connor PM, et al. Constititive expression of B-myb can bypass p53-induced Waf1/Cip1-mediated G1 arrest. Proc Natl Acad Sci USA 1994; 91: 10079–10083.

148. Peng HQ, Hogg D, Malkin D, et al. Mutations of the p53 gene do not occur in testis cancer. Cancer Res 1993; 53:3574–3578.

149. Heindal K, Lothe RA, Lystad S, et al. No germline TP53 mutations detected in familial and bilateral testicular cancers. Genes Chromosomes Cancer 1993; 6:92–97.

150. Fleischhacker M, Strohmeyer T, Imao Y, et al. Mutations of the p53 gene are not detectable in human testicular tumours. Mod Pathol 1994; 7:435–439.

151. Chresta CM, Masters JR, Hickman JA. Hypersensitivity of human testicular tumours to etoposide-induced apoptosis is associated with functional p53 and a high Bax: Bcl-2 ratio. Cancer Res 1996; 56:1834–1841.

152. Zamble DB, Mikata Y, Eng CH, et al. Testis-specific HMG-domain proteinalters the responses of cells to cisplatin. J Inorg Biochem 2002; 91:451–462.

153. Koberle B, Masters JRW, Hartley JA, et al. Reduced repair of cisplatin-induced DNA damage in testicular germ cell tumours due to a specific protein defect. Curr Biol 1999; 9:273–276.

154. Mueller T, Voigt W, Simon H, et al. Failure of activation of caspase-9 induces a higher threshold for apoptosis and cisplatin resistance in testicular cancer. Cancer Res 2003; 63:513–521.

155. Spierings DC, de Vries EGE, Vellenga E, et al. Loss of drug-induced activation of the CD95 apoptotic pathway in a cisplatin-resistant testicular germ cell tumor cell line. Cell Death Differ 2003; 10:808–822.

156. Rao PH, Houldsworth J, Palanisamy N, et al. Chromosomal amplification is associated with cisplatin resistance of human male germ cell tumours. Cancer Res 1998; 58: 4260–4263.

27

Radiotherapy: Scientific Principles and Practical Application in Urogical Malignancies

Angela Swampillai, Rachel Lewis, Mary McCormack, and Heather Payne

Department of Oncology, University College Hospitals, London, U.K.

INTRODUCTION

Radiotherapy is the therapeutic use of ionizing radiation. X rays were first used in the treatment of cancer over 100 years ago by Freund, a German surgeon. Since that time, our understanding of the effects of ionizing radiation on malignant and normal tissues has progressed through the field of radiobiology. In parallel with this, our knowledge of radiation physics has advanced together with significant technological developments in treatment planning and delivery.

This chapter outlines the underlying physical and radiobiological principles of radiotherapy and discusses the scientific practice of radiotherapy as applied to urological tumors.

RADIATION PHYSICS

Radiation used therapeutically is called ionizing radiation, as it causes its effects through the ionization of intracellular molecules. Ionizing radiation can be classified as electromagnetic or particulate.

Electromagnetic Radiation

The two types of electromagnetic radiation used in radiotherapy are X rays and γ rays. They are physically identical, but known by different names to distinguish their means of production. γ Rays are produced from the nuclear decay of radioactive isotopes. X rays are produced by interactions that occur outside the nucleus. Both types of radiation have short wavelengths, high frequencies and carry high energies that enable them to break chemical bonds and produce biological effects (Fig. 1). The term "photon" is another name that can be used to describe both X rays and γ rays.

X rays are usually produced artificially by electrical means, accelerating electrons to a high energy and then abruptly stopping them in a heavy metal target. Part or all of the kinetic energy of the electrons is converted into X rays. The energies necessary to generate therapeutic X-ray beams capable of penetrating human tissues are in the megavoltage (MV) range and are usually produced by a machine called a linear accelerator. This type of treatment is an example of teletherapy, where the source of radiation is distant from the body and is often referred to as "external beam radiotherapy."

As the energy of the treatment beam increases so does the penetration depth, as the X rays are less able to interact with superficial tissues (Fig. 2). Modern radiotherapy techniques use MV photons with beam energies typically greater than 8 MV to treat urological tumors such as carcinoma of the prostate or bladder. Prior to the introduction of MV treatment (cobalt machines and linear accelerators), the only available treatment energies were up to 300 kV, which gave inadequate penetration for the treatment of deep target tissues. The term "deep X-ray therapy" (DXT) is often mistakenly applied to all radiotherapy but historically refers specifically to energies in the 250 to 300 kV range. These beams deposit their maximum dose in the skin and have a therapeutic penetration of only 3 to -4 cm. Lower energy beams (90–300 kV) are now used mainly to treat lesions in the skin and superficial tissues.

The other common types of therapeutic radiation, γ rays, are produced by the nuclear decay of radioactive elements and represent the excess energy that is emitted as an unstable nucleus decays into a more stable form. The higher energy γ rays emitted from isotopes such as cobalt (^{60}Co) or cesium (^{137}Cs) can be used therapeutically if harnessed into beams for external radiotherapy treatment. Cobalt machines are still used in some centers, but since they produce a relatively low energy beam, their uses are limited for urological treatments.

Other isotopes such as radium (^{226}Ra), iridium (^{192}Ir) and iodine (^{125}I) can be used as temporary or permanent implants, a process known as brachytherapy. Sealed isotope sources can be placed into body cavities (intracavity brachytherapy) or directly into tissues (interstitial brachytherapy).

The main physical advantage of brachytherapy is that it allows a high tumor dose and considerable sparing of surrounding normal tissues. This occurs because of the inverse square law that governs the intensity of all electromagnetic radiation. As the distance from a radiation source doubles, the intensity falls to one-quarter, producing a rapid decline in effect that can be exploited therapeutically in brachytherapy.

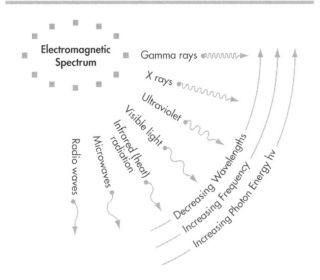

Figure 1   Illustration of the electromagnetic spectrum.

The isotopes used in brachytherapy are known as sealed sources because they are contained within protective coverings to stop physical contact between the body and the radioactive material while still allowing the radiation to escape. Radium is now no longer used because of the difficulty of ensuring adequate radiation protection. It decays into radon gas, which is difficult to contain and emits α particles, a highly damaging form of particulate radiation (see below).

A third therapeutic use for γ rays is as "unsealed sources" in which an isotope is exploited because of its metabolic effect on biological tissues. The isotope is usually incorporated into tissues because of its physical properties, radioactivity being released as the isotope decays. An example of this is administration of radioactive strontium for the palliation of painful bone metastases in metastatic prostate cancer. Strontium is taken up into bone, and the radioactive decay produces local tumor cell kill, resulting in pain relief.

Particulate Radiation

Particulate radiation consists of subatomic particles, including electrons, protons and α particles. In current radiotherapy, electrons are the only commonly used type of particulate radiation. Electrons are also generated by a linear accelerator, but instead of the beam hitting a target to generate X rays, the electrons are allowed to penetrate directly into the tissues to produce the therapeutic effect.

Electron beams differ from those of photons in that there is a much sharper decline in radiation dose (Fig. 2), sparing any underlying tissues. These properties make electron beams ideal for treating superficial tumors where a high dose if needed at or just below the skin surface, but it is necessary to spare the underlying tissues.

Linear accelerators are usually able to produce a range of electron beam energies of 4 to 20 MeV. The effective treatment depth in centimeters is about one-third of the beam energy in MeV (e.g., 4 cm for a 12-MeV electron beam). The electron energy used for treatment is chosen so that the tumor will typically receive 90% of the maximum dose (known as the 90% isodose). This allows for the best homogeneity of treatment dose across the tumor.

Interactions of X Rays with Matter

The process by which photons are absorbed depends principally on their energy and the chemical composition of the absorbing material. Three distinct

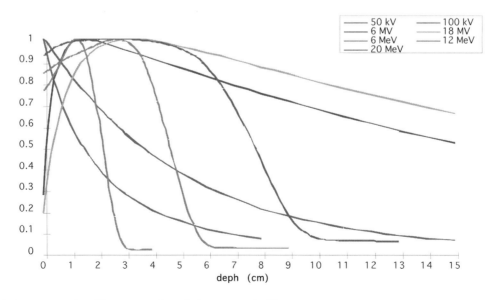

Figure 2   Depth dose curves for different energies of electrons and mV photons.

clinically relevant absorption mechanisms are recognized: the photoelectric effect, the Compton effect and pair production. As energy is being absorbed in these interactions, the SI unit of dose in radiotherapy measures the amount of energy in joules absorbed per unit mass in kilograms. The unit is the Gray (Gy) and 1 Gy is equal to 1 J of energy absorbed per kilogram of mass. To illustrate the amount of radiation energy absorbed in biological tissues, Hall has calculated that the same amount of energy is transferred in drinking one sip of hot coffee as is absorbed in a lethal 4-Gy dose of whole body radiation.

The absorption process for low energy X rays is called the photoelectric effect. The incident X ray interacts with an inner orbital electron shell of an atom within the absorbing material. The energy of the X ray is transferred to the electron as kinetic energy that causes the electron to be ejected from its orbit shell and the X ray to be dissipated. The ejected electron is now known as a "fast electron." These fast electrons can ionize other atoms in the absorbing material, breaking chemical bonds and initiating a sequence of changes that is ultimately expressed as biological damage. Mathematically, in this interaction, the energy absorbed is proportional to the cube of the atomic number (Z) of the material through which the beam passes (Fig. 3A).

The photoelectric effect is the major X-ray absorption process for diagnostic radiology. Absorption is preferential in bone because of its relatively high atomic number (Z), and this gives the characteristic white X-ray appearance of bone on standard diagnostic films (as X rays fail to reach and blacken the photoemulsion). This characteristic of the photoelectric effect is a disadvantage when used for radiotherapy, as bone and cartilage have a relatively high Z, and preferential absorption in these structures can cause radionecrosis. Because of the combination of poor penetration in tissue, the maximum deposition of energy in the skin and the preferential absorption in bone and cartilage, these lower-energy X rays are no longer routinely used except for the treatment of some skin and superficial cancers.

The absorption interaction for photons in the commonest therapy range of 1 to 10 MV is the Compton effect. In this interaction, the incident photon interacts with a more loosely bound outer electron in the atoms of the absorbing material. The photon gives up part of its energy to the electron as kinetic energy as before, and, deflected from its original path, proceeds through the material with corresponding decreased energy. The result of this interaction is also an ejected fast electron, which can ionize other atoms in the absorber. The deflected photon continues on its new path, interacting with further outer orbital electrons until all its energy is dissipated. Unlike the photoelectric effect the Compton process is independent of the atomic number of the absorbing material, and photons are not preferentially absorbed in bone and cartilage (Fig. 3B).

At treatment energies in excess of 10 MV, pair production predominates. The incident photon interacts with the nucleus of an atom, giving up all its

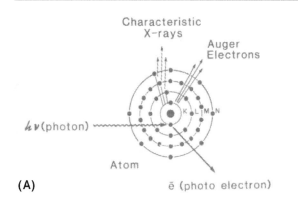

(A)

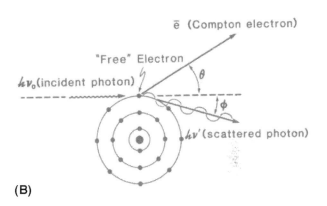

(B)

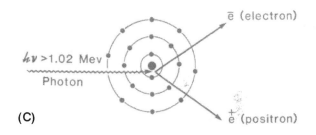

(C)

Figure 3 Interactions of photons with matter; (**A**) photoelectric effect, (**B**) Compton scatter, (**C**) pair production. *Source*: Adapted from Ref. 1.

energy in the process. This results in the production of a positron and a fast electron. The fast electron can go on to produce tissue ionizations, and the positron is quickly annihilated. Positron annihilation occurs as a further interaction with an adjacent electron of the absorbing material. This creates two new photons of 0.51 MeV energy each, both capable of producing additional tissue ionizations. Pair production, like the photoelectric effect, is also dependent on atomic number (Fig. 3C).

The resultant biological damage from fast electrons produced by all three different processes occurs in two ways. Direct ionization of atoms within target molecules may be produced, leading to chemical bond breakage and initiating the chain of events that leads to biological change. This is the dominant process when neutrons or α particles are used to irradiate tissues. X rays and γ rays interact mainly with target biological molecules in an indirect way. The interaction is initially with other atoms and molecules within the cells to produce free radicals. These are highly reactive molecules with an unpaired electron in the outer orbital shell and are able to diffuse far enough to reach and damage the critical targets.

Since approximately 80% of a cell is composed of water, it is necessary to consider what happens when radiation interacts with a water molecule. As a result of the interaction with a photon, the water molecule may become ionized.

$$H_2O - H_2O^+ + e$$

H_2O^+ is an ion radical—it is an ion because it is charged and a free radical because it has an unpaired electron in its outer shell. It is a highly reactive species with a very short lifespan in the order of nanoseconds. The ion radical can then interact with another water molecule to form the highly reactive hydroxyl radical (OH).

$$H_2O^+ + H_2O - H_3O^+ + OH$$

It is estimated that about two thirds of the damage to biological targets from X rays is produced by hydroxyl radicals. Free radicals can be inactivated by combining with sulphydryl molecules or they may interact with oxygen and form a highly reactive product, and by so doing, the damage may be fixed (i.e., made permanent). The interaction process is summarized in Figure 4.

Regardless of whether radiation effects occur because of the direct or indirect interaction, the main

biological target in tissues is believed to be DNA. Such interactions result in changes in DNA chemistry, leading to breaks within one or both helical strands. A single-strand break within DNA may be recognized and repaired as the complementary DNA strand is still present to act as a template. When several ionizations occur in close proximity, a double-strand DNA break may occur. It is thought that double-strand breaks are the lethal lesions that result in cell kill because of the inability of the cell to repair both damaged strands of DNA simultaneously. Apart from the physical characteristics of radiation beams, there are a number of other important features relating to cells and tissues themselves that influence their response to radiotherapy. These features are discussed below.

RADIOBIOLOGY

Radiobiology is the study of the actions of ionizing radiation on living things. The effects of radiation on both normal and malignant tissues evolve through a series of steps. This begins with the physical absorption of energy and ends with the biological effect, which results principally from damage to DNA. Classical radiobiology promotes the four "Rs" of the radiation response: repair, redistribution, reoxygenation, and repopulation (2). The development of tissue culture techniques has contributed enormously to our understanding of radiobiology in ways that are not possible to achieve in patients. With such techniques, it is possible to observe the effects of radiation on cells in vitro. The cell survival curve is a cornerstone of in vitro radiobiology and describes the relationship between radiation dose and the proportion of cells surviving (Fig. 5). Survival refers to the ability of a single cell to proliferate indefinitely to produce a large clone or colony. Such a cell is said to be clonogenic. Tumor cells are clonogenic, and if one cell survives after a course of radiotherapy, this may be sufficient for the tumor to regrow.

Repair

Radiation damage to mammalian cells can be divided into the following three categories.

Lethal damage—this is irreversible and irreparable leading irrevocably to cell death.

Sublethal damage (SLD)—this is damage that under normal circumstances can be repaired over a number of hours. SLD repair is inferred by the increase in survival observed when a dose of radiation is split into two fractions separated by a time interval.

Potentially lethal damage (PLD)—this refers to the component of radiation damage that can be modified by postirradiation environmental conditions.

The ability of cells to repair SLD was recognized by Elkind and colleagues, who demonstrated that the survival of Chinese hamster cells treated with a single dose of radiation was lower than that of cells given the same total dose of radiation, but split into two fractions separated by 30 minutes (Fig. 6) (3). Mechanisms

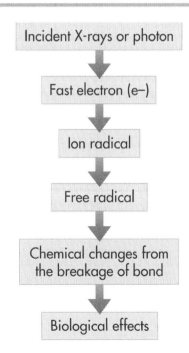

Figure 4 Summary of interaction of X rays or photons. *Source*: Adapted from Ref. 1.

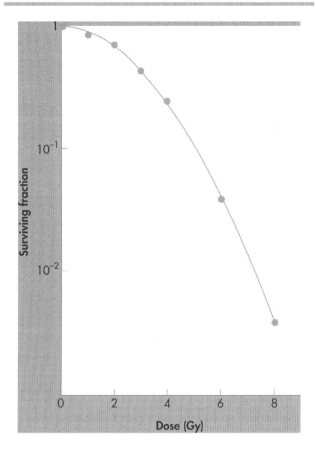

Figure 5 Clonogenic cell survival curve following radiation. A typical surviving fraction at 2 Gy is 0.6 with higher doses producing a lower surviving fraction. *Source*: Courtesy of Dr Gillian Duchesne.

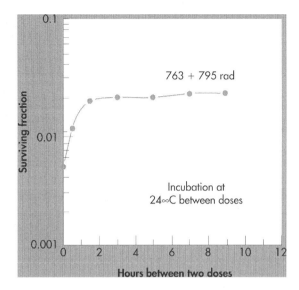

Figure 6 Survival of Chinese hamster cells exposed to two fractions of X rays with various time intervals between the two and incubated at room temperature. As the time interval is increased the surviving fraction increases until at about two hours, a plateau is reached corresponding to a surviving fraction of 0.02. *Source*: Courtesy of Ref. 3.

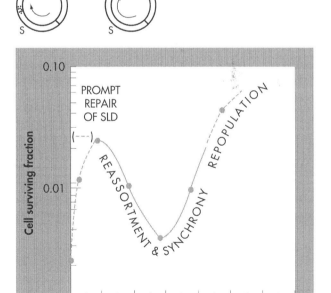

Figure 7 Survival of Chinese hamster cells exposed to two fractions of X rays with various time intervals between the two doses. This also illustrates three of the four Rs of radiobiology. *Source*: Courtesy of Refs. 1 and 3.

of DNA repair include nonhomologous end-joining and homologous recombination.

Redistribution

The radiosensitivity of cells also varies with the phases of the cell cycle (Fig. 7). Radiation damage to DNA is frequently not expressed until cell division. Cells that are in the G0 (resting) phase or only in a very slow cell cycle will not express damage immediately. The length of the cell cycle for most rapidly dividing tumors is approximately 24 hours. In such tumors, the interval between fractions of radiation may be critical to the cell kill achieved, as radiation sensitivity varies by at least two fold through the cycle. Cells located in the S phase of the cell cycle are said to be relatively radioresistant, while those in the G2 or M phase are said to be radiosensitive. In the experiments by Elkind et al. (3) described above, most of the surviving cells from the first dose of radiation were located in the S phase. When a second dose of radiation was given after an interval of six hours, this cohort of cells had progressed around the cell cycle and was now in the G2 or M phase (more sensitive) at the time of the second dose—a process called redistribution (or reassignment). If the increase in radiosensitivity in moving from late S to the G2-M period exceeds the effect of SLD repair, the surviving fraction will fall. In human tissues, the time intervals for cell cycles and SLD repair are generally less well defined, but maximal recovery appears to be complete after four to six hours.

While this phenomenon is relatively easy to demonstrate and manipulate in vitro, it has been difficult to exploit in routine clinical practice.

Reoxygenation

The importance of a good blood supply for radiosensitivity was first recognized by Mottram in 1924 (4). Further work by Thoday and Reed (5) demonstrated that the proportion of chromosome aberrations resulting from irradiation of root tips in oxygen was three times greater than those seen when irradiation was carried out in nitrogen. They concluded that the availability of oxygen is a very important factor in the production of radiation-induced chromosome aberrations. Experiments by Thomlinson and Gray (6) and Tannock (7) led to the conclusion that cells were present in only two states, which have radiobiological significance—oxygenated and hypoxic. Tumor cells closest to blood vessels are generally well oxygenated, and those at a distance greater than the oxygen-diffusion capacity are hypoxic.

Acute as well as chronic hypoxia occurs within tumors; intermittent blood flow within abnormal tumor vasculature was shown to be a cause of acute hypoxia and variability in radiation response by Chaplin et al. in 1986 (8). The proportion of hypoxic cells within solid tumors may vary considerably depending on the tumor type. Although a dynamic process, the hypoxic fraction is thought to remain relatively constant within a given tumor. Immediately after a radiation exposure, remaining viable cells are more likely to be hypoxic, as the well-oxygenated cells die. Over the following hours, oxygen diffuses into these previously hypoxic areas and reoxygenation occurs. The cells are now more sensitive to the next radiation exposure and the whole process is repeated again. Over a fractionated radiotherapy schedule of several weeks, it is likely that most cells will receive some radiation exposure while in the oxygenated state. Efforts to overcome tumor hypoxia have dominated radiobiological research for the past 40 years. The approaches investigated have included hyperbaric oxygen and hypoxic-cell radiosensitizing drugs, such as misonidazole, but they have met with only limited success.

Repopulation

During a course of fractionated radiotherapy, viable tumor cells continue to divide and repopulate the tumor. Repopulation is an important process for early-responding normal tissues, such as the gut and bone marrow. A protracted, fractionated regimen helps to spare these normal tissues but may compromise tumor cure. In the above experiment, when the interval between the split doses is 10 to 12 hours, there is an increase in the surviving fraction because of cell division (repopulation) because this time interval exceeds the length of the cell cycle of these rapidly growing cells.

Treatment with radiation or cytotoxic drugs can trigger surviving clonogens in a tumor to divide faster than tumor cells in an unperturbed state. This is known as accelerated repopulation. There is evidence that this phenomenon may occur in human tumors. Withers et al. (9) used the published literature on radiotherapy for head and neck cancer to estimate the dose of radiation required to achieve local control in 50% of cases [tumor control dose$_{50}$ (TCD$_{50}$)]. The analysis suggests that clonogen repopulation in this type of cancer accelerates at about day 28 after treatment begins. A dose increment of about 0.6 Gy/day is thought to be required to compensate for this repopulation. In clinical practice the dose of radiation per fraction is not usually increased after day 28 provided there are no unscheduled gaps over the course of the treatment. Cancers of the bladder, head and neck and cervix are tumors where gaps or delays in treatment are thought to have considerable significance for overall tumor control probability. It has been recommended that, if gaps in treatment occur in these types of tumors some form of compensation is required to ensure tumor control is not compromised (10). This may involve increasing the dose per fraction for part or all of the remaining treatment or hyperfractionation, where two fractions are given on the same day with an interfraction interval of at least six hours.

The Linear Quadratic Model

The duration of the cell cycle and the ability of cells to repair SLD, varies not only between different normal tissues but also between normal tissues and tumors. Normal tissues may be divided into those that are considered "early responding," such as skin, mucosal epithelium and bone marrow and those that are "late responding," such as the spinal cord and central nervous system tissue. Most tumors behave as early-responding tissues. Early-responding tissues are triggered to proliferate within a few weeks of starting a fractionated course of radiotherapy and tissue damage, such as skin desquamation or tumor shrinkage, will become apparent during the course of treatment. However, a conventional course of radiotherapy of six to seven weeks is never long enough to trigger proliferation in late-responding tissues; consequently, radiation effects on these tissues may not become apparent for months to years after the treatment.

Various mathematical models have been used to describe the shape of the cell survival curve and are useful for the theoretical interpretation of observed experimental changes. The linear quadratic (α/β) model is one model where α measures the probability of causing lethal damage by a single event (such as a double-stranded DNA break), and β estimates the probability of cell death from the interaction between two separate sublethal events. (α is a measure of the

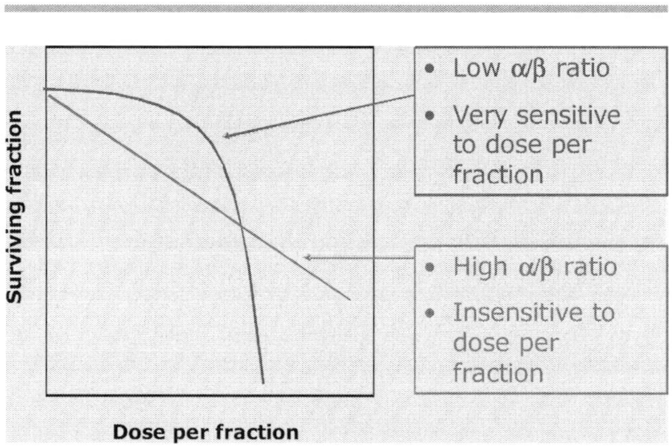

Figure 8 Cell survival curve for low and high α/β ratio.

width of the shoulder of the curve, while β indicates the curviness of the curve.) It is the ratio of α/β [i.e., the dose at which cell killing by linear (α) and quadratic (β) components is equal], rather than the individual values of each, which determines how tissues behave to changes in fractionation. Early-responding tissues and most tumors have a high α/β ratio (10–30 Gy), indicating that they are relatively insensitive to changes in radiotherapy fractionation. Late-responding tissues have a low α/β (1–4 Gy) indicating a higher degree of sensitivity to fractionation changes. By altering fractionation, it is possible to produce a differential in cell kill between tumors and late-responding normal tissues, modifying the therapeutic index (i.e., the tumor response for a fixed level of normal tissue damage) (Fig. 8).

Most tumors arise from epithelial cells and have a fairly high α/β ratio (10–25 Gy). Tissues that give rise to late reactions (months or years) in radiotherapy have relatively low α/β ratios and changes in fractionation can be made that improve the therapeutic ratio.

However, adenocarcinoma of the prostate has been estimated to have a low α/β ratio (approximately 1.5 Gy). This is even lower than the estimated α/β ratio of late bowel effects (3 Gy). If this data is correct, a hypofractionated schedule of radiotherapy (>2 Gy per fraction) could potentially achieve improved tumor control without increasing toxicity. The CHHIP [conventional or hypofractionated high-dose intensity-modulated radiotherapy (IMRT) for prostate cancer] trial (11) is a phase III randomized controlled trial comparing different fractionation regimes (60 Gy/20 fractions of radiotherapy and 57 Gy/19 fractions) against the standard (74 Gy/37 fractions) to look at local control rates and long-term side effects, and will also yield further radiobiological data.

Combined Modality Treatment

The combination of chemotherapy or biological agents with radiotherapy is increasingly used to try and improve local control rates and eradicate micrometastases. The effects of multimodality treatment can be additive, synergistic or independent. By using two treatment modalities, resistance mechanisms are

more likely to be overcome. The systemic agents may also radiosensitize tumor tissue and may favorably alter the tumor biology, for example, by reoxygenation, cell cycle redistribution, inhibiting DNA repair and impairing accelerated repopulation. This concept is being evaluated for bladder cancer in a randomized controlled trial comparing radical radiotherapy with radiotherapy plus concomitant 5 FU/mitomycin C. Theoretically, 5 FU would kill radioresistant cells in the S phase of the cell cycle. In addition, radiation induces the expression of thymidine phosphorylase in cancer tissues, which is the first enzyme involved in the activation of 5 FU (12).

PRINCIPLES OF RADIOTHERAPY TREATMENT

Radiation is an important modality for the treatment of cancer and can be used with radical, adjuvant or palliative intent. To justify treatment with radiotherapy it is important that patients have histological confirmation of cancer and relevant imaging. They should have all their treatment options discussed, be aware of treatment intentions, side effects and consent to treatment.

Radical radiotherapy aims to deliver a tumoricidal treatment dose to a well-defined target volume with curative intent, sparing the surrounding normal tissues as much as possible. Currently, most departments use 3-D conformal radiotherapy, which is achieved using modern linear accelerators with multileaf collimators. More recently a further development has been IMRT. This technique uses computer-assisted technology to modify and shape the intensity of radiotherapy beams during treatment to deliver very precise coverage of the target area, with even greater conformity. Radical radiotherapy is given as a fractionated course, usually over six to eight weeks for localized tumors of the bladder, prostate and penis.

Adjuvant radiotherapy is used to reduce the risk of tumor recurrence after primary surgery. The aim of treatment is to eradicate occult micrometastatic disease that cannot be demonstrated on imaging as occurs in a significant percentage of patients. An example of this is prophylactic, para-aortic radiotherapy after orchidectomy for stage 1 seminoma. Adjuvant treatment in this setting reduced relapse rates from approximately 20% to 3% to 4% (13).

Palliative radiotherapy can be used to alleviate symptoms of local disease (such as hematuria) or distant metastases (such as bone pain). Treatment is usually given with a small number of fractions, and effective results can also be achieved with a single fraction of radiotherapy.

The planning and delivery of radiotherapy is discussed below:

RADIOTHERAPY PLANNING

The initial phase of any radiotherapy is treatment planning, during which the following parameters are defined:

- Patient position and immobilization
- Definition of treatment volumes

- Choice of technique
- Calculation of dose distribution

Patient Position and Immobilization

The treatment position of the patient must be accurately reproducible throughout radiotherapy. Variation in daily positioning is a result of daily treatment setup and internal organ movement and as a result can alter external and internal anatomy of the patient. Ultimately, this can lead to underdosage of the tumor or an overdosage of the surrounding normal tissues.

To limit patient setup error they are immobilized in a comfortable position thereby minimizing movement. Treatment position varies with different tumor sites but for urological tumors, the patient is supine. Accurate patient setup on the planning machine is achieved by aligning fixed, wall mounted lasers to certain anatomical reference points such as bony landmarks or permanent skin tattoos applied during planning. An identical alignment system is then used on the treatment machine, ensuring that patient setup is fully reproducible.

There is also a need to limit variation in internal organ movement. For example, the position of the prostate is dependent on the relative positions of the bladder and rectum. Therefore tumors of the prostate are usually treated with a full bladder to reduce the volume of bladder tissue irradiated and also to move the small intestine out of the field. Patients are given dietary advice/ laxatives to keep the rectal volume as small as possible. To limit normal tissue toxicity it is also necessary to determine if any normal tissues need to be shielded. For example, in penile cancer, the penis is placed in a block and this

rests on a lead shield, which protects the underlying testis and skin.

Definition of Treatment Volumes

In delivery of radiotherapy treatment, parameters such as volume and dose have to be specified for the purposes of prescription, recording and reporting. This has been standardized by the International Committee of Radiation Units and Measurements (ICRU), allowing national and international comparison of treatments between different centers (14). This report defines the concepts of gross tumor volume (GTV), clinical target volume (CTV), and planning target volume (PTV).

The GTV is the demonstrable macroscopic extent of the tumor. To encompass subclinical or microscopic disease, one adds a margin to the GTV and this volume is defined as the CTV. During a course of radiotherapy there may be technical and physiological variations, which can cause movement of the CTV. To ensure that the prescribed dose is delivered to the CTV for every fraction of treatment, a further margin is added to form the PTV. This is a combination of a setup margin (SM) to allow for variation in patient positioning and an internal margin (IM) to account for normal organ movement.

Localization of the Target Volume

The target volume for internal tumors is usually localized by plain X rays on a machine called a simulator (conventional planning) or a computerized tomography (CT) scanner with an integrated computerized planning system (CT planning) (Fig. 9).

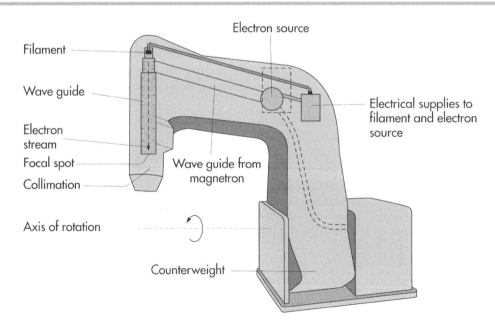

Figure 9 A simulator. This is a diagnostic X-ray unit which has an image intensifier linked to a closed-circuit television for the purpose of screening. It can reproduce treatment conditions.

For radical radiotherapy the target volume is localized using a CT planning scan and the data from this is sent to the radiotherapy planning computer for outlining. This has the advantage of providing anatomical detail about the tumor and surrounding normal tissues, allowing for 3-D conformal therapy or IMRT.

A simulator is a diagnostic X-ray machine used to reproduce the exact treatment arrangement for any MV therapy machine. It has the facility for screening by an image intensifier linked to a close-circuit television. In the simulator, the target volume is localized by using both clinical information (staging results, surface anatomy and palpable masses) and radiological information (image intensifier views and staging diagnostic X rays). The conventional method of planning a bladder cancer, for example, involves the introduction of contrast into the bladder through a urinary catheter. Anteroposterior and lateral X-ray films are then taken on the simulator and these are then used to outline the target volume.

Choice of Technique

In addition to the target volumes defined above, the other important considerations in the choice of technique are the types of normal tissues within the proposed treatment volume. During a course of radiotherapy it is inevitable that both the tumor and normal tissues will be irradiated. There is considerable variation in the tolerance of different normal tissues to radiotherapy, and the Therapeutic Index, which is the tumor response for a fixed level of normal tissue damage, is a major determination of both the total dose that can be delivered and the treatment technique. Therefore, it is important to outline and identify the important normal tissues within the target volume as well as the tumor.

The simplest technique for treatment is a single radiation field (Fig. 10). This is often used for palliative therapy, such as treatment of bone metastases. Another simple arrangement is the use of two opposing parallel fields (anterior and posterior or two lateral fields). This produces a more even dose distribution throughout the irradiated area than a single field and the combination of fields allows greater penetration at

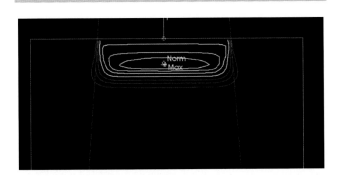

Figure 10 Electron isodose chart.

depth. This technique is used for the prophylactic treatment of the para-aortic lymph nodes in stage 1 seminoma (Fig. 11).

For radical treatment of the prostate or bladder it is necessary to use higher treatment doses and often three or four fields are used to allow the greatest sparing of normal tissues while maximizing the tumor dose (Fig. 12). This can be achieved with 3-D conformal radiotherapy, which allows closer, more accurate irradiation of irregularly shaped tumor volumes. Treatment beams are produced within the machine, which conform much more closely to the shape of the target volume. This produces greater sparing of normal tissues allowing higher and potentially more effective doses of radiation to be delivered to the tumor without increasing side effects (15).

An emerging technique is the use of high-precision radiotherapy in the form of IMRT. This allows closer matching of treatment doses to tumor volumes. Rather than having a single or a few radiation beams, the radiation with IMRT is effectively broken into thousands of tiny pencil-thin beams. These enter the body from many different angles and all converge on the tumor. This produces a high tumor dose and a lower dose to surrounding normal tissues. An example of this is the use of IMRT in the treatment of pelvic lymph nodes in prostate cancer.

Calculation of the Dose Distribution

Once the PTV and important normal organs are localized, a dose distribution across the target volume is calculated and a plan is produced. This is done using a computer software that manipulates dose data measured directly from treatment machines. On reviewing the plan, the oncologist will ensure that the target is covered by the 95% isodose line and according to ICRU that there is a maximum variation of dose distribution of from −5% to +7% in dose across the PTV (Fig. 13). The dose to the normal tissues is also checked to ensure that their tolerance is not exceeded.

Treatment Delivery

Once an acceptable treatment plan has been agreed on, planning information is transferred to the treatment machine and therapy is started. An essential part of all treatment is verification of the planning setup, which is achieved by comparison of X rays or scans taken during simulation and treatment. Each center will define an accepted degree of variation between the images taken at simulation and those taken during treatment. For radical plans of the pelvis this is usually between 3 and 5 mm.

Therapy doses may also be checked directly during treatment by measurements from the patient. The entire process from planning to verification of treatment delivery is governed by the principles of quality assurance. These define procedures that test all the technical aspects of radiotherapy systems to eliminate any inaccuracy or deficiency leading to suboptimal treatments and must be a routine part of treatment.

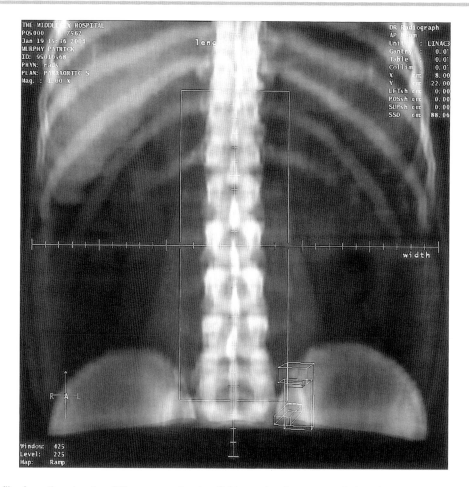

Figure 11   An AP film from the planning CT scanner, showing field margins for para-aortic lymph node irradiation.

Side Effects of Treatment

The side effects of radiotherapy may be divided into those that occur during or within a few weeks of treatment (acute reactions) and those that occur months to years later (late reactions). The severity of side effects depends principally on the normal tissues present in the treatment field, total dose and dose per fraction of treatment given. It is important to realize that the radiobiological principles defined in the previous section of the chapter are the basis for both the desirable therapeutic effects and the undesirable side effects that occur during a course of treatment.

During radical radiotherapy for prostate or bladder cancer patients principally experience a range of side effects to the normal bladder, bowel and skin within the treatment volume. These may include deterioration of urinary outflow symptoms, hematuria, proctitis and diarrhea. They are generally the effects of radiation on the normal acute-reacting tissues in the treatment volume. Acute side effects such as these are usually self-limiting and generally resolve within six to eight weeks after completing treatment. They can usually be successfully managed with supportive care during radiotherapy.

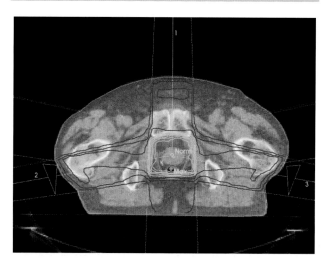

Figure 12   A three-field plan of the prostate showing an anterior and two posterior oblique wedged fields.

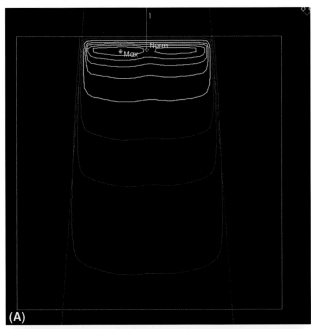

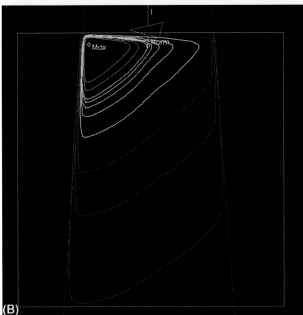

Figure 13 Isodose curves for a 6-MV linear accelerator (**A**) open field (**B**) wedged field.

The late effects of radiotherapy are usually more serious and may be irreversible. For pelvic radiotherapy, these local late effects include bladder fibrosis, chronic proctitis and impotence. Radiation carcinogenesis is another late effect that occurs within the site of the treatment volume and is believed to be due to radiation-induced genetic damage to normal tissues. It tends to occur after other late effects. In all radiotherapy treatments, the balance to be achieved lies between the desired beneficial effects (cure or palliation) and the level of acute and late effects that can be tolerated by the treated individual.

Brachytherapy

Brachytherapy has been used in the treatment of urological cancer for over 90 years, but it experienced a renaissance for the treatment of prostate cancer in the 1980s (16). This was due to improved prostatic imaging with transrectal ultrasound and technological advances in computerized planning systems, allowing better dosimetry and more accurate treatment.

The planning principles for brachytherapy are the same as for external beam treatment volumes (i.e., patient immobilization, definition of treatment volumes, choice of technique and calculation of the dose distribution). Selecting patients for brachytherapy is a combination of tumor characteristics and the ability of the patient to comply with radioprotection issues.

Brachytherapy can be used as a single modality to deliver a radical treatment alone (such a slow dose rate ^{125}I seed brachytherapy) or in combination with external beam radiotherapy to deliver a boost treatment (such as high dose–rate ^{192}Ir brachytherapy).

Permanent Iodine Seed Brachytherapy

Treatment with ^{125}I seeds is indicated for patients with low grade, organ confined tumors with a small volume (less than 50 cm^3) and no previous transurethral surgery (Fig. 14). Treatment has two stages, planning and therapy, both are carried out with the patient in the lithotomy position under anesthetic. Planning involves a transrectal ultrasound guided prostatic volume study that is done with reference to a fixable perineal positioning template. The prostate is positioned within the template grid and the urethra is centered in the middle row. Serial ultrasounds are taken from the apex to the base and the prostate is outlined. This information is sent to the planning

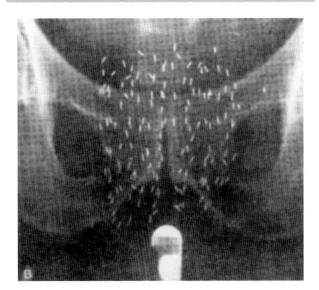

Figure 14 AP simulator film showing the distribution of ^{125}I seeds within the prostate.

computer and the relationship of the prostate to the surface template allows the exact number and position of each iodine seed to be planned and calculated with precision. In the second stage of the treatment applicator needles are inserted transperineally through the template into the corresponding planned position within the prostate. The iodine seeds are then inserted and the applicator needles withdrawn. A typical implant involves 60 to 120 seeds depending on prostatic volume and individual seed activity.

The aim of treatment is to deliver a dose of 145 Gy to the prostate plus margin and to limit the maximum rectal dose to < 200 Gy and urethral dose <220 Gy. The half life of ^{125}I is 59.4 days, with dose accumulation over the first few weeks and then a dose fall off to very low levels (17).

High–Dose Rate ^{192}Ir Brachytherapy

A temporary ^{192}Ir implant can be used in combination with external beam radiotherapy to escalate the dose of radiation to the prostate without significantly increasing normal tissue morbidity (Figs. 15 and 16) (18). The aim is improved local tumor control, and this treatment is mainly used for higher grade or locally advanced tumors. The implant procedure is similar to iodine seed therapy with a perineal template and applicator needles. In this case, instead of iodine seeds, which deliver the dose of radiation over many days, a very high activity (high dose rate) radioactive iridium source is used to deliver treatment over a period of minutes. Following insertion of the applicator needles a CT scan is done. The target volume and organs at risk are outlined on the planning system.

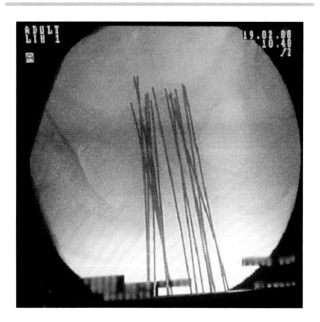

Figure 15 AP film of needles implanted in the prostate for ^{192}Ir high dose rate after loading brachytherapy.

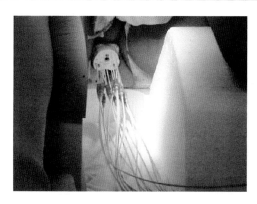

Figure 16 A patient in the lithotomy position attached to the microselectron unit while undergoing ^{192}Ir high dose rate after loading brachytherapy.

For treatment, flexible tubes link the template and applicator needles to a remote after-loading machine containing the iridium source. The iridium is driven under computer control into each successive applicator needle and moved within the needle in small steps for predetermined time periods (dwell times). This allows the total dose of treatment to the prostate to be built up over three to four fractionated treatments usually given over two days. There is also an advantage in allowing the dose to be optimized for the final resting position of each applicator needle in relation to all the others. At completion of treatment, the needles and template are removed and the patient proceeds to external beam radiotherapy after a 2-week break (Fig. 16).

CONCLUSION

Radiotherapy has an important role in both the radical and palliative treatment of urological tumors. The basic principles of physics and radiobiology are crucial to the optimization of treatment schedules and delivery. The science of radiation treatment continues to evolve with the aim of allowing higher and more effective doses of radiation to be delivered with minimal toxicity. The full potential of radiotherapy either alone or in combination with other therapies perhaps has yet to be fully realized.

REFERENCES

1. Hall EJ. The physics and chemistry of radiation absorption. In: Hall EJ, ed. Radiobiology for the Radiologist. Philadelphia: Lippincott Williams and Wilkins, 1994:1–14.
2. Withers HR. The four ''R''s of radiotherapy. Adv Radiat Biol 1975; 5:241–247.
3. Elkind MM, Sutton-Gilbert H, Moses WB, et al. Radiation response of mammalian cells in culture. V. Temperature dependence of the repair of X-ray damage in surviving cells (aerobic and hypoxic). Radiat Res 1965; 25:359–376.
4. Mottram JC. On the skin reactions to radium exposure and their avoidance in radiotherapy: an experimental investigation. Br J Radiol 1924; 29:1–8.

5. Thoday JM, Reed J. Effect of oxygen on the frequency of chromosome aberrations produced by X-rays. Nature 1947; 160:119.

6. Tomlinson RH, Gray LH. The histological structure of some human lung cancers and the possible implications for radiotherapy. Br J Cancer 1955; 9:59–549.

7. Tannock IF. The relation between cell proliferation and the vascular system in a transplanted mouse mammary tumour. Br J Cancer 1968; 22:258–273.

8. Chaplin DJ, Durand RE, Olive PL. Acute hypoxia in tumours: implications for modifiers of radiation effects. Int J Radiat Oncol Biol Phys 1986; 12:1279–1282.

9. Withers HR, Taylor JMG, Maciejewski B. Treatment volume and tissue tolerance Int J Radiat Oncol Biol Phys 1988; 14:751–759.

10. Royal College of Radiologists. Guidelines for the Management of the Unscheduled Interruption or Prolongation of a Radical Course of Radiotherapy. London, 1996.

11. CHHiP trial Conventional or Hypofractionated High dose Intensity Modulated Radiotherapy for Prostate cancer. Chief Investigator Professor David Dearnaley, Royal Marsden Hospital. Sponsored by Institute of Cancer Research.

12. Huddart RA, Hall EJ, James ND, et al. BC2001: a multicentre phase III randomized trial of standard versus reduced volume radiotherapy for muscle invasive bladder cancer. J Clin Oncol 2009; 27(suppl; abstr 5022):15s.

13. Fossa SD, Horwich A, Russell JM, et al. Medical Research Council Testicular Tumour Working Party. Optimal planning target volume for stage I testicular seminoma; an MRC randomised trial J Clin Oncol 1999; 17:1146–1154.

14. International Commission on Radiation Units and Measurements. Prescribing, recording and reporting photon beam therapy. ICRU 50. Washington DC: International Commission on Radiation Units and Measurements, 1993.

15. Dearnaley DP, Khoo VS, Norman AR, et al. Comparison of radiation side-effects of conformal and conventional radiotherapy in prostate cancer: a randomised trial. Lancet 1999; 353:267–272.

16. Holm HH, Juul N, Pedersen JF. Transperineal 125-iodine seed implantation in protatic cancer guided by transrectal ultrasonography. J Urol 1983; 10:283–286.

17. Hoskin P, Coyle C. Radiotherapy in Practice: Brachytherapy: Oxford: Oxford University Press, 2005:107–122

18. Mate TP, Gottesman JE, Hatton J, et al. High dose rate after loading iridium 192 prostate brachytherapy: feasibility report. Int J Radiat Oncol Biol Phys 1998; 41:525–533.

FURTHER READING

Radiation physics:

Williams JR, Thwaite DI, eds. Radiotherapy Physics in Practice. Oxford: Oxford University Press, 2000.

Khan FM. The Physics of Radiation Therapy. Linppincott Williams and Wilkins, 2003.

Radiobiology:

Steel GG. Basic Clinical Radiobiology. London: Arnold, 1997.

Radiotherapy planning:

Dobbs J, Barrett A, Ash D. Practical Radiotherapy Planning. London: Arnold, 1999.

28

Principles of Systemic Cancer Therapy

Christina Thirlwell and John Bridgewater
*University College London Cancer Institute, University College London
Medical School, London, U.K.*

Judith Cave
Southampton General Hospital, Southampton, U.K.

INTRODUCTION

Two-thirds of patients with cancer will develop metastatic disease during their illness. The most appropriate management for metastatic disease is systemic treatment, and this is most commonly chemotherapy or, more recently targeted, biological therapies. The potential benefit of systemic therapy for cancer has been proposed for sometime—in 1875 Cutler and Bradford induced remission in a patient with chronic myeloid leukemia by treatment with arsenic (1). During the First World War, soldiers who died of mustard gas poisoning were noted to have aplastic bone marrow suggesting a cytotoxic effect of mustard compounds (2). In 1946, Goodman and colleagues (3) successfully demonstrated that the cytotoxic effects of nitrogen mustard could treat a mouse transplanted with lymphosarcoma. The first human cancer to be cured by chemotherapy was choriocarcinoma, which has been cured with the drug methotrexate since the 1950s.

In this chapter the pharmacological, molecular, and biological basis of systemic anticancer treatment will be discussed, as well as some of the practical issues surrounding the administration of chemotherapy. Recent research has concentrated on improving response rates by the development of new molecularly targeted drugs and better supportive care.

CYTOKINETICS

The study of cytokinetics is central to oncological practice because of the observation that cells that are dividing more rapidly are usually more sensitive to chemotherapy (4). Choriocarcinomas and teratomas double in cell number in less than one month and are cured in more than 80% of cases, but colonic carcinomas double in over three months and are often resistant to chemotherapy (5–7). The relationship between cell doubling time and prognosis is not simple but for many types of tumor markers of high cell proliferation correlate with poor prognosis.

Tumor Growth

The relationship between cell cycle time and tumor doubling time is complex (Fig. 1). A proportion of cells will be in G0 or resting phase, either because they have differentiated into nondividing cells or because they are necrotic or apoptotic or because they are resting. Doubling time is therefore influenced by the growth fraction, the cells lost, and the cell cycle time.

Tumor growth has been modeled using tissue cultures and animals. The simplest model of tumor growth is exponential cell growth, which assumes that tumor doubling time is constant and therefore tumor size will increase exponentially with time (Fig. 2). An alternative is Gompertzian growth. In this model the growth fraction decreases as the tumor size increases, taking into account the effect of increased tumor size on blood supply, nutrients, and physical constraints. A Gompertzian growth curve is sigmoid in shape (8) and is a better reflection of the clinical scenario.

Cell Killing

There are numerous models of cell killing by treatment, and these are relevant to therapeutics. The first model is fractional cell kill, also known as the Skipper–Schabel–Wilcox model (9). Assuming that all cells in a tumor are equally sensitive to chemotherapy and that the tumor is growing exponentially, a given dose of a given drug will kill a constant fraction of the cells. If the treatment is repeated, or if another drug is given alongside the first drug, then the two fractional cell kills will be multiplied (Fig. 3). Adjuvant treatment (discussed later) of micrometastases after surgical removal of primary tumors is based on this hypothesis—the less the tumor load at the start of chemotherapy the higher the possibility of eradicating all the tumor and therefore curing a proportion of patients.

Unfortunately, it is not always true that adequate doses of chemotherapy will eradicate all tumor cells. The failure to completely eliminate even very small tumors with chemotherapy is largely due to drug resistance. If all cancers are clonal in origin (10), one would expect uniform sensitivity to drugs. However, as a tumor divides, spontaneous mutations occur and some of the cells will develop drug resistance. Consequently, most chemotherapy regimes include combinations of drugs in an attempt to avoid selecting out resistant cells in a heterogeneous tumor (Fig. 4).

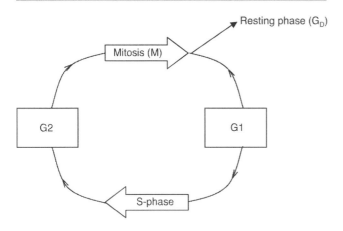

Figure 1 The cell cycle. Cells cycle between synthesis of DNA (S-phase) and mitosis or M-phase with variable gaps between protein synthesis and cell division (Gap 1 or G1 and Gap 2 or G2). Withdrawal into resting phase (G0) can be reversible or permanent. Progression around the cell cycle is dependent on cyclins and cyclin-dependent kinases.

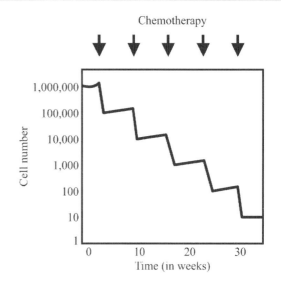

Figure 3 Cell kill.

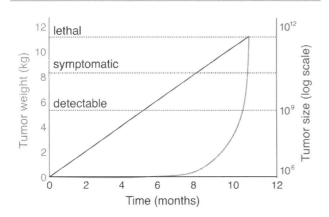

Figure 2 Exponential tumor growth.

PHARMACOLOGY

Scheduling and combining drugs correctly is crucial to the success of chemotherapy regimes. For example, some drugs work better when intermittently dosed than when given as continuous infusions (12–15). Intermittent dosing allows time for normal tissue recovery between doses, it is therefore both feasible and logistically sensible. In general, drugs with a short half-life ($T_{1/2}$) are more effective when given as an infusion to maintain steady state concentration, such as 5-fluorouracil (5-FU), which has a short half-life of seven minutes. In contrast, drugs with a longer $T_{1/2}$ such as cisplatin ($T_{1/2} = 7$ hours) are given as a shorter infusion. Toxicity also changes with scheduling. When 5-FU is given as a bolus, its toxicity is predominantly mucositis and neutropenia, whereas as an infusion it

is primarily hand-foot syndrome. When combination regimens are being designed, drugs with different mechanisms of action, resistance, and dose-limiting toxicities should be combined. All drugs in a regime should be active as single agents, and interactions should be considered.

Cytotoxic drugs have various mechanisms of action, and some of these are listed in Table 1. Some drugs act only on cells that are cycling and may even be specific to cells in a particular phase of the cell cycle. For example, microtubule poisons such as taxanes act during mitosis and cause metaphase arrest, but alkylating agents are cell cycle independent. Drug action is not always confined to one class; for example, mitomycin C is primarily an antitumor antibiotic, but it can also alkylate DNA.

DRUG RESISTANCE

Tumor cells may be resistant to drugs for reasons relating to the tumor, the drug, or the host. Some parts of a tumor may have such a poor blood supply that adequate doses of drug cannot reach the cells; nonreplicating cells may escape the cytotoxic effects of some drugs. In addition, there are "sanctuary sites" in the body where cytotoxic drugs cannot penetrate, classically the central nervous system and the testes. Individual patient characteristics can also cause tumor resistance (16); for example, if drugs are metabolized very efficiently or not absorbed adequately, then the dose reaching the tumor will not be effective. Inability of the patients to tolerate sufficient doses of drugs because of toxicity may also lead to ineffective dosage and lack of efficacy.

True resistance to adequate concentrations of drug can be either intrinsic or acquired. This often manifests clinically with disease progression while undergoing treatment.

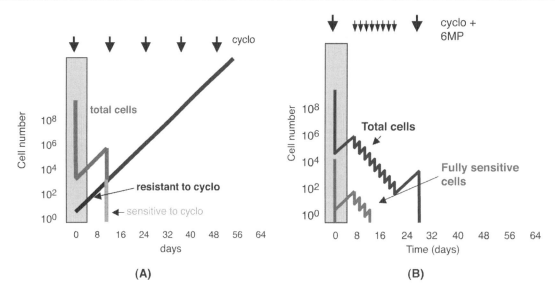

Figure 4 (**A**) Selection of a resistant clone by single agent cyclophosphamide chemotherapy. (**B**) Use of combination chemotherapy to overcome drug resistance. *Source*: Part A from Ref. 11.

Table 1 Mechanisms of Action of Chemotherapy

Class of drug	Examples	Target	Mechanism of action
Alkylating agents	Cyclophosphamide, thiotepa, carmustine, cisplatin	DNA	Create DNA cross-links that cannot be repaired
Antimetabolites	Methotrexate, cytarabine, flourouracil, fludarabine	Antifolates, purine, and pyrimidine analogues	Resemble normal substrates for RNA and DNA synthesis. Protein synthesis is aborted leading to cell death
Mitotic inhibitors	Vinca alkaloids Taxanes	Microtubules	Disrupt/stabilize microtubules leading to metaphase arrest
Topoisomerase drugs	Irinotecan/topotecan	Topoisomerase I	Binds to topoisomerase I–DNA cleavable complex and prevents re-ligation after cleavage
	Etoposide	Topoisomerase II	Produces double strand breaks in DNA an prevents entry of cells into mitosis
Antibiotics	Doxorubicin (and other anthracyclins)	DNA	Intercalation into DNA causes untwisting of DNA helix and strand breaks
	Bleomycin	DNA	Single- and double-strand DNA breaks
	Mitomycin	DNA	Cross-links DNA preventing function

Multidrug Resistance

Once a tumor is resistant to one drug, it is often also resistant to many other drugs. This discovery has led to the concept of "multidrug resistance," the best studied mechanism of which is P-glycoprotein over-expression. P-glycoprotein is a cell membrane glyco-protein pump coded for by the multidrug resistance (MDR-1) gene, which removes drugs from the cell (17). It is a naturally occurring glycoprotein that forms part of secretory epithelial structures similar to biliary canaliculi. Increased expression of MDR-1 (18) occurs when cells are cultured in the presence of cytotoxic drugs. MDR1a knockout mice, who cannot produce P-glycoprotein, have tumors that do not develop drug resistance. Similarly P-glycoprotein overexpression in vivo correlates with reduced responsiveness to drugs and reduced survival in some series (19).

It is possible to block P-glycoprotein and prevent the transmembrane protein from pumping drugs out of cells. Drugs available for this purpose include verapamil, quinidine, and cylcosporin A. Clinical trials using these drugs have demonstrated some success in altering pharmacokinetics (20), but in general clinical efficacy has not improved survival. It is likely that overexpression of P-glycoprotein is only one of many mechanisms involved in multidrug resistance (21–23).

Reduced apoptosis of DNA damaged cells may be an important mechanism of drug resistance. Apop-tosis in tumor cells is under the control of a complex pathway, which includes p53 and the Bcl-2 family of proteins (24). Cells with mutant p53 are more likely to be drug resistant than those with wild-type p53 (25–27), and there is interest in restoring wild-type p53 to cells in order to stimulate apoptosis after chemotherapy. Overexpression of the antiapoptotic protein Bcl-2 also contributes to chemoresistance, and modulation of Bcl-2 function may increase chemosensitivity (28). Bcl-2 antisense oligonucleotide therapy has also been tested in patients with non-Hodgkin's Lymphoma (29).

Resistance to Specific Drugs

Resistance mechanisms can be specific to a particular drug, a selection of these are outlined in Table 2. For example, anthracyclines and epipodophyllotoxins stabilize the cleavable complex formed by topoisomerase II and DNA. Topoisomerase II expression can be upregulated or topoisomerase II can mutate and change its intracellular location to avoid this effect (30,31). These mechanisms collectively are known as Topo II related drug resistance.

TOXICITY

Toxicities are generally divided into early and late, and while the majority are early toxicities, such as hair loss, which are entirely reversible, some late toxicities are not. The toxicity of a treatment often defines the doses at which a drug can be given, and therefore can be a key factor in limiting efficacy. Management of toxicity is clearly vital to the optimal delivery of chemotherapy.

Early Toxicity

Because stem cells in the bone marrow are dividing rapidly, all chemotherapy drugs have the potential to cause temporary bone marrow suppression. Marrow toxicity is very often the dose-limiting factor for chemotherapeutic agents, and both high-dose chemotherapy and prolonged chemotherapy can cause long-term marrow dysfunction.

Most chemotherapy regimes are given once every 3 weeks, and in general, bone marrow stem cells will recover within 10 days to 3 weeks of the dose being given. Because the life span of a circulating white blood cell is 4 to 5 days, the effects of bone marrow suppression on the peripheral blood are seen 4 to 12 days after the dose is given (the "nadir" or low point). Platelet nadirs are also drug specific, but as the lifespan of platelets is longer (9–10 days), they tend to occur later in the chemotherapy cycle. Red blood cells survive in the peripheral circulation for about three months, and so anemia is usually only seen with prolonged courses of chemotherapy, primarily with platinum-based compounds.

During periods of neutropenia, patients are prone to bacterial infections (32). Many studies have shown that broad-spectrum antibiotics covering aerobic gram-negative bacilli, especially *Pseudomonas aeruginosa*, should be introduced at the first sign of fever. Treatment should not be delayed until physical signs of infection are present or an organism is identified (33). The use of prophylactic oral quinolones has been shown to reduce the incidence of infections (34). Injection of recombinant granulocyte colony-stimulating factors (G-CSF) will reduce the duration and level of the neutropenia and the risk of developing a fever while neutropenic. To date, studies have failed to prove a survival advantage or reduction in significant infection rates for the use of G-CSF (35).

Other early side effects of chemotherapy are shown in Table 3.

Cytotoxic drugs are all potentially teratogenic, especially if given in the first trimester. Folate

Table 2 Mechanisms of Resistance to Chemotherapy

Drug class	Examples	Method of resistance
Topoisomerase I inhibitors	Irinotecan	Decreased expression of topoisomerase I
Spindle poisons	Vinca alkaloids	Reduced binding to microtubules
	Taxanes	
Platinum	Cisplatin	Increased DNA repair
Alkylating agents	Cyclophosphamide	Drug inactivation by aldehyde dehydrogenase
		Increased DNA repair
Antimetabolites	Methotrexate	Decreased reduced folate carrier expression
		Increased production of dihydrofolate reductase
		Increased thymidylate synthase levels
	5-Fluorouracil	

Table 3 Early Toxicities of Chemotherapy

Toxicity	Drugs	Comments
Alopecia	Anthracyclines and taxanes	Starts 2–3 wk after chemotherapy initiated. Reversible, usually starts growing back within 1–2 mo of end of treatment
Mouth ulcers	5-Flourouracil	Can be exacerbated by fungal or viral infections
Diarrhea	Capecitabine	Often associated with ulceration elsewhere in the GI tract
Constipation	Vinca alkaloids	Vinca alkaloids can cause gut neuropathy
Nausea	Most	Chemotherapy drugs can be directly emetogenic, but constipation and GI ulceration can exacerbate this. Usually well controlled with serotonin subtype 3 receptor blockers

antagonists such as methotrexate have the most consistently poor record (36). Observational studies of patients given chemotherapy during pregnancy reveal that chemotherapy can be administered relatively safely in the second and third trimester, but it is possible that miscarriage, intrauterine growth retardation, and premature labor may be increased (37). The incidence of long-term side effects among adults who have received chemotherapy while in utero are not known.

Late Toxicity

Male and female fertility are commonly reduced after chemotherapy (38), and there is a substantial literature on the effects of individual drugs (39). In the male, sperm production takes place constantly, and chemotherapy reduces or stops production by damaging the germinal epithelium. Azoospermia is therefore not always associated with diminished or absent hormone production. During intensive treatment, 96% of men will become azoospermic (40). Depending on the regime, a proportion of them will regain fertility after chemotherapy. In women, as ovarian germ cells are present at birth, the mechanism of infertility is different. Estrogen levels are depleted by treatment, and an early menopause can be induced. The extent of the toxicity is related to the underlying diagnosis, dose and type of drugs used, and age of patient at time of treatment (39).

Because chemotherapeutic drugs work by damaging DNA, they carry a risk of latent carcinogenesis. Alkylating agents are associated with a significant risk of myelodysplasia and acute myeloid leukemia (41), and after combination chemotherapy, the risk of many solid malignancies is increased: After treatment for Hodgkin's disease, the relative risk of any cancer is 6.4 times population risk, and the relative risk of AML is 144 (42,43). The risk of second malignancy is highest when chemotherapy and radiotherapy are used in combination.

Drug-Specific Toxicities

All chemotherapy drugs have specific side effects in addition to the generic effects described (Table 4). Specific side effects can either be related to cumulative dose (e.g., anthracyclines and cardiac toxicity) or be idiosyncratic. The mechanisms of toxicity vary but are not necessarily directly related to the cytotoxic action of the drugs. As management of toxicity improves, for example, with the use of peripheral blood stem cell rescue, bone marrow suppression is less likely to be the dose-limiting toxicity and some of the toxicities mentioned in Table 4 may become dose limiting. This list is not intended to be comprehensive, but to indicate the wide range of possible side effects of chemotherapy.

The toxicity of certain drugs can be reduced by techniques to protect normal tissue. For example, cyclophosphamide and ifosfamide produce acrolein, which is an irritant metabolite excreted through the

Table 4 Drug-Specific Toxicities

Drug	Examples of toxicities
Anthracyclines	Cardiotoxicity
Cytosine arabinoside	Cerebral/cerebellar dysfunction
Methotrexate	Hepatitis
	Nephrotoxicity
Vinca alkaloids	Neurotoxicity
	Constipation
5-Flourouracil	Palmar-plantar erythrodysesthesia
Taxanes	Neurotoxicity
	Hypersensitivity or anaphylaxis
Bleomycin	Pulmonary fibrosis
	Skin pigmentation
Cyclophosphamide	Hemorrhagic cystitis due to excretion of metabolites
	Bladder tumors
Cisplatin	Nephrotoxicity
	Deafness

bladder. Mesna is a thiol compound that acts as a reducing agent, and when given with cyclophosphamide reacts with acrolein in the urinary tract and helps prevent chemical cystitis (44).

MEASURING EFFICACY

Before prescribing a course of chemotherapy, a method of assessing the success or failure of the treatment should be identified. The method will obviously depend on the tumor type and site. For tumors that produce markers (e.g., prostate-specific antigen for prostate cancer and alpha-fetoprotein for germ cell tumors), serum levels can be readily measured. Symptomatic improvement can also often indicate response, for example, by a reduction in analgesic requirement by the patient. However, even in the palliative setting, symptomatic improvement alone is rarely considered adequate to prove response, and for solid tumors, demonstration of radiological response is the gold standard.

The common practice in assessing radiological response is to obtain an image of a measurable tumor site before and after treatment. The World Health Organization, the National Cancer Institute, and the European Organisation for Research and Treatment of Cancer have issued guidelines for tumor response criteria (45).

Response to treatment is a reasonable surrogate for the only true measure of treatment efficacy, overall survival.

Minimal Residual Disease

At a complete radiological response (or after radical surgery), there will be no evidence of disease as measured by any standard marker. Unfortunately, there will often be residual viable tumor cells present in these patients (Fig. 5). Currently, imaging does not allow us to detect microscopic disease, but using real-time quantitative polymerase chain reactions (PCR),

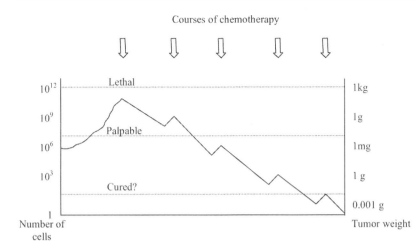

Figure 5 Minimal residual disease. *Source*: Modified from Ref. 9.

residual disease at the molecular level can be detected. The absence of minimal residual disease (MRD) could theoretically be used as an end point for radical therapy. In acute promyelocytic leukemia (APML), evidence of MRD in the bone marrow correlates well with outcome (46). It is likely that the absence of evidence of t15:17 in the bone marrow, as measured by real-time PCR, will also correlate with long-term survival after chemotherapy.

INTENSIFYING TREATMENT

In vitro evidence suggests that for some drugs such as cisplatin, there is a clear relationship between dose of chemotherapy and proportion of cells killed (16,47). In potentially curable tumors, there has been a great deal of interest in escalating treatment doses to improve survival, but, as mentioned above, dose is commonly limited by bone marrow suppression. Supportive care has improved significantly in recent years, and since the 1970s, it has been possible to perform peripheral blood stem cell rescue (48,49). This is a procedure whereby the patient's stem cells are collected from the peripheral blood and stored so that they can be returned after a high dose of chemotherapy, thus shortening the duration of neutropenia. The introduction of 5-HT3 antagonists has enabled nausea to be controlled more effectively (enabling the majority of chemotherapy regimens to be given as outpatient), and for some drugs the use of colony-stimulating factors alone is enough to significantly increase the tolerated dose (50).

NEW ANTICANCER DRUGS

Understanding of the molecular biology of malignant cells has increased dramatically in recent years. Therefore, there is scope for developing drugs that are targeted at malignant cells (51,52). The principle is that drugs are developed that target abnormal biology specific to tumors, thus increasing efficacy and reducing normal tissue damage. This section aims to mention some of the new drugs that are either in use in the clinic or are undergoing trials, to illustrate the range of possible new therapeutic strategies becoming available.

Immune Modulators

Immune modulation is an attractive anticancer therapeutic option. It has been noted that prolonged periods of immunosuppression predispose to malignancies (53) and also that spontaneous regression of metastatic tumors (classically renal cell cancers) can occur (54). What is more, regression of tumors can occasionally be induced by deliberate inoculation with pus or bacterial toxins (55). The immune system can be stimulated nonspecifically or by generation of specific antitumor immunity.

Cytokines

The immune system can be nonspecifically stimulated with supraphysiological doses of naturally occurring cytokines. Examples include tumor necrosis factor (TNF), interferons, and interleukins. This method has been shown to have some efficacy in the treatment of renal cell carcinoma, melanoma, and chronic leukemias (56–58).

Antibody Therapy

In the 19th century, investigators attempted to treat patients with the sera of animals that had been inoculated with human cancers (59), and since the discovery of the monoclonal antibody in 1975 (60), it has been possible to produce antibodies to specific tumor antigens.

The exact means by which monoclonal antibodies mediate cell killing is complex and not completely understood. Nevertheless, significant advances have been made with the recent introduction of anti-c-erbB2 (trastuzumab) for breast cancer and anti-CD20 (rituximab) for B-cell lymphoma (61). The human epidermal growth factor receptor 2 (HER2neu) antigen is overexpressed on the cell surface of 25% to 30% of breast cancers (62) and is associated with a poor prognosis (63). Patients can be tested for the presence of c-erbB2 on the tumor cell surface, and if the antigen is found, anti c-erbB2 antibodies induce responses in patients who have failed treatment with conventional chemotherapy, or in whom conventional chemotherapy is contraindicated (64,65). There is a higher response rate to chemotherapy plus anti-c-erbB2 antibodies than to chemotherapy alone (66). The side effect profile of monoclonal antibodies is very favorable when compared with conventional chemotherapy, and antibodies to other cell surface markers are under investigation. Unfortunately, resistance to monoclonal antibodies invariably develops, and discovering the mechanism of this resistance is going to be vital in terms of improving immune-based therapies.

Targeting Mediators of Malignancy

Receptors on the cell surface require intracellular signaling pathways to translate receptor ligand binding into cell proliferation or other end points. These intracellular signaling pathways are potential targets for anticancer drugs. For example, the epidermal growth factor receptor (EGFR also known as HER-1) is over-expressed in many cancers and seems to be responsible for malignant behavior of tumor cells (67–69). The EGFR has an intracellular tyrosine kinase (TK) domain that is activated by phosphorylation. TK activation can be blocked by specially designed small molecules. Over the past five years, TK inhibitors (TKIs) and monoclonal antibodies have been introduced for treatment of several solid cancer types including renal, colorectal cancer, squamous cell carcinoma of head and neck, and breast and ovarian cancer. Currently, there are monoclonal antibodies directed against the

extracellular domain of the EGFR receptor (cetuximab and panitumumab) and also the intracellular TK domain (erlotinib, lapatinib, and gefitinib).

A potential problem with blocking intracellular signaling pathways is that the effect may be short-lived if the cell can bypass the point in the intracellular pathway cascade at which the drug is acting. This can either occur by upregulation of alternative pathways or by mutation of target proteins. Individuals whose tumors harbor *k-RAS* mutations do not respond to EGFR inhibition as the downstream pathway is continuously "switched on" by the mutated k-ras oncogene (70).

Anti-Angiogenesis Agents

The ability to metastasize is a defining feature of malignant tissue, and metastasis cannot occur without angiogenesis. Angiogenesis is under the control of multiple cytokines, enzymes, and proteins (71). The concept of angiogenesis as a therapeutic target was suggested by Folkman in 1972 (72). Thalidomide is an anti-angiogenesis drug currently in use, originally marketed as a sedative but was withdrawn because of teratogenic effects, primarily amelia and phocomelia. It was proposed that these effects were due to degeneration of major limb arteries (73), and it was subsequently found that thalidomide inhibits the angiogenic cytokines, basic fibroblast growth factor (bFGF) and vascular endothelial growth factor (VEGF) (74,75). Clinical efficacy has been variable (76,77).

VEGF has been identified as a particularly important angiogenic cytokine (78).

A significant impact on both the overall survival and time to progression in renal and colorectal cancer has been achieved by using VEGF inhibitors alongside mTOR (hypoxia-driven rapamycin pathway) and *RAF* inhibitors (79). Several TKIs now inhibit more than one pathway (see Table 5 for an overview of molecularly targeted drugs). It is now accepted that VEGF

Table 5 Overview of Molecularly Targeted Therapies Used in Solid Tumors

Cancer type	Agent	Molecular targets	Trial phase
Breast	Trastuzumab (Herceptin)	HER-2 mAb	III
	Lapatinib		
		EGFR TKI	
Colorectal	Cetuximab	EGFR mAb (IgG1)	II/III
	Panitumumab	EGFR mAb (IgG2 humanized)	II/III
	Bevacizumab (Avastin)	VEGF	II/III
Non–small cell lung cancer	Erlotinib	EGRF TKI (intracellular)	II/III
Renal	Bevacizumab (Avastin)	VEGF mAb	II,III
	Sorafenib	VEGFR2,3, PDGFR, FLT-3,	II,III
		BRAF, CRAF	II,III
	Sunitinib	VEGF2, PDGFR, FLT-3, c-kit	II,III
	Temsirolimus	mTOR	II
	Everolimus	mTOR	II
	Axitinib	VEGFR1, 2, PDGFR, c-kit	II
	Pazopanib	VEGFR1–3, PDGFR	II
Squamous cell carcinoma of head and neck	Cetuximab	EGFR mAb	II/III

Abbreviations: mAb, monoclonal antibody; TKI, tyrosine kinase inhibitor; VEGFR, vascular endothelial growth factor receptor; BRAF, B-raf proto-oncogene serine/threonine protein kinase; CRAF, C-raf proto-oncogene serine/threonine protein kinase; EGFR, epidermal growth factor receptor.
Source: Adapted from Ref. 80.

inhibition should be the first-line therapy in advanced and metastatic renal carcinoma; outcome data are awaited for the use of these therapies in the adjuvant setting.

Toxicities and Scheduling of Targeted Therapy

Novel targeted therapies have resulted in novel toxicities. Common side effects of EGFR inhibition include fatigue, facial acneiform rash, and diarrhea. VEGF inhibition can lead to hypertension, renal impairment, and thromboembolic events. These toxicities are generally managed symptomatically. In the majority of cases these side effects are managed through treatment breaks and dose reduction where necessary.

Scheduling is critical in the use of targeted therapies. The recommended scheduling of sunitinib in renal cell carcinoma is four-weeks-on therapy followed by two weeks off to give the body time to recover between cycles. However, it is also possible to take daily sunitinib at a lower dose without significant toxicity.

Mechanisms of Resistance to EGFR and VEGF Inhibitors

Resistance to targeted agents is a significant clinical problem. Preclinical studies have determined several mechanisms of developing resistance to angiogenesis inhibition (VEGF/mTOR pathways) namely, upregulation of bFGF, overexpression of matrix metalloproteinase 9, increased levels of stromal cell–derived factor-1α and hypoxia-induced factor-1α, and recruitment of bone marrow CD45+ cells.

Studies in development of resistance to EGFR inhibition have found that several processes are involved, including activation of alternative TKIs that bypass the EGFR pathway (c-MET and IGF-1R), increased angiogenesis, activation of downstream mediators (PTEN and *k*-RAS), and the presence of EGFR mutations (81).

CONCLUSIONS

Conventional chemotherapy along with radiotherapy has formed the mainstay of curative and palliative treatment of solid malignancies in the past 40 years. All conventional cytotoxic drugs damage normal tissue as well as having a therapeutic effect by killing tumor cells. Combining different types and doses of cytotoxic drugs has lead to significant improvements in survival from some important cancers in the last 50 years.

Over the past five years, novel molecularly targeted agents have emerged through improved understanding of the molecular basis of many cancers. Molecularly targeted agents are now in routine use as single therapies or more commonly alongside chemotherapy and radiotherapy. The introduction of molecularly targeted inhibition of the VEGF, RAS, BRAF, and mTOR pathways has had a significant impact on the time to progression and overall survival in renal cancer.

It is expected that in the future, systemic treatment of cancer will include targeted therapies alongside chemotherapy and radiotherapy with associated improval in survival rates and reduction in associated toxicities. It will also be possible to "personalize" cancer therapy through the identification of individuals who are likely to respond to certain therapies.

REFERENCES

1. Burchenal JH. The historical development of cancer chemotherapy. Semin Oncol 1977; 4(2):135–146.
2. Krumbhaar EB, Krumbhaar HD. The blood and bone marrow in yellow gas (mustard gas) poisoning: changes produced in bone marrow of fatal cases. J Med Res 1919; 40:497.
3. Goodman LS, Wintrobe MM, Dameshek W, et al. Nitrogen mustard therapy: use of methyl-bis(beta-chloroethyl)amine hydrochloride and tris(bets-chloroethyls)amine hydrochloride for Hodgkin's disease, lymphosarcoma, leukaemia and certain allied and miscellaneous disorders. JAMA 1946; 132:126–132.
4. Twentyman PR, Bleehen NM. Changes in sensitivity to cytotoxic agents occurring during the life history of monolayer cultures of a mouse tumour cell line. Br J Cancer 1975; 31(4):417–423.
5. Steel GG, ed. Growth Kinetics of Tumours. Oxford: Oxford University Press, 1977.
6. Shackney SE, McCormack GW, Cuchural GJ Jr. Growth rate patterns of solid tumors and their relation to responsiveness to therapy: an analytical review. Ann Intern Med 1978; 89(1):107–121.
7. Modulation of fluorouracil by leucovorin in patients with advanced colorectal cancer: evidence in terms of response rate. Advanced Colorectal Cancer Meta-Analysis Project. J Clin Oncol 1992; 10(6):896–903.
8. Schabel FM Jr. The use of tumor growth kinetics in planning "curative" chemotherapy of advanced solid tumors. Cancer Res 1969; 29(12):2384–2389.
9. Skipper HE. Biochemical, biological, pharmacologic, toxicologic, kinetic and clinical (subhuman and human) relationships. Cancer 1968; 21(4):600–610.
10. Friedman JM, Fialkow PJ. Cell marker studies of human tumorigenesis. Transplant Rev 1976; 28:17–33.
11. Goldie JH, Coldman AJ. The genomic origin of drug resistance in neoplasms: implications for systemic therapy. Cancer Res 1984; 44(9):3643–3653.
12. Selawry OS, Henanian J, Wolman IJ. New treatment schedule with improved survival in childhood leukaemia. Intermittent parenteral versus daily oral administration of methotrexate for maintenance of induced remission. Acute leukaemia group B. JAMA 1965; 194(1):75–81.
13. Reiter A, Schrappe M, Ludwig WD, et al. Chemotherapy in 998 unselected childhood acute lymphoblastic leukemia patients. Results and conclusions of the multicenter trial ALL-BFM 86. Blood 1994; 84(9):3122–3133.
14. Devita VT Jr., Serpick AA, Carbone PP. Combination chemotherapy in the treatment of advanced Hodgkin's disease. Ann Intern Med 1970; 73(6):881–895.
15. Wolfrom C, Hartmann R, Fengler R, et al. Randomized comparison of 36-hour intermediate-dose versus 4-hour high-dose methotrexate infusions for remission induction in relapsed childhood acute lymphoblastic leukemia. J Clin Oncol 1993; 11(5):827–833.
16. Teicher BA, Herman TS, Holden SA, et al. Tumor resistance to alkylating agents conferred by mechanisms operative only in vivo. Science 1990; 247(4949 pt 1):1457–1461.

17. Riordan JR, Deuchars K, Kartner N, et al. Amplification of P-glycoprotein genes in multidrug-resistant mammalian cell lines. Nature 1985; 316(6031):817–819.

18. Gottesman MM, Hrycyna CA, Schoenlein PV, et al. Genetic analysis of the multidrug transporter. Annu Rev Genet 1995; 29:607–649.

19. Pogliani EM, Belotti D, Rivolta GF, et al. Anthracycline drugs and MDR expression in human leukemia. Cytotechnology 1996; 19(3):229–235.

20. Belpomme D, Gauthier S, Pujade-Lauraine E, et al. Verapamil increases the survival of patients with anthracycline-resistant metastatic breast carcinoma. Ann Oncol 2000; 11 (11):1471–1476.

21. Solary E, Witz B, Caillot D, et al. Combination of quinine as a potential reversing agent with mitoxantrone and cytarabine for the treatment of acute leukemias: a randomized multicenter study. Blood 1996; 88(4):1198–1205.

22. Wilson WH, Bates SE, Fojo A, et al. Controlled trial of dexverapamil, a modulator of multidrug resistance, in lymphomas refractory to EPOCH chemotherapy. J Clin Oncol 1995; 13(8):1995–2004.

23. Wishart GC, Bissett D, Paul J, et al. Quinidine as a resistance modulator of epirubicin in advanced breast cancer: mature results of a placebo-controlled randomized trial. J Clin Oncol 1994; 12(9):1771–1777.

24. Reed JC. Bcl-2 family proteins. Oncogene 1998; 17 (25):3225–3236.

25. Cho Y, Gorina S, Jeffrey PD, et al. Crystal structure of a p53 tumor suppressor-DNA complex: understanding tumorigenic mutations. Science 1994; 265(5170):346–355.

26. Chin KV, Ueda K, Pastan I, et al. Modulation of activity of the promoter of the human MDR1 gene by Ras and p53. Science 1992; 255(5043):459–462.

27. Lowe SW, Ruley HE, Jacks T, et al. p53-dependent apoptosis modulates the cytotoxicity of anticancer agents. Cell 1993; 74(6):957–967.

28. Konopleva M, Zhao S, Hu W, et al. The anti-apoptotic genes Bcl-X(L) and Bcl-2 are over-expressed and contribute to chemoresistance of non-proliferating leukaemic CD34+ cells. Br J Haematol 2002; 118(2):521–534.

29. Waters JS, Webb A, Cunningham D, et al. Phase I clinical and pharmacokinetic study of bcl-2 antisense oligonucleotide therapy in patients with non-Hodgkin's lymphoma. J Clin Oncol 2000; 18(9):1812–1823.

30. Pommier Y, Leteurtre F, Fesen MR, et al. Cellular determinants of sensitivity and resistance to DNA topoisomerase inhibitors. Cancer Invest 1994; 12(5):530–542.

31. Beck WT, Danks MK, Wolverton JS, et al. Resistance of mammalian tumor cells to inhibitors of DNA topoisomerase II. Adv Pharmacol 1994; 29B:145–169.

32. Bodey GP, Buckley M, Sathe YS, et al. Quantitative relationships between circulating leukocytes and infection in patients with acute leukemia. Ann Intern Med 1966; 64(2):328–340.

33. Schimpff S, Satterlee W, Young VM, et al. Empiric therapy with carbenicillin and gentamicin for febrile patients with cancer and granulocytopenia. N Engl J Med 1971; 284(19):1061–1065.

34. Engels EA, Lau J, Barza M. Efficacy of quinolone prophylaxis in neutropenic cancer patients: a meta-analysis. J Clin Oncol 1998; 16(3):1179–1187.

35. Messori A, Trippoli S, Tendi E. G-CSF for the prophylaxis of neutropenic fever in patients with small cell lung cancer receiving myelosuppressive antineoplastic chemotherapy: meta-analysis and pharmacoeconomic evaluation. J Clin Pharm Ther 1996; 21(2):57–63.

36. Doll DC, Ringenberg QS, Yarbro JW. Antineoplastic agents and pregnancy. Semin Oncol 1989; 16(5):337–346.

37. Berry DL, Theriault RL, Holmes FA, et al. Management of breast cancer during pregnancy using a standardized protocol. J Clin Oncol 1999; 17(3):855–861.

38. Chapman RM, Sutcliffe S. The effects of chemotherapy and radiotherapy on fertility and their prevention. In: Whitehouse JMA, Willams CJW, ed. Recent Advances in Clinical Oncology. Edinburgh: Churchill Livingston, 1986:239–251.

39. Sieber SM, Adamson RH. Toxicity of antineoplastic agents in man, chromosomal aberrations antifertility effects, congenital malformations, and carcinogenic potential. Adv Cancer Res 1975; 22:57–155.

40. Drasga RE, Einhorn LH, Williams SD, et al. Fertility after chemotherapy for testicular cancer. J Clin Oncol 1983; 1 (3):179–183.

41. Reimer RR, Hoover R, Fraumeni JF Jr., et al. Acute leukemia after alkylating-agent therapy of ovarian cancer. N Engl J Med 1977; 297(4):177–181.

42. Tucker MA. Solid second cancers following Hodgkin's disease. Hematol Oncol Clin North Am 1993; 7(2):389–400.

43. Henry-Amar M, Dietrich PY. Acute leukemia after the treatment of Hodgkin's disease. Hematol Oncol Clin North Am 1993; 7(2):369–387.

44. Brock N, Pohl J, Stekar J. Detoxification of urotoxic oxazaphosphorines by sulfhydryl compounds. J Cancer Res Clin Oncol 1981; 100(3):311–320.

45. Therasse P, Arbuck SG, Eisenhauer EA, et al. New guidelines to evaluate the response to treatment in solid tumors. European Organization for Research and Treatment of Cancer, National Cancer Institute of the United States, National Cancer Institute of Canada. J Natl Cancer Inst 2000; 92(3):205–216.

46. Venditti A, Buccisano F, Del Poeta G, et al. Level of minimal residual disease after consolidation therapy predicts outcome in acute myeloid leukemia. Blood 2000; 96 (12):3948–3952.

47. Skipper HE, Schabel FM. Quantitative and cytokinetic studies in experimental tumour systems. In: Holland JF, Frei FE, ed. Cancer Medicine. Philadelphia: Lea and Febiger, 1988:663–684.

48. Gorin NC, Najman A, Salmon C, et al. High dose combination chemotherapy (TACC) with and without autologous bone marrow transplantation for the treatment of acute leukaemia and other malignant diseases: kinetics of recovery of haemopoiesis. A preliminary study of 12 cases. Eur J Cancer 1979; 15(9):1113–1119.

49. Appelbaum FR, Deisseroth AB, Graw RG Jr., et al. Prolonged complete remission following high dose chemotherapy of Burkitt's lymphoma in relapse. Cancer 1978; 41(3):1059–1063.

50. Gianni AM, Bregni M, Siena S, et al. Granulocyte-macrophage colony-stimulating factor or granulocyte colony-stimulating factor infusion makes high-dose etoposide a safe outpatient regimen that is effective in lymphoma and myeloma patients. J Clin Oncol 1992; 10(12):1955–1962.

51. Garrett MD, Workman P. Discovering novel chemotherapeutic drugs for the third millennium. Eur J Cancer 1999; 35(14):2010–2030.

52. Gibbs JB. Anticancer drug targets: growth factors and growth factor signaling. J Clin Invest 2000; 105(1):9–13.

53. Penn I. Cancers complicating organ transplantation. N Engl J Med 1990; 323(25):1767–1769.

54. Oliver RT, Nethersell AB, Bottomley JM. Unexplained spontaneous regression and alpha-interferon as treatment for metastatic renal carcinoma. Br J Urol 1989; 63(2):128–131.

55. Coley-Nauts HC, Fowler GA, Bogatko RN. A review of the influence of bacterial infection and of bacterial products (Coley's toxins) on malignant tumours in man. Acta Med Scand Supp 1953; 274:29–97.

56. Rosenberg SA, Yang JC, Topalian SL, et al. Treatment of 283 consecutive patients with metastatic melanoma or

renal cell cancer using high-dose bolus interleukin 2. JAMA 1994; 271(12):907–913.

57. Bukowski RM, Goodman P, Crawford ED, et al. Phase II trial of high-dose intermittent interleukin-2 in metastatic renal cell carcinoma: a Southwest Oncology Group study. J Natl Cancer Inst 1990; 82(2):143–146.

58. Quesada JR, Reuben J, Manning JT, et al. Alpha interferon for induction of remission in hairy-cell leukemia. N Engl J Med 1984; 310(1):15–18.

59. Hericourt J, Richet C. De la serotherapie dons la traitment du cancer. Comptes Rendues du l'Academie des Sciences 1895; 121:567–569.

60. Kohler G, Milstein C. Continuous cultures of fused cells secreting antibody of predefined specificity. Nature 1975; 256(5517):495–497.

61. Coiffier B, et al. CHOP chemotherapy plus rituximab compared with CHOP alone in elderly patients with diffuse large-B-cell lymphoma. N Engl J Med 2002; 346(4): 235–242.

62. Hynes NE, Stern DF. The biology of erbB-2/neu/HER-2 and its role in cancer. Biochim Biophys Acta 1994; 1198 (2–3):165–184.

63. Slamon DJ, Godolphin W, Jones LA, et al. Studies of the HER-2/neu proto-oncogene in human breast and ovarian cancer. Science 1989; 244(4905):707–712.

64. Cobleigh MA, Vogel CL, Tripathy D, et al. Multinational study of the efficacy and safety of humanized anti-HER2 monoclonal antibody in women who have HER2-overexpressing metastatic breast cancer that has progressed after chemotherapy for metastatic disease. J Clin Oncol 1999; 17(9):2639–2648.

65. Vogel CL, Cobleigh MA, Tripathy D, et al. Efficacy and safety of trastuzumab as a single agent in first-line treatment of HER2-overexpressing metastatic breast cancer. J Clin Oncol 2002; 20(3):719–726.

66. Slamon DJ, Leyland-Jones B, Shak S, et al. Use of chemotherapy plus a monoclonal antibody against HER2 for metastatic breast cancer that overexpresses HER2. N Engl J Med 2001; 344(11):783–792.

67. Aaronson SA. Growth factors and cancer. Science 1991; 254 (5035):1146–1153.

68. Salomon DS, Brandt R, Ciardiello F, et al. Epidermal growth factor-related peptides and their receptors in human malignancies. Crit Rev Oncol Hematol 1995; 19 (3):183–232.

69. Tysnes BB, Haugland HK, Bjerkvig R. Epidermal growth factor and laminin receptors contribute to migratory and invasive properties of gliomas. Invasion Metastasis 1997; 17(5):270–280.

70. Karapetis CS, Khambata-Ford S, Jonker DJ, et al. K-ras mutations and benefit from cetuximab in advanced colorectal cancer. N Engl J Med 2008; 359(17):1757–1765.

71. Risau W. Mechanisms of angiogenesis. Nature 1997; 386 (6626):671–674.

72. Folkman J. Anti-angiogenesis: new concept for therapy of solid tumors. Ann Surg 1972; 175(3):409–416.

73. Parman T, Wiley MJ, Wells PG. Free radical-mediated oxidative DNA damage in the mechanism of thalidomide teratogenicity. Nat Med 1999; 5(5):582–585.

74. D'Amato RJ, Loughnan MS, Flynn E, et al. Thalidomide is an inhibitor of angiogenesis. Proc Natl Acad Sci U S A 1994; 91(9):4082–4085.

75. Kruse FE, Joussen AM, Rohrschneider K, et al. Thalidomide inhibits corneal angiogenesis induced by vascular endothelial growth factor. Graefes Arch Clin Exp Ophthalmol 1998; 236(6):461–466.

76. Baidas SM, Winer EP, Fleming GF, et al. Phase II evaluation of thalidomide in patients with metastatic breast cancer. J Clin Oncol 2000; 18(14):2710–2717.

77. Figg WD, Dahut W, Duray P, et al. A randomized phase II trial of thalidomide, an angiogenesis inhibitor, in patients with androgen-independent prostate cancer. Clin Cancer Res 2001; 7(7):1888–1893.

78. Ferrara N. Vascular endothelial growth factor: molecular and biological aspects. Curr Top Microbiol Immunol 1999; 237:1–30.

79. Motzer RJ, Basch E. Targeted drugs for metastatic renal cell carcinoma. Lancet 2007; 370(9605):2071–2073.

80. Chowdhury S, Larkin JM, Gore ME. Recent advances in the treatment of renal cell carcinoma and the role of targeted therapies. Eur J Cancer 2008; 44(15):2152–2161.

81. Dempke WC, Heinemann V. Resistance to EGF-R (erbB-1) and VEGF-R modulating agents. Eur J Cancer 2009; 45(7): 1117–1128.

29

Embryology

David F. M. Thomas

Department of Paediatric Urology, St James's University Hospital, Leeds, U.K.

INTRODUCTION

In recent years Embryology has undergone a remarkable transformation from being a largely descriptive science to its current status at the forefront of innovative therapeutic research. Many of the advances in this field, including the cloning of mammalian embryos, can be traced back to early work on assisted conception and in vitro fertilization (IVF), but perhaps the greatest impetus for embryo research came from the isolation and culture of pluripotent embryonic stem cells from early embryonic tissue (1). The ambitious and costly embryo and stem cell research programs that are now being undertaken across the world are underpinned by the expectation that this work will ultimately pave the way to the development of a wide range of clinical applications, including cell transplantation, tissue regeneration, and tissue engineering. More controversially, research is also underway to explore the feasibility of creating artificial gametes using genetic material derived from somatic cells. The creation of human–animal hybrid embryos is being explored as a potential source of (human) pluripotent embryonic stem cells to circumvent the problems created by the scarcity of donated human oocytes. In some controversial areas the pace of scientific advance threatens to outstrip the ability of legislators to adapt regulatory frameworks in a way that is acceptable to the scientific community and society as a whole. In the United Kingdom, responsibility for regulating embryo and stem cell research lies with the Human Fertilisation and Embryology Authority (HFEA).

A more detailed consideration of the current status of the embryo and stem cell research would be outside the scope of this chapter and, in any event, would almost certainly be rapidly overtaken by further advances. However, this chapter will encompass some of the relevant advances in less controversial areas of developmental biology that are shedding new light on the genetic and environmental basis of congenital malformations.

The advent of research methods such as polymerase chain reaction and fluorescent in situ hybridization have greatly facilitated the study of the genetic mechanisms regulating the complex and tightly ordered anatomical sequence that characterizes normal embryological development. As well as mapping and sequencing genes, research methodology is identifying many of the gene products responsible for implementing the genetic "program" encoded on DNA at a cellular and molecular level. Moreover, the function of specific genes is being extensively studied in experimentally induced null or "knockout" gene deletions in experimental rodents. Relevant examples will be cited throughout the chapter.

With the benefit of information being derived from new methodology, it is becoming increasingly apparent that the traditional account of the embryological development of the urinary tract and other systems was oversimplified. For example, on the basis of this interpretation of sequential serial sections at different stages in development, concepts such as the division of the foregut and "partition" of the cloaca by the descent of the urorectal septum and lateral ingrowth are now thought to be a conceptual artifact. There is growing evidence that many of the structural changes observed in the developing embryo reflect a process of dynamic remodeling in situ, which is a consequence of simultaneous growth, differentiation, and apoptosis, rather than three-dimensional interactions between different structures. Nevertheless, for the clinician, as opposed to the embryologist, the conventional three-dimensional descriptive accounts of embryology simplify understanding of the development of the genitourinary tract. In turn, these descriptive models can be invoked to explain many of the congenital abnormalities encountered in clinical practice. For this reason, this chapter provides a largely conventional, practical, and clinically orientated account of developmental anatomy of the genitourinary tract, accompanied, where appropriate, by consideration of genetics and relevant aspects of developmental biology.

FERTILIZATION AND EARLY DEVELOPMENT OF THE HUMAN EMBRYO

Human gestation spans the period from fertilization to birth, which averages 38 weeks. Obstetricians conventionally subdivide pregnancy into three 3-month trimesters. Embryogenesis, the formation of organs and systems, occurs principally between the 3rd and 10th weeks. Subsequent development throughout the

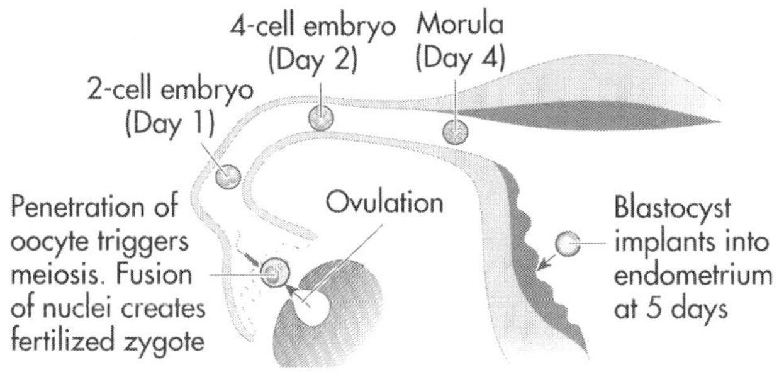

4-cell embryo (Day 2) Morula (Day 4)

2-cell embryo (Day 1)

Penetration of oocyte triggers meiosis. Fusion of nuclei creates fertilized zygote

Ovulation

Blastocyst implants into endometrium at 5 days

Figure 1 Key stages in the five to six days from fertilization to implantation.

rest of fetal life is characterized by the processes of differentiation, branching, maturation, and growth.

Fertilization is defined by fusion of the nuclear material of the fertilizing spermatozoon and the oocyte. The process of gametogenesis, whereby spermatozoa and oocytes develop from their germ cell precursors, is considered hereafter. In males, spermatogenesis is a continuing process initiated at puberty whereas the initial phase of female gametogenesis occurs in fetal life, and primary oocytes remain dormant in the prophase of the first meiotic division until the onset of puberty.

During each ovulatory cycle, under the influence of follicle-stimulating hormone, a small number of primary oocytes resume meiotic activity, but, of these, only one usually progresses to maturity as a Graafian follicle. At the mid-point of the menstrual cycle, the primary oocyte destined for ovulation transforms into a secondary oocyte by proceeding into the remaining phases of the long-arrested first meiotic division. Protected by the zona pellucida, the secondary oocyte is extruded from the surface of the ovary, from where it is drawn into the reproductive tract by the fimbriae of the fallopian tube. From an ejaculate totaling perhaps 40 to 100 million spermatozoa, only a few hundred are destined to complete the journey up the female reproductive canal to come into potential contact with the ovulated oocyte.

Penetration by the fertilizing spermatozoon of the zona pellucida surrounding the secondary oocyte triggers the second meiotic division, which results in the formation of the definitive oocyte and an aggregate of nonfunctional DNA termed the polar body.

The normal human karyotype comprises a total of 23 pairs of chromosomes, that is, 22 pairs of autosomes and one pair of sex chromosomes, either XX (female) or XY (male). As a result of the two meiotic divisions, each gamete (the spermatozoon or oocyte) carries only half the normal complement of chromosomes, that is, 22 unpaired autosomes and either an X or Y sex chromosome. Fusion of the haploid nuclei of the two gametes at the time of fertilization imparts diploid status (i.e., 22 pairs of autosomes plus 2 sex chromosomes) to the nucleus of the fertilized zygote. From the time of fertilization, the journey down the fallopian tube to the site of implantation in the primed uterine endometrium takes five to six days (Fig. 1). During this time, the

fertilized zygote has undergone a series of cell divisions termed cleavage. By the fourth day, sequential cleavage has created a 32-cell embryo, classically likened to a mulberry (hence the Latin-derived term "morula"). Further cell division is accompanied by structural differentiation and the formation of a sphere-like blastocyst. It is at this stage in development that the embryo is implanted into the uterine endometrium, six days after fertilization.

CHROMOSOMAL ABNORMALITIES: CLINICAL CONSIDERATIONS

A detailed account of the pathogenesis and clinical manifestations of chromosomal abnormalities arising during gametogenesis and cleavage is outside the scope of this chapter. Major chromosomal abnormalities are common, but mostly result in the death of the embryo and spontaneous abortion at an early stage in pregnancy. The most serious chromosomal abnormalities consistent with survival to term are the trisomies, notably trisomy 21 (Down's syndrome.) A trisomy state occurs when an additional chromosome or portion of a chromosome becomes incorporated into the nucleus of a gamete by nondisjunction or translocation. Nondisjunction refers to the faulty separation of a pair of chromosomes during meiotic or mitotic cell division. In translocation, paired chromosomes separate completely, but one of the pair, or a fragment thereof, becomes inadvertently attached to another unrelated chromosome and is thus retained within the haploid nucleus. Trisomic states are also associated with the formation of a gamete that is lacking a copy of the affected chromosome, and any zygote arising from fertilization will therefore have only one copy of this chromosome—termed monosomy. Although complete monosomic states involving autosomes are uniformly lethal, some partial monosomies created by deletion of part of a chromosome are compatible with survival. Some have been identified in association with specific syndromes; for example, deletion of a particular portion of chromosome11 has been implicated in the etiology of some cases of Wilms tumor. Apart from translocation and nondisjunction, other structural defects involving identifiable segments of chromosomes include deletion, inversion, duplication, and substitution.

Nondisjunction of the X and Y sex chromosomes during gametogenesis accounts for a number of genetically determined syndromes, notably Klinefelter's syndrome (47 XXY) and Turner's syndrome (45X). Complete monosomic forms of Turner's syndrome (45X) account for approximately 50% of cases, while "mosaicism" (45X/46XX) is present in approximately 30% of cases and a structural deletion on one of the X chromosomes accounts for the remaining 20% of cases.

Unsurprisingly, the gross genetic imbalance created by the presence of additional replicated DNA within the zygote nucleus results in profound disturbances of embryogenesis, affecting a number of systems including the genitourinary tract. The incidence of coexistent renal anomalies ranges from

Table 1   Chromosome Defects Associated with Urinary Tract Anomalies

Chromosome defect or syndrome	Frequency (%)	Genitourinary anomalies
Turner's syndrome 45X	60–80	Horseshoe kidney Duplication
Trisomy 18 (Edwards' syndrome)	70	Horseshoe kidney Renal ectopia Duplication Hydronephrosis
Trisomy 13 (Patu syndrome)	60–80	Cystic kidney Hydronephrosis Horseshoe kidney Ureteric duplication
4p (Wolf–Hirschorn syndrome)	33	Hypospadias Cystic kidney Hydronephrosis
Trisomy 21 (Down's syndrome)	3–7	Renal agenesis Horseshoe kidney

approximately 5% in Down's syndrome (trisomy 21) to 75% in Turner's syndrome (45 X) (Table 1).

Nondisjunction and translocation anomalies are not confined to gametogenesis, but can also occur during the early mitotic cell divisions in the process of cleavage. In the resulting state, termed mosaicism, the embryonic tissues contain a varying ratio of cell lines with differing karyotypes depending on the phase of cleavage at which nondisjunction occurred, such as two-cell, four-cell, and eight-cell embryo. Abnormalities of the sex chromosomes are often found in mosaic form. Ovotesticular disorders of sex development (previously termed true hermaphroditism) (2) can be explained on this basis. Affected individuals possess both ovarian (XX) and testicular (XY) tissues that coexist in streak-like gonads termed ovotestes. Gonadal mesenchyme carrying a Y chromosome differentiates as testicular tissue, whereas tissue derived from the original population of non–Y embryonic cells differentiates passively down the female (ovarian) pathway. Karyotypes show a varied pattern, including 45 X/46 XY and 46 XX/47 XXY.

Turner's syndrome and Klinefelter's syndrome are often associated with mosaic karyotypes.

IMPLANTATION AND EARLY EMBRYONIC DEVELOPMENT

On the fifth or sixth day after fertilization, the blastocyst implants into the endometrium of the uterine cavity in which the endometrium has been primed by progesterone secreted by the corpus luteum. Over the ensuing 10 days, two cavities develop within the spherical mass of rapidly proliferating embryonic cells. The embryonic disc, from which the early embryo is derived, forms in the three-layered interface between the amniotic cavity and definitive yolk sac. The amniotic surface of the trilaminar embryonic disc gives rise to the ectodermal tissues of the embryo, whereas the endodermal derivatives originate from the yolk sac–derived surface. The intraembryonic mesoderm is formed by the inpouring of cells on the amniotic surface of the disc via the primitive streak (Fig. 2). The layer of intraembryonic mesoderm

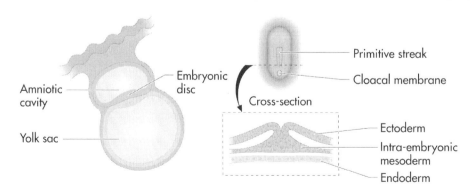

Figure 2   The embryonic disc at 16 days. Inpouring of cells at the primitive streak creates the intra-embryonic mesoderm from which the genitourinary tract is formed.

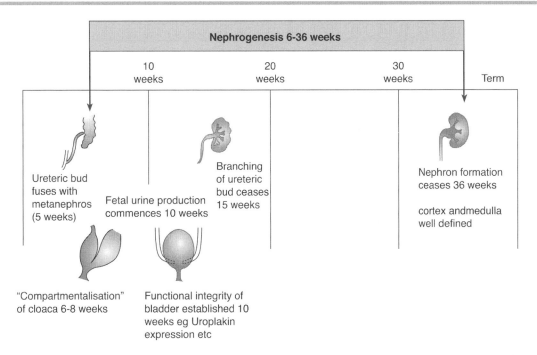

Figure 3 Timescale of key events in the development of the upper and lower urinary tracts.

created by the inpouring process soon subdivides into three components, comprising the paraxial mesoderm, intermediate mesoderm and lateral plate mesoderm. It is from the blocks of intermediate mesoderm on either side of the midline that much of the genitourinary tract is ultimately derived. The third and fourth weeks of gestation are dominated by the processes of segmentation and somite formation that characterize all vertebrate embryogenesis, which are closely regulated by expression of the Hox group of genes. At this stage, folding of the expanding embryonic disc imparts recognizable shape to the growing embryo.

UPPER URINARY TRACT (FIG. 3)

The kidneys develop from the caudal zones of the paired columns of intermediate mesoderm on either side of the midline. The formation of the metanephros, the precursor of the definitive kidney, is preceded by the formation of the pronephros and mesonephros in the cephalad and mid-zones, respectively. During the fourth week of gestation, the primitive pronephros appears in the cervical (cephalad) portion of the intermediate mesoderm but then rapidly regresses and disappears. Later in the fourth week, primitive nephron-like tubular structures appear in the mesonephros (Fig. 4A).

Linear rod-like condensations of mesenchyme develop concurrently in areas lateral to the developing mesonephros, and these then canalize to give rise to the mesonephric ducts—which advance caudally to fuse with the cloaca (the terminal portion of hindgut destined to give rise to the bladder by a process termed compartmentalization). Canalization of the mesonephric ducts, which are in communication with the primitive mesonephric tubules, creates a patent excretory unit that is believed to function transiently between 6 and 10 weeks. The beginning of the fifth week sees the appearance of the ureteric buds (Fig. 4B), arising from the most distal portion of the paired mesonephric ducts.

Normal embryological development of the upper urinary tract is crucially dependent on the role of the ureteric bud. Faulty or failed interaction between the ureteric bud and metanephric mesenchyme results in renal agenesis or differing patterns of renal dysplasia, whereas abnormal budding results in ureteric duplication (which in the case of complete duplication may also be associated with dysplasia in the renal relevant moiety). Abnormalities of early ureteric development are also implicated in the etiology of vesicoureteric reflux (VUR) and vesicoureteric junction obstruction.

At around 32 days, the advancing ureteric bud makes contact with the metanephros, thus initiating the interactive process of nephron formation (nephrogenesis). During the sixth to ninth weeks, the lobulated embryonic kidneys ascend up the posterior abdominal wall from their caudal sites of origin to their definitive lumbar position (Fig. 5).

In human, the process of nephron formation (nephrogenesis) within the embryonic and fetal kidney spans a period of approximately 30 weeks, from weeks 6 to 36 of gestation, whereas in some other species nephrogenesis continues postnatally. The ureteric bud and the metanephric mesenchyme each make specific contributions to the definitive structure

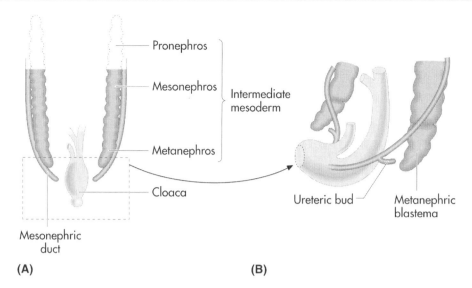

Figure 4 (**A**) Following the regression of the pronephros, the mesonephros assumes prominence before the emergence of the metanephros as the definitive embryonic kidney. (**B**) At around 28 days, the ureteric buds appear and advance toward the metanephric mesenchyme.

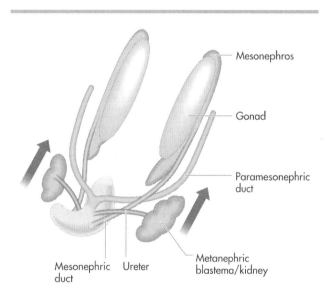

Figure 5 At Five to seven weeks: penetration of the metanephric mesenchyme promotes nephrogenesis by a process of mutual induction. Mesonephric tissues support the development of the embryonic gonads in the genital ridges. The paramesonephric ducts develop in the mesenchyme adjacent to the mesonephric ducts.

of the kidney. Sequential budding and branching of the ureteric bud gives rise to the renal pelvis, the major calices, the minor calices, and the collecting ducts. Within the metanephric mesenchyme, differentiating cells aggregate to form the glomeruli, convoluted tubules, and loop of Henle. At around the 10th week, the distal convoluted tubules (derived

from metanephric mesenchyme) establish continuity with the collecting ducts (of ureteric bud origin) to form functional excretory units. The definitive architecture of the kidney, with cortex and medulla, is established by 15 weeks gestation although new generations of nephrons continue to appear within the cortex up to 36 weeks. The rate of nephrogenesis is greatest toward the end of this period. At around 36 weeks nephrogenesis ceases and the number of nephrons then remains fixed throughout life, ranging between 0.7 and 1.4 million per kidney. The process of tubular differentiation within the metanephric mesenchyme is initiated by contact with the ureteric bud. Similarly, proliferative budding and branching of the ureteric bud tissues are dependent on induction by the metanephric mesenchyme. Nephrogenesis represents one of many examples of reciprocal induction occurring in embryological development. When cultured independently neither ureteric bud tissue nor metanephric has the capacity to differentiate into nephron-like structures. However, when cultured together, nephrogenesis is observed.

MOLECULAR BIOLOGY OF NORMAL AND ABNORMAL UPPER TRACT DEVELOPMENT

In view of the pivotal role played by the ureteric bud and embryonic ureter in regulating normal and abnormal upper tract development, it is not surprising that the genes expressed in these structures and the identity of the gene products responsible for mediating the cell-to-cell signaling at a molecular level have been intensively studied. The methodology employed includes immunohistochemistry, scanning electron microscopy, tissue culture and organ culture, and the use of targeted mutations in "knock out" mice.

Embryonic urothelium has been shown to induce differentiation of adjacent mesenchyme by secretion of sonic hedgehog (Shh), a signaling growth factor that orchestrates the activity of a number of other proteins and transcription factors (3). Secretion of Shh and similar gene products by embryonic urothelium stimulates differentiation of the adjacent mesenchyme into detrusor muscle and ureteric smooth muscle. Urinary tract abnormalities attributed to faulty development of ureteric and bladder smooth muscle are observed in "knock out" mice lacking Shh. Similar phenotypes arise from deletion of the gene for the transcription factor teashirt 3 (4).

Uroplakin 3 (UP3) is one of the structural proteins expressed in the asymmetric unit membrane on the urothelial surface, and targeted ablation of the UP3 gene in embryonic mice results in high-grade VUR associated with dilated kidneys (5). The UP3 "knock out" mouse provides the most convincing experimental model for VUR yet described—raising the possibility that this gene might be implicated in the etiology of familial VUR in humans. However, genetic screening studies to identify possible UP3 mutations in patients with non–syndromic VUR have been uniformly negative (6) and likewise no evidence of abnormal UP3 expression is present in the urothelium of patients undergoing surgery for high-grade VUR (7).

Nevertheless, UP3 mutations have been identified in a small number of patients with a combination of VUR and severe renal dysplasia (8). Similarly mutations of the PAX 2 gene have been implicated in rare familial cases of VUR (9). The renin-angiotensin system (10) is also known to play an important role in regulating early differentiation and development of the urinary tract. Two types of receptor are responsible for mediating the actions of angiotensin II in target tissues. Stimulation of the angiotensin 1 (AGTR 1) receptor in the embryo promotes cellular proliferation, matrix deposition, and the release of growth factors in the mesenchymal precursors of the kidney and ureter. By contrast, the angiotensin 2 (AGTR2) receptor, which is expressed principally in the embryo and fetus, is responsible for inducing apoptosis and decreased cell growth. "Knockout" deletions of the AGTR1 and AGTR2 genes in mice result in different patterns of urinary tract malformations. While deletion of the AGTR1 gene is characterized by progressive dilatation of the collecting system in postnatal life, deletion of AGTR2 gene gives rise to varying degrees of congenital renal hypoplasia, dysplasia, and ureteric dilatation. Some of the many genes now known to be involved in early ureteric development include Gdnf, c-ret, Rara, Agtr2, L1-CAM, Bmp4, Foxc1, Foxc2, Slit 2 Slit 3, Robo, and Pax2 (11).

The process of nephron formation within the kidney has also been extensively studied and a large number of gene products have already been demonstrated to play a role in regulating the different phases. The actions of positive growth factors, such as fibroblast growth factor 2 and glial cell line–derived neurotrophic factor (GDNF), are balanced by other molecules, such as tumor necrosis factor, that act as negative growth factors by promoting apoptosis (programmed cell death).

Transcription factors constitute another important group of signaling molecules. These DNA-binding proteins are involved in regulating gene expression. Examples of transcription factors closely involved in nephrogenesis include the gene products of the Pax2 gene and Wilms' tumor suppressor gene (WT1 gene), both of which play a central role in branching of the ureteric bud and in the induction of metanephric mesenchyme. Other signaling molecules include those responsible for cell-to-cell adhesion and cell-to-cell matrix adhesion, such as laminins and integrins.

CONGENITAL RENAL MALFORMATIONS: CLINICAL CONSIDERATIONS

For convenience, congenital anomalies of the kidney and urinary tract (CAKUT) can be arbitrarily grouped in the following broad morphological categories:

1. Renal agenesis—total absence of the kidney
2. Renal dysplasia—a kidney is present, although it is often reduced in size. The internal architecture is disordered and the histological appearances are characterized by immature, primitive, "undifferentiated" tubules, and the inappropriate presence of tissues such as cartilage and fibromuscular tissue within the renal parenchyma
3. Cyst formation
4. Gross developmental anomalies, such as duplication, horseshoe kidney, and pelvic kidney

Ureteric duplication can be explained by bifurcation of the ureteric bud, and according to the level of the original bifurcation, the duplication may be complete or incomplete. In cases of complete ureteric duplication, the upper pole ureter paradoxically enters the urinary tract at a more distal (caudal) level than the lower pole ureter. In the accepted conceptual model this anatomical pattern (described by the Meyer Weigert law) arises when the mesonephric duct separates from the embryonic ureter and its terminal portion descends toward the primitive posterior urethra, drawing the upper pole ureter with it.

Gross renal anomalies such as horseshoe kidney, pelvic kidney, and crossed ectopia date from the 6th to 10th week of gestation when the developing kidneys may fuse (horseshoe kidney), cross the midline (crossed fused ectopia), or fail to ascend (pelvic kidney).

EMBRYOLOGY OF THE LOWER URINARY TRACT (BLADDER AND URETHRA) (FIG. 3)

The bladder and urethra originate from the anterior portion of the cloaca, the common terminal section of hindgut into which the mesonephric ducts and embryonic ureters drain. The cloaca also contributes the urogenital sinus—which in turn contributes to the vagina. Conventionally the urorectal septum has been likened to a shutter that descends to subdivide the

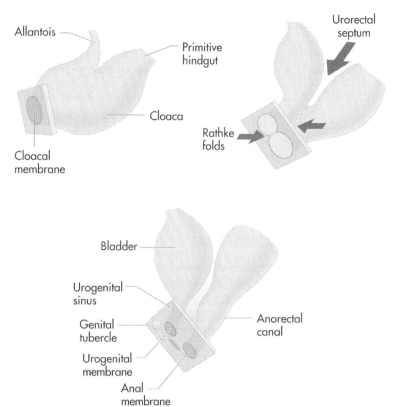

Allantois

Primitive
hindgut

Urorectal
septum

Cloaca

Rathke
folds

Cloacal
membrane

Bladder

Urogenital
sinus

Genital
tubercle

Urogenital
membrane

Anal
membrane

Anorectal
canal

Figure 6 Descent of the urorectal septum between four and six weeks divides the cloaca into an anterior urogenital compartment, the precursor of the bladder, urethra, prostate and distal vagina, and a posterior anorectal canal.

cloaca into the urogenital canal anteriorly and the anorectal canal posteriorly between the fourth and sixth weeks of gestation (12). This process is aided by the lateral ingrowth of the folds of Rathke (Fig. 6). Our understanding of this mechanism is based on historical interpretation of sequential sections of embryos at different stages in early gestation. More recently, however, this mechanism (and indeed the very existence of the urorectal septum and Rathke's folds) has been called into question by the results of studies employing modern methodology such as scanning electron microscopy and immunostaining for apoptosis. It is now thought that partitioning of the cloaca results from in situ deposition of mesenchyme in the cloaca and urogenital sinus coupled with simultaneous apoptosis and changes in the curvature of the adjacent abdominal wall and spine (13).

As the bladder becomes more clearly defined in the upper portion of the urogenital canal, the points of entry of the ureter and mesonephric ducts begin to separate (Fig. 7). When the distance between them increases, the mesonephric ducts descend caudally to open into the developing posterior urethra. By contrast, the ureters retain their original position with respect to the developing bladder. Although the triangular plate of mesoderm enclosing the ureteric orifices and openings of the mesonephric ducts is covered by the endodermal lining of the urogenital canal, its outline is retained as the trigone. It should be noted, however, that as with the compartmentalization of the cloaca the conventional account of the

translocation of the mesonephric ducts and formation of the trigone has been challenged by studies employing modern methodology (14). It now seems more probable that apparent changes in relative anatomy are a consequence of remodeling because of laying down of new tissue and apoptosis in situ rather than actual three-dimensional movement of anatomical structures in the early embryo. The most distal (perineal) portion of the urogenital canal gives rise to the entire length of the female urethra and to the posterior urethra in the male. The anterior portion of the male urethra is created by closure of the urogenital groove, described below. Meanwhile the allantois, an elongated diverticulum protruding from the dome of the fetal bladder into the umbilicus, is gradually obliterated but persists as the median umbilical ligament.

CLINICAL CONSIDERATIONS

Despite recent changes in our understanding of the process of compartmentalization of the cloaca, the concept of failed or incomplete descent of the urorectal septum, nevertheless, provides a simple and readily understood model to account for the spectrum of anomalies that includes urogenital sinus and complete, persistent cloaca. The etiology of bladder exstrophy and epispadias is less well understood, but these anomalies are believed to reflect underlying defects of the cloacal membrane. Persistence of all or part of the allantois gives rise to the various urachal abnormalities.

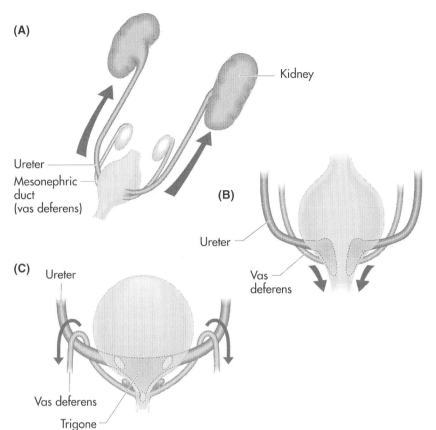

(A)

Kidney

Ureter

Mesonephric duct (vas deferens)

(B)

Ureter

Vas deferens

(C) Ureter

Vas deferens

Trigone

Figure 7 (**A**, **B**): Although the ureters maintain their position in relation to the developing bladder, the mesonephric ducts are drawn distally to enter the proximal urethra. (**C**) Testicular descent causes the mesonephric ducts (vasa deferentia) to loop over the ureters.

FUNCTIONAL DEVELOPMENT OF THE FETAL URINARY TRACT

Around the 9th to 10th week of gestation, fetal urine is excreted into the amniotic cavity. At this stage the urothelium adopts the morphology associated with its barrier function, notably the expression of uroplakins on the luminal surface. The embryonic urothelium also induces smooth muscle differentiation in surrounding pelvic and ureteric mesenchyme by secretion of Shh and other signaling molecules. Initially, urine composition closely resembles that of plasma filtrate. In the fetus, the excretory and homeostatic functions of the kidney are fulfilled by the placenta, and the principal role of the fetal kidneys is to contribute urine to amniotic fluid. The volume of amniotic fluid reaches its maximum of around 1000 mL at 38 weeks' gestation—at which point 90% of the amniotic fluid is derived from fetal urine. In addition to providing a protective fluid environment for the fetus, amniotic fluid plays a vital role in fetal lung development. Reduction in fetal urine output as a consequence of either renal agenesis or infravesical obstruction results in oligohydramnios, which in turn is associated with pulmonary hypoplasia. Molding or compression deformities such as talipes and characteristic facial molding (Potter's facies) occur as a consequence of the compressive effect of the surrounding uterus.

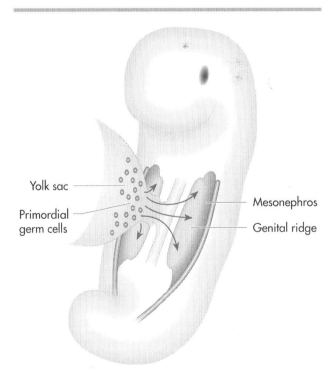

Yolk sac

Primordial germ cells

Mesonephros

Genital ridge

Figure 8 Migration of the primordial germ cells from the yolk sac across the coelomic cavity to colonize the mesoderm of the genital ridges during the fifth week.

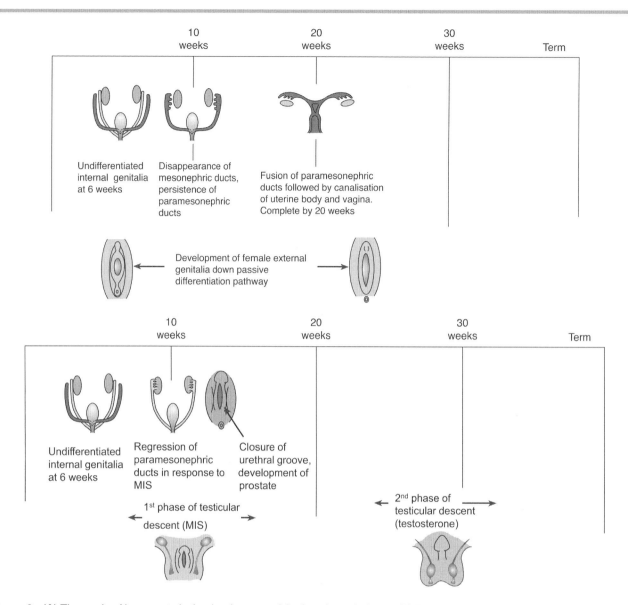

Figure 9 (**A**) Timescale of key events in the development of the female genital tract. (**B**) Timescale of key events in the development of the male genital tract.

GENITAL TRACTS

The internal and external genitalia of both sexes share identical embryonic precursors, and it is only from the 6th week onward that differences become apparent. In both sexes, the formation of the gonads and genital tracts is initiated by the migration of primordial germ cells from the base of the yolk sac, across the coelomic cavity to condensations of mesenchyme flanking the midline of the lumbar region of the embryo (the genital ridge) (Fig. 8). By a process of reciprocal induction (analogous to nephrogenesis), the interaction of the germ cells and surrounding mesenchyme results in the formation of the primitive sex cords within the embryonic gonad. It is around this time that a second pair of genital ducts (the paramesonephric ducts) makes its appearance. Derived from condensations

of coelomic epithelium and lying lateral to the mesophric ducts, these ducts fuse distally at their point of attachment to the urogenital canal. From the sixth week onward, the paths of male and female differentiation diverge and will be considered separately in the following subsections;

The timescale of key events in the development of both female and male genital tracts is summarized Figure 9A and B.

Female (Fig. 9A)

Internal Genitalia

It is widely accepted that without the genetic information carried by the testis-determining gene (*SRY*), the gonads and genital tract of the embryo are

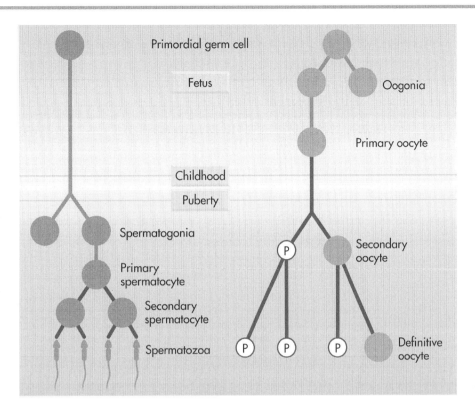

Figure 10 Gametogenesis. Mitotic division of the primordial germ cells in the male embryo is suppressed by the Sertoli cells of the embryonic germinal epithelium. Gametogenesis recommences at puberty. The gametes (spermatozoa) are the product of two meiotic divisions, that is, primary spermatocyte to secondary spermatocyte to spermatozoa. Immediately after the second meiotic division, the immature haploid gametes are termed spermatids. The morphological maturation to spermatozoa occurs during passage through the seminiferous tubule. In the female, the initial phases of gametogenesis occur in the first five months of fetal life. Primary oocytes remain in arrested meiotic division until meiosis recommences in the maturing Graafian follicle. The two meiotic divisions culminate in the production of a single definitive oocyte and three polar bodies (P).

programmed to differentiate down a female pathway. However, it is probably an oversimplification to view differentiation of the female gonads as an entirely passive or "default" process. For example, females with Turner syndrome (45X) have dysplastic or streak gonads—indicating that normal ovarian development requires the presence of two X chromosomes and is not simply determined by the absence of genetic material carried on the Y chromosome.

Within the genital ridges the primitive sex cords degenerate, but secondary sex cords derived from mesoderm enclose the primordial germ cells to form the primitive follicles. In the female, gametogenesis commences in intrauterine life with the transition from primordial germ cells to primary oocytes being completed in the fetal ovary. These primary oocytes then proceed into the first phase of meiosis before entering a long phase of arrested division, which only resumes again after puberty (Fig. 10). Persistence of the mesonephric ducts in male embryos is dependent on local stimulation by testosterone; therefore, in the absence of androgen stimulation in the female, the mesonephric ducts regress (with the exception of vestigial remnants of the epoophoron and paroophoron

and Gartner's cysts) (Fig. 11). The paramesonephric ducts persist and develop to become the fallopian tubes, and their fused distal portions give rise to the uterus and upper two-thirds of the vagina. At their point of attachment to the urogenital sinus, the fused tips of the paramesonephric ducts induce a condensation of tissue—the sinuvaginal bulb. Downward growth of the sinuvaginal bulb in the direction of the fetal perineum between weeks 10 and 20 has the effect of separating the vagina from the urethra. The vagina is initially represented by a solid plate of paramesonephric tissue, but this canalizes to create the vaginal lumen before the 20th week. The distal third of the vagina is derived from the urogenital sinus (endoderm), whereas the introitus and external genitalia are ectodermal in origin (Fig. 12).

External Genitalia

The external genitalia of the embryo and fetus are "programmed" to differentiate passively down a female pathway unless exposed to androgenic stimulation. Thus, the genital tubercle forms the clitoris, the introitus and vestibule of the vagina are derived from the urogenital sinus, the urogenital folds evolve into

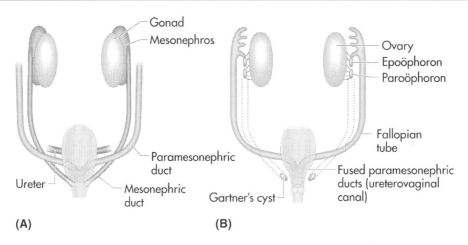

Figure 11 (**A**) The genital tract of both male and female embryos remains in the same undifferentiated state until the sixth week of gestation. (**B**) Paramesonephric duct a b derivatives in the female embryo.

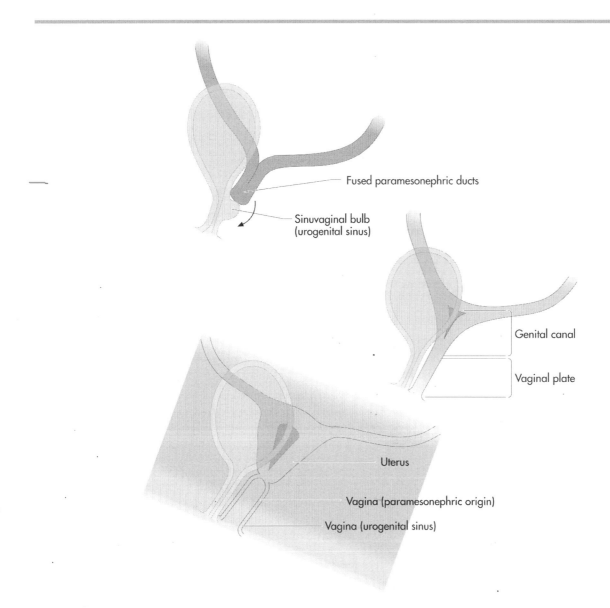

Figure 12 Development of the lower female genital tract between 10 and 20 weeks. Migration of the sinuvaginal bulb toward the fetal perineum results in formation and elongation of the vaginal plate and separation of the vagina from the urethra.

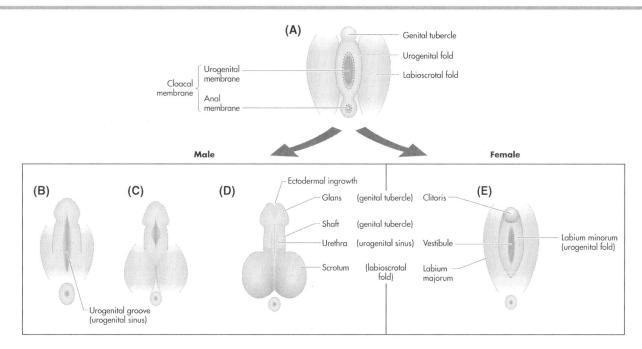

Figure 13 (**A**) Undifferentiated precursors of male and female external genitalia. (**B–D**) Androgen (testosterone-derived dihydrotestosterone)-induced differentiation of the male external genitalia between 12 and 16 weeks. (**E**) In the absence of androgenic stimulation, the external genitalia are programmed to differentiate along a female pathway.

the labia minora, and the labioscrotal folds persist as the labia majora (Fig. 13).

Male (Fig. 9B)

Internal Genitalia

Although many aspects of the male differentiation pathway are mediated by "downstream" genes located on the Y chromosome and on autosomes, the process is initiated by the testis-determining gene (*SRY*) located on the Y chromosome. In experiments in transgenic mice, the insertion of DNA carrying the *SRY* gene into the genotype of an XX (female) mouse results in differentiation of a male genital phenotype (15). The *SRY* gene product (a transcription factor) stimulates the medullary sex cords of the embryonic gonad to differentiate into secretory Sertoli cells. From the seventh week onward, the Sertoli cells secrete a glycoprotein—anti-Müllerian hormone or Müllerian-inhibiting substance (MIS)—that switches differentiation down the male pathway. At least three key functions have been ascribed to MIS:

1. It causes regression of the paramesonephric ducts, which disappear completely in the male with the exception of vestigial remnants (the appendix, testis, and the utriculus).
2. It stimulates the Leydig cells of the embryonic testis to produce testosterone from the ninth week of gestation.
3. It induces the first stage of testicular descent by its action on the gubernaculum, which anchors the

testis in the vicinity of the developing inguinal canal.

Further division of the primordial germ cells is inhibited in the male embryonic gonad. Until recently, it was believed that the testis is quiescent throughout childhood and that the subsequent sequence of gametogenesis is resumed again only at puberty. This concept is now being challenged by evidence pointing to the occurrence of two maturational steps in the prepubertal testis. The first, occurring around two to three months of age, consists of the switch from gonocytes (fetal stem cells) to adult-type spermatogonia (the adult stem cell pool). The second step, at approximately 5 years of age, is marked by a transient phase of meiosis, which can be detected histologically by the appearance of primary spermatocytes. Information obtained from biopsy studies of undescended testes has revealed that cryptorchidism has a major impact on prepubertal germ cell maturation—with obvious implications for the timing of orchidopexy.

Regression of the paramesonephric ducts in response to MIS is accompanied by the development of mesonephric duct derivatives under the influence of testosterone secreted by the fetal testis (Fig. 14A). During the period between the 8th and 12th week of gestation, the mesonephric ducts give rise to the epididymis and rete testis, vas deferens, ejaculatory ducts, and seminal vesicles (Fig. 14B). Within the testis, the seminiferous tubules take their origin from the primitive sex cords of the genital ridge mesoderm with the rete testis and epididymis being derived from the mesonephric tubules.

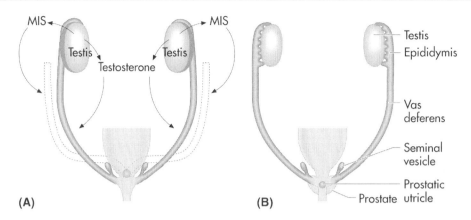

Figure 14 (**A**) Differentiation of male internal genitalia. Secretion of Müllerian-inhibiting substance (MIS) by pre-Sertoli cells induces regression of the paramesonephric ducts between 8 and 10 weeks. (**B**) MIS also stimulates the embryonic Leydig cells to secrete testosterone, which in turn stimulates the mesonephric ducts to differentiate into the definitive male internal genitalia.

The development of the prostate gland provides another example of reciprocal induction. At around week 12, in response to androgenic stimulation, a condensation of mesenchyme in the fetal pelvis induces the outgrowth of endodermal buds on the adjacent region of the developing urethra (16). In the experimental setting it has been shown that transitional epithelium from the adult rat can be induced to differentiate into prostatic glandular epithelium when cultured in contact with the appropriate embryonic mesenchyme. In normal fetal development, however, the endodermal proliferation and branching that give rise to the ducts and glandular acini of the prostate gland cease after the 15th week. The glandular tissue of the prostate is derived from the urethral endoderm (urogenital sinus); the capsule and smooth muscle are mesenchymal in origin, whereas the mesonephric ducts form the intraprostatic vas deferens and ejaculatory ducts.

External Genitalia (Fig. 13)

Prior to the compartmentalization of the cloaca to form the urogenital and anorectal canals between the sixth and seventh weeks, the primitive perineum consists of little more than the cloacal membrane and genital tubercle. Separation of the cloaca into the urogenital canal and anorectal canal is accompanied by subdivision of the cloacal membrane into the urogenital membrane anteriorly and the anal membrane posteriorly. Urogenital folds surround the urogenital membrane, flanked by the labioscrotal folds. From the seventh week onward, the urogenital sinus advances onto the perineum anteriorly and onto the penis as the urethral groove. Ingrowth of the urethral groove creates a solid urethral plate, which subsequently canalizes to form the definitive urethra. Differentiation of the male external genitalia is dependent, first, on the enzymatic conversion of testosterone to dihydrotestosterone and also requires the presence of the appropriate receptors in the target tissues. During the 12th to 14th week, the external genitalia begin to adopt a distinctively male configuration in response to androgenic stimulation (17). Closure of the urethra is complete by around 15 weeks, the terminal portion being formed by ingrowth of ectoderm from the tip of the glans.

Testicular Descent

As already described, the fetal testis originates from the interaction of primordial germ cells, with the mesenchyme of the genital ridge and tubular mesonephric duct derivatives. Testicular descent occurs in two phases. The first stage occurs in response to exposure to MIS, the second being stimulated by testosterone. Between weeks 8 and 15, the cord-like gubernaculum extending down from the testis enlarges at its distal end in the region of the labioscrotal swellings (Fig. 15A). Because the length of the gubernaculum remains relatively fixed during a period of active fetal growth, this has the effect of anchoring the testis in the region of the future inguinal canal (Fig. 15B). The second, more active, phase of testicular descent occurs around 25 to 30 weeks of gestation when testosterone causes the gubernaculum to shrink and contract, thus guiding the testis down the inguinal canal into its final scrotal position (Fig. 15C) (18). On its route of descent, the testis is preceded by a sac-like protrusion of peritoneum, the processus vaginalis, which normally closes spontaneously prior to delivery or in the early months of life.

GENITAL ANOMALIES: CLINICAL CONSIDERATIONS

A number of mechanisms can give rise to abnormalities of genital development, including chromosomal defects, abnormalities of gonadal development, and impaired synthesis of sex hormones or defects of their corresponding receptors.

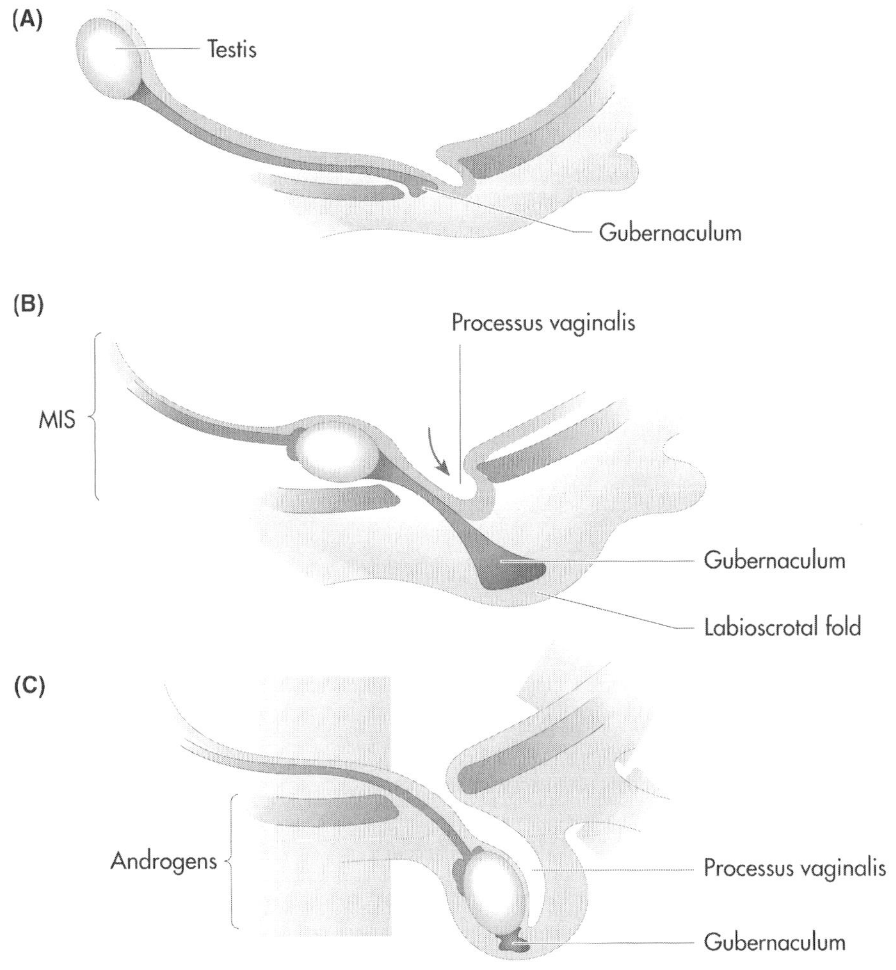

Figure 15 (**A**) Formation of the gubernaculum. (**B**) 10 to 15 weeks: enlargement of the caudal end of the gubernaculums (in response to MIS) anchors the fetal testis at the developing inguinal canal. (**C**) 25 to 30 weeks: testosterone-induced second stage of a testicular descent.

Defective development of the paramesonephric ducts results in a variety of clinical manifestations. At its most fundamental level the unilateral absence of paramesonephric duct derivatives, which is also associated with ipsilateral unilateral renal agenesis, points to a fundamental defect dating from the original intermediate mesoderm. Agenesis of the upper two-thirds of the vagina (Rokitansky syndrome) results from failure of the paramesonephric ducts to fuse distally and merge with the urogenital sinus. Incomplete fusion of the distal ends of the paramesonephric ducts accounts for anomalies such as bicornuate uterus, while defective canalization of the vaginal plate results in transverse vaginal septa and short atretic segments.

Approximately 80% of infants with ambiguous genitalia are 46 XX females with congenital adrenal hyperplasia whose external genitalia have virilized in response to high levels of circulating androgens of adrenal origin. In this condition, however, the internal reproductive tract develops normally down the female pathway. Individuals with a 46 XY karyotype and complete androgen-insensitivity syndrome (previously termed "testicular feminization") have a female external genital phenotype because of a genetically determined peripheral receptor insensitivity to dihydrotestosterone, which causes the external genitalia to fail to virilize despite exposure to androgens secreted by the fetal testes.

Incomplete closure of the urethral groove accounts for moderate and severe forms of hypospadias, while distal (glanular) hypospadias probably represents failure of ectodermal ingrowth from the glanular tip. Severe forms of proximal hypospadias are often associated with cryptorchidism and a persistent utriculus (Müllerian remnant). While these features point to the presence of an underlying virilization defect, attempts to identify specific endocrinopathies in boys with severe hypospadias have generally proved unrewarding.

There is some epidemiological evidence to suggest that the incidence of hypospadias and cryptorchidism is increasing and exposure of male fetuses to estrogenic or antiandrogenic environmental pollutants has been postulated as a possible cause.

Cryptorchidism affects 1% to 2% of the male infant population, but there is no single unifying etiology. Endocrinopathy or imbalance of the pituitary-gonadal axis can be implicated in cases of bilateral cryptorchidism, particularly when associated with hypospadias. By contrast local mechanical factors (possibly related to the gubernaculum or the processus vaginalis) are likely to play a more important role in unilateral cryptorchidism. In the rare, genetically determined syndrome of MIS deficiency, intra-abdominal testes are found in conjunction with persistent paramesonephric duct structures, including fallopian tubes and uterus. Although deficiency of MIS accounts for a proportion of cases, this condition is misnamed since it is more commonly because of a receptor defect for MIS.

Simple mechanical factors provide the most obvious explanation for unilateral cryptorchidism, but the reported finding of histological abnormalities in the contralateral descended testis suggests that endocrinopathy may also play a role in unilateral cryptorchidism. The presence of a blind-ending vas and spermatic vessels in most cases of testicular "agenesis" is widely interpreted as evidence of intrauterine testicular torsion rather than a defect of embryogenesis.

THE GENETIC BASIS OF GENITOURINARY MALFORMATIONS (TABLE 2)

Malformations of the urinary and genital tracts are relatively common and are estimated to account for one-third of all congenital anomalies. Although the importance of genetic factors is being increasingly recognized, it remains the case that most CAKUT occur on a sporadic basis resulting from defective embryogenesis or faulty development in fetal life.

The adult and infant forms of polycystic renal disease provide the most convincing examples of genetically determined structural renal disease. Genetic factors have also been implicated in the etiology of renal agenesis, VUR, and upper tract duplication. Genitourinary malformations with a recognized familial tendency are most commonly inherited as autosomal traits of variable penetrance and expression. Although some conditions, such as polycystic kidney disease, have their origins in a single gene mutation, the etiology of most structural anomalies of the urinary tract is more complex—as illustrated by the fact that upper tract anomalies are often expressed unilaterally or asymmetrically even when genetic factors are clearly implicated. When genitourinary anomalies occur within the context of a recognized syndrome, it is probable that the affected gene (or genes) encodes for gene products that play a fundamental molecular role in the regulation and development of a number of systems. For example, the KAL gene implicated in X-linked Kallmann's syndrome (microphallus, renal agenesis, and anosmia) is known to code for an adhesion molecule that is expressed during the migration of olfactory neurons in the brain and also in the developing genitor urinary tract. Other examples include renal–coloboma syndrome (VUR and the ophthalmic anomaly, coloboma), which is because of a mutation of the PAX-2 gene encoding for a transcription factor.

IN VITRO FERTILIZATION AND OTHER APPLICATIONS OF DEVELOPMENTAL BIOLOGY IN UROLOGY

The availability of techniques for IVF has given many urological patients the potential for parenthood whereas previously their outlook for fertility would have been bleak. Examples of patients who might benefit from IVF techniques include men with oligospermia or azoospermia because of cryptorchidism and men with impaired ejaculation associated with a history of posterior urethral valves or bladder exstrophy. In the technique of intracytoplasmic sperm injection, spermatozoa are harvested directly from the testis or epididymis and a single spermatozoan is selected and injected into an oocyte. The fertilized zygote is then implanted into the uterus. Other variants of IVF such as gamete intrafallopian transfer (GIFT) or zygote intrafallopian transfer (ZIFT) may also be applicable for urological patients with a range of congenital or acquired causes of infertility.

Table 2   The Genetic Basis of Common Urinary Tract Abnormalities

Adult polycystic kidney disease	Autosomal dominant	Chromosome 16p Chromosome 4
"Infantile" polycystic kidney disease	Autosomal recessive	
Vesicoureteric reflux	Autosomal dominant, variable penetrance and expression	(*Pax-2* gene in renal–coloboma syndrome)
Renal agenesis	Various, i.e., autosomal dominant, recessive and X-linked patterns identified	
Ureteric duplication	Autosomal dominant—variable penetrance and expression	
Pelviureteric junction obstruction	When familial behaves as autosomal dominant	Documented familial evidence as isolated anomaly or pelviureteric junction obstruction in association with specific syndromes (e.g., Schinzel–Giedion and Johanson–Blizzard syndromes)

Embryo Research

The concept of therapeutic cloning is based on aspects of the methodology originally developed for IVF. The key steps are as follows:

1. The nucleus of a harvested or donated oocyte is removed by micropuncture. A diploid nucleus extracted from a somatic cell is then injected into the enucleated oocyte. For the purposes of therapeutic cloning, it is envisaged that the somatic cell would be derived from the patient.
2. The cell thus created is induced to divide, as for example, by an electrical charge.
3. A sequence of doubling divisions then ensues, which mirrors that of the fertilized zygote. Proteins within the cytoplasm of maternal oocyte are thought to be responsible for inducing the cloned cell to behave as a fertilized zygote rather than the mature somatic cell from which its nucleus was derived.

Human embryo research has focused on the extraction of pluripotent embryonic stem cells from early embryonic tissue. Tissue derived by inducing differentiation of pluripotent stem cells would share the same genetic identity as the somatic nucleus used to create the cloned embryo and would therefore not provoke rejection by the immune system when reintroduced into the individual (patient) from whom the nuclear material had been obtained.

Clinical indications envisaged for such forms of treatment include tissue reconstruction, the treatment of degenerative disease—particularly neurodegenerative disorders such as Parkinson's disease—and islet cell transplants to treat type 1 diabetes.

At present the potential application of early human embryonic tissue for therapeutic purposes is constrained by practical considerations such as the scarcity of donated oocytes and the invasive nature of oocyte donation. One of the more controversial proposals to overcome this hurdle envisages injecting a human diploid nucleus into an enucleated oocyte derived from another species to create a human–animal hybrid embryo from which (human) stem cells would be extracted at a very early stage to create stem cell lines in tissue culture. Another approach being explored would obviate the use of oocytes by manipulating differentiated cells in vitro to cause them to revert to an undifferentiated state to create induced pluripotent stem cells.

In the light of current knowledge, it seems most likely that within the field of Urology the applications of embryo research will lie mainly in reproductive medicine—notably in the development of innovative treatments for male infertility. By contrast, the treatment of renal impairment by reactivating nephrogenesis to stimulate new nephron formation in poorly functioning kidneys or alternatively the creation of tissue engineered kidneys for use in transplantation must be seen as highly futuristic prospects.

REFERENCES

1. Thomson JA, Itskovitz-Eldor J, Shapiro SS, et al. Embryonic stem cell lines derived from human blastocysts. Science 1998; 282:1145–1147.
2. Houk CP, Hughes IA, Ahmed SF, et al. Summary of consensus statement on intersex disorders. International Intersex Consensus Conference. Pediatrics 2006; 118(2):753–757.
3. Haraguchi R, Motoyama J, Sasaki H, et al. Molecular analysis of coordinated bladder and urogenital organ formation by Hedgehog signalling. Development 2007; 134:525–533.
4. Caubit X, Lye CM, Martin E, et al. Teashirt 3 is necessary for ureteral smooth muscle differentiation downstream of SHH and BMP4. Development 2008; 135(19):3301–3310.
5. Hu P, Deng FM, Liang FX, et al. Ablation of uroplakin III gene results in small urothelial plaques, urothelial leakage, and vesicoureteral reflux. J Cell Biol 2000; 151(5):961–972.
6. Jiang S, Gitlin J, Deng FM, et al. Lack of major involvement of human uroplakin genes in vesicoureteral reflux: implications for disease heterogeneity. Kidney Int 2004; 66: 10–19.
7. Garthwaite MA, Thomas DFM, Subramaniam R, et al. Urothelial differentiation in vesicoureteric reflux and other urological disorders of childhood: a comparative study. Eur Urol 2006; 49:154–160.
8. Jenkins D, Bitner-Glindzicz M, Malcolm S, et al. Mutation Analysis of Uroplakin II in children with renal tract malformations. Nephrol Dial Transplant 2006; 21: 3415–3421.
9. Feather S, Woolf AS, Gordon I, et al. Vesicoureteric reflux—is it all in the genes? Lancet 1996; 348:725–728.
10. Yerke EB. The new renal angiotensin system and its impact on upper urinary tract development. Dialogues Pediatr Urol 2000; 23:4–5.
11. Stahl DA, Koul HK, Chacko JK, et al. Congenital anomalies of the kidney and urinary tract (CAKUT): a current review of cell signaling processes in ureteral development. J Pediatr Urol 2006; 2:2–9.
12. Thomas DFM. Cloacal malformations: embryology, anatomy and principles of management. In: Spitz L, Wurnig P, Angerpointner TA, eds. Progress in Paediatric Surgery. Vol 23. Berlin: Springer-Verlag, 1989:135–143.
13. Pennington EC, Hutson JM. The absence of lateral fusion in cloacal partition. J Pediatr Surg 2003; 38(9):1287–1295.
14. Oswald J, Schwentner C, Lunacek A, et al. Reevaluation of the fetal muscle development of the vesigal trigone. J Urol 2006; 176:1166–1170.
15. Larsen WJ. Development of the urogenital system. In: Larsen WJ, ed. Human Embryology. 3rd ed. Philadelphia: Churchill Livingstone, 2001:265–313.
16. McNeal JE. Anatomy and embryology. In: Fitzpatrick JM, Kane RJ, eds. The Prostate. Edinburgh: Churchill Livingstone, 1989:3–9.
17. Kurzrock AE, Jeyatheesan P, Cunha GR, et al. Urethral development in the fetal rabbit and induction of hypospadias: a model for human development. J Urol 2000; 164(5):1786–1792.
18. Hutson JM, Terada M, Baiyun Z, et al. Normal Testicular Descent and the Aetiology of Cryptorchidism. Advances in Anatomy, Embryology and Cell Biology. Vol. 132. Berlin: Springer-Verlag, 1996:

30

Urological and Biochemical Aspects of Transplantation Biology

David Talbot

Department of Hepatobiliary and Transplant Surgery, Freeman Hospital, Newcastle upon Tyne, U.K.

Naeem Soomro

Department of Urology, Freeman Hospital, Newcastle upon Tyne, U.K.

INTRODUCTION

The first successful human renal allograft was performed in Boston by Merrill and Murray on December 23, 1954. Preceding this had been many unsuccessful animal and even human transplants. Only two things had been learned from this early work; firstly, how vessels could be successfully anastomosed, and, secondly, that transplantation between nonrelated individuals was impossible. The Boston transplant was successful because it was between identical twin brothers, and it was not until immunosuppressive drugs became available that transplantation could really develop.

ORGAN DONATION

The early transplants were all performed from live donors; then, with the advent of immunosuppression, nonrelated cadaver donors could be used. These initially were simply cadavers and therefore were "non–heart beating" donors, but later, with legislation and acceptance of brain death, heart-beating but brain-dead donors were used. More recently, with the limited supply of brain-dead donors, there has been significant expansion of both live donation and non–heart beating donation.

BRAINSTEM DEATH

Though death is an unavoidable aspect of life, all countries have their own procedures and legislation connected with it. With the advent of transplantation and possible use of organs, most countries were forced to consider and thereby distinguish between cardiac and brain death. In some countries, such as Austria, donation was extremely easy because legislation had been introduced many years previously giving the state more roles after death so postmortems were compulsory to minimize health risks to the living. In many countries, criteria were established for the diagnosis of brain death. In the United Kingdom, the tests had to be performed on two occasions by two experienced medical practitioners. Certain prerequisite conditions had to be fulfilled;

namely, normothermia and absence of sedative drugs. Furthermore, the subject had to be shown to be ventilator dependent with elevated carbon dioxide levels and have absent cranial nerve reflexes, notably the gag, corneal and vestibulocochlear reflexes, by two experienced medical practitioners on two occasions (1). When the patient was diagnosed as being brain dead, the issues of donation and transplant could be discussed with the relatives. The posts of transplant coordinators evolved in the mid-1980s, in part to act as bereavement counselors and to coordinate the multiple teams involved in a multiorgan donor. Their role has been essential in maintaining donor numbers in the face of reduced death rates from road traffic accidents and improved outcome of neurosurgery.

NON–HEART BEATING DONATION

Because of the increasing shortage of kidneys for donation, there is a need to increase the pool of organs. Therefore, the option of non–heart beating donoration, which had been utilized before brain death legislation, was explored again. These donors have been subjected to a varying amount of primary warm ischemia, during the time between cardiac arrest and perfusion with cold preservation solution. Different categories can be defined (Maastricht), which have implications for the degree of warm ischemia, simply these are controlled (awaiting cardiac arrest, Maastricht III and IV) and uncontrolled (failed resuscitation in the emergency setting, Maastricht I and II) (2). Because there is damage to the organs after cardiac arrest (warm ischemia), care must be taken to establish which kidneys are safe to transplant (3). If such steps are taken and the kidneys are used, delayed graft function is common (4). However, after a time, the function recovers, and the long-term outlook is the same as for kidneys transplanted from brain-dead donors (4,5) Livers and pancreata have all been transplanted from such donors, but greater care must be taken, as delayed graft function, if it occurs, in a liver transplant is usually fatal (6).

The proportion of kidneys from such donors is increasing year on year such that in 2007 20.4% of kidney donors were from non–heart beating donors. The increase has in the main been because this is a different source of cadaver donors but to a lesser extent there have been brain-dead donors that have come to donation via the non–heart beating route for different reasons.

LIVE RELATED AND UNRELATED DONATION

As cold ischemia is considerably reduced in live donation, the long-term graft survival is better than with cadaveric donor kidney grafts. Formerly, centers with large cadaver-kidney programs have generally had small live donor programs, presumably indicating that supply is sufficient for demand. However, with the generally declining cadaver programs, live donor numbers have increased. Commercialization of transplantation has created a huge ethical issue, and many countries have "solved" this by banning the practice.

There are countries that embrace commercialization such as Iran where it is usual to keep a panel of potential donors who are called up when a potential recipient is identified the donors being subsequently compensated financially. Most Western countries though they have made donation for money illegal often use some financial support such as for transport costs but compensation for lost income is difficult. In the United States, tax concessions for donors and a reduction their health insurance have been proposed. Regulation of live donor transplantation has evolved but is country specific, so, for example, the United Kingdom formerly required proof of first degree relatives by Tissue typing/ DNA analysis or approval by Unrelated Live Transplant Regulatory Authority (ULTRA) for all others. This has recently changed with the establishment of the Human Tissue Authority (HTA). This means that any potential live donor after they have been assessed and are judged to be suitable have to have an assessment by an "independent" assessor. These assessors have all been trained and are approved by the HTA and establish that the potential donor has not been coerced. All documents are then submitted and approval granted by the HTA. This mechanism means that all related and unrelated are managed the same. It has also enabled paired donation (swopping donor/recipient combinations when the transplant cannot occur between pairs, e. g., with ABO incompatible combinations or donor specific antibodies) and completely altruistic donation. Full details on the legal requirements within the United Kingdom for live donation can be found at www.hta.gov.uk.

Kidney donation from live donors carries a low mortality rate and is preferably conducted in parallel with the recipient surgery, which minimizes ischemia. It is also useful for the occasional difficult recipient such that the kidney is not removed until the recipient vessels are confirmed to be suitable. From the live donors perspective undoubtedly the preferable method of donation is with a laparoscopic approach. From the recipients point of view the warm ischemic time to the kidney is slightly longer (usually about five minutes) during the kidney extraction but this has been shown to have no significant affect on outcome. However, laparoscopic right-kidney donation carries some risk of caval or duodenal injury and should be done routinely only after considerable experience has been obtained from left-kidney donation.

ORGAN PRESERVATION

In the early days of renal transplantation, there was considerable uncertainty as to how to store the organ. The two methods were simple static cold storage and dynamic machine perfusion, which was also performed at cold temperature. Most groups stopped machine preservation when it was discovered that, generally, the longer the kidney remained in storage, the worse was the outcome (7). Certain groups, principally Belzer et al. from the United States, persisted with machine perfusion, and when the solutions were improved, it was found that the kidney preservation was better with this method than with static storage (8). This was principally the case with marginal donor kidneys, and this method had the added benefit of allowing the surgeons to improve their viability assessment by assessing the resistance and flow through the kidney (3,9).

The "holy grail" of preservation, however, is being able to do it at normal temperature, as this allows more accurate viability assessment and recovery of the organ. However, it is extremely difficult because of the metabolic demands of the organ, and only limited success has been possible so far (10).

PRESERVATION SOLUTIONS

The first aim of preservation fluid is to replace blood, which, if allowed to stand within the organ, will clot and thereby render it useless. The second aim is to reduce the temperature of the organ to near freezing point to minimize the metabolic demands of the organ (hence, the solutions are kept cold). At cold temperatures, the normal cell-membrane electrolyte pumps fail, and cellular swelling occurs. The early solutions were essentially hyperosmolal mannitol, and though they prevented swelling, the intracellular electrolyte concentrations changed; therefore, acute tubular necrosis was common, particularly when cold storage was prolonged. The solutions were therefore modified to preserve the intracellular milieu; hence, Marshalls, Collins, and Euro-Collins were developed. Though acute tubular necrosis still occurred with these solutions, it was not as common. However, other organs, notably the liver, that had to work immediately on transplantation had to have a very restricted cold ischemic time with these solutions. This improved with the development of University of Wisconsin, or Belzer I, solution that contained the inert sugar lactobionate and starch, which was very effective in preventing cell swelling (11). Both kidneys and livers preserved with this solution could be cold stored for longer with an increased chance of primary function on reperfusion (12). After cold storage, reperfusion with blood generates oxygen free radicals, and these further damage the graft. Though the University of Wisconsin solution contains glutathione, which is a free radical scavenger, its slightly acid pH means that the glutathione is not stable, and so damage on reperfusion is a problem. Other solutions have been developed, notably histidine, tryptophane-ketoglutarate, and celsior, all of which contain inert buffers and free radical scavengers that could confer some advantages on reperfusion (13).

ASSESSMENT OF THE LIVE DONOR

Live donation in the United Kingdom is now governed by the 2004 Human Tissue Act, which became law from September 2006. There is a legal requirement in setting the transplant up (see above) and they can only be performed in registered establishments.

Initial Assessment

This is usually performed by the nephrologist and transplant coordinator, the former often referring the potential donor to another nephrologists to avoid conflict of interest. At the first consultation the following are established:

Medical, surgical and anesthetic fitness for surgery
Ensure the potential donor has two kidneys
Identify risk factors for the future development of renal disease
Exclude the presence of diseases transmissible to the recipient (e.g., infection or malignancy)
Provide information preferably both verbal and written on the procedure
Determine blood group compatibility (transplanting across ABO barrier is possible but difficult)
Human leukocyte antigen (HLA) typing and cross-matching of the donor and recipient (determination of donor specific antibodies present in the donor)

Subsequent Assessment

The perioperative mortality rate for living donor nephrectomy is reported as between 1 in 1600 and 1 in 3300. The major perioperative complication rate for donor nephrectomy is 2%.

Informed consent is undertaken with discussion about the potential risks of donor nephrectomy, including death and the general complications of surgery with specific mention of venous thrombo-embolism, intra-abdominal bleeding and infection, chest complications, urinary tract infections, and the possible need for blood transfusion.

The primary aim of the donor evaluation process is to ensure the suitability, safety and well-being of the patient. All potential soonors have their ABO and HLA compatibility with the donor checked. In addition, the

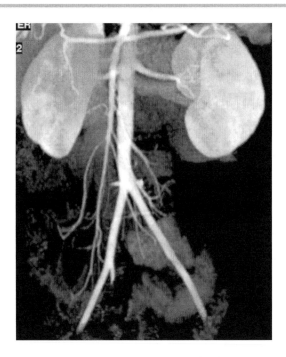

Figure 1 Magnetic resonance angiography for donor vessel assessment.

recipient's serum is tested against the donor cells by cross-match.

In the past, renal anatomy was defined in the donor by abdominal ultrasound, intravenous urography and renal angiography. This meant several hospitals visit with potential morbidity from anaphylaxis and vascular damage from angiography. Now, in most centers, either spiral computerized tomography (CT) or magnetic resonance (MR) angiography with 3-D reconstruction has replaced the need for all these tests. The procedure requires one visit to the hospital, and the visualization of the renal venous anatomy is excellent (Fig. 1).

Assessment of glomerular function rate (GFR) is done in all the potential donors. Serum creatinine is often used as a surrogate marker, and the Cockcroft-Gault equation is widely used.

Male GFR (mL/min) 5 (140, age) 3 ideal body weight (kg)/0.8 3 serum creatinine (lmol/L) (Female GFR 3 0.85)

A creatinine clearance of 80 mL/min/73 m² is a reasonable lower limit for kidney donation. The radio-isotope glomerular filtration rate obtained with ^{51}Cr EDTA is a more reliable measure, and this test can also provide information about split renal function. A minimum level of acceptable GFR is stipulated to prevent the donor from being put at risk) (Table 1). This level depends on the age, and it has to be above two standard deviations below the mean for the age (BTS guidelines) (Fig. 2).

The absolute and relative contraindications for live donations are tabulated in Table 2 (14–16).

Table 1   Acceptable GFR Prior to Donation

Donor age (yr)	GFR (mL/min/1.73m^2)
Up to 40	86
50	77
60	68
70	59
80	50

On the basis of British Transplant Society guidelines (www.BTS.org.uk/standards).

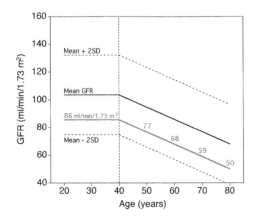

Figure 2   Diagram showing the variation with age of mean GFR (*solid black line*). The outer dashed lines show the ± 2 population standard deviation limits. GFR is constant up to the age of 40 years and then declines at the rate of 9mL/min/1.73 m^2 per decade. The reference plot is based on an analysis of data for 428 live renal transplant donors who had 51Cr-ETDA GFR measurements performed according to the method described in the British Nuclear Medicine Society GFR guidelines. The solid gray line shows the safety limit of 86 mL/min/1.73 m^2 for young adults declining to 50 mL/min/1.73 m^2 at age 80. For transplant donors with preoperative GFR values above the solid gray line the GFR of the remaining kidney will still be greater than 37.5 mL/min/1.73 m^2 at age 80. *Source*: From Ref. 2.

Table 2   Contraindications to Donation for Renal Transplantation

Absolute contraindications
Evidence of coercion
Inability to give informed consent
Most malignancies
HIV
Major respiratory or cardiovascular disease
Hypertensive end-organ damage
Body-mass index 35 kg/m^2
Pregnancy
Intravenous drug use
Thrombophilia
Renal disease
Relative contraindications
Age below 18 yr
Age over 70 yr
Body-mass index of 30–35 kg/m^2
Cigarette smoking
Psychiatric disorder
Risk factors for type 2 diabetes
Hepatitis B infection
Hypertension

Source: From Ref. 15.

ASSESSMENT OF CADAVERIC DONOR

In the United Kingdom, cadaveric donor rates are 24 per million population. This is the largest source of kidneys for transplantation. The number of potential donors is much higher, but lack of awareness among the staff and donors' relatives about donation means that these numbers have not increased.

The two main goals of donor evaluation are to exclude donors with severe disease, which can be transmitted to the recipient and to exclude kidneys with severe anatomical or functional changes, which could compromise allograft function.

All donors with malignancy are excluded except those who have cutaneous basal cell carcinoma or primary brain tumors with no metastases. Because of the risk of transmitting choriocarcinoma, chorionic gonadotrophin is estimated in all females of childbearing age who have died from cerebral hemorrhage.

The presence of HIV should preclude the use of organs. Donors with active hepatitis B and C infection are generally excluded, although organs can be transplanted safely into recipients who have already been exposed to these viruses. Measuring viral gene loads can be useful to assess the donor's infectivity. Any possibility of new variant Creutzfeldt-Jacob disease always precludes donation. Donors who have had adequate treatment of bacterial or fungal infection can be used, but a cautious approach is mandatory.

Kidneys from old ($<$70 yr) or young ($<$2 yr) donors or those with a body weight of less than 15 kg perform poorly. Prolonged hypotension, profound use of inotropic drugs, disseminated intravascular coagulation and diabetes mellitus in donors are relative contraindications. Those with high serum creatinine levels can be used safely as kidney donors provided they have a reversible cause of their kidney failure, such as hepatorenal failure. When the renal impairment is established it is unwise to transplant the kidney into a high demand recipient, that is, young recipient, particularly male, with a large muscle mass. Male donor to elderly female is more appropriate and dual transplant better still. In general, the GFR of the recipient will not be better than the donor and is likely to be worse.

ASSESSMENT OF THE RECIPIENTS

Ideally, patients with chronic renal failure should receive a transplant at precisely the time that they require a transplant. Unfortunately, this is rarely possible. The timing of the transplant work-up is based on the assumption that most patients would wait for cadaveric transplant for up to two years, and it takes approximately three months to prepare for a living donor transplant.

The assessment aims to look at recipient suitability to undergo a surgical procedure, and to identify any underlying disease or condition that may delay or would need to be rectified prior to transplantation. It is also an opportunity for the recipient to know what transplantation involves and the pitfalls and possible side effects of immunosuppression.

Cancer is generally a contraindication to immunosuppression, and patients who have active or recent evidence of malignancy, except for some skin cancers, may need to postpone or cancel transplant evaluation. It would be prudent to wait for some time to exclude patients who would develop a recurrence. Delay of longer than five years would exclude 87% of patients who would develop a recurrence, whereas a two-year wait would eliminate about 53% of recurrences. Generally, in most malignancies, patients should be free from recurrence for two years before transplantation, but a longer waiting time is required for malignant melanomas, breast cancer and colorectal cancer. No waiting time may be necessary in most skin cancers.

Cardiovascular disease is one of the leading causes of death after renal transplantation. Specific indicators of underlying cardiac disease are a definite history of acute myocardial infarction within the past six months, angina, ventricular arrhythmia, or left bundle branch block. Unfortunately, the ability of these indicators to predict a postsurgical cardiac event is not reliable.

The accepted risk factors for cardiovascular disease are as follows:

1. Family history of premature coronary artery disease
2. Hypertension
3. Diabetes
4. Men over the age of 45
5. Women over the age of 55
6. Decreased high-density lipoprotein
7. Increased low-density lipoprotein

For asymptomatic patients who are at high risk or have a history of IHD, a noninvasive test is quite useful to screen patients who might require coronary artery angiography. Thallium scintigraphy and dobutamine echocardiography have been used to screen such patients. All patients who have critical lesions on coronary angiography should undergo revascularization before transplantation.

Patients with a history of transient ischemic attacks or other evidence of cerebral vascular disease within the previous six months should have further evaluation. Patients with autosomal dominant polycystic kidney disease (ADPKD) have an increased risk of ruptured intracranial aneurysms. They should have MR angiography, and patients who have an aneurysm larger than 7 mm would probably benefit from prophylactic surgery.

Hepatitis A and E are not known to cause chronic liver disease in renal transplant recipients. However, recipients who are hepatitis B surface antigen positive, or are e antigen positive (HbeAG), or who have serological evidence of active viral replication are at a higher risk of disease progression in the posttransplant period. Patients who are hepatitis C positive have an increased incidence of chronic active hepatitis.

Extensive work-up is recommended for children and also adults who have a history of urological abnormalities or urinary tract infections. Renal ultrasonography and video-urodynamic studies may be indicated to look into the possibility of reflux and bladder physiology.

The risk of recurrent disease to the transplant kidney is real, but only around 5% graft loss is attributed to recurrent disease. There is a 10% to 25% risk of recurrence of hemolytic uremic syndrome and 10% to 30% risk of recurrence of focal segmental glomerulosclerosis; 40% to 50% of patients with recurrence will experience graft loss, and there is a 10% to 25% risk of recurrence in recipients whose original disease was membranous glomerulonephritis. In some cases, the type of immunosuppression used can affect the probability of disease recurrence; for example, calcineurin antagonists (ciclosporin and tacrolimus) promote recurrence of hemolytic uremic syndrome. NB it is important to have conducted genetic testing for HUS as disease recurrence can be inevitable no matter what the immunosuppression in which case there are a growing number of patients offered combined liver and kidney transplant for this condition to minimize any chance of this happening.

When recipients have met the criteria, they are put on the waiting list to receive a cadaveric organ through the national sharing scheme. At the time of the availability of a suitably matched kidney, a final cross-match is done before transplantation.

MATCHING DONOR AND RECIPIENTS

From the first successful renal transplant, it has been known that for the best results the recipient should have tissue similarities with the donor. This tissue similarity is essentially the ABO blood group and the major histocompatibility complex also known as the HLA (carried by chromosome 6). For major blood group matching, the same rules apply as blood transfusion, as the endothelium of the kidney is thrombogenic in an ABO mismatched combination. The major histocompatibility complex is subdivided into classes I and II, which, in man, comprise the HLAs A, B, C (I), and D (II), respectively. Though class I is expressed by all cells, the role of the professional antigen-presenting cells is more important, and these express class II. Therefore, matching for class II between donor and recipient is more important. Matching has a significant impact on long-term graft survival; therefore, most organ-sharing schemes have this as the principal philosophy. However, paradoxically, in live unrelated donation, usually spouse to spouse, where cold ischemic time is minimized, the normal milieu of the kidney has minimal disruption, and therefore the recipient's immune system does not become aware that any change has occurred. As a consequence, maximal mismatched kidney transplants can be tolerated without inevitable rejection. This state of affairs is also improved by the use of more successful modern immunosuppressive drugs.

Prior to transplantation, the recipients are tested for their immune sensitivity to the donor. This is done by incubating the donor lymphocytes with the recipients' sera to determine whether or not antibodies are present. This is usually detected by the addition of complement and viability stains for cell death. Flow cytometry can also be used to detect lower concentrations of antibody and to determine the type of antibody. When present, IgG is suggestive of memory and therefore has alloreactive potential, whereas IgM is more nonspecific. To transplant in the face of a positive cytotoxic cross-match carries the risk of hyperacute rejection when intravascular thrombosis can occur within minutes of reperfusion.

RENAL TRANSPLANTATION

The surgical technique of transplantation is quite standard and uses the extraperitoneal iliac fossa approach. The vessels are accessible at this point, and the ureter can be kept short, thereby minimizing the risk of ischemia. With careful surgical technique, no ureteric stent is required, but in large transplant units with many surgeons of different grades, most units utilize a ureteric stent, as it guarantees at least a minimal level of anastomotic technique. It also means the incidence of leak is extremely low. The external iliac artery is the commonest artery used, but the internal and common iliac arteries are also used (Figs. 3 and 4). In children with small vessels, it is important to utilize the common iliac artery or aorta to ensure a good pressure inflow, as arterial thrombosis is a common reason for graft failure. In those recipients of numerous previous renal allografts, an intraperitoneal approach and even an orthotopic approach with native nephrectomy at the time of transplant have been used successfully.

IMMUNOSUPPRESSION

Transplantation could not develop until the immune system was tamed by drugs. These initially were very nonspecific—radiotherapy, steroids and 6-mercaptopurine—but when used in conjunction with good donor-recipient matching, they produced 10-year graft survival not dissimilar to those achieved today.

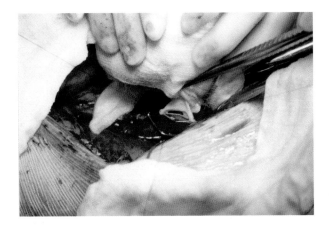

Figure 3 Anastomosing the transplant renal vein to the recipient external iliac vein.

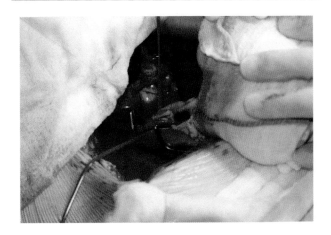

Figure 4 Anastomosing the transplant renal artery to the recipient external iliac artery.

Azathioprine, derived from 6-mercaptopurine, was developed in the 1960s. It is an antimetabolite and therefore produces marrow suppression. Antithymocyte globulin is a polyclonal antibody initially derived from the horse and later from the rabbit. This antibody was introduced in 1968; it lyses human leukocytes and thereby produces a cytokine "storm," giving the recipient a self-limiting temperature and rigors. This was found to be of particular benefit in steroid-resistant rejection. OKT3, which is a monoclonal antibody directed against T lymphocytes, was developed to supersede ATG. Lymphoma, recognized as a particular problem of strong immunosuppression, was slightly more common with OKT3. The calcineurin antagonists ciclosporin and later tacrolimus were derived from soil organisms and were found to be very effective in minimizing the immunological response; that is, IL2 production was inhibited. These drugs produced a spectacular improvement in graft survival up to five years. Beyond this, chronic graft dysfunction produced steady graft attrition, so that at 10 years, graft survival was similar to that seen with the more primitive agents. Mycophenolate mofetil and mycophenolic acid inhibit the purine pathway, most cells except lymphocytes have an escape pathway, so lymphocyte proliferation is inhibited. Animal work has suggested that these agents have benefit in chronic graft dysfunction, though human data have not yet confirmed this. Rapamycin, which is also derived from soil organisms, downregulates IL2 production, but in a slightly different way from ciclosporin and tacrolimus, and it therefore is not complicated by the calcineurin nephropathy that may in part contribute to chronic graft dysfunction. Rapamycin could possibly therefore also have benefits for long-term graft function.

In most transplant units combination therapies of the above agents are used; increasingly popular is antibody induction using IL2 receptor blockers, which allows the oral medication to be used more sparingly.

Serious bacterial infection is not a common problem now as it was in early transplant experience, where excessive immunosuppression was often used. Viraemia is now more of an issue as a consequence of immunosuppression, particularly with Epstein-Barr virus or herpes 6, the former giving rise to neoplasia and the latter to Karposi's sarcoma. BKV and JCV, which are related to SV40, and belong to the polyoma virus group, can be troublesome after transplant. BKV causes interstitial nephritis and ureteric strictures, while JCV can cause leucoencephalopathy in the immunosuppressed patient.

POSTTRANSPLANT MANAGEMENT

In the early postoperative period, fluid management and blood pressure are the most important aspects, as vascular thrombosis and pulmonary edema are serious consequences of both extremes of fluid state. Immunosuppression should be modified to obtain suitable levels of calcineurin antagonists. The patients have generally been on antihypertensive agents, and these may not be suitable after a transplant. ACE inhibitors can often be used safely later, but renal impairment at this time complicates the recipients' management. Antiviral prophylaxis is common for cytomegalovirus (CMV), especially if the donor has been exposed to this infection before and the recipient has not. Gangciclovir, valacyclovir, or valganciclovir can be used in this situation, though many units choose to monitor for CMV by PCR and treat only when viremia develops.

The recipients are supported until such time as the kidney starts to work, and graft dysfunction is monitored by graft biopsy to identify acute rejection early. Acute rejection is usually treated by augmented steroids, with or without altering the baseline regimen. Steroid-resistant rejection is still often managed by poly- or monoclonal antibody therapy. Urinary tract infections are managed with appropriate antibiotics, and the ureteric stent is often removed early in this situation.

LONG-TERM MANAGEMENT

This is essentially a balancing act, retaining renal function while trying to minimize potentially harmful medication and avoiding rejection. Early after transplantation, immunosuppression is maximal. The primary aim at this time is to reduce steroid augmentation without incurring rejection to baseline levels. Fluid management is usually only relevant in the first few weeks before it stabilizes, unless other problems arise. Blood pressure needs to be optimized initially by non-ACE inhibitor drugs, though they can be used later, especially if proteinuria is detected.

Hypercholesterolemia can be a problem, particularly in recipients receiving ciclosporin or rapamycin, and they may require treatment with statins. Diabetes mellitus, if present, usually worsens with steroids. In addition, diabetes can develop where it was not present before; this is especially the case with tacrolimus, and it can be reversed by switching immunosuppression to rapamycin. There is a great propensity in the early phase for recipients to put on weight by excessive eating. This occurs because they are suddenly recovering from renal failure and feel fitter, and the dietary restrictions of fluid and potassium are lifted. In addition, steroids increase their appetites. Good dietary care is needed in this early phase because reversing excessive weight gain later is difficult.

The renal function must be monitored together with immunosuppressive drug levels. Graft dysfunction must be investigated after elimination of obvious courses by ultrasound scans and biopsy. Ureteric stenosis should be managed appropriately, usually by, initially, ureteric stent and later ureterotomy or reimplantation, though there is a role for revolving ureteric stents.

Acute rejection should be managed by steroid augmentation and drug manipulation if necessary. Consideration should always be given to patient compliance with immunosuppression, as this is a significant cause of graft failure, particularly in adolescent recipients that are graduating to adult clinics. Osteoporosis and atherosclerosis from protracted steroid use give rise to significant morbidity later; therefore, steroids should be limited as much as is safe to do. Similarly the use of steroids in child hood can have irreversible affects on long bone development. The small stature of children with renal failure though still a problem is not as acute as was the case formerly due to the common use of growth hormone.

Vigilance for skin tumors, cervical cancer, Karposi's sarcoma, and hypernephroma, particularly in polycystic kidneys and posttransplant lymphoproliferative disease, should always be practiced.

RESULTS

In the early days of renal transplantation in the 1950s, the only successful transplants were those between identical twins, obviously a very select group. With the advent of azathioprine and steroid, one-year outcome was of the order of 35% to 40%. This figure improved dramatically with the advent of ciclosporin. Since that time, a one-year recipient death rate of 5% and graft survival of greater than 80% have become usual. These improved figures extend to 10 years after the transplant, but because of a steady attrition rate from chronic rejection, the outcome after 10 years is similar with modern immunosuppressive agents to that seen in the preciclosporin era (17) at 40%. The best results are generally seen in the recipients of live donor kidneys with minimal cold ischemia, among whom there is a graft half-life of 15 years. Those grafts which experience initial delayed function have a significantly worse long-term outcome. In addition, donor morbidity, such as hypertension, and death from cerebrovascular disease have a negative impact on graft survival. Poor tissue match between donor and recipient, and recipient hypertension and smoking habits all have a negative impact on outcome. The hidden issues of noncompliance with immunosuppressive medication could potentially have an enormous impact on outcome (18), though one can take the contrary view that certain drugs promote the cytokine TGFb, which promotes fibrosis and therefore potentially chronic rejection (19).

REFERENCES

1. Security DoHaS. Cadaveric organs for transplantation. A code of practice including the diagnosis of brain death. London: Health Departments of Great Britain and Northern Ireland, 1983.
2. Transplantation. EBPGfR. Nephrol Dial Transplant 2000; 15(suppl 7):46–47.
3. Balupuri S, Buckley P, Snowden C, et al. The trouble with kidneys derived from the non heart beating donor: a single centre 10 year experience. Transplantation 2000; 69:842–846.
4. Gok M, Buckley P, Shenton B, et al. Long-term renal function in kidneys from non-heart-beating donors: a single-center experience. Transplantation 2002; 74:664–669.
5. Nicholson M, Metcalfe MS, White SA, et al. A comparison of the results of renal transplantation from non-heart-beating, conventional cadaveric and living donors. Kidney Int 2000; 58:2585–2591.
6. D'Alessandro A, Hoffmann R, Knechtle S, et al. Successful extrarenal transplantation from non-heart-beating donors. Transplantation 1995; 59:977–982.
7. Newman C, Baxby K, Hall R, et al. Machine-perfused cadaver kidneys. Lancet 1975; 2:614.
8. Burdick J, Rossendale J, McBride M, et al. National impact of pulsatile perfusion on cadaveric kidney transplantation. Transplantation 1997; 64:1730–1733.
9. Light J. Viability testing in the non-heart-beating donor. Transplant Proc 2000; 32:179–181.
10. Brasile L, Stubenitsky B, Booster M, et al. Overcoming severe renal ischemia: the role of ex vivo warm perfusion. Transplantation 2002; 73:897–901.
11. Hoffman R, Stratta R, D'Alessandro A, et al. Combined cold storage-perfusion preservation with a new synthetic perfusate. Transplantation 1989; 47:32–37.
12. Groenewoud A, Thorogood J. Current status of the Eurotransplant randomized multicenter study comparing kidney graft preservation with histidine-tryptophane-ketoglutarate, University of Wisconsin and EuroCollins. Transplant Proc 1993; 25:1582–1585.
13. Muhlbacher F, Langer F, Mittermayer C. Preservation solutions for transplantation. Transplant Proc 1999; 31:2069–2070.
14. Association BTSaR. United Kingdom Guidelines for Living Donor Kidney Transplantation, 2000.
15. Kasiske B, Ravenscraft M, Ramos E, et al. The evaluation of living renal transplant donors: clinical practice guidelines. J Am Soc Nephrol 1996; 7:2288–2313.
16. Kasiske B, Ramos E, Gaston R, et al. The evaluation of renal transplant candidates. Clinical practice guidelines. Patient Care and Education Committee of the American Society of Transplant Physicians. J Am Assoc Nephrol 1995; 6:1–34.
17. Beveridge T, Calne R. Cyclosporin (Sandimmun) in cadaveric renal transplantation. Ten-year follow up of a European multicenter trial group. Transplantation 1995; 59:1568–1570.
18. de Geest S, Borgermans L, Gemoets H, et al. Incidence, determinants, and consequences of subclinical noncompliance with immunosuppressive therapy in renal transplant recipients. Transplantation 1995; 59:340–347.
19. Mohamed M, Robertson H, Booth T, et al. TGF-b expression in renal transplant biopsies. A comparative study between cyclosporin-A and tacrolimus. Transplantation 2000; 69(5):1002–1005.

31

Tissue Transfer in Urology

Daniela E. Andrich and Anthony R. Mundy
Institute of Urology, University College Hospital, London, U.K.

INTRODUCTION

Two types of tissue transfer are common in urology, firstly, the use of skin and buccal mucosa for urethral reconstruction and, secondly, the use of bowel for bladder reconstruction. The three factors that require some consideration in relation to the subject of tissue transfer in these contexts are the general subject of wound healing, the use of grafts and flaps, and the consequences of incorporating bowel into the urinary tract.

The final section of this chapter will give a brief overview of tissue engineering. In recent years there has been a great deal of progress in tissue engineering in urology with the aim of developing alternative tissue sources for urethral and bladder reconstruction, amongst other things. The most recent and exciting developments in this field overall have been in the use of pluripotent stem cells although their application in urology is still in its infancy.

WOUND HEALING

This is the replacement of destroyed tissue by living tissue. In certain reptiles, it includes the ability to replace a tail or limb. This occurs because of the ability of cells to dedifferentiate and then redifferentiate (1), which does not occur in human adults.

Healing in adults is limited to the fibrous obliteration of dead space and limited regeneration. In the embryo, scarless healing has been noted and this is currently the focus of intense research. Fetal wounding shows less inflammatory infiltrate with less content of the inflammatory cytokine transforming growth factor β (TGF-β) compared with the adult (2) and fetal fibroblasts have been shown to be of particular importance in scarless wound healing (3).

The Phases of Wound Healing

Wound healing is traditionally divided into three phases—an inflammatory phase, a proliferative phase and a maturation phase. These phases overlap to some degree, but as a general rule the inflammatory phase lasts for about the first five days, the proliferative phase lasts from about day 3 to about day 14, and the maturation phase starts on about day 8 and lasts about three months. Each of these phases is controlled and regulated by growth factors.

The first phase of wound healing is the hemostatic response to the injury itself and the inflammation that follow immediately afterward. At the site where blood vessels and the surrounding tissues are injured, circulating blood comes into contact with extracellular collagen and platelets aggregate and are activated and the intrinsic component of the coagulation cascade is activated as well. The platelets release the contents of their granules, including cytokines, growth factors, fibronectin, thromboxane and serotonin. The thromboxane and serotonin promote vasoconstriction at the site of the injury, whereas vasodilatation occurs around that site to allow other important healing factors to get to the wound. The vasodilatation is mediated by histamine, which is also released from platelets but other cells as well such as mast cells and basophils.

At the same time, both the intrinsic and the extrinsic coagulation systems are activated, leading to the formation of a fibrin clot. This serves as a scaffolding to allow inflammatory cells such as neutrophils, macrophages and lymphocytes to move into the injured area. The neutrophils arrive first. Selectin receptors on the endothelial cell surface cause neutrophil adhesion to the endothelium, and integrin receptors on the neutrophil cell surface bind to the extracellular matrix, thus bringing the neutrophils into the damaged area. Neutrophils, however, are not essential to wound healing except to deal with bacterial contamination when that exists. The next cells to arrive, the macrophages, are essential. They arrive on about the third day after injury and act as the principal cell controlling the wound-healing process. The main functions are as follows:

1. An antimicrobial effect caused by the release of oxygen radicals and nitric oxide, and by phagocytosis
2. Wound debridement by phagocytosis and by the release of various enzymes
3. Matrix synthesis regulation by the release of growth factors, cytokines, enzymes and prostaglandins
4. Cell recruitment and activation by the release of growth factors, cytokines and fibronectin
5. Angiogenesis by the release of growth factors and cytokines

The principal cells recruited and activated are fibroblasts and lymphocytes, which migrate in toward the end of the inflammatory phase. The principal enzyme released is collagenase. The principal growth factors released are TGF-β, EGF, PDGF and the angiogenesis growth factors bFGF and VEGF (4). The principal cytokines are TNF-α, IL-1, IFN-c and ILC.

Lymphocytes are attracted by the cytokines released by activated macrophages, and these in turn release interferons and interleukins. They also produce nitric oxide. The arrival of the fibroblasts heralds the second, or "proliferative" phase. Their number increases, so the number of neutrophils decreases.

Fibroblasts, together with macrophages, then start the process of matrix formation and collagen synthesis. At the same time, endothelial cells proliferate from the margin of the wound to form new capillaries by the process of angiogenesis (5). At this stage, the inflammatory phase is over, and any remaining inflammatory mediators are inactivated and removed from the wound by diffusion or by the macrophages. The fibroblasts are activated by PDGF and FGF, and also by complement and fibronectin, which binds fibroblasts and helps them to move into the wound in the same way that integrins in the extracellular matrix bound neutrophils in the early inflammatory phase.

As activated fibroblasts begin the process of matrix deposition, largely by replacing the fibrin and fibronectin originating from hemostasis and macrophages with collagen, epithelial cells start to proliferate from the wound edges. Again, macrophages are important, producing appropriate cytokines and growth factors. As the proliferative phase comes to an end and the maturation phase becomes established, macrophages (and neutrophils) start to leave the area.

The cardinal feature of the maturation phase is the deposition of collagen. It is the rate, quality and total amount of collagen deposition that determines the strength of the scar, and most of the problems of healing that arise are secondary to poor collagen deposition.

Initially, in the inflammatory phase, the matrix deposited in the wound was composed principally of fibrin and fibronectin that originated from hemostasis and from macrophages, respectively. Other extracellular microproteins, such as glycosaminoglycans and proteoglycans, come next. Collagen follows after this.

In the intact dermis, collagen I predominates, forming 80% to 90% of the total collagen. The remaining 10% to 20% is collagen III. In the granulation tissue of the maturation phase, there is rather more type III collagen—as much as 30%—although this reduces in time to about 10%. Collagen III production actually peaks during the inflammatory phase, while collagen I production, which starts about the first day after injury, continues for about four to five weeks. Initially, the collagen is laid down in thin collagen fibers, parallel to the skin and organized along the stress line of the wound. In time, the collagen fibers become thicker, but they never develop the basket-weave-like pattern characteristic of normal dermis. It is perhaps for this reason that the breaking strength of a scar never quite equals the breaking strength of normal skin. At one week, the breaking strength of a wound is about 3% to 5% of its final strength; by three weeks, it has reached 20% of its final strength; by three months, it reaches 80% of the strength of unwounded skin, and this is about as strong as it ever gets.

Wound contraction is the name given to the final approximation of the wound edges and the shortening of the scar that is typically seen. In the process of healing by first intention—which is what we have been describing so far—contraction is less marked than in healing by second intention. In both circumstances, the process is the same and poorly understood. One theory proposes that the myofibroblast—a special type of fibroblast—is responsible for this (6). The other main theory is that the movement of cells with reorganization of the cellular cytoskeleton is responsible for contraction. In summary, the exact mechanism is not clear.

Healing by secondary intention (where the wound edges are widely separated) differs in two respects.

1. Epithelialization occurs from the basal cells of the epidermis at the margins of the wound. These cells lose their attachment to the basement membrane and send out cytoplasmic projections, becoming flatter as they do so. As they change, they become more like phagocytes in appearance. Within a day or two of injury, the basal cells show mitosis at an increasing rate and continue to replicate until the defect is covered. When coverage is complete and the epidermis (or other epithelium) has reconstituted itself, the basal cells regain their normal appearance and synthesize their own basement membrane constituents.
2. Contraction plays a far more important role in healing by secondary intention. Animal models have demonstrated contraction of up to 80% (7). However, the pathological process involved in contraction is the same.

Complications of Wound Healing

Complications include infection, wound dehiscence, excessive granulation, keloid, pigmentation, pain, weak scars, circatrization, implantation cyst and neoplasia. Factors influencing healing are listed in Table 1.

Table 1 Factors Influencing Wound Healing

Local factors	Poor blood supply
	Adhesion to underlying structures
	Direction of wound
	Infection/foreign body
	Movement
	Drying
	Neoplasia
General	Age
	Nutrition (protein, vitamin C, zinc)
	Hormones
	Temperature

GRAFTS AND FLAPS

Most surgical trainees gain their first experience of grafting in the use of thin split-skin grafts to cover a granulating open wound. The open wound, which is secreting collagen and actively generating small new vessels, is covered by a nutrient-rich layer of serum, from which the thin split-skin graft gains its nutrition by a process known as "imbibition." This is sufficient to nourish a split-skin graft for a day or two, but to nourish it beyond that time, as well as to fix it and incorporate it into the healing wound, there must be a link-up between the capillary bed on the undersurface of the graft and the developing capillaries in the open wound, together with interlinking of collagen, and this process is known as "inosculation." During the 48 hours of imbibition and the 48 hours of inosculation, the graft must be immobilized and if the host bed is well vascularized, then the graft will "take." At the end of 96 hours, blood flow into the graft should be established. Eventually, lymphatic vessels will grow in as well. The "tie-over" dressing commonly used for immobilizing a skin graft clearly produces some pressure. However, too much pressure, sufficient to inhibit completely the formation of small hematomas and seromas, would probably be sufficient to impair blood flow in the host bed (8,9). In other words, the dressing is to immobilize the graft; it is not supposed to be hemostatic.

Thus far, we have been considering the simple split-skin graft, and at this stage we should draw attention to the difference between grafts and flaps. A graft is tissue transferred from a donor site to a recipient site without a blood supply, whereas a flap is tissue that is transferred from a donor site with its own blood supply intact, although one type of flap is the free flap in which tissue is transferred with its blood supply disconnected and then reconnected by means of microvascular surgery at the recipient site.

In urology we are principally concerned with split-thickness skin grafts, full-thickness skin grafts, buccal mucosal grafts, bladder epithelial grafts and flaps of local genital skin for urethral reconstruction. In addition, the urologist may wish to use a dermal graft for the correction of Peyronie's disease, and some have used a graft of tunica vaginalis for this purpose (9–11).

Other than the use of genital skin flaps for urethral reconstruction, simpler advancement, rotation and transposition flaps are commonly used for wound closure, although we do not often think of them as such, except in the specific case of the Z-plasty.

Less commonly, flaps may be used for perineal and genital reconstruction, and in this way a simple scrotal flap may be used to cover a perineal defect, or the infinitely more complex radial or ulnar forearm flap may be transferred by microvascular techniques for phalloplasty (12).

Grafts

Skin has an epidermal layer and a dermal layer, under which lies a subcutaneous, fatty layer. At the interface between the dermis and the subcutaneous layer is the subdermal plexus, which is fed from deeper segmental vessels and which in turn feeds the dermal and epidermal layers above through a second, more superficial, plexus within the dermis itself, called the intradermal plexus (Fig. 1). The outermost layer of the epidermis is the cornified layer, and the inner layer—the epidermis proper—contains the skin appendages, some of which extend into the dermal layer. The principal skin appendages are the sweat glands, sebaceous glands and hair follicles, and in urological practice it is worth noting that the glans and prepuce in the male and the skin of the labia minora and introitus in the female are free of skin appendages. The same areas also have skin in which the dermis is thin. The dermis consists of the more superficial "papillary" or "adventitial" dermis and the deeper "reticular" dermis. The papillary dermis has a fairly constant thickness, and fibroblasts and capillaries predominate. The deeper reticular dermis is thicker but more variable and here collagen and elastin predominate. The subdermal plexus lies on the deep aspect of the reticular dermis, and the intradermal plexus lies between the reticular and the papillary dermis.

A full-thickness skin graft includes both the epidermis and the dermis with the vessels of the subdermal plexus exposed on its undersurface, and it is to these vessels that the new vessels developing within the host bed must connect by inosculation.

Full-thickness skin grafts, because of their high content of dermal collagen, contract very little during healing and tend to give the most satisfactory long-term results as a consequence, but there are two problems associated with their use. Firstly, the amount of suitable skin is restricted and, secondly, the subdermal plexus is less extensive than the intradermal plexus and, because of this and also because the graft is relatively thick, it is only slowly revascularized and takes only under the most favorable conditions. A postauricular full-thickness skin graft (or in fact any facial skin graft harvested from above the jaw line) has a denser subdermal plexus and therefore takes more readily than other extragenital skin.

The split-thickness skin graft contains the epidermis and a portion of the adventitial dermis with the vessels of the intradermal plexus exposed on its undersurface. The graft is thinner and the vessels of the intradermal plexus are more plentiful and so a split-thickness graft is more likely to take and will do so under less favorable circumstances than a full-thickness skin graft. On the other hand, because there is less dermal collagen, a split-thickness graft tends to contract and, lacking the collagen and elastin of the reticular dermis, the graft tends to be more brittle and fragile than a full-thickness graft.

Bladder epithelial grafts and buccal mucosal grafts are harvested and behave as full-thickness grafts. Bladder epithelium has the disadvantage that it is very prone to desiccation, which leads to hypertrophic changes when, for example, it is used at the urethral meatus (13). Buccal mucosa is far more resistant to desiccation, and there is the additional advantage that it is easier to open the mouth than the

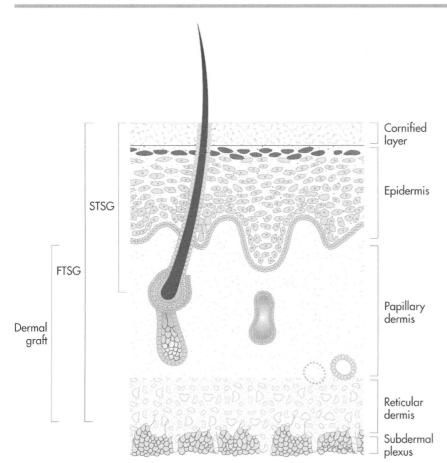

Figure 1 Cross-sectional diagram of the skin. *Abbreviations*: STSG, split-thickness skin graft; FTSG, full-thickness skin graft.

bladder. The particular advantages of buccal mucosa are its thickness and toughness (which contrast markedly with the thinness and fragility of bladder epithelium), and the density of the intradermal and subdermal plexuses (14) (Fig. 2).

Grafts were the first sort of tissue to be used for urethral reconstruction but fell into disfavor because of their unpredictability until just recently, with the advent of buccal mucosal grafting for "patch" urethroplasty of strictures that are too long for excision and end-to-end anasthromosis (15). Until then, grafts had become virtually restricted to the use of meshed split-skin grafts for the salvage repair of extensive urethral strictures (16,17). This is a technique that is only rarely indicated nowadays. A free preputial skin graft might be used by specialist reconstructive surgeons for anterior urethroplasty, particularly for hypospadias repair, but grafting had become almost entirely superseded by the use of flaps for hypospadias repair and for urethroplasty in the penile urethra, largely under the influence of Duckett (18). Preputial and postauricular full-thickness skin grafts are now being used more frequently again, particularly for the two-stage reconstruction of the penile urethra (19). Postauricular full-thickness skin grafts have a particularly rich subdermal plexus and, although the amount of tissue is relatively restricted, the take is far more predictable than with other extragenital skin.

Thus, preputial or postauricular full-thickness skin grafts or buccal mucosal grafts, which behave like full-thickness grafts, may be used to reconstruct the anterior urethra. Buccal mucosal grafts are particularly useful for the repair of urethral strictures because of lichen sclerosus (also known as balanitis xerotica obliterans or BXO) as buccal mucosa is not commonly affected by this skin disease. Buccal mucosal grafts and bladder epithelial grafts have also been used as tube grafts in the anterior urethra (20) although tube grafts of any sort are unreliable because of difficulties with circumferential revascularization.

Flaps

The use of skin flaps in reconstructive surgery dates back to northern India at about 600 BC, when Susruta developed forehead rhinoplasty after a traumatic nasal amputation—a form of punishment at that time (21). Then, in the 16th century, Gaspare Tagliacozzi from Bologna successfully transposed skin pedicles from the arm to the face to reconstruct the nose of patients who had lost theirs because of syphilis. Tagliacozzi's work was disregarded by his peers and it was not until World War One and Two when surviving war veterans with shrapnel wounds, traumatic amputations and severe burns provided both the opportunity and the need for advancements in

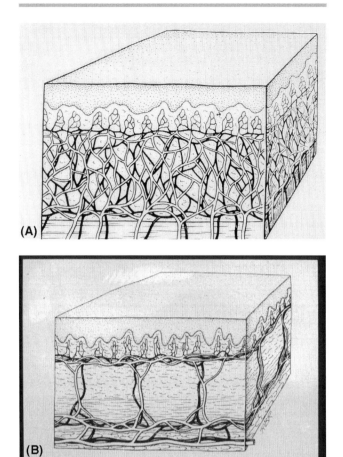

Figure 2 Subdermal plexus of buccal mucosal graft compared with skin graft. (**A**) BMG. Dense subdermal capillary plexus. (**B**) Skin. Less extensive subdermal capillary plexus, separate intradermal plexus.

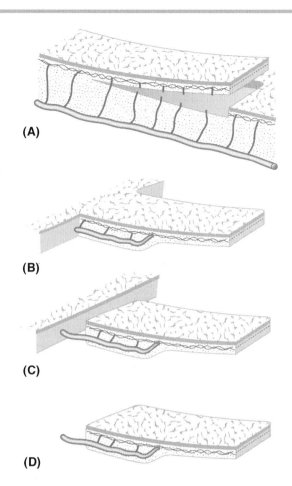

Figure 3 Diagrammatic representation of: (**A**) a random peninsular flap; (**B**) an axial peninsular flap; (**C**) an axial island flap; and (**D**) a free microvascular flap.

reconstructive surgery that led to the redevelopment of such skin flap techniques (22) During the First World War, Harold Gillies laid the foundations of reconstructive plastic surgery. His cousin Archibald McIndoe continued to perfect reconstructive techniques during World War 2, culminating (urologically) in the first phallic reconstruction in the 1960s using a staged tubed pedicled skin flap technique (23).

In urology we are principally concerned with skin flaps for urethral and genital reconstruction, omental and labial fat pad flaps to help support vesicovaginal fistula closure, gracilis muscle flaps to support urorectal fistula closure and intestinal flaps for bladder reconstruction. Flaps may be classified in two ways (8,9). Firstly, according to their method of elevation, into: peninsular flaps, in which the base of the flap remains in continuity; island flaps, in which the flap is only in continuity through the arteriovenous pedicle; and free flaps, in which all continuity of the flap is interrupted and the vascularity is reestablished at the recipient site. The second way of classifying flaps is by vascular classification, which distinguishes between: random flaps, in which there

is no identifiable arteriovenous pedicle and survival is dependent entirely on the dermal and intradermal plexuses; axial flaps, which have an identifiable artery and vein entering through the base; and two special forms of axial flap known as myocutaneous and fascio-cutaneous flaps. Random flaps are restricted in use by a length to width ratio whereas axial flaps are not, being restricted in length only by the nature of the feeder vessels. A peninsular flap may be either a random or an axial flap, but island flaps are all axial flaps (Fig. 3). Peninsular flaps are used for advancement, rotation and transposition but are relatively restricted in scope. Axial island flaps have a much greater range of application. Island flaps are somewhat fragile and have to be handled with care, as the vascular pedicle provides both structural and vascular continuity—with such a fragile structure that vascular continuity is threatened unless great care is taken. Sometimes, however, the continuity of an island flap is maintained through a muscle or fascial flap, giving rise to the two particular forms of axial flap referred to above. In the myocutaneous flap, the arteriovenous pedicle is within the muscle itself and the skin island (or "paddle") retains its attachment to the muscle. Examples include gracilis and rectus abdominis muscle flaps, both of which have applications in urology (24,25). Similarly, the fasciocutaneous flap transmits the arteriovenous pedicle in close relation to a defined layer of fascia to which the skin paddle is attached. In both the myocutaneous and the fasciocutaneous flaps, the muscle and fascia, respectively, support and protect the arteriovenous pedicle, making the flap more robust.

Free flaps, to be transferred by microvascular anastomosis to the recipient site, can be elevated as axial cutaneous, axial myocutaneous, or axial fasciocutaneous flaps and are the most versatile flaps of all because they can be transferred anywhere. The limitations in their use are firstly technical—they are difficult to learn how to perform—and they tend to leave large donor sites that may leave ugly scars (26) although this is usually more than offset by a satisfactory end result from the flap itself. Most flaps are mobilized with a defined sensory nerve to provide sensibility to the flap. The best example of the use of a free flap in urology is the ulnar forearm flap used for phalloplasty (12). A radial artery flap is easier to raise but has considerable donor-site morbidity because the many tendons in the forearm are exposed and, even if these can be covered, the donor site leaves an unsightly scar. The ulnar forearm flap exposes fewer, if any, tendons and the donor site is more easily concealed and has the additional advantage that the skin on the ulnar side of the forearm is much less hirsute, but the flap is more difficult to raise. Both flaps are innervated by the lateral and medial antebrachial cutaneous nerves, which are easily identified and mobilized with the flap to provide sensibility.

Gracilis and rectus myocutaneous flaps have also been used for phallic reconstruction, but are more commonly used for covering large skin defects in and around the groins and perineum. The gracilis muscle can also be used purely as a muscle flap for filling dead space and holding suture lines apart, in the same way that the labial fat pad and omentum are used.

Intestinal Flaps in Bladder Reconstruction

These days there are probably more urologists using bowel for bladder reconstruction or replacement by continent or conduit urinary diversion than there are urologists using skin for urethral reconstruction.

Bowel is always carried on its blood supply and, as long as there is no undue tension on the vascular pedicle, the bowel heals well in its new circumstances and ischemia is rare, except when the bowel and its blood supply are compromised by previous radiotherapy. The purpose of this section is not to discuss the more technical aspects related to mobilizing gut segments for use in the urinary tract, but to discuss the metabolic, infective, histological and other consequences of incorporating the gut into the urinary tract. Such matters have been extensively studied by certain

groups in experimental models (27), and the clinical consequences have been extensively scrutinized by other groups in humans, but it is still not yet clear how we should apply the theoretical knowledge gleaned from such studies in clinical practice, as that knowledge is currently very incomplete.

Bowel has been used in urology for many years and this has engendered an attitude that it can be freely deployed within the urinary tract without significant consequence. On the other hand, intestine was never meant to serve either as a conduit for urine or as a storage vessel for it, and a more likely explanation for the fact that it appears to be capable of being used freely without complication is that in most circumstances only a small section of bowel is incorporated and, in most patients in whom such procedures are performed, there are compensatory mechanisms to deal with any adverse consequences that might otherwise result. Furthermore, many of these patients have only a short life expectancy, as when an ileal conduit or substitution cystoplasty is used after cystectomy for bladder cancer, and the short duration of use in a patient who is expected to die before long in any case might lead one to overlook consequences that might be apparent in younger patients with longer life expectancy.

Even with this proviso, it was recognized many years ago that patients with ureterosigmoidostomy were prone to the specific metabolic problem of hyperchloraemic acidosis from the absorption of urinary constituents by the colon (28), and prone also to the development of tumors at the site of implantation of the ureters into the colon (29). For these reasons, ureterosigmoidostomy fell into relative disuse some years ago (30). Other than the consequences of incorporating a segment of gut into the urinary tract, there may be consequences from removing it from its natural situation. In practice, the only problem that commonly arises is a degree of bowel dysfunction (31), for reasons that are not entirely clear. There is, in any case, a strong association between detrusor instability and the irritable bowel syndrome (32) and neuropathic bowel and neuropathic bladder dysfunction, (33) and it is these two groups that are most prone to notice disturbance of bowel function after augmentation cystoplasty. Bowel dysfunction is far less commonly noted after substitution cystoplasty for conditions such as bladder cancer.

Removal of the terminal ileum or of the ileocaecal valve can interfere with the absorption of bile salts (34) and lead to bacterial colonization of the terminal ileum, both of which may give rise to diarrhea. For this reason, the terminal ileum is avoided whenever possible during such surgery. There has been concern that the removal of the terminal ileum can give rise to vitamin B12 deficiency and other forms of anemia, but these rarely seem to occur in practice. It is not clear how much ileum has to be removed from the intestinal tract before bile acid malabsorption is sufficiently severe to cause malabsorption of fat and fat-soluble vitamins, but malnutrition and steatorrhea are rarely, if ever, seen in clinical practice. Diarrhea may occur more frequently in patients after ileal conduit diversion or continent diversion after previous bowel excision or when the bowel is diseased or deficient in any other way. Removing the right side of the colon may cause diarrhea, although this does not seem to be a long-term problem. Removal of the sigmoid colon may be a problem in neuropathic patients in whom the sigmoid colon is an important storage organ, but it does not usually cause bowel problems otherwise. In short, other than in those with previously abnormal bowel, problems rarely arise from taking the bowel out of continuity, and all we need really consider are the problems that arise from incorporating it into the urinary tract.

THE CONSEQUENCES OF INCORPORATING THE BOWEL INTO THE URINARY TRACT

The first point to make is that bowel continues to behave like bowel even when it is in the urinary tract and has been there for many years. It continues to produce mucus—the only overt abnormality that most patients are aware of—and it continues to secrete and absorb just as it does in its natural situation. There is a tendency for both the ileal and colonic epithelium to atrophy with time (35), and it is not clear whether this represents the consequence of loss of the normal stimulation that it receives during fecal transport in its normal situation or whether, alternatively, it represents some toxic effect of urine. However, the atrophy is less when the intestine is in contact with urine than when it is not in contact with anything at all, so it appears that urine tends to maintain ileal integrity, if anything, albeit less so than does the fecal stream. The atrophic appearance is therefore likely to represent a true, albeit partial, atrophy rather than a toxic effect.

Metabolic Changes

The principal metabolic abnormality is a tendency to a respiratory-compensated metabolic acidosis, usually of mild degree (36). This may influence bone metabolism to a sufficient degree to cause demineralization of the skeleton in growing children (37). Changes otherwise tend to be subtle, particularly, it is thought, if renal function is normal. Thus, only young patients are prone to any sort of problems in most circumstances.

Why people seem to suffer less from metabolic acidosis these days with a substituted intestinal bladder than they used to suffer with a ureterosigmoidostomy is almost certainly related, at least in part, to the recurrent sepsis that they also suffered with refluxing ureterosigmoidostomies (38). The nature and severity of the electrolyte anomalies that patients can suffer from depend on the segment of bowel used in the urinary tract. If stomach is used, hypochloremic metabolic alkalosis can occur. This is rarely significant in the presence of normal renal function, but may be when renal function is severely limited.

When jejunum is used, hyponatremic, hyperchloraemic, hyperkalemic metabolic acidosis occurs, and this is both common and potentially serious,

Table 2 Metabolic Changes Using Different Gut Segments for Bladder Reconstruction or Replacement

Stomach	Hypochloraemic metabolic alkalosis
Jejunum	Hyponatremic, hyperchloremic, hyperkalemic metabolic acidosis
Ileum, colon	Hyperchloraemic acidosis

resulting in lethargy, nausea, vomiting, dehydration, muscular weakness and an elevated body temperature and, if uncorrected, death. This is the "jejunal conduit syndrome" (39). If ileum or colon is used, hyperchloraemic acidosis may occur (Table 2).

The reported incidence varies and to a certain extent depends on how it is looked for. If the plasma chloride level is the parameter used to make the diagnosis, then about 15% of patients suffer; if arterial blood gas analysis is performed, then a respiratory-compensated metabolic acidosis is found far more commonly—indeed, in the majority (36). The mechanism of the metabolic acidosis when ileum or colon is interposed in the urinary tract is not entirely clear. What is known is largely derived from the work of McDougall and coworkers (27). Water transport across the intestinal epithelium normally follows its osmotic gradient and is dependent on the permeability of the intercellular junctions of the luminal cells. If these junctions are tight, there is very little leakage; when they are not so tight, water follows its osmotic gradients. Generally, the tightness of the intercellular junctions increases the further down the intestinal tract the segment is taken from. Stomach is very leaky, but there are bidirectional fluxes that cancel each other out. Jejunum is leaky and jejunal conduits lose large amounts of water. Ileum is better but is still somewhat leaky. Colon is the most efficient segment of gut because its intercellular junctions are tighter, and colon segments therefore have a much lower tendency to lose water.

Most electrolyte shifts in the gut are transcellular, although paracellular movement of ions does occur. Furthermore, most electrolyte movements in one direction are coupled with movement of other electrolytes in the opposite direction. Thus, when sodium is absorbed, hydrogen is excreted and when chloride is absorbed, bicarbonate is excreted. Under certain circumstances, these transport processes can be reversed.

Sodium absorption is much the same in the ileum and in the colon and, in general, ileum absorbs less chloride but more potassium than colon. In neither ileal nor colonic segments is either sodium or potassium loss a problem, although in extreme metabolic acidosis, hypokalemia can occur, as can hypocalcaemia and hypomagnesaemia.

The mechanism for the development of hyperchloraemic acidosis appears to be primarily because of ammonia absorption. Ammonium ions may dissociate into ammonia and hydrogen, in which case the ammonia diffuses into the cell and the hydrogen ion is actively absorbed in exchange for sodium. Alternatively, ammonium may be absorbed as a substitute for potassium through potassium channels. Either way, ammonium enters the ileal or colonic luminal cell and this is balanced by chloride absorption in exchange for bicarbonate secretion. Thus, ammonium and chloride are absorbed, causing hyperchloraemic acidosis, and bicarbonate is lost.

When hypokalemia does occur it is usually in ureterosigmoidostomy (40) or as a result of osmotic diuresis. Hypocalcaemia is usually due to bone demineralization. Hypomagnesaemia may be associated with hypocalcaemia but is more commonly due to nutritional depletion or renal wasting.

In most patients this metabolic acidosis is of little consequence but growing children with intestine incorporated into the urinary tract have been shown to be more prone to orthopedic problems and to pathological fractures, and there was a tendency for them to drop off the growth curve that they were previously following (41). Exactly why acidosis should lead to skeletal demineralization in growing children and not in adults is not clear, but postmenopausal women who might also be prone to skeletal demineralization do not show this abnormality after enterocystoplasty or urinary intestinal diversion. However, this is controversial, as more recently a large cohort study of 123 children followed up into their adolescence after childhood enterocystolasty. The distribution of percentile positions before and after enterocystoplasty showed normal configuration and 85% of children either remained on the same or reached a higher centile (42).

Again, the mechanism by which acidosis causes demineralization of the skeleton is not clear, but chronic acidosis is buffered predominantly by muscle protein and by bone. In bone, in chronic metabolic acidosis, hydrogen ions are buffered in exchange for calcium. The main buffer is thought to be bicarbonate or carbonate derived from skeletal carbon dioxide stores, and the utilization of this buffer system is accompanied by an efflux not only of calcium but of divalent phosphate as well, because of dissolution of the mineral phase. Calcium efflux is dependent on the bicarbonate concentration as well as on the pH, and compensated chronic metabolic acidosis, in which there is a systemically reduced bicarbonate concentration, will have an adverse effect on skeletal mineralization even though the pH is within the normal range because of the compensation mechanism.

It should again be emphasized that it is growing children who are vulnerable to skeletal demineralization in this way. Once the skeleton has reached maturity, it appears to be resistant to this mechanism. In practice, it means that growing children should have any identifiable metabolic acidosis corrected, but in adults it need not be corrected if it is asymptomatic (37). It is frequently reported that patients with renal function below a certain level should not undergo any form of enterocystoplasty or urinary intestinal diversion because metabolic problems are far more likely. Although frequently reported, there is little evidence to support this except in ureterosigmoidostomy patients who have continuing fecal reflux to contend with as well as hyperchloraemic acidosis. In practice,

most patients with impaired renal function undergoing enterocystoplasty or urinary diversion have an obstructive nephropathy, either due to frank outflow obstruction at sphincter level or to high intravesical pressure. If these two problems are eliminated by enterocystoplasty, whatever the level of renal function, there will be at least a temporary stabilization, if not an overt improvement in renal function, and this usually amounts to a window of 18 months to two years before intrinsic renal disease causes further deterioration in renal function on the downward slope to renal replacement therapy.

Urinary Infection and Malignant Transformation

Bacterial colonization of the urinary tract is very common after bowel interposition. Although one or two authors report sterile urine in their patients, the majority of surgeons find that the urine is usually, if not always, colonized.

Very often this is with a mixed growth of bacteria and less than the usual 100 000 organisms/mL associated with a "classic" urinary infection. Not only is this bacteriuria common, there is also an increased incidence of both local and systemic infection in such patients. Average reported figures are that 80% of patients suffer bacteriuria (43) with a diverse bacterial flora and that 15% of patients will suffer acute pyelonephritis at some stage (44). The highest incidence appears to be during the first year. This incidence is higher than in those who are on clean, intermittent self-catheterization with a normal bladder (41). Unlike urothelium, bowel does not attempt to sterilize its luminal content. When bowel is distended, it becomes relatively ischemic and the mucosal barrier preventing bacterial translocation from mucosa to blood is disrupted. Urine from a substitute bladder is less bacteriostatic because the concentration of urea is lower and the pH higher than in normal urine. These three points probably account for the increased incidence of infection in such patients.

This infection is difficult, if not impossible, to eliminate and most patients suffer asymptomatic bacteriuria even if they are completely unaware of it. Although asymptomatic, it may be nonetheless important in the long run as there is a theoretical link between infection and cancer.

Patients with ureterosigmoidostomy were noted to have an incidence of cancer at the ureterointestinal anastomosis of between 6% and 29%, with a mean of 11% (29). Generally speaking, there is a lag time of 10 to 20 years between the surgery and the development of the tumor. These tumors are extremely aggressive and one-third of patients die from them. They appear to be adenocarcinomas in the main, although other histological types have been reported. Overall, this represents a 500-fold increase in the incidence of tumors in the sigmoid colon in this patient group, and it has been reported that, in patients diverted by this means before the age of 25, the increased risk is 7000-fold (45). The etiology of these tumors is not clear. Presumably, as most are adenocarcinomas, they arise in intestinal epithelium adjacent to the anastomosis, although adenocarcinoma has been shown to arise from transitional epithelium exposed to feces in experimental animals (46). Furthermore, histological assessment of the ureters in patients with ureterosigmoidostomies shows a high incidence of dysplasia as judged by biopsies or surgical specimens from close to the anastomosis (47). Stewart suggested that these tumors arose as a result of the conversion of nitrates and secondary amines in the urine into nitrosamines due to the action of fecal bacteria (48). Nitrosamines are known carcinogens and certainly patients with ureterosigmoidostomies show high concentrations of nitrosamines in the fecal/urinary slurry that they pass.

Patients with enterocystoplasties or urinary diversions show dysplastic changes, and malignant change has been reported, albeit infrequently (49). Most patients show chronic inflammatory changes in their bladder on biopsy, and nitrosamines are present in the urine, in this case produced by the bacteriuria that they have rather than by exposure to feces. The greater the degree of the bacteriuria, the greater the degree of the pyuria associated with it, the higher the nitrosamine levels in the urine and the higher the incidence of histological changes, which in some instances would be classified as premalignant if they were found in the bowel in its natural situation. Such changes include keratinizing squamous metaplasia and transitional epithelial mucin distribution—changes similar to the alterations in colonic mucin secretion demonstrated in patients with ureterosigmoidostomy. Other factors have been suggested for the development of these tumors, including superoxide radicals and epidermal growth factor receptor proliferation, induced by the urothelial-colonic juxtaposition. Whatever the cause, there seems to be little doubt that some patients, at least, will develop tumors in the long run. Patients should therefore not be lost to follow-up so that such tumors can be detected at the earliest possible moment. Patients usually are enrolled to surveillance investigations around 10 years after their enterocystoplasty. Traditionally cystsocopy is used for this purpose, but recently MRI cystogram has shown the advantage that this noninvasive imaging technique has adequate resolution to pick up small bladder lesions and at the same time screens the upper tact for incidental pathology (50).

Stones

Patients with ileal conduits were found to have a 20% incidence of renal calculus formation if followed for more than 20 years (41). Up to one-third of patients with Kock pouches were found to have stones in their pouch, in this instance related to nonreabsorbable staples. More recently, stones have been noted in the absence of foreign material in patients with diversions and orthotopic substitutions and these have been attributed to acid renal tubular fluid, an increased excretion of calcium, and a high incidence of infection with urease-producing bacteria, as well as to the presence of mucus and almost universal bacteriuria.

Robertson has shown that metabolic and dietary factors are present in stone forming enterocystoplasty patients, which may be as important in the etiology of stone formation as the already recognized factors of infection and poor reservoir drainage. The majority of enterocystoplasty patients have risk factors for at least three different types of stone although 86% are of infective origin. Stone formers have a higher pH, and sodium and protein excretion and a lower calcium and citrate excretion (51). Nonstone formers have a higher fluid intake, higher citrate excretion, a lower urinary pH and higher dietary magnesium and phosphate intake (52).

However, it should be noted that patients with ileal conduits and with orthotopic substitution cystoplasties that empty their bladders spontaneously and with little or no residual urine have a low incidence of stone formation. An orthotropic substitution that has to be emptied by clean intermittent self-catheterization has a higher incidence. The highest incidence of all occurs in patients with continent diversions being emptied by clean intermittent self-catheterization from the top of the bladder via a Mitrofanoff channel, rather than from the bottom through the urethra—suggesting that stagnation is the most important factor in stone formation, with mucus presumably acting as a nidus and bacterial colonization as the catalyst.

Other Problems

It has already been noted, when discussing metabolic abnormalities, that the primary abnormality leading to acidosis is the increased absorption of ammonia. This ammonia is normally converted into urea by the liver. If the liver is in any way abnormal, then hyperammonemic encephalopathy may result (53), and is particularly common in patients with chronic liver disease such as cirrhosis. In healthy patients however, the hepatic reserve to clear ammonia is high, so this is not a common problem unless liver disease is fairly advanced.

Certain drugs may be absorbed from the urine when bowel is interposed, and phenytoin (54) and certain antimetabolites such as methotrexate (55) have been reported to reach toxic levels in such patients. Perhaps more importantly, glucose can be reabsorbed from the urine in diabetic patients and control of their diabetes may be made more difficult as a result (56).

TISSUE ENGINEERING IN UROLOGY

Tissue engineering is defined as "an interdisciplinary field which applies the principles of engineering and life sciences toward the development of biological substitutes that aim to maintain, restore or improve tissue function" (57). There are three current strategies for tissue engineering: integrating biomaterials such as cell-seeded or nonseeded matrices into diseased tissues to promote the development of functional new tissue; nuclear transfer for reproductive or therapeutic cloning; and stem cell induced tissue regeneration.

Cell-Seeded or Cell-Nonseeded Matrices

There are different classes of biomaterials: natural derived materials, such as collagen and alginate; tissue matrices, such has bladder submucosa and small intestinal submucosa (cell-seeded or nonseeded); and synthetic polymers such as polyglycolic acid, polylactic acid and polylactic-co-glycolic acid. These biomaterials slowly disintegrate and are replaced by extracellular matrix relying on ingrowths of healthy cells and remodeling into regenerated tissue. Several nonseeded biomaterials have been used in animal models for urethral reconstruction (58–61).

In clinical practice, nonseeded materials have been used with some success in substitution urethroplasty for relatively short strictures (62) potentially replacing buccal mucosal grafts in similar circumstances, but have failed in longer strictures requiring circumferential repair (63), presumably because the maximum distance cells can travel from the healthy urethral edges is only only 1 cm. For longer strictures, matrices seeded with urethral epithelial or buccal mucosal cells are required, but the larger the mass of cells, the more it becomes important to have an adequate vascular network to deliver nutrients and oxygen to each cell. To overcome this problem, it has been proposed to prevascularize the matrix before seeding the cells onto the scaffold (64).

The application of tissue-engineered tissues in bladder replacement is also still experimental and results of studies using acellular matrices have been disappointing resulting in graft contraction and loss of capacity (65–67). Bladder augmentation with cell-seeded matrices appear to be more promising achieving a composite graft of normal bladder architecture (68) but the goal of a bio-engineered bladder becoming a clinical reality is still some way into the future (69).

Nuclear Transfer for Reproductive or Therapeutic Cloning

Cloning involves transfer of a donor nucleus with its genetic material into an enucleated oocyte, which will produce an embryo with identical genetic material as its cell source (reproductive cloning). The embryo can be implanted into a female to develop into a clone of the donor, as demonstrated with "Dolly the sheep" in 1997. Therapeutic cloning (somatic cell nuclear transfer) is used to only produce autologous embryonic stem cells for tissue regeneration after a patient's nuclear DNA from a somatic cell was transferred into an enucleated (donated) oocyte. Therapeutic cloning is in its infancy but a degree of renal tissue regeneration has been achieved in a large animal model (70).

Stem Cells–Induced Tissue Regeneration

Ethical issues concerning the use of cloned human embryos for the derivation of stem cells have stimulated the search for methods of harvesting stem cells or reprogramming differentiated cells into pluripotent stem cells.

There are several sources of stem cells provision, principally autologous adult stem cells harvested mainly from bone marrow biopsy (but also from adipose and other tissues) and human embryonic stem cells, which are ethically more controversial. Both have the potential to differentiate into derivatives of all three embryonic germ layers (71). Pluripotent embryonic stem cells are separated during the blastocyst stage at five days after fertilization and if used clinically would have the disadvantage of requiring immunosuppression apart from the potential risk to transdifferentiate into a malignant phenotype. Adult autologous stem cells avoid these problems but the quantity of harvested cells is limited. Another source are fetal stem cells derived from amniotic fluid or placental tissue which could be stored for later potential future self-use, avoiding immunosuppression and malignant transformation (72).

New strategies to generate a source of patient-specific pluripotent stem cells is focusing on reprogramming technologies which requires resetting of the gene expression program of a somatic cell to a state consistent with embryonic development (73). Amazing progress had been made recent years in cell and developmental biology. Undoubtedly further developments in finding the ideal source of stem cells for tissue regeneration will evolve in the not too distant future (74).

REFERENCES

1. Brockes JP, Kumar A. Appendage regeneration in adult vertebrates and implications for regenerative medicine. Science 2005; 310(5756):1919–1923.
2. Adzick NS, Lorenz HP. Cells, matrix, growth factors, and the surgeon. The biology of scarless fetal wound repair. Ann Surg 1994; 220(1):10–18.
3. Lorenz Hp, Lin RY, Longaker MT, et al. The fetal fibroblast: the effector cell of scarless fetal skin repair. Plast Reconstr Surg 1995; 96(6):1251–1259.
4. Kingsnorth AN, Slavin J. Peptide growth factors and wound healing. Br J Surg 1991; 78:1286–1290.
5. Furcht LT. Critical factors controlling angiogenesis: cell products, cell matrix and growth factors. Lab Invest 1986; 55:505–509.
6. Skalli O, Gabbiani G. The biology of the myofibroblast relationship to wound contraction and fibrocontractive disease. In: Clark RAF, Henson PM, eds. The Molecular and Cellular Biology of Wound Healing. New York: Plenum Press, 1988:373.
7. Blair GH, Slome D, Walter JB. Review of experimental investigations on wound healing. In: Ross JP, ed. British Surgical Practice: Surgical Progress. London: Butterworth, 1961.
8. Converse JM, McCarthy JG, Brauer RO, et al. Transplantation of skin. Grafts and flaps. In: Reconstructive Plastic Surgery. Vol. 1. 2nd ed. Philadelphia: WB Saunders, 1977:152–182.
9. Grabb WC, Smith JW. Plastic Surgery. 2nd ed. Boston: Little Brown, 1973:1–122.
10. Devine CJ Jr, Horton CE. Surgical treatment of Peyronie's disease with dermal graft. J Urol 1989; 142:1223–1226.
11. Perlmutter AD, Montgomery BT, Steinhardt G. Tunica vaginalis free graft for the correction of chordee. J Urol 1985; 134:311–313.

12. Gilbert DA, Horton CE, Terzis J, et al. New concepts in phallic reconstruction. Ann Plast Surg 1987; 18:128–136.

13. Ehrlich RM, Reda EF, Koyle MA, et al. Complications of bladder mucosal graft. J Urol 1989; 142:626–627.

14. Baskin LS, Duckett JW. Mucosal grafts in hypospadias and stricture management. AUA Update Series 1994.

15. Burger RA, Muller SC, El-Damanhoury H, et al. The buccal mucosal graft for urethral reconstruction: a preliminary report. J Urol 1992; 147:662–664.

16. Horton CE, Devine CJ Jr. A one stage repair of hypospadias cripples. Plast Reconstr Surg 1970; 45:425–430.

17. Schreiter F, Noll F. Meshgraft urethroplasty using split thickness skin graft of foreskin. J Urol 1989; 142:1223–1226.

18. Duckett JW. The island flap technique for hypospadias repair. Urol Clin North Am 1981; 8:503–511.

19. Morehouse DD. Current indications and technique of two stage repair for membraneous urethral strictures. Urol Clin North Am 1989; 16:325–328.

20. Mundy AR. Results and complications of urethroplasty and its future. Br J Urol 1993; 71:322–325.

21. Brain DJ. The early history of rhinoplasty. Facial Plast Surg 1993; 9:81–89.

22. Backstein R, Hinek A. War and medicine: the origins of plastic surgery. Univ Toronto Med J 2005; 3:217–219.

23. Williams P, Harrison T. McIndoe's Army. 2nd ed. London: Sphere, 1981.

24. McCraw J, Massey F, Shaiklin K, et al. Vaginal reconstruction with gracilis myocutaneous flaps. Plast Reconstr Surg 1976; 58:176–183.

25. Horton CE, Sadore RC, Jordan GH, et al. Use of the rectus abdominis muscle and fascia flap inreconstruction of epispadias/exstrophy Clin Plast Surg 1988; 15:393–397.

26. Taylor GI, Daniel RK. The anatomy of several free flap donor sites. Plast Reconstr Surg 1975; 56:243–253.

27. Koch MO, McDougal WS, Thompson CO. Mechanisms of solute transport following urinary diversion through intestinal segments: an experimental study with rats. J Urol 1991; 146:1390–1394.

28. Fern DO, Odel HM. Electrolyte pattern of the blood after bilateral ureterosigmoidostomy. JAMA 1949; 142:634–641.

29. Zabbo A, Kay R. Ureterosigmoidostomy and bladder extrophy: a long-term follow-up. J Urol 1986; 136:396–398.

30. Fisch M, Wammack R, Muller SC, et al. The Mainz 11 (sigma rect um pouch). J Urol 1993; 149:258–263.

31. Singh G, Thomas DG. Bowel problems after enterocystoplasty. Br J Urol 1997; 79:328–332.

32. Whorwell PJ, Lupton EW, Erdiran D, et al. Bladder smooth muscle dysfunction in patients with irritable bowel syndrome. Gut 1986; 27:1014–1017.

33. Spirnak SP, Caldamone AA. Ureterosigmoidostomy. Urol Clin North Am 1986; 13:285.

34. Durrans D, Wujanto R, Carrol RN, et al. Bile acid malabsorption: a complication of conduit surgery. Br J Urol 1989; 64:485–488.

35. Dean AM, Woodhouse CRJ, Parkinson MC. Histological changes in ileal conduits. J Urol 1984; 132:1108–1111.

36. Nurse DE, Mundy AR. Metabolic complications of cystoplasty. Br J Urol 1989; 63:165–170.

37. Mundy AR, Nurse DE. Calcium balance, growth and skeletal mineralisation in patients with cystoplasties. Br J Urol 1992; 69:257–259.

38. Wear JB Jr, Barquin OP. Ureterosigmoidostomy. Urology 1973; 1:192–200.

39. Klein EA, Montie JE, Montague DK, et al. Jejunal conduit urinary diversion. J Urol 1989; 64:412.

40. Geist RW, Ansell JS. Total body potassium after ureteroileostomy. Surg Gynaec Obstet 1961; 113:585–589.

41. McDougall WS, Koch MO. Impaired growth and development and urinary intestinal interposition. Trans Am Assoc Genitourin Surg 1991; 105:3.

42. Gerharz EW, Preece M, Duffy PG, et al. Enterocystoplasty in childhood: a second look at the effect on growth. BJU Int 2003; 91:79–83.

43. Guinan PD, Moore RH, Neter E, et al. The bacteriology of ileal conduit urine in man. Surg Gynaec Obstet 1972; 134:78–82.

44. Schwarz GR, Jeffs RD. Ileal conduit urinary diversion in children: computer analysis of follow-up from 2 to 16 years. J Urol 1975; 114:285–288.

45. Husmann DA, Spence HM. Current status of tumour of the bowel following ureterosigmoidostomy: a review. J Urol 1990; 144:607–610.

46. Aaronson IA, Constantinides CG, Sallie LP, et al. Pathogenesis of adenocarcinoma complicating ureterosigmoidostomy. Experimental observations. Urology 1987; 29:538–543.

47. Aaronson IA, Sinclair-Smith CC. Dysplasia of ureteric epithelium: a source of adenocarcinoma in ureterosigmoidostomy? Z Kinderchir 1984; 39:364–367.

48. Stewart M, Hill MJ, Pugh RC, et al. The role of N-nitrosamine in carcinogenesis at the uretero-colic anastomosis. Br J Urol 1981; 53:115–118.

49. Filmer RB, Spencer JR. Malignancies in bladder, augmentations and intestinal conduits. J Urol 1990; 143:671–678.

50. Andrich DE, Hirst JP, Kirkham APS, et al. Feasibility of Magnetic Resonance Cystography in the surveillance of augmentation and substitution cystoplasty. BJU Int 2008; 101:45.

51. Robertson WG, Woodhouse CR. Metabolic factors in the causation of urinary tract stones in patients with enterocystoplasties. Urol Res 2006; 34:231–238.

52. Hamid R, Robertson WG, Woodhouse CR. Comparison of biochemistry and diet in patients with enterocystoplasty who do and do not form stones. BJU Int 2008; 101:1427–1432.

53. McDermott WV Jr. Diversion of urine to the intestines as a factor in ammoniagenic coma. N Engl J Med 1957; 256:460–462.

54. Savarirayan F, Dixey GM. Synope following ureterosigmoidostomy. J Urol 1969; 101:844–845.

55. Bowyer GW, Davies TW. Methotrexate toxicity associated with an ileal conduit. Br J Urol 1987; 60:592.

56. Sridhar KN, Samuell CT, Woodhouse CRJ. Absorption of glucose from urinary conduits in diabetics and nondiabetics. Br Med J 1983; 287:1327–1329.

57. Atala A. Tissue engineering and cell therapy: perspectives for urology. In: Wein AJ, Kavoussi LR, Novick AC, et al., eds. Campbell-Walsh Urology. Vol. 1. 9th ed. Philadelphia: Saunders Elsevier, 2007:553–573.

58. Bazeed MA, Thürhoff JW, Schmidt RA, et al. New treatment for urethral strictures. Urology 1983; 21:53–57.

59. Kropp BP, Ludlow JK, Spicer D, et al. Rabbit urethral regeneration using small intestinal submucosa onlay grafts. Urology 1998; 52:138–142.

60. Chen F, Yoo JJ, Atala A. Acellular collagen matrix as a possible 'off the shelf' biomaterial for urethral repair. Urology 1999; 54:407–410.

61. Sievert KD, Bakircioglu ME, Nunes L, et al. Homologous acellular matrix graft for urethral reconstruction in the rabbit: histological and functional evaluation. J Urol 200; 163:1958–1965.

62. Atala A, Guzman L, Retik A. A novel inert collagen matrix for hypospadias repair. J Urol 1999; 162:1148–1151.

63. DeFilippo RE, Yoo JJ, Atala A. Urethral replacement using cell-seeded tubularized collagen matrices. J Urol 2002; 168:1789–1793.

64. Fontaine M, Schloo B, Jenkins R, et al. Human hepatocyte isolation and transplantation into an athymic rat, using prevascularized cell polymer constructs. J Pediatr Surg 1995; 30:56–60.

65. Kropp BP, Sawyer BD, Shannon HE, et al. Characterization of small intestinal submucosa regenerated canine detrusor: assessment of reinnervation, in vitro compliance and contractility. J Urol 1996; 156:599–607.

66. Sutherland RS, Baskin LS, Hayward SW, et al. Regeneration of bladder urothelium, smooth muscles, blood vessels, and nerves into an acellular tissue matrix. J Urol 1996; 156:571–577.

67. Yoo JJ, Meng J, Atala A. Bladder augmentation using allogenic bladder submucosa seeded with cells. Urology 1998; 51:221–225.

68. Oberpenning F, Meng J, Yoo J, et al. De novo reconstitution of a functional urinary bladder by tissue engineering. Nat biotechnol 1999; 17:149–155.

69. Bolland F, Southgate J. Bio-engineering urothelial cells for bladder tissue transplant. Expert Opin Biol Ther 2008; 8:1039–1049.

70. Lanza RP, Chung HY, Yoo JJ, et al. Generation of histocompatible tissues using nuclear transplantation. Nat Biotechnol. 2002; 20:689–696.

71. Tomson JA, Kalishman J, Golos TG, et al. Isolation of a primate embryonic stem cell line. Proc Natl Acad Sci U S A 1995; 92:7844–7848.

72. Siddiqui MM, Atala A. Amniotic fluid-derived pluripotential cells. In: Lanza RA, ed. Handbook of Stem Cells. Vol. 2. Philadelphia: Academic Press, 2004:175–179.

73. Jaenisch R, Young R. Stem cells, the molecular circuitry of pluripotency and nuclear reprogramming. Cell 2008; 132(4):567–582.

74. Hipp J, Atala A. Sources of stem cells for regenerative medicine. Stem Cell Rev 2008; 4(1):3–11.

32

Energy Sources in Urology

Andy Symes and Ken M. Anson
Department of Urology, St George's Hospital, London, U.K.

INTRODUCTION

In every operating theater around the world, an energy source of some description will be available to help the surgeon perform procedures with as limited morbidity as possible. The move toward less invasive therapeutic interventions has also resulted in energy sources moving out of the operating theater into the outpatient department. Advances in energy delivery have arisen alongside and often in tandem with advances in surgery. The introduction of extracorporeal shock wave lithotripsy (ESWL) remains the most potent example of the impact of technology upon surgical practice. The liaison between industry and health care professionals remains critically important both to the understanding of present day devices, and for the development of the surgical tools of the future.

It is our aim in this chapter to present the physical principles that underpin the various energy sources that are currently commercially available to urologists. It is hoped that this will provide a "working knowledge" that will help the clinician not only to choose the tool best suited to the job at hand, but also to be able to use it appropriately and safely. We have divided the energy sources into four broad families: electrosurgical, electromagnetic, acoustic, and mechanical (Table 1). We shall examine the physical characteristics of each, explain their tissue interactions, outline the delivery systems available, and provide a brief description of their clinical applications.

ELECTROSURGICAL ENERGY

Cauterizing wounds to stop bleeding was recorded as early as Hippocrates—"Those diseases which medicines do not cure, iron cures; those which iron cannot cure, fire cures; and those which fire cannot cure, are to be reckoned wholly incurable" (1). It was not until the 19th century that a physicist called Becquerel first demonstrated electrocautery. He showed that passing electrical current through a needle generated heat, which could be used as a controllable source of heat to stop bleeding via coagulation (the process by which blood forms solid clots). Jacques-Arsene d'Arsonoval (1891) subsequently discovered that high-frequency alternating electric current could be passed through

the body without an electric shock, creating heat but not neuromuscular excitation (2). The term diathermy, "heating through," was coined in 1907 by German physician Carl Franz Nagelschmidt, and one year later, Vincenz Czerny used this process to cut tissue (3). The first electrosurgical device, the surgical Bovie knife, was not developed commercially until 1928 (4). The general principles of this device apply today and surgical diathermy remains an essential tool for all surgeons.

Basic Principles

To understand how diathermy works, it is important to be aware of the basic principles governing any electrical circuit (Table 2). Electric current flows when electrons pass from one atom to another, with flow expressed in amperes (A). The greater the current, the larger are the number of electrons that are moving, and to allow flow an electric circuit must be formed between a positive and negative electrode. Voltage, measured in volts, is the force that enables electrons to move around a circuit. If electrons meet resistance (impedance) to their flow, then heat is generated at that point and resistance is measured in ohms. The overall power of an electric circuit is measured in watts and is an interaction between current, voltage, resistance, and time. Standard mains electric current is alternating (flows in both directions) and oscillates at around 60 cycles per second. The speed of oscillation is measured in hertz (Hz) (Fig. 1).

Applied Physics

A generator is the source of flow and voltage to an electrosurgical circuit. In clinical practice the completed circuit comprises a generator, the active electrode (handpiece), the patient and the return electrode, with the connecting cables in between. The patient's tissue impedes flow of the current, leading to the production of heat. At 60 Hz, electricity interferes with the normal conduction of nerves and leads to electrocution: ventricular fibrillation, nerve stimulation, and muscular seizures (5). However, nerve and muscle stimulation cease at around 100,000 Hz, and it is then possible to pass high power through the body without causing

Table 1 Energy Sources in Urology

Electrosurgical energy	Diathermy
	Radio waves
Electromagnetic energy	Microwaves
	Lasers
	Extracorporeal shock wave lithotripsy
Acoustic energy	Ultrasound
Mechanical energy	Kinetic energy

Table 2 The Properties of Electricity

Current	Flow of electrons during a period of time (measured in amperes)
Circuit	Pathway for the uninterrupted flow of electrons
Voltage	Force pushing current through the resistance (measured in volts)
Resistance	Obstacle to the flow of current, measured in ohms (impedance = resistance)

electrocution. Modern electrosurgical generators produce current at greater than 300,000 Hz.

There are currently two ways in which an electrosurgical circuit can be formed—bipolar or monopolar circuits.

Bipolar electrosurgery. In bipolar electrosurgery both the active and return electrodes are enclosed in one instrument, usually a pair of forceps. The two tines of the forceps perform both the active and return electrodes. The current enters the patient's body only in the tissue between the two tines. No patient return electrode is therefore required and because only a small amount of tissue is exposed to the current a relatively low power can be used.

Monopolar electrosurgery. Monopolar electrosurgical circuits are the most commonly used. The active and return electrodes are separated by a part of the patient's body, with the active electrode usually an electrosurgical probe or pair of forceps, and the return electrode in the form of a much larger, flat plate in contact with the patient's skin. The current flows through the circuit and is concentrated (current density) at the narrow active electrode, resulting in heat deposition at this point.

Tissue Interactions

The only variable that determines the effect electrosurgical current has on tissues is the rate at which it produces heat. High levels of heat generated rapidly will cut tissues; low levels of heat generated slowly will coagulate tissues and result in hemostasis. The ability of the electrosurgical current to produce heat in the tissues can be changed by manipulating several factors: current density, power, time, and waveform.

1. Electrosurgical generators are able to produce a variety of electrical *waveforms*. As the waveform changes, the effects on surgical tissue alter and a different surgical effect is produced. The three waveforms are traditionally termed CUT, COAG, and BLEND, and cause the surgical effects of cutting, fulguration (destruction of tissue by high-frequency electric current), and desiccation (Fig. 2).

CUT waveform: This is a continuous high-current, low-voltage waveform. The high current helps it

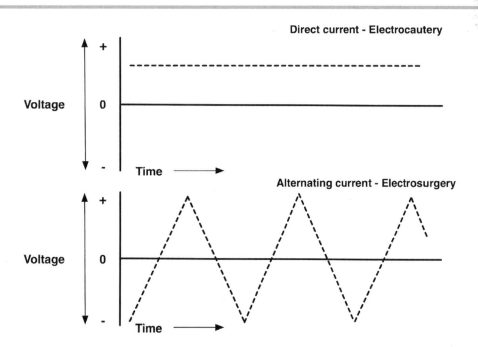

Figure 1 Electrosurgery differs from electrocautery in its use of alternating current.

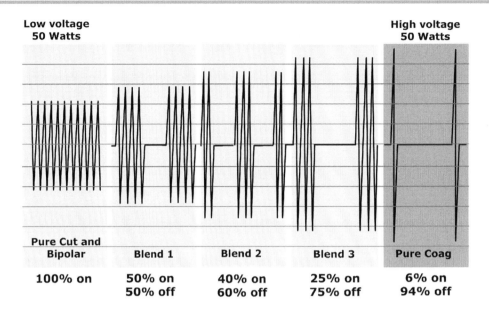

Figure 2 Alteration of power and waveform affects tissue interaction.

to heat tissues quickly and the low voltage prevents the formation of sparks, which would dissipate the heat. The tissues heat quickly, swell, and explode and the effect can be very clean, with the electrode acting like a scalpel.

COAG waveform: COAG is an intermittent low-current, high-voltage waveform. The low current causes a slow heating effect and the high voltage causes the production of sparks, dissipating the heating effect over a large area. At low power this leads to desiccation or drying out of the tissues, with formation of a coagulum. At higher powers the sparks cause a burning effect, leading to necrosis and fulguration of tissues. This is sometimes referred to as "spray." At very high power the COAG waveform will produce enough current density for cutting.

BLEND waveform: This combines the effect of COAG and CUT by altering the parameters of the waveform, with an increasing coagulation effect and a relative reduction in the cutting effect.

2. *Current density* is the ratio of the power of the current to the area of the tissue it affects. Thus, current density will be high at the active electrode and low at the return electrode for a given power of current.
3. *Power* of the current can affect the surgical effects it produces. For example, a high-power COAG waveform can be used to cut tissue; similarly, a low-power CUT waveform can be used very effectively to desiccate tissue.

The size and position of electrode will also impact on current density. A small electrode will produce a higher current density than a large electrode. Eschar is relatively high in resistance to current;

therefore, keeping electrodes clean and free of eschar will enhance performance by maintaining lower resistance within the surgical circuit.

Delivery Systems and Clinical Applications

Argon-enhanced electrosurgery. Electrosurgical current easily ionizes argon gas, making it more conductive than air. As argon gas is inert and noncombustible, it is a safe medium through which to pass current. Applying a stream of argon gas to the electrosurgical current creates a bridge between the electrode and tissue, which allows use in a noncontact fashion. This reduces surrounding tissue damage, causes less smoke and odor, and is said to produce a flexible eschar.

Vessel-sealing technology[TM]. Vessel-sealing technology combines electrosurgical energy and pressure to create a seal. The LigaSure[TM] device (ValleyLab, Colorado, U.S.) utilizes a specialized generator/instrument system that can be used in open or minimally invasive surgery. Vessels (<7 mm) or tissue bundles are placed between the jaws of the instrument, which are closed under pressure, and a bipolar current is applied (6). Upon release of the blades, the coagulated/sealed tissue is divided by sharp dissection. Thermal spread is reduced and seals have been proven to withstand 3× normal systolic blood pressure. The potential benefits of this technology are reduced blood loss, time saving compared to suturing, reduced needle stick injuries, avoidance of thermal damage to surrounding structures, and avoidance of foreign bodies (sutures).

Bipolar resection. The Gyrus[TM] bipolar resectoscope applies bipolar electrosurgical current across a specialized TUR loop, with the active and return electrode on the same axis, separated by a ceramic insulator (7). The Olympus system also utilizes a bipolar system, allowing transurethral resection in saline (TURis™). Benefits include better hemostasis, and avoidance of dilutional hyponatremia, as isotonic saline is the irrigation solution used. Measurable outcomes appear similar to conventional monopolar TURP (7,8), although long-term data are awaited.

Safety

When first introduced in the 1920s, surgical diathermy machines converted grounded mains electricity to grounded electrosurgical current. The current would return to ground, which was the common earth, via the return electrode. If the return electrode were to fail, then the current would find an alternative way to earth via a contact between the patient and any other earthed object. This was called current division and could lead to an accidental patient burn. Isolated electrosurgical systems were introduced in 1968 with the isolated generator, creating a separate circuit not referenced to the common earth but with its source in the generator itself. In other words the circuit is completed not by the ground but by the generator itself. Current division is therefore minimized and the potential for alternative site burns reduced. If the circuit is broken—the return electrode falls off—then current will cease to flow. Return electrode burns, however, may still occur and burns still occur through inappropriate use. All operators should therefore be familiar with the equipment in use in theater. Electrosurgery should not be used in the presence of flammable agents, and oxygen-enriched environments should be avoided, as there is a very real risk of ignition. When not in use, active electrodes should be kept in a clean, dry, and well-insulated nonconductive holster. Cords should not be wrapped around metal instruments, nor bundled together. This can lead to reactive coupling, generating electromagnetic energy [radio frequency (RF)], which is not always confined by insulation.

Minimally invasive surgery. Electrosurgery used with minimally invasive surgery has its own hazards: insulation failure, direct coupling of current, and capacitively coupled current (9). Breaks in insulation can create an alternate route for current to flow, and this is often not apparent with minimally invasive surgery where the views may be limited. Direct coupling occurs when the user activates the generator near another metal instrument. The secondary instrument becomes energized, with current seeking a pathway back to the return electrode, with potential for patient injury.

A capacitor occurs when a nonconductor separates two conductors, and may create an electrostatic field between them, thus passing current between them. During minimally invasive surgery, an "inadvertent" capacitor may be created by the surgical instruments. The conductive active electrode is surrounded by nonconductive insulation, which in turn is surrounded by a conductive metal cannula. Burns may occur from the outer metal cannula, and plastic sheaths are now favored.

Smoke. Surgical smoke is created when tissue is heated and cellular fluid is vaporized by the thermal action of the energy source. Viral DNA, bacteria, carcinogens, and irritants are known to be present in electrosurgical smoke, and where possible a smoke evacuation system should be used (10).

Tissue density feedback. Modern electrosurgical generators measure tissue impedance at the electrode contact and adjust settings according to the tissue involved. Voltages are kept lower and theater staff are not required to frequently change power settings.

Return electrode monitoring (REM™, ValleyLab). Pad site burns are caused by inadequate contact of the return electrode on the patient. REM-equipped generators actively monitor the amount of impedance at the patient/pad interface. If the generator detects a high level of impedance at the interface, then the system will deactivate.

ELECTROMAGNETIC ENERGY

Many urological instruments use sources that provide energy in the form of electromagnetic radiation (EMR). At first sight, they appear to be very disparate devices with varied delivery systems, but, on closer inspection, they share many common principles that arise from the use of the electromagnetic wave source. Their tissue effects may also seem unrelated but in fact are similar (i.e., the deposition of heat within tissues), and often they can be separated only by the speed and depth of energy absorption. However, some of these sources (particularly lasers) have very specific tissue effects, which are wavelength dependent and vary greatly from one wavelength to another.

EMR is a self-propagating wave in space with electric and magnetic components. These components oscillate at right angles to each other and to the direction of propagation, and are in phase with each other. EMR is classified into types according to the frequency of these waves: in order of increasing frequency, radio waves, microwaves, terahertz radiation, infrared radiation, visible light, ultraviolet radiation, X rays, and gamma rays (Fig. 3). EMR carries energy and momentum, which may be imparted when it interacts with matter.

Basic Science

Visible light, X rays, microwaves, radio waves, and lasers are all part of the electromagnetic spectrum and are members of the same family. All travel through space at the same velocity (v) of 3×10^8 m/sec (the speed of light (c)—about 186,000 miles per second). When they travel through a material medium, their speed is reduced but with no evidence of movement of the medium to indicate their passage. There is a constant relationship between velocity ($v = c$, the speed of light through an empty space), wavelength (k), and frequency (f), such that $v = fk$. It follows that the relationship between wavelength and frequency is inversely proportional.

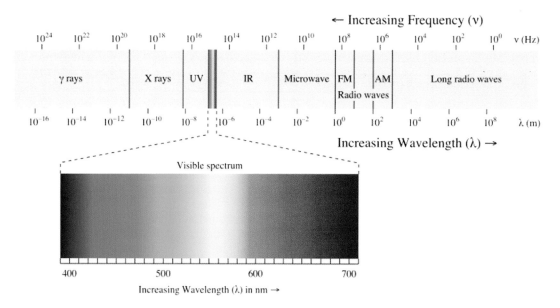

Figure 3 The electromagnetic spectrum.

Quantum Physics—Wave-Particle Duality

Theories about light stem back to the fifth to sixth century BC, when ancient Indians, Greeks, and Romans all put forward theories bearing striking resemblance to the modern theories of light—"The light and heat of the sun; these are composed of minute atoms which, when they are shoved off, lose no time in shooting right across the interspace of air in the direction imparted by the shove" (11). In the 15th and 16th centuries, Gassendi, and then Robert Hooke and Christian Huygens, proposed opposing theories of light, as either particulate or wave. In 1845, Michael Faraday discovered that the angle of polarization of a beam of light could be altered by a magnetic field as it passed through a polarizing material, an effect now known as Faraday rotation (12). This was the first evidence that light was related to electromagnetism. Faraday proposed in 1847 that light was a high-frequency electromagnetic vibration, which could propagate even in the absence of a medium such as the "ether" (12). This wave theory was successful in explaining nearly all optical and electromagnetic phenomena, and was a triumph of 19th century physics. By the late 19th century, a handful of experimental anomalies remained that could not be explained by or were in direct conflict with the wave theory. Experimental evidence led to three main observations: first, when light was directed at a metal surface, electrons were instantaneously ejected; second, when light intensity was increased, more electrons were ejected, but their velocity remained the same; and third, changing the color of the light toward the blue end of the visible spectrum (increasing the frequency) increased the maximum velocity of the ejected electrons (the photoelectric effect) (13). The wave theory of light could not explain these phenomena, as metals would have to reach high temperatures before electrons were ejected, and some time delay would be required to allow sufficient energy transfer. Similarly, increasing the intensity would increase the speed of the ejected electrons, and the frequency of light would not be expected to change these findings, since intensity, and not color, determines the energy of waves. In 1905, Einstein solved this puzzle by resurrecting the particle theory of light to explain the observed effects (14). Einstein's ideas were met initially by great skepticism, but his explanation of the photoelectric effect would triumph, ultimately forming the basis for wave-particle duality and much of quantum mechanics.

These findings led to the quantum theory of light, which states that light (or any other EMR) exists in the form of quanta known as photons, which are tiny "packets" of energy with no mass traveling through space at the speed of light (3×10^8 m/sec). The energy of each photon is given as $E = hf$, where E is the energy in joules, f is the frequency, and h is a universal constant (Planck's constant, 6.63×10^{-34} J/sec). The fundamental concept that energy is dependent on the frequency of the radiation applies to all parts of the electromagnetic spectrum. Therefore, it can be seen that as the frequency increases, so does the energy of the EMR. Thus, microwaves and radio waves are of low energy, while X-ray photons have a high energy enabling them to ionize matter that they come into contact with.

Applied Physics

Although electromagnetic waves share many physical characteristics, varying only in frequency and wavelength, their effect upon living tissue is very different. For example, the human body is transparent to radio waves, opaque to visible light, and mostly transparent to X rays. The quantum theory states that to raise an atom from ground to excited state, a photon of a given frequency and hence given energy ($\Delta E = hf$, where ΔE is the energy difference) is required. Thus, for a photon to be absorbed (to transfer its energy), it must interact with an atom that will be excited only by that corresponding packet of energy. Radio waves can pass through the body with little effect, while microwaves cause molecular rotation and torsion, and induce tissue heating. The infrared band causes molecular vibration, and X rays cause tissue ionization.

At the microscopic level, the electrical response of soft tissues to EMR is dependent on the frequency of the energy. This phenomenon is known as the dielectric property of tissues. At low frequencies [i.e., below several hundred kilohertz (kHz)], conductivity is determined by electrolytes in the extracellular space, and tissues have a high permeability to EMR at these frequencies. In the low-kilohertz range, tissues exhibit a dispersion (the alpha dispersion) because of several processes. These include polarization of counter ions near charged surfaces and membrane-bound structures within tissues. In the RF band, the tissues exhibit a dispersion (the beta dispersion) centered on the 0.1 to 10-MHz range, because of charging of cell membranes through the intracellular and extracellular media. At microwave frequencies (above 1 GHz and centered around 20 GHz), gamma dispersion occurs because of rotational relaxation of tissue water.

Tissue Interactions

In urological practice, nonlaser EMR is commonly used to induce thermal damage in tissues. Radio wave and microwave generators have been designed to heat the prostate, bladder, and kidney to different temperatures to achieve varying degrees of tissue damage. Some laser techniques have also been developed to obtain similar thermal effects. In each case, the energy inherent within the EMR is converted to heat within tissues. Each different energy source will vary between the amount of energy that can be delivered and the depth to which that energy can reach, but the basic tissue effect desired is the same. The response of tissues to heating varies with the temperature achieved at the target area. At temperatures around 45°C, tissue retracts because of macromolecular conformational changes, bond destruction, and membrane alterations. Beyond 60°C, protein denaturation occurs, and this is commonly called "coagulation" and results in coagulative necrosis. Carbonization of tissues occurs at approximately 80°C along with membrane permeabilization and collagen denaturation. Finally, at temperatures in excess of 100°C, vaporization of water occurs, and in combination with carbonization, yields decomposition of tissue constituents. Below temperatures of 45°C, there is virtually no histological change in tissue following heating. The World Health Organization (WHO) has defined heat treatments as hyperthermia for temperatures of 37°C

to 45°C, and as thermotherapy when temperatures exceed 45°C.

Many other factors influence the degree of heat deposition at a particular area including the locoregional blood supply, the thermal conductivity of the target and adjacent tissue, and the histopathological nature of the target tissue.

Radio waves and Microwaves

Microwave and RF radiation is EMR that is lower in frequency and therefore longer in wavelength than infrared radiation. "Radio frequency" is the name given to that section of the electromagnetic spectrum from frequencies of 300 kHz to 300 GHz. In general, the section of the electromagnetic spectrum from frequencies of approximately 300 MHz to 300 GHz and wavelengths of approximately 1 m to 1 mm are called microwaves. As a result of its low energy, RF, unlike other forms of nonionizing EMR, requires direct contact with tissues to exert an effect. As the RF energy attempts to pass into tissue, transference of energy occurs in a concentrated area. RF energy is efficient with minimal wastage; consequently, low-wattage energy (up to 15 W) can achieve temperatures approaching 100°C within a short time (typically 5 minute) without the need for interruption and cooling. RF devices are therefore often small and compact. Because of the low energy of RF, adjacent structures are relatively spared from heat dissipation.

Microwaves occupy the electromagnetic band at frequencies of 300 MHz to 300 GHz. These higher frequencies result in higher energy, and therefore greater tissue penetration than RF. The effect of microwave energy on tissue is predominantly because of molecular torsion and rotation (oscillation) and polarization of small molecules, especially water, resulting in tissue heating. In clinical practice, frequencies of 915 or 1296 MHz are used.

Clinical Applications

Transurethral Needle Ablation of the Prostate

Transurethral needle ablation (TUNA) of the prostate is a procedure used to treat benign prostatic hyperplasia (BPH). It is performed by placing interstitial RF needles through the urethra and into the lateral lobes of the prostate, causing heat-induced coagulation necrosis. The tissue is heated to 110°C at an RF power of 456 kHz for approximately 3 minutes per lesion. A coagulation defect is created. The TUNA device consists of an RF generator and monitor where energy, ablation time, lesion temperature, urethral temperature, and tissue impedance are displayed. In this device, the 465 to 490-kHz RF signal is transmitted directly into the prostate via two needles delivered via the TUNA catheter (Fig. 4). The delivery system has a disposable cartridge, a resterilizable handpiece, and a zero-degree fiberoptic lens. The TUNA cartridge contains two retractable needles, each surrounded by a protective retractable Teflon shield, except at the needle tips. When extended, the needles leave the body of

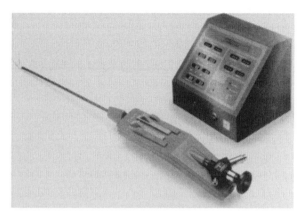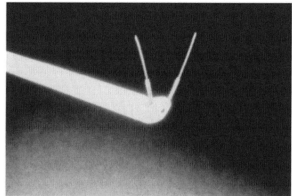

Figure 4   TUNA catheter with retractable needles and sheaths.

the catheter and diverge at an angle of 40° between each other and perpendicular to the catheter. Thermocouples are located at the tips of the protective shields and near the tip of the catheter for temperature monitoring of the lesion and prostatic urethra, respectively. The catheter tip is clear in order to allow visualization of the needles during penetration into the prostate. The procedure can be performed under local anesthesia and sedation (15). Lesions produced by the TUNA device are well-defined, ellipsoid necrotic lesions as a result of coagulative necrosis. The exact mechanism whereby relief of symptoms occurs is debated. The concept of anatomical debulking is flawed, as prostate volume changes following TUNA treatment are minimal (16). There is increasing evidence that the therapeutic effect of TUNA is explained by intraprostatic neuromodulation, which alters the physiologic function of voiding (dynamic component of BPH). Thermal neural ablation, including surgical alpha-receptor blockade, has been demonstrated by various researchers (17,18). There has been concern about the durability of this procedure, with up to 20% of patients requiring a TURP within two years (19). One study has provided good long-term clinical improvement at five-year follow-up with more than 75% of the patients not requiring additional treatment (20).

Radio Frequency Ablation of Renal Tumors

This technology was initially developed for treating primary and metastatic liver lesions (21). Zlotta et al. (22) first described the use of RF ablation (RFA) as the primary treatment for small renal tumors. It is used in patients with small renal tumors who have poor renal reserve, multiple bilateral renal cell carcinomas (RCC) in von Hippel–Lindau or hereditary RCC, or in those who are poor surgical candidates (23). A high-frequency electrical current is transmitted through an electrode placed directly into the renal tumor either percutaneously, under USS/CT/MRI guidance, or under direct vision laparoscopically (24,25).

Alternating current delivered through the probe causes ions in the surrounding tissues to vibrate, creating frictional heat that results in heat-induced tissue damage. Target temperatures of 105°C are achieved by generators of greater than 200 W (Cool-Tip ValleyLab, Radionics). The heat generated by RFA causes tissue destruction in three phases. Immediately postablation, molecular friction produces destruction of cellular structure, protein denaturation, membrane lipid melting, and cellular vaporization (26). Coagulative necrosis follows days later with surrounding areas of cellular edema and inflammation leading to tumor destruction (26). The final evolution of the ablated tissue is reabsorption of the necrotic foci with the resulting fibrotic scar nonenhancing on contrast imaging (27). For the cellular changes to occur as described earlier, temperatures above 50°C must be achieved. The success of tumor ablation with RFA depends on factors including probe temperature, generator power, temperature distribution, and targeting of the tumor (28).

Microwave Prostatic Therapies

Microwave energy may be applied transrectally and transurethrally to the prostate, and may induce hyperthermia or thermotherapy, depending on the target tissue temperature achieved. Transrectal hyperthermia, originally described in the treatment of prostate cancer (29) and subsequently BPH (30), has failed to show relief of the obstructive component of BPH and has largely been abandoned. Transurethral microwave thermotherapy (TUMT) aims to achieve high temperatures (45–80°C) in the prostate and involves the insertion of a specially designed Foley-type catheter into the bladder, allowing a microwave antenna to be positioned within the prostatic fossa (Fig. 5—ProstaLund Operations AB, Lund, Sweden; marketed by ACMI). Microwaves are then passed into prostate tissue to induce thermal coagulative necrosis.

Energy sources may be monopolar or bipolar. The Prostatron™ device uses a monopolar antenna. The initial software program, Prostasoft 2.0, was a

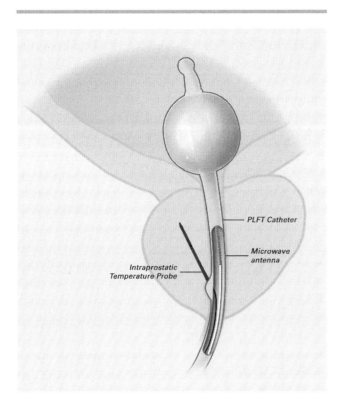

Figure 5 The ProstaLund CoreTherm® catheter (PLFT—ProstaLund Feedback Treatment).

low-energy protocol with maximum energy of 60 W. Treatment took 60 minutes, and noticeable symptomatic but not objective improvement occurred. Later, the higher-energy Prostasoft 2.5 was introduced, which allowed a stepwise increase in energy without interruptions to achieve intraprostatic temperatures of 75°C (167°F), and used urethral cooling with 20°C (68°F) water. The treatment also took 60 minutes, and results were better than with the initial software (31). The most current and powerful software is Prostasoft 3.5 (32). Only 30 minutes of treatment is required. Rectal temperature is monitored, and an alarm system is set that causes a cutout if excessive rectal temperatures occur. The therapy is contraindicated in patients with prostate or bladder cancer, urethral stricture, or claudication, or in patients with a pacemaker, defibrillator, or other metallic implants. Studies have compared TUMT with TURP, revealing greater symptomatic improvement with TURP than TUMT, as well as better objective response as measured by flow rate (33). Complications were lower with TUMT and it may be an alternative to surgery in patients who are deemed a high surgical or anesthetic risk and not controlled with pharmacotherapy.

Microwave Bladder Therapies

Human and animal studies have proven that microwave-induced hyperthermia combined with intravesical mitomycin C is a feasible, effective, and safe conservative approach for those patients with (high

risk) multiple and recurrent superficial bladder tumors, when other treatment strategies have failed, and/or when cystectomy is contraindicated or the patient refuses to undergo radical surgery (34,35). The Synergo® system employs a 915-MHz microwave applicator inserted into the bladder via a special catheter. Thermocouples are also inserted to control the temperature of the bladder wall layers, which are heated to a temperature of 42°C (±2°). Intravesical Mitomycin is pumped out and reinstilled, to avoid overheating. Each treatment lasts one hour, and no anesthesia is required. Side effects are minimal and largely related to the sensation of heat, which is temporary, and the effects of mitomycin.

Lasers

The invention of the laser, an acronym for "light amplification by stimulated emission of radiation," can be dated to 1958 with the publication of *Infrared and Optical Masers*, by Schawlow (36). It was Albert Einstein, however, in his 1917 paper "Zur Quantentheorie der Strahlung," who laid the theory for the invention of the laser and its predecessor the "maser." His theoretical model postulated that when a photon interacted with an excited atom, another photon would be released with identical wavelength. In 1960, Theodore Maiman invented the ruby laser considered to be the first successful optical or light laser (37). He used a ruby rod, excited by a helical flash lamp, to produce a beam of red laser light. A number of lasers were subsequently produced in the 1960s including the carbon dioxide (CO_2) and the neodymium: yttrium-aluminium-garnet (Nd:YAG) laser, which remain the most popular lasers used in medicine today. Initially called "an invention looking for a job," the laser now represents an entire scientific field and a multibillion dollar industry.

Basic Principles

Absorption and spontaneous emission. Atoms consist of a positively charged core (nucleus), which is surrounded by negatively charged electrons. The electrons can be thought of as orbiting the nucleus, with those with the largest energy orbiting furthest from the nuclear core. There are many energy levels that an electron within an atom can occupy; however, electrons usually rest at lower energy levels. Normally, when a photon of light is absorbed by an atom in which one of the outer electrons is initially in a low-energy state, the energy of the atom is raised to an upper energy level, and remains in this excited state for a very short period. It then spontaneously returns to the lower state, with the emission of a photon of light. These common processes of absorption and spontaneous emission cannot give rise to the amplification of light. The best that can be achieved is that for every photon absorbed, another is emitted.

Stimulated emission. This is a very uncommon process in nature but it is central to the operation of lasers. If a photon of light interacts with an excited atom, at a higher energy state, it can stimulate a return to the lower state. One photon interacting with an excited atom results in two photons being emitted. Furthermore, the two emitted photons are said to be in phase. Stimulated emission is the process that can give rise to the amplification of light and results in the laser beam produced having the property of coherence. Under most conditions, stimulated emission does not occur to a significant extent, as under conditions of thermal equilibrium, there will be far more atoms in the lower energy level than in the higher level. Absorption, therefore, will be much more common than stimulated emission. For stimulated emission to predominate there must be more atoms in the higher energy state than in the lower one. This unusual condition is referred to as a population inversion and is necessary for laser action to occur.

Population inversion. Population inversion is the state of a medium where a higher-lying electron level has a higher population than a lower-lying level. Finding substances (gain medium) in which a population inversion can be set up is central to the development of new kinds of laser. The first material used was synthetic ruby, and lasers today use argon, CO_2, semiconductors, Nd:YAG, among others. To stimulate most of the electrons to the high-energy states, an initial energy is delivered to the atoms in the laser medium in the form of light, heat, or electricity.

Laser Design

Once stimulated emission occurs, photons are generated exponentially provided population inversion is maintained. The light from a typical laser emerges in an extremely thin beam with very little divergence. Another way of saying this is that the beam is highly "collimated." The high degree of collimation arises from the fact that the cavity of the laser has very nearly parallel front and back mirrors, which constrain the final laser beam to a path perpendicular to those mirrors. The back mirror is made almost perfectly reflecting while the front mirror is about 99% reflecting, letting out about 1% of the beam (Fig. 6). This 1% is the output beam, which you see. The light has passed back and forth between the mirrors many times in order to gain intensity by the stimulated emission of more photons at the same wavelength. The light from a laser typically comes from one atomic transition with a single precise wavelength. So the laser light has a single

Table 3 Properties of Laser Light

Coherent (in phase)
Collimated (nondivergent)
Monochromatic (of a single wavelength)

spectral color and is almost the purest monochromatic light available. This wavelength is entirely dependent on the laser medium present.

Applied Physics

These three unique properties of laser light (beam coherence, collimation, and monochromaticity) (Table 3) separate it from the widely divergent, confused, and multiple wavelength light emitted from conventional light sources. Because of the high spatial coherence of laser light, the beam is remarkably collimated and therefore of low divergence. This property allows the full power of the generated light energy to be coupled into, and transmitted down, fine fiberoptic cables to the operative site. As a result, very high-power densities (power per unit cross-sectional area) can be achieved at the tissue surface. Furthermore, the beam can be focused to produce even greater power densities with more pronounced tissue effects. The interaction of the light with tissue is dependent both on the laser wavelength and the color of the tissue irradiated; thus, the single wavelength nature of the beam confers a high selectivity of action. One single laser will not be suitable for all clinical applications. A number of different laser wavelengths are available for clinical use. They are named after the medium used to generate the laser energy (Table 4).

Laser energy can be continuous or pulsed. Pulsing of lasers delivers a higher peak power (the maximum rate of energy delivery during the time of the pulse) and is commonly used to fragment calculi [pulsed dye, holmium:YAG, and frequency-doubled potassium-titanyl-phosphate (KTP)/Nd:YAG]. Pulsing is achieved either by applying intermittent energy to the active medium or by a process known as Q switching, in which a fast shutter is placed between the active/using medium and the exit mirror (partial reflector). When the shutter is closed, the photons are trapped within the active medium, resulting in a rapid buildup of energy. When the shutter opens, there is an instantaneous release of energy with a very large peak power.

Tissue Interactions

Boulnois has proposed a classification for the possible types of "photomedical processes" that can occur when laser light interacts with biological tissue (38). The four photobiological laser processes are thermal, photochemical, electromechanical, and photoablative. As with the use of microwaves and RF, the predominant tissue effect with lasers in urology is thermal.

Thermal interactions. When laser light interacts with tissue, it is reflected, transmitted, scattered, and absorbed, depending on the tissue type. When

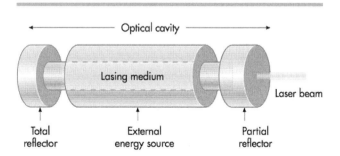

Figure 6 Basic laser design.

Table 4 Characteristics of Medical Lasers

Laser type	Mode	Wavelength (nm)	Visibility	Tissue penetration (mm)	Tissue absorption	Effects	Clinical Uses
Carbon dioxide	CW	10600	Invisible	0.1	Water, proteins, nucleic acids, fat	Intense carbonization, vaporization. Minimal penetration	Superficial skin lesions (penile warts). Bowens disease
Argon	CW	488 + 514(dual wavelength)	Blue	1	Hemoglobin, melanin	Tissue coagulation, vaporization	Nephron-sparing surgery, laparoscopy
Nd:YAG	CW P	1064	Invisible	3–8	Protein	Protein denaturation, coagulative necrosis	BPH & TCC therapy, interstitial therapy to solid tumors
KTP-532	CW P	532	Green	0.3–1	Hemoglobin	Tissue coagulation, vaporization	Photoselective vaporization prostate (PVP)
Holmium:YAG	P	2100	Invisible	0.5	Water	Mechanical pressure wave fragmentation Thermal	Urinary tract calculi. Enucleation of prostate
Pulsed dye laser (coumarin green)	P	504	Green	Minimal	Hemoglobin, but pulses too short for HB to absorb	Pressure effects. Plasma formation. Minimal damage to urothelium; little thermal effect	Urinary tract calculi
Semiconductor diode lasers	CW	800–900	Invisible	3–7	Protein	Protein denaturation, coagulative necrosis, vaporization	BPH therapy, interstitial therapy to solid tumors
Thulium	CW	2013	Invisible	0.002	Water	Tissue coagulation, vaporization	BPH therapy, vaporization prostate

CW, continuous wave; P, pulsed.

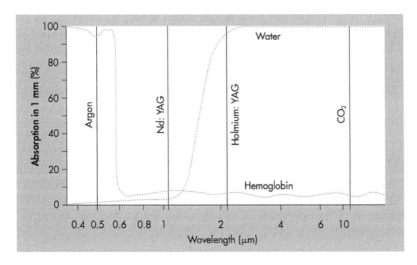

Figure 7 Laser wavelength absorption by hemoglobin and water.

absorbed, the electromechanical energy of the incident beam is converted into thermal energy within the tissues. Scattering of the beam results in widespread distribution of the energy at all angles to the incident beam; the energy is subsequently absorbed and converted into thermal energy. Both the wavelength of the interacting light and the color of the tissue irradiated determine the relative amount of absorption and scattering within tissue components (Fig. 7). The CO_2 laser has a wavelength of 10,600 nm and is therefore highly absorbed by water, proteins, nucleic acids, and fat; thus, its depth of penetration is very small at 0.1 mm. The high absorption by water makes this laser light unsuitable for endoscopic procedures (39), and it is used for the treatment of superficial lesions (skin/external genitalia). There is intense and instantaneous tissue vaporization and carbonization with a very shallow thermal damage front, and healing is achieved with minimal scarring. In contrast, the Nd:YAG wavelength (1064 nm) has little effect on water, but proteins absorb it. It is, therefore, widely scattered to a depth of up to 0.8 cm, as the predominantly water-containing tissue is transparent. The scattering results in a wider distribution of the energy at all angles away from the incident beam. The energy is therefore absorbed within a larger volume of tissue. The power of a laser is related to the power density, that is, the power per surface area, and is given as $PD = W/\pi r^2$ [W (watts) is the power emitted from the laser]. The total energy delivered multiplies the power density by duration of exposure; thus, total energy = $Ws/\pi r^2$ (measured in joules). It can be seen that doubling of the spot size reduces the power fourfold. The rate of ablation varies with the total energy delivered; the higher the total energy, the faster is the ablation. At low power, heat is conducted into deeper tissues. Consequently, at a higher power density, there is less thermal damage to underlying tissues. A highly focused beam results in a shallow zone of thermal damage below the target tissue, "the thermal damage front," and results in minimal scarring. A defocused beam results in a reduction of power density at the lesion, but a thick zone of thermal damage front beneath the target's surface.

Photoablative and electromechanical interactions. Pulsing of lasers (such as holmium:YAG) has the additional benefit of a very high peak pressure, causing fragmentation by erosion, shattering, and plasma bubble formation with cavitation. When the pulse is very short, thermal damage is minimized (39), although the holmium:YAG laser will damage ureteric tissue if in contact (40). This property endows the laser with a dual purpose, as it can be used to incise tissue such as the prostate and bladder neck (HoLEP) (41).

Photochemical effects—photodynamic therapy. Low-power laser light can photochemically activate a photosensitizing dye such as a hematoporphyrin derivative. This dye is chemically inert until exposed to specific laser wavelengths; this exposure results in energy release in the form of free radicals that are cytotoxic (42). Tissues that take up these dyes can be destroyed when laser energy is directed at them. Endothelial cells are most sensitive to the effects of free radicals and have increased density within tumors. The injured endothelium also releases interleukin and tumor necrosis factor, causing additional damage to malignant epithelium. This technique is being used in the treatment of carcinoma in situ of the bladder and is being investigated in the treatment of both benign and malignant prostatic disease (42).

Tissue-welding effects. Laser energy can induce interdigitation of collagen, resulting in a tissue-welding effect. Albumin has been used as a tissue solder, particularly in vasovasostomy (43).

Laser Delivery Systems

Laser light can be focused to diameters near 50% of its wavelength. This allows laser light to be transmitted along single quartz fiberoptic fibers. Laser energy is conducted along the fiber by a process known as internal reflection where the light is reflected from one side to the other, as the beam travels along the fiber. The beam must be reflected at a specific angle, known as the critical angle of reflection. If the fiber is displaced, or bent too far, the beam will no longer strike the sidewall at the critical angle and will escape from the fiber, causing injury to the user, the endoscope, or both. Once the beam exits the fiber tip, it is no longer coherent, as it is driven out of phase during internal reflection, and divergence occurs (about 17%, assuming a flat fiber tip). Therefore, the highest power density is at the tip of the fiber.

Clinical Applications

The Nd:YAG laser has been used to cause widespread coagulative necrosis within the benign prostate (endoscopic laser ablation of the prostate) (44), and it can also be used to coagulate superficial bladder tumors. Q-switching of Nd:YAG lasers may be used to fragment calculi, although it is less effective than the holmium laser, since it relies primarily on the photochemical mechanism for lithotripsy. Addition of a KTP crystal doubles the frequency (therefore halving the wavelength—532 nm) and causes the beam to become visible in the green band of visible light. Its use has recently become popular in photoselective vaporization of the prostate (45). This wavelength is highly absorbed by oxyhemoglobin and penetrates the prostatic tissue only 1 to 2 mm deep. These important characteristics allow the laser energy to be confined in a small volume of tissue, eliminating the risks caused by excessive coagulation. The high-power KTP laser instantly removes tissue by vaporization of cellular water, leaving only a thin 1- to 2-mm rim of coagulated tissue remaining. The KTP laser is thought to ablate prostate tissue more efficiently than the Nd:YAG laser. The Nd:YAG laser can also be used for ablation of skin lesions (including penile carcinoma), and in removal of hair post urethral reconstruction. However, the significant depth of penetration means that there is a risk of injury to the underlying tissues and subsequent scar/stricture formation.

The holmium:YAG laser is widely used in endoscopic surgery both for stone fragmentation (46) as well as resection of the prostate (HoLEP) (47). The beam falls in the near infrared portion of the electromagnetic spectrum (2100 nm). The Ho:YAG laser has 350-μsec pulse duration. The laser energy is absorbed in <0.5 mm of fluid, making it an ideal surgical laser for endourological applications such as laser lithotripsy. The laser energy is delivered to the surface of stones using flexible quartz fibers with multiple different diameters (200, 365, 550 μm). During the pulse of laser energy, there is a microscopic air bubble on the tip of the fiber that allows the laser energy to travel further than through the fluid medium directly transmitting the laser energy into the stone. In addition, the Ho:YAG laser has been used to incise urethral strictures, ureterocoeles, and obstructing pelviureteric junctions.

The Indigo laser is a diode laser with a wavelength between 800 and 850 nm. It penetrates deep into tissues, up to 3 mm, and thus produces thermal lesions several centimeters in diameter. It has been used primarily for prostate tissue ablation via interstitial laser coagulation.

The CO_2 laser is an infrared laser with a very long wavelength (10,640 nm), which results in a relatively short depth of penetration (40 to 240 μm). Its zone of thermal tissue injury is small and it is used to treat superficial skin lesions, such as condyloma.

Laser Safety

Strict protocols regarding the use of lasers in the theater are mandatory. All personnel in the theater must wear protective goggles. Different goggles are required for different wavelengths, and the wearer should check that the goggles protect against the wavelength in use. The area where the laser is being used must be clearly marked with warning notices and the theater doors locked when the laser is in use. An illuminated light must be on during laser firing. Black curtains should be applied above eye level to all windows. The retina is susceptible to laser light in the range 400 to 1400 nm. Accidental exposure can lead to injury, ranging from small scotomata to optic nerve burns. Wavelengths beyond 1400 nm may cause corneal injuries. There is a greater chance of an accidental burn to the skin than the eye. Laser safety rules should be available in all areas where lasers are in use, and the local laser safety officer will be able to advise on these.

ACOUSTIC ENERGY

The word "acoustic" is derived from the ancient Greek word ακουστός, meaning pertaining to hearing. Audible sound waves travel at frequencies of 50 to 20,000 Hz. Frequencies above this range (30,000 Hz to 1 MHz) are termed ultrasonic, with frequencies below termed infrasonic (100 kHz to 0.1 Hz). The word "acoustic" refers to the entire frequency range without limit. The introduction of ESWL and high-intensity focused ultrasound (HIFU) into clinical practice has ushered in a new generation of treatment modalities for a variety of benign (stones) and malignant (prostate) conditions. Shock wave and ultrasonic therapies will be discussed here with HIFU mentioned elsewhere.

Basic Principles

Waves carry vibrations through a medium (solid, liquid, gas) and are created whenever an object moves within a fluid (either gas or liquid). Waves have a measurable speed, wavelength, and frequency and are created when an object moves, compressing molecules adjacent to it. This compression is in turn transmitted to further adjacent molecules and so on. The compression is therefore relieved in the original region but is propagated onward to a new region with the formation of a wave. The speed of this wave is dependant on the characteristics and temperature of the medium within which it travels (solids > liquids > gases). It is independent of pressure, frequency, and amplitude. Acoustic waves differ from electromagnetic waves in that individual molecules do not travel with acoustic waves. Electromagnetic energy displays wave-particle duality with particles (photons) physically traveling through space. Acoustic energy therefore requires a medium where as electromagnetic energy does not: light can travel through a vacuum but sound cannot.

When an object moves within a medium, it moves to (compresses) and moves away from the medium (rarefaction) creating a compressive and tensile wave. In most cases these waves propagate similarly and move at the same sound speed. Wave forms may be sinusoidal in nature; however, many are not, for example, shock waves.

Extracorporeal Shock Wave Lithotripsy

Shock waves are high-energy waves with high amplitude, characterized by extremely short buildup times. Using shock waves, the first kidney stone was successfully disintegrated in Munich in 1980, and now ESWL is accepted as a first-line treatment in the management of renal and ureteric stones (48). Lithotripsy has undergone numerous technological advances; however, the fundamentals of shock wave generation and delivery have changed little.

Applied Physics

A typical shock wave is shown in Figure 8. It is characterized by a short wave of about 5 μsec with a near-instantaneous leap to a peak-positive pressure of about 40 MPa (compressive phase) (MPa, MegaPascal—the metric unit of pressure). This is known as a shock. The pressure falls rapidly to zero and then below with a peak-negative pressure of 10 MPa (tensile phase), which is always much less than the positive pressure. The majority of lithotripters produce a similar shock wave; however, the peak pressures may vary (peak positive: 30 to 110 MPa; peak negative: −5 to −15 MPa). Thus, the main difference is the amplitude of wave.

When a shock wave encounters a medium, part of the wave will continue (transmitted wave) and part will be reflected (reflected wave). The density and sound speed of a medium determine its specific acoustic impedance. The transmission from water to tissue is very efficient (99%), as is water to stone (75–95%). The transmission from water to air is very poor and 99.9% of energy will be reflected. Shock wave generators in lithotripsy are therefore water filled, with both patient and generator in water (most efficient), or with water-filled pads directly applied to the patient, with care taken to eliminate air from the contact. Thus, the flank provides the best "acoustic window" with a pure tissue path to the kidney.

The shock wave is focused onto the stone to concentrate acoustic energy and minimize damage to the surrounding tissues. This is achieved by differing means depending on machine. The acoustic pressure is greatest at one point and is surrounded by an area of high amplitude. This is known as the focal zone, which is ellipsoid in shape and ranges from a few to tens of millimeters. The focal length is the distance from the mouth of the therapy head to the focus (stone). The power of a lithotripter is related to the volume and peak pressure at the focal point. The energy delivered is measured in joules and is greatest

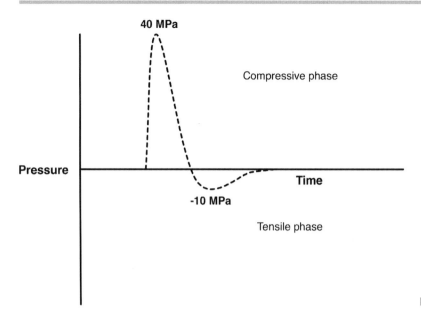

Figure 8 Acoustic shock wave.

for spark-gap lithotripters, because of their large focal points and high peak pressures (49).

Tissue Interactions and Stone Fragmentation

There are thought to be numerous ways in which shock waves fragment stones. When applied to a stone, the positive pressure phase part of the shock wave is reflected at the stone surface, causing erosion at the entry and exit points because of a high-pressure gradient. A compressive wave continues through the stone, causing shattering (Fig. 9). Shear stress on the stone will be generated by both shear and compressive waves as they enter the stone. Superfocusing is the amplification of stresses inside the stone either by refraction or diffraction of the shock wave dependent on the geometry of the stone. Squeezing occurs

because of differing sound speeds of waves between the stone and surrounding fluid, resulting in tensile stress and stone breakage. During the negative-pressure phase cavitation occurs (50), causing rapid expansion of gas bubbles in the liquid medium at the stone surface (Fig. 10). This phenomenon occurs when a negative pressure greater than the ambient pressure exists in a liquid, which then fails under stress (50). These unstable bubbles collapse, forming microjets that strike the stone surface. Microjet velocities range from 130 to 170 m/sec.

Lithotripter Design

Lithotripters require an energy source, a focusing mechanism for the shock wave, a coupling medium, and a stone localization system.

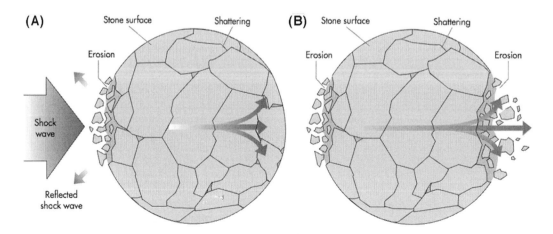

Figure 9 (**A**) Positive-pressure phase effect of a shock wave upon a calculus. Surface erosion occurs at entry and exit points. (**B**) Negative-pressure phase effect of a shock wave upon a calculus. The effect of cavitation.

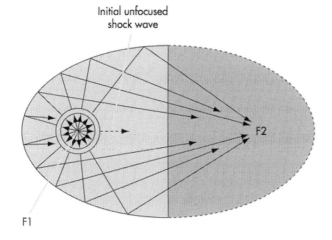

Figure 10 Model stone located at the focal point. Cavitation bubbles exist 540 μsec after the shock wave is released.

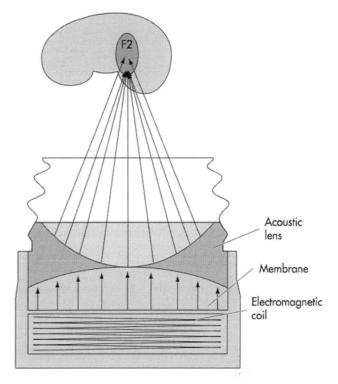

Figure 12 Electromagnetic lithotripter. Application of an electric current to the coil results in a strong magnetic field that repels a metallic disk upward to strike a fixed metal plate. Shock waves are focused by an acoustic lens or parabolic reflector.

Figure 11 Spark-gap lithotripter. A spark, generated at F1, causes a hydrodynamic pressure wave that is focused at a set distance to the target area (F2) by an ellipsoid reflector.

Electrohydraulic lithotripters. Spark-gap lithotripters use an underwater spark that generates a hydrodynamic pressure wave (Fig. 11). The point of spark generation (F1) is placed in front of an ellipsoid mirror, which focuses the pressure waves at a set distance to the target area (F2). Position of the spark relative to the ellipse is critical, with displacement by only 1 mm resulting in loss of focusing and lengthening and broadening of the focal zone (51). Although frequent changing and or replacement of the electrodes can overcome this, there can still be significant variability from shock to shock.

Electromagnetic lithotripters. Electromagnetic lithotripters require the application of an electric current to a coil. This generates a strong magnetic field that repels and thrusts a metallic disk upward to strike a fixed metallic plate, thus generating an acoustic shock wave (Fig. 12). The shock waves are focused either by an acoustic lens (such as the Siemens LITHOSTAR®) or by a parabolic reflector (such as the Storz MODULITH®). Electromagnetic shock wave sources can deliver several hundred thousand shock waves before servicing, in contrast to spark-gap machines.

Piezoelectric lithotriptor. Piezoelectric lithotriptors have a number of piezoceramic crystals aligned on a fixed metallic concave surface (Fig. 13). The application of simultaneous high-voltage electrical current to the piezoceramic crystals causes a sudden conformational change that generates an acoustic shock wave. As a result of the focusing mechanism, piezoceramic lithotriptors produce shock waves with not only a very high-peak pressure at F2 but also small focal points. This type of lithotriptor is said to be safe for use in patients with pacemakers.

As previously mentioned the shock wave is coupled to the body using water, which results in efficient transfer of energy. The first-generation lithotripters (e.g., Dornier HM3) used an open water bath in which the patient was immersed and had excellent results. Most current machines have the shock wave head mounted in a therapy head, which is filled with water. A thin rubber membrane is pressed against the patient with a coupling jelly or oil to reduce air. This design is more convenient for the clinic; however, it is less effective at allowing energy transfer because of reflection from the rubber and the inevitable small air bubbles.

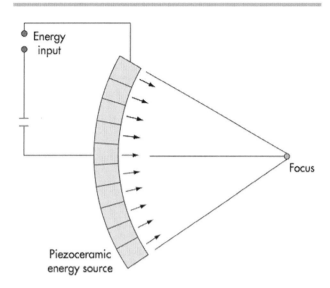

Figure 13 Piezoceramic lithotripter. Application of an electric current to piezoceramic crystals causes a sudden conformational change, resulting in the generation of an acoustic shock wave.

Localization is essential for effective lithotripsy and currently either ultrasound or X rays are used. Ultrasound is either in-line or off-line with relation to the therapy head. In-line is more accurate than off-line, where the targeted zone may not correspond with the treated zone. Ultrasound is preferable to X ray localization, as it allows real-time monitoring and avoids radiation exposure. It is poor at localizing upper and mid-ureteric stones where fluoroscopy is preferred.

Tissue Damage

Severe adverse effects are well documented with ESWL and therefore it is not true that shock waves pass harmlessly through the body (52). Focal zones from lithotripters may reach up to 5 cm and thus the entire kidney may be subject to mechanical forces. Tissue is, however, far less susceptible to damage than kidney stones as shock waves pass through tissue (like water) without significant reflection resulting in far less tensile forces. Cavitation driven by negative pressure has been shown to cause vascular trauma to the kidney and is thought to be responsible for tissue damage (53). There is evidence that patients with impaired renal function treated with ESWL may experience late-onset hypertension and worsening of renal function (54), and this is the subject of an on going Food and Drug Administration (FDA) sponsored multicenter study.

Clinical Applications

ESWL is well described in the fragmentation of urinary calculi, but its effect on both benign and malignant tissue has also been studied. The effects of ESWL on in vitro and in vivo tumor cell lines (55–57), and in particular, whether enhancement of chemotherapeutic effect occurs on ESWL-treated tissue, have been the subject of much study (58,59). ESWL has been shown to cause cellular damage regardless of the cell's doubling time. The mitochondria are most sensitive to its effect (59), although damage also occurs at the cell membrane, within the nucleus, along the endoplasmic reticulum, and in other cell organelles (such as lysosomes). Cellular damage may be mechanical or because of the generation of free radicals (60,61) caused by homolytic cleavage of the molecule within the collapsing bubble. Extracorporeal shock wave techniques have been described in the treatment of Peyronie's plaques (62) although outcomes are mixed.

Ultrasonic Probe for Stone Fragmentation

The ultrasound probe used to fragment calculi consists of an ultrasound energy source coupled to a long metal probe (Fig. 14). The application of about 100 W to the piezoceramic elements results in oscillation at a frequency of 23 to 27 MHz (63). The probe oscillates in both transverse and longitudinal directions with a displacement of 20 μm. At displacements of >50 μm, soft-tissue disintegration occurs, and such machines may be useful in renal sparing surgery. Heat is generated at the point of stone disintegration, and therefore irrigation is required for cooling. This heat can reach temperatures of 50°C; therefore, ultrasound contact lithotripsy is unsuitable for use in the ureter, although its direct effects on tissue are minimal. The metal probe is usually hollow to allow suction of irrigant and small stone fragments. Some hard stones are resistant to ultrasound lithotripsy, but lithotripsy appears particularly useful for soft stones that are difficult to treat with mechanical intracorporeal lithotripters.

Harmonic Scalpel

The Harmonic Scalpel™ is a device consisting of an ultrasonic source that causes vibration of forceps or a blade. Typically, the displacement is 50 to 80 μm, and the vibrational frequency approaches 55,500 Hz (64). Heat is generated, with tissue temperatures ranging from 50°C to 100°C and a depth of penetration of 1 to 2 mm. Coagulation occurs by means of protein denaturation when the blade couples with protein, forming a coagulum that seals small coapted vessels. When the effect is prolonged, secondary heat is produced that seals larger vessels. Blood and tissue are desiccated and oxidized (charred), forming eschar that covers and seals the bleeding area. Rebleeding can occur when blades removed during electrosurgery stick to tissue and disrupt the eschar. The surgeon controls the precision of cutting and coagulation by adjusting the power level, blade edge, tissue traction, and blade pressure. This device has proved particularly useful in laparoscopic surgery.

MECHANICAL ENERGY

The adjective "kinetic" to the noun energy has its roots in the Greek word for motion (kinesis). Lord Kelvin is credited with coining the term "kinetic energy" circa

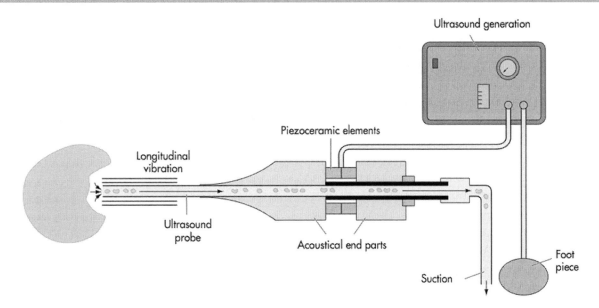

Figure 14 Ultrasound probe. Piezoceramic elements oscillate, causing longitudinal and transverse vibration of the probe.

1849. In Urological surgery there are a few devices that utilize this source of energy; one of the most widely available is the Swiss Lithoclast™.

Basic Principles

Work is a force acting upon an object to cause displacement. When work is done upon the object, that object gains energy. Mechanical energy is the energy possessed by an object because of its motion (kinetic energy) or position (potential energy). An object that possesses mechanical energy is able to do work, by being able to apply a force to another object to cause it to be displaced.

Clinical Applications

Mechanical Lithotripsy

The Swiss Lithoclast was developed by the departments of medical electronics and urology at the University Teaching Hospital in Lausanne, Switzerland (65). The device utilizes compressed air, derived from the operating theater supply (66,67). This pressure, in the range 3 to 5 bar, is delivered in a pneumatic blast of short duration to the inside of a hollow metal cylinder. This causes a metal projectile to be rapidly fired to the opposite end of the cylinder, where it collides and transfers kinetic energy to a metal probe (Fig. 15) (68). The distal end of the probe is in direct

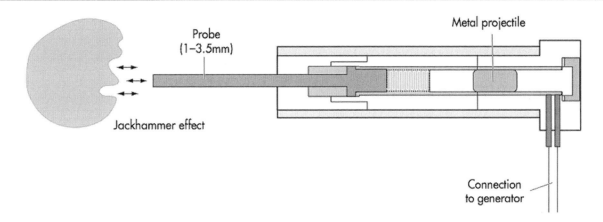

Figure 15 Mechanical lithotripsy. A compressed-air jet propels the metal projectile to strike the base of the probe (pneumatic lithotripsy). An electromagnetic field may be substituted for compressed air (electrokinetic lithotripsy).

contact with the stone. Transference of kinetic energy from probe to stone causes highly effective fragmentation. Analogy has been made with the jackhammer used to fragment parts of the pavement during road construction. The device is simple, cheap, and very effective. One major problem is the propulsion effect upon stones, which is much more marked with this form of energy than with laser lithotripsy. More recently the StoneBreaker™ (LMA Urology, Gland, Switzerland) device has been released, offering a more compact and ergonomic design, as well as greater contact pressures. Early reports are encouraging (69).

CONCLUSION

It is hard to think of an area of urological practice that does not involve an energy source. With the increasing number of technologies available (each with their own unique advantages and disadvantages), it is important that clinicians understand the basic principles of the equipment that they wish to use. This chapter aims to provide the reader with the relevant information to enable them to make the best use of the technology available today to offer safe and efficacious surgery for our patients.

REFERENCES

1. Cruse JM. History of medicine: the metamorphosis of scientific medicine in the ever-present past. Am J Med Sci 1999; 318:171–180.
2. Culotta CA. Dictionary of Scientific Biography. New York: Charles Scribners' Sons, 1970:302.
3. Sachs M, Sudermann H. [History of surgical instruments: 7. The first electrosurgical instruments: galvanic cauterization and electric cutting snare]. Zentralbl Chir 1998; 123:950–954.
4. O'Connor JL, Bloom DA, William T. Bovie and electrosurgery. Surgery 1996; 119:390–396.
5. Fraser-Darling A. Electrocution, drowning, and burns. Br Med J (Clin Res Ed) 1981; 282:530–531.
6. Heniford BT, Matthews BD, Sing RF, et al. Initial results with an electrothermal bipolar vessel sealer. Surg Endosc 2001; 15:799–801.
7. Botto H, Lebret T, Barre P, et al. Electrovaporization of the prostate with the Gyrus device. J Endourol 2001; 15: 313–316.
8. Dunsmuir WD, McFarlane JP, Tan A, et al. Gyrus bipolar electrovaporization vs transurethral resection of the prostate: a randomized prospective single-blind trial with 1 y follow-up. Prostate Cancer Prostatic Dis 2003; 6:182–186.
9. Tucker RD, Voyles CR. Laparoscopic electrosurgical complications and their prevention. AORN J 1995; 62:51–53, 55, 58–59 passim; quiz 74–77.
10. Giordano BP. Don't be a victim of surgical smoke. AORN J 1996; 63:520, 522.
11. Brown PM. Lucretius: De Rerum Natura. Bristol: Bristol Classic Press, 1984.
12. Hamilton J. Faraday: The Life. London: Harper Collins, 2002.
13. Serway RA. Physics for Engineers and Scientists. Philadelphia: Saunders College Publishing, 1990.
14. Greiner W. Quantum Mechanics: An Introduction. Berlin: Springer-Verlag, 2001.
15. Issa MM. Transurethral needle ablation of the prostate: report of initial United States clinical trial. J Urol 1996; 156: 413–419.
16. Isa MM, Wojno KJ, Oesterling JE, et al. Histopathologic and biochemical study of the prostate following transurethral needle ablation (TUNA): insights to the mechanisms of improvement in BPH symptoms. J Endourol 1996; 10: 109.
17. Zlotta AR, Raviv G, Peny MO, et al. Possible mechanisms of action of transurethral needle ablation of the prostate on benign prostatic hyperplasia symptoms: a neurohistochemical study. J Urol 1997; 157:894–899.
18. Perachino M, Bozzo W, Puppo P, et al. Does transurethral thermotherapy induce a long-term alpha blockade? An immunohistochemical study. Eur Urol 1993; 23:299–301.
19. Schatzl G, Madersbacher S, Djavan B, et al. Two-year results of transurethral resection of the prostate versus four "less invasive" treatment options. Eur Urol 2000; 37: 695–701.
20. Hill B, Belville W, Bruskewitz R, et al. Transurethral needle ablation versus transurethral resection of the prostate for the treatment of symptomatic benign prostatic hyperplasia: 5-year results of a prospective, randomized, multicenter clinical trial. J Urol 2004; 171:2336–2340.
21. Lau WY, Leung TW, Yu SC, et al. Percutaneous local ablative therapy for hepatocellular carcinoma: a review and look into the future. Ann Surg 2003; 237:171–179.
22. Zlotta AR, Wildschutz T, Raviv G, et al. Radiofrequency interstitial tumor ablation (RITA) is a possible new modality for treatment of renal cancer: ex vivo and in vivo experience. J Endourol 1997; 11:251–258.
23. Gervais DA, McGovern FJ, Wood BJ, et al. Radio-frequency ablation of renal cell carcinoma: early clinical experience. Radiology 2000; 217:665–672.
24. Pavlovich CP, Walther MM, Choyke PL, et al. Percutaneous radio frequency ablation of small renal tumors: initial results. J Urol 2002; 167:10–15.
25. Jacomides L, Ogan K, Watumull L, et al. Laparoscopic application of radio frequency energy enables in situ renal tumor ablation and partial nephrectomy. J Urol 2003; 169:49–53; discussion 53.
26. Crowley JD, Shelton J, Iverson AJ, et al. Laparoscopic and computed tomography-guided percutaneous radiofrequency ablation of renal tissue: acute and chronic effects in an animal model. Urology 2001; 57:976–980.
27. Matsumoto ED, Watumull L, Johnson DB, et al. The radiographic evolution of radio frequency ablated renal tumors. J Urol 2004; 172:45–48.
28. Rehman J, Landman J, Lee D, et al. Needle-based ablation of renal parenchyma using microwave, cryoablation, impedance- and temperature-based monopolar and bipolar radiofrequency, and liquid and gel chemoablation: laboratory studies and review of the literature. J Endourol 2004; 18:83–104.
29. Mendecki J, Friedenthal E, Botstein C, et al. Microwave applicators for localized hyperthermia treatment of cancer of the prostate. Int J Radiat Oncol Biol Phys 1980; 6: 1583–1588.
30. Yerushalmi A, Fishelovitz Y, Singer D, et al. Localized deep microwave hyperthermia in the treatment of poor operative risk patients with benign prostatic hyperplasia. J Urol 1985; 133:873–876.
31. Ahmed M, Bell T, Lawrence WT, et al. Transurethral microwave thermotherapy (Prostatron version 2.5) compared with transurethral resection of the prostate for the treatment of benign prostatic hyperplasia: a randomized, controlled, parallel study. Br J Urol 1997; 79:181–185.
32. Gravas S, Laguna P, Kiemeney LA, et al. Durability of 30-minute high-energy transurethral microwave therapy

for treatment of benign prostatic hyperplasia: a study of 213 patients with and without urinary retention. Urology 2007; 69:854–858.

33. Hoffman RM, Monga M, Elliot SP, et al. Microwave thermotherapy for benign prostatic hyperplasia. Cochrane Database Syst Rev 2007:CD004135.

34. Gofrit ON, Shapiro A, Pode D, et al. Combined local bladder hyperthermia and intravesical chemotherapy for the treatment of high-grade superficial bladder cancer. Urology 2004; 63:466–471.

35. Colombo R, Da Pozzo LF, Salonia A, et al. Multicentric study comparing intravesical chemotherapy alone and with local microwave hyperthermia for prophylaxis of recurrence of superficial transitional cell carcinoma. J Clin Oncol 2003; 21:4270–4276.

36. Schawlow AL. Lasers. Science 1965; 149:13–22.

37. Maiman T. Stimulated optical radiation in ruby. Nature 1960; 187:493–494.

38. Boulnois JL. Photophysical processes in revent medical laser developments: a review. Lasers Med Sci 1985; 1:47–66.

39. Dretler SP. Laser lithotripsy: a review of 20 years of research and clinical applications. Lasers Surg Med 1988; 8:341–356.

40. Zorcher T, Hochberger J, Schrott KM, et al. In vitro study concerning the efficiency of the frequency-doubled double-pulse Neodymium:YAG laser (FREDDY) for lithotripsy of calculi in the urinary tract. Lasers Surg Med 1999; 25:38–42.

41. Dushinski JW, Lingeman JE. Urologic applications of the holmium laser. Tech Urol 1997; 3:60–64.

42. Fried NM. Therapeutic applications of lasers in urology: an update. Expert Rev Med Devices 2006; 3:81–94.

43. Mingin GC, Ditrolio JV. Vasovasostomy using albumisol solder with an argon laser. Br J Urol 1998; 81:628–629.

44. Anson K, Nawrocki J, Buckley J, et al. A multicenter, randomized, prospective study of endoscopic laser ablation versus transurethral resection of the prostate. Urology 1995; 46:305–310.

45. Te AE, Malloy TR, Stein BS, et al. Photoselective vaporization of the prostate for the treatment of benign prostatic hyperplasia: 12-month results from the first United States multicenter prospective trial. J Urol 2004; 172:1404–1408.

46. Matsuoka K, Iida S, Nakanami M, et al. Holmium: yttrium-aluminum-garnet laser for endoscopic lithotripsy. Urology 1995; 45:947–952.

47. Le Duc A, Gilling PJ. Holmium laser resection of the prostate. Eur Urol 1999; 35:155–160.

48. Lingeman JE, Kim SC, Kuo RL, et al. Shockwave lithotripsy: anecdotes and insights. J Endourol 2003; 17:687–693.

49. Pfister RC, Papanicolaou N, Yoder IC. Urinary extracorporeal shock wave lithotripsy: equipment, techniques, and overview. Urol Radiol 1988; 10:39–45.

50. Crum LA. Cavitation microjets as a contributory mechanism for renal calculi disintegration in ESWL. J Urol 1988; 140:1587–1590.

51. Cathignol D, Mestas JL, Gomez F, et al. Influence of water conductivity on the efficiency and the reproducibility of electrohydraulic shock wave generation. Ultrasound Med Biol 1991; 17:819–828.

52. Evan AP, Willis LR, Lingeman JE, et al. Renal trauma and the risk of long-term complications in shock wave lithotripsy. Nephron 1998; 78:1–8.

53. Ueda S, Matsuoka K, Yamashita T, et al. Perirenal hematomas caused by SWL with EDAP LT-01 lithotripter. J Endourol 1993; 7:11–15.

54. Bataille P, Cardon G, Bouzernidj M, et al. Renal and hypertensive complications of extracorporeal shock wave lithotripsy: who is at risk? Urol Int 1999; 62:195–200.

55. Russo P, Stephenson RA, Mies C, et al. High energy shock waves suppress tumor growth in vitro and in vivo. J Urol 1986; 135:626–628.

56. Randazzo RF, Chaussy CG, Fuchs GJ, et al. The in vitro and in vivo effects of extracorporeal shock waves on malignant cells. Urol Res 1988; 16:419–426.

57. Kohri K, Uemura T, Iguchi M, et al. Effect of high energy shock waves on tumor cells. Urol Res 1990; 18:101–105.

58. Berens ME, Welander CE, Griffin AS, et al. Effect of acoustic shock waves on clonogenic growth and drug sensitivity of human tumor cells in vitro. J Urol 1989; 142:1090–1094.

59. Clayman RV, Long S, Marcus M. High-energy shock waves: in vitro effects. Am J Kidney Dis 1991; 17:436–444.

60. Morgan TR, Laudone VP, Heston WD, et al. Free radical production by high energy shock waves—comparison with ionizing irradiation. J Urol 1988; 139:186–189.

61. Suhr D, Brummer F, Hulser DF. Cavitation-generated free radicals during shock wave exposure: investigations with cell-free solutions and suspended cells. Ultrasound Med Biol 1991; 17:761–768.

62. Lebret T, Loison G, Herve JM, et al. Extracorporeal shock wave therapy in the treatment of Peyronie's disease: experience with standard lithotriptor (Siemens-multiline). Urology 2002; 59:657–661.

63. Marberger M. Disintegration of renal and ureteral calculi with ultrasound. Urol Clin North Am 1983; 10:729–742.

64. Lee SJ, Park KH. Ultrasonic energy in endoscopic surgery. Yonsei Med J 1999; 40:545–549.

65. Lanquetin JM, Jichlinski P, Favre R, et al. The Swiss lithoclast. J Urol 1990; 143:179A.

66. Denstedt JD, Eberwein PM, Singh RR. The Swiss Lithoclast: a new device for intracorporeal lithotripsy. J Urol 1992; 148:1088–1090.

67. Schulze H, Haupt G, Piergiovanni M, et al. The Swiss lithoclast: a new device for endoscopic stone disintegration. J Urol 1993; 149:15–18.

68. Vorreuther R, Klotz T, Heidenreich A, et al. Pneumatic v electrokinetic lithotripsy in treatment of ureteral stones. J Endourol 1998; 12:233–236.

69. Rane A, Kommu SS, Kandaswamy SV, et al. Initial clinical evaluation of a new pneumatic intracorporeal lithotripter. BJU Int 2007; 100:629–632.

33

Instrumentation in Urology

Rashmi Singh
Department of Urology, Kingston and St. George's Hospital, London, U.K.

Ken M. Anson
Department of Urology, St. George's Hospital, London, U.K.

INTRODUCTION

The remarkable developments in endoscopy over the years have allowed access to virtually all areas of the genitourinary system. Advances in technology and miniaturization have enabled diagnostic and therapeutic options which up until recently were unimaginable.

The urologist was the first surgical specialist to explore and evaluate the field of minimal access surgery. Long before other surgeons awoke to the possibilities and impact of minimally invasive surgery, urologists had demonstrated and established the unquestionable benefits of transurethral bladder and prostate surgery compared with open surgery. The progress in technology during the late 20th century made laparoscopic surgery and minimally invasive surgery a reality. These technologies included development of the charge coupling device (CCD) chip that allowed the transmission of high-resolution video images, high-intensity light sources that enhanced visualization of the surgical field and improved instrumentation design for endoscopic and laparoscopic approaches. The advent of laser and fiberoptic technology together with advances in endoscope miniaturization have revolutionized upper tract endoscopy, resulting in increased efficiency and safety of these procedures.

The phenomenal advances in minimally invasive surgery have resulted in a shift toward day case and laparoscopic surgery. Recent years have seen the advent of robotic and computer-assisted surgery, which in the future promises to facilitate complex endoscopic procedures through voice control over the networked operating room, enhancement of dexterity and development of virtual simulator trainers.

ENDOSCOPY

History of Endoscopy

The history of endoscopy (1) dates back to the 19th century when surgeons such as Phillip Bozzini developed a long thin funnel attached to a candle proximally to provide a source of illumination. The instrument known as the "Lichtleiter" or light conductor (Fig. 1) could be used to inspect a number of anatomical cavities including the vagina, bladder and rectum, using funnels of varying sizes. Segalas and Desormeaux tried to refine the illumination of this instrument further by using either mirrors to focus the light or alcohol and turpentine burning kerosene lamps. Despite their attempts, the use of these instruments remained limited because of the problems associated with externally placed illumination.

The invention of the light bulb in 1880 by Thomas Edison enabled German urologist Nitze to overcome this problem. He developed the electric light cystoscope which had a small lamp mounted at the end which could then be used to visualize the inside of the bladder (Fig. 1). During the 20th century, further modifications to the optical system of the cystoscope continued. Otis produced the spherical prism in collaboration with Wappler and Bausch and Lomb, which enabled the wide-angle lens cystoscope. In 1907 the Amici prism was launched which allowed a vertical, brighter and sharper image.

Despite these various modifications, limitations in image quality and light intensity still compromised safety. It was the work of Harold Hopkins that revolutionized endoscopy. His development of the rod lens system in the late 1940s enabled the transmission of light to the end of the endoscope, thus illuminating the lumen of interest and simultaneously allowing transmission of the image from the end of the endoscope to the eyepiece of the scope for viewing.

Despite significant improvements in light transmission with the rod lens system, illumination still depended on a filament lamp at the tip of the cystoscope. Hopkins therefore joined forces with Karl Storz of Germany who had developed a system of transmitting light by glass fibers called the cold light. In 1967 the Storz-Hopkins instrument was launched which combined the Hopkins optical system and the Storz cold light.

Paralleling these advances in light technology were developments in instrument design (Fig. 1). The original cystoscope was modified by adding a

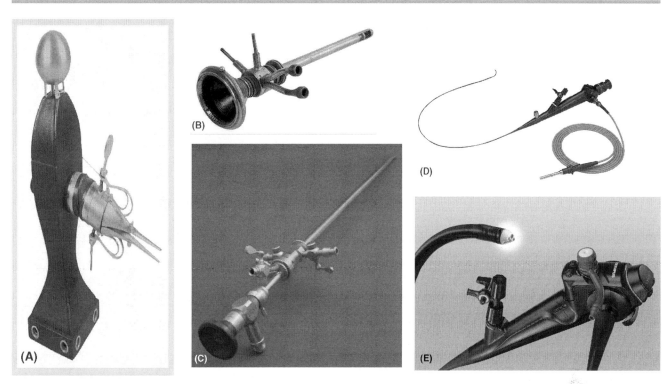

Figure 1 Historical development of endoscopes. (**A**) Bozzini Lichtleiter, (**B**) late 1880s cystoscope, (**C**) rod lens modern day cystoscope, (**D**) flexible ureterorenoscope, and (**E**) distal mounted CCD videocystoscope.

working sheath separate from the lens system, the incorporation of irrigation systems, and the addition of a deflecting (Albarran) mechanism. Brown developed the first 24-F double-catheterizing cystoscope and in 1906 Bransford Lewis designed the "universal cystoscope" through which operating instruments could be passed. Buerger, an American urologist combined many of the features developed by his predecessors including the 24-F Brown sheath, the Otis wide-angle lens and the Albarran deflecting lever to produce the Brown-Buerger cystoscope which became the most popular instrument for performing cystoscopy in the United States. This cystoscope was further refined with time to enable fulguration via a probe. The use of cautery for treatment of bladder tumors was illustrated by surgeons such as Nitze and Bottini, while Beer pioneered the use of monopolar fulguration under water. Wappler further advanced the use of electrocautery with the development of a dual generator capable of producing both cutting and coagulation current.

Early methods described for removal of prostatic tissue include the Young "cold punch technique." However, it was Maximilian Stern who developed the first resectoscope, which enabled electroresection. Joseph McCarthy designed the lever mechanism for controlling the resection loop, which formed the prototype for the resectoscope as we know it today. The Sachse cold knife optical urethrotome was designed with a similar handle mechanism to the resectoscope but had a reverse thrust.

Attention then turned to the development of camera systems to allow a record of the surgery to be taken. Although camera systems had been in use as early as 1875, it was Nitze who advanced the technique of endoscopic photography and first published his images. The next step was color photography 40 years later followed by the launch of television cameras.

The late 20th century heralded the digital revolution. Significant advances in digital imaging technology in combination with modern endoscopes have made it possible to now attain images with unparalleled detail and clarity.

Rod Lens, Fiber-Optic and Digital Technology

The original cystoscopes used between 1886 and 1951 were made up of a series of thin glass lenses positioned within a long narrow tube separated by annular spacers which held the lenses apart at measured distances. The limitations in precisely grinding these lenses meant that stray images occurred from their surface resulting in degradation of image quality and poor contrast. The light was provided by tiny lamps, which had a short life and often burnt out midprocedure particularly if there was a surge in current. To replace the lamp, the scope would have to be removed from the bladder and then reinserted resulting in longer operating times and also ran the risk of an electric shock to the patient. Hopkins overcame some of these problems by using long solid rod-shaped

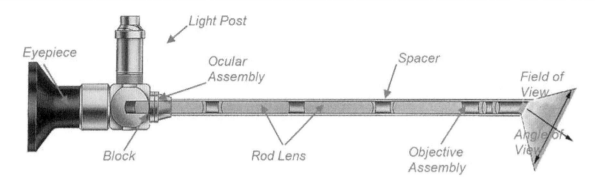

Figure 2 Rod lens cystoscope.

glass cylinders within the telescope, which could be ground and aligned with greater precision within the scope. The air gaps in between were the lenses. Adding an antireflective coating to both ends of the rod significantly increased the light available at the eyepiece (Fig. 2).

The introduction of fiber-optics in the 1960s led to the next revolution in endoscope design. Hopkins developed a method of transmitting images and light down a bundle of transparent fibers assembled as a cable, which are then coated with another transparent material with a different refractive index. The light then undergoes multiple total internal reflection. The fiber bundles can be either coherent whereby the position of a fiber at its proximal end mirrors its position at the distal end or incoherent where many fibers are assembled in a random arrangement and transmit high-density light throughout the cable.

In the early fiber-optic endoscopes, the illumination channel was coupled to an external xenon light source, while the imaging channel transmitted an image created by a lens at the distal end of the endoscope to a connected camera unit or display device (Fig. 3).

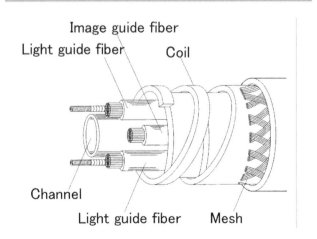

Figure 3 Cross-section of flexible cystoscope.

The Digital Revolution

One of the most significant advances in imaging technology has been the process of digitalization. The improved image quality with digital technology is secondary to the unique ability to adjust the characteristics of an image on a pixel-by-pixel basis. This is in contrast to older analogue systems where changes in image variables affected other image characteristics simultaneously causing analogue signals to be prone to interference. Digital images are processed by a CCD consisting of a silicone chip that absorbs light energy (Fig. 4). The CCD converts the various light intensities within an image into corresponding continuous voltage signals. A digital converter then captures each voltage signal and converts the voltage values into discreet numbers such as 0 or 1. The encoded numbers for each image element or pixel include information on color, contrast or light intensity. These stable variables can then be modified using image-processing software and can recombine on the video screen to create an exact replica. They can also be stored on computer hard drives or digital tape drives.

With the advent of digital technology and miniature CCDs, endoscope designers have moved to placing the imaging chip at the distal tip of the endoscope just behind the objective lens system. Because of the higher pixel count produced compared with fiber-optic bundles these "chip on the tip" endoscopes are able to produce higher resolution images. Unlike fiber-optic scopes, these endoscopes do not have a lens system running through them. The image is captured by the chip and transmitted via cables running through the scope to the camera. Digital video systems (2) are being applied in several areas in urology in particular flexible cystoscopy, laparoscopy and ureterorenoscopy. Miniature complementary metal oxide semiconductors (CMOS) imaging chips as small as 1 mm are now emerging as competitors to CCD chips (Fig. 4) because they are simple, their cost is decreasing, they are inherently all-digital and they provide comparable or possibly superior image quality. The advantages of digital flexible scopes with distal CMOS video sensors and built in LEDs for illumination are that a separate snap-on camera head with white balancing and

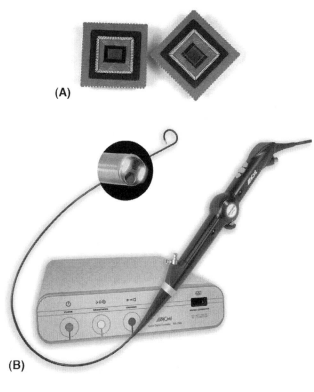

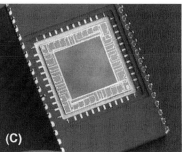

Figure 4 (**A**) CMOS chip, (**B**) distal sensor digital flexible ureterorenoscope, and (**C**) CCD chip.

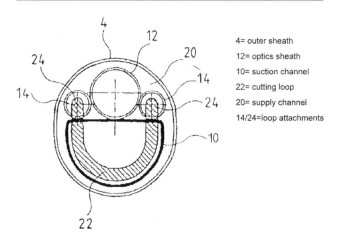

4= outer sheath
12= optics sheath
10= suction channel
22= cutting loop
20= supply channel
14/24=loop attachments

Figure 5 Cross-sectional view of distal end of continuous flow resectoscope.

Resectoscopes

The continuous flow resectoscope was first described by Iglesias in 1975 and was developed in response to the concerns that TURP syndrome is related to high intraoperative intravesical pressures. Unlike the standard intermittent flow resectoscopes, it has a fixed inlet channel for continuous irrigation and an outlet channel to which low-pressure continuous suction can be applied (Fig. 5). This allows continuous, simultaneous irrigation and suction, reducing the need for intermittent bladder emptying that is required with standard resectoscopes and enables sterile and safe evacuation of fluids (3). Studies of the continuous flow resectoscope have shown it to be superior to the conventional resectoscope in terms of operating rate and time, blood loss and irrigant absorption (4). Other advantages include less interruption during the procedure, better endoscopic vision due to a continuous clear inflow of more than 600 mL/min and low intravesical pressures of less than 10 mmHg. Since the entire amount of irrigating fluid is collected blood loss can be calculated and the amount of absorption can be determined. Despite these reported advantages, preference of the surgeon still tends to dictate the choice of system used for TURP with many urologists still using intermittent flow resectoscopes.

Ureteroscopes

Hugh Hampton Young performed the first endoscopy of a dilated ureter in a child in 1912 using a cystoscope. The first rigid ureteroscopy was performed in the 1970s by Goodman. The tips of the earliest ureteroscopes were as large as 13 to 16 F. The second-generation ureteroscopes became smaller at 8.5 to 11 F but often still required dilation of the ureteric orifice to enable atraumatic intubation. The developments in fiber-optic technology in the 1960s together with the demands of proximal upper tract anatomy led to the development of the modern

focusing issues is no longer necessary and there is no bulky light source requiring connection and adjustment. This enables systems like the Gyrus ACMI DUR-D to be an all-in one plug and play device, which is user friendly (Fig. 4).

Unlike fiber-optic scopes, images from distal sensor digital scopes appear not to be affected by pixelation, glare or Moiré effect and there is minimal loss of information during image transmission (3).

Rigid and Flexible Instruments

The entire upper and lower urinary tract can now be accessed endoscopically using either rigid endoscopes (which are based on the rod lens system) or flexible scopes which employ fiber-optic technology. "Chip on the tip" technology is rapidly being incorporated into these endoscopes.

small-caliber ureteroscopes used today, which are usually between 6 and 8.5 F. These instruments have moved away from being fully rigid to "semi-rigid" because of the subtle flexibility of the metallic shaft, which allow gentle deflection without deterioration in vision. Other design enhancements include an offset eyepiece to provide a straight working channel for rigid lithotripsy and beveled tips to minimize trauma to the ureteric orifice and mucosa. As the shaft progresses proximally, its caliber gradually increases giving the ureteroscope more strength and stability.

The need to access the proximal ureter and pelvi-calyceal system both for diagnosis and therapy led to the creation of flexible ureterorenoscopes. Design of these instruments has rapidly evolved over the years, particularly with regards to miniaturization to produce a generation of flexible ureteroscopes which are steerable and fully flexible through to 270° with nearly one to one torque and limited loss of image clarity at a magnification of 30 to 50 times. The present scopes are 6.8 F in diameter with a 3.6 F working channel for irrigation and the introduction of working elements such as guidewires, baskets, graspers, laser fibers and biopsy forceps. Their bi-directional active deflection near the distal tip significantly aids maneuverability particularly for accessing lower pole calyces. Deflection can either be primary active controlled by a lever or secondary passive. Dual active deflection ureteroscopes have an active secondary deflection mechanism controlled by a second lever instead of a passive mechanism enabling up to 360° downward deflection. Miniaturization of ancillary devices such as baskets and laser fibers has improved the efficacy of flexible ureterorenoscopy bringing the inner recesses of the pelvi-calyceal system into focus for both diagnostic and therapeutic interventions.

The latest flexible ureteroscopes such as the DUR-D by Gyrus/ACMI have the added advantage of "chip on the tip" technology with integrated camera and light within the scope. It has a CMOS imaging sensor at its distal tip replacing the previous generation's highly susceptible and lower resolution fiberoptics. It also employs a cool light LED, which is associated with fewer burns and lasts longer than xenon lamps.

However, an important limiting factor remains the fragility of these instruments. Their small diameter sheaths with even smaller working channels and deflection mechanisms are at risk of degradation and damage. Limited durability of the scopes (approximately 40–50 uses prior to significant damage) has significant economical implications. Common causes for damage include degradation through repeated use, excessive torquing/twisting, inadvertent firing of the laser fiber within the working channel, improper advancement of ancillary devices through a deflected ureteroscope and inadvertent damage during cleaning/processing. The use of nitinol instruments, smaller laser fibers and ureteral access sheaths can help to improve the life of the scopes.

Nephroscopes

As with other rigid endoscopes in urology, the design of the nephroscope is based on a stainless steel sheath, a port for light transmission, eyepiece for direct vision, irrigation ports and a working channel. The main difference is the large caliber of the sheath, which is usually 24 to 26 F and the large 13.5-F working channel. The nephroscope can either be used with an outer working sheath to enable continuous irrigation or more commonly without the outer sheath but using an Amplatz sheath for irrigation. Most nephroscopes have an angled offset eyepiece to accommodate rigid instruments through the working channel.

Flexible nephroscopes, similar in design to the flexible ureterorenoscopes but shorter and larger are becoming available to further enhance access during PCNL.

Laparoscopes

The most commonly used laparoscopes have either 0° or 30° lenses and similarly to cystoscopes are composed of an objective lens, a rod lens system and a fiber-optic cable. An offset working laparoscope is also available which comprises a working channel for the passage of basic laparoscopic instruments. The advantage of this scope is that it allows the surgeon to work in direct line with the image and potentially reduces the number of ports required. However, the space taken up by the working channel compromises the optical system resulting in inferior image quality.

The size of the earlier laparoscopes ranged from 2.7 to 12 mm with a usual size of 10 mm. The larger laparoscopes provided a wider view, better optical resolution and brighter image. Now miniaturization has resulted in the development of new generation laparoscopes of 2 to 5 mm, which provide comparable visualization to the original 10-mm laparoscopes. Other advances in laparoscope technology include flexible mobile tips, "chip on the tip" technology and all-in-one EndoEye (Olympus) laparoscopes.

IMAGING

Light Sources

The quality of the image obtained in endoscopy is very dependent on the quantity and quality of light available. A typical light source consists of a lamp, a heat filter, a condensing lens, an intensity control unit and a light guide cable.

Lamps

The lamp or bulb is the most important component of the light source and the quality of light will depend on the type of lamp used. The main types of lamp in use are quartz halogen, xenon, incandescent bulbs, and metal halide vapor arc lamps. The former two are the most frequently used in the commercially available light sources.

Halogen bulbs produce a highly efficient, almost crisp white light source with excellent color rendering (ability of a light source to reproduce the colors of an object compared with an ideal or natural light source). The electrodes in halogen lamps are made of tungsten. These bulbs are low voltage and use halogen gas, which enables them to burn more intensely with a long life (average 2000 hours).

Xenon lamps consist of a spherical or ellipsoidal envelope made of quartz glass, which can withstand high thermal loads and internal pressure. For superior image quality, highest-grade clear fused silica quartz is used. It is typically doped, although not visible to the human eye, to absorb harmful UV radiation during use. The light emitted by a xenon lamp is more natural compared with halogen, but the colors obtained with xenon tend to have a slightly bluish tint. Most modern cameras, however, analyze and compensate for these variations by automatic equalization of whites enabling the same image to be obtained with both light sources. A proper white balancing at the start of the procedure is therefore critical for obtaining a natural color. White light is composed of equal proportions of red, blue, and green colors. At the time of white balancing using a white target, the camera sets its digital coding for these primary colors to equal proportion. If during the white balance, the telescope is not seeing a perfectly white object then the setup of the camera will be impaired resulting in poor color perception.

Heat Filter

For 100% of energy consumed, a normal light source uses approximately 2% in light and 98% in heat. A heat filter is therefore needed to prevent the light cable from becoming extremely hot. The newer xenon light sources are defined as "cool light," in other words the heat to light ratio is lowered by creating more light. They are still not completely heat free and still have ignition hazards. Precautions must be taken to reduce such risks including avoiding contact between active light cables and drapes or the patient's skin and using standby mode wherever possible.

Condensing Lens

The purpose of the condensing lens is to converge the light emitted by the lamp to the area of the light cable input. In most light sources it is used for increasing the light intensity per square centimeter area.

Manual or Automatic Intensity Control Circuit

Manual adjustment allows the light source to be adjusted to a power level defined by the surgeon. This may be useful sometimes when close-up viewing is hampered by too much light or distant views are too dark.

Modern light systems use automatic intensity adjustment technology. Electronic signals produced by the camera are coded to be transported. Coding dissociates the luminance and chrominance of the image. It is the luminance (quantity of light signal) that dictates the quality of the final image. When there is too much light for the image, for example, when the endoscope is very close to tissue, the luminance signal increases. Conversely, when the light is low (distant view or blood in the field), the luminance is low and the electronic signal is much weaker. A good quality luminance signal is calibrated to 1 mV. Overexposed images will cause the electronic signal to increase to greater than one, while underexposed images drop the signal to less than one. Light sources analyze these signals and appropriately lower or increase their intensity to bring the signal back to the reference point.

Light Guide Cables

Light guide cables transmit the light output of the light source to the viewing endoscope. They consist of flexible glass fiber bundles encased in a cable jacket with appropriate connectors on either end. The efficiency of light transmission is reduced as the length of the cable increases. The cables need to be handled with care as if mishandled or broken, damage to the fiber bundles or outer coating can result in poor quality transmission and loss of light. When assessing the quality of a light guide cable, one must never look directly at the light with the naked eye, but instead shining the light on the ceiling or floor can indicate the number of damaged fibers. Damaged/old cables are relatively cheap to replace and should be done as required otherwise the quality of endoscopy will be significantly compromised.

Camera Systems

The early "tube" cameras used for endoscopy before the 1990s were based on cathode ray tube technology and were heavy and cumbersome to use. They have now been replaced with chip cameras, which are based on CCD and analogue technology. A CCD is an electrical silicon device that is used to create images of objects and to store information. It converts light or electrical input into an electronic signal (the output). The output is then processed and reconstructed on the television monitor into a video image. The high resolution achieved is related to the large number of pixels in the CCD array-the more pixels the finer the detail. Typically, modern CCDs contain anything from 1000 to 500,000 pixels.

A three-chip camera contains three separate CCDs, each one taking a separate measurement of red, green, and blue lights. Light coming into the lens is split by a trichroic prism assembly, which directs the appropriate wavelength ranges of light to their respective CCDs. By taking a separate reading of red, green, and blue values for each pixel, three-CCD cameras achieve much better precision than single-CCD cameras. Although three CCD cameras are generally regarded to provide superior image quality to one CCD cameras in terms of color, crispness of image and resolution, they are bulky and cannot be coupled directly to the endoscope because of size. They are also generally more expensive. Such cameras tend to be used predominantly in laparoscopic surgery. For most other procedures, urologists tend to employ single-chip cameras, which are small enough to couple directly with the endoscope without making it bulky to use.

High-Definition Video Technology

High-definition (HD) imaging systems are an exciting new development and take digital technology a step further. The main feature that makes them superior to standard-definition (SD) systems is the ability to capture and display more imaging data enabling much more clarity and detail (5).

Image resolution describes the detail an image holds. It quantifies how close structures can be to each other and still be visibly apart. An established measuring unit regarding image resolution is the number of pixels that make up the image. Pixel counts can be expressed as a single number, for example, "3-megapixel" digital camera, which nominally has three million pixels or a pair of numbers, as in a "640 by 480" computer display, which has 640 pixels from side to side and 480 from top to bottom. The more pixels used to represent an image, the closer the result can resemble the original. Increasing the number of pixel lines increases the quality of the picture and subsequently provides the surgeon with a more detailed and realistic impression. Pixel density or pixels per inch (PPI) is a measurement of the resolution of a computer/television display, related to the size of the display in inches and the total number of pixels in the horizontal and vertical directions. For example, a display that is 11 inches wide by 8.5 inches high, capable of a maximum 1024 by 768 pixel resolution, can display about 93 PPI in both the horizontal and vertical directions. This figure is determined by dividing width (or height) of the display area in pixels, by width (or height) of the display area in inches. The apparent PPI of a monitor therefore depends on the screen resolution (number of pixels) and the size of the screen in use; a monitor in 800 by 600 mode has a lower PPI than the same monitor at 1024 by 768 mode.

A key component of HD systems is the high-capacity CCD chips, which capture much more data, thus producing more pixels, which with the benefit of digital output result in a more reliable picture with significantly greater detail and clarity.

The other key component of HD technology is high-resolution video screens. HD pixels are smaller and squarer than SD pixels so are sharper and more of them can be fitted onto the screen. HD screens have four times the resolution of standard SD screens enabling them to show all of the fine detail that the high-capacity chips can deliver (Fig. 6).

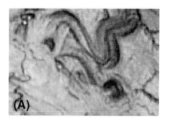

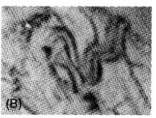

Figure 6   Image seen with (**A**) HDTV and (**B**) SDTV.

HD imaging has also been reported to offer better-depth perception, which is particularly important in laparoscopic intracorporeal suturing.

Fluorescent Cystoscopy

Fluorescent cystoscopy forms the basis of the photodynamic diagnosis and therapy of bladder tumors. When light is targeted at a tissue, some of the photons will be absorbed by the molecules in the tissue. If the energy produced by the photon results in the movement of an electron to a higher energy shell, when the electron returns to it original position, energy is emitted in the form of light (fluorescence). This fluorescent light can then be detected either with the naked eye as a change in color or by a sensor. Exogenous fluorescence involves the use of an external chemical to induce fluorescence (6). One such agent is the photosensitizing agent 5-aminolevulinic acid (5-ALA). 5-ALA is the starting point of the heme biosynthesis pathway. The metabolite immediately before heme in this pathway is protoporphyrin IX (PPIX), which is fluorescent, appearing red under blue-violet light. Photodynamic diagnosis works on the basis that malignant cells accumulate up to ten times more PPIX than normal cells. During fluorescent cystoscopy, exogenous 5-ALA is instilled into the bladder via a urethral catheter two hours pre cystoscopy but can also be given intravenously. The procedure uses the D-light imaging system (Karl Storz) which includes a short-arc xenon light source and filter turret capable of generating light in three operational modes: conventional white light, fluorescence and autofluorescence mode. It is possible to manually change from blue to white light during the procedure. Specially modified cystoscopes with lenses that maximally enhance the contrast between benign tissue autofluorescence and tumor fluorescence are used. Papillary tumors are seen to appear intensely red under blue light as do areas of mucosa involved with CIS (Fig. 7).

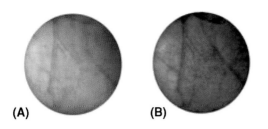

Figure 7 Cystoscopic views seen under (**A**) white and (**B**) blue light.

Narrow Band Imaging

Narrow band imaging (NBI) is a high-resolution endoscopic technique using optical filter technology. It enhances the fine structure of mucosal surfaces, for example, vascularity by optimizing the absorbance and scattering characteristics of light. It is based on the phenomenon that the depth of light penetration depends on wavelength-the longer the wavelength, the deeper the penetration. Blue light penetrates only superficially while red light is able to reach the deeper layers. The first prototype NBI system (Olympus) is based on a light source with sequential red-green-blue (RGB) illumination. White light from a xenon source is passed through a rotatory RGB filter which separates the white light into the three separate colors, which are then used to sequentially illuminate the mucosa. The red-, green-, and blue-reflected light is detected separately by a monochromatic CCD at the tip of the endoscope and the three images are integrated into a single color image by the video processor. In addition to the conventional RGB filters for white light endoscopy (WLE), the narrow band imaging system has special RGB filters of which the band-pass ranges have been narrowed and the relative contribution of blue light has been increased. This narrow bandwidth is strongly absorbed by hemoglobin thus increasing the clarity of vascular structures, for example, capillaries. The technology has been widely used in gastroscopy, where results have been reported as superior to WLE especially for the diagnosis of Barrett's esophagus. A small study looking at the application of NBI in cystoscopy showed increased detection rate of urothelial carcinoma compared with WLE (7).

Although the technique is still in its infancy and the details of further larger studies are needed, the future appears promising.

Three-Dimentional Imaging

The advances in HD and digital technology discussed earlier have been successfully applied to laparoscopic surgery resulting in improved image technology and clarity. The introduction of three-dimentional (3-D) video imaging systems or stereoscopic imaging in the last decade has the potential for safer, faster laparoscopy with a reduced learning curve (8). During normal vision, information on depth perception is interpreted by the visual cortex in response to binocular horizontal disparity or stereoscopy. This occurs when the left and right eyes view an object from slightly different angles. The difference between the resulting images transmitted to the two retinas is interpreted in the cortex as depth information. During laparoscopic surgery, both eyes see exactly the same image and stereoscopic depth information is lost. With time and experience, surgeons are able to overcome this by extracting "pictorial" depth cues from conventional images though this does not substitute for full 3-D perception of the operating field. Stereoscopy, stereoscopic imaging or 3-D video imaging is any technique capable of recording three-dimensional visual information or creating the illusion of depth in an image thus restoring depth perception by simulating binocular horizontal disparity. The illusion of depth in a two-dimensional image is created by presenting a slightly different image to each eye. Images are acquired via a single or dual lens/camera system and then presented to the surgeon on a head-mounted display (HMD) or on a video monitor. With a 3-D video monitor, the two images are separated by displaying a sequence of alternating left and right images which is synchronized with the surgeon's vision in the left and right eyes, enabling depth perception.

Synchronization can be via liquid crystal shutter glasses worn by the surgeon, which will let light through in synchronization with the images on the display. Alternatively synchronization can be achieved if the surgeon wears polarized 3-D glasses whereby a polarizing filter rotates the alternating left and right images by 90° to achieve image separation. With an HMD system a small display optic in front of one (monocular HMD) or each eye (binocular HMD) displays images (Fig. 8). Head-mounted displays may also be coupled with head-tracking devices, allowing the user to "look around" the operative field by moving their head which can help overcome the loss of hand-eye axis which can occur during complex maneuvers.

Second generation 3-D imaging systems include autostereoscopy, which obviates the need for HMDs or glasses altogether. Eye tracking systems are used to automatically adjust the displayed images and 3-D field by tracking the surgeon's pupils.

Virtual retinal displays create images by scanning low-power laser light directly onto the retina.

ANCILLARY INSTRUMENTATION

Instrument Channels

Instrument channels enable the influx and efflux of irrigant solutions and the delivery of ancillary devices into the operating field for therapeutic and diagnostic interventions. The first generation ureteroscopes had no working channel unlike the modern endoscopes, which have been designed to have as large an instrument channel as is practically possible or two separate working channels. Fiber-optic technology and

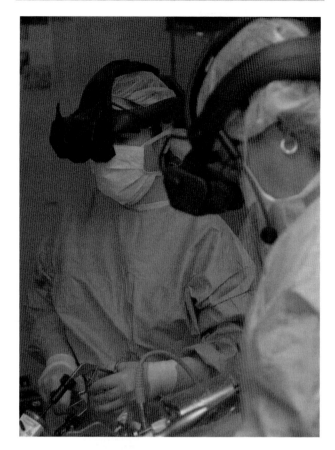

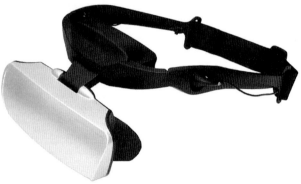

Figure 8   Head-mounted display for 3-D imaging.

increased miniaturization has enabled the incorporation of instrument channels as large as 75% of the total diameter of the scope. As a result it is possible to pass a grasping device and lithotripsy probe simultaneously through the single channel of some scopes. Although the ideal instrument channel should be as large as possible, the larger the instrument passed through the channel, the greater the reduction in flow of irrigant resulting in impaired visibility. To overcome this limiting factor, as for resectoscopes, some semi-rigid ureteroscopes now have dual channel functionality allowing a continuous flow irrigation system to be set up. By keeping the outlet open, it is possible to balance the hydrostatic pressure within the ureter

to enhance the view particularly when performing laser procedures.

As flexible ureteroscopes have only one working channel for irrigation and instrumentation, poor flow can impede visibility. The use of small (<3 F) instruments can help overcome this limitation.

Ancillary Devices

Guidewires

Guidewires are pivotal to any endourological procedure. Wires vary in material composition, size, tip design, rigidity, surface coating, and length (9).

Wires are composed of an inner stainless steel core, known as the mandrel, which is covered by a tightly coiled thin spring wire (spring guide). The mandrel may be round or flat in cross-section. Round mandrels have a standard stiffness, while flat mandrels are used for stiffer wires providing greater rigidity for the same diameter. The size and stiffness of the mandrel determines the rigidity and strength of the wire, while the spring guide acts as a track for the smooth passage of scopes and catheters. Recently wires have been developed with a mandrel made of nickel titanium alloy (Nitinol). Unlike stainless steel these wires are kink resistant and can be designed with a stiffer core. They also have the added advantage of "memory" enabling coil and recoil as will be discussed in more detail below.

The typical range for guidewires is 0.018 (1.4 F) to 0.038 inch (2.9 F) in diameter and 80 to 260 cm in length. Tips vary in their length, shape and flexibility. The distal tip is designed to be soft and flexible (floppy tip) to minimize trauma to the ureter.

The frictional resistance of the wire is determined by its stiffness and coefficient of friction. The coating of the wire determines the friction along its surface. The standard coating on most wires is PTFE (Teflon), which reduces the coefficient of friction by 50%. The friction coefficient of hydrophilic wires is only 16% enabling almost frictionless passage. These latter wires are therefore particularly useful for negotiating an impacted calculus or tortuous ureter.

Some of the newer wires combine the properties of both standard and hydrophilic wires, for example, Sensor® (Boston Scientific) making them universal for almost all endourological procedures (Fig. 9). The Sensor wire has a distal hydrophilic tip, which enables negotiation in difficult situations, combined with a Nitinol PTFE coated body, which makes the wire kink resistant.

Retrieval Devices

A variety of baskets and graspers are available for stone retrieval during endoscopic stone surgery (Fig. 10). They vary in their size, design and opening mechanisms. They range in size from 1.9 to 7 F with an average size of 3 F to fit down the working channel of most ureteroscopes. The device consists of a handle and a plastic sheath. Within the sheath is a thin shaft of metal, which forms the basket and comes in various

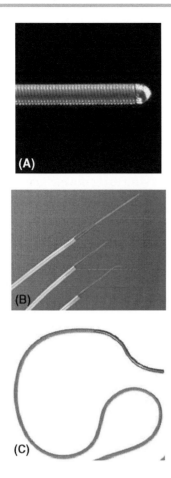

Figure 9 Guide wires. (**A**) Stiff PTFE guidewire, (**B**) hydrophilic guidewire, and (**C**) PTFE guidewire with hydrophilic tip.

shapes. The handle controls the opening mechanism of the basket and can be detachable.

Baskets are made from either stainless steel or nitinol usually with an outer PTFE sheath. In certain baskets, the sheath can be detached to reduce the overall size of the instrument of the basket in the working channel. Most baskets have a variable length tip extending beyond the basket. Hollow core baskets have a central channel to accommodate a laser fiber or guide wire. All baskets have a minimum of three wires, and the configuration of the wires affects its retrieval properties.

Similar to baskets, graspers are also made from stainless steel or nitinol wires, contained in an outer sheath and controlled by a release handle. They are typically three-pronged with distal hooks and vary in diameter from 1.9 to 5 F. Forceps/grasping devices have teeth to enable grip. They can be reusable or single use and semi-rigid or flexible depending on where they are being deployed within the collecting system.

Shape Memory Alloys

Nitinol is known as a shape memory alloy (SMA), in other words an alloy that remembers its shape. SMAs

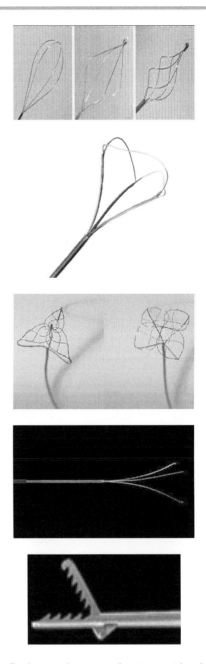

Figure 10 Baskets and graspers for stone retrieval.

are able to undergo a molecular rearrangement in the solid phase (Fig. 11). This means that during a solid-state phase change a molecular rearrangement occurs, but the molecules remain closely packed so that the substance remains a solid (10). These phase changes, known as martensite and austenite, involve the rearrangement of the position of particles within the crystal structure of the solid. Below the transition temperature, Nitinol is in the martensite phase and can be bent into various shapes. To fix the "parent shape," the metal must be held in position and heated to about 500°C. The high temperature causes the atoms to arrange themselves into the most compact and regular pattern possible resulting in a rigid cubic

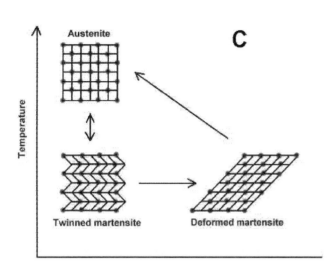

Figure 11 Shape memory alloy molecular rearrangements: transformation from the austenite to the martensite phase and shape memory effect.

arrangement known as the austenite phase. Above the transition temperature, Nitinol reverts from the martensite to the austenite phase that changes it back into its parent shape. This cycle of shape deformation and recovery can be repeated multiple times. The use of a SMA in urology is well illustrated by the Memokath™ range of stents.

In addition to its excellent shape memory, Nitinol is thinner and more elastic than conventional stainless steel. This has led to the commercial introduction of nitinol as an exciting technology in endourology enabling greater miniaturization of devices. This in turn means greater irrigant flow and less limitation to scope deflection during flexible ureterorenoscopy.

Port Technology

One of the critical areas of importance in laparoscopy has been the development of an optimal access port system. Characteristics of an ideal trocar include decreased tissue trauma and bleeding, decreased pain at the trocar site, ease of entry, a tight fascial seal to prevent frequent dislodgement during the operation, low risk of herniation and elimination of time-consuming wound closures. In the infancy of laparoscopy, most trocar systems employed metal, cutting tips and were reusable. Ease of entry through tissue was one of the main advantages. However, reports started to emerge describing complications associated with trocar systems. These included vascular and visceral injury, abdominal wall hematomas, trocar site pain and hernias.

As a result of these complications, new trocar systems were developed to try and minimize some of these complications. Recent systems have employed noncutting obturator tips, which dilate or separate

tissue, thus decreasing trauma to the tissues as they enter the abdominal cavity. Studies examining the benefits of radially expanding, noncutting trocar systems have documented decreased pain, less port-site bleeding, shorter wound scars and higher patient satisfaction. However, noncutting trocar systems typically require greater force to insert into the abdominal cavity, potentially increasing the risk of vascular injury.

In addition to the issue of cutting versus noncutting, the shape of the trocar tip has also been shown to be important. Conical tips pose less risk to intra-abdominal structures during insertion compared with pyramidal tips. Thus the optimal trocar system seems to be a noncutting trocar with a conically shaped tip.

In recent years disposable radially dilating noncutting complex trocar systems have been marketed but cost is a significant issue (Fig. 12). A further advancement has been the use of optical dilating bladeless trocars, which have an additional visual component thus combining radial dilatation with visual control. This allows safe and controlled placement of the first port during laparoscopy.

MECHANICAL ASSISTANCE DEVICES

Robotic Technology

Urology has been one of the leading specialities to pioneer robotic surgery, particularly with the DaVinci robot for radical prostatectomy. The technique is rapidly being taken up and developed internationally.

The first described use of robotic technology in the United Kingdom was in the 1980s by the urologist John Wickham at Guy's hospital (11). He designed the "PROBOT." This was essentially a TURP robotic frame, which could carry out automated transurethral prostate resection. The frame supported a six-axis Unimate Puma robot together with a Wickham Endoscope liquidizer, which rotated at 40,000 rpm and an aspirator. Although the technique was proven to be safe, effective and successful it was not embraced or developed any further by the urological world. The next generation of robot to follow was the Automated Endoscopic System for Optimal Positioning (AESOP) in the 1990s. In this system a voice or pedal-controlled robotic arm holds and navigates a laparoscopic camera in response to commands. The EndoAssist is similar but is controlled by infrared signals from the surgeon's headset. Though cheaper than the AESOP it requires more space to set up in the operating theater.

The ZEUS and the DaVinci (Fig. 13) robotic devices were the next "master-slave" systems to become commercially available. It is the latter system that has been widely adopted in urology, with an increasing number of prostatectomies being performed robotically in the United States and more recently in the United Kingdom. The system consists of a remote operating console from which the surgeon controls the robots arms and energy sources, for example, diathermy using manual or pedal controls (12). The robot only translates the surgeon's

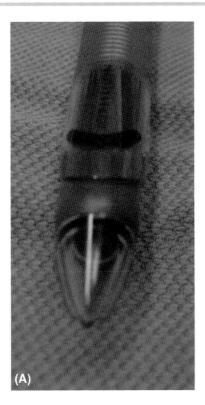

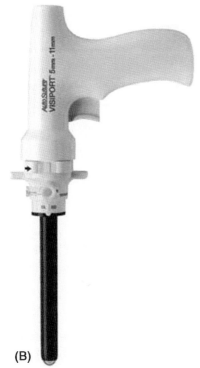

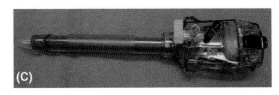

Figure 12 (**A**) Laparoscopy trochar, (**B**) optical trocar system, and (**C**) noncutting radially dilating trochar system.

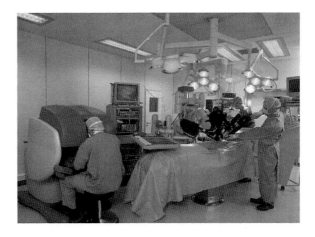

Figure 13 Robotic surgery.

movements as opposed to following preprogrammed set movements. At the console the surgeon can adopt a more suitably ergonomic position than is often possible when operating at the patient's side. Hand and foot controls allow more intuitive rather than fulcrum movements over the instruments as occurs in laparoscopy. This has led to the theory that the learning curve for robotic surgery is shorter and less demanding than for laparoscopy making the transition from open surgery to robotics easier. Up to 10× magnification, 3-D stereoscopic vision and motion scaling greatly enhance the image projected at the console. Motion scaling and the EndoWrist technology minimize tremor enabling smooth precise surgical movements. The other advantage of the EndoWrist instruments is that they enable seven degrees of freedom of movement compared with only four with standard laparoscopy, thus reproducing natural human wrist movements more accurately. The other components of the system include a patient side-cart which supports the robotic arms and the 3-D endoscope and a stack system housing the camera unit, recording equipment, television screen and a laparoscopic insufflator.

The main disadvantages of the DaVinci system at present include purchase and maintenance costs, long setup time and lack of haptic (tactile) feedback. However, it is anticipated that as the technique is increasingly embraced and refined over the next few years, these issues may be less of a problem particularly as surgeons increasingly incorporate virtual reality (VR) simulators into their training.

FUTURE TRENDS

Virtual Endoscopy

Virtual endoscopy (VE) is a technique in which computer-simulated 3-D viewing of hollow structures based on high-resolution anatomical imaging is conducted. VE is based on the careful integration of three

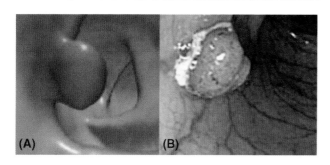

Figure 14 (**A**) Virtual colonoscopy image and (**B**) conventional colonoscopy image showing 8-mm polyp.

components—image acquisition, processing, and analysis (13). Image acquisition obtains a volumetric data set using various radiological modalities such as ultrasound, MRI, or helical CT. Uninterrupted image volumes are required which are free from motion artefact and have a high degree of spatial resolution. Volumetric data are then transferred to a workstation via a fiber-optic connection for processing images using perspective projection and real-time 3-D rendering computer techniques. The 3-D images created are then carefully analyzed. using an endoscopic "fly-through" simulation where a computer mouse is used to control the speed and direction of image presentation. The lumen wall can be made transparent to view adjacent structures. In this way VE images enable endoluminal navigation through hollow organs, simulating conventional endoscopy (Fig. 14). A specific point in the lumen wall can be targeted and axial, coronal and sagittal images displayed simultaneously to define the anatomy in more detail. Software programs can also be used to calculate wall thickness in combination with convexity and curvature information. Thus it is possible to identify "hot-spot" regions, which may harbor pathology.

VE has been used to inspect a number of anatomical regions in particular in the gastrointestinal tract where virtual colonoscopy has been extensively studied and has recently received NICE approval. The virtual colonoscopy experience has shown the technique to be well tolerated, requiring no sedation and is noninvasive or minimally invasive (14). The applications of VE in urology, which have been described to date include virtual CT ureteroscopy in the diagnosis of ureteric disease and virtual CT cystoscopy for mapping bladder wall thickness. Several clinical studies have validated the use of virtual cystoscopy in the diagnosis of bladder tumors with high sensitivity and specificity (15). Although encouraging, the published experience in this area of urology remains sparse at present.

Other Developments

Urological surgery is continuing to evolve rapidly particularly in the realms of minimally invasive surgery. It is likely that technological advances will continue at an explosive pace with increased miniaturization of equipment and digitalization of images.

Robotic surgery brings the potential for telesurgery and telementoring from a remote, even international site via portable laptop control stations and wireless connectivity (16). The ability to communicate with colleagues and experts during procedures increases training possibilities and patient safety.

VR simulators will become central to the future training of endoscopic surgeons. Although currently in its infancy, with refinements in software enabling tactile as well as visual reality, VR simulation models will become more lifelike. The operating theater of the future is likely to undergo radical change to accommodate the shift toward new-age surgery (17). Current operating rooms are cluttered by stack systems and trolleys bearing insufflators, light sources and camera control units. Further electrical and biological hazards are posed by tubing, video cables, light leads, diathermy sources and foot pedals scattered through the theater.

Dedicated minimally invasive operating suites are now available with design elements to facilitate endoscopic surgery and overcome some of these problems (Fig. 15). Procedures performed in dedicated minimally invasive surgical suites have been shown to be shorter and more efficient compared with a standard operating theater (18). Poor ergonomics has always been one of the major limiting factors in endoscopic surgery. Use of retractable arms, pendant workstations and voice command navigation systems to control equipment will improve these ergonomic issues. Further development of intraoperative imaging including real-time 3-D reconstructions of patients

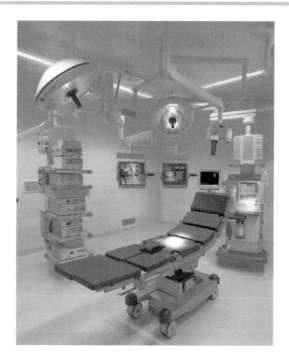

Figure 15 State of the art theater.

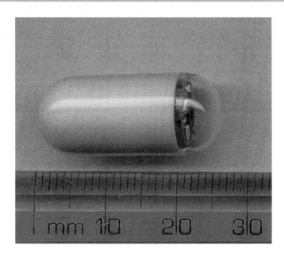

Figure 16 Wireless capsule endoscopy.

and computer-assisted surgery offer surgeons the opportunity for more accurate surgical planning.

Over the next decade, nanotechnology may see the development of nanorobots with tiny integrated circuit processors measuring just 50 μm, which can operate on individual cells and vessels rather than organs. Advancements in microchip and wireless technology may also allow the development of implantable cameras (Fig. 16), sensors and datasets as well as magnetically controlled implants that can be navigated remotely. The technology has arrived and carries exciting potential. Future research is likely to focus on the delivery of diagnostic and therapeutic modalities through natural orifices so that truly "noninvasive" surgery can become a reality.

ACKNOWLEDGMENT

We would like to thank the many manufacturers, in particular Olympus/ACMI who contributed material toward this chapter.

REFERENCES

1. Shah J. Endoscopy through the ages BJU Int 2002; 89(7):645–652.
2. Borin J, Abdelshehid C, Deane L, et al. The distal sensor digital flexible ureteroscope: an optical evaluation. Urotrends 2006; 11(2):4.
3. Notley RG. Transurethral resection of the prostate with and without continuous irrigation. J R Soc Med 1982; 75(11):871–874.
4. Iglesias JJ, Sporer A, Gellman AC, et al. New Iglesias resectoscope with continuous irrigation, simultaneous suction and low intravesical pressure. J Urol 1975; 114(6): 929–933.
5. Olympus. Home page. Available at: www.keymed.co.uk/optimised.
6. Zaak D, Karl A, Knüchel R, et al. Diagnosis of urothelial carcinoma of the bladder using fluorescence endoscopy. BJU Int 2005; 96(2):217–222.
7. Bryan RT, Billingham LJ, Wallace DM. Narrow-band imaging flexible cystoscopy in the detection of recurrent urothelial cancer of the bladder. BJU Int 2008; 101(6):702–705.
8. Pietrzak P, Arya M, Joseph JV, et al. Three-dimensional visualization in laparoscopic surgery. BJU Int 2006; 98(2):253–256.
9. Patel U, Ghani K, Anson K. Equipment used in endourology. Chapter 3 in Endourology A Practical Handbook. Taylor and Francis Group.
10. NDC. Home page. Available at: http://www.nitinol.com.
11. Challacombe BJ, Khan MS, Murphy D, et al. The history of robotics in urology. World J Urol 2006; 24(2):120–127.
12. Murphy D, Challacombe B, Khan MS, et al. Robotic technology in urology. Postgrad Med J 2006; 82:743–747.
13. Assimos DG, Vining DJ. Virtual endoscopy. J Endourol 2001; 15(1):47–51.
14. David Burling, James E East, Stuart A Taylor. Investigating rectal bleeding. BMJ 2007; 335:1260–1262.
15. Tsampoulas C, Tsili AC, Giannakis D, et al. 16-MDCT cystoscopy in the evaluation of neoplasms of the urinary bladder. AJR Am J Roentgenol 2008; 190(3):729–735.
16. Agarwal R, Levinson AW, Allaf M, et al. The RoboConsultant: telementoring and remote presence in the operating room during minimally invasive urologic surgeries using a novel mobile robotic interface. Urology 2007; 70(5):970–974.
17. Reijnen MM, Zeebregts CJ, Meijerink WJ. Future of operating rooms. Surg Technol Int 2005; 14:21–27.
18. Hsiao KC, Machaidze Z, Pattaras JG. Time management in the operating room: an analysis of the dedicated minimally invasive surgery suite. JSLS 2004; 8(4):300–303.

34

Minimally Invasive Technologies in the Treatment of Renal and Prostate Cancer

Hashim U. Ahmed, Caroline Moore, Manit Arya, and Mark Emberton
Department of Urology, Division of Surgical and Interventional Sciences, University College London, London, U.K.

INTRODUCTION

The use of minimally invasive ablative therapies in localized prostate and renal cancer offers the potential to reduce side effects and the healthcare burden associated with traditional surgical modalities. This article reviews outlines the therapeutic dilemmas facing patients with localized low volume prostate cancer and renal tumors and provides a comprehensive review of the basic science of cryotherapy, high-intensity focused ultrasound (HIFU), radiofrequency ablation and emerging technologies such as photodynamic therapy. These ablative technologies can deliver a minimally invasive, day case treatment with low morbidity. This chapter reviews the results of each modality in each of prostate cancer and renal tumors both in terms of side effects and cancer control.

Renal Tumors

Renal parenchymal tumors represents approximately 3.5% of all malignancies, but are the third most common cancer of the urinary tract. In the United States, there was an estimated incidence of 51,190 cases in 2007 with 12,890 renal cell carcinoma related deaths (1). In the United Kingdom, the incidence was 4622 with 3777 deaths in 2005. Worldwide, there are about 208,500 new cases per year (2). The rising incidence is exemplified in the United Kingdom with the number of new cases rising from about 5 per 100,000 population in 1975 to about 10 per 100,000 population in 2005. Similar patterns have been shown in the United States (3,4). This has predominantly been due to the increased use of diagnostic imaging for those who have abdominal symptoms leading to incidentally discovered small renal masses (5). Incidentally diagnosed renal tumors now account for between half and two thirds of renal cancer diagnoses (6) and have lead to a stage migration to lower risk tumors. However, although there has been an associated increase in surgical intervention there has been no concomitant increase in cancer-specific survival (CSS) (7).

Advances in the speed and precision of cross-sectional and ultrasound imaging have led to greater use in investigating abdominal symptoms. Ultrasound, computed tomography (CT), and magnetic resonance imaging (MRI) are currently being used for evaluation of abdominal complaints, virtual colonography, lung cancer screening, and follow-up of various benign and malignant conditions. This has brought with it a rise in the detection of small (<4 cm) solid renal masses, such that the majority of newly diagnosed renal masses are incidentally found (8). As a result, according to the U.S. SEER (Surveillance, Epidemiology, and End Results) database over the last 18 years, renal tumor size at presentation has steadily and consistently decreased (9). The majority (65–80%) of these tumors are renal cell carcinomas (RCCs) when histology is evaluated (10). Although radical nephrectomy was routinely offered for small renal masses, a nephron-sparing approach is increasingly offered. Despite this, extirpative surgery is not without shortcomings. Open partial nephrectomy for instance requires a large flank incision and has a long postoperative recovery period with complications in up to one-third (11). Recent publications on laparoscopic partial nephrectomy have reported complication rates that are not too dissimilar to the open approach (12,13). Nonetheless, the standard of care for clinically localized RCC remains surgical resection because of the favorable prognosis associated with surgery and the relative ineffectiveness of systemic therapy to give adequate clearance. Patients undergoing radical or partial nephrectomy for tumors, which are localized and 4 cm or less in size have demonstrated five-year CSS rates in excess of 95% (14). Laparoscopic approaches to nerve-sparing surgery have shown equally good early results (15).

However, because of the nature of incidental tumors, which are small and likely to progress slowly, observation or active surveillance of selected small renal masses in elderly populations may be a recommended strategy. A meta-analysis of clinically localized renal tumors showed an overall median growth rate of 0.28 cm/yr for observed lesions across multiple series (16). While growth rates vary considerably among reports, only 1% of observed lesions in this meta-analysis progressed to metastatic disease after a median follow-up of almost three years.

Prostate Cancer

The management of localized prostate cancer has centered on surveillance or radical therapy such as prostatectomy or radiotherapy. Furthermore, because of the reduction in disease severity as a result of early detection it is likely that the small absolute risk reduction—of approximately 5% over 10 years that has been demonstrated in a randomized controlled trial comparing surgery with watchful waiting—in men with low to moderate risk disease is likely to be reduced even further (17). The overtreatment problem is further exemplified by two recent randomized controlled trials assessing the role of PSA screening. The U.S. PLCO trial showed no difference in mortality between the screened and nonscreened arms with a mean follow-up of 7 years, while the European ESPRC study showed that 1400 men would need to be screened and 48 men treated to save one life within 10 years. The advent of active surveillance with selective delayed intervention is also likely to make this difference in mortality between surveillance and radical therapy less significant. As radical treatments carry significant morbidity with operative complications (wound infection, hemorrhage, hospital stay) and can cause significant long-term toxicity (incontinence, impotence, rectal problems) there has been a demand to develop ablative therapies that attempt to reduce treatment burden while retaining cancer control and avoiding the psychological morbidity associated with surveillance. Although a number of minimally invasive therapies have been described—cryosurgery, HIFU, photodynamic therapy (PDT)—each one is at a different stage in its evaluation and diffusion into clinical practice.

MINIMALLY INVASIVE TECHNOLOGIES: BASIC SCIENCE

Cryotherapy

Cryotherapy is the ablation of tissue by extremely cold temperatures. The first written report of its use was in 19th-century London, where Arnott applied ice-salt mixtures to breast and cervical cancers (18). Cryotherapy exerts its effects via a number of pathways, namely,

1. direct cytolysis through extracellular and intracellular ice crystal formation,
2. intracellular dehydration and pH changes,
3. ischemic necrosis via vascular injury,
4. cryoactivation of antitumor immune responses,

5. induction of apoptosis,
6. endothelial damage leads to platelet aggregation and microthrombosis, and
7. injury also occurs during warming because of osmotic cellular swelling and vascular hyperpermeability.

A number of factors affect the efficiency of tissue destruction, namely,

1. velocity of cooling,
2. nadir temperature,
3. freezing duration,
4. velocity of thawing,
5. number of freeze-thaw cycles, and
6. presence or otherwise of large blood vessels, which can act as heat sinks.

Overall, a minimum freezing temperature of $-40°C$ for duration of three minutes is sufficient for tumor eradication (19). It has also been demonstrated that complete cell death is unlikely at temperatures greater than $-20°C$, although cells not destroyed by initial freezing to $-20°C$ were destroyed with a second freeze cycle (20). Histopathological changes after cryotherapy in the prostate is divided into an early degenerative phase—because of coagulative necrosis—and a later phase of repair—fibrosis, calcification and hyalinization (21,22).

Renal tissue needs exposure to or below $-19.4°C$. Clinical protocols err on the side of caution and freeze to $-40°C$ with ultrasound monitoring of the evolving cryolesion. For renal tumors, in the absence of direct puncture into the collecting system with the cryoprobe, the collecting system heals without leading to urinary fistulas. This is in contrast to radiofrequency ablation, which has been associated with a greater risk of urinary leakage.

High-Intensity Focused Ultrasound

Ultrasound refers to mechanical vibrations above the threshold of human hearing (16 kHz) and has the ability to interact with tissue to produce biological changes. Ultrasound is generated by applying an alternating voltage across a piezoelectric material such as lead zirconate titanate. These materials oscillate at the same frequency as the alternating current causing ultrasound wave that can propagate through tissues. This in turn causes alternating cycles of increased and reduced pressure (compression and rarefaction, respectively). Diagnostic ultrasound usually uses frequencies in the range of 1 to 20 MHz, but therapeutic HIFU uses frequencies of 0.8 to 3.5 MHz with delivery of energy within the ultrasound beams that are several times greater than the energy levels within diagnostic ultrasound. Therapeutic ultrasound can be conveniently divided into two broad categories: ''low'' intensity $(0.125–3 \ W/cm^2)$ and ''high'' intensity $(>5 \ W/cm^2)$. The former can stimulate normal physiological responses to injury, and accelerate other processes such as the transport of drugs across the skin. High-intensity ultrasound can selectively destroy tissue if delivered in a focused manner (23).

HIFU relies on the physical properties of ultrasound, which allow it to be brought into a tight focus either using an acoustic lens, bowl shaped transducer or electronic phased array. As ultrasound propagates through a tissue, zones of high and low pressure are created. When the energy density at the focus is sufficiently high (during the high pressure phase), tissue damage occurs. The volume of ablation (or lesion) following a single HIFU pulse or exposure is small and varies according to transducer characteristics. It is typically shaped like a grain of rice or cigar with dimensions in the order of 1 to 3 mm (transverse) × 8 to 15 mm (along beam axis). To ablate larger volumes of tissue for the treatment of solid cancers, these lesions are placed adjacent to each other. The two predominant mechanisms of tissue damage are by the conversion of mechanical energy into heat and "inertial cavitation." If tissue temperatures are raised above 56°C, then immediate thermal toxicity can occur provided the temperature is maintained for at least one second. This will lead to irreversible cell death from coagulative necrosis. In fact, during HIFU the temperatures achieved are much greater than this, typically above 80°C, so even short exposures, can lead to effective cell death. Inertial cavitation occurs at the same time but is neither as controllable nor predictable. It occurs because of the alternating cycles of compression and rarefaction. At the time of rarefaction, gas can be drawn out of solution to form bubbles, which then collapse rapidly. The mechanical stress and a degree of thermal injury induce cell necrosis (24). Histologically, the tissue changes that occur are homogeneous coagulative necrosis, with an inflammatory response that follows leading to formation of granulation tissue—indicated by the presence of immature fibroblasts and new capillary formation—at the periphery of the necrotic area at about a week after treatment. Polymorphonuclear leukocytes migrate deep into the treated tissue and then at two weeks, the boundary of the treated region is replaced by proliferative repair tissue. The repair process has not been investigated in detail at the cellular level beyond this time, but imaging techniques using contrast enhanced ultrasound or magnetic resonance imaging show an eventual shrinkage of treated volumes indicating that the necrotic area has been replaced by fibrous scar tissue.

The placement of the small HIFU lesions requires precise planning for an entire tumor to be ablated reliably. Furthermore, patient movement can lead to areas of viable malignant tissue remaining after treatment and even in ideal situations other factors can prevent a successful treatment. The most important of these include the heat sink effect and calcification. The heat sink effect relates to one area that overheats in the HIFU pulses pathway and thus prevents adequate ultrasound propagation to the targeted area—such a phenomenon occurs if the time between HIFU pulses is inadequate for tissue cooling or if an area is high in water content, such as a cyst. In addition, highly vascularized tissues might be more resistant to thermal ablation owing to the heat sink effect of their blood supply. Calcification simply leads to reverberation and shielding of the targeted area from parts of the HIFU pulse leading to inadequate heating of the tissue.

Radiofrequency Ablation

RFA acts by converting RF waves to heat, resulting in thermal damage. High-frequency current flows from the needle electrode to target tissue with the resultant ionic agitation and heat-producing molecular friction, denaturation of proteins and cell membrane disintegration. The cellular and tissue effects of RFA vary with the duration of ablation and the local temperature achieved. This temperature-time dependence was demonstrated by in vitro studies in which irreversible cell injury of benign and malignant human cell lines were heated to 45°C for 60 minutes, 55°C for 5 minutes, and 70°C for 1 minute. These changes take four to six minutes at temperatures >50°C and occur almost immediately above 60°C. Temperatures >105°C result in vaporization of tissue, resulting in gas formation and inefficient creation of RF lesion. The goal of RFA is to induce temperatures of 50°C to 100°C throughout the tumor. Histological analysis after RFA demonstrates typical coagulative necrosis characterized by cell membrane disruption, protein denaturation and vascular thrombosis. Exophytic tumors that are surrounded by perirenal fat are better treated than central tumors in which vascular structures can act as a heat sink.

In practice, a grounding pad is placed on the patient, and the radiofrequency probe is inserted in the ablation zone. A computer-controlled generator provides an alternating current in the radiowave frequency of the electromagnetic spectrum. Bipolar RFA decreases the risk of accidental burns associated with monopolar RFA. The impedance of the tissue to this monopolar current leads to local tissue hyperthermia, which is the basis for cell kill effect. The temperatures reached during RFA depend on the generator's power, tissue impedance, heat conductivity and heat dissipation via the local circulation. Commercially available RFA units are classified into temperature-based or impedance-based systems. This means that the computer-controlled generator provides energy to the probe on the basis of either the average temperature achieved or the measured impedance of the tissue monitored during ablation. Impedance rises toward infinity when tissues are desiccated during ablation or when there is charring. RFA technology can also be classified by dry and wet RFA. The latter allow constant infusion of saline during ablation to reduce the degree of charring and thus premature rise in impedance.

Photodynamic Therapy

PDT uses a photosensitizing drug activated, after a given drug light interval, by light of a specific wavelength. It requires tissue oxygen for the treatment effect, with the activated drug forming reactive

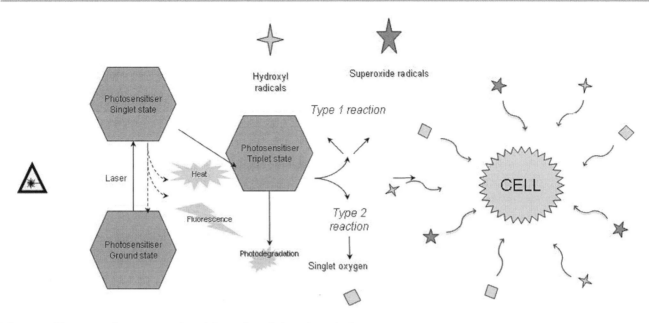

Figure 1 Diagrammatic representation of the action of photodynamic therapy.

oxygen species, which are directly responsible for damage to the treated volume (Fig. 1). The photosensitizing drugs are activated while either in the tissue or in the vasculature. Tissue activated drugs have long drug light intervals (typically hours to days) which means that the drug and light are given in separate treatment sessions. They usually take a long time to be cleared from the body, and can accumulate in the skin, requiring patients to be covered from sunlight (which could activate the drug and cause a sunburn like reaction) for a few weeks. Some of the tissue-activated photosensitizers accumulate preferentially in tumor tissue. This includes amino levulinic acid (ALA), which is used in the diagnosis of bladder tumors, and has also been assessed for use in the treatment of prostate cancer. Vascular activated drugs have the advantage of a short drug light interval (e.g., minutes), which allows the whole treatment to be done in a single session. They are usually cleared rapidly from the circulation, without accumulation in the skin, such that light restrictions are not necessary after a few hours.

Light delivery for prostate cancer, along with other interstitial tumors, uses low power laser light directed to the treatment site by optical fibers. These fibers can deliver light only at the end of the fiber (like a torch) or along a cylindrical diffuser (like a striplight). For prostate cancer, a transperineal approach is currently used, with hollow plastic needles placed in the prostate using transrectal ultrasound imaging. Cylindrical diffusers of the desired length are then placed within the hollow plastic needles, and low power laser, at a wavelength determined by the individual photosensitizer, is delivered to the prostate. Other approaches that have been used are transurethral light delivery, and open insertion of fibers at laparotomy.

PROSTATE CANCER: CLINICAL OUTCOME

Cryotherapy

Cryotherapy Devices

In 1966, probes cooled by liquid nitrogen in a closed circulation was the advent of modern cryotherapy and one of the very first applications of probe delivered cryotherapy was transurethral treatment for benign prostatic hyperplasia, soon followed by prostate cancer treatment using an open perineal approach (25). The transperineal percutaneous route came about a few years later (Fig. 2). The first-generation cryosurgery techniques for prostate cancer ablation were carried out without transrectal ultrasound guidance and urethral warmers. As a result of accurate monitoring of needle placement and ice ball, this inevitably led to a high incidence of complications (urinary incontinence, urethral sloughing, and rectourethral fistulae) (26). Transrectal ultrasound guidance and urethral warmers were introduced in second-generation cryosurgery leading to more precise probe placement as well as real-time monitoring of the ice ball. The urethral warmers decreased the risk of urethral sloughing. Third-generation devices has seen the introduction of probes in which pressurized gas is used to both freeze (argon gas) and then actively thaw (helium gas), allowing for smaller probes (17-gauge) which could enable more precise treatment a reduction in secondary structure damage, such as the external sphincter.

Clinical Cryotherapy Series

Thirteen series reporting extractable outcome data on the treatment of primary prostate cancer using cryosurgery were identified (Table 1) (27–39). These series have a wide range of patients treated

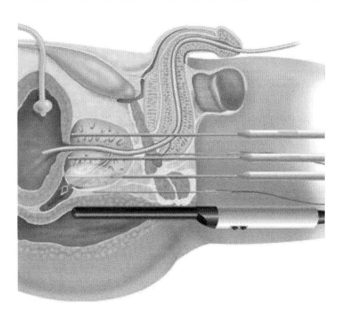

Figure 2 Diagram demonstrating percutaneous prostate cryoablation.

(N = range 22–975) with a wide range of follow-up (mean range nine months to 12 years). It was not clear whether there was double reporting of series from previous reports. Seven series reported on D'amico risk categories, while four reported on high and low risk categories using a different definition with no comment on why such criteria were used or whether they were validated. Two reported no risk stratification. Generation of device also varied but this was always reported. Hormonal use was reported on nine series and varied from 0% to 91.5% and was usually in the form of neoadjuvant treatment to reduce the size of the gland although the reason for hormonal ablation was not always given. PSA outcome data showed the greatest variation. A number of PSA nadirs were used including <1 ng/mL, <0.5 ng/mL, <0.4 ng/mL, and <0.2 ng/mL. Those series in which follow-up allowed also reported biochemical control according to the American Society for Therapeutic Radiology and Oncology (ASTRO) criteria. Three series also had salvage cryosurgery cases embedded within the data and it was not always possible to differentiate between the two salvage and primary outcomes. One series modified the ASTRO criteria to determine failure (PSA < 0.5 ng/mL with increase of at least 0.2 ng/mL on two consecutive occasions). Again, there were no reasons given as to why these criteria were used. Biopsy data was extractable from only nine series, and in those where biopsies were carried out the majority of series justified this on the basis of a "clinically significant" PSA increase or an inability to obtain a "satisfactory" PSA nadir rather than doing biopsies for all men after treatment. Three series reported on cryosurgery retreatments as part of the

overall outcome data with mean number of sessions ranging from 1.14 to 1.2.

Morbidity data demonstrate a similar variation in reporting with five series not reporting potency rates and four series not reporting incontinence rates. Where these were mentioned, most series did not clearly outline definitions of potency used, while incontinence grading was similarly poor. Impotence rates ranged from 49% to 95% and incontinence rates (all types) ranged from 0.4% to 16.7%. Fistulae rates varied from 0% to 0.5%. Other side effects and complications of treatment were not reported consistently with only three series demonstrating clear morbidity data and others either not reporting such outcomes or doing so selectively.

High-Intensity Focused Ultrasound

High-Intensity Focused Ultrasound Devices

Currently, there are two commercially available transrectal devices that can treat the prostate gland.

Ablatherm high-intensity focused ultrasound device. The Ablatherm® device (Edap-Technomed, Lyon, France) and the Sonablate®500 (Focus Surgery, Indiana, U.S.). The Ablatherm® device until very recently had separate imaging (7 MHz) and therapy transducers (3 MHz) which had a fixed focal length of 4 cm. Prostate imaging during treatment was not possible but performed between treatment zones by inserting the imaging transducer through the therapeutic transducer. The latest modification to the Ablatherm combines treatment and planning probes so that visual feedback is possible during treatment. However, because the Ablatherm uses algorithm-driven treatment protocols with preset energy levels, individual pulse energy levels cannot be modified by the operator. Other features include the incorporation of the probe into a table, which holds the pump and cooling mechanism and on which the patient is placed in the right lateral position. Treatment is to each lobe in turn and performed anterior to posterior within a complete block that incorporates the full anterior-posterior height of the prostate. A number of safety features that monitor the rectal wall energy deposition are in place to prevent damage to this area. Many centers that use the Ablatherm combine transurethral resection of the prostate or bladder neck incision to reduce gland size and stricture formation.

Sonablate 500 high-intensity focused ultrasound device. The Sonablate® system consists of a rectal probe (containing the transducer) with an operating frequency of 4 MHz that attempts to optimize the combined imaging and therapy roles of the transducer (Fig. 3). This has the advantage of allowing visualization of treatment effect following each pulse of the treatment cycle. Degassed water is pumped through the system and is chilled to temperatures of 17°C to 20°C to prevent rectal wall injury by heat build-up. Rectal wall monitoring features are also in place with this probe. Treatment planning, execution and monitoring are controlled using an user interface which allows the surgeon to precisely target the area of

Table 1 Biochemical and Biopsy Outcome in Series Reporting Treatment of Localized Prostate Cancer Using Cryosurgery

Study	Type, N	D'amico risk groups (unless otherwise specified)	Median follow-up	Biochemical control	Positive biopsy	Incontinence	Erectile dysfunction	Fistulae
Cohen et al. (34)	2nd N = 204	Low 18%; inter 39%; high 43%	12.55 yr	56% (old ASTRO); 62.4% (nadir plus 2 ng/mL)	25.6%	Not reported	Not reported	Not reported
Polascik et al. (35)	3rd N = 50	Low 72%; inter 18%; high 10%	18 mo	90% (PSA < 0.5 ng/mL)	4%	3.7% (1–2 pads/day)	Not reported	0
Ellis et al. (36)	3rd N = 416	Low 39.5%; inter 39.5%; high 21%	20.4 mo	79.7% < 0.4 ng/mL; 79.6% 4-yr biochemical disease-free survival[a]	10.1%	3.4% (stress incontinence) 0.6% (total incontinence)	100% impotent after procedure. 49% "predicted probability of impotence"	0
Cresswell et al. (37)	3rd N = 31	Low 55%; high 45%[b]	9 mo	79% (PSA < 0.5 ng/mL); 3% metastases	1 positive biopsy (only one biopsied)	Not reported	86%	0
Prepelica et al. (30)	3rd N = 65	High 100%[b]	35 mo	81.7% (old ASTRO); 50% (PSA < 4 ng/mL); 35% (PSA < 1 ng/mL)	8 patients biopsied, 1/8 positive	3.1% (any daily pad use)	Not reported	0
Han et al. (32)	3rd N = 122	Low 48.4%; high 51.6%[b]	12 mo	75% (PSA < 0.4 ng/mL)	Not reported	3% (pad use) 5% (no pads)	87%	0
Cytron et al. (33)	3rd N = 22	Primary group not reported separately	13 mo	Primary group not reported separately	Not reported separately	Not reported	80% overall	0
Aus et al. (29)	2nd N = 54	Low 24%; inter 24%; high 52%	58 mo	35% (PSA < 1 ng/mL)	28%	16.7% mild 2% severe	72%	2%
Bahn et al. (31)	2nd/3rd N = 590	Low 15.9%; inter 30.3%; high 53.7%	5.43 yr	89.5% (old ASTRO); 76% (PSA < 1 ng/mL); 62% (PSA < 0.5 ng/mL)	13%	15.9% (stress incontinence) 4.3% (pad usage)	95%	0.004%
Donnelly et al. (38)	3rd N = 76	Low 17%; inter 30%; high 52%[c]	5.1 yr	48–77% (PSA < 0.3 ng/mL); 75–89% (PSA < 1 ng/mL); 1.3% metastases; 1.3% mortality	14%	1.3%	53%	0
Long et al. (28)	2nd N = 975	Low 25%; inter 34%; high 41%	24 mo	63% (PSA < 1 ng/mL); 52% (PSA < 0.5 ng/mL)	18%	7.5% (not graded)	93%	0.5%
Koppie et al. (39)	2nd N = 141	Low 12.5%; high 87.5%[b]	3 yr	49%[d]	Not reported	Not reported	Not reported	Not reported
Cohen et al. (27)	2nd N = 383	Not reported	21 mo	69–77% (PSA < 1 ng/mL); 40–60% (PSA < 0.4 ng/mL)	18%	0.4%	Not reported	Perineal fistula 0.2% Urethrorectal fistula 0.4%

[a]Old ASTRO modified: three consecutive rises with final PSA > 1 ng/mL
[b]Low risk: PSA < 10 ng/mL and Gleason grade ≤7; high risk: PSA > 10 ng/mL or Gleason grade >7
[c]Low risk: Gleason ≤6, PSA < 10 ng/mL, stage ≤ T2a; intermediate risk: any one of Gleason ≥7 or PSA≥10 ng/mL or stage ≥ T2b; high risk: two to three of moderate risk factors
[d]PSA nadir ≥0.5 ng/mL or PSA nadir <0.5 ng/mL with increase of at least 0.2 ng/mL on two consecutive occasions

treatment, adjust the focal length of the transducer (currently 3 cm, 4 cm, or 4.5 cm) and alter the power intensity delivered to each focal zone individually. Rather than a protocol driven treatment, the power intensity of each pulse is guided by greyscale changes within the targeted area that represent steam, so that greater certainty about cell kill is obtained (Fig. 4) (40). In other words, the power is raised to obtain what we have deemed "Uchida" changes (or greyscale "popcorning"), named after the Japanese urologist who pioneered work using the Sonablate 500. The Sonablate 500 delivers treatment to the prostate in three separate blocks. The anterior portion of the prostate is treated initially, followed by midzone and then posterior gland (Fig. 5). The probe requires adjustment between each of these blocks. The posterior block is always treated using the 3-cm focal length and with lower energy levels. Within each zone, multiple overlapping lesions are created to enhance ablation.

Other high-intensity focused ultrasound devices include extracorporeal, transperineal, and transurethral.

Clinical High-Intensity Focused Ultrasound Series

The use of HIFU for the treatment of prostate cancer has until very recently been nested within a small number of enthusiasts over the last ten years. These have refined the indications, developed the technology

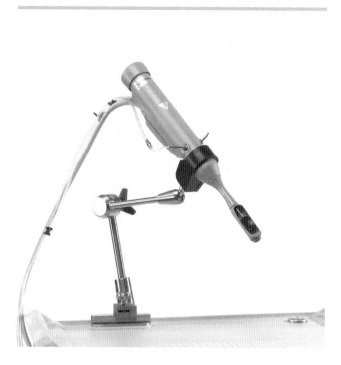

Figure 3 The Sonablate 500 transrectal HIFU probe and transducer. *Source*: Courtesy of UKHIFU Ltd., U.K.

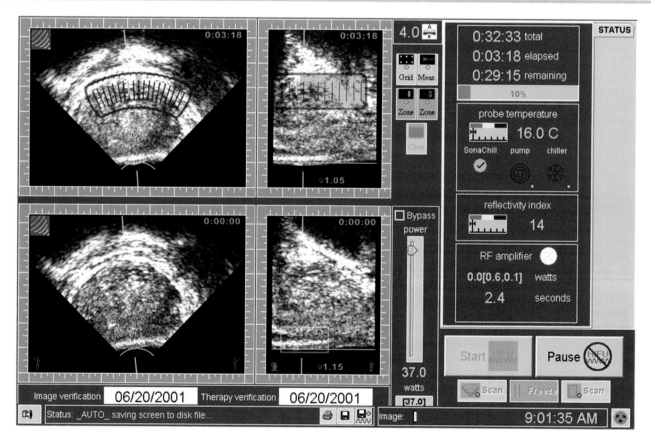

Figure 4 Screen capture demonstrating what the operator sees during a Sonablate 500 treatment. *Source*: Courtesy of UKHIFU Ltd., U.K.

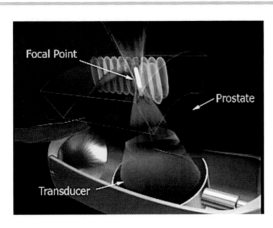

Figure 5 Diagrammatic representation of HIFU pulses delivered. Rows of pulses adjacent to each other are used to ablate larger areas of prostate. *Source*: Courtesy of UKHIFU Ltd., U.K.

and disseminated their early experience. Fourteen series have so far reported outcome data, with four using the Sonablate 500 and the remainder using the Ablatherm device (Table 2) (41–54). There was double reporting of a number of series, but this was not always made explicit in the papers. The number of patients treated ranged from 30 to 402, and mean follow-up ranged from 11 to 76.8 months. Morbidity data was inconsistently reported (Table 1). Incontinence rates were 0.5% to 15.4% and impotence rates ranged from 13% to 53%. These did not always grade the incontinence and where grading was used, these differed and were therefore not comparable across series. Definitions of impotence and potency had similar problems. Fistulae rates ranged from 0% to 2%, although most of the fistulae were nested in the early experience of most users with prototype machines. Other symptoms were inconsistently and selectively reported in most series. Neoadjuvant hormonal therapy was primarily used for cytoreduction of gland size but represented a possible confounding factor for cancer control rates. D'amico risk stratification was reported in six series, while one series categorized all patients as high risk using another definition (stage $\geq$ T3a, Gleason score 8–10, PSA > 20 ng/mL). Biochemical outcome was reported using either mean PSA values at longest follow-up, PSA nadir values (<1 ng/mL, <0.5 ng/mL, <0.2 ng/mL, <0.3 ng/mL, and 0.1 ng/mL), old ASTRO criteria as well as ASTRO Phoenix criteria (validated for radiotherapy only). Biopsies were not carried out in all men in all series, but only one series did not report on biopsy data. Most series included HIFU retreatments within the overall outcome data with the mean HIFU sessions ranging from 1.17 to 1.4 (Table 1). Second HIFU therapies were regarded as part of the treatment protocol rather than treatment failures per se, since one of the advantages of HIFU has been purported to be its repeatability sometimes up to three times for men who have residual prostate cancer.

The exact follow-up protocol to be used and criteria for success or failure are yet to be ascertained in HIFU therapy of prostate cancer, as is the case with cryosurgery. A number of groups have demonstrated that the use of gadolinium contrast enhanced MRI may be of use in the early determination of cancer control. Areas of necrosis are obvious through lack of enhancement and areas of residual undertreated tissue can be shown as early as two weeks after treatment with good correlation to biochemical outcome. The exact role for contrast enhanced MRI in follow-up of patients after HIFU is yet to be determined (55,56).

The natural history of prostate cancer prevents the use of mortality as an outcome measure in most short to medium term reports of prostate cancer therapy, so surrogates in the form of biochemical failure have emerged. However, the optimal definition of biochemical failure is far from clear. Indeed, because of this lack of certainty the reporting of minimally invasive modalities has shown little consistency. The variability in biochemical outcome is demonstrated by the differing PSA nadirs used to define successful outcome with groups using any one of PSA < 1 ng/mL, < 0.5 ng/mL, 0.4 ng/mL, < 0.3 ng/mL, < 0.2 ng/mL, and < 0.1 ng/mL. PSA of <0.2 ng/mL has evidence within radical prostatectomy series demonstrating its effectiveness to predict long-term outcome but such evidence is insufficient for HIFU (57). A number of series use three successive PSA rises to define treatment failure according to the old ASTRO criteria to define biochemical failure after radiotherapy (58). This has its own drawbacks since the old ASTRO criteria are not appropriate for evaluating PSA elevations sooner than three to five years after treatment and were only developed for use in radiotherapy. Indeed, with the emergence of the ASTRO Phoenix criteria (nadir + 2 ng/dL) (59), the old definition is in itself questionable, although some HIFU series have attempted to use this new definition. Indeed, the Phoenix definition of failure is being used by the Federal Drug Administration as the key determinant of success against which HIFU will be assessed in FDA Phase II/III trials in the United States, so this may need to be adopted as a reasonable standard for the foreseeable future.

Equally, morbidity data are reported poorly. Most series do not define incontinence or impotence, while the majority show inconsistent reporting of other perceived minor complications. As the premise of minimally invasive ablative therapies is to reduce the morbidity of therapy for men with localized prostate cancer while retaining cancer control and thus overcome the therapeutic dilemma that such men presently face, such lack of open reporting regarding morbidity data is disappointing. Although such data are difficult within the constraints of retrospective case series, it is important that a minimum dataset is agreed on for reporting complications.

Assessing health technology outcomes is difficult because of the hardware and software developments that occur as well as improved treatment delivery from overcoming the initial learning curve. For this reason, comparison with other series utilizing transrectal HIFU and other modalities is problematic, since not all publications make such changes explicit. The impact of these changes as well as the introduction of rectal cooling is evident by a reduction in the

Table 2 Biochemical and Biopsy Outcome in Series Reporting Treatment of Localized Prostate Cancer Using HIFU

Study	Device, number/ sessions	D'amico risk groups (unless otherwise specified)	Mean follow-up (mo)	Biochemical control (PSA, ng/mL)	Positive biopsy	Incontinence	Erectile dysfunction	Fistulae
Ahmed et al. (89)	Sonablate 500 N = 172	Low 28%; inter 38%; high 34%	12	92.4% no evidence of residual disease 61% (PSA < 0.2) 83% (PSA < 0.5)	7.6%	7.0% (grade 1, no pads) 0.6% (grade 3)	70% (sufficient for penetrative sex) IIEF-15 33.8–28.1	0
Mearini et al. (42)	Sonablate 500 N = 163	Low 49%; inter 29%; high 9%	23.8	78.2% (Phoenix) median PSA nadir 0.15	33.9%	16% mild, mixed; 0.6% grade 3	IIEF decreased from 16 to 12	0.6%
Uchida et al. (43)	Sonablate 200/500 N = 63	Low 35%; inter 41%; high 24%	22	70.3% (PSA < 0.4) 75% (ASTRO)	13%	2% grade 1	17% ("sexually active")	2%
Uchida et al. (44)	Sonablate 200/500 N = 181	Low 29%; inter 45%; high 26%	18	84%, 80%, and 78% [at 1, 3, and 5 yr (ASTRO)]	Not reported	0.5% (grade 1)	13% ("erectile dysfunction")	1%
Blana et al. (45)	Ablatherm N = 163	Low 51.5%; inter 48.5%	57.6	75% (Phoenix) 86% (PSA < 1.0) 64% (PSA < 0.2)	7.3% ("vital prostate cancer")	6.1% (grade 1); 1.8% (grade 2); 0 (grade 3)	55.3% (erections sufficient for intercourse)	0
Misraï et al. (46)	Ablatherm N = 119	Low 55%; inter 42%; high 3%	46.8	56.3% (Phoenix)	65%	Not reported	Not reported	Not reported
Blana et al. (52)	Ablatherm N = 140	Low 51.4%; inter 48.6%	76.8	68.4% (PSA < 0.5); 66% and 59% at 5 and 7 yr (Phoenix)	13.6%	5.8% grade 1. No grade 2/3 incontinence	53%	0.6%
Poissonnier et al. (53)	Ablatherm N = 227	Not reported	27	84% (PSA < 0.5); 66% disease-free survival at 5 yr[a]	14%	12% grades 1 and 2; 1% grade 3	39%	0
Ficarra et al. (54)	Ablatherm N = 30	High 100%[b]	12	90% (PSA < 0.3); 100% (PSA < 1)	23%	7%	Not reported	0
Vallancien et al. (47)	Ablatherm N = 30	Not specified	20	Mean PSA 0.9	14%	3%	32%	0
Blana et al. (48)	Ablatherm N = 146	Not specified	22	92% (PSA < 1); 83% (PSA < 0.5); 56% (PSA < 0.1)	7%	6% (5% grade I, 0.7% grade II)	43%	0
Thuroff et al. (49)	Ablatherm N = 402	Low 28%; inter 48%; high 23.6%	11	Median PSA 0.6; mean PSA 1.8	13%	10.6% grade 1; 2.5% grade 2; 1.5% grade 3	Not evaluable	1%
Chaussy and Thuroff (51)	Ablatherm N = 271	Not available	19	80–84% (old ASTRO)	29–34%	15.4% pre-HIFU TURP; 6.9% HIFU only	Not reported	Not reported
Gelet et al. (50)	Ablatherm N = 102	Not specified	19	66% (3 consecutive increases in PSA + velocity >0.75/yr or positive biopsy); 80–84% (ASTRO)	25%	Not available	Not available	Not available

[a]Any positive biopsy or a PSA > 1 ng/mL with three consecutive rises
[b]Clinical stage of ≥T3a or Gleason score 8–10, or total PSA > 20 ng/mL

recto-prostatic fistula rate. It was not always clear, especially from the HIFU series whether software modifications occurred and to what proportion of patients it was applied. Using the Sonablate 500, our own group has demonstrated that by changing power levels in a real-time fashion so as to visualize grey-scale changes (so called "visually directed HIFU") within each focal treatment zone leads to significantly lower PSA levels postoperatively in the primary setting (60). This was the first attempt at standardizing HIFU treatment. Future reports should report outcome data from just one clearly defined technique, device and software and to state otherwise if they have to report with numerous variables in the technique. Ideally, outcome data should be reported for the various modifications if possible.

Another difficulty in comparing HIFU with other treatments for localized prostate cancer is best illustrated by examining the demographic features of published trials. Most HIFU reports include patients in their late seventies and mid-eighties as the technology was initially used on men who were not suitable for other radical therapies. Heterogeneity of risk categories also exists in the cryosurgical groups and many series report risk categories using criteria that have yet to be validated. A number of studies do not include such data, but do include Gleason scores and PSA level. Such heterogeneity makes interpretation of disease-free survival and overall survival between studies difficult. The majority of published series on HIFU used in a primary setting include patients who were medically unfit for surgery or for a variety of reasons did not wish to have standard radical therapies. This group may be the group that benefit least from treatment and suffer a greater amount of morbidity from ablative techniques.

Photodynamic Therapy Series

The first report of PDT for prostate cancer was in a letter to the Lancet in 1990 (61). Two patients, whose prostate cancer was discovered after transurethral resection of the prostate, had a second resection, to ensure as complete a resection as possible. The residual prostate was then treated, using a transurethral approach, with a tissue based photosensitizer (either hematoporphyrin derivative or the polyporforin Photofrin). The drug light interval was either 48 or 72 hours. One patient died six months later of a previously undiagnosed lung tumor, and prostate histology at post mortem showed no evidence of residual disease. The second patient had a reduction in PSA and follow-up biopsy at three months showed no evidence of residual disease. The next reported use of PDT is as a salvage treatment following the failure of external beam radiotherapy. Nathan and colleagues report the treatment of 14 patients using the tissue based photosensitizer meso-tetra-hydroxy-phenyl-chlorin (mTHPC, Foscan) (62). This was a phase I/II study at given drug dose (0.15 mg/kg), with a range of drug light intervals (3–5 days), and a variety of light doses, using both bare fibers and cylindrical diffusers. Post procedure CT and MRI scanning showed devascularized areas, which correlated with the volume of intended treatment. One patient had a rectal biopsy to assess an area of abnormal rectal mucosa, following the procedure, and developed a rectourethral fistula, which required surgical intervention. Other side effects included urinary retention in three patients, and temporary stress incontinence in a further two patients. PSA was reduced in ten out of 14 treatments, by up to 96%. The same group reports primary treatment in a group of six men, who received a total of ten treatments (63). Each treatment was designed to treat either the right or left lobe, depending on biopsy and imaging results. The treatments were well tolerated, with side effects including irritative voiding symptoms for two weeks, temporary recatheterization (for less than two weeks) after two treatments, and one episode of gram-negative sepsis, despite prophylactic antibiotics. Post-treatment imaging showed devascularized areas in up to 51% of the gland. PSA levels fell after eight out of ten treatments.

A group in Germany have looked at the use of ALA in prostate cancer (64). Their initial work assessed the distribution of the tissue based photosensitizer ALA following oral administration, four hours prior to radical prostatectomy. Fluorescence distribution studies showed that the ALA was present in areas of prostate cancer, but not in benign tissue. Following this, they went on to perform photodynamic therapy in six patients, with previously untreated prostate cancer, using either a transurethral, transperineal or open surgical approach. No side effects are reported. Posttreatment monitoring was done using PSA, which fell by an average of 55%; unfortunately, there is no report of posttreatment imaging or biopsies. Hahn and colleagues have assessed another photosensitizer, motexafin lutetium (MLu, LuTex) in patients requiring salvage treatment following either external beam radiotherapy or brachytherapy (65–67). The study of 17 men used a variety of drug doses, drug light intervals and light doses (Table 3). Those men receiving high-dose PDT (2 mg/kg MLu, drug light interval of three hours and 150 J/cm light dose), showed a marked increase, followed by a decrease, in PSA. The effects were much less marked, and PSA rises post baseline were earlier, in the men receiving low-dose PDT (e.g., 0.5 mg/kg MLu, 24-hour drug light interval and 25 J/cm light dose). Side effects included mainly grade I urinary symptoms, with catheter related grade II urinary symptoms in one patient only. Again, no posttreatment imaging is reported.

A vascular acting photosensitizer, (Tookad or WST-11), one of the palladium bactereopheophorbide family, has been reported in both primary and salvage groups. A Canadian group initially performed a drug dose escalation study, followed by a light-dose escalation study, in men who had previously had external beam radiotherapy (68–71). They showed that around 60% of men receiving whole-gland treatment at the maximal drug and light dose, had a complete response to treatment, as shown by almost complete nonenhancement of the prostate on one week posttreatment dynamic gadolinium enhanced MRI, and prostate biopsies negative for prostate cancer at six months. This group used computer-aided light delivery planning

Table 3 Studies Using Photodynamic Therapy in the Treatment of Prostate Cancer

Study	Photosensitizer (drug dose)	Light delivery: route, dose, wavelength	Drug light interval	Target volume	Patient characteristics (Gleason, PSA, primary/salvage)	No. patients	Imaging results	PSA response	Adverse effects
Windahl et al. (61)	Hematoporphyrin derivative (1.5 mg/kg); Photofrin 2.5 mg/kg, IV	Transurethral, 15 J/cm², 638 nm	48 hr, 72 hr	Post TURP remnant	Post TURP (primary)	2	Not assessed	Reduction (10–2.5 ug/L; 6.0–0.2 ug/L)	None reported
Nathan et al. (62)	mTHPC 0.15 mg/kg IV	Transperineal, freehand insertion, 20 or 50 J/cm², 652 nm	3 days	Less than whole gland	Post radiotherapy for T2/3 cancer; PSA pre-RT up to 37	14	Up to 91% necrosis on cross-sectional imaging; 3/14 negative biopsies	10/14 PSA reduction (up to 96%)	Rectourethral fistula after rectal biopsy; 2 stress incontinence; 3 acute retention
Moore et al. (63)	mTHPC 0.15 mg/kg IV	Freehand transperineal insertion; 50 or 100 J or J/cm, 652 nm	2–5 days	Less than whole gland	Gleason 3 + 3 in all; PSA 1.9–15; 6 primary, 4 repeat treatments	6 (10)	≤51 cm³ necrosis; necrosis/fibrosis on biopsy; residual cancer in all	PSA reduction in 8/10 treatments	1 gram-negative sepsis; irritative voiding symptoms for 2 wk; 2 recatheterization (1 mild stress/urge incontinence)
Zaak et al. (64)	ALA 20 mg/kg orally	1 cm CD—perineal (N = 2); transurethral (N = 3), 1 at RP, 633 nm	4 hr	Variable	Primary: Gleason sum 5–8, PSA 4.9–10.6 ng/mL	6	None reported	Yes (average decrease 55%)	None
Pinthus et al. (65); Verigos et al. (66) Patel et al. (67)	Motexafin lutetium (MLu, LuTex) 0.5/1/2 mg/kg IV	Perineal template, 25–150 J/cm², 732 nm Computer-aided light-dose planning	3/6/24 hr	Whole gland	Post radiotherapy (8 external beams, 9 brachy-therapies)	17	Posttreatment imaging not reported	Transient rise; posttreatment PSA fall with high-dose PDT only	1/14 patients grade II urinary urgency (catheter related); grade I GU symptoms in many
Weersink et al. (68) Trachtenberg et al. (69, 70) Haider et al. (71)	WST-09 (Tookad) 0.1–2 mg/kg IV	Perineal template, computer-aided light-dose planning	10 min	Whole gland in multi fiber patients	Organ-confined recurrence after definitive radiotherapy	24 (2 light fibers); 28 multiple fibers	Complete response (MRI and biopsy) in 60% at high drug/light dose	Yes	2 rectourethral fistuale; intraoperative hypotension; decreased urinary function until 6/12

software to help to determine the optimal positions of the fibers on the basis of pretreatment imaging and average optical properties of the prostate. Side effects included two rectourethral fistulae, one of which required surgical intervention. Urinary side effects tended to last for up to six months. The same photosensitizer has been used by a group in London, in men with no previous treatment for prostate cancer (72). The first part of the study involved one optical fiber in each of the right and left lobes, to assess the effect of different light doses. The second part assessed the effect of multiple optical fibers. Posttreatment MRI showed nonenhancing lesions in the treatment volume, for those patients receiving optimal light doses. Publication of the full results is awaited.

A number of ways of improving PDT for prostate cancer have been suggested, including the modification of photosensitizers to allow more accurate targeting of cancer within the gland and more complex ways of monitoring and adjusting the treatment in real time (by assessment of intraprostatic drug, light and oxygen levels). Further studies will show whether these developments will allow the development of photodynamic therapy from its current status as an experimental procedure, to one that is an established technique for both primary and salvage treatment of organ-confined prostate cancer.

FUTURE PERSPECTIVES: FOCAL THERAPY

Focal therapy involves treatment directed only at the cancer focus and a margin of tissue surrounding the cancer (73,74). Most treatment related side effects are due to injury to the immediate surroundings of the prostate and not due to treatment of the prostate per se. Damage to prostate capsule, pelvic nerves/ganglia, bladder neck, bladder, seminal vesicles, rhabdosphincter, Denonvilliers fascia, and rectum cause erectile dysfunction, ejaculatory dysfunction, stress-related urinary incontinence, urge-related urinary incontinence, reduced bladder functional capacity, urethral or bladder neck strictures and bowel dysfunction (75,76).

Since unifocal or unilateral disease is present in up to one-third of men who are diagnosed in the PSA-screened era, it is feasible to attempt focal therapy. The modalities of cryosurgery, HIFU and photodynamic therapy are ideally placed to take on this new therapeutic strategy since they are capable of creating localized focal necrosis within the prostate of a predetermined size in a relatively controlled manner.

To date, only case series carried out in single institutions have reported as full publications although prospective trial data is starting to emerge at the time of writing (Tables 4 and 5). Onik et al. (86) first reported their results on hemiablation using cryotherapy. These results have recently been updated with the results of 55 men completing at least one-year follow-up (77). 95% (52/55) had a stable PSA (as defined by ASTRO criteria) and of the 51 potent prior to the procedure, 44 (86%) remained potent after hemiablation. Four (7%) required retreatment because of cancer remaining in the untreated area. Transperineal template biopsies were used to verify unilateral cancer and data using transperineal 5 mm spaced template biopsies shows that just under half of patients deemed to have unilateral disease by TRUS biopsy actually have cancer in

Table 4 Series Evaluating Focal Therapy of Prostate Cancer Using Cryotherapy

	Onik et al. (77) (Endocare)	Ellis et al. (78) (Endocare)	Lambert et al. (79) (Oncura)	Bahn et al. (80) (Endocare)	Crawford/Barqawi (81) (Endocare)	COLD registry (82) (Endocare)
Number	112	60	25	31	100	795
Therapy	Hemi	Hemi	Hemi	Hemi	Focal	"Focal/partial"
Biopsy	Template	TRUS	TRUS	TRUS + Doppler	Template	TRUS
Mean PSA (ng/mL)	8.3	7.2 +/− 4.7	6 (range 1–13)	4.95	5.2 +/− 4.1	
Gleason score	≤6	</= 8	</= 7	</= 7	</= 7	</= 8
Potency	85%	70.6%	70.8%	89%	83%	65%
Incontinence	0%	3.6%	0%	0%	–	2.8%
F/U (mean, mo)	43.2	15.2	28	70	–	12
Disease control	93% NED	76.7% (biopsy)	88% (>50% nadir reduction)	96% (biopsy) 92% (ASTRO)	97% (biopsy at 12/12)	4.5% (36/295) 25% (36/199) 83% (ASTRO)

Table 5 Series Evaluating Focal Therapy of Prostate Cancer Using HIFU

	Muto et al. (83) (Sonablate 500)	Barret (84) (Ablatherm)	Ahmed/Emberton (85) (Sonablate 500)
Number	29	12	20
Therapy	Hemiablation	Hemiablation	Hemiablation
Biopsy	TRUS biopsy	TRUS biopsy	Template
Mean PSA (ng/mL)	5 (range 2–25)	<10	<15
Gleason score	</= 8	</= 7	</= 7
Potency	Not reported	Not reported	95%
Incontinence	Not reported	0%	5%
Disease control	76.5% (biopsy)	58% (10 yr)	10% (any cancer) (0% significant cancer) (biopsy)

both lobes (87,88). Bahn et al. (80) have recently reported another series in which hemiablation was carried out using cryosurgery. At a mean follow-up of 70 months, biochemical disease-free status, according to the ASTRO definition, was maintained by 92.8% of patients (26/28) and a 96.0% negative-biopsy rate (24/25) was observed. Potency was retained by a total of 88.9% of those potent prior to treatment. The investigators used color doppler-guided TRUS biopsies to verify unilateral disease as well as posttreatment success. Since this technique does not carry the necessary accuracy for cancer detection significant under-treatment was a major problem. Another group demonstrated in 60 men who underwent focal cryosurgery followed by penile rehabilitation with a vacuum device, that 73% of those potent prior to treatment maintained potency alongside a low incontinence rate of 3.6% (78). After therapy, 35 patients underwent biopsy, with 14 showing positive findings (40.0%) at a mean of 12.0 months post treatment. Thirteen out of fourteen were actually from the untreated side. This was not surprising since this group do not report on using any further evaluation beyond TRUS biopsy to establish location of cancer. Lambert et al. (2007) reported on a small series of 25 who underwent hemiablation cryosurgery for presumed unilateral disease, although again this was based on TRUS biopsy at diagnosis only (79). Of the 24 patients potent prior to hemiablation cryosurgery, 17 (71%) were potent postoperatively. There was no rectal toxicity or incontinence. Recurrent cancer was detected in 3, with two recurrences on the contralateral side and one recurrence on the ipsilateral side of the cryosurgery. All were retreated successfully. Finally, Muto et al. (2008) report on hemiablation using the Sonablate 500 HIFU device (83). 29 patients who were found to have unilateral disease on the basis of TRUS biopsy were treated to ablation of both peripheral zones and one half of the transition zone. 10% (3/28) had positive biopsies at six months whereas 23.5% (4/17) had further positive biopsies at 12 months. There was no significant change in the IPSS score for urinary symptoms, although there was one urethral stricture and one urinary tract infection. Although demonstrating feasibility of focal therapy using a transrectal HIFU device, the reporting in this series was very poor and the group tried to make comparison with a nonrandomized group that were treated with whole-gland HIFU. Indeed, they made no comment on the erectile function rate.

This very limited data from uncontrolled case series suggests that treatment related toxicity could be reduced by treating malignant areas while preserving a significant amount of prostate tissue. Equally, the data suggests it might be possible to obtain clinically important periods of remissions from disease progression. Nonetheless, what is now required is a standardized assessment of a focal therapy intervention in a well-characterized group of men with a follow-up regimen under ethical prospective trial conditions. Two prospective National Cancer Research Network (U.K.) HIFU trials using the Sonablate 500 device evaluating the role of hemiablation of unilateral disease and focal ablation of bilateral, low volume disease verified by

template transperineal prostate biopsies, are being undertaken at our center (87). At the time writing, interim results have demonstrated preservation of genitourinary function in 95% of men with residual low volume cancer in the treated areas of approximately 10% (89). Prospective ethically approved trials evaluating hemiablation cryosurgery are underway in Colorado, U.S.A. (90), Memorial Sloan Kettering Cancer Center and MD Anderson Cancer Center.

Focal therapy can be delivered in a patient-specific manner as described below:

Hemiablation of Unilateral Cancer

The entire lobe affected, regardless of volume or position of cancer foci.

Focal Ablation of Unilateral or Bilateral Disease

Only cancer areas will be ablated with a margin (2–3 mm) of normal tissue and at least one neurovascular bundle will be preserved. Focal ablation, rather than hemiablation, of unilateral disease will be used if the cancer is confined to just one quadrant.

Index Lesion Ablation

Ablation of the largest focus of cancer alone with a 2- to 3-mm margin, provided the remaining lesions are small (total volume <0.2 cc) and low grade (Gleason score ≤6) (Figs. 6 and 7A, B).

What is the justification for the inclusion of the third intervention, index lesion ablation? First, there is good evidence that disease progression is determined by the volume of a tumor and that this volume equates to about 0.5 cc. Second, about 80% of men have a

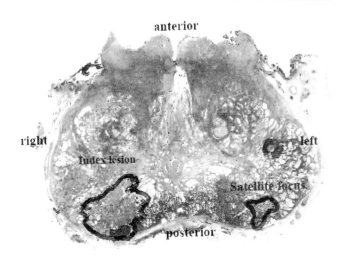

Figure 6 Whole-mount section of a prostate showing an index lesion in the right peripheral zone with a smaller low volume (<0.5 cc) lesion with Gleason score 6. This would be a typical example of a man who may have been suitable for index lesion ablation.

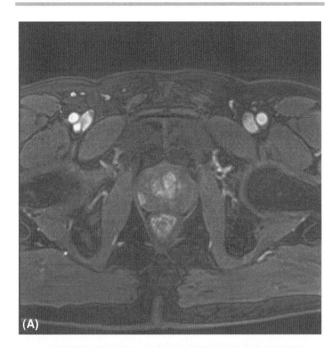

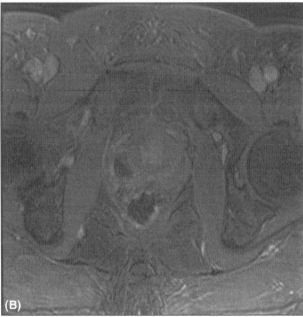

Figure 7 (**A**) Pretreatment dynamic gadolinium contrast enhanced axial MRI demonstrating a malignant lesion in right peripheral zone of prostate at the midgland. Template transperineal biopsies with sampling every 5 mm demonstrated two biopsies positive in that area (Gleason 3 + 4) with 1 mm Gleason 3 + 3 in one biopsy from the left side of the gland. (**B**) Post-HIFU ablation of the right peripheral zone index lesion dynamic contrast enhanced axial MRI at the same level demonstrating necrosis (*dark area*).

dominant tumor such as this, which also gives rise to most of the extracapsular extension. Third, 80% seem to have a dominant lesion with the remaining lesions of low grade (≤Gleason score 6) and a total volume of secondary lesions <0.5 cc. It seems reasonable therefore

to propose that ablation of the dominant lesion will give rise to disease control provided the remaining lesions can be well characterized in the pretreatment evaluation. We would propose a lower volume threshold (<0.2 cc) to ensure that this minimizes the risk from such a therapeutic strategy.

RENAL TUMORS

Cryotherapy

There are currently four cryoablation manufacturers: Endocare (California, U.S.), Galil Medical (Yokneam, Israel), Oncura (Illinois, U.S.), and Cryomedical Sciences (Maryland, U.S.). The first three-use argon gas to cause rapid freezing at the probe tip was based on the Joule-Thomson effect. The Cryomedical Sciences unit is a nitrogen-based system and is currently only used for prostate and liver applications. The recent development of third-generation cryotechnology using argon/helium gas circulation and ultra-thin 17-gauge needles has improved the procedure with reduced traumatic penetration of the renal capsule and precise insertion of the cryoprobes into the tumor under intraoperative ultrasound guidance. Multiple small probes can also be placed into the tumor so minimizing blood loss when the probes are removed as would happen with larger probes. Currently, renal cryoablation is performed laparoscopically or percutaneously. Surgeon preference and experience are crucial for choosing the optimal approach because each has advantages and limitations. Laparoscopic renal cryoablation offers the advantage of precise cryoprobe positioning and monitoring of the ice ball under real-time ultrasound as well as vision. Ultrasound shows the ice ball as a hyperechoic advancing area with a posterior acoustic shadow. Anterior or medial tumors, which would be difficult to target percutaneously can be approached laparoscopically. Percutaneous renal cryoablation is performed with the use of open gantry magnetic resonance imaging or CT guidance, although there has been a report of percutaneous cryoablation under general anesthesia with ultrasound guidance alone.

RFA

Open, laparoscopic, and percutaneous techniques have been used for renal RFA. Laparoscopic RFA has the advantage of mobilization of the tumor and avoidance of adjacent organ damage, and placement of the probe under direct vision, whereas percutaneous RFA, which is most popularly used, is better tolerated, can be performed under sedation on an outpatient basis and fits the minimally invasive criteria more closely. Probes are inserted under ultrasound, CT, and MRI guidance although cross-sectional imaging is by far more recommended since formation of microbubbles and the hyperechoic rim make ultrasound for real-time imaging of RFA problematic. The success of RFA is usually assessed typically by CT scan one month after treatment by demonstrating the absence of enhancement in the ablated tissue as early scans usually show a false positive enhancing rim.

RFA is suitable for tumors that are <4 cm which are >1 cm from the pelviureteric junction, and >1 cm from segmental renal vessels without abutting the pyelocalyceal system. Tumor location is the most important determinant for the choice of surgical approach since posterior or laterally based tumors are best served with the percutaneous approach and anterior tumors using a laparoscopic method. The feasibility of RFA for the treatment of renal tumors was reported in 1997 with only three patients who then underwent surgical resection after ablation. Several case series using percutaneous RFA have been published, but with large variation in patient selection, technique, follow-up and outcomes.

A meta-analysis conducted in 2008 evaluated forty-seven studies (1375 kidney lesions in total) treated by cryoablation or RFA. Cryoablation usually was performed laparoscopically (65%), whereas 94% of lesions treated with RFA were approached percutaneously. The study found no differences between ablation modalities with regard to mean patient age, tumor size or duration of follow-up. However, pretreatment biopsy was performed significantly more often for cryoablated lesions (82.3%) compared with RFA (62.2%; $P < 0.0001$), while unknown pathology occurred at a significantly higher rate for small renal masses that underwent RFA (40.4%) as opposed to cryoablation (24.5%; $P < 0.0001$). Repeat ablation treatment was required more often after RFA (8.5% vs. 1.3%; $P < 0.0001$) and the rates of local tumor progression were significantly higher for RFA (12.9% vs. 5.2%; $P < 0.0001$) compared with cryoablation. Metastasis was reported less frequently for cryoablation (1.0%) versus RFA (2.5%) although this did not reach statistical significance $P = 0.06$). The meta-analysis concluded that short-term data on tumor ablation, retreatment and local tumor progression supported cryoablation over RFA although development of metastases and long-term survival were yet to be shown to be superior, especially with lack of randomized comparative trials.

SUMMARY

The therapeutic dilemma between surveillance and radical therapy for those with early low risk prostate cancer and renal tumors combined with the significant morbidity associated with radical therapies has led to development of minimally invasive procedures that attempt to achieve effective cancer control while reducing the treatment burden. HIFU, RFA and cryosurgery have emerged as forerunners in this field and mature datasets now exist showing effective cancer control in the medium term with good side-effect profiles. PDT may follow suit. However, there is still much to determine. There is yet to be any agreement on what constitutes a successful treatment until long-term data are available.

CONFLICT OF INTERESTS

Hashim Uddin Ahmed and Mark Emberton receive funding from the Medical Research Council, Pelican Cancer Foundation, The Prostate Research Campaign, U.K. (charity) and Prostate Cancer Research Centre, U.K. (all charities) for work in focal therapy of prostate cancer. In addition, Mark Emberton and Caroline Moore receive funding and are Consultants for Negma Lerads, France (manufacturers of TOOKAD, a photodynamic agent used in prostate cancer therapy). Mark Emberton is a Consultant for Misonix/Focus Surgery/UKHIFU (manufacturers and distributors of the Sonablate 500 HIFU device). Mark Emberton and Hashim Ahmed receive funding from the Pelican Cancer Foundation charity (U.K.) and Misonix/Focus Surgery/UKHIFU (manufacturers and distributors of the Sonablate 500 HIFU device). Mark Emberton and Hashim Ahmed are approved proctors for training other surgeons in the use of the Sonablate 500 machine and have received fees for this activity.

Manit Arya has no conflict of interest.

REFERENCES

1. Jemal A, Siegel R, Ward E, et al. Cancer statistics, 2007. CA Cancer J Clin 2007; 57:43–66.
2. Lindblad P, Adami HO. Kidney Cancer in Textbook of Cancer Epidemiology. New York: Oxford University Press, 2002:467–485.
3. Office for National Statistics, Registrations of cancer diagnosed in 2005, England 2008.
4. Chow WH, Devesa SS, Warren JL, et al. Rising incidence of renal cell cancer in the United States. JAMA 1999; 281(17):1628–1631.
5. Jayson M, Sanders H. Increased incidence of serendipitously discovered renal cell carcinoma. Urology 1998; 51:203–205.
6. Volpe A, Panzarella T, Rendon RA, et al. The natural history of incidentally detected small renal masses. Cancer 2004; 100:738–745.
7. Hollingsworth JM, Miller DC, Daignault S, et al. Rising incidence of small renal masses: a need to reassess treatment effect. J Natl Cancer Inst 2006; 98:1331–1334.
8. Lightfoot N, Conlon M, Kreiger N, et al. Impact of non-invasive imaging on increased incidental detection of renal cell carcinoma. Eur Urol 2000; 37:521–527.
9. Nguyen MM, Gill IS, Ellison LM. The evolving presentation of renal carcinoma in the United States: trends from the Surveillance, Epidemiology and End Results program. J Urol 2006; 176(6 pt 1):2397–2400.
10. Frank I, Blute ML, Cheville JC, et al. Solid renal tumors: an analysis of pathological features related to tumor size. J Urol 2003; 170(6 pt 1):2217–2220.
11. Pasticier G, Timsit MO, Badet L, et al. Nephron-sparing surgery for renal cell carcinoma: detailed analysis of complications over a 15-year period. Eur Urol 2006; 49:485–490.
12. Matin SF, Gill IS, Worley S, et al. Outcome of laparoscopic radical and open partial nephrectomy for the sporadic 4 cm or less renal tumor with a normal contralateral kidney. J Urol 2002; 168:1356–1360.
13. Ramani AP, Desai MM, Steinberg AP, et al. Complications of laparoscopic partial nephrectomy in 200 cases. J Urol 2005; 173:42–47.

14. Frank I, Blute ML, Leibovich BC, et al. Independent validation of the 2002 American Joint Committee on cancer primary tumor classification for renal cell carcinoma using a large, single institution cohort. J Urol 2005; 173:1889–1892.

15. Moinzadeh A, Gill IS, Finelli A, et al. Laparoscopic partial nephrectomy: 3-year follow up. J Urol 2006; 175:459–462.

16. Kunkle DA, Egleston BL, Uzzo RG. Excise, ablate or observe: the small renal mass dilemma–a meta-analysis and review. J Urol 2008; 179(4):1227–1233.

17. Bill-Axelsen A, Holmberg L, Mirrja Ruuth, et al. Watchful waiting and prostate cancer. NEJM 2005; 352:1977–1984.

18. Arnott J. On the Treatment of Cancer by the Regulated Application of an Anesthetic Temperature. London: Churchill, 1851.

19. Hoffmann NE, Bischof JC. The cryobiology of cryosurgical injury. Urology 2002; 60(2 suppl 1):40–49.

20. Tatsutani K, Rubinsky B, Onik G, et al. Effect of thermal variables on frozen human primary prostatic adenocarcinoma cells. Urology 1996; 48:441–447.

21. Borkowski P, Robinson MJ, Poppiti RJ Jr, et al. Histologic findings in postcryosurgical prostatic biopsies. Mod Pathol 1996; 9:807–811.

22. Grampsas SA, Miller GJ, Crawford ED. Salvage radical prostatectomy after failed transperineal cryotherapy: histologic findings from prostate whole-mount specimens correlated with intraoperative transrectal ultrasound images. Urology 1995; 45:936–941.

23. Hill CR, ter Haar GR. Review article: high intensity focused ultrasound–potential for cancer treatment. Br J Radiol 1995; 68(816):1296–1303.

24. Kennedy JE. High-intensity focused ultrasound in the treatment of solid tumours. Nat Rev Cancer 2005; 5(4):321–327.

25. Soanes WA, Gonder MJ. Use of cryosurgery in prostatic cancer. J Urol 1968; 99(6):793–797.

26. Merrick GS, Wallner KE, Butler WM. Prostate cryotherapy: more questions than answers. Urology 2005; 66(1):9–15.

27. Cohen JK, Miller RJ, Rooker GM, et al. Cryosurgical ablation of the prostate: two-year prostate-specific antigen and biopsy results. Urology 1996; 47:395–401.

28. Long JP, Bahn D, Lee F, et al. Five-year retrospective, multi-institutional pooled analysis of cancer-related outcomes after cryosurgical ablation of the prostate. Urology 2001; 57:518–523.

29. Aus G, Pileblad E, Hugosson J. Cryosurgical ablation of the prostate: 5-year follow-up of a prospective study. Eur Urol 2002; 42:133–138.

30. Prepelica KL, Okeke Z, Murphy A, et al. Cryosurgical ablation of the prostate: high risk patient outcomes. Cancer 2005; 103:1625–1630.

31. Bahn DK, Lee F, Badalament R, et al. Targeted cryoablation of the prostate: 7-year outcomes in the primary treatment of prostate cancer. Urology 2002; 60:3–11.

32. Han KR, Cohen JK, Miller RJ, et al. Treatment of organ confined prostate cancer with third generation cryosurgery: preliminary multicenter experience. J Urol 2003; 170:1126–1130.

33. Cytron S, Paz A, Kravchik S, et al. Active rectal wall protection using direct transperineal cryo-needles for histologically proven prostate adenocarcinomas. Eur Urol 2003; 44:315–321.

34. Cohen JK, Miller RJ Jr, Ahmed S, et al. Ten-year biochemical disease control for patients with prostate cancer treated with cryosurgery as primary therapy. Urology. 2008; 71(3):515–518.

35. Polascik TJ, Nosnik I, Mayes JM, et al. Short-term cancer control after primary cryosurgical ablation for clinically localized prostate cancer using third-generation cryotechnology. Urology 2007; 70(1):117–121.

36. Ellis DS, Manny TB Jr, Rewcastle JC. Cryoablation as primary treatment for localized prostate cancer followed by penile rehabilitation. Urology 2007; 69(2):306–310.

37. Cresswell J, Asterling S, Chaudhary M, et al. Third-generation cryotherapy for prostate cancer in the UK: a prospective study of the early outcomes in primary and recurrent disease. BJU Int 2006; 97(5):969–974.

38. Donnelly BJ, Saliken JC, Ernst DS, et al. Prospective trial of cryosurgical ablation of the prostate: five-year results. Urology 2002; 60:645–649.

39. Koppie TM, Shinohara K, Grossfeld GD, et al. The efficacy of cryosurgical ablation of prostate cancer: the University of California, San Francisco experience. J Urol 1999; 162:427–432.

40. Haar GT, Coussios C. High intensity focused ultrasound: physical principles and devices. Int J Hyperthermia 2007; 23(2):89–104.

41. Zacharakis E, Ahmed HU, Dudderidge T, et al. Transrectal High Intensity Focused Ultrasound in the treatment of localised prostate cancer – the first UK series. J Urol 2008; 179(4 suppl 1):493.

42. Mearini L, D'Urso L, Collura D, et al. Visually directed transrectal high intensity focused ultrasound for the treatment of prostate cancer: a preliminary report on the italian experience. J Urol 2009; 181(1):105–111.

43. Uchida T, Ohkusa H, Nagata Y, et al. Treatment of localized prostate cancer using high-intensity focused ultrasound. BJU Int 2006; 97:56–61.

44. Uchida T, Ohkusa H, Yamashita H, et al. Five years experience of transrectal high-intensity focused ultrasound using the Sonablate device in the treatment of localized prostate cancer. Int J Urol 2006; 13(3):228–233.

45. Blana A, Rogenhofer S, Ganzer R, et al. Eight years' experience with high-intensity focused ultrasonography for treatment of localized prostate cancer. Urology 2008; 72(6):1329–1333.

46. Misraï V, Rouprêt M, Chartier-Kastler E, et al. Oncologic control provided by HIFU therapy as single treatment in men with clinically localized prostate cancer. World J Urol 2008; 26(5):481–485.

47. Vallancien G, Prapotnich D, Cathelineau X, et al. Transrectal focused ultrasound combined with transurethral resection of the prostate for the treatment of localized prostate cancer: feasibility study. J Urol 2004; 171:2265–2267.

48. Blana A, Walter B, Rogenhofer S, et al. High-intensity focused ultrasound for the treatment of localized prostate cancer: 5-year experience. Urology 2004; 63:297–300.

49. Thuroff S, Chaussy C, Vallancien G, et al. High intensity focused ultrasound and localized prostate cancer: efficacy results from the European multicentric study. J Endourol 2003; 17:673–677.

50. Gelet A, Chapelon JY, Bouvier R, et al. Transrectal high intensity focused ultrasound for the treatment of localised prostate cancer: factors influencing the outcome. Eur Urol 2001; 40:124–129.

51. Chaussy C, Thuroff S. The status of high-intensity focused ultrasound in the treatment of localized prostate cancer and the impact of a combined resection. Curr Urol Rep 2003; 4:248–252.

52. Blana A, Murat FJ, Walter B, et al. First analysis of the long-term results with transrectal HIFU in patients with localised prostate cancer. Eur Urol 2008; 53(6):1194–1201.

53. Poissonnier L, Chapelon JY, Rouvière O, et al. Control of prostate cancer by transrectal HIFU in 227 patients. Eur Urol 2007; 51(2):381–387.

54. Ficarra V, Antoniolli SZ, Novara G, et al. Short-term outcome after high-intensity focused ultrasound in the treatment of patients with high-risk prostate cancer. BJU Int 2006; 98(6):1193–1198.

55. Kirkham AP, Emberton M, Hoh IM, et al. MR imaging of prostate after treatment with high-intensity focused ultrasound. Radiology 2008; 246(3):833–844.

56. Rouvière O, Lyonnet D, Raudrant A, et al. MRI appearance of prostate following transrectal HIFU ablation of localized cancer. Eur Urol 2001; 40(3):265–274.

57. Ganzer R, Rogenhofer S, Walter B, et al. PSA nadir is a significant predictor of treatment failure after high-intensity focussed ultrasound (HIFU) treatment of localised prostate cancer. Eur Urol 2008; 53(3):547–553.

58. American Society for Therapeutic Radiology and Oncology Consensus Panel: consensus statement: guidelines for PSA following radiation therapy. In J Radiat 1997; 37:1035–1041.

59. Roach M 3rd, Hanks G, Thames H Jr, et al. Defining biochemical failure following radiotherapy with or without hormonal therapy in men with clinically localized prostate cancer: recommendations of the RTOG-ASTRO Phoenix Consensus Conference. Int J Radiat Oncol Biol Phys 2006; 65(4):965–974.

60. Illing RO, Leslie TA, Kennedy JE, et al. Visually directed HIFU for organ confined prostate cancer – a proposed standard for the conduct of therapy. BJU Int 2006; 98(6):1187–1192.

61. Windahl T, Andersson So, Lofgren L. Photodynamic therapy of localised prostate cancer. Lancet 1990; 336:1139.

62. Nathan TR, Whitelaw DE, Chang SC, et al. Photodynamic therapy for prostate cancer recurrence after radiotherapy: a phase I study. J Urol 2002; 168:1427–1432.

63. Moore CM, Nathan TR, Lees WR, et al. Photodynamic therapy using meso tetra hydroxyl phenyl chlorin (mTHPC) in early prostate cancer. Lasers Surg Med 2006; 38:356–363.

64. Zaak D, Sroka R, Hoppner M, et al. Photodynamic therapy by means of 5 ALA induced protoporphyrin IX in human prostate cancer—preliminary results. Med Laser Appl 2003; 18:91–95.

65. Pinthus JH, Bogaards A, Weersink R, et al. Photodynamic therapy for urological malignancies: past to current approaches. J Urol 2006; 175:1201–1207.

66. Verigos K, Stripp DC, Mick R, et al. Updated results of a phase I trial of motexafin lutetium mediated interstitial photodynamic therapy in patients with locally recurrent prostate cancer. J Environ Pathol Toxicol Oncol 2006; 25:373–388.

67. Patel H, Mick R, Finlay J, et al. Motexafin lutetium-photodynamic therapy of prostate cancer: short- and long-term effects on prostate-specific antigen. Clin Cancer Res 2008; 14(15):4869–4876.

68. Weersink RA, Forbes J, Bisland S, et al. Assessment of cutaneous photosensitivity of TOOKAD (WST09) in preclinical animal models and in patients. Photochem Photobiol 2005; 81:106–113.

69. Trachtenberg J, Weersink RA, Davidson SR, et al. Vascular-targeted photodynamic therapy (padoporfin, WST09) for recurrent prostate cancer after failure of external beam radiotherapy: a study of escalating light doses. BJU Int 2008; 102(5):556–562.

70. Trachtenberg J, Bogaards A, Weersink RA, et al. Vascular targeted photodynamic therapy with palladium-bacteriopheophorbide photosensitizer for recurrent prostate cancer following definitive radiation therapy: assessment of safety and treatment response. J Urol 2007; 178(5):1974–1979.

71. Haider MA, Davidson SR, Kale AV, et al. Prostate gland: MR imaging appearance after vascular targeted photodynamic therapy with palladium-bacteriopheophorbide. Radiology 2007; 244(1):196–204.

72. Moore CM, Hoh I, Mosse C, et al. Vascular-targeted photodynamic therapy in organ confined prostate cancer—report of a novel photosensitiser. European Association of Urology Annual Meeting abstract, 2006, AM06-1094.

73. Ahmed HU, Pendse D, Illing R, et al. Will focal therapy become a standard of care for men with localized prostate cancer? Nat Clin Pract Oncol 2007; 4(11):632–642.

74. Eggener SE, Scardino PT, Carroll PR, et al. International Task Force on Prostate Cancer and the Focal Lesion Paradigm. Focal therapy for localized prostate cancer: a critical appraisal of rationale and modalities. J Urol 2007; 178(6): 2260–2267.

75. Nilsson S, Norlen BJ, Widmark A. A systematic overview of radiation therapy effects in prostate cancer. Acta Oncol 2004; 43(4):316–381.

76. Meraney AM, Haese A, Palisaar J, et al. Surgical management of prostate cancer: advances based on a rational approach to the data. Eur J Cancer 2005; 41(6):888–907.

77. Onik G, Vaughan D, Lotenfoe R, et al. "Male lumpectomy": focal therapy for prostate cancer using cryoablation. Urology 2007; 70(6 suppl):16–21.

78. Ellis DS, Manny TB Jr, Rewcastle JC. Focal cryosurgery followed by penile rehabilitation as primary treatment for localized prostate cancer: initial results. Urology 2007; 70(6 suppl):9–15.

79. Lambert EH, Bolte K, Masson P, et al. Focal cryosurgery: encouraging health outcomes for unifocal prostate cancer. Urology 2007; 69(6):1117–1120.

80. Bahn DK, Silverman P, Lee F Sr, et al. Focal prostate cryoablation: initial results show cancer control and potency preservation. J Endourol 2006; 20(9):688–692.

81. Barqawi AB, Crawford ED. The current use and future trends of focal surgical therapy in the management of localized prostate cancer. Cancer J 2007; 13(5):313–317.

82. Jones JS, Rewcastle JC, Donnelly BJ, et al. Whole gland primary prostate cryoablation: initial results from the cryo on-line data registry. J Urol 2008; 180(2):554–558.

83. Muto S, Yoshii T, Saito K, et al. Focal therapy with high-intensity-focused ultrasound in the treatment of localized prostate cancer. Jpn J Clin Oncol 2008; 38(3):192–199.

84. Barret E, Prapotnich D, Cathelineau X, et al. Focal therapy with HIFU for prostate cancer in elderly: feasibility study with 10 years follow up. P-68. Focal therapy and imaging in prostate cancer workshop, Amsterdam, 2009.

85. Ahmed HU, Emberton M. Is focal therapy the future for prostate cancer? Future Oncol 2010; 6(2):261–268.

86. Onik G, Narayan P, Vaughan D, et al. Focal "nerve-sparing" cryosurgery for treatment of primary prostate cancer: a new approach to preserving potency. Urology 2002; 60:109–114.

87. Ahmed HU, Stevens D, Barbouti O, et al. Prostate cancer risk stratification and cancer mapping—template transperineal prostate mapping biopsies. European Association of Urology Annual Meeting, 2008.

88. Barqawi A, Lugg J, Wilson S, et al. The role of 3dimensional systematic mapping biopsy of the prostate in men presenting with apparent low risk disease based on extended transrectal biopsy. 439, AUA 2008.

89. Ahmed HU, Sahu M, Govindaraju SK, et al. High intensity focused ultrasound (HIFU) hemiablation trial in localised unilateral prostate cancer: interim results. Abstract 863. European Association of Urology Annual Meeting, 2009.

90. Barqawi AB, Lugg JE, Crawford ED. Target Focal therapy in early prostate cancer: initial single institution results. ASCO annual meeting, 2007.

35

Stratified Risk Assessment for Urological Surgery

Thiru Gunendran
Department of Urology, University Hospital of South Manchester, Manchester, U.K.

Nicholas A. Wisely
Department of Anaesthesia, University Hospital of South Manchester, Manchester, U.K.

Nicholas J. R. George
Department of Urology, Withington Hospital, University Hospitals of South Manchester, Manchester, U.K.

INTRODUCTION

Urological surgery covers a wide range of interventions and operations that may be offered to a broad spectrum of patients with a variable ability to respond to the stresses induced by such treatment. Hence, one of the most challenging aspects of surgery—setting aside technical ability and competence to undertake the procedure—is correctly to select and match the patient's pathophysiological reserves to the stresses inherent in any planned operative intervention. Thus, while a total cystectomy with neobladder formation would be a reasonable proposal in a 58-year-old, the same procedure would demand a very different risk analysis in a patient 20 years older. Even minor interventions are subject to the same constraints: an overweight diabetic patient requiring minor groin surgery might well be considered unsuited to otherwise routine day-case surgery.

A stratified risk assessment implies therefore an accurate appraisal of both the patient's *initial reserves* and the *ability to respond* to any particular stress as well as a detailed understanding of the basic physiological requirements that will be necessary for any organ or system to regain normal function following operative interventions. Clearly, a successful outcome to the intervention can be anticipated only by careful matching of these parameters (Fig. 1). In this chapter, the generic response to stress will initially be reprised followed by a consideration of risk according to the severity of the surgical procedure (low, intermediate, or high); finally risk assessment will be examined in terms of system-based criteria (i.e., cardiovascular, pulmonary), which will determine safe intervention either as a day case or as an inpatient for minor, intermediate, or major surgery.

Although there are many (often counter-productive) pressures on the modern NHS it will not be forgotten that the primary purpose of risk assessment is **patient safety**; hospital "efficiency," and other logistical considerations (e.g., same day admission for major surgery) must never override the absolute requirement to manage the patient so as to minimize risk (e.g., previous day admission for critical preoperative measurements). For all types of patient, minimal risk is paramount.

STRESS RESPONSE TO SURGERY (1,2)

The stress response is the name given to the hormonal and metabolic changes that follow any injury or trauma. This response can also be initiated by acute blood loss, shock, hypoxia, tissue ischemia, acidosis, hypothermia, pain, and altered immune function. It can be both adaptive and destructive. The physiologic response that ensues following injury encompasses a wide range of neuroendocrinologic, hematologic, and immunologic effects. There is also simultaneous activation of the sympathetic nervous system. The magnitude and duration of the response are proportional to the surgical insult and the development of complications such as sepsis. This response to injury has classically been grouped into the ebb phase and the flow phase (Fig. 2).

The initial *ebb phase*, typically characterized by clinical features of shock, develops quickly and is primarily due to autonomic and neuroendocrine mechanisms. The features are related to preservation of blood volume and redirection of blood flow to reduce tissue ischemia. During the *flow phase* that follows, there is an increase in catabolic activity and consumption of body fuels. This helps promotes wound healing and resolution in inflammation by transferring amino acids and fuel from muscle and adipose tissue to the site of injury. In the *recovery phase* attempts are made to restore the body's depleted stores. This process is slow and prolonged.

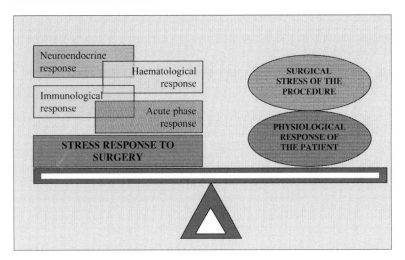

Figure 1   Various factors affecting outcome of surgery.

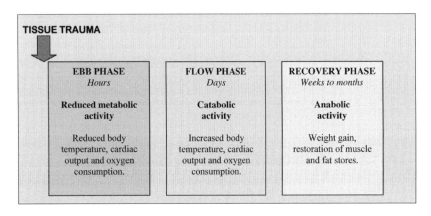

Figure 2   Physiologic response to injury.

Neuroendocrine Response to Surgery

This is characterized by increased secretion of pituitary hormones (hypothalamic-pituitary-adrenal axis) and activation of the sympathetic autonomic nervous system (Fig. 3). It is regulated by the central nervous system that functions as part of a complex reflex arc. In the initial phase (*ebb phase*) catecholamines, cortisol, aldosterone, growth hormone, and glucagon secretion increases, while insulin levels may decline. The suppression of insulin secretion is presumed to be secondary to the effects of catecholamines and autonomic stimulation of the pancreas. After some time (*flow phase*), blood levels of catecholamines also decline despite relatively maintained levels of the other hormones. A degree of insulin resistance may also follow despite elevated glucose levels resulting in increased oxygen requirement. The overall metabolic effect is one of increased catabolism with substrate mobilization, muscle protein loss coupled with retention of sodium and water. The resultant breakdown of polysaccharides, lipids, proteins, and nucleic acids into smaller units provides energy sources necessary for maintenance of

cell growth and repair. Generally, the magnitude of this response is proportional to the severity of the surgical trauma. The increase in metabolic rate varies from 10% in elective surgery to 60% with multiple trauma and 150% in major burns.

Immunological and Hematological Response to Surgery

The local release of cytokines has a major role in the inflammatory response to surgery and tissue trauma. Cytokines are produced from activated leucocytes, fibroblasts, and endothelial cells as an early response to tissue injury. The activated cells release interleukin-1 and tumor necrosis factor-α. This then stimulates the production of more cytokines, in particular interleukin-6, which then mediates the acute phase response. Cytokines can broadly be grouped into pro-inflammatory and anti-inflammatory cytokines (Fig. 4). They can influence cell proliferation, differentiation, and survival, and actively promote wound healing. Pro-inflammatory cytokines promote the inflammatory

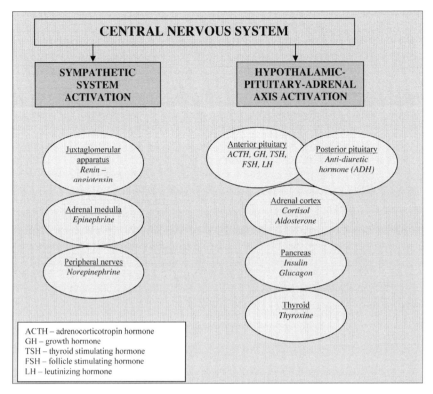

CENTRAL NERVOUS SYSTEM

SYMPATHETIC SYSTEM ACTIVATION

HYPOTHALAMIC-PITUITARY-ADRENAL AXIS ACTIVATION

Juxtaglomerular apparatus
Renin – angiotensin

Anterior pituitary
ACTH, GH, TSH, FSH, LH

Posterior pituitary
Anti-diuretic hormone (ADH)

Adrenal medulla
Epinephrine

Adrenal cortex
Cortisol Aldosterone

Peripheral nerves
Norepinephrine

Pancreas
Insulin Glucagon

Thyroid
Thyroxine

ACTH – adrenocorticotropin hormone
GH – growth hormone
TSH – thyroid stimulating hormone
FSH – follicle stimulating hormone
LH – leutinizing hormone

Figure 3 Neuroendocrine response in the initial phase of surgery.

Pro-inflammatory cytokines	Anti-inflammatory cytokines
Tumor necrosis factor-α	Tumor necrosis factor-β
Interleukin-1	Interleukin-4
Interleukin-2	Interleukin-10
Interleukin-6	Interleukin-13
Interleukin-8	Interleukin-16
Interleukin-12	Interferon-α
Interleukin-18	
Interferon-γ	
Granulocyte-macrophage colony-stimulating factor	

Figure 4 Pro-inflammatory cytokines and anti-inflammatory cytokines.

Positive acute phase proteins	Negative acute phase proteins
Fibrinogen	Albumin
Serum amyloid A	Transferrin
C-reactive protein	Insulin growth factor 1
Complement factors	Retinol-binding protein
Alpha 1-antitrypsin	
Alpha 1-antichymotrypsin	
Alpha 2-macroglobulin	
Ferritin	

Figure 5 Positive and negative acute phase proteins.

response to trauma and infection, while anti-inflammatory cytokines may be associated with immunosuppression and enhanced susceptibility to infections. The net effect of an inflammatory response is determined by the balance between pro-inflammatory cytokines and anti-inflammatory cytokines.

The Acute Phase Response

The acute phase response (APR) is initiated in response to inflammation, infection, or tissue trauma, resulting in the production of acute phase proteins by the liver. One of the key mediators of this response is related to the stimulation of hepatocytes in the liver by cytokines, in particular interleukin-6. The APR is characterized by fever, granulocytosis, and changes in the plasma concentrations of various acute phase proteins (Fig. 5). These proteins act as inflammatory mediators to prevent ongoing tissue damage, isolate and destroy the infective organism, and activate the repair process.

RISK STRATIFICATION

Surgery results in tissue trauma, which initiates many of the responses mentioned in the preceding text. Although the stress response can be beneficial as it leads to wound healing, restoration, and repair, it can be quite morbid for older patients and those with a compromised physiological reserve. This can be particularly significant when major abdominal, thoracic, or pelvic surgery is being performed. In most cases however, where operations are minor and the procedure is short with minimal tissue injury, limited blood loss, or fluid shifts, the accompanying physiologic response is mild and transient. Hence by looking at the surgical stress of the procedure and identifying the physiological reserve of the patient, a decision can be made on the ideal setting (e.g., day case, short stay, or inpatient) of surgery and the necessary preoperative intensification that needs to ensue.

SURGICAL STRESS OF PROCEDURE

The key pathogenic factor is the surgical stress of the procedure and likelihood for increased demands on organ function and tissue oxygen delivery. The choice of the surgical technique according to the patient's risk profile is also important.

Low-Risk Procedures

There is minimal tissue damage with no significant fluid shifts, negligible blood loss, low risk of postoperative complications, minor postoperative pain, and little requirement for postoperative oxygen demand.

Patients who fall into the low-risk group probably require minimal preoperative investigations. Generally, for the majority of endoscopic and inguinoscrotal cases, routine tests would suffice on the basis of set hospital criteria. Most patients would tolerate a short procedure under general or regional anesthesia.

Intermediate to High-Risk Procedures

These include procedures that involve moderate to extensive tissue damage, significant intra- and extracellular fluid shifts, increased demand for postoperative oxygen consumption, and procedures where moderate pain is expected or recovery is unpredictable.

When a more demanding procedure is planned, baseline fitness and coexisting illness will determine what further tests are necessary to establish if the patient will be able to tolerate the physiological stresses associated with surgery. Despite reducing tissue trauma, laparoscopic procedures carry a number of challenges because of the effects of pneumoperitoneum and patient positioning.

Laparoscopic- and Robotic-Assisted Laparoscopic Surgery

Laparoscopic surgery has gained increasing popularity within the urological community. It aims to reduce the surgical stress response by avoiding large incisions and minimizing tissue trauma, which correlates to reduction in pain, blood loss, postoperative pulmonary complications, and hospital stay. Laparoscopic surgery causes less tissue injury than conventional procedures with a lesser rise in the levels of interleukin-6, tumor necrosis factor-α, interferon-γ, and acute phase proteins

(3,4). However, this is at the expense of increased intra-abdominal pressure, systemic absorption of carbon dioxide, and reduced venous return, which if prolonged carries its own risk of cardiopulmonary and thrombotic complications. Additionally, one has to predict how the patient might react to positive pressure ventilation, fluid challenges, and other mechanisms normally employed to counter rises in intra-abdominal pressure (5). The steep head down position in robotic-assisted laparoscopic surgery carries the added risk of cerebral edema, intraocular edema, and pulmonary interstitial edema. Some experts view a history of significant cardiovascular comorbidity, pulmonary disease, or cerebrovascular disease as contraindications for laparoscopic pelvic procedures such as prostatectomy and cystectomy due to the head down position (6). Selection for such procedures will thus depend on clinical judgment and assessment of the patients' ability to withstand the physiological changes associated with patient positioning.

PHYSIOLOGICAL RESERVE OF THE PATIENT

Clearly, it will be necessary initially to estimate and if indicated later to measure objectively the patient's physiological functional capacity and reserves. For example, the cardiopulmonary reserve is determined by the patient's cardiopulmonary functional capacity and the ability to support postoperative demand for increased oxygen consumption. Cardiac output and myocardial ischemia are important determining factors in this equation. For these purposes assessment protocols are widely utilized, and frequently these may be found to vary significantly between departments and hospital units. Such variation however is not of concern as long as the proforma addresses specific risk associated with each type of surgery, for example, day case or intermediate inpatient surgery. The requirements for construction of a valid proforma to cover differing orders of clinical risk for various forms of surgery are detailed by physiological system as noted later.

RISK ASSESSMENT FOR DAY-CASE SURGERY

Patients with reasonable cardiopulmonary functional capacity and physiological reserve undergoing low-risk procedures should ideally be undertaken as a day case. Such patients should be selected according to their physiological status and not limited by arbitrary restrictions such as age and weight (7). In fact, day surgery should be the norm unless there is a specific contraindication. Assessment should be performed well in advance of their surgery to correct any abnormalities and allow the patient to be adequately informed and prepared for surgery.

In the United Kingdom, the Department of Health has stated its aim for 75% of elective procedures to be performed on a day-case basis within the next decade (8). In 2001 the Audit Commission produced a list of urological procedures thought to be suitable for day surgery (orchidopexy, circumcision, meatotomy, and transurethral resection of bladder tumor) (9,10), while the British Association of Day Surgery (BADS) (11) proposed that at least 50% of urethrotomies, bladder neck incisions, and laser prostatectomies could be done as day case. Ideally any quick, simple procedures with minimal risk of prolonged bleeding, little analgesic requirements, and prompt recovery would fall into this category. There is some recent evidence suggesting that slightly more complex, minimally invasive surgical procedures, such as laparoscopic nephrectomy, can safely and successfully be undertaken on a day-case basis (12). However, this is significantly dependant on the institution, surgeon's expertise, appropriate staffing support, and facilities for overnight stay. A number of factors may deem day-case surgery to be inappropriate, unsafe or impossible although ultimately such decisions are at the discretion of the anesthetist, urologist, and local hospital policy.

Exclusion for Day Surgery (7,9,13,14)

Operation Factors

- Moderate to high risk of postoperative hemorrhage
- Significant risk of airway compromise following surgery
- Analgesic requirements likely to be moderate or uncontrolled with oral analgesia
- Continued requirement for intravenous fluids postoperatively
- Long recovery period is likely

Patient Factors

- Respiratory—poorly controlled asthma or chronic obstructive pulmonary disease (COPD), for example, needing oral steroids often or within last three months; dyspnea at rest or mild exertion; obstructive sleep apnea; requirement for home oxygen or non invasive ventilation
- Cardiovascular—myocardial infarction (MI) within last six months; uncontrolled or poorly controlled angina, cardiac failure, or hypertension (blood pressure greater than 100 to 110 mmHg diastolic, or systolic greater than 170 to 180 mmHg regardless of diastolic pressure); orthopnea, significant valvular or congenital heart disease
- Cerebrovascular—recent cerebrovascular accident or transient ischemic event
- Hematological—hemophilia; coagulopathy; patients on warfarin (relative contraindication); sickle cell disease (not trait)
- Endocrine—poorly controlled diabetics (HbA_{1c} >10% or 86 mmol/mol); insulin-dependent diabetics (although many day surgery units now consider stable diabetics maintained on oral hypoglycemic drugs or insulin suitable for most day-surgery procedures); untreated thyrotoxicosis; adrenal insufficiency

- Renal—moderate to severe renal failure; patients on dialysis
- Liver—advanced liver failure
- Neurological—uncontrolled epileptics or history of recent fits; myasthenia gravis; muscular dystrophies
- Anesthetic factors—suxamethonium apnea; malignant hyperpyrexia; difficult intubation; previous anesthetic reactions
- Others—pregnant patients

Social Factors

- Lives alone or no responsible person at home for 24 hours following surgery (excludes local anesthetic procedures)
- Transport problems—no suitable transport home (must be non-public transport for general anesthetic procedure/regional anesthesia)
- No ready access to a telephone

RISK ASSESSMENT FOR INPATIENT SURGERY

Patients deemed unsuitable for day case will have to be admitted for their procedure as inpatients. Other factors may also need to be taken into account depending on their social circumstances, coexisting illness, and cooperation. Increasingly, short-stay wards with a 23-hour model of care have been developed as an intermediate between true day-case surgery and inpatient surgery. Suitable patients have been carefully selected as appropriate cases and are treated using anesthetic techniques that allow rapid recovery with minimal pain. The episode of care can generally be delivered within an envelope of 23 hours during which time patients may require pain relief, some intravenous fluids, and monitoring in a supervised setting until fit for discharge.

PREOPERATIVE AND SYSTEM SPECIFIC ASSESSMENT

Cardiovascular Assessment and Optimization (15)

Assessment of the cardiovascular reserve is predominantly aimed at looking for the presence of congestive heart failure, valvular heart disease, myocardial ischemia, uncontrolled hypertension and arrhythmias. Patients with vascular impairment often have coronary artery disease risk factors and the usual symptomatic presentation of angina in these patients may be obscured by exercise limitations imposed by intermittent claudication. Ideally, surgery should be delayed until the cardiac condition has been optimized, either medically or surgically. In patients with angiographically proven coronary artery disease, revascularization should be undertaken first if moderate- to high-risk elective urological surgery is contemplated (16,17). By comparison, patients undergoing low-risk operations only have a very small risk of postoperative death (<1%) or MI that is unaffected by prior coronary treatment (17).

METs	Equivalent type of activity
< 4 METs (poor)	Activities of daily living (e.g. eating, dressing), house work
4–7 METs (moderate)	Climbing two flights of stairs, gardening, cycling
> 7 METs (excellent)	Running, squash, singles tennis

Figure 6 Assessment of functional capacity using metabolic equivalents (METs).

The early assessment of surgical risk was directed at indentifying individuals at high risk of perioperative ischemic events with transurethral prostate resections being considered intermediate risk (17). Preoperative cardiac risk assessment was initially popularized by Goldman et al. (18) and later modified by Detsky et al. (19). It was proposed that MI within six months, unstable angina, recent pulmonary edema, critical aortic stenosis, and emergency surgery carried a significant risk of perioperative cardiac complications. Although highly specific, they had a low sensitivity. The Revised Goldman Cardiac Risk Index was much simpler but still misleading and could not always reliably identify patients with severe cardiopulmonary abnormalities.

Prior to surgery, the subjective assessment of patient's exercise tolerance is thought to be a reasonable indicator of fitness for anesthesia. A patient's functional capacity can be measured in metabolic equivalents (METs), although assessment is limited by mobility (Fig. 6). A patient with an exercise tolerance of four METs or more is thought to be at low risk of perioperative morbidity.

However, METs do not provide an accurate or objective measure of cardiopulmonary functional capacity. Stress testing (exercise electrocardiogram monitoring) has also probably outlived its time as the most useful discriminator for predicting adverse cardiac events. This is because such assessments are unable to predict the ability of the cardiopulmonary system to deliver oxygen to the tissues under conditions of surgical stress. Cardiopulmonary exercise (CPX) testing is being used increasingly to assess patients' fitness prior to major urological surgery. CPX can risk stratify patients into low, higher, and unacceptably high-risk groups prior to surgery. Low-risk groups can be safely managed on the ward after surgery leaving more critical care capacity to manage the higher risk patients. The objective data provided by CPX allow those patients with unacceptably high risk to be counseled into nonsurgical management, and the test may also identify cardiac or respiratory problems that can be optimized prior to surgery. Further details about CPX testing is described on page 529.

Disease Modifying Interventions

Recent myocardial infarction. MI may be the first presenting feature of ischemic heart disease in up to 50% of patients. Patients with a previous MI have an overall risk of perioperative reinfarction of 30% to 40% within three months and 15% to 25% at three to six months (20,21). The mortality rate with reinfarction can be 30% to 50% (20). As such, elective urological procedures should be postponed for at least six months after an MI where possible (22). Uncontrolled angina is also associated with a high risk of intra-operative MI if the symptom is not controlled preoperatively. Following MI, a β-blocker can be beneficial as it protects the ischemic myocardium, promotes recovery, and lowers the risk of death by decreasing the heart's demand for oxygen (23).

Congestive cardiac failure. Patients with diastolic heart failure or a left ventricular ejection fraction of less than 30% on echocardiography are at an increased risk of cardiovascular events during surgery. Angiotensin-converting enzymes are increasingly being used to manage congestive cardiac failure as they increase cardiac output, improve exercise tolerance, and prolong survival (24). These drugs may, however, precipitate renal failure in patients with marked renal artery stenosis by reducing the efferent arteriole vascular resistance with a resultant fall in glomerular filtration pressure.

Valvular heart disease.
1. Aortic stenosis—There is risk of myocardial ischemia due to increased demand from the hypertrophied ventricle. Intra-operative hypotensive periods can be very poorly tolerated in severe stenosis because of fixed cardiac output, and such patients should be referred for valve surgery (replacement) first prior to major surgery.
2. Mitral stenosis—The risk of pulmonary edema is increased in patients undergoing elective surgery depending on the severity of stenosis.
3. Aortic regurgitation and mitral regurgitation—Generally surgery is reasonably better tolerated than with valve stenosis.
4. Endocarditis prophylaxis—Antibiotic prophylaxis against infective endocarditis is no longer recommended for people undergoing genitourinary tract procedures (25).

Cardiomyopathy. A cardiological opinion should be sought if hypertrophic obstructive cardiomyopathy is present.

Pacemakers. Pacemaker checks should be verified. Single or dual chamber pacemakers can be reprogrammed in fixed rate mode to avoid risks associated with diathermy use. Bipolar diathermy is generally safe, but if monopolar diathermy is used it should be employed in short bursts and the patient plate sited so as to avoid transmission through the thorax.

Implantable converter defibrillator. Any pacemaker that has the ability to cardiovert or overpace should be deactivated prior to surgery to avoid erroneous discharge in case diathermy noise is interpreted as a tachyarrhythmia; reactivation is required immediately following the procedure.

Hypertension. Hypertension is the leading cause of congestive heart failure, and in untreated patients, the five-year mortality rates approach 50% (26).

Degree of hypertension	Suggested management
Mild diastolic hypertension (diastolic <100 mmHg)	Minimal increase in risk. Proceed with surgery
Moderate diastolic hypertension (diastolic 100-115 mmHg)	Control over a few days or weeks and proceed with surgery. If end organ damage is present, than re-list after 4 weeks of treatment
Severe diastolic hypertension (diastolic >115 mmHg)	Cancel surgery if possible and investigate. Control and re-list after 4 weeks of treatment

Figure 7 Recommendations for control of hypertension prior to surgery.

Treatment has been shown to be associated with decreased death rates from stroke and coronary heart disease in a nonsurgical setting. Hypertension should be treated to the currently recommended target of 140/90 mmHg or lower (27). Patients with relevant comorbidities, for example, diabetes or renal disease, should be treated to a lower blood pressure target. Blood pressures greater than recommended values on assessment should be referred to the general practitioner or physician for control prior to surgery (Fig. 7). Approximately 3% to 5% of hypertensive patients have a surgically correctable cause for their elevated blood pressure such as renal artery stenosis, Cushing's disease, pheochromocytoma or aldosteronoma. Phaeochromocytoma patients often have severe hypertension and carry an operative death rate in excess of 50% if untreated.

Laparoscopy in cardiac disease. Patients with severe congestive cardiac failure and valvular insufficiency are more prone to develop cardiac complications than patients with ischemic heart disease (28).

CARDIOPULMONARY TESTING

Although cardiovascular and respiratory assessment is often undertaken as a separate entity comprising of individual system assessment, it is probably of much greater relevance if they are assessed as a combined unit. CPX testing is a cost-effective, noninvasive and objective method of evaluating the pathophysiology of both the cardiovascular and respiratory systems. It classifies cardiac failure on the basis of oxygen consumption at the anaerobic threshold (AT) and the maximal aerobic capacity. As postoperative mortality following major surgery is closely related to preexisting cardiac failure, CPX is arguably now the "gold standard" for evaluation of cardiopulmonary function. CPX-derived data of cardiovascular and respiratory limitation have repeatedly emerged as precise predictors of survival rate and CPX concentrates on measurement of ventricular function, respiratory function, and cellular function via measurement of gas exchange, as well as detection of myocardial ischemia.

During the test a patient performs an increasing amount of work on an electronically braked cycle ergometer while their oxygen consumption (VO_2), carbon dioxide production (VCO_2), and tidal volumes (V_t) are measured through a tight fitting mask or mouthpiece. A 12-lead electrocardiogram (ECG) is also analyzed throughout the test to detect ECG evidence of exercise-induced myocardial ischemia and arrhythmias. After a two-minute period of rest, the subject starts to cycle at around 60 revolutions per minute (rpm) with no added load for three minutes. The work load is increased at the rate of between 5 and 20 W/min depending on the fitness of the subject. The test should last between 8 and 15 minutes and stops when the subject is unable to maintain 60 rpm.

Critical Data Derived from the Test

Anerobic Threshold

AT is the oxygen consumption of the subject at the point when the work that he or she is performing just exceeds his or her body's capacity to achieve this without the accumulation of lactic acid in the blood. It is also referred to as the lactate threshold. AT is reproducible and is effort independent (29). Work above AT results in increasing anerobic metabolism, lactic acidosis, and is nonsustainable. Carbon dioxide production increases relative to oxygen uptake at work levels in excess of AT as more carbon dioxide is generated from bicarbonate buffering of lactic acid. The AT can be identified by plotting VCO_2 against VO_2 in the V slope method (Fig. 8). The AT is the VO_2 at the break point in the relationship between VCO_2 and VO_2.

Peak VO2

Peak VO_2 is the highest value of VO_2 during the test. It is clearly effort dependent but values of over 20 mL/kg/min have been associated with a reduced mortality after major surgery.

VE/VCO2

VE/VCO_2 is the ventilatory efficiency for carbon dioxide. It reveals how efficient the lungs are at removing carbon dioxide and is increased in disorders that increase the amount of lung dead space such as COPD, cardiac failure, and pulmonary vascular diseases.

ΔVO2/Δwork rate

$\Delta VO_2/\Delta$work rate is the relationship between oxygen uptake and work. The normal subject will increase their oxygen consumption by 10 mL/min/watt. Cardiorespiratory pathology will reduce this.

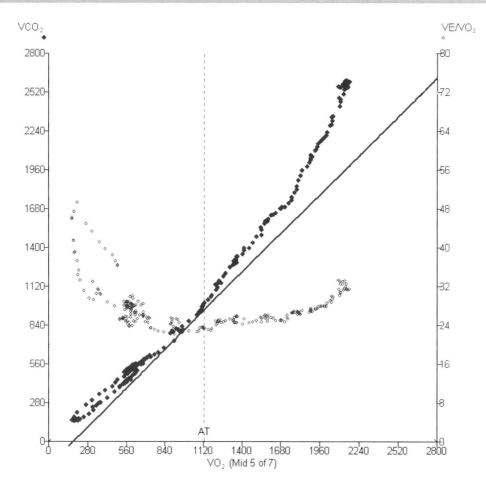

Figure 8 "V-slope" method for determining the VO_2 anaerobic threshold (AT). VCO_2 (mL/min) is plotted against VO_2 (mL/min) as represented by the solid blue points. Initially the slope is unity up to the AT as marked by the dashed green line. The gradient of the slope then increases from this deflection point as more CO_2 is produced from bicarbonate buffering of lactic acid. The VE/VO_2 as shown by the purple circles also rises after AT is passed.

O₂ pulse

O_2 pulse is the oxygen consumption per heart beat and is the product of stroke volume and the arterial-venous oxygen difference. It is reduced in conditions such as coronary artery disease, heart failure, and pulmonary vascular disorders.

AT and mortality in elderly patients

Older's group in Melbourne found that if patients above 60 years had an AT over 11 mL/kg/min then they had a much lower postoperative mortality compared to those with an AT below 11 mL/kg/min (30). Postoperative mortality was particularly high at 42% if myocardial ischemia was identified from the ECG prior to the patient reaching their AT. They went on to use CPX testing in elderly patients for major surgery to determine where they would be best managed postoperatively. Those patients deemed fit with an AT above 11 mL/kg/min and sent to the general ward had a 0% cardiovascular mortality (31). Hence, CPX testing is increasingly being used to assess fitness and predict mortality following major urological surgery

and is currently the most accurate indicator of physiological reserve.

Respiratory Assessment and Optimization

Postoperative pulmonary complications are an important cause of perioperative morbidity, mortality, and increased length of stay. The incidence of complications depends on coexisting risk factors, type, and site of surgery as well as mode of anesthesia (Fig. 9) (21,32).

A chest radiograph is indicated if active or advanced lung disease is suspected. Peak flow measurement can be useful in COPD or asthma. A baseline blood gas can also help predict the likelihood for postoperative ventilation following major surgery. It should be checked if the patient is breathless on minimal exertion or at rest, has an oxygen saturation of less than 95% on room air or is cyanosed. A resting P_aCO_2 >6.0 kPa suggests respiratory failure and is predictive of pulmonary complications.

Chronic lung disease

Anatomical chest wall deformity e.g., kyphoscoliosis, ankylosing spondylitis

Physiological restrictive lung disease e.g., neuromuscular disease

Congestive heart failure

Heavy smoking

Malnutrition

Severe obesity—this tends to reduce ventilatory compliance and functional residual capacity. Gas exchange is also impaired by altering the ventilation/perfusion relationship in the lungs.

Obstructive sleep apnea—this can result in difficulty with airway management

Duration of surgery—prolonged operations carry a higher risk although the definition of prolonged surgery ranges from two to four hours

Surgical incision site—thoraco-abdominal incisions carry a much higher risk followed by upper and lower abdominal incisions

Figure 9 Factors influencing respiratory complications following major surgery.

Pulmonary function tests (PFTs) have long been used in an attempt to stratify pulmonary risk in patients with significant respiratory disease. While no single test can effectively predict morbidity and mortality from pulmonary complications, the forced expiratory volume in the first second of forceful exhalation (FEV_1) can be a useful tool. When the FEV_1 is greater than 2 L or 50% of predicted, major complications are rare. However, routine pulmonary function testing prior to abdominal surgery has been shown to be of no additional benefit when compared with a thorough history and physical examination (33). Moreover, one of the most useful surrogate markers for respiratory outcome is adequate postoperative analgesia with movement and maintaining the ability to cough. Protecting and facilitating this ability is more valid than PFT or any other clinical markers in predicting outcome. The analgesia provided by a thoracic epidural analgesia is preferable especially if an upper abdominal or thoracoabdominal incision is utilized.

Disease Modifying Interventions

Smoking cessation. Smoking has been linked to peri- and postoperative complications with increased risk of respiratory, cardiac, wound, and infectious complications (34–36). Cessation of smoking 10 to 20 hours preoperatively lowers carboxyhemoglobin concentrations and may reduce heart rate, blood pressure, and catecholamine concentrations. The incidence of chest infections can be reduced by 50% if the patient stops smoking eight weeks before surgery with the risk falling to that of nonsmokers if cessation was for six months prior to surgery. Sputum production also declines over a six-week period if smoking is stopped. An effective smoking intervention program applied six to eight weeks before surgery has been shown to halve the frequency of postoperative complications especially those related to wound healing and the

cardiovascular insufficiency (37). Prescription of nicotine replacement therapy (transdermal patch, gum, nasal spray, and sublingual tablets) increases the rate of quitting by 50% to 70%, regardless of setting.

Medical therapy. In patients with chronic lung disease and poorly controlled asthma, the use of preoperative inhalers, nebulized bronchodilators, and/or corticosteroids may be beneficial. It may also help prevent respiratory exacerbations in the postoperative period.

Chest physiotherapy. Preoperative physiotherapy helps clear sputum and secretions. It can also educate patients to undertake regular postoperative breathing exercises.

Oxygen delivery. There is reasonable evidence supporting the benefits of preoperative oxygenation in high-risk surgical patients. When oxygen delivery falls, tissue oxygenation becomes physiologically inadequate. Optimizing such high-risk patients with fluids and inotropes can also enhance tissue perfusion and promote oxygen delivery prior to surgery (38). Currently, only about 5% of all planned elective surgical admissions to intensive care are admitted preoperatively (39).

Laparoscopy and respiratory disease (5,40). Laparoscopy results in multiple postoperative benefits allowing for quicker recovery and shorter hospital stay. However, severe lung disease is generally believed to be a contraindication to laparoscopic surgery, partly due to concerns over impaired gas exchange, hypercarbia, and pneumoperitoneum. The partial pressure of carbon dioxide in the blood ($PaCO_2$) increases because of carbon dioxide absorption from the peritoneal cavity. In compromised patients, cardiopulmonary disturbances aggravate this increase in $PaCO_2$. Adequate pain control with a thoracic epidural, careful attention to ventilation parameters, and the combination of an experienced anesthesiologist and advanced laparoscopic surgeon can enable the safe management of patients with end-stage lung disease (41).

Renal Disorders and Assessment

Renin is synthesized and stored in the juxtaglomerular apparatus of the kidney. Fall in blood pressure, ACTH, ADH, glucagon, potassium, and prostaglandins can all increase renin secretion. Through the generation of angiotensin II, it helps preserve extracellular fluid volume. Patients with renal impairment however may experience problems with fluid and electrolyte imbalance and metabolic waste product elimination. The lower the glomerular filtration rate (GFR), the more problems to be anticipated. Impaired immune function, delayed wound healing, as well as coagulation defects may also be encountered. Every effort should be made to optimize the renal function leading up to surgery.

Individuals on renal replacement therapy should undergo preoperative dialysis to improve their electrolyte and fluid balance. Close liaison with the patient's renal physician is vital. These patients often have a creatinine clearance of less than 15 mL/min resulting in fixed renal excretion of salt and water, which does not cope with acute changes. A sudden increase in fluid volume or salt concentration can lead to hypertension and congestive cardiac failure. With such a low number of functional nephrons, thiazide monotherapy is ineffective and loop diuretics are often indicated.

Drugs that may potentially affect or worsen the renal function should be utilized with caution, for example, angiotensin-converting enzyme inhibitors, nonsteroidal anti-inflammatory drugs, radiocontrast agents, metformin, and aminoglycosides. Drug doses will need to be carefully titrated on the basis of the GFR, and, as noted in the preceding text, careful attention to fluid balance and asepsis will be required to avoid deterioration in remaining renal function.

Metabolic Assessment and Optimization

Diabetes

Insulin is a key anabolic hormone. After induction of anesthesia and during surgery (ebb phase), insulin secretion is suppressed despite rising blood glucose presumably due to the effects of catecholamines and α-adrenergic inhibition of β-cell secretion within the endocrine pancreas. During the postoperative period however, in the flow phase, expression of insulin increases and insulin levels rise. Tolerance for exogenous glucose is reduced and in general, glucose levels are higher than normal resulting in the so called "insulin resistance." The resistance to insulin during the flow phase is thought to be secondary to the effect of glucocorticoids.

In diabetics undergoing surgery, optimal control of blood glucose is crucial. Hyperglycemia is associated with electrolyte disturbances, altered collagen formation, abnormalities in leukocyte function, reduced granulocyte adherence, impaired phagocytosis, delayed chemotaxis, depressed bactericidal capacity, and suppressed immune function. Ketoacidosis may develop, leading to increased carbon dioxide production and ventilatory requirements. Recent evidence suggests that perioperative hyperglycemia is the main risk factor for the development of postoperative infection in critically ill surgical patient and that intensive glucose control lowers this risk (42). Tight glycemic control in critically ill patients has also been shown to reduce mortality and hospital length of stay (43).

Hyper- and Hypothyroidism

Patients who are found to be thyrotoxic must be deferred until adequate control of the disease is achieved by medical or surgical therapy. Under normal circumstances, concentrations of total and free triiodothyronine (T_3) usually fall after surgery and normalize within a few days. Thyroid hormones stimulate the oxygen consumption of tissue resulting in increased metabolic rate and heat production. Surgery in the presence of uncontrolled thyroid disease can precipitate a thyrotoxic crisis or thyroid storm, which can be fatal. Postoperative complications (e.g., sepsis, persistent tachycardia, hypertension, hemorrhage, pyrexia) can mimic the thyrotoxic state and a high index of suspicion coupled with early recognition is paramount. In an emergency setting, the use of β-adrenergic blockers for tachycardia and α-adrenergic blockers for hypertension may be necessary.

Hypothyroidism may sometimes be difficult to identify clinically but if present should be treated by replacement therapy with thyroxine before surgery.

Adrenal Failure

The daily basal dose of corticosteroid is equivalent to 7.5 mg of prednisolone or 30 mg of hydrocortisone (44). In patients with a normal endocrine response, cortisol secretion usually rises immediately after the start of surgery and can be modified by anesthetic intervention. In primary or secondary adrenal failure, the body's physiological response to stress is impaired, and increases in cortisol levels will not occur. Patients who have been on long-term high dose steroids will also lack such a response because of suppression of the hypothalamic corticotropin-releasing hormone and pituitary adrenocorticotropic hormone secretion. Such individuals may have mild symptoms of adrenal insufficiency such as fatigue, malaise, arthralgia, depression, nausea, and low-grade fever. These patients usually respond poorly to stress. Failure of cortisol secretion may result in the circulatory collapse and hypotension characteristic of an "Addisonian" crisis.

Pre- and perioperative steroid cover will be required in the following group of patients:

1. Patients who are currently on daily dose of ≥10 mg prednisolone (or equivalent). Equivalent doses include methylprednisolone 4 mg, dexamethasone 6 mg, and hydrocortisone 20 mg.
2. Patients who have received longer than one-week course of ≥10 mg prednisolone daily in the last three months. This is because adrenal suppression can occur after one week and may take up to three months to recover (45).
3. Patients on high-dose inhaled corticosteroids, for example, beclomethasone 1.5 mg daily)

Equivalent daily doses are also recommended in the postoperative period until the patient is able to resume their usual oral medication (Fig. 10).

	On induction	Post operative
Minor surgery	Continue with usual regime	
Intermediate surgery	25 mg hydrocortisone parenteral	Resume usual regime if able to eat and drink
Major surgery	25 mg hydrocortisone parenteral	25 mg six hourly for 3 days followed by maintenance dose

Figure 10 Suggested regime for steroid replacement in adrenal insufficiency.

Liver Disorders and Assessment

One of the most useful indicators of surgical risk in liver failure patients is the Child-Pugh score (46,47) (Figs. 11, 12), although the newer MELD (Model for End-Stage Liver Disease) score takes into account serum creatinine as well and may be a better predictor of survival (48). The cornerstones of perioperative management are medical treatment of the complications of liver disease, including coagulopathy, ascites, encephalopathy, and malnutrition. These individuals are at an increased risk of bleeding, sepsis, acute renal failure, respiratory distress syndrome, and postoperative hepatic decompensation including hepatic coma or death. Therefore, the decision to perform surgery in these patients must be carefully weighed.

Measure	A	B	C
Points (per field)	1	2	3
Bilirubin (μmol/l)	< 34	34–50	> 50
Albumin (g/L)	> 35	30–35	< 30
INR	< 1.7	1.70–2.20	> 2.20
Ascites	None	Slight	Moderate
Neurological state	None	Minimal	Coma

Figure 11 Relative risk of a surgical procedure for patients with liver cirrhosis (Child-Pugh score). *Abbreviation*: INR: International normalized ratio.

Total score	5–6	7–9	10–15
Operative mortality	0–5%	10–15%	> 25%

Figure 12 Prediction of operative mortality based on Child-Pugh scores.

Neurological Disorders and Assessment

Specific consideration should be given to assessment of any associated respiratory impairment including weakness of the respiratory muscles and the inability to clear secretions. Patients who suffer from autonomic dysfunction may have a labile blood pressure and in such patients, urinary retention, arrhythmias, delayed gastric emptying, and sudden cardiac arrest may be triggered by sympathetic stimulation, blood loss, and postural change. Useful bedside tests of autonomic function include orthostatic hypotension (a drop of >30 mmHg systolic pressure indicates autonomic dysfunction) and reduced heart rate in response to the Valsalva maneuver.

Patients with dementia, learning difficulties, and Alzheimer's disease can become extremely confused, agitated, and disorientated in a surgical ward. They may also not be able to give a coherent history and attempts to speak to relatives, next of kin or carers are mandatory.

Musculoskeletal Disorders and Assessment

Patients with rheumatoid arthritis can have unstable necks, limited neck movement, or reduced mouth opening, and flexion/extension radiographs of the neck are required before general anesthesia. Similarly, patients with severe ankylosing spondylitis can experience problems with intubation, and the anesthetist should be warned in advance in case a fiberoptic intubation is necessary.

Muscular dystrophy can pose a problem postoperatively because of excessive secretions and respiratory problems. Preoperative chest physiotherapy and nebulizers may be beneficial if major surgery is planned.

Hematological Disorders and Assessment

A careful history may reveal features of excessive bleeding after previous surgery, nose bleeds, spontaneous bruising, or a family history of bleeding disorders. A coagulation screen is necessary for all such patients. If this is normal and the index of suspicion is high for an inherited or acquired defect of coagulation, more sophisticated clotting studies may be required, including a factor VII assay.

In a study of patients with idiopathic thrombocytopenic purpura, bleeding after trauma was uncommon unless the platelet count was less than $60,000/\mu L$. Surgical bleeding due solely to a reduced platelet count does not generally occur until the platelet count is less than $50,000/\mu L$, while clinical or spontaneous bleeding does not occur until the platelet count is less than 10,000 to $20,000/\mu L$ (49).

Patients with hematological malignancy, hemoglobinopathies (e.g., sickle cell disease, thalassemia), or other blood dyscrasias may require no additional intervention prior to surgery but if in doubt a hematological opinion should be sought. In the case of known multiple red cell antibodies, appropriately cross-matched blood products will be required well in advance of any procedure where significant blood loss is likely. If a patient is known to have severe clotting factor deficiencies, 4 to 6 units of fresh frozen plasma should be administered prior to surgery.

Most anesthetists would regard a preoperative hemoglobin of greater than 10 g/dL as adequate, although lower levels may be accepted in chronic disease or procedures where minimal blood loss is expected. One alternative would be to consider autologous predeposit (blood banking) if the patient is fit enough and there is a greater than 50% chance of significant blood loss requiring blood products. Arrangements for intraoperative red blood cell salvage during major surgery offer an alternative to allogeneic or predonated autologous blood transfusion.

In patients who object to blood transfusion on religious or other grounds, the use erythropoietin may be considered. It should be administered at least four weeks before elective surgery and requires careful monitoring.

Immunological Disorders and Assessment

Immunological conditions like immune thrombocytopenic purpura, Guillain–Barré syndrome, and Lambert–Eaton (myasthenic) syndrome require discussion with the anesthetist and responsible physician before surgery. Pre-anesthetic treatment with intravenous immunoglobulins may be advised in some cases. Immunosuppressed patients, either as a result of disease or medical therapy, are potentially at higher risk of sepsis. They may require additional antibiotic prophylaxis in the pre-, peri-, and postoperative period depending on the surgical procedure undertaken.

Microbiological Assessment and Antibiotic Prophylaxis

Urine

Routine preoperative testing and treatment of urine is advisable in patients undergoing endoscopic, percutaneous, or open stone surgery. However, bladder urine culture has been found to correlate poorly with infection in the upper urinary tract (50), while positive stone culture and renal pelvic urine culture are better predictors of potential urosepsis (51). The antibiotic of choice depends on surgeon preference and local protocol.

During the last decade, community-acquired extended-spectrum β-lactamase (ESBL)-producing *Escherichia coli* have been increasingly recognized in the community. These organisms are most often isolated from the urinary tract but have also been isolated from the blood. Advancing age, female gender, foreign travel, requirement for hemodialysis, urinary incontinence, bladder cancer, prostate cancer, urolithiasis, urethral catheter, diabetes mellitus, prior ESBL colonization, and recent hospitalization are important risk factors for developing ESBL-producing bacterial infections (52,53). In addition, previous urological operations and fluoroquinolone or cephalosporin use during the last three months were found to be independent risk factors (53). This is of great importance in planning empirical antibiotic therapy.

Methicillin-Resistant Staphylococcus aureus

In United Kingdom, the Department of Health has indicated that methicillin-resistant staphylococcus aureus (MRSA) screening for all elective admissions should be introduced by March 2009 (54). This excludes elective day-case endoscopic procedures. The specific sites have not been stated although all screening must include the nose with consideration to groin, perineum, axilla, urine from catheterized patients and skin lesions or wounds. Ideally, this should be undertaken at the preoperative clinic at least six to nine weeks before admission.

Antibiotic Prophylaxis (55)

Endoscopic surgery. No prophylaxis is required for uncomplicated procedures unless there is a history of genitourinary infection, recent instrumentation, institutionalization, bacterial colonization, or other risk factors like diabetes mellitus, malnutrition, and immunosuppression. All patients undergoing transurethral resection (TUR) of the prostate, ureteroscopy for proximal or impacted stone and percutaneous nephrolithotomy should be given antibiotic prophylaxis peroperatively. Antibiotics may also be used in patients who have an indwelling urinary catheter, ureteral stent, or nephrostomy tube. Routine, uncomplicated procedures like cystoscopy, bladder tumor resection, and ureteroscopy for distal stone do not typically require antibiotic cover.

Open and laparoscopic surgery. No prophylaxis is required for clean procedures. Surgery involving opening of the urinary tract should receive a single or one-day dosage of antibiotic prophylaxis, while a slightly longer course is recommended in procedures using bowel segments or implantation of prosthetic devices.

Typically, cephalosporins, fluoroquinolones, and aminoglycosides are used, although the choice of antimicrobials should be based on procedure type, knowledge of the local pathogen profile, antibiotic sensitivity, and patient allergies.

Nutritional Status Assessment

All patients should have their height and weight measured to calculate their body mass index (BMI). Obesity may be defined as a BMI >30 kg/m^2, while morbid obesity refers to those with a BMI >40 kg/m^2. These patients may have problems with reduced respiratory functional residual capacity and desaturation, obstructive sleep apnea, impaired glucose tolerance (or undiagnosed diabetes), difficult intubation, and uncontrolled hypertension (56). They are also at much higher risk of thromboembolism and should receive both mechanical and pharmacological thromboprophylaxis. A supervised exercise program and dietician referral may be beneficial, leading up to surgery.

On the other hand, poor nutritional status is often a neglected condition that is only addressed in the postoperative period. A weight loss of more than 10% is a risk factor for increased postoperative morbidity and mortality rates. Chronic hypoalbuminemia with serum albumin levels less than 30 g/L are associated with visceral protein mass depletion. Malnutrition can predispose to delayed ambulation, respiratory complications, wound infection, and poor wound healing. It is important to identify at-risk patients early to facilitate recovery following major abdominal and pelvic surgery. Perioperative nutritional support in these patients decreases postoperative complications such as wound infections and sepsis (57), and preoperative nutritional support should also be considered in patients with loss of >20% of their normal body weight. In general, enteral feeding is preferred to total parenteral nutrition (TPN). Dietician referral in conjunction with high-calorie build-up drinks prior to surgery may be beneficial in mild to moderately malnourished patients.

OTHER SPECIFIC CONSIDERATIONS

Thromboprophylaxis (58,59)

Patients undergoing urological surgery can be stratified according to low, medium, or high risk of developing venous thromboembolism (60) (Fig. 13). Contributory risk factors include increasing age, high BMI, poor mobility, multiple medical problems, and surgical factors. Open pelvic, perineal, and abdominal surgery of longer than 30 minutes duration carry significantly higher risk than a short inguinal,

scrotal, or endoscopic case. Patients who have been on long haul travel of more than four hours duration within the last week as well as those on the combined oral contraceptive are also at higher risk. Patients should be advised to stop such hormone medication four weeks before elective surgery if major surgery is contemplated.

Depending on the patients' risk category several modalities can be utilized to reduce the chance of a thromboembolic event. Most hospitals will have a local policy that can be consulted. Below is a suggested guideline (Fig. 14).

In a recently published guideline, the American Urological Association recommends early ambulation for the vast majority of patients undergoing transurethral procedures, with the use of compression stockings, mechanical prophylaxis, and low-dose unfractionated

		Distal DVT (%)	Proximal DVT (%)	PE (%)
Low risk	Minor surgery Operation time < 30 minutes duration Age < 40 No other risk factors	<10	<1	<0.01
Moderate risk	Moderate surgery Operation time > 30 minutes duration Age > 40 Presence of risk factors such as obesity, active malignancy, sepsis, use of combined estrogen oral contraceptives, varicose veins or immobilization Major medical illness (chronic heart failure, chronic lung disease, inflammatory bowel disease, malignancy)	10-40	1-10	0.1-1
High risk	Major surgery Operation time > 30 minutes duration Major abdominal or pelvic surgery for malignancy Previous DVT or PE Hypercoagulable state (Factor V Leiden mutation, deficiencies in protein S, protein C and antithrombin III, prothrombin gene mutation, anti-phospholipid antibody syndrome) Trauma to thorax, abdomen, pelvis, spine or lower limbs	40-80	10-20	1-5

Figure 13 Risk factors and incidence of postoperative thromboembolism in patients undergoing elective surgery. *Abbreviations*: DVT, deep vein thrombosis; PE, pulmonary embolism. *Source*: Modified from Ref. 60.

	Low risk	Moderate risk	High risk
Early ambulation	Yes	Yes	Yes
Graduated anti-embolism stockings[a]	Yes	Yes	Yes
Subcutaneous low molecular weight heparin (LMWH)		Yes, at standard dose (e.g. enoxaparin 20mg subcutaneous)	Yes, but at higher dose (e.g. enoxaparin 40mg subcutaneous)
Intermittent pneumatic compression or foot impulse devices		Yes	Yes
Postoperative LMWH and mechanical prophylaxis			Consider

[a] *Unless contraindicated e.g. established peripheral arterial disease or diabetic neuropathy*

Figure 14 Risk stratification and surgical thromboprophylaxis.

Hypercoagulable state (Factor V Leiden mutation, deficiencies in protein S, protein C and antithrombin III, prothrombin gene mutation, anti-phospholipid antibody syndrome)
Recent thromboembolic episode within the last 1 to 3 months
Mechanical heart valve
Atrial fibrillation with a history of cardioembolism
Recurrent pulmonary emboli or deep vein thrombosis

Figure 15 High-risk patients where bridging from warfarin to subcutaneous low molecular weight heparin or intravenous unfractionated heparin is required.

heparin (LDUH) or low molecular weight heparin (LMWH) reserved for high-risk patients (61). For open urologic surgery, complex anti-incontinence, and pelvic reconstructive surgery, a combination of mechanical and pharmacologic prophylaxis (LDUH or LMWH) is recommended. However, due to some concerns about the risk of retroperitoneal bleeding at time of urologic laparoscopic and/or robotically assisted surgery, the use of mechanical prophylaxis is recommended intra-operatively other than in the high risk group where additional pharmacologic prophylaxis may be useful.

Anticoagulation Therapy Dicontinuation

The peak effects of warfarin occur two to three days after a dose with the overall effect lasting up to five days. In atrial fibrillation, the risk of stroke doubles when international normalized ratio (INR) falls to subtherapeutic levels. A systematic review from 2003 showed that discontinuation of warfarin without administration of intravenous unfractionated heparin carries a 0.6% risk of perioperative thromboembolic event (62). High-risk patients should be administered subcutaneous LMWH once the INR falls below therapeutic levels (Fig. 15). Bridging from warfarin to intravenous heparin is recommended in patients with mechanical heart valves and those with a recent venous thromboembolic episode (within the previous 4 weeks) (63). Where possible, surgery should be postponed for three to six months if there has been a recent thromboembolic event. In low risk patients, warfarin can be stopped three to five days before surgery and resumed the same day once surgery is complete unless there is excessive bleeding.

Antiplatelet Therapy Discontinuation

The use of antiplatelet agents in primary and secondary prevention of MI is increasingly common. The effect of antiplatelets are irreversible for the life of the platelet (14 days), and its function returns to normal only once new platelets are released into the circulation.

Current guidelines published by the U.K. National Institute for Health and Clinical Excellence (NICE) recommend that antiplatelet therapy (aspirin and clopidogrel) should be continued for one year after a non-ST-segment elevation acute coronary syndrome and for four weeks after an ST elevation MI (64). This combination should also be continued for one year following any percutaneous coronary intervention (e.g., stenting, angioplasty), as it reduces risk of death, MIs, in-stent thrombosis, and stroke (65). Clopidogrel is regarded as mandatory until the coronary stents are fully endothelialized, which takes 3 months for bare metal stents, but up to 1 year for drug-eluting stents. Patients who stop clopidogrel within 30 days of stent placement are 10 times more likely to die especially as stent thrombosis carries a 20% risk of mortality (66). Late stent thrombosis rates are relatively low with short-term discontinuation of clopidogrel in patients with drug-eluting stents providing aspirin therapy is maintained (67).

There is currently insufficient evidence to suggest that low-dose aspirin (75 mg) significantly increases morbidity or mortality after TURP or other urological procedures. One study has, however, shown that aspirin at a dose of 150 mg daily carries a higher risk of bleeding after TURP and recommends that it should be discontinued 10 days before surgery (although transfusion rates were not significantly higher) (68).

The risk of bleeding with dipyridamole (antiplatelet and vasodilator) is thought to be less and probably not clinically significant. There was no statistically significant difference between the incidences of major (combination 3% vs. aspirin alone 4%) or minor (both 12%) bleeding (69).

In all cases, antiplatelet therapy should be restarted as soon as it is safe so to do. Early aspirin initiation after lower urinary tract surgery has not been shown to carry an increased risk of postoperative bleeding. In summary, the decision to discontinue these agents needs to be weighed against the risk of serious or life-threatening cardiac events (70). Such judgment depends on the type of surgery and merits discussion between the surgeon, anesthetist, and cardiologist.

Substance Abuse

Patients with a history of substance abuse (drugs or alcohol) undergoing surgery are likely to experience withdrawal symptoms while in hospital. All patients should be asked about the number of units of alcohol consumed in a typical week. The current medically recommended units of alcohol per week are 14 for women and 21 for men. A more detailed history should be taken if their intake is above that recommended. A simple, quick method is to use the Fast Alcohol Screening Test (FAST) that consists of four simple questions (71). Signs of alcohol withdrawal such as tremor, sweating, intoxication, confusion, or stigmata of liver disease should heighten awareness and under these circumstances appropriate, timely inpatient prescription of benzodiazepines can be extremely useful in managing the condition. A reducing chlordiazepoxide regime over a three- to five-day period may be necessary if prolonged recovery and inpatient stay is likely.

Allergy and Drug Intolerance

The estimated risk of anaphylaxis in the general population is 1% to 2% for insect stings and foods, with a lower reported prevalence for drugs and latex (72), but in spite of being so uncommon intraoperative anaphylactic reactions are a constant concern to the anesthesiologist. The incidence of such reactions in anesthetized patients ranges between 1 per 5000 and 1 per 25,000, mortality being 3% to 4% (73). A thorough assessment includes adequate knowledge of known allergies, drug sensitivities, and past reactions to anesthetics. There may be a documented allergy to anesthetic drugs, analgesics, local anesthetics, muscle relaxants, or latex. A family history of malignant hyperpyrexia, pseudocholinesterase deficiency, and porphyria may warn the anesthetist of future potential problems. Allergy history may be obtained from a number of sources, for example, the patient or their carers, general practitioners, care homes, and hospital notes. This should be clearly recorded according to trust documentation policy.

The incidence of latex allergy is slightly higher in health care workers, rubber industry workers, and patients with neural tube defects (including spina bifida) due to recurrent bladder catheterizations. Patients with latex allergy require special preparation of the operation theater and such cases should be undertaken first on the morning list to allow latex dust to settle. Depending on the number of air changes within the room, sufficient time should be allowed to reduce any aerosolized natural rubber latex proteins in the atmosphere. Adequate coordination of the entire surgical staff together with replacement of any anesthetic and surgical material containing latex are all mandatory to prevent severe hypersensitivity reactions.

Pregnancy

In a large study of nonobstetric surgery undertaken during pregnancy, an operative rate of 0.75% was reported (74). Surgery and anesthesia in pregnancy increase the risk of miscarriage in the first trimester from 5% to 8%, and the risk of premature labor from 5% to 7.5% (75). Where possible, it is sensible to delay nonurgent surgery until the second trimester.

RISK ASSESSMENT FOR EMERGENCY SURGERY

Assessment of patients requiring emergency surgery depends on their current presenting condition and associated background comorbidities. As time is often the greatest limiting factor for successful optimization of any risk factors present, two questions need to be addressed from the outset.

- Can surgery be delayed until their medical condition has been optimized?
- Do the risks of surgery outweigh the benefits?

Clearly if the risk of significant morbidity or death from the patient's condition outweighs the risk of surgical related mortality, then it may be deemed appropriate to proceed with surgery providing the surgeon, anesthetist, and patient are all in agreement. Often, a degree of medical optimization can occur prior to surgery, and the conditions that can be improved by medical management should be identified and targeted. Particular attention to adequate oxygenation, optimal fluid resuscitation, and correction of electrolyte and blood gas abnormalities (e.g., acidosis, hypercarbia) will be required and it is helpful to inform and involve the critical care team (and the anesthetist) from the outset if resuscitation with invasive monitoring is required. Such patients are best managed in the high dependency or intensive care unit. Diabetic patients require tight glycemic control with a sliding scale to avoid ketoacidosis, reduce sepsis, and decrease mortality. In patients with renal failure, there is no evidence to suggest that measures used to protect the kidneys during the perioperative period are beneficial. There is no difference in morbidity (renal failure) or mortality following the use of various perioperative interventions including the use of dopamine and its analogues, diuretics, calcium channel blockers, angiotensin-converting inhibitors, or hydration fluid (76). Immediate assessment and prompt recognition of comorbidities coupled with timely intervention will enable the patient to tolerate the hemodynamic insults imposed by surgery as much as possible, and this can make the difference between a successful outcome and mortality.

SPECIFIC SURGICAL PROBLEMS

Transurethral Resection Syndrome

TUR syndrome is most commonly associated with transurethral resections of the prostate and has an incidence of 0.5% to 2%. It can also occur following large bladder tumor resections and percutaneous nephrolithotomy. It occurs because of the adverse effects of excessive irrigation fluid absorption when glycine 1.5% is used. Prolonged resection time (>60–90 minutes), large vascular gland resection, presence of capsular perforation, and continuous flow resection are thought to predispose to this complication.

The osmolality of 1.5% glycine is 230 mosm/L compared to serum osmolality of 290 mosm/L and hence dilutional hyponatremia and fluid overload will occur with excessive glycine absorption (Fig. 16). Glycine itself is toxic to the heart, central nervous system, and retina and may lead to hyperammonemia. The inclusion of 1% ethanol in the glycine bags allows detection of excessive absorption by measuring the ethanol concentration in expired breath (77). Although a rising breath ethanol level suggests absorption, it is unpredictable and does not prevent TUR syndrome. Early signs of glycine absorption include prickling sensations and facial warmth. A spectrum of symptoms and signs can follow ranging from nausea, tachycardia, restlessness, dyspnea, arrhythmias, hyper- or hypotension, transient blindness, confusion, seizures, coma and death (78).

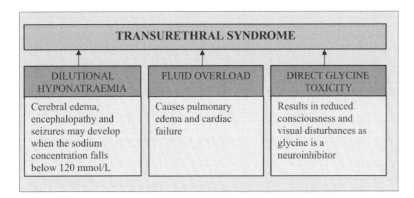

Figure 16   Pathophysiology of TUR syndrome.

Investigations

Low serum sodium can confirm the diagnosis; levels below 120 mmol/L commonly cause symptoms and a rapid fall is most likely to lead to problems. At sodium levels below 115 mmol/L, electrocardiography may show QRS widening, ST segment elevation and T wave inversion. A low-serum osmolality and high anion gap may be present.

Management

If possible, stop further resection and control the bleeding. Patients may need to be sedated and ventilated if awake. Slow correction of hyponatremia with intravenous furosemide to promote a diuresis is recommended although some authorities maintain that intravenous hypertonic saline is the treatment of choice (79). The serum sodium should be increased by about 1 mmol/L/hr as rapid correction has been implicated with central pontine myelinolysis. In the presence of intractable seizures or encephalopathy, the sodium level may be corrected more rapidly at a rate of up to 8 to 10 mmol/L/hr, and this level should be checked every few hours.

Undoubtedly, the best management is prevention: limiting resection time, careful surgical technique, and appropriate patient selection are important factors to consider. Newer techniques, such as bipolar resection, laser ablation, and photoselective vaporization, which use saline as the irrigating fluid, can prevent the risk of TUR syndrome.

Sepsis

Sepsis following urological procedures may present with unexplained hypotension, rigors, shock, or systemic inflammatory response syndrome (leucocytosis or leucopenia, fever or hypothermia, tachycardia, tachypnea). Early recognition is paramount as these signs may be the first event in a cascade to multiorgan failure. Once established, aggressive fluid resuscitation in conjunction with early transfer to a high dependency or intensive care unit for invasive monitoring, inotropic support, and organ support can be the difference between life and death. Mortality is considerably increased when severe sepsis or septic shock are present (up to a 50%).

Gas Embolism

Laparoscopic urological surgery has increasingly become accepted as an alternative to open surgical techniques. Carbon dioxide (CO_2) is the most commonly used gas to create a pneumoperitoneum and inadvertent rapid insufflation directly into the blood stream or solid organ can result in gas embolism. Most cases occur immediately after the pneumoperitoneum is established. A large embolus can cause a "gas lock" resulting in ineffective right ventricular contraction, arrhythmias, profound hypotension, and cardiac arrest. Although rare it is potentially fatal with a reported incidence of 15 per 100,000 cases per year (80). Signs include cyanosis, hypoxia, a mill-wheel cardiac murmur and sudden hypotension in the setting of reduced end-tidal CO_2, and decreased chest compliance. Transesophageal echocardiography may help confirm the diagnosis. The mainstay of treatment is to remove the pneumoperitoneum, hyperventilate with 100% oxygen, and place the patient in a head down left lateral decubitus position. A central venous catheter should be placed into the right atrium if not already present and blood withdrawn (typically foamy blood) to aspirate the embolus.

Problems Due to Inappropriate Patient Positioning

The lithotomy position may cause nerve compression, dislocation of hip prostheses, lower leg compartment syndrome, and respiratory compromise in patients with preexisting lung disease. Postoperative injuries to the common peroneal nerve (especially from pressure effects exerted by the stirrups), ulnar nerve, sciatic nerve, brachial plexus, obturator nerve, and lateral cutaneous nerve of the thigh have also been described.

The steep head down Trendelenburg position utilized during robotic prostatectomy can cause shoulder and nerve palsies. If shoulder braces are used to prevent the patient sliding, the clavicle can be pushed up into the brachial plexus. Also when the hip is abducted more than 30°, obturator nerve strain and leg pain is more likely to occur although the addition of 45° hip flexion or greater can alleviate the strain (81). Rhabdomyolysis has been reported after prolonged positioning in the extended lateral decubitus position for nephrectomies. The use of a subaxillary roll is important to prevent excessive traction of the brachial plexus. Care must be taken to avoid excessive arm abduction and rotation and to ensure that all pressure points are adequately padded (81).

Intraoperative Priapism

Priapism during a cystoscopic procedure can occur because of surgical stimulation when depth of anesthesia is inadequate. It is usually sufficient to stop the stimulus for a few minutes and deepen the general anesthesia. A small dose of intravenous ketamine or β-blocker (e.g., propranolol 1 mg) can also be useful. If such measures fail, it may be necessary to aspirate corporeal blood or administer a small intracavernosal dose of an alpha-adrenergic agonist (250 µg of phenylephrine). Resolution usually occurs within 5 to 20 minutes.

Obturator Spasm

Obturator spasm occurs when the obturator nerve is directly stimulated by diathermy current. The nerve runs adjacent to the lateral walls of the bladder, and resection of lateral wall bladder tumors can cause direct stimulation of the nerve resulting in sudden, violent adduction of the hip (adductor jerk). This increases the risk of bladder perforation, incomplete tumor resection, and obturator hematomas. Reducing the diathermy current, transpositioning of inactive electrode from buttock to thigh, using combined general anesthesia and muscle relaxants, resection of tumor in smaller chips, shifting to saline irrigation and preventing over distension of the bladder can all help reduce the magnitude of adductor spasm. Obturator nerve blocks (3 cm lateral and 3 cm inferior to the pubic tubercle) can also be beneficial.

REFERENCES

1. Palmer QB. Physiologic responses to surgery and injury. In: John DC, Robin CNW, eds. Surgery. London: Mosby, 2001:section 1:3.1–3.18.
2. Desborough JP. The stress response to trauma and surgery. Br J Anaesth 2005; 85:109–117.
3. Kehlet H. Multimodal approach to control postoperative pathophysiology and rehabilitation. Br J Anaesth 1997; 78:606–617.
4. Burgos FJ, Linares A, Pascual J, et al. Modifications of renal blood flow and serum interleukin levels induced by laparoscopic and open living donor nephrectomies for kidney transplant: an experimental study in pigs. Transplant Proc 2005; 37:3676–3678.
5. Conacher ID, Soomro NA, Rix D. Anaesthesia for laparoscopic urological surgery. Br J Anaesth 2004; 93:859–864.
6. Vallencian G, Guillonneau B, Fournier G, et al. Laparoscopic Radical Prostatectomy: Technical Manual. Paris: Les Editions, 2002.
7. Department of Health. Day surgery: Operational Guide. Waiting, Booking and Choice. London: DoH, 2002.
8. The NHS Plan—A plan for investment, A plan for reform. HMSO, The Copyright Unit, St Clements House, 2–16 Colegate, Norwich NR3 1BQ, 2000.
9. Audit Commission. Day surgery: Review of national findings. Audit Commission, London 2001.
10. Cahill CJ. Basket cases and trolleys—day surgery proposals for the millennium. J One Day Surg 1999; 9:11–12.
11. British Association of Day Surgery. BADS directory of procedures. London: British Association of Day Surgery, 2007.
12. Golash A, Luscombe C, Rajjayabun P, et al. The expansion of laparoscopic day case major urological procedures; an initial experience. J One Day Surg 2007; 17(suppl):B1.
13. Department of Health. NHS Modernisation Agency. Day surgery: A Good Practice Guide. London: DoH, 2004.
14. Department of Health. NHS Modernisation Agency. National Good Practice Guidelines on Pre-Operative Assessment for Day Surgery. London: DoH, 2002.
15. Fleisher LA, Beckman JA, Brown KA, et al. ACC/AHA 2007 Guidelines on Perioperative Cardiovascular Evaluation and Care for Noncardiac Surgery: Executive Summary: A Report of the American College of Cardiology/American Heart Association Task Force on Practice Guidelines (Writing Committee to Revise the 2002 Guidelines on Perioperative Cardiovascular Evaluation for Noncardiac Surgery) Developed in Collaboration With the American Society of Echocardiography, American Society of Nuclear Cardiology, Heart Rhythm Society, Society of Cardiovascular Anesthesiologists, Society for Cardiovascular Angiography and Interventions, Society for Vascular Medicine and Biology, and Society for Vascular Surgery. J Am Coll Cardiol 2007; 50:1707–1732.
16. Foster ED, Davis KB, Carpenter JA, et al. Risk of noncardiac operation in patients with defined coronary disease: The Coronary Artery Surgery Study (CASS) registry experience. Ann Thorac Surg 1986; 41:42–50.
17. Eagle KA, Rihal CS, Mickel MC, et al. Cardiac risk of noncardiac surgery: influence of coronary disease and type of surgery in 3368 operations. CASS Investigators and University of Michigan Heart Care Program. Coronary Artery Surgery Study. Circulation 1997; 96:1882–1887.
18. Goldman L, Caldera DL, Nussbaum SR, et al. Multifactorial index of cardiac risk in noncardiac surgical procedures. N Engl J Med 1977; 297:845–850.
19. Detsky AS, Abrams HB, Forbath N, et al. Cardiac assessment for patients undergoing noncardiac surgery. A multifactorial clinical risk index. Arch Intern Med 1986; 146:2131–2134.
20. Tarhan S, Moffitt EA, Taylor WF, et al. Myocardial infarction after general anesthesia. Anesth Analg 1977; 56:455–461.
21. Rao TL, Jacobs KH, El-Etr AA. Reinfarction following anesthesia in patients with myocardial infarction. Anesthesiology 1983; 59:499–505.
22. Falter F, Martinelli G. Perioperative care of the patient with cardiovascular disease undergoing non-cardiac surgery. Surgery (Oxford) 2005; 23:246–250.
23. Radford MJ, Krumholz HM. Beta-blockers after myocardial infarction—for few patients, or many? N Engl J Med 1998; 339:551–553.
24. Foex P. Pharmacology of cardiovascular drugs. Clin Anaesthesiol 1989; 3:131–161.
25. Richey R, Wray D, Stokes T. Prophylaxis against infective endocarditis: summary of NICE guidance. BMJ 2008; 336:770–771.
26. Kannel WB, Castelli WP, McNamara PM, et al. Role of blood pressure in the development of congestive heart

failure. The Framingham study. N Engl J Med 1972; 287:781–787.

27. National Collaborating Centre for Chronic Conditions. Hypertension: Management in Adults in Primary Care: Pharmacological Update. London: Royal College of Physicians, 2006.

28. Midgley S, Tolley D. Anaesthesia for Laparoscopic Surgery in Urology. EAU-EBU Update Series. 2006; 4:241–245.

29. Kothmann E, Danjoux G, Owen SJ, et al. Reliability of the anaerobic threshold in cardiopulmonary exercise testing of patients with abdominal aortic aneurysms. Anaesthesia 2009; 64:9–13.

30. Older P, Smith R, Courtney P, et al. Preoperative evaluation of cardiac failure and ischemia in elderly patients by cardiopulmonary exercise testing. Chest 1993; 104:701–704.

31. Older P, Hall A, Hader R. Cardiopulmonary exercise testing as a screening test for perioperative management of major surgery in the elderly. Chest 1999; 116:355–362.

32. Smetana GW, Lawrence VA, Cornell JE. Preoperative pulmonary risk stratification for noncardiothoracic surgery: systematic review for the American College of Physicians. Ann Intern Med 2006; 144:581–595.

33. Lawrence VA, Page CP, Harris GD. Preoperative spirometry before abdominal operations. A critical appraisal of its predictive value. Arch Intern Med 1989; 149:280–285.

34. Morton HJV. Tobacco smoking and pulmonary complications after operation. Lancet 1944; 1:368–370.

35. Jorgensen LN, Kallehave F, Christensen E, et al. Less collagen production in smokers. Surgery 1998; 123:450–455.

36. Bluman LG, Mosca L, Newman N, et al. Preoperative smoking habits and postoperative pulmonary complications. Chest 1998; 113:883–889.

37. Moller AM, Villebro N, Pedersen T, et al. Effect of preoperative smoking intervention on postoperative complications: a randomised clinical trial. Lancet 2002; 359:114–117.

38. Wilson J, Woods I, Fawcett J, et al. Reducing the risk of major elective surgery: randomised controlled trial of preoperative optimisation of oxygen delivery. BMJ 1999; 318:1099–1103.

39. Intensive Care National Audit and Research Centre. Annual report from the national case mix programme database. London: Intensive Care National Audit and Research Centre, 1998.

40. Kaba A, Joris J. Anaesthesia for laparoscopic surgery. Current Anaesthesia and Critical Care 2001; 12:159–165.

41. Linden PA, Gilbert RJ, Yeap BY, et al. Laparoscopic fundoplication in patients with end-stage lung disease awaiting transplantation. J Thorac Cardiovasc Surg 2006; 131:438–446.

42. Ramos M, Khalpey Z, Lipsitz S, et al. Relationship of perioperative hyperglycemia and postoperative infections in patients who undergo general and vascular surgery. Ann Surg 2008; 248:585–591.

43. van den Berghe G, Wouters P, Weekers F, et al. Intensive insulin therapy in the critically ill patients. N Engl J Med 2001; 345:1359–1367.

44. Byyny RL. Preventing adrenal insufficiency during surgery. Postgrad Med 1980; 67:219–225, 228.

45. LaRochelle GE Jr, LaRochelle AG, Ratner RE, et al. Recovery of the hypothalamic-pituitary-adrenal (HPA) axis in patients with rheumatic diseases receiving low-dose prednisone. Am J Med 1993; 95:258–264.

46. Child CG, Turcotte JG. Surgery and portal hypertension. In: The liver and portal hypertension. Philadelphia: Saunders, 1964:50–64.

47. Pugh RN, Murray-Lyon IM, Dawson JL, et al. Transection of the oesophagus for bleeding oesophageal varices. Br J Surg 1973; 60:646–649.

48. Malinchoc M, Kamath PS, Gordon FD, et al. A model to predict poor survival in patients undergoing transjugular intrahepatic portosystemic shunts. Hepatology 2000; 31:864–871.

49. Lacey JV, Penner JA. Management of idiopathic thrombocytopenic purpura in the adult. Semin Thromb Hemost 1977; 3:160–174.

50. Mariappan P, Tolley DA. Endoscopic stone surgery: minimizing the risk of post-operative sepsis. Curr Opin Urol 2005; 15:101–105.

51. Mariappan P, Smith G, Bariol SV, et al. Stone and pelvic urine culture and sensitivity are better than bladder urine as predictors of urosepsis following percutaneous nephrolithotomy: a prospective clinical study. J Urol 2005; 173:1610–1614.

52. Laupland KB, Church DL, Vidakovich J, et al. Community-onset extended-spectrum beta-lactamase (ESBL) producing Escherichia coli: importance of international travel. J Infect 2008; 57:441–448.

53. Yilmaz E, Akalin H, Ozbey S, et al. Risk factors in community-acquired/onset urinary tract infections due to extended-spectrum beta-lactamase-producing Escherichia coli and Klebsiella pneumoniae. J Chemother 2008; 20: 581–585.

54. MRSA—Operational Guidance (Gateway reference 10324), Department of Health, Crown copyright. 2008. Available at: http://www.dh.gov.uk/en/Publicationsandstatistics/Lettersandcirculars/Dearcolleagueletters/DH_086687.

55. Grabe M, Bishop MC, Bjerklund-Johansen TE, et al. Guidelines on the management of urinary and male genital tract infections: Peri-operative antibacterial prophylaxis in urology. Arnhem, The Netherlands: European Association of Urology (EAU), 2008:90–99.

56. The Association of Anaesthetists of Great Britain and Ireland. Peri-operative management of the morbidly obese patient, 2007.

57. Torosian MH. Perioperative nutrition support for patients undergoing gastrointestinal surgery: critical analysis and recommendations. World J Surg 1999; 23:565–569.

58. Hill J, Treasure T. Reducing the risk of venous thromboembolism (deep vein thrombosis and pulmonary embolism) in inpatients having surgery: summary of NICE guidance. BMJ 2007; 334:1053–1054.

59. Fitzmaurice DA, Murray E. Thromboprophylaxis for adults in hospital. BMJ 2007; 334:1017–1018.

60. Salzman EW, Hirsh J. Prevention of venous thromboembolism. In: Colman RW, Hirsh J, Marder V, et al., eds. Hemostasis and thrombosis: basic principles and clinical practice. New York: Lippincott, 1982:986.

61. Forrest JB, Clemens JQ, Finamore P, et al. AUA Best Practice Statement for the prevention of deep vein thrombosis in patients undergoing urologic surgery. J Urol 2009; 181:1170–1177.

62. Dunn AS, Turpie AG. Perioperative management of patients receiving oral anticoagulants: a systematic review. Arch Intern Med 2003; 163:901–908.

63. Kearon C, Hirsh J. Management of anticoagulation before and after elective surgery. N Engl J Med 1997; 336: 1506–1511.

64. National Institute for Health and Clinical Excellence. Clinical guideline 48: MI: secondary prevention in primary and secondary care for patients following a myocardial infarction. London: NICE, 2007.

65. Steinhubl SR, Berger PB, Mann JT, et al. Early and sustained dual oral antiplatelet therapy following percutaneous coronary intervention: a randomized controlled trial. JAMA 2002; 288:2411–2420.

66. Jones JS. Urologists: be aware of significant risks to stopping anticoagulants in patients with drug-eluting coronary stents. BJU Int 2007; 99:1330–1331.

67. Eisenberg MJ, Richard PR, Libersan D, et al. Safety of short-term discontinuation of antiplatelet therapy in patients with drug-eluting stents. Circulation 2009; 119:1634–1642.

68. Nielsen JD, Holm-Nielsen A, Jespersen J, et al. The effect of low-dose acetylsalicylic acid on bleeding after transurethral prostatectomy-a prospective, randomized, double-blind, placebo-controlled study. Scand J Urol Nephrol 2000; 34:194–198.

69. Halkes PH, van Gijn J, Kappelle LJ, et al. Aspirin plus dipyridamole versus aspirin alone after cerebral ischaemia of arterial origin (ESPRIT): randomised controlled trial. Lancet 2006; 367:1665–1673.

70. Spahn DR, Howell SJ, Delabays A, et al. Coronary stents and perioperative anti-platelet regimen: dilemma of bleeding and stent thrombosis. Br J Anaesth 2006; 96:675–677.

71. Hodgson R, Alwyn T, John B, et al. The FAST Alcohol Screening Test. Alcohol Alcohol 2002; 37:61–66.

72. American Academy of Allergy and Immunology Board of Directors Position Statement. J Allergy Clin Immunol 1994; 94:666–668.

73. Withington DE. Allergy, anaphylaxis and anaesthesia. Can J Anaesth 1994; 41:1133–1139.

74. Mazze RI, Kallen B. Reproductive outcome after anesthesia and operation during pregnancy: a registry study of 5405 cases. Am J Obstet Gynecol 1989; 161:1178–1185.

75. Wheeler D. Perioperative management of challenging comorbid conditions. Surgery (Oxford) 2006; 23:262–266.

76. Zacharias M, Conlon NP, Herbison GP, et al. Interventions for protecting renal function in the perioperative period. Cochrane Database Syst Rev 2008; (4):CD003590.

77. Hahn RG. Ethanol monitoring of irrigating fluid absorption in transurethral prostatic surgery. Anesthesiology 1988; 68:867–873.

78. Olsson J, Nilsson A, Hahn RG. Symptoms of the transurethral resection syndrome using glycine as the irrigant. J Urol 1995; 154:123–128.

79. Hahn RG. Fluid absorption in endoscopic surgery. Br J Anaesth 2006; 96:8–20.

80. Orebaugh SL. Venous air embolism: clinical and experimental considerations. Crit Care Med 1992; 20:1169–1177.

81. Van Appledorn S, Costello AJ. Complications of robotic surgery and how to prevent them. In Patel VR ed. Robotic urologic surgery. New York: Springer, 2007:169–178.

36

Screening in Urology

Nicholas J. R. George

Department of Urology, Withington Hospital, University Hospitals of South Manchester, Manchester, U.K.

INTRODUCTION

Screening has been defined as the identification of unrecognized disease or defect by the application of tests, examinations, or other procedures that can be applied rapidly. The process may be broadly divided into "one-shot" screening exercises and procedures applied to chronic diseases or conditions that may be repeated at intervals. The second category may be further subdivided into mass screening, selective screening, and case finding. In the context of urological surgery, the debate concerning screening programs chiefly concerns the search for chronic disease, typically urological neoplasia, usually by means of case finding or, at best, selective screening programs.

"ONE-SHOT" SCREENING

One-off screening procedures are most frequently employed to detect defects typified by congenital malformation or inherited metabolic disorders, such as phenylketonuria and galactosemia, for which treatments are available. Screening for disorders that are untreatable has generally been avoided (see sect. "Fundamentals of Screening"), although this basic concept has been challenged over the last 15 years (1,2). Programs involving sophisticated tests for rare diseases (3,4) may not, at a superficial glance, seem cost-effective; however, the long-term costs of supporting the patient to adulthood with undetected disease may be the crucial factor in determining public-health policy (5).

"Single-shot" screening of a blood specimen originally replaced the "nappy test" for phenylketonuria 40 years ago and introduced the possibility of detecting galactosemia, cystic fibrosis, and others although testing for congenital hypothyroidism remained the only other official recommendation in the early days. Recent advances in tandem mass spectrometry with DNA extraction from dried blood spots in the newborn have greatly expanded the analytical possibilities although major questions relating to laboratory technique, quality control, health policy, and ethics have not been fully addressed (6,7). As ever, the development of effective treatments for

hitherto untreatable disorders remains at the heart of this debate.

SCREENING FOR CHRONIC DISEASE

Mass (Population) Screening

Mass screening is the identification of preclinical disease within the population by procedures that have been carefully assessed and validated as part of public health policy.

Mass-screening programs demand a precise cost-benefit analysis closely linked to the ethical and cultural ethos of the country and government concerned. In general, programs initiated by the departments of health in the West address only health issues that are both common and, at least in part, preventable, such as heart disease or certain types of neoplasia. Within this politico-medical process, certain groups, such as young women with disease, inevitably attract more political support than other groups such as older men with disease.

Selective Screening

In an attempt to boost the effectiveness of screening programs in relation to cost, the specified test may be directed at selected groups within the overall population. In fact, nearly all programs are selective in terms of age and sex, as in the case of breast-cancer screening, where high-risk groups of women are targeted in terms of age and menopausal status.

Genetic and racial variables are further examples of factors that may be selectively targeted in screening programs. Within urology, the risks of prostate cancer are known to be increased in certain families with a history of the disease, and epidemiological studies clearly demonstrate the differing racial incidence of the disease both worldwide and, most dramatically, within the United States itself.

Selective screening may also be undertaken by targeting groups exposed to various industrial or social risks. The lifelong follow-up of workers from aniline dye factories and the association of various diseases with heavy smoking are examples of this type of selectivity.

Case Finding

Case finding is widely interpreted as "screening" by both the general public and the medical profession. In essence, case finding is no more than sporadic attempts by interested doctors and patients to detect disease or establish that disease is not present. As will be described below, chronic urological disease does not, in general, attain criteria sufficient to support full public-health screening programs. In the absence of such programs—often interpreted by critics as a "lack of interest" by the Department of Health—case finding becomes the predominant mode of preclinical disease identification, usually widely, and often inaccurately, reported by both the lay and medical press. Case finding is, however, a genuine and valid attempt by concerned doctors and patients to solve a medical dilemma, but the process should not be confused with scientifically designed and validated mass-screening programs.

In this chapter, the issues and principles of screening will be described in general terms. The process will then be analyzed with reference to the generally accepted criteria for screening, and finally the application of these principles to chronic urological disease will be discussed.

LIFETIME EVENTS AND SCREENING TERMINOLOGY

When mass-screening programs for chronic diseases are developed, it is common practice to describe episodes that occur during the patient's lifetime by an accepted terminology that describes and defines the evolving events up to the point of death. These lifetime periods may be illustrated as in Figure 1.

Assuming initial health, the first event is the initiation of a biological disease process. This continues until, in the absence of a screening program, symptoms appear, leading to presentation and eventual clinical diagnosis.

The time from disease initiation to clinical diagnosis is defined as the total preclinical phase (TPCP) (8). Clearly, the TPCP is a theoretical concept, as the time at which the disease is initiated can never be known with certainty; indeed, with reference to neoplasia, it is likely that multiple events are required to establish the cancerous process, making it almost impossible to define precisely the start time of the disease.

If a mass-screening test has been developed for a disease, it becomes possible to detect its presence during the TPCP. The period between the earliest time at which the disease is detectable by the test and the time at which clinical symptoms become apparent is defined as the detectable preclinical phase (DPCP), also known as the "sojourn time" (9). Clearly, the length of the DPCP depends on the sensitivity of the screening test, and this is likely to be different for each disease under consideration. It is also apparent that different forms of screening tests for any one disease will be associated with different DPCP times; thus, breast self-examination will have a shorter DPCP than mammography, and digital rectal examination will have a shorter DPCP than a prostate-specific antigen (PSA) screening test. Naturally, the effectiveness of any proposed mass-screening program will be determined by the ratio of DPCP to TPCP—the longer the detectable phase, the more effective the program. Occasionally, DPCP is mistakenly understood to stand for precancerous phase. This is misleading, as a variable portion of the correctly

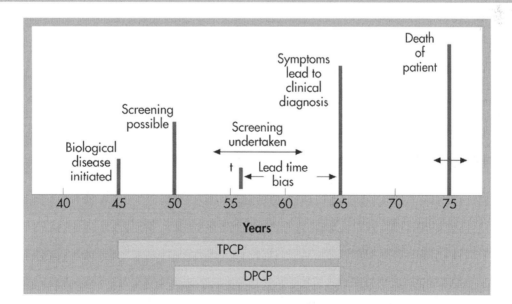

Figure 1 Lifetime events and terminology of screening programs. DPCP: detectable preclinical phase; TPCP: total preclinical phase. Depending on the sensitivity of the test, screening may be undertaken at any time *t* during the DPCP. Lead-time bias is defined as the time between the initiation of the test and the time of symptomatic clinical presentation. The death of the patient may occur earlier or later depending on whether the screening process is harmful or beneficial to the individual.

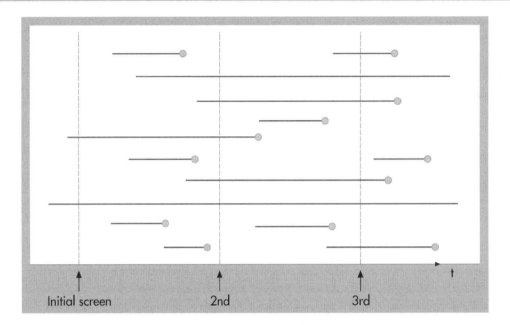

Figure 2 Length bias. Solid lines indicate duration of detectable preclinical phase. Biologically active tumors develop and present more quickly than indolent tumors that progress over long periods. Some tumors may never present clinically. Screening events (vertical dotted lines) automatically select a preponderance of the more indolent tumors. *Source:* Refs. 12 and 13.

defined DPCP may be related to invasive (i.e., not precancerous) yet asymptomatic cancerous growth. Hence, screening for diseases that have a significant invasive asymptomatic period during the DPCP (perhaps breast) is likely to be less effective than screening for diseases with extensive noninvasive periods during the DPCP (perhaps prostate).

The detection of disease during the DPCP by the screening test itself results in difficulties when attempts are made to judge the effectiveness of any single program. The time between the positive result of the screening test and the time at which clinical symptoms would have appeared is defined as the lead-time bias. It will be evident that if treatment for the disease is ineffective, the patient will die at the same point as if it had originally been detected because of clinical symptoms. Survival, however, will apparently have been increased by the amount of time between the positive screening test and the clinical presentation; hence, it is necessary to account for lead-time bias when assessing the efficacy of screening for any particular disease (10). For severe chronic disease such as cancer, the elimination of lead-time bias is best achieved by randomized controlled trials of the screening program, as described below.

The death of the patient is an event that is determined by the severity of the disease and the efficacy of treatment. As noted above, it is necessary to demonstrate that a screening program results in prolonged survival after lead-time bias and other distortions have been taken into account. It should not be forgotten that screening programs may also lead to a shortening of the patient's life—if, for instance, death occurs because of septicemia following transrectal biopsy for presumed prostate cancer suspected on the basis of a

screening test, the program (depending on the frequency of the complication) will be judged as being of questionable value with regard to public health.

A further distortion that may be observed when mass screening for chronic disease is described as length bias (11). In the case of neoplasia, different tumors grow at different rates, and, thus, fast-growing cancers are characterized by a short DPCP. A screening test undertaken during the DPCP will, of necessity, detect more slow-growing cancers than fast-growing cancers (Fig. 2); thus, the disease so detected will have a more favorable outcome than the disease detected by standard clinical tests. This length-bias effect may be reduced by repeat screening, but once again it can be seen that improved prognosis in the screening group may not necessarily be related to a real improvement in survival for the disease in question.

It is often difficult to persuade the general public—and occasionally the medical profession—that earlier detection of disease is not automatically associated with a better prognosis. Figures 1 and 2 well illustrate the complexity of the issues raised when mass screening is undertaken for chronic disease.

FUNDAMENTALS OF SCREENING

Before describing other issues concerned with mass-screening programs, one should emphasize that there are certain situations in which it is not possible or necessary to offer a screening test.

- If there is no preclinical phase (TPCP), it is clearly not possible to offer a test which can detect that phase of disease.

- If there is no possible treatment for the disease, conventional wisdom suggests that screening should not be offered, as, by definition, no improvement in morbidity and mortality will be achieved. Interestingly, this principle has recently been questioned in relation to single-shot screening of the newborn for rare inherited disorders. Duchenne's muscular dystrophy is an X-linked lethal disorder of delayed onset with no effective treatment. It has been argued (14) that screening for the disease should be undertaken on the grounds that it would lessen parental distress by alerting them to risks before the disease became apparent in their older children. Clearly, such a proposition raises highly complex ethical arguments that need to be carefully considered before any such program could be adopted (14).

- If it is possible to cure a disease when it presents clinically, there is no need to offer a screening test for the disease. Examples of neoplastic diseases that conform to this definition are clearly few and far between, but testicular tumor might be cited as an example of a cancer that is curable if efficiently detected in stage one by the patient himself.

ETHICAL CONSIDERATIONS AND ATTITUDES TO SCREENING

It will be realized that in a mass-screening program for disease, different forces are at work that depend on individual expectation of the enterprise. It is often assumed that satisfactory outcomes would, by definition, be acceptable to everybody concerned with the program. To assess this matter, it is necessary to look at any screening program from the point of view of both the Department of Health, "the screener," and the individual member of the general public, "the screenee," who is required to undertake the specified test.

The attitude and perspective of those offering a mass-screening program—usually the Department of Health—are principally influenced by their primary directive to improve the health of the nation as a whole. The screener does not promise or imply that every individual screened will be better off as a result of taking the test, although this point is rarely emphasized in the accompanying publicity that suggests that "screening must be good for you." In this context, the death of a patient following prostatic biopsy (as noted above) would be an acceptable if regrettable incident were mass screening for prostate cancer to be confirmed as a beneficial program for the nation as a whole. The individual suffering disadvantage, as inevitably occurs in the best-validated screening programs, will have a different perspective on the matter. The dichotomy between these two points of view is in part related to the generalized belief noted above that early diagnosis must be good—"catch the disease early." It is perhaps understandable how this entrenched view of health and disease may lead to disappointment both for the screener (15) and the screenee who suffers an adverse event following the screening test.

Cost issues are also a major factor for those considering ways of improving the public health. In developing countries, it is by no means certain that screening for certain diseases would be of greater advantage to the population than money put into other aspects of public health such as water supplies and sewage systems. In the West, cost-benefit analysis raises highly complex issues requiring scientific resolution, often in an atmosphere made obscure by the prominent opinions of vested-interest groups. An example, discussed below, is the ongoing controversy surrounding prostate cancer screening. Critical analysis of diagnostic and mortality data shows that this disease is not the commonest cause of cancer death in males (12.6%, 1:8 cancer deaths) and particularly for younger males a case might be made for expending valuable resource on other noncancer causes of mortality (Figs. 6 and 7)—the debate continues in both medical and lay press.

The expectations and aspirations of those screened are very different. Persons selected by a program or those who elect to go to their general practitioner naturally hope that disease will not be detected. Asymptomatic persons who visit their practitioner do so in the expectation that they will be found to be healthy—what normal person would attend a physician in the expectation that cancer would be found? The screener is looking for disease, but the screenee expects a healthy outcome. These attitudes explain in part the problems that occur when a screening test "goes wrong"—when either the test induces morbidity or the test reveals disease. Success or failure of the process is a value judgment based on point of view. In practice, of course, the vast majority of people who undergo screening tests are found to be negative (true negative—see below). When diseases are of low prevalence, a negative predictive value is both very accurate and very reassuring for the person concerned. A negative screening test for a rare but serious disease is, in fact, one of the greatest benefits that can accrue from a screening program.

Ethical considerations in screening programs are of major importance to both health departments and the population as a whole. Clinicians readily acknowledge ethical problems in routine medical practice, but in this case the patients have almost invariably sought the help of the physician to deal with their disease. In the case of mass screening, selected people who consider themselves to be healthy have been approached by physicians on behalf of the Department of Health and asked to undertake tests which, as has been seen, will usually, but not necessarily, be of benefit to them. Initiation of the screening process deems that the ethical burden on the screener is as great or greater than that resting on colleagues in clinical medicine.

VALIDITY OF SCREENING

Conventionally, the validity of screening is measured in terms of both the test, or tests, utilized in the procedure and the validity of the program itself in

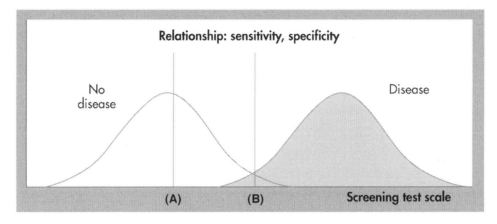

Figure 3 Sensitivity and specificity of a screening test and the effect of variation of the cut off value. (**A**) high sensitivity, low specificity; (**B**) low sensitivity, high specificity.

its entirety. Each of these aspects may be measured by means of two indicators: Sensitivity relates to the positive identification of preclinical disease, and specificity is associated with establishment of healthy persons within the general population. Naturally, the validity of screening in terms of sensitivity and specificity can be known only if the true disease rate in the population is known—a follow-up diagnostic test is required to confirm or refute the result of the screening test.

The Validity of Screening Tests

In terms of the test, sensitivity is defined as the percentage of persons with a positive test among those who are later found to have the disease. Specificity is defined as the percentage of persons screening negative among people who are genuinely free of disease. The relationship between the indicators and the presence or absence of disease is usually depicted as in Table 1. As noted above, the calculations demand that an independent diagnostic test is able to determine which of the screened population has or does not have the disease itself. It has already been seen that application of this diagnostic test may induce significant morbidity in persons who are other wise genuinely well. Sensitivity is the ratio between true positives and true positives with false negatives. Specificity is the ratio between true negatives and false positives with true negatives.

Table 1 Possible Outcomes of Screening Examinations

Screening Test Result	Diagnosis	
	Disease present	Disease absent
Positive	A (True positive)	b (False positive)
Negative	C (False negative)	d (True negative)

Sensitivity = a/a + c; specificity = d/d + b; positive predictive value = a/a + b; negative predictive value = d/d + c.

It is unusual for the screening test itself to demarcate exactly between those with and without disease. Almost invariably, the population groups (healthy and diseased) overlap considerably; hence, variably specified test results will give rise to different levels of calculated sensitivity and specificity.

Conventionally, these difficulties are depicted by means of a bimodal graph, as illustrated in Figure 3. The screening test scale is shown on the horizontal axis, and the distribution of the healthy and diseased populations overlaps to a greater or lesser extent. Selection of different discriminant values of the test results (known as the "cutoff point") demonstrates the inverse association between the sensitivity and specificity of the screening test. Selection of cutoff point A determines that the test will have high sensitivity and low specificity—all those with the disease will be identified by the test, but a high proportion without disease will also be identified (false positive). Altering the cutoff point to B results in a test with low sensitivity but high specificity—a small number of persons with the disease are missed (false negative), although the great majority of people without disease are correctly identified as screen negative.

Selection of an appropriate cutoff point and hence particular values of sensitivity and specificity is a complex process involving considerable degrees of subjective judgment related to the disease in question. Some disorders, such as cervical cancer, can afford a high sensitivity for the screening test, as diagnostic clinical confirmation is reliable and relatively inexpensive, while in others, high specificity would be of greater desirability. Value judgments concerning the disease in question, the cost of diagnostic tests, and its place in society are required, and the results of such judgments will determine the levels of false-positive and false-negative screening tests that will be tolerated.

Urologists well appreciate the effect a variable cutoff may have on the sensitivity and specificity of disease. Difficulties in calculating effective "cutoffs" for prostate cancer "screening" have been widely reported, and the advent of newer, more sophisticated PSA tests ("free and bound") have not lessened the debate on the ideal discriminant value between benign and malignant disease.

A further attempt to refine and optimize values of sensitivity and specificity involves the construction of a receiver operating characteristic (ROC) curve. Such curves can be drawn if the screening test result is both quantitative and variable. Sensitivity on the vertical axis and 1/- specificity on the horizontal axis are plotted for a range of values (Fig. 4A), and the optimal point is that which lies furthest from the diagonal. Although, strictly speaking, ROC curves are difficult to construct for subjective tests such as digital rectal examination, this form of analysis reinforces the impression that PSA is the best predictor of the presence of prostatic carcinoma (16).

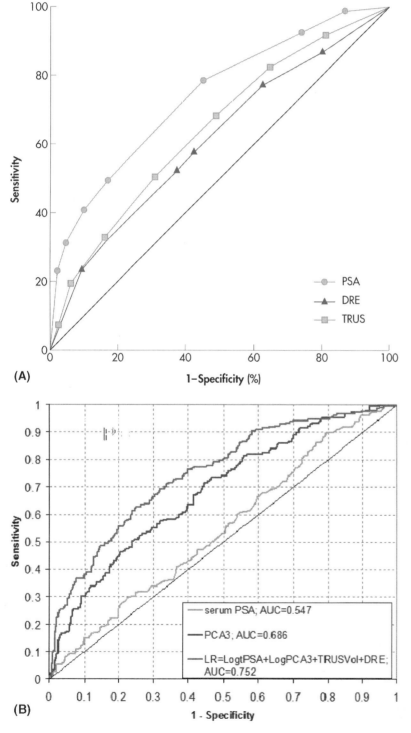

Figure 4 (**A**) Receiver–operator characteristic curve for serum PSA, transrectal ultrasonography (TRUS) and digital rectal examination (DRE). *Source:* Data from Ref. 16. (**B**) Receiver–operator characteristic curve analysis from 553 men suggesting that addition of a logistic regression algorithm could further enhance prediction of biopsy outcome over and above serum PSA and urine PCA3 alone. *Source:* Data from Ref. 17.

Checking the Sensitivity of a Test

The screening test has already been defined as a measurement that is able to identify disease in the preclinical period (DPCP). Unfortunately, because the true prevalence of disease during this stage must, by definition, be unknown, the sensitivity of the test cannot with certainty be calculated. To overcome this problem, screening tests are occasionally tested on populations with known clinical disease. Experience has shown, however, that this may be highly misleading, in that the test may perform exceptionally well when offered such a relatively gross challenge but will perform indifferently in the true DPCP screening situation. Hence, sensitivity and specificity may vary widely according to the stage of the disease.

A further theoretical approach to the problem of defining sensitivity might be to perform a diagnostic test on every person offered the screening test. Clearly, however, the morbidity of the diagnostic test applied to large numbers of asymptomatic people would preclude this approach on ethical grounds alone. The estimation of test sensitivity therefore rests imperfectly with the test itself and the diagnostic measures that are subsequently undertaken to confirm or deny the presence of disease. The emergence of new clinical cases (called in cancer screening programs "interval cancers") from a previously screened population, as well as information gathered from rescreening exercises, eventually leads to a reasonable estimate of the sensitivity of a particular screening test. By contrast, the estimation of specificity is less problematical. As the ratio of people with disease to the general population is usually very low, an accurate estimation may be obtained by calculating the proportion of those testing negative to the sum of those with negative or false-positive tests.

The predictive value is an important measure of a screening test of interest to both the screener and the screened population (Table 1). A positive predictive value is the proportion of those with preclinical disease relative to those with a positive screening test. A negative predictive value is the proportion of persons who are healthy among the population with a negative test. Predictive values vary and relate not only to the validity of the test itself (see above) but also to the prevalence of the disease in the general population. These effects are illustrated in Table 2. A high positive predictive value clearly indicates satisfactory test performance, but as disease prevalence declines, so does the positive predictive value until, with a disease of

Table 2 The Effect of Preclinical Prevalence of Disease on Positive and Negative Predictive Values

Prevalence (%)	Predictive value (%)	
	Positive	Negative
10 (high)	68	99.4
1	16	99.9
0.1 (low)	2	99.99

Sensitivity: specificity: 95%.

Table 3 The Effect of Repeat Screening on the Prevalence of Disease

Cancer	Survey	Prevalence (per 10^3)	
		1st Pass	2nd Pass
Cervix	Females Age 20+ Rescreen <3 years	3.9	1.3
Breast	Females Age 20–64 Rescreen 1 year	2.7	1.5
Lung	Males Age 40–65 Rescreen 6 months	1.0	0.4

Source: Abstracted from Ref. 18–20.

low prevalence, only a very small percentage of those with a positive test actually have preclinical disease—2% in the example given in Table 2. By contrast, under the same circumstances of low prevalence, a negative test clearly indicates that it is very unlikely indeed that the person has the disease. As has been stated above, this is an ideal result from the point of view of screenees, who have attended in the hope that their impression of good health will be supported by the test.

Effect of Repeat Screening

It might be expected that disease "pickup" rates would be maximal during the first screening exercise and reduced thereafter. Table 3 illustrates this effect for early studies involving programs for cervix, breast and lung cancers. More recently, similar effects have been noted during "screening" for prostate cancer in the United States where, additionally, the incidence of metastatic disease in bone has fallen steadily, perhaps indicating detection of disease earlier in the DPCP.

PROGRAM VALIDITY

The performance of the screening test itself is naturally but one part of the overall efficacy of any particular screening program. Other factors that will be crucial to the outcome of the enterprise include the screening request response rate, the interval between screens, and the ability to accurately process those people found to be screen positive. Most recently, in the United Kingdom, such problems have been vividly illustrated in the case of screening for cervical carcinoma. Allegedly inexperienced and underfunded laboratories have led to significant doubts concerning the interpretation of large numbers of smear tests. Clearly, the efficacy of a program is no greater than the efficacy of its weakest link.

Overall evaluation of a screening program depends therefore not only on sensitivity and specificity indicators but also on the entire screening infrastructure and most particularly on outcome measures as judged by objectives laid down at the commencement of the program. Apart from these problems with infrastructure, resources, diagnostic quality control, etc., it has been noted that screening programs contain

Trial of screening

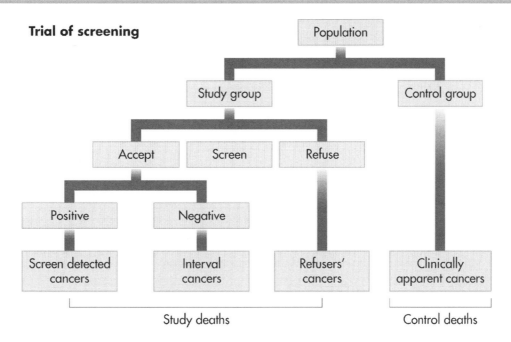

Figure 5 Ideal design of a randomized controlled trial to evaluate the benefits or otherwise of a screening program. Refusers: people who refuse to undertake screening tests despite randomization to the screening arm. Interval cancers: cancers arising by conventional clinical symptoms between screening tests.

a degree of bias that may significantly affect outcome measures, such that those persons identified with screen-positive disease will almost invariably survive longer than those detected by standard clinical criteria. Some of these biases have already been mentioned but are restated below to emphasize their importance in the overall evaluation of screening programs:

Lead-time bias: Lead-time bias is that proportion of the DPCP by which survival will be increased even if the screening program has no effect on disease mortality.

Length bias: Length bias determines that the screening process will naturally select persons with more indolent or biologically inactive disease. Length bias is most pronounced at the initial screen and is in part mitigated by subsequent screening.

Selection bias. Despite attempts to screen broad sections of the community, the process itself is inevitably voluntary; thus, those who attend screening programs are generally more interested in their own personal health than those who refuse. As stated above, these health-conscious people expect to be told that they do not have serious disease and to this end have usually spent their lives avoiding risk factors such as unhealthy diets and smoking. Additionally, even if these persons are found to have disease, their attitude to personal health means that it is likely that they will have a better outcome from the disease than those who neglect themselves.

Overdiagnosis bias. A number of chronic conditions, particularly cancers, may have a semi-indolent phase that may not lead to clinical disease in the natural lifetime of the patient. Overdiagnosis of this

form of disease—perhaps best illustrated by the case of prostate cancer—will again lead to false estimates of survival. This bias can be seen to be an extreme form of length bias, as illustrated in Figure 2.

These forms of bias, acting individually and together, almost invariably mean that patients with screen-detected disease survive longer than those detected in the normal way. To eliminate effectively, the combined influence of these factors requires a randomized controlled trial of the screening process itself (15). The basic design for such a trial is illustrated in Figure 5. It can be seen that not only is the population randomly allocated to a study or control group, but also all cancers are followed whether screen detected or refusal detected. Although it is generally agreed that randomized trials offer the most objective test of a screening process, ethical issues may prevent establishment of a formalized trial structure. While such trials have been established for prostate cancer (see page 556), these issues may cause significant problems for diseases such as breast cancer, where randomization to the control arm may meet with consumer resistance. To circumvent these problems, a number of complex methodologies has been proposed, the details of which are beyond the scope of this account.

SCREENING AND CONTROL OF DISEASE

Screening is but one method of controlling disease in the population. Others include prevention or the application of curative methods once the disease has become manifest. Of these options, screening is a relative newcomer, and its role in the control of mass disease remains somewhat controversial. It is convenient to consider disease control in terms of both mass screening and selective screening.

Encouraged by successes in eliminating chronic inflammatory disease, health departments within the past 25 years have turned their resources toward an attempt to eradicate other chronic diseases such as cancer. However, inspection of mortality-reduction targets shows that screening is expected to contribute only a small proportion of the target total—it has gradually become clear that the complexities and problems involved in mass screening preclude utilization of this methodology as a significant means of disease control.

Several factors underlie this failure to achieve specified goals. The Wilson and Junger criteria (described below) dictate that disease must be common and an important health problem. Yet, careful analysis of mortality data (Figs. 6 and 7) demonstrates clearly that this is often not the case despite public perception to the contrary. Presently, programs are in place for cervical and breast cancer and certain aspects of cardiovascular disease (hypertension), although organization of programs varies widely between countries and, within time, in any one country. There remain significant problems related to population compliance. No better example of the discrepancy between expectation and achievement is provided by the prostate cancer "screening" policy in the United States. Despite enormous publicity and guidelines provided by bodies such as the American Cancer Society, significant screening test take-up rates are to be found only within the Anglo-Saxon population. Take-up within the black community, although improving, is acknowledged to be low and difficult to achieve. Black men have a 60% higher incidence of the disease than whites and the disease presents at an earlier age (23), often at a more advanced stage (24). In a recent study by Catalona investigating high-risk populations in Washington, Missouri, only 1200 black men were available to compare with nearly 16,000 whites (25). It is very clear that, in this group of people, screening is presently of limited value as a method of disease control.

However, selective screening has been more successful at reducing disease rates in the last few decades. Targeting populations exposed to risk factors such as asbestos and tobacco has been in part successful in reducing disease because of these agents. Nevertheless, prevention strategies are at least as important as a means of disease control. Urine screening of workers who were in the past exposed to aniline dyes continues, but, undoubtedly, the main factor responsible for the reduction in industrial disease–related transitional cell carcinoma is the exclusion of carcinogenic substances from the manufacturing process in the mid-1950s.

In summary, mass screening for chronic disease is effective as a means of disease control in certain carefully defined groups of patients. For the majority, however, other programs of disease control are required. By contrast, single-shot screening of the newborn is an effective method of disease containment, which, even in the case of rare disease, may prove to be cost-effective in the long term.

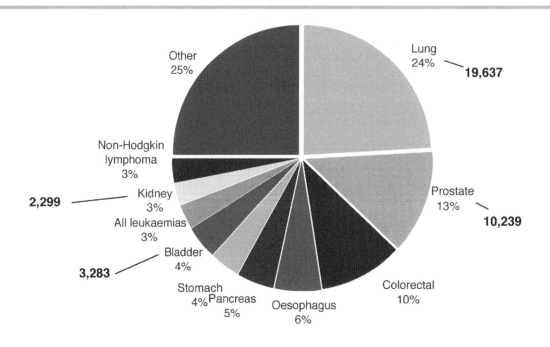

Total male deaths 2007   80,907

Figure 6 System-specific cause of death for males England and Wales 2008. *Source:* Data from Ref. 21.

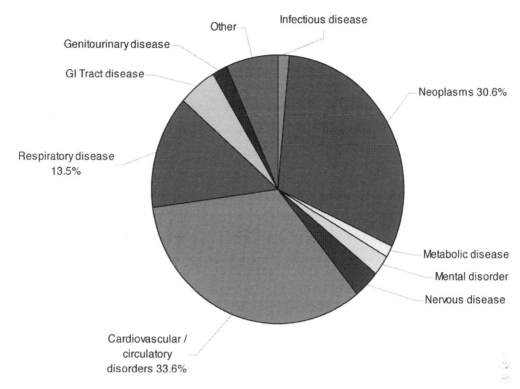

Figure 7 The 10 commonest causes of cancer death in men in the United Kingdom (2007). Prostate deaths (10,239) at any age constitute 12.6% of the whole. *Source:* Data from Ref. 22.

GENERAL PRINCIPLES RELATING SCREENING PROGRAMS

During the past 30 years, the general principles that underpin a successful screening program have been analyzed and refined. A broad consensus has emerged from individuals and international workshops (26,27) regarding the criteria that should be met to establish a successful screening program. Of these criteria, the most widely quoted at the present time are those published in the public health papers of the World Health Organization (28) by Wilson and Junger (Table 4). It is instructive to discuss each individual principle in turn.

The condition should be an important health problem. Clearly, this statement refers to the point of view of the health department of the country concerned. Accurate mortality statistics (Figs. 6 and 7) will be required for that country, although these may well reveal that problems considered by the general public to be of major importance may well not be significant in public health terms. Clearly, in the northwest of England, cardiovascular disease is the preeminent public-health problem, whereas in males each organ-specific cancer site, with the possible exception of lung, contributes little to the overall picture. For women, breast cancer assumes a significant position in the public-health priority list, not only because of the numbers involved but also because the disease affects younger women whose economic and social lives are important to the nation. By the same token, disorders that affect older men—for

Table 4 Accepted Criteria for Successful Population Screening Programs

1. The condition sought should be an important health problem
2. The natural history of the condition should be adequately understood
3. There should be a detectable latent or preclinical stage
4. A test of suitable sensitivity and specificity should be available
5. There should be an accepted mode of treatment for patients discovered to have the disease
6. Adequate facilities for both diagnosis and treatment should be available
7. The tests must be acceptable to the population
8. The benefits should outweigh any adverse effects of screening
9. The cost of screening must be acceptable in relation to overall medical expenditure
10. Screening for chronic disease is an ongoing process requiring critical analysis and audit of results

Source: From Ref. 28.

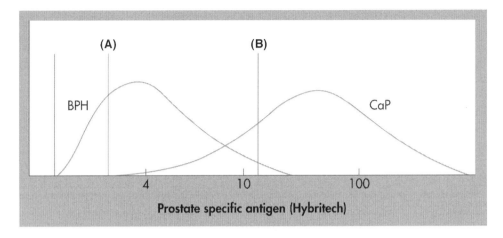

Figure 8 Sensitivity and specificity as applied to PSA testing. Conventionally a cut off of 4 ng is accepted as the best compromise although significant numbers of cancers may be identified with PSA values below that level. **(A)** Theoretical ideal sensitivity, poor specificity; **(B)** good specificity, unacceptable sensitivity.

example, colorectal and prostate tumors—score less heavily in terms of being an "important health problem" in the eyes of the Department of Health. The controversy that surrounds prostate cancer screening at the present time is further discussed below.

The natural history of the condition should be adequately understood. It is naturally very important that the biological progress of the disease should be known with reasonable certainty. This matter is not always as simple as it might seem. In the case of single-shot antenatal screening for hydronephrosis and urinary tract obstruction, significant numbers of babies with hydronephrosis were detected as the sophistication of interuterine ultrasound increased. Subsequently, it became clear that physiological changes at and after birth restored many of these upper urinary tracts to normal, and it was clear that the "screening test" was overestimating the incidence of significant pathology in these children. Prostate cancer provides the best example of a chronic condition whose natural history is incompletely understood. Evidence from well-known postmortem studies from the 1950s indicates that the disease is extremely common in old age—men die "with" rather than "of" prostate cancer. The inability to distinguish indolent from aggressive cancers in younger men continues to generate heated debate.

There should be a detectable latent or preclinical stage. It has already been mentioned that it is impossible, by definition, to perform a screening test on a disease that does not have a detectable preclinical stage. Hence, while cervical dysplasia permits consideration of effective programs for cervical cancer sputum, cytology and chest X ray have been found wanting in terms of their ability to reduce mortality from lung cancer (15).

A test of suitable sensitivity and specificity should be available. The measures that describe the validity of any particular screening test have been

described above, and the difficulties of agreeing an acceptable cutoff point have been emphasized. This problem is particularly well illustrated by reference to PSA and the ability of this marker to distinguish between benign and malignant prostate disease (Fig. 8). Although 4 ng is generally accepted as an adequate cutoff, significant numbers of men with PSA results under this value are found to have tumors, and some authorities argue that a lower cutoff, as illustrated, should be employed.

There should be an accepted mode of treatment for patients discovered to have the disease. Of course, early diagnosis of an untreatable disease is not a cost-effective public-health policy, although the debate surrounding such conditions as Duchenne's muscular dystrophy has been noted. The proposed treatment should be effective in terms of reducing mortality, and the ideal methodology for evaluation of screening programs has been described.

Adequate facilities for diagnosis and treatment should be available. It is self-evident that there is no point in establishing an expensive screening process if facilities to confirm diagnosis and confer treatment are not readily available.

The test must be acceptable to the population. The poor take-up rate in some screening programs testifies to the fact that there is a limit to the discomfort that the public is willing to suffer to detect asymptomatic disease (from which, in any case, they believe they are not suffering). Mammography is not usually a comfortable procedure, and there is no doubt that in North America the thought of a rectal examination and perhaps transrectal ultrasound is the primary reason for poor attendance at screening sessions by certain segments of society. The paradoxical situation of the Afro-American in the United States has already been mentioned.

The benefits should outweigh any adverse effect of screening. "Benefits" in this context are taken to refer to those as observed from the public-health point of view. Clearly, from the individual standpoint, there may be significant morbidity (and perhaps, rarely, mortality) from a screening test; hence, personally, the individual would be unlikely to recognize any benefit. Judged overall, the benefits to the general population should outweigh the adverse effects within the same population, and outcome measures should indicate a real advantage to the screened populations, ideally in terms of increased survival times.

The cost of screening must be acceptable in relation to overall medical expenditure. It has been emphasized that screening is but one part of health policy aimed at containing disease. Furthermore, disease containment is but one part of overall medical strategy for the population, and, as such, screening costs have to be considered side by side with all other claims on the health-service purse.

Screening for chronic disease is an ongoing process requiring critical analysis and audit of results. Self-evidently, disease is an ever-present threat emerging constantly during the life years of the population. Hence, effective screening programs must be ongoing, as must continuing audit and evaluation of the process.

In general, the Wilson and Junger criteria (28) provide a very good framework for discussion of disease as a matter of public-health policy. The principles are naturally more applicable to some diseases than others, and the opportunity is now taken to discuss screening programs in terms of organ-based uropathology.

SCREENING FOR UROLOGICAL DISEASE

Single-Shot Screening

Congenital abnormalities of the urogenital system are relatively common, as such abnormalities are not invariably fatal for the fetus. Within the past 15 years, increasingly sophisticated ultrasound technology has been able to pick up urological abnormalities in utero with increasing confidence. Most normal fetal kidneys are visible before 20 weeks, and hydronephrosis may be detectable as early as 16 weeks. With such technology, the incidence of congenital renal abnormalities has been reported as approximately 1 in 800 live births (29), which compares favorably with the 1 in 650 reported from autopsy series (30).

Good-quality pictures may be obtained of both hydronephrosis and hydroureter when present (Fig. 9A and B). Although not all cases of simple hydronephrosis may need intervention after birth, the screening process undoubtedly identifies at-risk babies, allowing the pediatric service to concentrate its efforts in a cost-effective and efficient manner.

SCREENING FOR UROLOGICAL ASPECTS OF INFECTIOUS DISEASE

Screening During Pregnancy

Within the United Kingdom, testing is made available to pregnant women (i.e., "selective" screening) for rubella antibody, syphilis, HIV, and hepatitis B infections (31). Informed consent is required but the assays are run from a single blood test that is also used for other routine monitoring under pregnancy.

Screening for Infectious Disease

Overall, because of successful immunization and public health programs, the infectious diseases of the past no longer constitute a major mortality threat to the population. By contrast, the incidence of certain sexually transmitted diseases has increased dramatically in recent years leading, if not to death, to chronic morbidity, pelvic pathology, and infertility.

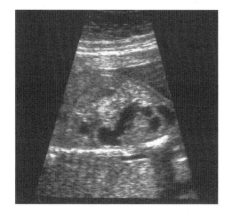

(A)

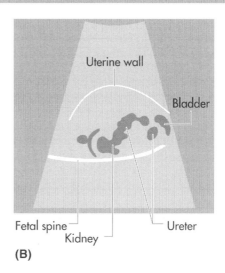

Uterine wall

Bladder

Fetal spine

Kidney

Ureter

(B)

Figure 9 **(A)** Antenatal ultrasound of a fetus with hydronephrosis and hydroureter but a normal bladder. **(B)** Diagramatic representation to illustrate scan.

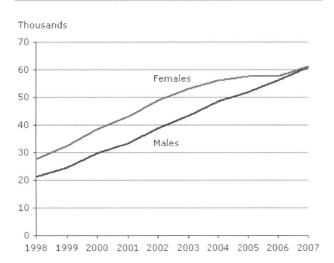

Thousands

Figure 10 New diagnoses of *Chlamydia trachomatis* England and Wales 1998–2007, totaling 113,585 cases in 2006. Rates in women consistently greater than men but stabilizing in 2005 perhaps as a result of the NCSP. Effective screening in infectious diseases might be expected to impact more rapidly when compared to screening for chronic (neoplastic) disease as discussed in Ref. 47. *Source:* Data from Health Protection Agency. Available at: www.hpa.org.uk/infections/chlamydia.

Table 5 The Benefits and Disadvantages of Screening for Cancer

Benefits	Disadvantages
Improved prognosis for some cases detected by screening	Longer morbidity for cases whose prognosis is unaltered
Less radical treatment needed to cure some cases	Overtreatment of borderline abnormalities
Reassurance for those with negative test results	False reassurance for those with false-negative results. Unnecessary morbidity for those with false-positive results Hazard of screening test
Resource saving	Resource costs

Source: From Ref. 15.

The vaccination programs to counter the oncological effects of sexually transmitted HPV 16 and 18 are mentioned in chapter 9. The incidence of *Chlamydia trachomatis* in younger adults (Fig. 10) reached 113,585 cases per year in 2006, with girls (16–24) and men (18–29) predominantly effected. It is acknowledged that the observed increase might be due not only to increased prevalence but also to greater health awareness, sporadic screening, more sensitive tests, and more complete national statistics (32). To counter this epidemic, an opportunistic screening program was rolled out across England (NCSP, National Chlamydia Screening Programme) initially commencing at certain locations in 2004 (33). Previous studies, however, had revealed patchy uptake with limited engagement in deprived areas, so there is concern that the scheme might lead to further inequalities in health (32). Nevertheless, compared to the earlier cumbersome culture techniques, the evolution of rapid point of care tests for both men (VB1 urine) (34) and women (vaginal swab) (35) has allowed immediate specific treatment and, most valuably, rapid contact tracing.

SCREENING FOR CHRONIC UROLOGICAL DISEASE

Screening programs are directed toward the eradication of serious chronic disease such as cancer (Table 5). Therefore, if such programs are to be applied to the urogenital system, neoplastic disease is most likely to be the target of the enterprise. Serious chronic inflammatory disease, such as tuberculosis, is no longer a significant health problem from a screening point of view. However, as will be seen in terms of numbers, urological cancers, with the possible exception of prostate, do not recommend themselves as ideal subjects for screening protocols.

Renal Cancer

Kidney cancer is relatively uncommon. Ranked as the 11th most common neoplasm diagnosed in the United Kingdom by crude rate, 7000 cases were observed in 2004, 2.5% of all detected neoplasms (excluding non-melanoma skin cancer) (36). Although clearly not, in these terms, a cancer of the highest political priority, cancer-specific mortality nevertheless was 3500 cases in 2005 (37) and the great majority of these deaths were from advanced stage metastatic disease. Advances in uroradiological diagnosis suggest that a case might be made for earlier stage detection of the disease by ultrasound, and while such a program would not meet with strict political approval in terms of Wilson and Junger criterion 1 (Table 4), other criteria could be accepted by both screeners and screenees who would hopefully benefit from diagnostic down-staging enabling active surveillance (38) followed by excision as indicated utilizing modern laparoscopic techniques. Such an approach might eventually eliminate or at least reduce significantly the need for the hyperexpensive ethically challenging new oncological therapies now associated with advanced stage disease. It would seem that a politically astute overall cost-benefit analysis would be the key to population screening for these diseases of apparently lesser numerical importance yet escalating therapeutic complexity, particularly when the test is as innocuous and as acceptable for the screenee as renal ultrasound.

A form of selective screening might apply to patients with von Hippel–Lindau disease, who have multiple abnormalities, including a 30% incidence of renal cell carcinoma. However, the symptoms and signs of the disorder are so characteristic and the association with kidney cancer so strong that the term "selective screening" is unnecessary for what is in effect a practical clinical surveillance program.

Bladder (Urothelial) Cancer

Although more common than kidney cancer, bladder cancer is again not perceived as a critical public health problem with 3% (4700) cancer deaths reported by Cancer Research UK (CRUK) in 2005 (37). Hence, the question as to whether symptom-free members of the public should be population screened for bladder cancer has not as yet been addressed other than in the context of selective studies for particular at-risk groups, that is, for workers previously exposed to Aniline dyes.

It is accepted that bleeding usually arises from established urothelial tumor rather than a preclinical phase. The debate continues as to the ideal diagnostic protocol that should be employed following such a symptom bearing in mind that only approximately three quarters of patients with bladder cancer have hematuria (39) and the many other disorders that may manifest as blood in urine. Urine cytology has been widely utilized, but it is acknowledged that, while the test has good specificity, it has a relatively low sensitivity for detecting low- and intermediate-grade transitional cell carcinoma (40). Cystourethroscopy is the accepted gold standard for identifying urothelial tumor, although even direct vision does not result in perfect sensitivity and specificity for the test.

The imperfections of these modalities have led to a search for additional novel markers and techniques to improve detection rates in bladder cancer (41–43). In this context it is very important to distinguish between test performance when used in the broader "diagnostic" mode (i.e., at the hematuria clinic) and performance when applied to the more selective screening mode that involves patients already known to have the disease (surveillance protocols). Not surprisingly, complicating conditions such as inflammation, being more prevalent in the former group, have led to relatively disappointing results as a diagnostic test (relating both to sensitivity and specificity), and thus recent enthusiasm for the new markers has tended to concentrate on their performance as part of surveillance protocols for tumor recurrence (43,44). Few studies report test performance exclusively in the "diagnostic" screening group, most series including both diagnostic and recurrent tumor patients (45). Hence, current urothelial "screening" is a good example of the confounding problems referred to earlier, whereby a potential screening test is evaluated in patients who are already known to suffer from the clinical disease (see page 548). As has been emphasized, the real test of such screening techniques occurs when the procedure is appropriately applied to a truly unselected population.

Prostate Cancer

Prostate cancer is acknowledged at the present time to be the second commonest cause of cancer death in males, with 10,239 patients dying of the disease in 2007 (22) (Fig. 7). However, from the public-health point of view, these figures are relatively unimpressive. Taken together, Figures 6 and 7 show that, despite the marked increase (39%) in age standardized incidence rate recorded between 1995 and 2004 (36), such deaths only account for approximately 4% (12.6% of 31%) of male mortality, and hence it is not surprising that health care policy targets excess mortality and deprivation relating to lung cancer (8%) and cardiovascular/respiratory disease that together presently account for nearly half (47%) of all male deaths in England and Wales (21).

CRUK figures (22) show (Fig. 11) that the majority of these deaths occur in men over 65, 85% of cases being over 70 years old; indeed, recorded death

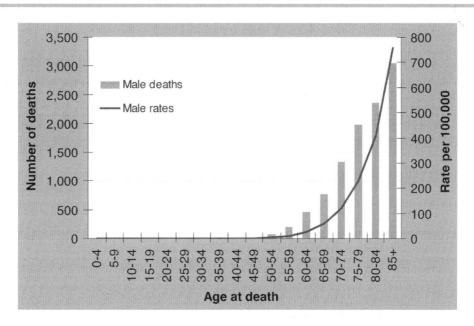

Figure 11 Quinquennial deaths from prostate cancer in the UK (2007). Of 10,239 deaths, 85% occurred in men over 70 years old. *Source:* Data from Ref. 22.

because of prostate cancer in the over 85 years group has actually increased in recent years, probably because of more accurate information on death certificates. Similarly, the median age of death because of the disease in white Americans is 80 years (46). Age-adjusted mortality increased gradually in both the United Kingdom and the United States up to the early 1990s, but then fell in both countries, more so in the United States by a factor of 4 (47)—despite the dramatic rise in incidence noted above. Hence, in terms of public and thus political perception and notwithstanding spirited efforts to raise the disease profile (48), this image of an elderly disease with a declining mortality is always likely to suffer compared to a "high impact" disease (mortality), particularly in younger members of the opposite sex.

Leaving politics and vested interest groups to one side, it can be seen that a critical examination of prostate cancer in terms of Wilson and Junger criteria raises two fundamental questions that touch on most aspects of any screening process. First, is it possible to design and carry out a randomized controlled trial of screening (see page 549) with the death rate from prostate cancer as the primary outcome, and second, for those cases identified, is there an effective treatment available?

The European Randomised Study of Screening for Prostate Cancer (ERSCP) was instituted in the early 1990s to answer the first question by means of PSA-based screening (49) (Fig. 12A). 182,000 men were identified in seven different European countries including a core group of 162,387 men between 55 and 69 years of age. Variations in schedule, screening interval, PSA cutoff value (50), and other factors (Fig. 13) occurred between centers (51,52), but interim analysis of the common core protocol identified 5990 cancers in the screened group and 4307 in the control group, corresponding to a cumulative incidence of 8.2% and 4.8%, respectively (Fig. 12B).

In an intention to screen analysis after a median follow-up of 9 years and an average screening interval of 4 years, the study identified a relative reduction of 20% in the death rate from prostate cancer in men between 55 and 69 years. It was calculated that to prevent death, 1410 men would need to be screened and 48 additional men would have to be treated. While noting the "positive" outcome for the trial, the authors commented on the major issues raised in terms of overdiagnosis, overtreatment, quality of life, overall cost, and cost-effectiveness, recalling memories of Schroder's own earlier editorial comments on overtreatment (53).

The Prostate, Lung, Colorectal and Ovarian (PLCO) screening trial in the United States reported interim results published in the same issue of the *New*

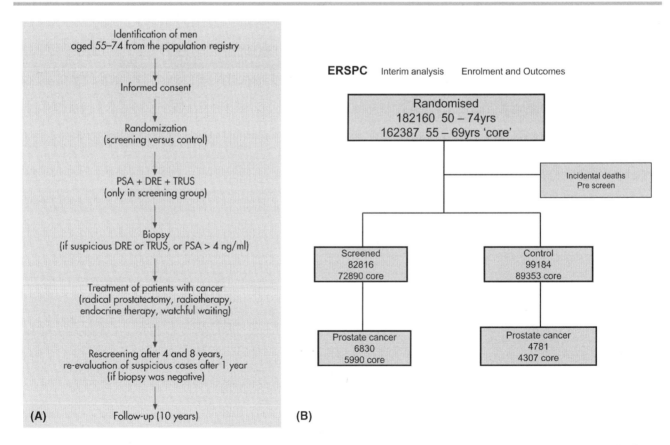

Figure 12   **(A)** Details of the Rotterdam randomized controlled trial, screening acceptance arm. Basic RCT design as illustrated in Figure 5. *Source:* Data from Ref. 50. **(B)** Enrolment and outcomes of ERSPC according to age group at randomization. Predefined core group of 162,387 males identified. *Source:* Data from Ref. 49.

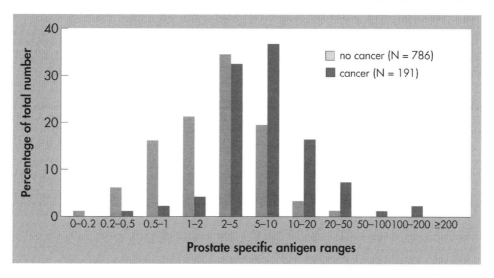

Figure 13 Sensitivity, specificity, and cutoff values illustrated by early data obtained from the Rotterdam screening study. The difficulty of establishing a cutoff between health and disease can be appreciated. *Source:* Data from Ref. 50.

England Journal (54). In a smaller study of the prostate arm, 38,343 men were followed for 6 years with annual PSA screening and a cutoff of 4 ng/mL. At interim analysis the death rate was very low but did not differ significantly between the study groups. The authors considered that this lack of separation might be due to a number of reasons: the screening protocol with a 4-ng cutoff might not be effective; the high level of "peer pressure" screening in the control group might dilute any observable effect; "pretrial" PSA tests might have already eliminated significant tumors from the entire group (high background PSA testing in the United States); and finally, the possibility that therapeutic improvements during the period of the study might have altered outcomes in both trial arms.

The simultaneous publication of these two conflicting, large trials (49,54) mandated a period of reflection for the urological community (55): on one hand an apparently negative result, on the other an encouragingly positive outcome in terms of lives saved yet tinged with the promise of significant overtreatment and questionable cost-effectiveness. More than a decade of intensive investigation seemed to have obscured rather than clarified the question as to whether screening for prostate cancer does more good than harm.

Originally dissatisfied with prospects for screening and particularly with a poor evidence base for treatment modalities, Neal, Donovan and coworkers (56,57) addressed the 5th postulate relating to acceptable/ideal treatment for screen-detected disease that, of course, remained unanswered by the recently reported studies. As a result of their evidence the UK Health Technology Assessment Programme funded another approach that sought to answer the second question relating to efficacy of treatment. The ProtecT (Prostate Testing for Cancer and Treatment) feasibility study (58) is a multicenter trial in which patients with suitable early disease are randomized to radical surgery, radical radiotherapy, or watchful waiting (active surveillance). The randomization and counseling process is reported to take 20 minutes, but in practice can last much longer, a significant problem that has led to reevaluation of the processes involved in the trial (59). This and other studies of patient preference (60) should eventually determine whether screening for this disease will be valuable, but it is apparent that even if ProtecT identifies an ideal therapy the high overtreatment rate implied by the ERSPC will confound the purpose of the public health exercise.

As has been known for some time, to merely identify histologic prostate cancer is not in itself an adequate goal; to be of value the screening process must be able to select out the minority subset of disease that carries an excess mortality risk to the patient within his own lifespan.

Testis Cancer

The rarity of this condition precludes a national screening effort, but all urologists will be aware of the importance of self-examination and self-referral in preventing presentation of patients with advanced disease. Publicity about self-examination may be likened to that surrounding breast disease, but, clearly, diagnostic confirmation and treatment are both easier and cheaper for cases of testis cancer, with the added benefit of excellent long-term outcome measures.

CONCLUSION

Screening, as noted above, remains a relatively novel and somewhat unproven mechanism for disease control. With time, the common-sense view that "it must be good for you" appears to become more rather than less controversial. Recent studies questioning the value of screening for Down's syndrome (61) and cervical cancer (62) have generated heated debate while the latest trend of whole body screening with computerized tomography (63) ("the ideal gift for a 50th birthday") has led to accusations of a screening industry feeding off "simple-minded enthusiasm"—a charge clearly directed at the medical profession as a whole. Nevertheless, the issues are and will remain within the public domain, so the urologist must advise according to the evidence taking care to ensure that the patient is not deceived by the apparent simplicity of the available information.

REFERENCES

1. Bowman JE. Screening new-born infants for Duchenne muscular dystrophy. BMJ 1993; 306:349.
2. Parsons EP, Clarke AJ, Hood K, et al. Newborn screening for Duchenne muscular dystrophy: a psycho-social study. Arch Dis Child Fetal Neonatal 2002; 86:F91–F95.
3. Bogart MH, Pandian MR, Jones OW. Abnormal maternal serum chorionic gonadotrophin levels in pregnancies with fetal chromosome abnormalities. Prenat Diagn 1987; 7: 623–630.
4. Wald NJ, Cuckle HS, Densem JW, et al. Maternal serum screening for Down's syndrome in early pregnancy. BMJ 1988; 297:883–887.
5. Rosenberg T, Jacobs HK, Thompson R, et al. Cost effectiveness of neonatal screening for Duchenne muscular dystrophy: how does this compare to existing neonatal screening for metabolic disorders? Soc Sci Med 1993; 37:541–547.
6. Downing M, Pollitt R. Newborn blood spot screening in the UK—past, present and future. Ann Clin Biochem 2008; 45:11–17.
7. Parsons EP, Clarke AJ, Hood K, et al. Newborn screening for Duchenne muscular dystrophy: a psycho-social study. Arch Dis Child Fetal Neonatal 2002; 86:F91–F95.
8. Cole P, Morrison AS. Basic issues in cancer screening. In: Miller AB, ed. UICC Technical Report Series, 40. Geneva: UICC, 1978:7.
9. Day NE, Walter SD. Simplified models for screening: estimation procedures from mass screening programmes. Biometrics 1984; 40:1–7.
10. Hutchison GB, Shapiro S. Lead time gain by diagnostic screening for breast cancer. J Natl Cancer Inst 1968; 41: 665–669.
11. Feinleib M, Zelen M. Some pitfalls in the evaluation of screening programmes. Arch Environ Health 1969; 19: 412–417.
12. Prorok PC, Connor RJ, Baker SG. Statistical considerations in cancer screening programmes. Urol Clin North Am 1990; 17:699–708.
13. Prorok PC, Connor RJ. Screening for the early detection of cancer. Cancer Invest 1986; 4:225–238.
14. Bradley DM, Parsons PE, Clarke AJ. Experience with screening new-borns for Duchenne muscular dystrophy in Wales. BMJ 1993; 306:357–360.
15. Prorok PC, Chamberlin J, Day NE, et al. UICC workshop on the evaluation of screening programmes for cancer. Int J Cancer 1984; 34:1–4.
16. Ellis WJ, Chetner MP, Preston SD, et al. Diagnosis of prostatic carcinoma: the yield of serum prostate specific antigen, digital rectal examination and transrectal ultrasonography. J Urol 1994; 152:1520–1525.
17. Deras Il, Aubin SMJ, Blase A, et al. PCA3: a molecular urine assay for predicting prostate biopsy outcome. J Urol 2008; 179; 1587–1592.
18. Christopherson WM. The control of cervix cancer. Acta Cytol 1966; 10:6–10.
19. Shapiro S. Evidence on screening for breast cancer from a randomised trial. Cancer 1977; 39:2772–2782.
20. Brett GZ. The value of lung cancer detection by 6 monthly chest radiographs. Thorax 1968; 23:414–420.
21. Office of National Statistics: data from England and Wales, 2008.
22. Cancerresearch.org/cancerstats. 2007.
23. Smith DS, Carvalhal GF, Mager DE, et al. Use of lower prostate specific antigen cut-offs for prostate cancer screening in black and white men. J Urol 1998; 160:1734–1738.
24. Powell IJ, Meyskens FL. African–American men and hereditary/familial prostate cancer: intermediate-risk populations for chemo-prevention trials. Urology 2001; 57: 178–181.
25. Catalona WJ, Antenor JA, Roehl KA. Screening for prostate cancer in high-risk populations. J Urol 2002; 168:1980–1984.
26. Whitby LG. Screening for disease: definitions and criteria. Lancet 1974; 2:819–821.
27. Miller AB. Screening in cancer: a report of the UICC workshop in Toronto. UICC Technical Report Series 40. Geneva: UICC, 1978.
28. Wilson J, Junger G. Principles and practice of screening for disease. World Health Organization Public Health Paper No. 34. Geneva: WHO, 1968.
29. Thomas DFM, Whitaker RH. Prenatal diagnosis. In: Whitaker RH, ed. Current Perspectives in Paediatric Urology. New York: Springer-Verlag, 1989:45–53.
30. Ashleigh DJB, Mostofi FK. Renal agenesis and dysgenesis. J Urol 1960; 83:211–230.
31. Department of Health. Screening for infectious diseases in pregnancy: standards to support the UK antenatal screening programme. Available at: http://www.dh.gov.uk/dr_consum_dh/groups/dh_digitalassets/@dh/@en/documents/digitalasset/dh_4092049.pdf
32. Macleod J, Salisbury C, Low N, et al. Coverage and uptake of systematic postal screening for genital *Chlamydia trachomatis* and prevalence of infection in the United Kingdom general population: cross-sectional study. BMJ 2005; 330:940–943.
33. Low N, McCarthy A, Macleod J, et al. Epidemiological, social, diagnostic and economic evaluation of population screening for genital chlamydial infection. Health Technol Assess 2007; 11(8):1–165.
34. Nadala EC, Goh BT, Magbanua JP, et al. Performance evaluation of a new rapid urine test for *Chlamydia* in men: prospective cohort study. BMJ 2009; 339: b2655.
35. Mahilum-Tapayl, Laitila V, Wawrzyniak JJ, et al. New point of care *Chlamydia* rapid test—bridging the gap between diagnosis and treatment: performance evaluation study. BMJ 2007; 335:1190–1194.
36. Cancer Research UK. Cancer Stats London: Incidence, 2008.
37. Cancer Research UK. CancerStats London: Mortality, 2007.
38. Chawla SN, Crispen PL, Hanlon AL, et al. The natural history of observed enhancing renal masses: meta-analysis and review of the world literature. J Urol 2006; 175: 425–431.
39. Boman H, Hedelin H, Jacobsson S, et al. Newly diagnosed bladder cancer: the relationship of initial symptoms, degree of micro haematuria and tumour marker status. J Urol 2002; 168:1955–1959.
40. Pfister C, Shautard D, Devonec M, et al. Immunocyt test improves the diagnostic accuracy of urine cytology: results of a French multicentre study. J Urol 2003; 169:921–924.

41. Parekattil SJ, Fisher HAG, Kogan BA. Neural network using combined urine nuclear matrix protein-22, monocyte chemoattractant protein-1 and urinary intercellular adhesion molecule-1 to detect bladder cancer. J Urol 2003; 169:917–920.

42. Kipp BR, Halling KC, Campion MB, et al. Assessing the value of reflex fluorescence in situ hybridisation testing in the diagnosis of bladder cancer when routine urine cytological examination is equivocal. J Urol 2008; 179: 1296–1301.

43. van Rhijn BWG, van der Poel HG, van der Kwast TH. Urine markers for bladder cancer surveillance: a systematic review. Eur Urol 2005; 47:736–748.

44. Grossman HB, Soloway M, Messing E, et al. Surveillance for recurrent bladder cancer using a point of care proteomic assay. JAMA 2006; 295:299–305.

45. Konety BR. Molecular markers in bladder cancer: a critical appraisal. Urol Oncol: seminars, original investigations 2006; 24:326–337.

46. Ries LAG, Melbert D, Krapcho M, et al. SEER Cancer Statistics Review 1975–2005. Bethesda, MD: National Cancer Institute, 2008.

47. Collin SM, Martin RM, Metcalfe C, et al. Prostate cancer mortality in the USA and UK in 1975–2004: an ecological study. Lancet Oncol 2008; 9:445–452.

48. Kirby RS. Prostate cancer diagnosis: strengths and weaknesses of prostate specific antigen and evaluation of prostate cancer gene 3 (PCA3). 2009. Available at: http://www.prostateuk.org/prostatenews/20090301_article_pca3_rsk.htm.

49. Schröder FH, Hugossson JH, Roobol MJ, et al. Screening and prostate cancer mortality in a randomised European study. N Engl J Med 2009; 360:1320–1328.

50. Bangma CH, Rietbergen JBW, Schroder FH. Prostate specific antigen as a screening test—The Netherlands experience. Urol Clin North Am 1997; 24:307–314.

51. de Koning HJ, Liem MK, Baan CA, et al. Prostate cancer mortality reduction by screening: power and time frame with complete enrolment in the ERSPC trial. Int J Cancer 2002; 98:268–273.

52. Schroder FH, Roobol-Bouts M, Vis AN, et al. Prostate specific antigen based early detection of prostate cancer—validation of screening without rectal examination. Urology 2001; 57:83–90.

53. Schroder FH. Prostate cancer—to screen or not to screen. BMJ 1993; 306:407–408.

54. Andriole GL, Grubb RL, Buys SS, et al. Mortality results from a randomised prostate cancer screening trial. N Engl J Med 2009; 360:1310–1319.

55. Barry MJ. Screening for prostate cancer—the controversy that refuses to die. N Engl J Med 2009; 360:1351–1354.

56. Neal DE, Donovan JL. Prostate cancer: to screen or not to screen? Lancet Oncol 2000; 1:17–24.

57. Neal DE, Leung HY, Powell PH, et al. Unanswered questions in screening for prostate cancer. Eur J Cancer 2000; 36:1316–1321.

58. Donovan J, Hamdy F, Neal D, et al. Prostate testing for cancer and treatment (ProtecT) feasibility study. Health Technol Assess 2003; 7(14):1–88.

59. Donovan JL, Mills N, Smith M, et al. Quality improvement report: improving design and conduct of randomised trials by embedding them in qualitative research: ProtectT. BMJ 2002; 325:766–770.

60. Sculpher M, Bryan S, Fry P, et al. Patient preferences for management of non-metastatic prostate cancer: discrete choice experiment. BMJ 2004; 328:382–386.

61. Wellesley D, Boyle T, Barber J, et al. Retrospective audit of different antenatal screening policies for Down's syndrome in 8 district general hospitals in one health region. BMJ 2002; 325:15–19.

62. Raffle AE, Alden B, Quinn M, et al. Outcomes of screening to prevent cancer: analysis of cumulative incidence of cervical abnormality and modeling of cases and death prevented. BMJ 2003; 326:901–904.

63. Editorial. Screening for cancer with computed tomography. BMJ 2003; 326:894–895.

37

Evidence-Based Medicine

Kieran J. O'Flynn

Department of Urology, Salford Royal Foundation Trust, Salford, Manchester, U.K.

INTRODUCTION

Evidence-based medicine is broadly defined as using the best available evidence to guide decision making in the care of patients (1). It has become a hugely popular movement in medicine over the past decade and the term "evidence base" is frequently used to inform decision making in other disciplines. The rise of the evidence-based movement reflects a number of key changes in society over the past two decades. First, there is a vast and daily growing medical literature that makes it virtually impossible for a dedicated clinician to keep up-to-date in his or her own chosen field. Second, with increased investment in health care in most economies, governments, health care providers, and the public wish to be assured that new monies are spent appropriately and not wasted on treatments, whose efficacy is in doubt. Third, the global increase in Internet access has meant that information, once limited to academic journals can now be sourced through a suitable search engine by anyone with access to a modem.

Sackett, regarded as one of the founding fathers of the EBM movement, defined evidence-based medicine as the "conscientious, explicit, and judicious use of current best evidence in making decisions about the care of individual patients" (2). This definition is appropriate for urologists as it emphasizes the importance of both diagnostic, clinical expertise and judgment, which is so important in a craft specialty. Evidence-based medicine is meant to complement, not replace, clinical judgment tailored to the individual patients, recognizing that patients will potentially make different choices, based on their own belief and prejudices, when presented with unbiased accurate information (3).

EVIDENCE-BASED UROLOGY IN PRACTICE

There are many types of questions that a urologist needs to ask (or be asked in turn by a patient or relative). These may include questions concerning etiology, diagnosis, prognosis, harm, effectiveness, and qualitative outcomes. Different questions require different study designs. To find out what living with a condition (e.g., advanced prostate cancer) is like, a qualitative study that explores the patient experiences is required. In contrast, a qualitative study relying only on the subjective experiences of individuals could be unhelpful when trying to establish whether an intervention or treatment works. The best design for effectiveness is the randomized controlled trial (RCT), which is discussed later in the chapter. A hierarchy of evidence exists (Fig. 1), published by the Oxford Centre for Evidence-Based Medicine, by which different methods of collecting evidence are graded as to their relative levels of validity. The design of a study (such as a case report for an individual patient or a double-blind randomized control trial) and the end points measured (such as survival or quality of life) affect the strength of the evidence. A cross-sectional survey is a useful design to determine the frequency of a particular condition. However, when determining an accurate prognosis for someone diagnosed with, say, lower urinary tract symptoms, a cross-sectional survey (that observes people who have the disease and describes their condition) can give a biased result. A design more suited for a prognosis in question is an inception cohort—a study that follows up a recently diagnosed patient and records what happens to them over an extended period of time. The most up-to-date hierarchy of evidence for the five themed areas (diagnosis, therapy, prognosis, economic, and decision analysis) can be accessed at www.cebm.net.

It is important to recognize that different questions require different study designs for critical appraisal; first, because you need to choose a paper with the right type of study design for the question that you are seeking to answer and, second, to realize that different study designs are prone to different biases. Thus, when critically appraising a piece of research it is important to first ask: did the researchers use the right sort of study design for their questions? It is then necessary to check that the researchers tried to minimize the biases (i.e., threats to internal validity) associated with any particular study design. These differ between studies.

An evidence-based approach can be practiced in any situation where there is doubt about an aspect of clinical diagnosis, prognosis, or management. The process comprises five distinct steps (2):

1. The information required is converted into an answerable question.
2. The literature is searched with maximum efficiency for the best evidence with which to answer the posed question. In an ideal world, the best

Levels of evidence	Therapy/Prevention/Etiology/Harm
1a	Systematic review with homogeneity of RCTs
1b	Individual RCT with narrow confidence interval
1c	All or none*
2a	Systematic review (with homogeneity) of cohort studies
2b	Individual cohort study (including low quality RCT; (e.g., follow-up <80%)
3a	Systematic review (with homogeneity) of case controlled study
3b	Individual case control study
4	Case series (and poor quality cohort and case control studies)
5	Expert opinion without explicit critical appraisal or based on physiology, bench research or 'first principles'

*Met when all the patients died before the treatment became available, but some now survive on it, or when some patients died before the treatment became available, but now none die on it.

Figure 1 Levels of evidence for therapeutic studies. *Source*: Adapted from http://www.cebm.net.

quality evidence would come from properly conducted randomized trials and/or well constructed meta-analyses.

3. The evidence obtained from the literature search is critically appraised for its validity (closeness to the truth) and usefulness (clinical applicability).
4. The results of the appraisal are implemented into clinical practice.
5. The clinician evaluates his or her own performance.

FINDING THE EVIDENCE

Online Searching

Until recently clinicians depended on the printed word for their information. Books, including this one, are likely to be out of date by the time they are printed. Scanning specialty journals offer only a limited sample of new developments and is a particular problem for the inquisitive urologist as the best clinical research is most likely to be published in journals with a large impact factor. It is impossible for a clinician to keep up with all important new developments simply by reading a few journals. A urologist (even if he had the time), reading most of the high-yield journals (e.g., New England Journal of Medicine, Lancet, Journal of Urology, European Urology, Urology, British Journal of Urology International) would still miss some of the scientific and clinically relevant articles in the specialty.

Colleagues may not be available when advice is required, and the information obtained tends to be overtly reliant on personal experience, possibly biased, with anecdote being no substitute for hard data!

Ideally, a busy clinician requires rapid access (within minutes) so that the information can guide clinical questions as they arise, and learning is promoted by the answers coming soon after the questions ("just in time learning"). Ideally information should be targeted to a specific clinical question, with potential solutions derived from the best and most current research information.

The advent of the personal computers and personal digital assistants (PDAs) means that information is easy to come by and the potential hits are almost limitless. Clinicians who want to keep up with the medical literature and source the most relevant information will need to invest time in developing their electronic searching capabilities and learn to rapidly appraise the information for its validity. "Knowledge management," the effective and efficient way of finding and organizing the best available information, is an undisputable core skill for the 21st century clinician. Internet sites and resources that can be used include the following:

Medline

Medline (Medical Literature Analysis and Retrieval System Online) is a bibliographic database of life sciences and biomedical information. It includes bibliographic information on articles from academic journals covering the entire field of health care. Compiled by the United States National Library of Medicine, MEDLINE is freely available on the Internet. The quality of the information retrieved depends on the search criteria used, and the occasional user may be frustrated as most searches will turn up information that is not clinically relevant and important articles may be missed. Searching may be made more sensitive by using specific MESH headings, although the process can be tedious. Online tutorials are available and Medline can be accessed at www.ncbi.nlm.nih.gov/pubmed/.

Google Scholar

Google Scholar is a freely accessible Web search engine at www.scholar.google.co.uk that indexes the full text of scholarly literature across an array of publishing formats and disciplines. Released in November 2004, the Google Scholar index includes most peer-reviewed online journals of the world's largest scholarly publishers. A significant problem with Google Scholar is the secrecy about its coverage. Some publishers do not allow it to access their journals. Google Scholar does not publish a list of scientific journals crawled, and the frequency of its updates is unknown. It is therefore impossible to know how current or exhaustive searches are in Google Scholar.

Clinical Practice Guidelines

When done well, guidelines are comprehensive synthesis of the best available evidence, upon which the guidance is based. In urology, important guidelines have been produced by the European Urology Association (www.uroweb.org) and the American Urological Association (www.auanet.org). Standards for the production of guidelines are discussed later and there remains a great variation in how guidelines meet these standards. With ever emerging new data, guidelines may quickly become out of date, and it is worthwhile checking when they were last revised.

The Cochrane Collaboration

The Cochrane Collaboration is a group of over 15,000 volunteers in more than 90 countries who review the effects of health care interventions tested in biomedical RCTs. It was founded in 1993 by Iain Chambers and named after Archie Cochrane (1909–1988), a prominent epidemiologist with the Medical Research Council in Cardiff who argued for up to date systematic reviews of all RCTs of clinical care. This collaboration comprises an ever expanding international group of clinicians, epidemiologists, statisticians, and consumers who have come together to produce systematic reviews, which are updated each time an important new trial is published. Abstracts of these reviews are made available on the web at www.cochrane.org and complete reports are available by subscription.

RSS

RSS ("Really Simple Syndication") is a family of web feed formats used to publish frequently updated works in a standardized format allowing users to aggregate information from multiple websites as it is published. Examples of websites that might be useful to clinicians are those for news, MEDLINE, AUA, EAU, other Societies, Journals, and government supporting agencies. By subscribing to any one of a large number of software options, clinicians can get timely updates, tailored to their needs, on a personal desktop computer.

UpToDate©

UpToDate© is an evidence-based, peer-reviewed information resource available via the Web, desktop computer, and PDA. Currently it covers more than 7700 topics in 15 medical specialties (including urology) and includes more than 80,000 pages of text, graphics, links to Medline abstracts, more than 260,000 references, and a drug database. The content is peer reviewed and an updated version is released every four months.

The National Institute for Clinical Excellence

The National Institute for Clinical Excellence (accessed at www.nice.org.uk) was established in the United Kingdom in April 1999. As one of the key elements of the NHS in England and Wales, NICE aims to provide patients and the health care industry with authoritative, robust, and reliable guidance on best-practice procedures in health care. Appraisal of new and existing pharmaceutical interventions and medical technologies is a key function of NICE, with emphasis on the demonstration of the value that these products and devices can bring to the NHS on the basis of proven clinical and cost-effectiveness. NICE is also involved in the development and implementation of evidence-based guidelines for appropriate clinical practice, and in the production of tools that can be used for clinical audit within the NHS.

Journals of Secondary Publication

These journals make a useful contribution by identifying high-quality research from a number of different sources. Articles in these publications are screened for relevance to clinical practice and have passed critical appraisal filters and are methodologically sound. *ACP Journal Club* (www.acpjc.org) is published by the American College of Physicians/American Society of Internal Medicine in Annals of Internal Medicine. It reviews the world's English-language medical journals in internal medicine, selects scientifically strong articles by explicit criteria, and summarizes those meeting these criteria as structured abstracts with commentary by an expert, one article per page. Typically, a structured abstract of the paper occupies one page of the journal along with a commentary from an established clinician in the field, giving the bottom line. *Evidence-Based Medicine*, published by the BMJ, performs a similar function and has a greater emphasis on recently published surgical trials.

APPRAISING THE EVIDENCE

Principles of Critical Appraisal

Urologists should have the ability to do an in-depth analysis of research articles that are especially important to their practice. The basic elements of critical reading are centered on three main areas: validity, results, and clinical relevance.

Internal validity

Internal validity assesses if the results of clinical research are correct for the patients in the study. Internal validity is threatened by two processes, bias and chance. Bias is any systematic error (e.g., in assembling and allocating participants to comparison groups, following them up, and measuring outcomes) that might distort the observed result relative to the true situation. Chance is a random error, inherent in all observations. The probability of chance effects can be minimized by studying a large number of patients and is described by p values (the probability of a false-positive result), power (the probability of a false-negative result), and by confidence intervals for the range that is likely to include the true effect size.

The urologist will need to ask if the results of the study apply to his patients? This concept of external validity (generalizability) emphasizes the potential differences between study patients and those seen on a daily basis in clinical practice. Study patients are typically highly selected. Trials are most commonly published from academic centers, with patients, who fulfill clearly defined criteria, are rarely elderly, do not have other coexisting diseases, and are willing to cooperate. As part of the trial participants are encouraged to be compliant with the treatment and will be reviewed frequently by interested enthusiastic clinicians. As a result treatment effectiveness reported from clinical studies may be higher than that achieved in later routine clinical. In interpreting research findings, the reader must make a well-informed judgment about whether the study results can be applied in his own practice.

Studies of the care of patients in many settings have consistently shown a gap between the evidence base, as derived from carefully performed trials or observational studies, the recommendations of experts in clinical practice guidelines, and actual practice (4). Reasons include a lack of knowledge of research results, clinician concern about applying the results of large studies to individual patients, financial constraints, and failure to organize care in a way that fosters use of evidence.

Assessing a Systematic Review and Meta-Analysis

Any urologist attempting to keep abreast of current developments must find ways of dealing with the huge amount of published literature. One commonly used solution to this problem is to track down and appraise a review article. Reviews are frequently written by experts in their field and by virtue of this are prone to be selective in their appraisal of the current literature. Reviews may generate incorrect conclusions and clinical recommendations, potentially delaying the introduction of efficacious treatment. A systematic review is an overview of primary studies in which the authors have systematically searched for, appraised, and summarized all of the medical literature for a specific topic. Its goal is to minimize bias, by seeking out published and unpublished reports in every language. Systematic reviews may include some statistical methods for combining the results of individual studies. A meta-analysis is a systematic review that uses quantitative methods to summarize the results. The rationale for systematic reviews and meta-analysis is based on a number of premises. Firstly, in some therapeutic areas (e.g., drug treatment in the management of detrusor overactivity), there exist numerous trials attempting to answer questions about clinical efficacy. These trials are frequently carried out in diverse settings and may show different net effects or uncertainty (because of small trial size) with some studies showing little effect (or harm) while others showing benefit.

Sound methodology is at the heart of systematic review and meta-analysis. In a systematic review, the questions to be answered and the methods used must be clearly stated. Thorough data collection is of vital importance in the preparation of a systematic review, whether or not a meta-analysis is a part of the review. Complete identification of all relevant studies (published or unpublished) is particularly important and where possible the original patient data should be reassessed (5). Some studies may not have been published for reasons related to the findings. Authors are less likely to submit RCTs with negative results for

publication and when submitted, trials with negative results are less likely to be published. A comprehensive review of RCTs relying solely on Medline searches will omit about half of the available studies. The reasons for this are multifactorial. Part of this problem results from inadequate indexing. For example, it was only in 1990 that the term *"randomized control trial"* was introduced as a descriptor term and in 1991 as a publication type. Further problems arise in that some authors may not have described their methodology clearly enough to allow accurate indexing. Retrieval of high-quality studies will depend on the searching skills of the authors. A rigorous systematic review will include hand-searching journals, conference proceedings, theses, and the databases of pharmaceutical companies.

Ideally the methods section of a systematic review should include a section describing the inclusion criteria for papers in the systematic review and the criteria used for assessing the validity of individual studies. A systematic review in which multiple independent reviews of individual studies were carried out, with good agreement between the reviewers, lends credence to the outcome. Where possible the use of individual patient data (rather than summary data or published reports) is important as it enables the reviewer to look in greater detail at combined subgroups form different trials. This was used with great effect in the meta-analysis of total androgen blockade (TAB) in advanced prostate cancer where the individual details of 5710 patients were individually assessed (6). This meta-analysis showed five-year survival rates 22.8% and 26.2% for castration and maximum androgen blockade, a nonsignificant improvement of 3.5%, leading to a shift in patient management. A good meta-analysis should allow readers to determine for themselves whether the decisions taken by the reviewers were reasonable and the likely impact on the final estimate of effect size. There are many checklists for the assessment of the quality of systematic reviews; the QUOROM statement (quality of reporting of meta-analyses) provides a benchmark against which a meta-analysis can be assessed (7). Because of the many ways in which decisions taken about selection, inclusion and aggregation of data may affect the main findings, it is usual for authors to carry out some sensitivity analysis on the meta-analysis. A proper sensitivity analysis should explore, among other things, the effect of excluding various categories of studies; these might include unpublished studies perhaps because of negative findings, or those of poor quality. If a sensitivity analysis is not performed, the reader is left guessing whether the excluded studies might have led to a different conclusion.

Calculating Effect Sizes

Clinical trials commonly present their results as the frequency of some outcome (e.g., stone passage in the intervention groups and the control group). For meta-analysis, these are usually summarized as a ratio of the frequency of the events in the intervention to that in the control group. Either the odds ratio or the risk

Odds ratio (OR) The ratio of the odds of having the target disorder in the experimental group relative to the odds in favor of having the target disorder in the control group (in cohort studies or systematic reviews) or the odds in favor of being exposed in subjects with the target disorder divided by the odds in favor of being exposed in control subjects (without the target disorder). This is expressed as OR = AD/BC

	Adverse event		Totals
Study Group	**Did occur**	**Did not occur**	
New intervention	A	B	A + B
Standard intervention	C	D	C+D
Totals			

Confidence Intervals (CI) quantifies the uncertainty in measurement. It is usually reported as 95% CI, which is the range of values within which we can be 95% sure that the true value for the whole population lies. For example, for an NNT of 10 with a 95% CI of 5 and 15, we would have 95% confidence that the true NNT value was between 5 and 15. The width of the confidence interval is determined by the sample size (larger samples will give more precise results with a narrower CI) and the variability of the characteristic being measured (between subjects, within subjects, measurement error, etc.)

Homogeneity and heterogeneity Clinical homogeneity means that, in trials included in a review, the participants, interventions and outcome measures are similar or comparable. Studies are considered statistically homogeneous if their results vary no more than might be expected by chance. Clinical heterogeneity may arise as trials differ in their patient selection, disease severity, operative management and duration of follow-up.

Figure 2 Commonly used terminology in meta-analysis. *Source*: Adapted from http://www.consort-statement.org.

ratio can be used (Fig. 2). Although they are technically different, the odds ratios and relative risks are usually interpreted in the same way. A ratio of 2 implies that the defined outcome happens about twice as often in the intervention group as in the control group; an odds ratio of 0.5 implies around a 50% reduction in the defined event in the treated group compared with the controls. The findings from individual studies can be combined using an appropriate statistical method. Separate methods are used for combining odds ratios, relative risks, and other outcome measures such as risk difference or hazard ratio. The methods use a similar approach in which the estimate from each study is weighted by the precision of the estimate.

The results of meta-analysis tend to be presented graphically in a Forest plot or blobbogram (Fig. 3). Each trial is represented by a horizontal line, the length of which represents the uncertainty of the estimate of the treatment effect in that individual study (the 95% confidence interval) of the estimate. The "blob" in the middle represents the point estimate of the difference between the groups. The vertical line down the middle is the line of no effect,

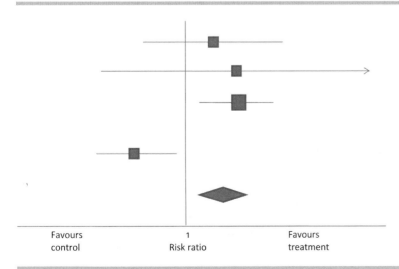

Favours control — 1 Risk ratio — Favours treatment

Figure 3 Forest plot. In a forest plot, each trial is represented by a horizontal line, the length of which is the confidence interval for the study. The graph may be plotted on a natural logarithmic scale when using odds ratios, so that the confidence intervals are symmetrical about the means from each study and to ensure undue emphasis is not given to odds ratios greater than 1 when compared to those less than 1. The area of each square is proportional to the study's weight in the meta-analysis. A vertical line representing no effect is also plotted. If the confidence intervals for individual studies overlap with this line, it demonstrates that at the given level of confidence their effect sizes do not differ from no effect for the individual study. The combined measure of effect is commonly plotted as a diamond, the lateral points of which indicate confidence intervals for this estimate.

Are the results valid?
Is this a systematic review of randomized trials?
How likely is it that relevant articles were missed?
Were the individual studies assessed for validity?
Were individual patient data (or aggregated data used in the analysis?
Was the assessment of the results reproducible?
Were the results similar from study to study?

Are the valid results of the systematic review of therapy important?
Are the results consistent across studies?
What is the magnitude of treatment effect?
How precise is the treatment effect?

Figure 4 Assessing an systematic reviews.

representing a relative risk of 1 (i.e., no difference between the two groups). If the confidence interval of the result crosses the vertical line, this means that either the sample size was too small to detect a difference between the two groups or there was no significant difference between the treatments. The aggregate effect size for certain sub-groupings and the overall effect size are usually displayed in the same figure. The tiny diamond below the horizontal lines represents the pooled data from all the trials, the lateral points of which indicate confidence intervals for this estimate.

Systematic reviews have the advantage that they are generally more reliable and accurate because of the explicit methods used. Thus, large amounts of information can be quickly assessed by the discerning reader. Results of different studies can be formally compared to see if the findings are consistent, and if this is not the case, new hypotheses may be generated about particular subgroups (Fig. 4).

On a cautionary note, the finding of some meta-analysis have later been contradicted by other later systematic reviews or large RCTs. Eysenck (8) and others argue that the results of meta-analysis are only applicable if the data summarized is homogeneous, that is, treatment, patients, and end points must be similar or at least comparable. The key difficulty lies in deciding which trials are combinable. Good meta-analyses will use explicit and objective criteria for inclusion or rejection of studies on the grounds of quality. Misleading meta-analysis may arise because of the existence of publication bias and other biases that are introduced in the process of finding, selecting, and combining studies.

A good meta-analysis of badly designed studies may result in a misleading outcome. Because of the risk of publication bias, many meta-analyses now include a "failsafe N" statistic that calculates the number of studies with null results that would need to be added to the meta-analysis in order for an effect to no longer be reliable (9). Use of a funnel plot may enable the identification of possible bias (10). Funnel plots display the included trials in a meta-analysis in a

plot of size effect against sample size. As smaller studies have greater heterogeneity, the expected picture is that of an inverted funnel. If the plot is asymmetrical, this may support the view that some trials may have been missed in the original analysis.

Assessing a Randomized Controlled Trial

In an oft-quoted editorial in 1995, Richard Horton, then editor of the Lancet castigated surgery for its over-reliance on case series in the surgical literature, with insufficient evidence derived from RCTs (11). The situation has improved over the past decade, yet many new surgical advances are not adequately scrutinized under trial conditions.

The purpose of randomization is to avoid selection bias and to generate groups that are comparable to each other. For this reason, evidence from a randomized control trial is the soundest we can obtain about causation (whether it concerns etiology, therapeutics, or the outcome of a new surgical procedure). A number of criteria must be met for the proper conduct of an RCT; clinical equipoise (a genuine uncertainty of the researcher as to whether there is a real difference between the treatments), no foreknowledge, no bias in patient management, no bias in the outcome assessment of the patient, and an intention to treat analysis of the data, with no post randomization exclusions.

CONSORT (Consolidated Standards of Reporting Trials), first published in 1996, describes various initiatives developed by the group to improve the quality and standards of RCTs (12). The CONSORT statement is an evidence-based, minimum set of recommendations for reporting randomized trials. It offers a standard way for authors to prepare reports of trial findings, facilitating their complete and transparent reporting, reducing the influence of bias on their results, and aiding their critical appraisal and interpretation. The CONSORT Statement comprises a 22-item checklist and a flow diagram, along with some brief descriptive text (Fig. 5). The checklist items focus on reporting how the trial was designed, analyzed, and interpreted; the flow diagram displays the progress of all participants through the trial (Fig. 6). Considering an evolving document, the CONSORT Statement is subject to periodic changes as new evidence emerges. The current definitive version of the guidance may be accessed at www.consort-statement. org/. The CONSORT statement is endorsed by most of the world's most cited medical journals.

In a properly controlled trial, the decision to enter a patient is made, in ignorance of which of the trial treatments the patient will be allocated (13). Known prognostic factors should be recorded for all patients before the treatment is allocated. There should be no bias in patient management, although this can obviously pose significant problems in surgical trials. In an *intention to treat analysis*, the randomization not only decides the allocated treatment, but also how the patients' data will be analyzed (14). If a medical therapy is being compared with surgery, all the surgical program is included (e.g., delay prior to surgery, death

CONSORT Checklist

Items to include when reporting a randomized trial

Item	PAPER SECTION	Description
1	**TITLE & ABSTRACT**	How participants were allocated to interventions (*e.g.*, "random allocation", "randomized", or "randomly assigned").
2	**INTRODUCTION**	Scientific background and explanation of rationale.
3	**METHODS** Participants	Eligibility criteria for participants and the settings and locations where the data were collected.
4	Interventions	Precise details of the interventions intended for each group and how and when they were actually administered.
5	Objectives	Specific objectives and hypotheses.
6	Outcomes	Clearly defined primary and secondary outcome measures and, when applicable, any methods used to enhance the quality of measurements (*e.g.*, multiple observations, training of assessors).
7	Sample size	How sample size was determined and, when applicable, explanation of any interim analyses and stopping rules.
8	Randomization – Sequence generation	Method used to generate the random allocation sequence, including details of any restrictions (*e.g.*, blocking, stratification)
9	Randomization – Allocation concealment	Method used to implement the random allocation sequence (*e.g.*, numbered containers or central telephone), clarifying whether the sequence was concealed until interventions were assigned.
10	Randomization – Implementation	Who generated the allocation sequence, who enrolled participants, and who assigned participants to their groups.
11	Blinding (masking)	Whether or not participants, those administering the interventions, and those assessing the outcomes were blinded to group assignment. If done, how the success of blinding was evaluated.
12	Statistical methods	Statistical methods used to compare groups for primary outcome(s); Methods for additional analyses, such as subgroup analyses and adjusted analyses.
13	**RESULTS** Participant flow	Flow of participants through each stage (a diagram strongly recommended). For each group report the numbers of participants randomly assigned, receiving intended treatment, completing the study protocol, and analyzed for the primary outcome. Describe protocol deviations from study as planned, together with reasons.
14	Recruitment	Dates defining the periods of recruitment and follow-up.
15	Baseline data	Baseline demographic and clinical characteristics of each group.
16	Numbers analyzed	Number of participants (denominator) in each group included in each analysis and whether the analysis was by "intention-to-treat". State the results in absolute numbers when feasible (*e.g.*, 10/20, not 50%).
17	Outcomes and estimation	For each primary and secondary outcome, a summary of results for each group, and the estimated effect size and its precision (*e.g.*, 95% confidence interval).
18	Ancillary analyses	Address multiplicity by reporting any other analyses performed, including subgroup analyses and adjusted analyses, indicating those pre-specified and those exploratory.
19	Adverse events	All important adverse events or side effects in each intervention group.
20	**DISCUSSION** Interpretation	Interpretation of the results, taking into account study hypotheses, sources of potential bias or imprecision and the dangers associated with multiplicity of analyses and outcomes.
21	Generalizability	External validity of the trial findings.
22	Overall evidence	General interpretation of the results in the context of current evidence.

Figure 5   CONSORT checklist. Adapted from www.consort-statement.org.

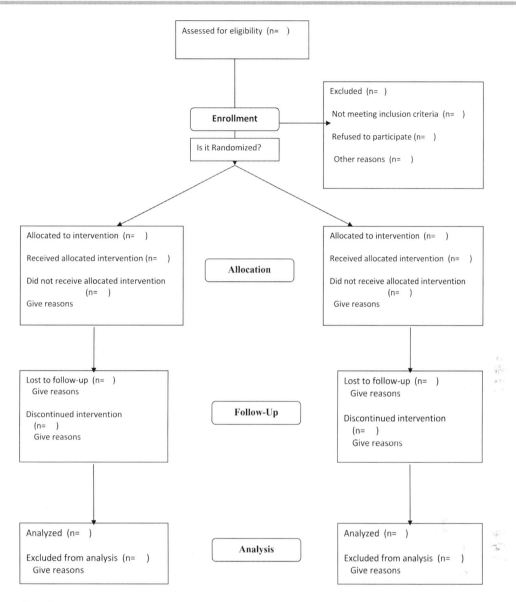

Figure 6 Consort flow diagram.

before surgery), and the data is analyzed irrespective of whether or not the patient received the prescribed treatment. In essence by the end of a trial there are four groups of patients and the trial will compare the total number assigned to receive one treatment compared with the other.

Although improving, there remains a relative paucity of high quality RCTs in the surgical literature. RCTs in surgery pose particular problems. By its very nature, the practice of surgery is highly technical, and surgeons invest a great deal of time and effort in acquiring operative skills and may be reluctant to trial a new technique that truly assesses its efficacy. In urological surgery, the uptake of laparoscopic and robotic surgery (despite the expense) had been enormous, untroubled by an evidence base attesting to its efficacy. In most medical trials, all patients receive

standardized treatments (e.g., a fixed dosage of a drug). The treatment is independent of any particular skill of the physician. The operating skill of the surgeon and his experience clearly affect the outcome, and care needs to be taken that surgeons participating in RCTs are adequately trained during a prerandomization period that should ideally last until the surgeon is fully conversant with the new technique. The surgeon should have an acceptable rate of postoperative complications from the procedure. It follows that whenever a new surgical technique, which requires training, undergoes evaluation, it is unlikely that any surgeon would be willing to randomize his first few patients! These precautions, designed to reduce bias in the surgical trial, may however lead to a restriction in the number of participating surgeons. Yet, the more surgeons participate in a trial, the more convincing the results, and ideally the trial should aim at obtaining results that can be generalized. Proper randomization is pivotal in the conduct and assessment of an RCT as nonrandomized trials tend to overestimate the effects of treatment.

Clearly, it is ethical to randomize patients in surgical trials when we are uncertain as to whether a specific procedure might do more harm than good. Conversely, patients cannot have their treatment chosen at random, if either they or their surgeons are already reasonably certain about what treatment they prefer. Such an attitude has lead to the widespread acceptance of radical prostatectomy by patients and doctors as the treatment of choice for localized prostate cancer in the United States despite good randomized controlled trial evidence. As a consequence, the PIVOT trial designed to assess the efficacy of radical prostatectomy versus watchful waiting has struggled to enroll participants, since its inception in 1994 (15).

When surgery is being compared to a nonsurgical treatment it is impossible to blind the carers or the patients at the time. Unblinded studies overestimate the effects of treatment, and ideally the outcome assessment should be performed by a clinician who is unaware of the procedure, and the patient should not divulge these details to the assessor. An attempt to recruit a patient into an RCT may dramatically alter the surgeon-patient relationship. Surgeons with their extrovert and optimistic approach may have difficulty explaining to their patients the basis for their uncertainty and the need for a randomized trial. Likewise patients, used to the benign paternalism of the surgical fraternity, may not readily accept their surgeon's (well founded) clinical uncertainty.

A properly conducted RCT should have an explicit methodology section, with evidence of credible patient enrolment, clear objectives, and clear outcome measures. It is important that the outcomes being measured are important to doctors and/or patients. Large studies with a prestudy calculation of the required sample size are essential, as small studies may not have sufficient size to show a true treatment effect. Studies with large number of dropouts should probably be treated with circumspection, as their absence from the analysis my lead to an overestimation of the effect of the treatment. Most of the world's leading journals will no longer publish RCTs with less than 80% follow-up.

A good RCT will have a clear statement adequately describing the statistical procedures used and conform to the CONSORT guidance. It should be remembered that a statistical significance of $p < 0.05$ is only 1:20. Any study where the authors choose a single positive statistic out of many should probably be discarded. Treatment effects are frequently recorded as relative risk reductions (RRRs) (Fig. 7). However, RRR fail to discriminate huge absolute treatment effects from small ones. This is because the RRR discards the underlying susceptibility or baseline risk of patients entering randomized trials.

With increasing commercial pressures, there is a pressing need to assess the efficacy of new (and almost always more expensive) surgical interventions. Despite its enhanced cost, approximately 35,000 robotic prostatectomies have been performed in the United States, yet to date there is no RCT attesting to its efficacy over conventional surgery. The message is clear. New technology should be carefully assessed and validated prior to its introduction into health care.

Assessing a Clinical Practice Guideline

Clinical Practice Guidelines

Clinical practice guidelines are documents produced with the aim of guiding decisions and criteria regarding diagnosis, management, and treatment in specific areas of health care. In contrast to previous approaches, which were often based on tradition or authority, modern medical guidelines are based on an examination of current evidence within the paradigm of evidence-based medicine. They usually include summarized consensus statements, but unlike the latter, they also address practical issues.

The United States and other countries maintain medical guideline clearinghouses. In the United States, the National Guideline Clearinghouse maintains a catalog of high-quality guidelines published by various organizations. In the United Kingdom, clinical practice guidelines are published primarily by the National Institute for Health and Clinical Excellence (NICE). Guidelines are also produced by the American Urological Association (AUA) and the European Association of Urology (EAU).

Modern clinical guidelines identify, summarize, and evaluate the best evidence and most current data about prevention, diagnosis, prognosis, therapy, risk benefit, and cost-effectiveness. They should define the most important questions related to clinical practice and identify all possible decision options and their outcomes (Fig. 8). Some guidelines contain decision or computation algorithms to be followed. Thus, they integrate the identified decision points and respective courses of action to the clinical judgment and experience of practitioners. Many guidelines place the treatment alternatives into classes to help providers in deciding which treatment to use. Additional objectives of clinical guidelines are to standardize medical care, to raise quality of care, to reduce several kinds of risk (to the patient, to the health care provider, to medical insurers, and health plans), and to achieve the best balance between cost and effectiveness. It has been demonstrated repeatedly that the use of guidelines by health care providers such as hospitals is an effective way of improving patient care.

Clinicians' concerns about the legal status of guidelines and potential litigation resulting from non-compliance may be a barrier to their implementation. In the United Kingdom, mere deviation from a guideline is unlikely to be accepted as evidence of negligence by a court, unless the deviation itself were of a type that no doctor acting under ordinary skill and care would make. Doctors cannot be found negligent simply because they follow a practice that is rejected by another school of medical thought.

Calculating relative risk reduction

Relative risk reduction (RRR) is the proportional reduction in rates of bad outcomes between the experimental and control participants in a trial, calculated below and accompanied by a 95% confidence interval. The RRR doesn't reflect the risk of the event without therapy (the CER or baseline risk) and therefore cannot large treatment effects from small ones.

Absolute risk reduction is the absolute difference in rates of outcomes between the experimental and control group in a clinical trial. ARR retains the underlying susceptibility of patients and provides more complete information than RRR

Number need to treat (NNT) is derived from 1/ARR and is the number of patients that we need to treat with the experimental therapy in order to prevent one additional bad outcome

	Disease	No disease	Total No of patients
Exposed	A	B	Number
Not exposed	C	D	Number

Experimental event rate (EER) $= A/A + B$
Control event rate (CER) $= C/C + D$
Relative risk $=$ EER/CER
Relative risk reduction $=$ EER$-$CER/CER expressed at a percentage
Absolute risk reduction (ARR) $=$ CER $-$ EER
Number needed to treat $=$ 1/ARR ($\times$100)

Outcome		Risk reduction		
Control %	Treatment %	Relative risk reduction %	Absolute risk reduction %	No needed to treat
50	40	20	10	10
5	4	20	1	100
0.5	0.4	20	0.1	1000

Figure 7 Treatment effects in a randomized control trial.

Are the recommendations of the guideline valid?
Did the developers carry our a reproducible literature review?
Is each of the recommendations tagged by the level of evidence upon which it is based and linked to a specific citation?

Will the recommendations help me care for my patient?
Is the burden of illness too low to warrant implemenatation?
Are the beliefs of the patient about the value of the intervention incompatible with the guideline?
Are resources available to implement the guideline?

Figure 8 Assessing a guideline.

In assessing a guideline, it is important to know the back round of the group who have developed it. If the guideline has not been developed by a fully multidisciplinary group that is representative of those who will be using it, the result may be a lack of ownership, with limited utilization. Recommendations that do not take due account of the evidence can potentially result in suboptimal, ineffective, or harmful practice. There is often a paucity of high-quality scientific information to guide clinical practice, and the authors of a good guideline will document the strength of their recommendation using the criteria espoused by the Centre for Evidence-Based Medicine (16) (Fig. 1).

Guideline development groups often lack the time, resources, and skills to gather and assess the evidence in detail. Value judgments made by a guideline group may be the wrong choice for individual patients. Recommendations are naturally influenced by the opinions, clinical experience, and composition of the guideline group, and if it is not truly multi-disciplinary or representative, incorrect conclusions may be promoted. Patients' needs may not be the only priority in making recommendations; those of doctors, risk managers or politicians may also be involved. Conflicting guidelines from different professional bodies can confuse and frustrate patients and clinicians alike. As of April 2009, the American Urological Association advises that the prostate-specific antigen (PSA) test should be offered to well-informed men aged 40 years or older who have a life expectancy of at least 10 years, a view not currently supported by the American Cancer Society.

In conclusion, the development of good clinical guidelines should consider all relevant disciplines and stakeholders as well as local circumstances. Guidelines should be firmly based on reliable evidence relating to clinical effectiveness and cost-effectiveness, and any recommendations should be linked to the evidence, with references and a grading of the supporting evidence. Active educational intervention should be adopted for the effective dissemination of the results.

Assessing a Case Series

Many interventions in medicine cannot be evaluated by a randomized control trial. The development of surgery as a craft specialty has largely depended on the reporting of carefully performed observational studies. Case series abound in the urological literature and although much derided occupy an important part of the surgical literature. A case series is a medical research study that tracks patients with a known exposure, given similar treatment, or examines their medical records for exposure and outcome. A case series can be retrospective or prospective and usually involves a smaller number of patients than more powerful case-control studies or RCTs. Case series may be consecutive or nonconsecutive, depending on whether all cases presenting to the reporting authors over a period of time were included, or only a selection. Accordingly, case series may be confounded by selection bias, which limits statements on the causality of correlations observed.

There is an important role for a carefully performed observational studies, which may be used to show clinical uncertainty, to generate a new hypothesis. Careful observation and reporting of the evaluation of a new surgical procedure is valid evidence, as it may reduce the learning curve of other surgeons eager to improve their skills. Case series have the advantage that they are cheap, quick and easy to perform. A case series will frequently provide important preliminary information, paving the way for a methodologically sound randomized control trial, where feasible. Some therapeutic interventions have an impact so large that observational data alone are sufficient to show it (e.g., urinary catheterization for relief of pain associated with urinary retention). Randomized control trials are frequently time limited and observational data provides a realistic means of assessing the long-term outcome of medical or surgical intervention.

While often thought provoking, particularly when describing an author's experience with a new surgical technique, case series are prone to overinterpretation by the authors and provide the weakest evidence for assessing the efficacy of a treatment as they are subject to uncontrolled biases, particularly in patient selection.

The reader of a case series will have to decide whether the evidence is the strongest that could have been obtained under the circumstances or if the intervention could have been assessed by means of a controlled trial.

Assessing a Case-Control Study

In a case-control study, the subjects are selected on the basis of whether they do or do not have the particular disease under study. The groups are then compared with respect to the proportion who have had a history of exposure or characteristic of interest. If those cases (patients) who have had an adverse outcome were more likely to have undergone the treatment, this may constitute some evidence that the treatment might cause or precipitate the adverse outcome.

Some of the advantages of case control studies are that they are easy to carry out and will become even easier in the future as more and more patient records are computerized. Case control studies also provide a feasible method for the evaluation of rare diseases and for assessing rare and late adverse effects of drugs. This study design is efficient in both time and costs relative to other analytical approaches.

For a case control study to provide sound evidence of whether there is a valid statistical link between an exposure and disease, comparability of cases and controls is essential. The major issues to be considered in the design and assessment of a case control study are the composition of the study group and the information about exposure and disease. Strict diagnostic criteria for the disease are mandatory. The individuals with the condition must be identified. Commonly, there are two sources, first, patients treated at a particular hospital (hospital-based case control study) and second, selecting persons in a defined population during a given period of time (population-based case control study). The advantage of a population-based study is that it avoids bias from whatever factor led the patient to be treated in a particular hospital by a particular physician (referral bias, medical expertise, etc.), and it allows a description of a disease in the population and direct assessment of rates of disease in exposed and nonexposed individuals.

For the control group, the crucial requirement is that they are comparable to the target population of the cases and that any exclusions or restrictions made in the identification of cases applies equally to the controls and visa versa (2). Case control studies cannot provide information about the absolute risk of an event but only about the relative risk. However, case control studies can provide useful information and are useful when the disease outcome is rare or the duration of follow-up is long.

Assessing an Article on Diagnosis

Making a clinical diagnosis is dependent on history taking, physical examination, and diagnostic tests. Urological practice is heavily reliant on diagnostic tests. We use laboratories with ever increasing frequency to order tests, sometimes inappropriately, so we should be concerned about their use and utility. Diagnostic data is used for several different but interrelated reasons. Diagnostic information is necessary to assess the severity of an illness and to predict the subsequent clinical course and prognosis of the

Are the results valid?

Was there an independent, blind comparison with the reference ('gold') standard of diagnosis

Was the diagnostic test evaluated in an appropriate spectrum of patients (like those it would be used in practice)?

Was the reference standard applied irrespective of the diagnostic test result?

Is this valid evidence important?

Will the result help me in patient care?

Is the diagnostic test available, accurate and precise in my practice?

Are the results applicable to my patients?

Will the test change my management?

Will my patients be better off because of this test?

Figure 9 Assessing an article on diagnosis.

condition (e.g., Gleeson grade in prostate cancer). Such information may also help estimate the potential for response to therapy (hormone manipulation) and to determine the actual response to therapy.

Appraising an article on diagnosis should aim to assess the validity and applicability of the test (Fig. 9) (14). The diagnostic test should in the first instance have been compared with the gold standard, that is, a definitive diagnosis attained by biopsy, surgery, autopsy, or other accepted standard to decide its validity. The test should be applied to patients known to have the target disorder and also applied to a second group of patients known not to have the target disorder, that is, all patients should have definitive verification of their disease status. The "true" situation is given independently by the reference test, so that the false-negatives and false-positive rates of the screening test can be obtained (Fig. 10). This can pose practical difficulties particularly in cancer screening. Changing the cutoff value for a test (e.g., PSA) will alter the sensitivity and specificity of the test. It may

	Disease present	**Disease absent**
Test positive	True positive (TP) = a	False positive (FP) = b
Test negative	False negative (FN) = c	True negative (TN) = d

Sensitivity = TP/TP + FN
Positive predictive value = TP/TP + FP
Specificity = TN/TN + FP
Negative predictive value = TN/TN + FN
Pre-test probability = TP + FN/ TP + FN + FP + TN
Likelihood ratios for a positive test result (LR +)
$= \frac{\text{Sensitivity}}{1-\text{specificity}} = \frac{a/(a+c)}{1-(d/b+d)}$
Likelihood ratios for a negative test result (LR−)
$= \frac{1-\text{sensitivity}}{\text{Specificity}} = \frac{c/(a+c)}{d/(b+d)}$

Figure 10 Calculating sensitivity, specificity, positive predictive value, and likelihood ratios.

be impossible to say if a cancer is present or not in those patients who are negative on screening, and accordingly the false-negative rate for the test cannot be directly measured. Where this occurs, positive samples may be over-represented in the verified sample leading to inflated estimates of sensitivity (verification bias). Some authors may get around this problem by continuing to follow up the patients for a period of time to identify cancers that may have been present despite a negative result on screening. In this kind of assessment using follow-up, estimates of sensitivity will decrease over time as more cases of cancer are discovered in patients who had negative test results; these are then counted as false-negative results. Some authors may make the erroneous assumption that all unverified patients are disease free and in situations where the proponderance of unverified patients have negative test results, this may results in an inflated estimation of the test's specificity.

The primary determinants of a diagnostic test benefit are its sensitivity and specificity. Sensitivity may be defined as the proportion of people with the target disorder who have a positive test and specificity as the proportion of people without the target disorder who have a negative test. Sensitivity and specificity are characteristics of the test alone and will depend on the artificial cutoff point that defines a positive and negative test result (Fig. 11). For example, in screening tests for prostate cancer, age specific serum PSA levels are frequently used. Reducing the cutoff level would increase the test's sensitivity but reduces the test's specificity. In clinical practice, this will increase the false test positives, creating anxiety for the patient (and surgeon) as a work-up is performed to decide if prostate cancer is present. Tests with high values of sensitivity may be very useful as a negative result effectively rule out the diagnosis. Similarly when a test has a very high specificity, a positive result effectively rules in the diagnosis.

The likelihood ratio (LR) is sometimes cited in articles on diagnostic tests (Fig. 10). It expresses the odds that a given finding would occur in a patient with, as opposed to without, the target disorder or condition. With the LR above 1, the probability of the condition or disease being present goes up; when it is below 1 the probability of the disease being present goes down and when the LR is 1, the probability is unchanged. LR can also be calculated for the negative as well as positive. Likelihood ratios can be used to support or exclude a diagnosis and can be used to generate posttest probability (i.e., the proportion of patients with that particular test result who have the target disorder). In assessing a diagnostic test, the clinician must decide if the test is applicable to the patient's clinical situation and if the test result will alter patient management.

Assessing an Article on Prognosis

Prognosis refers to the possible outcome of the disease and the frequency with which it is expected to occur (e.g., death, survival, etc.). Frequently, there are characteristics of the patient or the underlying condition

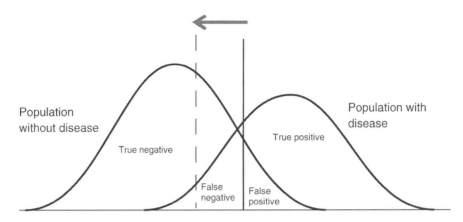

Figure 11 Importance of cutoff values on test performance. As the cutoff value is moved to the left, the true positive rate (sensitivity) increases, but specificity decreases.

that we use to predict the patients eventual outcome. Prognostic factors need not cause the outcome but may be associated with it strongly enough to predict their development. Ideally, the best study design to identify the presence of an increased risk associated with a prognostic factor is a cohort study. In an ideal cohort study, investigators follow a group of individuals who have not yet had the adverse event and monitor the number of outcome events over a long period of time.

In assessing an article about prognosis, it is important to determine if a well-defined sample of patients at a similar point in the course of their illness were included (Fig. 12). There are likely to be systematic differences in the results of population-based and speciality clinic–based studies on the clinical course and prognosis of a disease as referral may be influenced by disease severity. A hospital's reputation may result from its particular expertise in a specialized area of clinical care. "Referral bias" results from the referral of patients with a particular condition to a clinician or tertiary center with acknowledged expertise in the area concerned. This may increase the likelihood of adverse or nonfavorable outcomes. Inception cohorts at tertiary care centers yield useful information to other clinicians who work in such settings, but it may not be possible to generalize the results to the wider population. To allow a true assessment of outcome patients should be at a similar well-defined point in the course of their disease. The follow-up period of the study should be sufficiently long to detect the outcome of interest (e.g., late recurrence of tumor). Under ideal circumstances, the authors will report on all patients entered into the study, but in practice this rarely occurs. Patients may fail to return for follow-up for a wide variety of reasons (death, ill health, relocation, etc.). The larger the number of patients whose fate is unknown, the greater the treat to the study's validity. In general, fewer than 5% loss probably leads to little bias and greater than 20% probably threatens the validity of the study. The lower the risk of a prognostic outcome, the greater the potential effect of patients who are lost to follow-up (17).

The examination for important prognostic outcomes should be carried out by clinicians who were "blind" to the other features of these patients. This avoids bias on two counts. Firstly, a clinician who knows the patient has a prognostic factor may carry out a more detailed search for the relevant condition (diagnostic-suspicion bias). Secondly, clinicians (pathologists, radiologists, and surgeons) may have their judgment influenced by prior knowledge of the case (expectation bias). Ideally in a published report on prognosis, the diagnostic suspicion bias will have been avoided by subjecting all patients to the same diagnostic studies. In surgical studies on prognosis, the occurrence of death is frequently a cited outcome. Judging the cause of death is very prone to error (especially when based on death certification) and assigning a cause to death may be subject to both diagnostic-suspicion and expectation biases.

Is the evidence about prognosis valid?
Was a defined representative sample of patients assembled at a common point in the course of their disease?
Was follow-up of study patients sufficiently long and complete?
Were objective outcome criteria applied in a 'blind' fashion?
If subgroups were identified

- Was there adjustment for important prognostic factors?

Is the valid evidence about prognosis important?
How likely are the events over time?
How precise are the prognostic estimates?

Will the results help me care for my patient?
Were the study patients similar to my own?
Will this evidence make a clinically impact on decision about what to offer or tell our patient?

Figure 12 Assessing an article on prognosis.

Articles on prognosis in surgery frequently claim an altered prognosis for different subgroups. These groups' prognostic factors may be age, gender, disease grade, TNM stage, or comorbidity. It should be remembered that these prognostic factors need not cause the outcome, they may only be associated with its development strongly enough to predict it. When a "new" prognostic factor is identified, there is no guarantee that it hasn't resulted from a "quirk" in its distribution between patients with different prognoses. This initial group is called the "training set". In assessing articles on prognosis, there should be a statement (in the methods section of a paper) of a prestudy intention to examine this specific possible prognostic factor (the test set). If this second independent study confirms the prognostic finding in the test set, one can feel more confident about the validity of the evidence. One final point in studying prognosis: There are very few disorders for which medical interventions do not interfere with studying the natural history of the condition, and it should be clear from the publication what interventions the patients underwent.

CONCLUSION

Although evidence-based medicine has become as the "gold standard" for clinical practice, there are a number of limitations and criticisms of its use. There are 3 to 5 million new biomedical publications each year, and it is virtually impossible for a clinician to keep up to date in his field without a clear strategy to guide his reading. Large randomized double-blind placebo-controlled trials are expensive, so that funding sources play a role in what gets investigated. Government funding will inevitably flow toward high impact medical interventions, while pharmaceutical companies will fund studies intended to demonstrate the efficacy and safety of particular drugs, often avoiding head-to-head comparisons, when the outcomes may be in doubt. Surgical trials are expensive to set up and run and attract less funding. As a consequence many newer surgical treatments have established a place in the urologist's practice, with grade 4 evidence at best. Such is the position of emerging surgical techniques in urology that it might prove impossible to evaluate them with RCTs.

Evidence-based guidelines do not remove the problem of extrapolation of results to different populations or longer time frames. Even if several top-quality studies are available, questions always remain about how far, and to which populations, their results can be applied. Furthermore, skepticism about results may always be extended to areas not explicitly covered: for example, a drug may influence a "secondary endpoint" such as test result (PSA, symptom score, etc.) without having the power to show that it decreases overall morbidity or mortality or in a population. The quality of studies performed varies; certain groups have been historically under-researched (racial minorities, the elderly and people with many comorbid diseases). This makes comparison difficult and the clinician may be unsure if the results will apply to his patient.

It is recognized that not all evidence is made accessible and that efforts to reduce various forms of publication and retrieval bias and retrieval bias are required. Failure to publish negative trials is the most obvious gap, and moves to register all trials at the outset, and then to pursue their results, are under way. In response to the growing body of opinion in favor of prospective registration of controlled trials, Current Controlled Trials Ltd.) launched a website (http://www.controlled-trials.com) in late 1998, aiming to increase the availability, and promote the exchange, of information about ongoing RCTs worldwide. This project is committed to providing free and open access to information about ongoing trials. The rapid development of e-publishing should reduce the difficulty of accessing a trial that concludes it did not prove anything new, including its starting hypothesis.

For today's urologist, the laudable aim of making decisions based on evidence may be impaired by the quality and scope of the published literature. Tonelli (18) argued that "the knowledge gained from clinical research does not directly answer the primary clinical question of what is best for the patient at hand" and suggests that evidence-based medicine should not discount the value of clinical experience. Although EBM asserts the primacy of meta-analysis and randomized control trials over other evidence sources, the astute clinician will balance these factors, his personal experience and the patient's wishes, in deciding how best to treat the person in front of them.

REFERENCES

1. Evidence-Based Medicine Working Group. Evidence Based Medicine. A new approach to teaching the practice of medicine. JAMA 1992; 268:2420–2425.
2. Straus SE, Richardson WS, Glaziou P, et al. Evidence-based medicine. How to practice and teach EBM. 3rd ed. Edinburgh: Churchill Livingstone, 2005.
3. Sackett DL, Rosenberg WM, Gray JA, et al. Evidence-based medicine. What it is and what it isn't. BMJ 1996; 312:71.
4. Smith R. What information do doctors need? BMJ 1996; 313:1062–1068.
5. Dickersin K. The Existence of Publication Bias and Risk Factors for Its Occurrence. JAMA 1990; 263(10):1385–1389.
6. Maximum androgen blockade in advanced prostate cancer: an overview of the randomised trials. Prostate Cancer Trialists' Collaborative Group. Lancet 2000; 355(9214):1491–1498.
7. Moher D, CookDJ, Eastwood S, et al., for the QUOROM Group. Improving the quality of reports of meta-analyses of randomised controlled trials: the QUOROM statement. Lancet 1999; 354:1896–1900.
8. Eysenck HJ. Problems with meta-analysis. In: Chalmers I, Altman DG. Sytematic Reviews. London: BMJ Publishing Group, 1995:64–74.
9. Egger M, Smith GD. Misleading meta-analysis. BMJ 1995; 311(7007):753–754.
10. Egger M, Davey Smith G, Scheider M, et al. Bias in meta-analysis detected by a simple graphical test. BMJ 199; 315:629–634.
11. Horton R. Surgical Research or comic opera: questions but few answers. Lancet 1996; 347:984–985.

12. Moher D, Schulz KF, Altman DG. The CONSORT statement: revised recommendations for improving the quality of reports of parallel-group randomised trials. Lancet 2001; 357(9263):1191–1194.

13. Jadad AR, Moore RA, Carroll D, et al. Assessing the quality of reports of randomized clinical trials: is blinding necessary? Control Clin Trials 1996; 17:1–12.

14. Sackett DL, Haynes RB, Guyatt GH, et al. Clinical Epidemiology. A Basic Science for Clinical Medicine. Little, Brown and Company. 2nd ed. 1991;180–181.

15. Wilt TJ, Brawer MK, Barry MJ, et al. The Prostate cancer Intervention Versus Observation Trial:VA/NCI/AHRQ Cooperative Studies Program #407 (PIVOT): design and baseline results of a randomized controlled trial comparing radical prostatectomy to watchful waiting for men with clinically localized prostate cancer. Contemp Clin Trials 2009; 30(1):81–87.

16. Guyatt G, Rennie D, eds. Users' Guides to the Medical Literature. A Manual for Evidence Based Clinical Practice. Chicago: AMA Press, 2002.

17. Sackett DL, Haynes RB, Guyatt GH, et al. In Clinical Epidemiology, A Basic Science for Clinical Medicine. 2nd ed., 1991:180–181.

18. Tonelli MR. The limits of evidence-based medicine. Respir Care 2001; 46(12):1435–1440.

Index